EQUINE APPLIED AND CLINICAL NUTRITION

Content Strategist: Robert Edwards
Content Development Specialist: Nicola Lally/Veronika Watkins
Project Manager: Sruthi Viswam
Designer/Design Direction: Miles Hitchen
Illustration Manager: Jennifer Rose
Illustrator: Richard Tibbitts

EQUINE APPLIED AND CLINICAL NUTRITION

HEALTH, WELFARE AND PERFORMANCE

Edited by

RAYMOND J. GEOR BVSc, MVSc, PhD, Diplomate ACVIM (Large Animal), Diplomate ACVSMR, Diplomate ACVN (Honorary)

PATRICIA A. HARRIS MA, PhD, Diplomate ECVCN, VetMB, MRCVS

MANFRED COENEN Prof., Dr. med. vet., Diplomate ECVCN

Foreword by HRH Princess Anne

SAUNDERS

ELSEVIER

Edinburgh London New York Oxford Philadelphia St Louis Sydney Toronto 2013

SAUNDERS
ELSEVIER

Reprinted 2015, 2016

ISBN 978-0-7020-3422-0

British Library Cataloguing in Publication Data
A catalogue record for this book is available from the British Library

Library of Congress Cataloging in Publication Data
A catalog record for this book is available from the Library of Congress

Notices
Knowledge and best practice in this field are constantly changing. As new research and experience broaden our understanding, changes in research methods, professional practices, or medical treatment may become necessary.

Practitioners and researchers must always rely on their own experience and knowledge in evaluating and using any information, methods, compounds, or experiments described herein. In using such information or methods they should be mindful of their own safety and the safety of others, including parties for whom they have a professional responsibility.

With respect to any drug or pharmaceutical products identified, readers are advised to check the most current information provided (i) on procedures featured or (ii) by the manufacturer of each product to be administered, to verify the recommended dose or formula, the method and duration of administration, and contraindications. It is the responsibility of practitioners, relying on their own experience and knowledge of their patients, to make diagnoses, to determine dosages and the best treatment for each individual patient, and to take all appropriate safety precautions.

To the fullest extent of the law, neither the Publisher nor the authors, contributors, or editors, assume any liability for any injury and/or damage to persons or property as a matter of products liability, negligence or otherwise, or from any use or operation of any methods, products, instructions, or ideas contained in the material herein.

The publisher's policy is to use **paper manufactured from sustainable forests**

Printed and bound in the United Kingdom
Last digit is the print number: 12

Contents

SECTION C Applied Nutrition – Feeds

SECTION D Applied Nutrition

SECTION E Clinical Nutrition

Foreword

BUCKINGHAM PALACE

These days people are constantly being reminded of the link between diet and conditions such as food-related allergy, obesity, and heart disease. We are becoming increasingly aware that there is also a strong association between the feeding and the health status of our companion animals. As those responsible for their diet, it is our responsibility to ensure they are appropriately fed.

In the case of the horse, we need to be sure that any feeding practice is tailored towards a species which evolved for prolonged foraging on predominantly poor-quality forage in a seasonally variable environment. Whilst for horses and ponies used for pleasure activities, the mimicking of this circumstance is relatively easy to achieve, we face a particular challenge with respect to the feeding of high-performance competition horses. Here the challenge appears to be slightly different, in that we need to ensure sufficient energy and nutrients are provided to support optimal performance but in a way that avoids health risks, (particularly disturbances to digestive tract function), while still promoting positive behaviours.

With the increasing knowledge of the importance of diet in the health, welfare, performance and behaviour of the horse comes the responsibility of sharing this information so that all horses can benefit. I am therefore very pleased to provide the foreword for this book *Equine Clinical and Applied Nutrition*. It has been written by experienced clinicians, researchers and nutritionists from all over the world. Their united aim is to provide all those interested in the scientific basis and practical application of equine nutrition with the most current information available on the subject. I applaud their efforts to bring scientifically confirmed knowledge into daily use, for the benefit of the health as well as the welfare of horses and related species. I am happy to be associated with their efforts.

Anne

Preface

Knowledge pertaining to the nutrition and feeding management of horses and other members of the genus *Equus* (ponies, donkeys, and mules) continues to expand in concert with the growth in the use of these animals for a wide range of purposes, particularly competition and other recreational riding activities. Appropriate nutrition and feeding management is both a *science* and an *art*. The science encompasses understanding of (1) feeding behavior, (2) the physiology of nutrient digestion and utilization (especially digestive physiology), (3) the nutrient requirements of various physiological classes, and (4) the composition, digestibility and safety of feedstuffs available for use in horse rations. Other important areas are the role that nutrition in its broadest sense (i.e., not just overt deficiency or excess of one or more nutrients) plays in maintenance of health, welfare and behavior, as well as the effects of disease on nutrient requirements and the impact of nutrition on recovery from illness - although our understanding in these areas is lacking in comparison to the body of knowledge that underpins the feeding of healthy horses. The art of equine nutrition is especially relevant to feeding management, recognizing that in many situations a "one size fits all" approach does not work and tailoring to the individual animal is required to ensure attainment of nutritional goals. The art component also takes in the human side of the equation because ultimately it is the owner, trainer, barn manager, etc. who has responsibility for feeding management. We firmly believe that critical application of evidence-based information is essential for sound feeding management of equids. As such, a major impetus of this book was to accurately summarize and synthesize current scientifically-based information in the context of feeding management.

Although contemporary reference materials on equine nutritional requirements are available (e.g., German Equine Feeding Standards, Institut National de la Recherches Agronomique INRA, National Research Council [NRC] *Nutrient Requirements of Horses*, 6th revised edition), we recognized the need for a comprehensive source of information on equine nutrition and feeding management for nutritionists, veterinarians, undergraduate and graduate students in these fields, as well as well-informed lay horsemen and women. Our primary goal was to develop a book that spans from the basic foundations of equine nutrition (digestive and metabolic physiology; nutrient functions and requirements), to nutritional management by life stage or function, plus the assessment of feedstuffs and feeding programs, and finally to clinical nutrition. A second goal was for the book to be international in scope, drawing upon the knowledge and expertise of nutritionists and veterinarians from around the world and ensuring that reviews of scientific literature were truly comprehensive. We hope that we have succeeded in meeting the requirement for a comprehensive reference text that integrates the basic and applied aspects of equine nutrition. That said, we recognize that this book is far from perfect and will not meet the needs of all potential readers.

The book is divided into five major sections. In the first section on *Nutritional Foundations*, detailed reviews on digestive physiology, metabolic and endocrine physiology as well as factors affecting feed intake are followed by chapters that describe the function and requirements of each of the major nutrients (e.g., amino acids, minerals, etc.). The second section, *Nutrition for Life-stage, Type or Function*, has chapters on feeding broodmares and stallions, growing horses, athletic horses, and the older horse. In addition, this section contains a chapter devoted to the nutritional management of donkeys and mules. The third and fourth sections on *Applied Nutrition* cover a number of topics relevant to the development and assessment of feeding programs, including chapters on feedstuffs, pastures and pasture management, the assessment of feed quality and hygiene, ration evaluation, and the assessment of nutritional status, among others. The last main section, *Clinical Nutrition*, has 15 chapters that describe current knowledge of nutritionally-related conditions as well as recommendations for dietary management of horses with these conditions. Although it is recognized that there are many gaps in our knowledge of equine clinical nutrition, we are confident that this section provides a great deal of useful information on dietary management for the prevention or treatment of disease. Finally, there is an appendix that summarizes nutritional requirements and recommendations for different physiological states according to North American (NRC 2007) and German (GEH 2013) authorities, as well as more adjusted recommendations of the editors. Also included in the appendix are examples of typical "real-world" rations, with graphical depiction of how the nutrients provided match with the requirement data as well as a brief narrative on selected aspects of each ration.

Our sincere gratitude is extended to the authors of chapters in this book for their willingness to contribute knowledge in their area of expertise and in recognition of the considerable time and effort required to prepare a comprehensive review. We also thank Robert Edwards, Nicola Lally, and Veronika Watkins at Elsevier and, most importantly, our families for their assistance, support and tolerance during the development of this book.

Raymond J. Geor
Patricia A. Harris
Manfred Coenen

Contributors

Caroline McGregor Argo BSc, BVSc, PhD, Diplomate ECAR, MRCVS
Senior Lecturer, Veterinary School and Dept of Obesity and Endocrinology, University of Liverpool, Neston, UK

Ruth Bishop BSc(Hons), Dip Eq S
Ruth Bishop Consulting Limited, Shrewsbury, UK

Faith A. Burden BSc, PhD
Head of Research, The Donkey Sanctuary, Sidmouth, UK

Elizabeth A. Carr DVM, PhD, Diplomate ACVIM, Diplomate ACVECC
Associate Professor, Department of Large Animal Clinical Sciences, College of Veterinary Medicine, Michigan State University, East Lansing, MI, USA

Rebecca A. Carter PhD
Health & Nutrition Scientist, The Nutro Company, Franklin, TN, USA

Manfred Coenen Prof. Dr. med vet., Diplomate ECVCN
Professor of Animal Nutrition and Dietetics, Institute of Animal Nutrition, Nutrition Diseases and Dietetics, Faculty of Veterinary Medicine, University Leipzig, Leipzig, Germany

Derek Cuddeford BSc, MSc, PhD
Honorary Fellow, Royal (Dick) School of Veterinary Studies, University of Edinburgh, Roslin, UK

Nadia F. Cymbaluk BSc.Ag, MSc, DVM
Director, Veterinary Research/Field Compliance, Pfizer Canada Inc, Manitoba, Canada

Alexandra H.A. Dugdale MA, VetMB, DVA, Diplomate ECVAA, PhD, PGCert(LTHE), FHEA, MRCVS
Senior Lecturer in Veterinary Anaesthesia, School of Veterinary Science, University of Liverpool, Neston, UK

Catherine E. Dunnett BSc, PhD, R.Nutr
Independent Equine Nutrition, Mildenhall, UK

Andy E. Durham BSc, BVSc,CertEP, DEIM, Diplomate ECEIM, MRCVS, RCVS and European Specialist in Equine Internal Medicine Liphook Equine Hospital, Liphook, UK

Andrea D. Ellis Diplomate EuHum, BSc (Hons), PGCert Ed, PhD
Director, UNEQUI Ltd. Research Education Innovation, Southwell, UK

Raymond J. Geor BVSc, MVSc, PhD, Diplomate ACVIM, Diplomate ACVSMR, Diplomate ACVN (hon)
Professor and Chairperson, Department of Large Animal Clinical Sciences, College of Veterinary Medicine, Michigan State University, East Lansing, MI, USA

Patricia A. Harris MA, PhD, Diplomate ECVCN, VetMB, MRCVS
Director of Science for MARS Horsecare; Head of Equine Studies Group WALTHAM Centre for Pet Nutrition, Waltham-on-the-Wolds, UK; Adjunct Professor of Equine Studies at Virginia Polytechnic Institute and State University, USA; Visiting Professor, University of Liverpool, UK; Honorary Professor in Equine Nutrition, University of Nottingham, School of Veterinary Medicine and Science UK; Adjunct Professor at University of Queensland, Australia

Rhonda M. Hoffman PhD, PAS, Diplomate ACAN
Professor, Horse Science, Middle Tennessee State University, School of Agribusiness & Agriscience, Middle Tennessee State University, Murfreesboro, TN, USA

Becky Hothersall MSc, PhD
Research Assistant, School of Veterinary Science, University of Bristol, Langford, UK

Véronique Julliand DVM, MS, PhD
Professor of Animal Science, AgroSup Dijon; Head of the Research Unit "URANIE" equine nutrition, AgroSup Dijon; Head of the Master of Equine Science and Business, AgroSup Dijon, France

Josef Kamphues Prof. Dr. med. vet., MAgrSc, M.V. Sc, Diplomate ECVCN/ECPHM
INSTITUTE of Animal Nutrition, University of Veterinary Medicine, Hannover, Foundation; Hanover, Germany

John A. Keen BSc, Bvet.Med, MSc, CertEM(Int Med), Diplomate ECEIM, MRCVS
Senior Lecturer in Equine Medicine, Dick Vet Equine Hospital, Royal (Dick) School of Veterinary Studies and Roslin Institute, University of Edinburgh, Roslin, UK

Ellen Kienzle Dr. med. vet., Diplomate ECVCN
Professor of Animal Nutrition and Dietetics, Ludwig-Maximilians-University Munich, Veterinary Science Department, Oberschleißheim, Germany

Laurie M. Lawrence PhD
Provost's Distinguished Service Professor, Department of Animal and Food Sciences, University of Kentucky, Lexington KY, USA

Jan Erik Lindberg PhD
Professor, Swedish University of Agricultural Sciences, Department of Animal Nutrition and Management, Uppsala, Sweden

Annette C. Longland BSc, PhD, DIC
Head of Research, Equine and Livestock Nutrition Services, Tregaron, Ceredigion, UK

Nanna Luthersson DVM
Equine Practitioner, Hestedoktoren, Denmark

Tim Mair BVSc, PhD, DEIM, DESTS, Diplomate ECEIM, Assoc ECVDI, MRCVS
Partner, Bell Equine Veterinary Clinic, Mereworth, Maidstone, UK

Bruce McGorum BSc, BVM&S, PhD, CEIM, Diplomate ACVIM, MRCVS
Head of Equine Section, Dick Vet Equine Hospital, Royal (Dick) School of Veterinary Studies & Roslin Institute, Midlothian, UK

C. Wayne McIlwraith BVSc, PhD, DSc, FRCVS, Diplomate ACVS, Diplomate ECVS, Diplomate ACVSMR
University Distinguished Professor, Barbara Cox Anthony University Chair in Orthopaedics, Director Orthopaedic Research Center, Colorado State University, Ft. Collins, CO, USA

Alfred M. Merritt AB, DVM, MS, Diplomate ACVIM (hon)
Professor Emeritus, Department of Large Animal Clinical Sciences, College of Veterinary Medicine, University of Florida, Gainesville FL, USA

Jenifer A. Nadeau MS, PhD
Associate Professor of Animal Science, Department of Animal Science, University of Connecticut, Connecticut, USA

Christine J. Nicol, MA, DPhil
Professor of Animal Welfare, School of Veterinary Science, University of Bristol, Langford, UK

Brian D. Nielsen PhD, PAS, Diplomate ACAN
Professor, Equine Exercise Physiology, Department of Animal Science, Michigan State University, East Lansing, MI, USA

Robert S. Pirie BVM&S, PhD, Cert EP, Cert EM (Int Med), Diplomate ECEIM, MRCVS
Senior Lecturer in Equine Medicine, Dick Vet Equine Hospital, Royal (Dick) School of Veterinary Studies & Roslin Institute, University of Edinburgh, Roslin, UK

Sarah L. Ralston VMD, PhD, Diplomate ACVN
Associate Professor, Department of Animal Sciences, School of Environmental and Biological Sciences, Rutgers, the State University of New Jersey, New Brunswick, NJ, USA

José Luis L. Rivero DVM, PhD
Full Professor of Veterinary Anatomy, Departamento de Anatomía y Anatomía Patológica
Comparadas, Facultad de Veterinaria, University of Cordoba, Cordoba, Spain

Harold C. Schott II. DVM, PhD, Diplomate ACVIM
Professor and Equine Division Head, College of Veterinary Medicine, Michigan State University, Large Animal Clinical Sciences, East Lansing, MI, USA

David G. Smith PhD, MSc, BSc (Hons), Cert. Ed (FE), FHEA
Lecturer, School of Nursing, Midwifery and Social Care, Faculty of Health, Life and Social Science, Edinburgh Napier University, Edinburgh, UK

William B. Staniar, MS, PhD
Assistant Professor, The Pennsylvania State University, Department of Animal Science, The Pennsylvania State University, University Park, PA, USA

Sarah J. Stoneham BVSc, CertESM, MRCVS
Veterinary Surgeon, Lone Oak Stud, Hilborough, UK

Kristine L. Urschel PhD
Assistant Professor, Department of Animal and Food Sciences, University of Kentucky, Lexington KY, USA

Ingrid Vervuert Dr. med. vet.
Docent of Animal Nutrition and Dietetics, Faculty of Veterinary Medicine, University of Leipzig, Institute of Animal Nutrition, Nutrition Diseases and Dietetics, Leipzig, Germany

Kelly R. Vineyard MS, PhD, PAS
Research Equine Nutritionist, Land O'Lakes Purina Feed, Gray Summit, MO, USA

Lori K. Warren MS, PhD, PAS
Associate Professor, Department of Animal Sciences, Institute of Food and Agricultural Sciences, University of Florida. Gainesville, FL, USA

Carey A. Williams PhD
Associate Professor, Department of Animal Science, Rutgers, the State University of New Jersey, New Brunswick, NJ, USA

Annette Zeyner DAI, DNM, Dr.
Professor of Animal Nutrition, Professor of Animal Nutrition, Department of Animal Nutrition, Halle, Germany

Nutritional Foundations

SECTION A

Gastrointestinal physiology

Alfred M. Merritt, Véronique Julliand

This chapter is directed primarily at the normal function of the gastrointestinal tract (GIT) of the prototype 500 kg adult horse. Readers interested in the GIT of foals are advised to consult the various available texts on equine neonatology. The authors have focused on information that is specifically available for the horse and data applicable to other species is only presented to make *a point of* comparison or contrast. This chapter therefore differs in some aspects from previous reviews on this topic which inferred that certain mechanisms have been shown to be present in horses when, in fact, they are not. This chapter considers the different anatomical regions of the GIT in sequence (i.e. mouth, esophagus, stomach, small intestine, and large intestine). It must be remembered from the outset that the horse is a classic "hind gut fermenter" with a particularly large cecum and complex large colon structure in which digestion of plant fiber occurs (Fig. 1.1).

Each section starts with a short description of the respective anatomy and then covers secretion, digestion, motility and absorption, in that order, as appropriate. The initial introductory section presents a brief overview of the enteric nervous system (ENS) which is essential to the functioning of the entire GIT and, hopefully, emphasizes that, despite an arbitrary subdivision, to facilitate discussion, it is one integrated system. Specific effects of diet have been included, where appropriate, in the discussion of a particular process (e.g. gastric receptive relaxation; intragastric fermentation of a diet high in soluble CHO vs one high in fiber) rather than being considered as a separate section.

Enteric Nervous System

In mammals, all GIT function is constantly monitored and modified by the highly complex *enteric nervous system* (ENS), commonly referred to as the "brain of the gut". It functions both on an independent local level and in conjunction with modulatory input from the central nervous system (CNS) via the vagus nerve (parasympathetic) and the sympathetic ganglia. Essentially, the ENS itself is made up of intrinsic afferent neurons, ascending and descending interneurons and motor neurons. At least twenty different subtypes of these motor neurons have been identified (Furness 2006, 2008, Goyal & Hirano 1996).

Concerning GI motility, virtually all of the parasympathetic (vagal) input into the gastro intestinal tract (GIT) is processed through the ENS, with acetylcholine (ACh) playing a predominant role in intra-neuronal communication (Berthoud 2006, Furness 2006, Goyal & Hirano 1996). Parasympathetic input is stimulatory whereas sympathetic (adrenergic) input, with respect to controlling motility, is inhibitory. The majority of the sympathetic input is directly from the sympathetic ganglia, and mediated at the neuromuscular junction by norepinephrine (NE). There is a smaller component of the sympathetic input to the ENS that down-regulates ENS-mediated ACh stimulation via intrinsic α_2-adrenergic pathways (Scheibner et al 2002).

Synaptic transmission, paracrine signaling and hormonal signaling are forms of chemical information transfer within the ENS. Motor neurons that stimulate muscle contraction may express, in addition to ACh, either substance P (SP) or the peptide motilin at the neuromuscular junction. Those neurons from the ENS that inhibit contraction can express a variety of neurotransmitters including nitric oxide (NO), vasoactive intestinal peptide (VIP) or adenosine triphosphate (ATP). These three neurotransmitters, along with SP, comprise the non-adrenergic, non-cholinergic (NANC) component of the ENS (Burnstock 2009, Goyal & Hirano 1996, Kunz & Furness 1999). Calcitonin gene-regulated peptide (CGRP) and numerous subtypes (e.g. 5-HT_1, 5-HT_2, 5-HT_3, etc.) of serotonin (5-HT) act within the ENS to either up-regulate or down-regulate the activity (Berthoud 2006, Goyal & Hirano 1996, Kunz & Furness 1999). Various receptors within the GIT mucosa that constantly monitor the wall tension and the physicochemical characteristics of the digesta evoke either stimulatory or inhibitory responses via the ENS intrinsic afferent neurons; again, CGRP and 5-HT are important mediators in this process (Braun et al 2007, Cooke 1986, Holzer et al 2001, Lundgren 2004 Schemann & Mazzuoli 2010) (Fig. 1.2).

In horses, all of the mentioned neurotransmitters have been found, with varying degrees of expression depending upon the segment of the GIT (Ceccarelli et al 1995, Chiochetti et al 2009, Domenghini et al 2004, Fink et al 2006, Freytag et al 2008, Kotz & Van Aswegan 1990, Malone et al 1999, 2000, Merritt et al 1998, Pearson 1994; Rakestraw et al 1996, Rutkowski et al 1998, Sasaki & Yoshihara 1998, Sasaki et al 2000, Sellers et al 1984b, Solinger & Sonea 2008). There

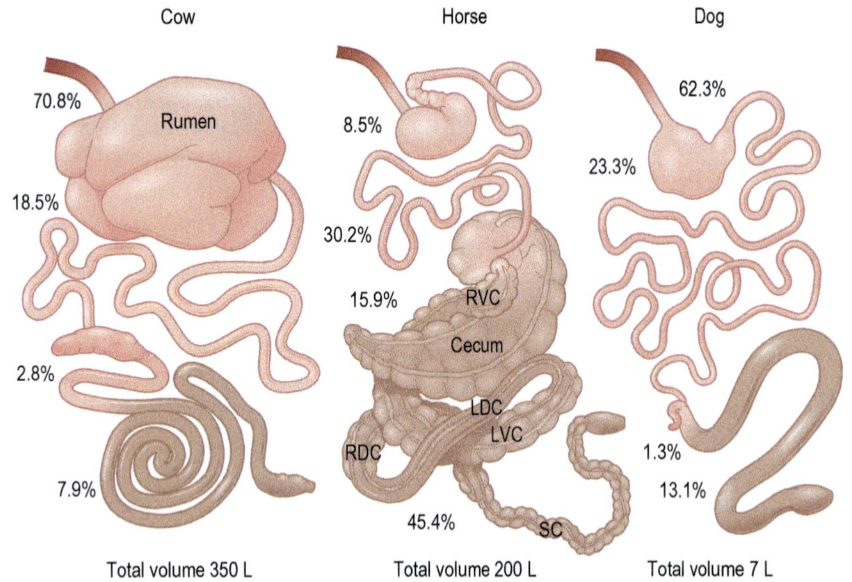

Figure 1.1 GIT anatomy of: 1) the cow, representing herbivores that ferment ingested plant fiber within the compartmentalized forestomach, primarily within the rumen; 2) the horse, representing herbivores that ferment plant fiber within the hindgut, primarily within the cecum and colon, and; 3) the dog, representing the carnivores. The percentage of total GIT volume that each of these sections comprises in each of the species is indicated. Total GIT volume values are for a 500 kg cow or horse, and a 20 kg dog. The major divisions of the doubly folded ascending (great) colon of the horse, starting at the cecocolic orifice, are: right ventral colon (RVC), left ventral colon (LVC), left dorsal colon (LDC) and, right dorsal colon (RDC). Final desiccation of the ingesta to form the fecal balls takes place in the descending (small) colon (SC).

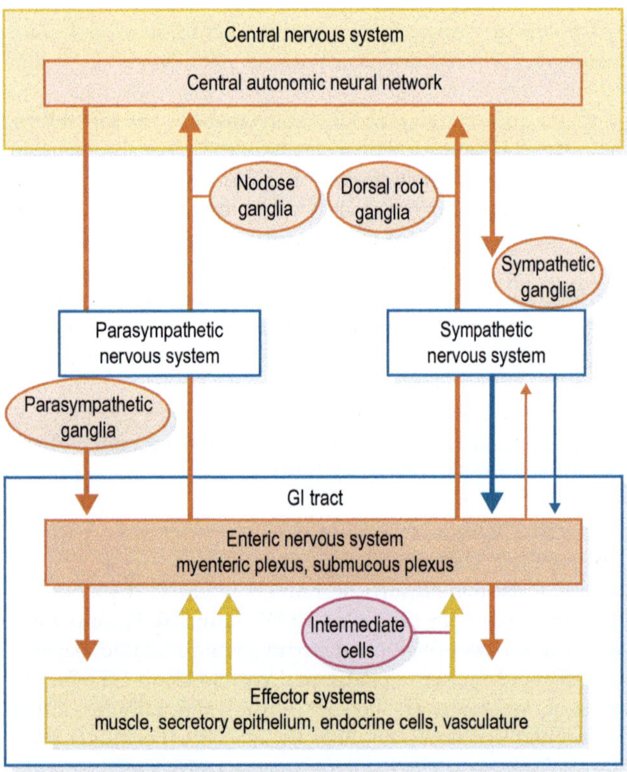

Figure 1.2 Schematic diagram of the general organization of the enteric nervous system (ENS) and its connections with central nervous system (CNS).
Adapted from Goyal & Hirano 1996.

may be some equine species specificity with respect to predominance of 5-HT subtype, which has important implications concerning the development of drugs to control GIT function in the horse, but this still needs further clarification (Delesalle et al 2008, Lippold et al 2004, Nieto et al 2000, Prause et al 2009).

In all species, secretory epithelia, endocrine cells and vasculature within the GIT are also under ENS control. Neurotransmitters involved, in addition to those mentioned above, include numerous well-known peptides such as cholecystokinin (CCK), somatostatin (SST), gastrin-releasing peptide (GRP), neuropeptide Y (NPY) and various opioids (Berthoud 2006, Cooke 1986, Furness 2006, Wood & Galligan 2004). Finally, orexin A, a neurotransmitter found to be involved in appetite control in rats, has also recently been found within the ENS of the horse (Dall'Aglio et al 2009).

Key Points

- The ENS monitors and modifies all aspects of equine GIT function, with modulatory input from the CNS via the vagus nerve and the sympathetic ganglia.
- Numerous neurotransmitters are involved in ENS function that manifest their effects by neurocrine, paracrine and hormonal routes.

Mouth

The horse has three main salivary glands, parotid, mandibular (submandibular), and sublingual, named according to their anatomical location. The parotid is the largest and most peripheral, the dorsal end being just in front of the ear and the ventral end being just behind the caudoventral margin of the ramus of the mandible. The mandibular gland lies underneath the ventral portion of the parotid gland and extends from the atlantal fossa to the hyoid bone. The sublingual gland, which is the smallest, is located just under the oral mucous membrane between the body of the tongue and mandible (Sisson & Grossman 1959).

Secretion

Equine saliva is >99% water (Alexander, 1966). In general it contains relatively more calcium and chloride, and less bicarbonate and sodium, than that of ruminants and is thus more similar in composition to that found in carnivora and omnivora (Alexander & Hickson 1970, Stick et al 1981). Resting electrolyte concentrations in parotid saliva, which is hypotonic to plasma, are listed in Table 1-1. Concentrations of Na^+, Cl^- and HCO_3^- increase in a linear relationship to the rate of secretion. Adult horses may secrete up to 35–40 liters/day with a pH of 8.6–9.1, the majority originating

Table 1-1 Parotid Salivary Composition as Reported by Various Investigators

Reference	Moore 1898	Alexander 1966	Alexander and Hickson 1970	Kolb 1975	Stick et al 1981	Eckersall 1984	Eckersall et al 1985	Coenen et al 1986
Origin	Total	Parotid	Parotid	Parotid	Total	Total	Total	Total
pH		7.49 ± 0.18		7.31–7.80		4.5 ± 0.15	6.83 ± 1.47	
Composition								
Water (%)	99							
MO (%)	0.21–0.60							
Sodium (mmol/l)		55.0 ± 14.7	55		62–90	25 ± 3.2	8.86 ± 5.26	67.0
Potassium (mmol/l)		14.5 ± 3.7	15		18–20	15 ± 2.7	17.47 ± 5.68	18.2
Chloride (mmol/l)		49.0 ± 13.0	50		60–85	22 ± 3.5	11.86 ± 5.75	60.0
Calcium (mmol/l)		13.0 ± 1.7	13			11.6 ± 2.0	6.24 ± 1.86	3.9
Magnesium (mmol/l)		3.3 ± 0.05				2.05 ± 0.42	1.57 ± 0.48	1.4
Bicarbonate (mmol/l)		48.0 ± 7.8						
Phosphate (mmol/l)		0.26 ± 0.008				1.75 ± 0.53	0.89 ± 0.49	
Urea (mmol/l)						1.6 ± 0.20	1.09 ± 0.47	
Protein (g/l)						2.5 ± 0.47	0.657 ± 0.16	0.6

Table 1-2 Saliva Production for Different Feeds and DM of Swallowed Boluses (Meyer et al 1986)

Feed	l/kg fresh feed	l/kg DM	DM of swallowed bolus %
Grass	0.59	2.95	12.6
Grass/alfalfa silage	2.35	4.49	15.2
Leaves	2.81	7.07	11.2
Hay	5.8	6.53	14.4
Straw	5.22	5.87	13.6
Pelleted compound feed	1.7	1.9	33.6
Sugar beet pulp 90*	2.23	2.34	29.0
SBP 49*	1.18	2.42	23.2
SBP 35*	0.63	1.87	20.6

SBP, sugar beet pulp.
*DM of fed SBP in dependence on soaking.

from the parotid (Meyer et al 1985, Moeller et al 2008, Stick et al 1981). As in other species, the rate of secretion in the horse is stimulated by food intake and mastication. The greater the dry matter within the food, the greater the amount of saliva secreted due in part to the physical composition of the meal and in part to the time needed for adequate mastication, with the latter being the major determinant (Meyer et al 1985, 1986). In one study using esophagofistulated horses, the DM content of swallowed material varied between 11–15% during intake of roughage and increased to 21–34% after intake of concentrates (Meyer et al 1986) (Table 1-2).

Finally, in contrast to carnivora and omnivora, equine saliva contains virtually no digestive enzymes: as an example, the average concentration of amylase was reported to be 0.44 U/ml in horses vs. the average data 77 U/ml in humans and 98 U/ml in swine (Varloud 2006). Therefore, its most important digestive functions appear to be the lubrication of swallowed ingesta and the buffering of gastric contents which would promote intra-gastric bacterial fermentative activity (see Stomach).

Host source enzymatic digestion

The mean value of α-amylase activity in equine saliva was reported to be very low as stated earlier. This concentration is considered to be insufficient, when linked to the extent of any mastication, to digest starch (Varloud 2006). There are no specific data in horses regarding the activity levels and properties of salivary lysozyme. Lysozyme is an antibacterial enzyme found in human saliva with activity against gram-positive bacteria.

Digestive ecosystem and digestion/fermentation

Saliva contains less than 10 cfu total bacteria/ml (Varloud 2006). The contribution of these bacteria to digestive processes is typically ignored. Lindner and his collaborators measured salivary lactate concentrations in exercising horses in an attempt to find a means to monitor lactate production during exercise without having to take blood samples. After continuous exercise, the average concentration sampled was 2.21 ± 1.97 mmol/l saliva at the upper site of sampling, close to the opening of the parotid duct (Lindner et al 1999). Considering the potential production 40 l of saliva per day, this could represent up to 160 mmol of lactate flowing into the stomach and helping to acidify the contents.

Motility

Anyone who has watched a horse eat is left with the impression that it chews its food quite thoroughly, which reduces the particle size of the ingesta and presumably provides a higher digestion from both enzymatic and microbial enzymes (Ellis & Hill 2005). In fact, however, horses may actually chew their food less thoroughly than do ruminants, based upon minutes of chewing per kg of DM of food ingested (Dulphy et al 1997). Bonin et al (2007) describe three phases of the equine chewing cycle: opening, closing, and power stroke. During the *opening phase* there is a downward hinge movement combined with a rolling motion around the rostrocaudal axis that separates upper and lower dental arcades on the chewing side. At the same time a yaw motion around the dorsoventral axis swivels the mandible away from the chewing side. During the *closing phase* a small amount of roll brings the upper and lower arcades into apposition on the chewing side, while the yaw swivels the mandible across the midline. For the *power stroke*, the lower dental arcade slides across the upper arcade in a lateral to medial direction. In their study where horses were fed either hay or pellets in random order, Bonin et al. found that the chewing cycle duration was significantly longer, and thus chewing frequency reduced, during intake of hay vs. pellets (Bonin et al 2007). Meyer et al report that after a typical mastication of a roughage meal, the particle size of about one-half of the contents of the swallowed bolus is <1.6 mm (Meyer et al 1985). It is presumed by many that teeth in poor condition or any other problem that may interfere with normal mastication can cause digestive disturbances and/or chronic weight loss in horses, but the validity of this association has been questioned (Ralston et al 2001, Ellis and Hill 2005, Carmalt and Allen 2006). However, Meyer et al. (1985) have shown that chewing releases a notable portion of the soluble components within ingested roughage, a function that could perhaps be reduced when there is malocclusion (Meyer et al 1993). After mastication food is moved into the pharynx where the pattern-elicited swallowing action occurs.

Key Points

- Equine saliva is ~99% water and is relatively high in Ca and Cl content compared to other species. It contains only a trace of amylase activity thus it serves primarily as a lubricant for ingested food.
- Horses secrete large amounts of saliva. The secretion increases in response to DM food intake and chewing duration. In general, forage intake, which requires more chewing, causes a larger volume of salivary secretion than does concentrate intake.
- Three phases of the equine chewing cycle have been described: opening phase, closing phase and power stroke. Chewing not only breaks ingested fiber down into smaller particles for optimal digestion, within the large intestine, but it also releases soluble nutrient components within the fiber which can be digested pre-cecally.

Esophagus

The esophagus is 1.2–1.5 meters long in the adult 500 kg horse. It is anatomically divided into cervical, thoracic and abdominal parts (Nickel et al 1979). It has a sphincter at either end, the upper (UES) marking the division between it and the pharynx, and the lower (LES) between it and the stomach. The musculature of the proximal two thirds of the equine esophagus is striated, while the distal third is smooth. It is, as in all mammalian species, lined with a modified stratified squamous epithelium. This mucosa has no significant secretory activity (Slocombe et al 1982).

Motility

When a swallow is induced by the presence of food in the caudal pharynx, both sensory and motor components of which are via the vagus nerve (Meyer 2009), the upper UES relaxes to allow the bolus of food to enter the esophageal lumen. The bolus is passed through the esophagus by classical peristaltic (propagating ring of contraction) motor activity. Contractions through the striated muscle region are of shorter duration and propagate more rapidly than those through the smooth muscle region (Clark et al 1987, Ruckebusch et al 1981, Stick et al 1983). In humans, the peristalsis within the striated muscle is centrally controlled solely by vagal afferent nerves whereas the smooth muscle is innervated by intramural inhibitory (nitric oxide releasing) and excitatory (ACh releasing) neurons that receive inputs from separate sets of preganglionic neurons located in the dorsal motor nucleus of the vagus (Goyal and Chadbury 2008). Once the bolus reaches the distal end of the esophagus, the LES relaxes, allowing the contents to enter the stomach. The rate at which swallowed material traverses the total length varies, according to physical content, but typically takes between 4 and 10 seconds (Greet 1982), with liquid passing more rapidly (Fig. 1.3).

Key Points

- The musculature of the proximal two thirds of the equine esophagus is striated, while the distal third is smooth.
- Motility is characterized by propagating rings of contraction (peristalsis), which are shorter in duration and more rapid in velocity of propagation in the striated muscle region.

Stomach

The volume of the equine stomach is about 8% of the total GIT; thus, in the adult 500 kg horse it is 8–15 liters (Nickel et al 1979). The proximal one-half of the stomach is lined with a modified stratified squamous epithelium essentially similar to that of the esophagus and contains no secretory glands. The esophagus opens into this part. Squamous and glandular portions are well demarcated by the *margo plicatus*. The glandular mucosa is divided into cardiac, fundic and pyloric portions. The *cardiac* region comprises only a thin strip right adjacent to the *margo plicatus;* little is known about its secretory products. The *fundic* mucosa contains parietal cells which secrete acid, zymogen cells which secrete pepsin and lipase, and enterochromaffin-like (ECL) cells that secrete histamine in response to gastrin and vagal stimulation. The *pyloric* mucosal region is the site of G-cells which synthesize gastrin. D-cells, which synthesize somatostatin, are found in both fundic and pyloric mucosas (Hersey

& Sachs 1995, Modlin & Tang 1996, Schubert and Peura 2008, Vuyyuru L et al 1995). The pyloric region, also known as the gastric antrum, is connected to the small intestine, with the point of delineation being the pyloric sphincter of the stomach.

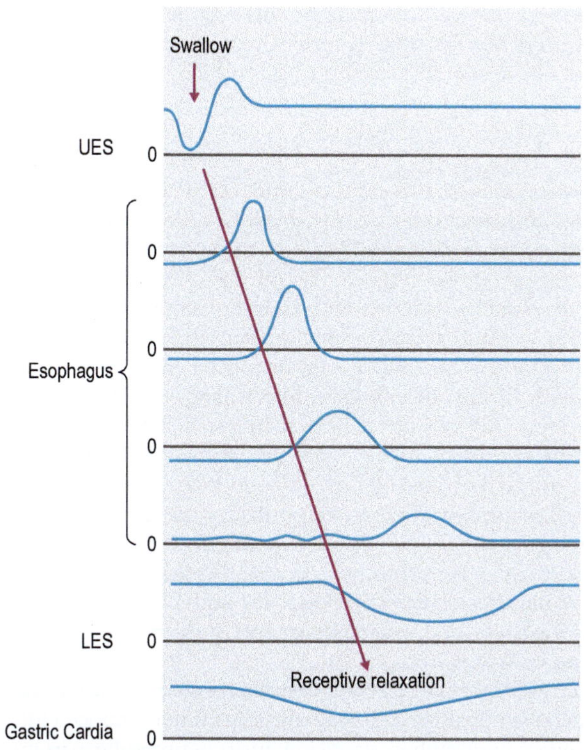

Figure 1.3 Schematic representation of the pressure changes within the upper esophageal sphincter (UES), esophagus, lower esophageal sphincter (LES) and gastric cardia in response to a swallow. The "0" indicates a zero pressure line within each section depicted.

Secretion

The major secretory product of the stomach in the horse, as in all species, is hydrochloric acid (HCl) (Andrews et al 1992, Baker & Gerring 1993, Campbell-Thompson & Merritt 1987, 1990, Murray & Schusser 1993, Sangiah et al 1988). As indicated in the anatomical review, HCl is secreted by the parietal cells which are located within the gastric glands of the fundic mucosa. Like any other bodily function, control of secretion involves a complex interaction between stimulatory and inhibitory signals. From the most elemental standpoint, the primary neural component for stimulation is vagally released acetylcholine, and the primary hormonal component is the peptide, gastrin, that is produced by G-cells located within pyloric mucosa. But this simple concept has now become much more complex in light of continuing discoveries. Current evidence suggests that the major stimulatory effect of both acetylcholine and gastrin on the parietal cells is indirect, by inducing ECL cells to release histamine that acts via the H_2 receptors, rather than by directly stimulating the muscarinic and gastrin receptors (Modlin & Tang 1996). Acid secretion is modulated by various feedback loops, mainly involving somatostatin, that are, in themselves, responsive to numerous factors, including intra-gastric pH and ingesta composition (Kidd et al 1996, Modlin & Tang 1996, Schubert and Peura 2008, Vuyyuru et al 1995) (Fig. 1.4).

In the equine, Olowo-okorun was the first to demonstrate the presence of gastrin in pyloric mucosa in 1975 (Olowo-okorun 1975). In 1990, Young and Smythe confirmed this and suggested that the posttranslational G-cell processing of progastrin in horses may differ from that of species previously studied (Young & Smythe 1990). This suggestion was confirmed by Johnsen et al (1998) who found that, in contrast to other species, equine antral gastrins are virtually non-sulfated due to low tyrosyl sulfotransferase activity

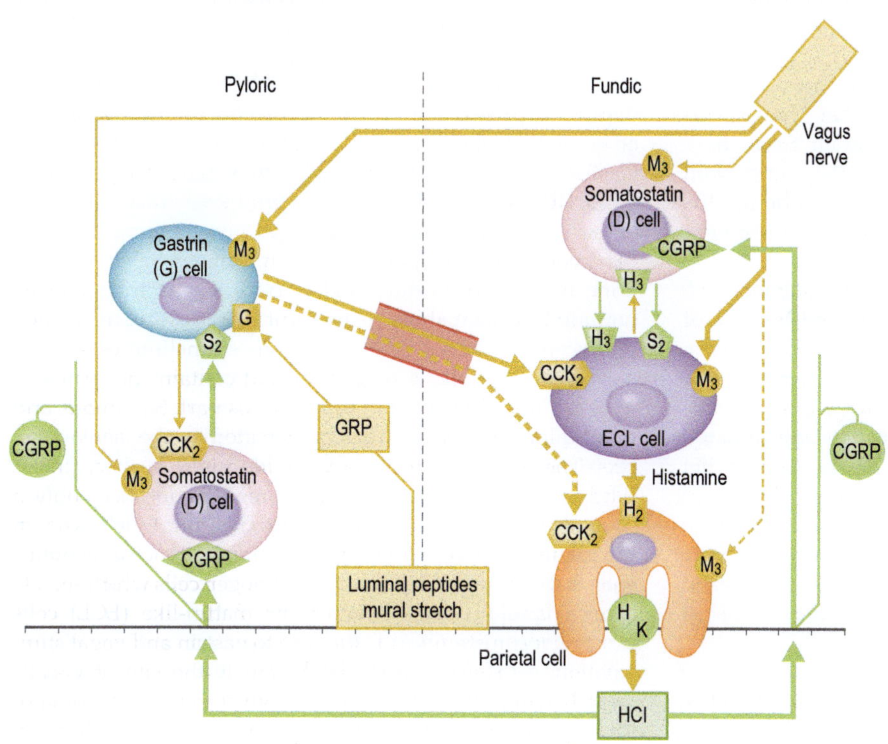

Figure 1.4 Diagrammatic representation of the major components of the control of gastric acid secretion. The orange arrows indicate inputs into the various cell types found within the pyloric and fundic portions of the gastric mucosa respectively that upregulate, and the green arrows indicate inputs that down-regulate, acid secretion by the parietal cells. The specific receptors are shown on each cell type for each of the agonists and antagonists. "M_3" are muscarinic sub-type 3 cholinergic receptors. The black lines at the bottom represent the mucosal surface. The H/K in the circle on the parietal cell represents the H^+/K^+-ATPase proton pump that is responsible for elaborating the acid secretion.

within the G-cells. This may explain why plasma gastrin in the horse is proportionally high in the "large" (G-34) vs the "small" (G-17) form, but the implications of this with respect to endogenous gastrin activity remain to be elucidated.

Horses, like pigs, monkeys, rats and humans, and in contrast to carnivora, continue to secrete HCl acid at a variable rate even when the stomach is empty (Andrews et al 1992, Campbell-Thompson & Merritt 1987, 1990, Merritt 1999, Merritt et al 2003, Murray & Schusser 1993, Orsini et al 1991, Sangiah et al 1988). This is commonly referred to as "basal" secretion and while it is reasonable to assume that a truly empty stomach is not a normal physiological condition in the horse, it is of comparative interest. Under this contrived condition, healthy horses have been found to secrete ~200 μeq/kg/hr of HCl (Campbell-Thompson & Merritt 1990) which is mixed with varying amounts of pancreatic and duodenal fluid that has refluxed into the stomach from the upper small intestine (Kitchen et al 2000). Whether or not such reflux occurs during fed conditions remains to be determined. Also, as in all mammalian species, acid secretion in the horse is stimulated by acetylcholine (Campbell-Thompson 1994), histamine (Kitchen et al 1998) and gastrin (Campbell-Thompson & Merritt 1990), and inhibited by somatostatin (Sojka et al 1992). However, the relative responses to these agents show some species-specific characteristics. For example, in vitro studies of isolated equine parietal cells conducted by Campbell-Thompson indicated that equine parietal cells are much more sensitive to histamine than to gastrin, whilst just the opposite is the case for canine parietal cells (Campbell-Thompson 1994). Two studies have specifically looked at the effects of food intake on plasma gastrin concentration in adult horses. Brown et al recorded a significant increase to ~2.5 times the fasting value within 15 minutes of ingestion of a pelleted meal of unstated amount. This increase was present until at least 75 minutes after feeding (Brown et al 1987). Sandin et al found there was an immediate and large increase in response to a large meal, whereas a small meal evoked a later and smaller response. They suggested that the degree of gastric distention may play a role in this discrepancy. Furthermore, grain meals evoked a slower and more prolonged response than hay meals (Sandin et al 1998). The obvious implication from these studies is that size and composition of a meal are important determinants of the amount of acid secreted, although the *specific* amount is very difficult to measure when food is present within the stomach.

In most monogastric animals, including the neonatal foal, the gastric contents are quite acidic throughout because of the uniform semiliquid to liquid consistency of the ingesta. In contrast, the contents of an adult equid on a regular hay/grain diet, *where the roughage is available on a free-choice basis*, vary in their pH depending upon where they are situated within the stomach. It is the roughage component of the diet that determines this since, as in the rumen, the lower density/larger particle size components tend to remain at the top of the mat of ingesta where they are minimally exposed to acid produced in the lower glandular region and maximally exposed to swallowed saliva which has a pH of ~7.5 (Stick et al 1981).

Thus, during the time when roughage intake is the highest in horses allowed free choice intake (Dulphy et al 1997, Houpt 1998), the mean pH of the contents just inside the lower esophageal sphincter vacillates between 5–7 over time, whereas the higher density, more liquid contents found in the bottom part of the stomach are consistently acidic at pH 2.0–3.0 (Husted et al 2008, Lorenzo-Figueras & Merritt 2002, Merritt 2003). When roughage intake is decreased either because it is withheld or because horses eat less during the early morning hours even if it is available, the mean pH in the upper part of the stomach drops markedly to 4.0 or less (Husted et al 2008, 2009) (Fig. 1.5). Furthermore, the ingesta within the stomach of horses fed pellets in the morning meal and no hay has been shown to coalesce immediately into a bowl shape remaining a couple of hours within the glandular region (Varloud et al 2007) where the surrounding liquid would be quite acidic.

This variance in the pH has an important implication with respect to the intensity of intra-gastric fermentation since the organisms involved within the stomach are more numerous and active at the higher pH values (Meyer et al 1980, Varloud et al 2007). Furthermore, when the pH drops below 4.0 within the nonglandular region, that mucosa is challenged and may ulcerate since it does not contain the elaborate mechanisms to protect it against HCl that are found within the glandular mucosa (see discussion of gastric mucosal protection below) (Andrews et al 2006, Widenhouse et al 2002). There is evidence that feeding alfalfa hay may provide some protection against this acid challenge of the nonglandular mucosa, perhaps through buffering effects of its high Ca and protein content (Lybbert et al 2007, Nadeau et al 2000).

The two digestive enzymes of note secreted by the equine stomach are pepsin and lipase, which is in concordance with most other mammalian species. Pepsin is proteolytic in an acid medium. The primary secretion by the zymogen (chief) cells found within fundic and pyloric mucosas is pepsinogen, which is converted to pepsin when the pH of the medium is <4.0. More than one biochemical form of equine pepsinogen exists, but the functional significance of this, with respect to intragastric proteolysis, is currently unknown (Gonchar et al 1984, Khittoo et al 1991, Sayegh et al 1999). Pharmacological suppression of gastric acid secretion with an agent such as omeprazole would be expected to result in depressed pepsin activity but this seems to have negligible effect on GIT function, at least in humans (McCarthy 2010). Gastric lipase is also produced by zymogen cells, primarily within the fundic mucosa. Horses produce a notable amount of gastric lipase which has a pH optimum ranging between pH 4.0 and pH 6.0 and is resistant to exposure at pH conditions as low as 1.5 (Moreau et al 1988), but as with pepsin, nothing is known about its role in the processing of ingesta in this species.

Finally, all regions of glandular gastric mucosa secrete mucus and bicarbonate, which stay close to the respective mucosal surfaces and are a very important component in the protection of these surfaces from destruction by gastric acid (Flemström & Isenberg 2001, Holzer 1998). Thus, under normal conditions, the pH of the medium just adjacent to the glandular mucosal surface is biologically neutral. As is well known, one of the most important inducers of mechanisms directed at protecting the glandular mucosa is prostaglandin-E_2 (PGE_2) that is up-regulated by cyclo-oxygenase-1 (COX-1) and 2 (COX-2) of the arachidonic acid cycle (Peskar 2001a, b). Both COX-1 and COX-2 are found throughout the equine GIT submucosa, in varying degrees

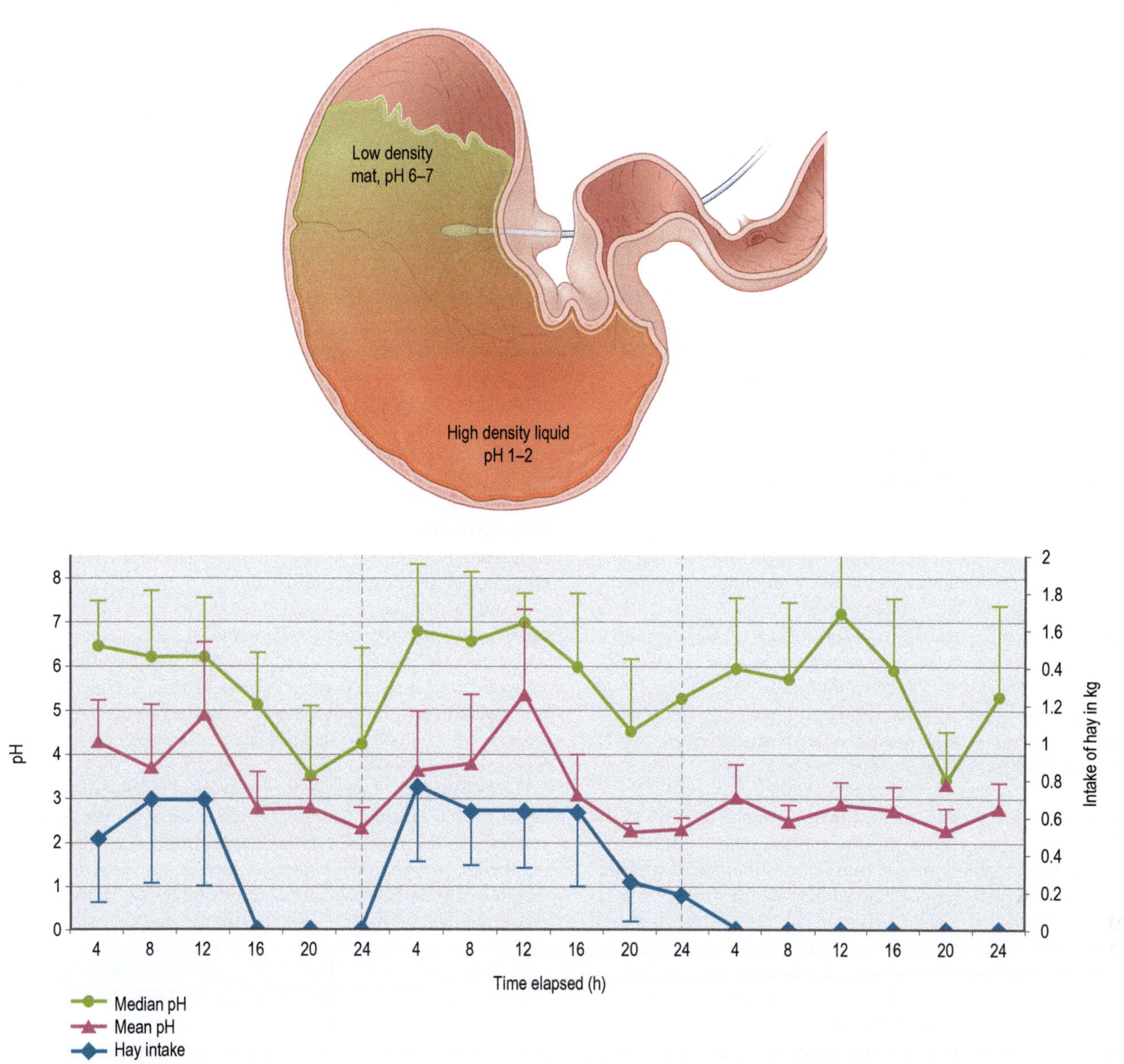

Figure 1.5 The top image represents the pH gradient of contents within the stomach of an adult horse fed forage ad libitum. The higher density, most recently swallowed food at the top maintains a median pH between 6 and 7 due to the fact that it has continuing exposure to saliva and, being in region of the non-glandular mucosa, has not been exposed to acid. The lower density contents and liquid within the lower part of the stomach, near where the acid is secreted, maintain a pH between 1–2.The graph at the bottom, published by Husted et al (2009), depicts pH changes within the non-glandular region near the opening of the lower esophageal sphincter (LES), as measured every 8 seconds via an in situ electrode shown in red. Three days of recording of median and mean pH and hay intake, broken into 4 hour blocks, are shown. During the first day, the horses, which were stalled, were allowed to eat hay ad libitum for the first 12 hours and it was taken away for the next 12 hours. During the second day, hay was available for the full 24 hours, and during the third day, it was taken away for the full 24 hours. Note that the pH of the region around the electrode trends much lower when hay is not available, thus exposing the non-glandular mucosa to a pH that could be detrimental to its integrity.

according to region (Morissey et al 2008, Morton et al 2008a, b). Probably one of the most important systems by which PGE_2 and other mediators involved in promoting mucosal protection are affected is the so-called "gastric neural emergency system" (Fig. 1.6) (Holzer 1998). This is a component of the ENS within the stomach, which is essentially a reflex arc, the afferent arm of which is constantly sampling the pH at the mucosal surface. A sufficient drop in pH results in the neural reflex up-regulation of PGE_2 expression, along with that of other mediators of protection, such as calcitonin gene-related peptide (CGRP) and constitutive nitric oxide synthase (cNOS) which increase mucosal blood flow to enhance mucus and bicarbonate secretion (Holzer 1998, Peskar 2001a) (Fig. 1.6). Another mucosal protective effect of PGE_2 is the direct inhibition of acid secretion by the parietal cell (Peskar 2001b, Peskar & Maricic, 1998). In a study done by Cargile et al, daily feeding to ponies of 20 ml/kg of corn oil, which is made up of ~40% of the arachidonic acid precursor linoleic acid, significantly increased PGE_2 and reduced gastric acid output, both before and during IV pentagastrin infusion. This indicates that this mechanism is present within the equine stomach (Cargile et al

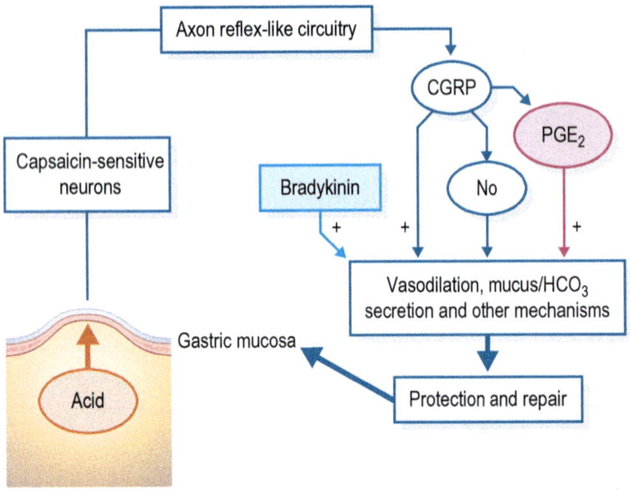

Figure 1.6 A schematic of the "neural emergency system" in the stomach as proposed by Holzer (1998) **whereby receptors reside within the gastric glandular mucosa that are sensitive to the presence of gastric acid. Their stimulation induces a neural reflex arc within the gastric component of the ENS that up-regulates mechanisms that protect the mucosa against destruction by the acid.** For instance, CGRP, as depicted in Fig. 1.3, causes somatostatin release which, in turn, down-regulates release of both gastrin and histamine. Nitric oxide (NO) causes submucosal vasodilation which, in turn, makes more HCO_3^- available to buffer the acid at the luminal surfaces of the mucosal cells, and PGE_2 invokes numerous protective actions such as increased mucus secretion and suppression of acid secretion. This schema is based upon studies done in small laboratory animals but the mediators shown have been found in the equine stomach.

2004). Additional evidence of the importance of PGE_2 to the protection of the equine glandular mucosa is the glandular ulcerogenic effects of nonsteroidal anti-inflammatory drugs (NSAIDs) which have strong antiprostaglandin activity (MacAllister et al 1993, Mackay et al 1983, Meschter et al 1990). *There is no evidence, however, that any of the mechanisms discussed above are operative in the non-glandular (squamous) gastric mucosa* (Andrews et al 2006, Widenhouse et al 2002). Bullimore et al described the presence of a thin layer of mucus on top of the gastric squamous mucosa but they proposed that its source was the glandular mucosa since they found no mucus-producing cells within the squamous mucosa (Bullimore et al 2001). However, in *in vitro* experiments Peretich et al. (2009) have described an increased expression of mRNA for sodium-potassium adenosinetriphosphatase (NAKA) within nonglandular mucosa that has been exposed to HCl and VFA. NAKA plays a critical role in maintaining intracellular Na-K homeostasis and could thus play an important role in protection of the non-glandular mucosa. Interestingly, this response was relatively greater in older than in younger horses. This interesting finding requires further study.

Digestion

Host source enzymatic digestion

In mammals, the conversion of pepsinogen to pepsin occurs within an acidic medium. Despite the relative importance of pepsin's role in protein digestion in the horse is currently unknown, it probably is similar to other mammals. The endogenous and microbial proteolytic activity has been measured in the gastric content of ponies in both the fundic and pyloric regions. It was negligible in the fundic region (0.14 μg of hydrolyzed protein/mg ingesta/min). Although greater in the pyloric region, it was still ten-fold less (2.43 μg of hydrolyzed protein/mg ingesta/min) than that of the small intestine content (Kern et al 1974).

We do not know the role of gastric lipase in the horse but, presumably, as in humans, it contributes to the partial digestion of feed triacylglycerols (TAG) to form diacylglycerols and free fatty acids (FFA). TAG are mainly composed of long-chain fatty acids (LCFA, number of carbons ≥ 16), plus phospholipids and sterols. The level of lipolytic activity was reported to be the highest in the fundic mucosae compared to the nonglandular, cardiac and pyloric mucosas (87 units per g of fresh tissue versus 8, 4, and 5 respectively). However, this value remained much lower than pancreatic lipase activity: the ratio of total lipase pancreatic/preduodenal activities was 61 (Moreau et al, 1988).

Digestive ecosystem: digestion/fermentation

Intragastric fermentative activity in the horse has been recognized since the early 1940, and in the early 1960s, lactobacilli and streptococci were detected in gastric contents (Alexander & Davies, 1963). However, no protozoa have been found in the stomach (Kern et al 1974). Recent work using culture-dependent and -independent techniques has revealed a diverse bacterial community in the gastric contents and confirmed that the acidic conditions do not prevent a large number of bacteria being present (Al Jassim 2005, Varloud et al 2006). The gastric biotope, in fact, offers a favorable environment for bacterial growth: dietary components that are barely digested prior to introduction into the stomach and are retained, in the most part, for 85–300 min postprandially; water content that varies from 98.9% in fasted animals (Nadeau et al 2000) to 69.3% after a meal (Wolter & Chaabouni, 1979). Temperature is widely recognized as being crucial for managing bacterial cultivation, but very few data are available about this characteristic in the gastric ecosystem. Varloud and collaborators reported temperatures that never exceeded 28°C with an average temperature of 24°C (Varloud et al 2007). No data are available regarding the aerobic–anaerobic status of the gastric environment but it is probable that the redox potential is compatible with the growth of facultative anaerobic bacteria that can tolerate small amounts of O_2. As for the intragastric pH, its values fluctuate largely depending on feed ingestion and region within the stomach, as previously described.

In fasting horses, the pH of gastric contents can periodically increase and even exceed neutrality due to duodenal reflux (Campbell-Thompson & Merritt 1990) which is favorable to bacterial colonization. This probably explains why Varloud et al found a large variation of the total anaerobe concentration that from 10^2 could reach 10^6 cfu/ml within the fundic glandular region (Varloud et al 2007). Similarly, concentration of total anaerobes were reported to be surprisingly high on the mucosa of non-glandular proventricular (10^4–10^6 cfu/ml) and glandular cardiac (10^5–10^7 cfu/ml) regions in the empty stomach (Varloud 2006). Despite the large densities of microbial communities, the end-product concentrations were low, confirming that bacterial fermentative activity is weak in the empty stomach (Varloud et al 2007).

In fed horses, saliva is secreted and contributes to increased pH mean values, which can reach up to 7.0 in the proximal stomach (Healy et al 1995, Husted et al 2008, 2009, Lorenzo-Figueras & Merritt, 2002). In one feeding study, from the first postprandial hour the concentrations of bacterial communities increased greatly whereas the inter-individual variability decreased (e.g. pH fluctuations were less pronounced and more homogeneous; Varloud et al 2007). After the first postprandial hour, the gastric microfloral concentration continued increasing with total anaerobe concentration from 9.5×10^6 to 2×10^8 cfu/ml in average at 60 and 210 min post ingestion of the meal respectively (Varloud et al 2007). Even higher values were reported in previous studies (de Fombelle et al 2003, Kern et al 1974). The total anaerobe concentration in the gastric content is equivalent to, or even higher than, that measured in the post-ileal compartments, such as the cecum or the colon (de Fombelle et al 2003). In some recent studies, lactobacilli concentration averaged 1.3×10^7 cfu/ml 210 min after ingestion of the meal (Varloud et al 2007) and from 1.3×10^7–2.5×10^8 cfu/ml 30 min later (de Fombelle et al 2003). As for streptococci, their concentration averaged 1.5×10^6 cfu/ml 210 min after ingestion of the meal (Varloud et al 2007) and varied from 2×10^7–3.2×10^8 cfu/ml thirty min later (de Fombelle et al 2003). The concentration of lactate-utilizing bacteria also increased and averaged 2.5×10^4 cfu/ml 210 min after the distribution of the meal (Varloud et al 2007) and varied from 6.5×10^6–4×10^7 cfu/ml 30 min later (de Fombelle et al 2003). Despite the decrease in intragastric pH when the meal contained more starch, the 240 min postprandial concentrations of the different bacterial communities were similar or even higher (de Fombelle et al 2003).

Merritt has suggested that microbes that convert ingested non-structure carbohydrates to VFA colonize, in particular, the coarser fibrous ingesta, which collects towards the top of the stratified mat of gastric contents. Here the pH of the contents is a more suitable environment for the microbes as the mat has not been fully penetrated by gastric acid (Merritt 2003). The marked increases in bacterial count observed postprandially cannot be explained purely by an influx from the small intestine, and the bacterial concentrations in the feed are too low to cause the effect. As mentioned above, total anaerobe concentration is very high on the mucosa of non-glandular proventricular (10^5–10^7 cfu/ml) and glandular cardiac regions (10^5–10^7 cfu/ml) in the empty stomach, which suggests that these bacteria are responsible for the inoculation of the ingested bolus. Also, three species of lactobacilli (*L. crispatus*, *L. salivarius* and *L. reuteri*) have been identified on the gastric mucosa (Yuki et al 2000) and within the gastric content (Al Jassim et al 2005, Fujisawa et al 1993), sustaining the hypothesis of an inoculation of the gastric contents by the desquamation of mucosal cells previously colonized by bacteria (Yuki et al 2000).

In the horse stomach, cellulolytic bacterial concentrations have been reported to be negligible (de Fombelle et al 2003, Kern et al 1974). Therefore, the contribution of gastric microflora to plant cell wall degradation is probably insignificant. On the contrary, there is a strong impact of the gastric microflora on starch digestion, due to the high proportion of amylolytic bacteria. Starch is degraded into lactate intragastrically whereas it would provide glucose in the small gut. These two nutrients do not contribute equally to the horse energetic provision. The impact of this starch disappearance in the stomach has not been quantified from a global nutritional point of view.

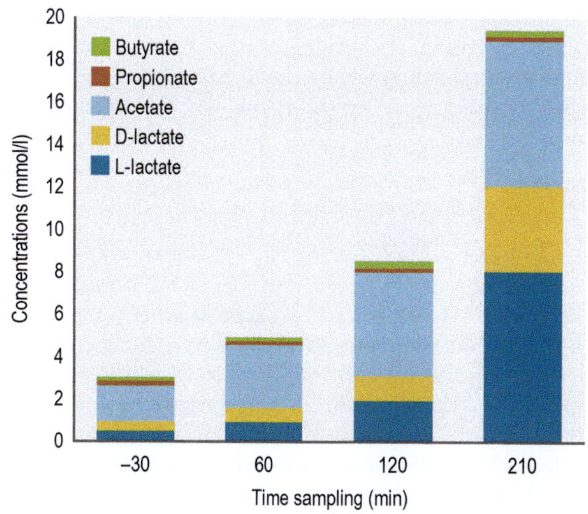

Figure 1.7 Concentrations of fermentation end-products in the gastric content before and 60, 120 and 210 minutes after intake of a complete pelleted meal.

Varloud et al found that, along with the bacterial densities, the intra-gastric lactate concentration increased linearly from the first postprandial hour and reached 8.0 mmol/L 210 min after the meal distribution (Varloud et al 2007) (Fig. 1.7). Lactate is the major end-product (Argenzio et al 1974b, de Fombelle et al 2003, Kern et al 1974, Varloud et al 2007, Wolter & Chaabouni 1979) and, depending on the studies, L-lactate (Nadeau et al 2000, Varloud et al 2007, Wolter & Chaabouni 1979) or D-lactate (de Fombelle et al 2003, Al Jassim 2006, Varloud et al 2006) represents the major isomer.

In the Varloud et al study, VFA concentration also increased linearly from the first postprandial hour to ~8.0 mmol/l 180 min after meal ingestion (Varloud et al 2007). Argenzio et al reported a maximal VFA concentration 4 h after the meal ingestion (Argenzio et al 1974b). However, others have indicated that the maximal intragastric VFA concentration is reached 1 h postprandially (Nadeau et al 2000). VFA concentrations within the gastric contents have varied from 4.4–51.3 mmol/l (Alexander and Davies 1963, Argenzio et al 1974b, de Fombelle et al 2003, Elsden et al 1946, Kern et al 1974, Morris et al 2002, Varloud et al 2007). Overall, acetate represents the highest molar proportion (70–80%). The second highest is propionate which represents less than 10% of the total VFA.

Varloud et al found that the ammonia concentration increased from 2 h postprandially and reached 3.51 mmol/l 3 h after meal ingestion (Varloud et al 2007) being probably the result of the protein degradation as this contributes to the production of the ionized form of NH_3 (Jouany et al 1995). In horses fed a hay-based diet, ammonia concentrations are low postprandially (0.17–0.23 mmol/l) (Kern et al 1974), in contrast to horses fed a starchy concentrate where ammonia can reach concentration levels tenfold higher (Wolter & Chaabouni 1979). As for D-glucose, an end-product of starch hydrolysis, in the Varloud et al study its concentration increased from 14.4 mmol/l to 41.2 mmol/l 3 h after the meal ingestion (Varloud et al 2007), indicating a strong starch-degrading activity of the microbial population.

In conclusion, it is important to remember that the intense fermentative activity that occurs within the stomach can lead to partial utilization of ingested starch which is therefore transformed into end-products other than glucose. The extent to which this impacts on the nutrition of the horse is currently ignored, but probably should be taken into account.

Motility

There are numerous ways that gastrointestinal motility has been studied and defined. With respect to the horse, these have included: (1) recording *myoelectrical activity* via electrodes implanted into muscle preparations in vitro, and either surgically implanted onto the serosa or by a transabdominal technique in vivo; (2) recording *mechanical activity* of muscle bath preparations in vitro, or via strain gauges implanted onto the serosa or intra-luminal pressure sensors in vivo; (3) measuring *actual transit time* by use of various markers; and, (4) undertaking *ultrasonographic imaging*. The best picture to date of normal GIT motility in the intact, conscious equid has been provided by myoelectrical and mechanical recordings done in numerous laboratories (Hudson & Merritt 2008).

Myoelectrical recordings are perhaps the most complex in terms of the information they can provide. There are essentially two different events that can be seen in GI smooth muscle: (1) the *slow wave* (SW), a regularly occurring subthreshold oscillation of the resting membrane potential with which there is no associated contraction; and, (2) the *action potential* (AP), which indicates muscle depolarization and, therefore, contraction. An AP can only occur associated with a SW (Bass et al 1961, Christensen 1971). Therefore, the inherent SW frequency within any given region determines the *maximal* contraction frequency of the muscle fibers within that region and during periods of time when there are only slow waves present, there is no motility.

The contractile events of the stomach are governed primarily by local myoelectrical activity and neural control through the vagus (Furness 2008). Myoelectrically, the slow wave frequency which, as mentioned above, determines the *maximum* frequency that the stomach can contract, is around 3/min in the horse and pig, whereas in dogs and ruminants it is closer to 6/min (Kelly et al 1969, Malbert & Ruckebusch 1989, Merritt et al 1989, Minami & McCallum 1984, Ruckebusch & Bueno, 1976). An interesting feature of equine and ruminant gastroduodenal motility is that just prior to the commencement of phase I of the migrating motility complex (MMC) in the proximal duodenum, the gastric antrum stops moving for a few minutes (Merritt et al 1989). During this time gastric emptying ceases which may allow backflow of duodenal contents into the stomach (see section on small intestinal motility for explanation of the MMC).

From the limited number of studies that have been done to date, it appears that equine gastric motility that results in emptying, per se, is not fundamentally different from that of other species. That is, the coarser contents are moved out primarily by peristaltic contractions that start at mid-fundic level and move through the pyloric region with increasing rate and strength ("antral systole") to force the contents into the upper duodenum. The finer, more liquid contents collect within the pyloric region and are forced into the upper duodenum by a combination of increased proximal gastric tone and antral systole (Camilleri et al 1985, Hinder and Kelly 1977, Kwiatek et al 2009, Tack 2000, Treacy et al 1990). Basically, the time it takes for a meal to leave the stomach is determined by the latency period between time of ingestion and the initiation of emptying and the rate of emptying itself. In general, ingested liquids empty significantly more rapidly than solids. The data available indicate a half time ($T_{1/2}$) for emptying of a small liquid meal in the horse is ±30 minutes, and for a small solid meal ±90 minutes (Lohmann et al 2000, Ringger et al 1996, Sutton et al 2003). Clearly, however, these values are dependent upon experimental procedure and the size and composition of the diets used for the studies. For instance, Metayer et al found that increasing the amount of starch in a solid concentrate meal significantly increased the $T_{1/2}$ value and that despite a greater rate of emptying when a large meal was fed the $T_{1/2}$ value was increased compared to a smaller meal of the same concentrate composition (Metayer et al 2004) (Fig. 1.8).

Conversely, the normal gastric wall increases in compliance in response to meal ingestion. This relaxation response has been divided into two phases - an initial "receptive relaxation" phase occurring as the meal is being eaten followed by a more prolonged "adaptive relaxation" phase (Kwiatek et al 2009, van den Berghe et al 2009). Some have referred to the whole process as "accommodation". What this means with respect to a maximal volume limitation in the normal equine stomach has not yet been determined. It has been proposed that the first phase is induced by mechanosensors within the pharynx and/or esophagus, whereas the second phase is controlled by sensors within the duodenum that are triggered by food entering it from the stomach (Schwizer et al 2002). Such a biphasic response has been documented in horses ingesting a hay meal of either 0.5 or 1 g/kg body weight. The duration of the receptive relaxation phase was directly related to the time it took to eat the meal, and was greatest during ingestion of the larger meal. Furthermore, the only significant degree of second phase adaptive relaxation above baseline was after the large hay meal (Lorenzo-Figueras et al 2002) suggesting that it

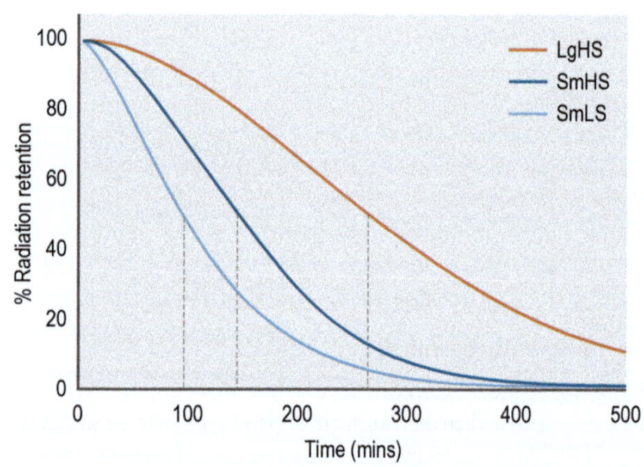

Figure 1.8 Gastric emptying, as measured by scintigraphy, of various meals labeled with Tc^{m99}. The horses had been adapted to one of 3 feeding regimens, designated as small high starch (SmHS), small low starch (SmLS), or large high starch (LgHS), over 15 days prior to the emptying study. The LS and HS pelleted rations had a digestible energy content of 2.47 kcal/g and 3.26 kcal/g respectively. The SmHS curve is significantly different from the SmLS curve, and from the LgHS curve. Where the vertical red lines intersect with the ordinate represents the $T_{1/2}$ value for the respective emptying curves.

Adapted from Metayer et al 2004.

surpassed a threshold whereby duodenal interaction was induced which could putatively down-regulate the delivery of gastric contents to the duodenum. Based upon studies done in rats, carnivores and humans, "duodenal interaction" includes the release of CCK which, in turn, increases gastric wall compliance and decreases gastric emptying rate. In these species, there is a direct relationship between the amount of CCK released and the amount of fat in the diet. Accordingly, a follow-up to this study was done by Lorenzo-Figueras et al where a commercial sweet feed meal, instead of hay, was given, supplemented isocalorically with either corn oil or glucose (Fig. 1.9). Interestingly, the glucose-supplemented meal induced a significantly more prolonged receptive relaxation phase than the fat supplemented meal, which is just the opposite of what was expected based upon results in other species as described above. But there was no significant difference in emptying time between the meals as determined by the ^{13}C-octanoic acid breath test technique (Lorenzo-Figueras et al 2005). Wyse et al found, however, that the addition of soybean oil to an oats and bran mixture significantly decreased gastric emptying rate in ponies, also determined by the ^{13}C-octanoic acid breath test, although they did not measure receptive relaxation (Wyse et al 2001). In conclusion, this an area of research that needs a much more standardized approach in the horse.

Absorption

In vitro the absorptive capacity of the gastric epithelium was studied and the data showed that the VFA produced within the equine stomach are not absorbed from the stomach into the bloodstream (Argenzio et al 1974b). This suggested that the normal nonglandular (squamous) mucosa is particularly resistant to VFA penetration. More recently, Nadeau et al have found, in in vitro studies also, that VFA can penetrate into the non-glandular submucosa if the mucosa is exposed to a pH of <4.0 (Nadeau et al 2003). As indicated above, this can be detrimental to the integrity of the mucosal barrier but whether it allows significant movement of VFA from lumen to blood in vivo remains to be determined.

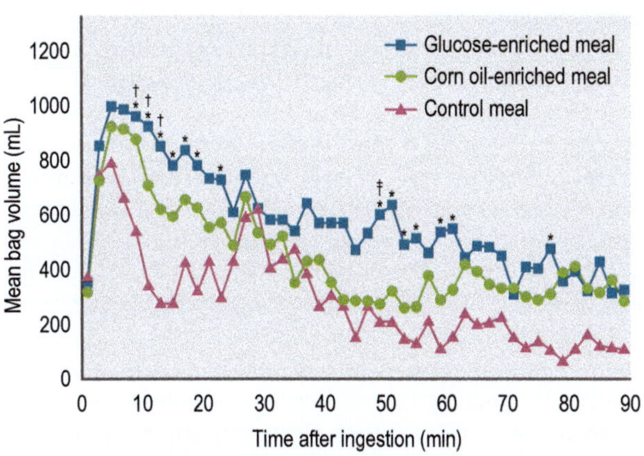

Figure 1.9 Gastric receptive relaxation, as measured by a barostatically controlled bag placed into the nonglandular region of six horses, expressed as mean bag volume. An increase in volume indicates relaxation. At time 0, the horses were fed either a control meal of 0.5 kg/kg body weight of a commercial 10% protein sweet feed mixture, or a control meal with 1.95 kcal/kg body weight of either glucose or corn oil mixed in. Each post-prandial volume represents a value from which the baseline value for that experiment has been subtracted. Bag volume was significantly higher than baseline during the entire length of the experiment after ingestion of each enriched meal, whereas it remained significantly higher than baseline for only 40 minutes after ingestion of the control meal. *Significant ($P < 0.5$) difference between glucose-enriched meal and control meal within the same period. †Significant difference between corn oil-enriched meal and control meal within the same period. ‡Significant difference between glucose and corn oil-enriched meals during the same period (Lorenzo-Figueras et al 2005).

Key Points

- The proximal one-half of the equine stomach is lined with a non-glandular, squamous, mucosa that is similar to esophageal mucosa. The distal one-half is lined with glandular mucosa comprised of the classical cardiac, fundic and pyloric portions.
- As in other species, the fundic mucosa is the site of HCl secretion and the pyloric mucosa is the production site of gastrin, a major HCl secretagogue. HCl secretion is stimulated by food intake but continues at a low level even if the stomach is empty.
- In the horse allowed roughage intake ad libitum, there is a distinct pH gradient within the contents, with it being notably higher in those in the proximal vs the distal stomach. Salivary secretion contributes to the higher pH in the proximal region.
- There is a diverse and active gastric bacterial population that, dependent upon prevailing pH, converts some of the non structural carbohydrate-based feeds into lactic acid essentially and volatile fatty acids to a lesser extent. How much, if any, of these end-products is absorbed across the gastric mucosa is not well understood.
- Size and composition of diet appear to be important determinants of degree of fermentation receptive relaxation and emptying rate of the equine stomach. Limited data available indicate that, as in other species, liquids empty more rapidly than solids, but retention times for concentrates and forage may differ.

Small intestine

As in other mammalian species, the small intestine of the horse is divided into three major regions: duodenum, jejunum, and ileum. Relative to its body size, the horse has a rather short small intestine – around 25 meters in length in the 500 kg adult, with the majority being the jejunum with the duodenum and ileum being about 1 and 0.7 meters long respectively. The bile duct and the primary pancreatic duct open into the duodenal diverticulum which is located ~15 cm aboral to the pyloric sphincter. Because of this location, it is common for bile and pancreatic juice to reflux back into the stomach, especially if it is empty, since the sphincter remains open during the intervals between antral contractions (Kitchen et al 2000). A secondary pancreatic duct opens into the duodenum very close to the duodenal diverticulum (Nickel et al 1979).

The small intestine is lined throughout by a mucosa composed of finger-like villi, each of which is surrounded by a group of crypts; the surface epithelial cells arise from the crypts and migrate up the villi as they mature (Fig. 1.10). During maturation numerous small projections, called microvilli, develop on the luminal (apical) surface of certain cells and it is within these microvilli, especially those in the cells lining the top one-third of each villus, that the

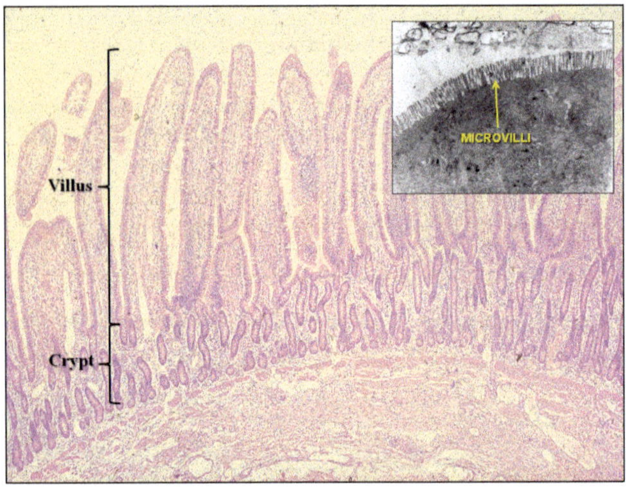

Figure 1.10 Typical equine jejunal mucosal architecture, as shown in the light micrograph of H&E stained tissue. The inset is an electron micrograph of a portion of an enterocyte on a villus showing the microvilli that line the luminal surface of these cells (intestinal lumen top left).

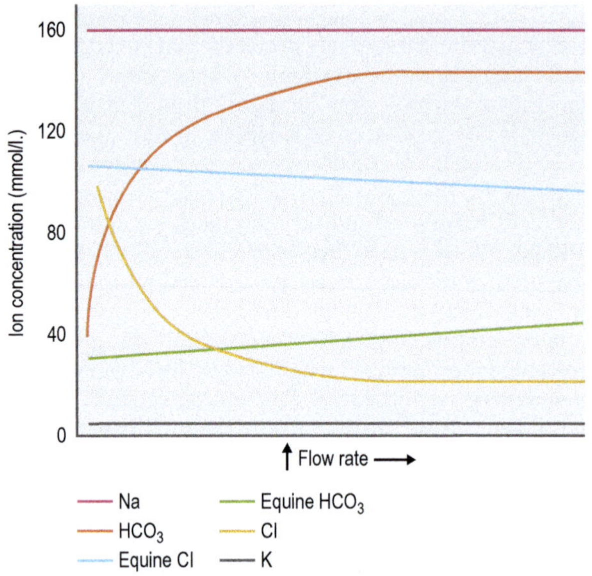

Figure 1.11 Trends in ion concentration in pancreatic juice in relation to flow rate. In humans, carnivora, swine and rats the chloride and bicarbonate concentrations reflect those of plasma at low rates of secretion but change dramatically as the secretory rate increases (yellow and red lines respectively), whereas in horses the changes are minor (blue and green lines respectively). In all species the sodium and potassium concentrations remain similar to those in plasma irrespective of flow rate.
Adapted from Alexander & Hickson 1970.

intestinal digestive enzymes are found. Those same cells incorporate the mechanisms involved in absorption of the digested nutrients, thus their designation as absorptive cells. Other cells that can be found within the surface epithelium are mucus (goblet) cells, enteroendocrine cells that interact with the ENS, Paneth cells and undifferentiated columnar cells. Within the center of each villus there is a circulatory network, the venous arm of which carries absorbed water soluble micronutrients into the portal vein system, and a lymphatic vessel into which the absorbed long-chain fats move to eventually attain their entrance into the blood stream via the thoracic duct (see section on small intestinal absorption). Enterocytes are connected to each other by tight junctions, which restrict the transmucosal flux of large molecules, although they are permeable to water and many low-molecular weight substances such as nicotinamide, ascorbic acid and biotin (Madara and Trier 1994).

Secretion

A considerable amount of fluid and other substances are secreted into the small intestine, predominantly from the liver and pancreas in order to aid digestion. In those species in which it has been studied, fat digestion is promoted by the interaction of bile salts secreted through the biliary system and lipase from the pancreas. Bile salt excretion in the equid appears to be dependent upon an intact enterohepatic circulation, as in other species (Engelking et al 1989). The only actual flow data available is from studies using ponies where the bile flow rate was 18.6 ± 1.7 µl/kg-min, with a bile acid excretion rate of 0.18 ± 0.02 µmol/kg-min (Gronwall et al 1975). It is presumed that this represents true original bile production since there is no gall bladder in the horse in which the bile might be stored.

With respect to the pancreas, in contrast to most other species, the nonstimulated (basal) secretion in the horse is profuse and apparently continuous. Alexander and Hickson reported a secretory rate of 10–12 l/day in a 100 kg pony (Alexander & Hickson 1970) and Kitchen et al estimated that the average size adult horse secretes 20–25 L/day (Kitchen et al 2000). When further secretion is stimulated with secretin the concentration of bicarbonate in equine pancreatic juice does not increase, with a corresponding decrease in chloride concentration, as it does in other species. Rather, both remain much closer to their resting concentrations (Alexander & Hickson 1970) (Fig. 1.11). Nonetheless, the pH of equine pancreatic juice is basic (~8.0) due to its bicarbonate content (~30 mEq/l) and it is an important source of buffering against the gastric acid entering the duodenum (Alexander & Hickson 1970, Kitchen et al 2000). *There is now some evidence that gastrin may also be a major stimulant of pancreatic water and electrolyte output in horses, comparable to the effect of secretin in equid and nonequid species* (Merritt et al 1996, Kitchen et al 2000).

The concentrations of those digestive enzymes within the pancreatic juice of horses that have been investigated (i.e., amylase and trypsinogen (trypsin)), are very low in comparison to other species (Alexander & Hickson 1970, Kienzle et al 1994). Of interest is that, on a relative basis, equine pancreatic tissue contains much more lipase than any of the other digestive enzymes (Lorenzo-Figueras et al 2007) (Table 1-3). Whether this is also true for the juice itself remains to be determined. It is presumed, but not yet shown, that CCK, which is produced by specialized cells in the small intestinal mucosa, plays a major role in stimulating enzyme secretion from the equine pancreas. In other species CCK release from these cells is stimulated by a specific CCK releasing factor (CCK-RF) secreted into the intestinal lumen by another cell type in the mucosa and CCK-RF secretion itself is stimulated by the presence of trypsin in the lumen (Liddle 1995). CCK, along with other GI peptides,

Table 1-3 Comparative Pancreatic Tissue Specific Activity Expressed as Mean IU/mg Protein (Lorenzo-Figueras et al 2007)

	A	L	E	Tr	Ch
Adult horse (n = 7)	2.3 (1)*	41.5 (18.04)	0.07 (0.03)	0.13 (0.06)	0.36 (0.16)
Adult pig (n = 12)	107 (1)	49 (0.46)	0.22 (0.002)	0.44 (0.004)	2.26 (0.02)
Adult rat (n = 20)	56 (1)	39 (0.69)	0.02 (–)	0.10 (0.001)	1.34 (0.02)
Calf 14 d 6 months (n = 4)	2.3 (1)	11 (4.78)	0.03 (0.01)	0.07 (0.03)	1.51 (0.66)

A = amylase; L = lipase; E = elastase; Tr = trypsin; Ch = chymotrypsin.
*Values in parentheses relative to amylase = 1.

is present within the equine small intestinal mucosa (Kitamura et al 1984), but Lorenzo-Figueras and Merritt found that, in contrast to other species, it is immeasurable in equine plasma, even after meal ingestion (Lorenzo-Figueras & Merritt 2006).

Under normal conditions, secretion of electrolytes by the small intestine itself, which occurs within the crypts, is normally out-paced by absorption so that net movement of water, which follows solute, is from lumen into bloodstream. Chloride is the major anion involved in this secretion (Hirota & McKay 2006, Venkatasubramanian et al 2010) and there is evidence that in horses its mechanism of secretion may be different from respective transport mechanisms in other species because it could not be blocked in vitro by the usual chloride channel blockers (Cehak et al 2009). There are two important sites where specific secretion of bicarbonate is very important: (1) in the duodenum from Brunner's glands to help protect the duodenal mucosa from acidic contents emptied from the stomach (Pfeiffer & Dabareiner 1992); and (2) in the distal ileum, thought to be a mechanism to help establish the necessary beneficial environment for the cecal microbes involved in fermentation (Argenzio & Stevens 1975).

Digestion

Host source enzymatic digestion

Pancreatic and intestinal brush border enzymes act by hydrolyzing dietary nonstructural carbohydrates and proteins as well as, in conjunction with bile salts, dietary fats.

Pancreatic and intestinal enzyme contribution

Enzymes involved in starch hydrolysis (Fig. 1.12)

The activity of the pancreatic endoenzyme α-amylase is highly variable and low, compared to other species (Kienzle & Radicke 1993, Kienzle et al 1994) but adequate for horses fed high proportion of forage in their ration (Roberts 1974). In response to increased dietary carbohydrate intake, the equine α-amylase activity can be enhanced: the activity of amylase which averaged 22.3 U/g wet weight in jejunal chyme was twice higher when horses were fed grain diets (30.8 ± 15.4 U/g chyme) for 24 h rather than maintained on an all-hay diet (15 ± 3.4 U/g) (Kienzle et al 1994). As suggested recently by Dyer and his collaborators, this enhancement requires a longer time for adaptation than the regulation of the Na+/glucose co-transporters (Dyer et al 2009). The optimal activity of pancreatic α-amylase occurs at pH 4–9 (Kolb 1975). In humans, pancreatic α-amylase expresses its optimal activity in the presence of chloride ions which act as co-factors (Feller et al 1996).

The α-amylase works by penetration of starch via formation of wells or cracks in the granule which is then hydrolyzed from the center to the periphery (Kienzle et al 1997, Lynn & Cochrane 1997). Pancreatic α-amylases randomly hydrolyse links α-(1,4) (Tester et al 2004) and liberate α-glucose and oligosaccharides from 2–7 units with a terminal α-glucose. The action of α-amylase is incomplete because it is stopped by links α-(1,6) which can only be hydrolyzed by unconnected enzymes such as pullulanase or isoamylase (Tester et al 2004).

Oligosaccharides liberated from amylose, amylopectin and residual α-dextrins initially produced by starch digestion are further hydrolyzed by the disaccharidases sucrase and maltase, both of which have been reported to be present on the brush border membrane of the equine small intestine (Dyer et al 2002). Sucrase is a α-glucosidase capable of hydrolyzing sucrose and ramification links α-(1,6) of residual α-dextrins in α-D-glucose and α-D-fructose. Sucrase activity is highest in the proximal small intestine of the horse on a grass-based diet, with activity levels of 0.187 ± 0.023, 0.470 ± 0.116 and 0.273 ± 0.061 μmol/min/mg protein in the duodenum, jejunum and ileum respectively. Maltase activity is also distributed throughout the equine small intestine, with activity levels of 0.317 ± 0.089, 0.929 ± 0.187 and 0.697 ± 0.151 μmol/min/mg protein in the proximal, mid and distal small intestine respectively, which is extremely high (Dyer et al 2002). Therefore, horses possess sufficient small intestinal disaccharidase activity to digest sucrose and maltose, particularly the latter (Dyer et al 2002, Roberts et al 1974).

The third major disaccharidase, lactase (which digests milk sugar, lactose), is also found in the brush border membrane of the equine small intestine. Its activity is highest in the jejunum (Roberts et al 1973, Dyer et al 2002). It is present in the equine small intestine in two forms: neutral and acid β-galactosidase. The activity of both forms diminishes with maturity, with the neutral form virtually disappearing after 4 years of age (Roberts et al 1973).

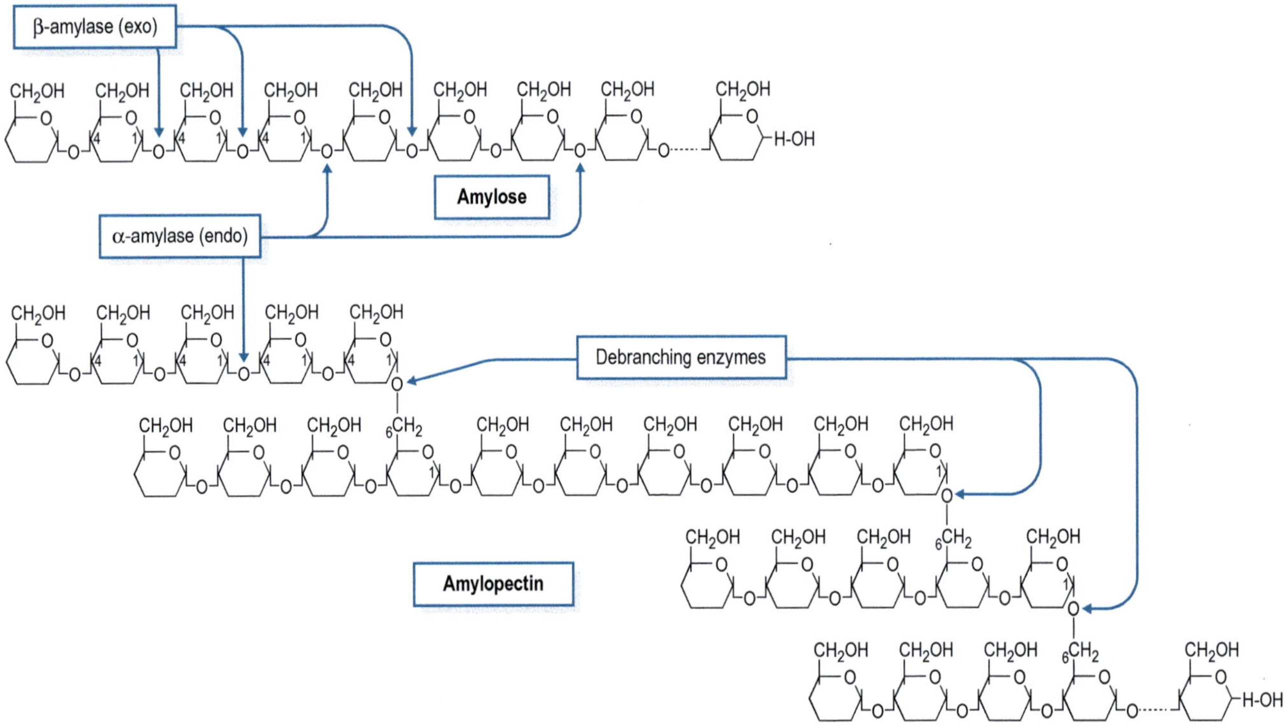

Figure 1.12 **The pancreatic α endo-amylase hydrolyses the α-(1,4) links of amylase and amylopectine of starch into α-glucose and oligosaccharides (from Tester et al 2004).**

Enzymes involved in fat hydrolysis

Surprisingly, recent data showed that the predominant digestive enzyme in equine pancreatic tissue is lipase (Lorenzo-Figueras et al 2007) (Table 1-3). In humans, pancreatic lipase is the main enzyme responsible for dietary fat digestion. It mainly breaks down the diacylglycerols liberated by the gastric lipase. It operates under a slightly alkaline pH, in contrast to gastric lipase. It leads to the release of 2-monoacylglycerides and long chain fatty acids (LCFA). In contrast to other nutrients, products of lipolysis are poorly soluble in an aqueous solution and need the presence of bile salts to be transported to the enterocytes (Lengsfeld et al 2004). However, pancreatic lipase cannot act alone in the presence of bile salts; it needs the presence of a proteinic co-factor, co-lipase, to form a complex that counteracts the effects of bile salts by permitting an interfacial binding of pancreatic lipase and subsequent triacylglycerol hydrolysis (Lengsfeld et al 2004). Molecular cloning has resulted in expression of cDNA encoded co-lipase A and B in the horse (Crenon et al 1994).

Bile salts contribution

In general, gastric and pancreatic lipases need an emulsification of their substrate for optimal activity. It is now recognized that bile salts do not constitute good emulsifiers of triacylglycerols, as previously thought, but play an essential role in the solubilization of lipolysis products by adsorbing at the triacylglycerol-water interface because they are amphiphilic molecules. Monoacylglycerols and LCFA interact with bile salts and phospholipids to form mixed micelles. The micellar solubilization makes it possible for the products of lipolysis to move through the intestinal brush border where they are absorbed by the enterocytes (Lengsfeld et al 2004). Within the enterocyte they are then re-formed into triacylglycerols, packaged in a lipoprotein envelope and moved into the lymphatic system. The mechanisms of fat digestion and absorption in the equine GIT remain to be elucidated.

Enzymes involved in protein hydrolysis

Endogenous and microbial proteolytic activity was reported to be highest in the ileum of the horse compared to other areas of the GIT (23.85 µg of hydrolyzed protein/mg ileal content/min) (Kern et al 1974). It been shown in a number of species, but not as yet in the horse, that pancreatic trypsinogen, is activated to trypsin by proteolytic cleavage by the brush border enzyme enterokinase, or by intraluminal trypsin itself. Trypsin is an endoprotease that hydrolyses the C-terminal peptide bonds of basic amino acids; it also activates all the other oligopeptidases (e.g. procarboxypeptidases and chymotrypsinogen) to their active forms. The smaller oligopeptides that have been broken down are then hydrolyzed by pancreatic carboxypeptidases that remove one AA at a time from the carboxyl end of the chain. Finally, brush border oligopeptidases break down the small neutral peptides yielded by pancreatic-derived peptidases into constituent di- and tripeptides [~25%] or amino acids [~75%] (Johnson 2001).

Unfortunately, there is also very little information available concerning intestinal digestion and absorption of protein in the horse. One group (Duckworth et al 1992) looked at glutamine by in vitro methods. They found the mean specific activity of jejunal and ileal glutaminase was 4.38 and 4.00 µmol/mg of protein/h respectively and that the basolateral sodium-dependent glutamine carrier transported glutamine at <5 nmol/mg of protein/min. Thus the

Table 1-4 Lactate Concentration in The Different Segments of The Small Intestinal Content Depending on The Diet at Various Hours Post-Feeding

Diet		Lactate concentration (mmol/l)						Reference
		3	4	5	6	7	8	
Complete pelleted feed	D	2.1	3.3	4.5	5.8	4.2	2.0	Wolter et al 1980
Complete semi expanded feed	D	2.5	3.9	6.3	8.6	7.8	4.7	Wolter et al 1980
Oats	J	10.4	17.5	28.7	26.3	14.5	7.5	Kleffken 1993
Corn	J	6.2	11.2	16.6	11.0	6.4	3.6	Kleffken 1993
Oats	J	0.6	3.8	6.9	15.7	21.2		Kleffken 1993
Corn	J	4.2	3.2	4.9	8.3	10.4		Kleffken 1993
Oats – pelleted feed	I	23.4		21.6		28.1		Kleffken 1993
Corn – pelleted feed	I	13.8		26.0		25.4		Kleffken 1993
Hay	I	0.2		0.2		0.1		Kleffken 1993

D = duodenum. J = Jejunum. I = Ileum.

capacity of glutaminase is considerably greater than that of the isolated transporter and would seem to be able to handle large loads of glutamine. Glutamine is taken up by intestinal cells at a rate equal to that of glucose uptake and is even more important than glucose as an oxidative fuel for enterocytes (Duckworth et al 1992, Windmueller & Spaeth 1974). Earlier studies that have looked at strictly N kinetics in the equine GIT indicate that 11–30% of whole tract apparent N digestion is attributed to the small intestine (Gibbs et al 1988, Reitnour and Salsbury 1972).

Digestive ecosystem and digestion/fermentation

The environmental characteristics of the small intestine are conducive to the presence of large densities some microorganisms are facultative anaerobes, either are strict anaerobes. The temperature is approximately 39°C. Water content is reported to vary from 86.7 (Wolter & Chaabouni 1979) to 96.5% (Freeman 2002). The pH values, particularly in the ileum, are among the highest to be found throughout the digestive tract (Argenzio et al 1974b, de Fombelle et al 2003, Jansen et al 2007, Respondek et al 2007, Wolter & Chaabouni 1979). For example, de Fombelle et al reported mean values of 6.3, 7.1 and 7.3 in the duodenum, jejunum and ileum respectively (de Fombelle et al 2003). As indicated above, this is probably due to the secretion of bicarbonate from the pancreas, duodenum and ileum (Alexander & Hickson 1970, Argenzio et al 1974b). To our knowledge, however, no one has yet measured the O_2 tension or the redox potential.

Bacteria represent the only microbial community within the small intestine of the horse, the presence of fungi or protozoa having not yet been reported. Recorded total anaerobic bacterial counts are: 2.9 cfu.ml^{-1} in the proximal duodenum (Mackie & Wilkins 1988), from 10^7–10^9 cfu.ml^{-1} in the jejunum (de Fombelle et al 2003, Kollarczik et al 1992, Mackie & Wilkins 1988) and from 10^6–10^9 cfu.ml^{-1} in the ileum (de Fombelle et al 2003, Kern et al 1974, Mackie & Wilkins 1988).

The presence of cellulolytic bacteria was also detected in the jejuno-ileum but their concentration did not exceed 3.0×10^2 cfu.ml^{-1} (de Fombelle et al 2003, Kern et al 1974). Bacteria such as lactobacilli, streptococci and lactate-utilizing bacteria are implicated in the breakdown of starch as well as other highly fermentable carbohydrates and constitute the predominant microflora. Recorded lactobacilli concentrations, in the small intestinal contents, range from 10^7–10^9 cfu.ml^{-1} (Alexander & Davies 1963, de Fombelle et al 2003, Kollarczik et al 1992) and streptococci counts from 10^7–10^8 cfu.ml^{-1} (de Fombelle et al 2003). The concentrations of lactobacilli declined from the stomach to the small intestine whereas streptococci counts increased and were higher in the small intestine than lactobacilli. This increase in streptococci is probably related to the higher pH values of the ileal contents (de Fombelle et al 2003). Two studies have found concentrations of lactate-utilizing bacteria ranging from 10^7–10^8 cfu.ml^{-1} in the small intestinal contents (Alexander & Davies 1963, de Fombelle et al 2003).

Jejunal total anaerobes and lactobacilli counts are sensitive to the composition of the ration (Kollarczik et al 1992). De Fombelle et al (2003) confirmed that the concentration of lactobacilli, as well as those of streptococci and lactate-utilizing bacteria, increased in the ileum of horses fed a high starch compared to those fed a high fiber diet, thus impacting the concentration of lactate and VFA (Table 1-4). However, no data are available about the involvement of these bacteria in carbohydrate, fat or protein digestion within the small intestine.

Motility

Small intestinal contents are ultimately moved aborally by motile events that involve both rapidly and slowly propagated contractions. Myoelectrical studies reveal that slow waves (SW) are at a much higher frequency in the small intestine than in the stomach – 9–18/min depending upon region and species, with the fastest rate always being in the duodenum and the slowest in the ileum (Christensen 1971, Ruckebusch 1977). In the horse the frequencies are ~14 in the duodenum and ~9 in the ileum (Berry et al 1986, Hudson et al 2001, Lester et al 1998, Merritt et al 1989). Again, an action potential (AP), which signals muscle depolarization and contraction, can only occur in association with a given SW, but there can be SW without any accompanying AP.

Built upon this is a basic pattern of action potential (AP) activity, referred to as the migrating myoelectrical (or motility) complex (MMC) (Code & Marlett 1974, Ruckebusch 1973, 1977). The MMC in the equine small intestine is qualitatively similar to that seen in other species, showing the three phases (I, II, III) (Berry et al 1986, Merritt et al 1989, Milligan et al 2007, Ruckebusch 1973). The most prominent of these phases, from both a myoelectrical and mechanical perspective, is phase III which is a sustained period of contraction of ~10 minutes duration that initiates in the duodenum on a recurring cycle of 90–120 minutes and slowly migrates aborally to end at the distal ileum. Each phase III is followed by phase I, a period of no motility lasting ~5 minutes in the horse that, in turn, is followed by phase II, a period of intermittent contractile activity lasting until a new phase III begins ~100 minutes later (Fig. 1.13). The classical peristalsis and segmentation occur within phase II and results of studies in other species indicate that it is during this phase that the bulk of ingesta transit occurs (Bueno et al 1975, Ruppin 1985). In dogs and humans, food intake induces a myoelectrical "fed pattern", essentially phase II-like activity, for up to 8 hours postprandially. In the horse, however, food intake does not disrupt the MMC to any great degree unless the animal is under a strict meal feeding regimen, such as a stalled environment with a defined amount of hay and grain given twice a day. Even then, a meal may only induce a "fed pattern" of variable duration which appears to be dependent upon the feeding intervals and the duration of active ingestion (Merritt et al 1989, Ruckebusch 1977).

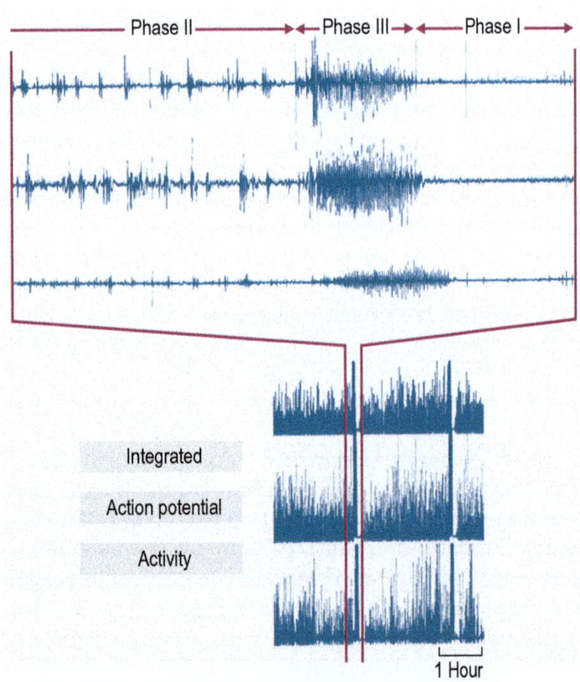

Figure 1.13 A myoelectrical recording of the proximal jejunum of a conscious horse demonstrating the migrating myoelectrical (motility) complex (MMC) that is seen in some variation in the small intestine of all mammalian species. The electrodes are 5 cm apart with the most proximal (orad) at the top. In the recording at the top, typical patterns of the three distinct phases of the MMC are shown. The most prominent is phase III which is a period of repetitive action potentials, one occurring with each slow wave. This is followed by phase I where there are no action potentials, and thus no motility. The subsequent phase II, a period of intermittent spike activity, comprises the majority of an MMC cycle and it is within this phase that most of the aboral movement of contents occurs. In the 5 hour long recording at the bottom in which the action potential (spike) activity has been simultaneously integrated, one full MMC cycle of about 120 minutes duration is seen, starting with the commencement of the phase III complex shown in the expanded recording above and ending with the commencement of the next.

Indications are that the transit rate of digesta through the small intestine of the horse is quite rapid. In one study, 50% of a liquid marker instilled into the stomach of a pony was found within the distal ileum by the end of one hour after intragastric instillation. By 90 minutes postinstillation, 25% of that liquid marker was within the cecum (Argenzio et al 1974a). However, particulate matter moves somewhat more slowly; in general, the larger the particle, the slower the transit rate (Argenzio et al 1974a, Drogoul et al 2000). When expressed as mean retention time (MRT), solid phase gastric and small intestinal transit combined appears to be between 4–7 hours, depending upon diet composition and amount eaten (Drogoul et al 2000, de Fombelle et al 2004, Medina et al 2002b). For instance, the pre-cecal MRT of a chopped hay diet was significantly longer than ground and pelleted hay diet in fistulated ponies (Drogoul et al 2000). Thus, as indicated by the few studies that have been currently done in horses, numerous factors including nutrient composition and quantity, liquid or solid phase, partial size, autonomic nervous activity, gastrointestinal hormone release and time between feedings, along with the character of the motile events, govern the rate at which digesta moves through the GIT. Strict control of motility is crucial to the promotion of efficient digestion and absorption within. Within the small intestine, control of all of this activity is predominantly by the ENS, with minimal input from the CNS (Furness 2008).

Absorption

Different end-products of carbohydrate, fat and protein digestion absorbed from the small intestine fulfil some, but certainly not all, of the basal energetic and nitrogenic requirements of the horse (Argenzio & Hintz 1972, Roberts 1975).

Absorption of carbohydrate end-products

In horses, D-glucose and galactose are transported across the brush-border membrane of the enterocytes by the SGLT1, Na+/glucose co-transporter (Fig. 1.14). In horses maintained on pasture forage, the major site of glucose absorption is in the proximal intestine (duodenum > jejunum), with lower expression of SGLT1 in the ileum (Dyer et al 2002). Shirazi-Beechey reported that there is a wide variation in SGLT1 expression between individuals and suggested that this may be significant in terms of their responsiveness to the diet type and susceptibility to digestive disorders and laminitis (Shirazi-Beechey 2008).

When horses on an all forage diet received a concentrate diet consisting of 60% hay, 40% grain for 1 month and then of 40% hay, 60% grain for a further month the nutrient carriers expressed on the apical membrane of intestinal absorptive cells were directly exposed to the gradually increased concentration of glucose. Consequently SGLT1 expression increased. In the duodenum no changes were observed in rates of D-glucose uptake (180.0 ± 28.5 pmol/s/mg protein). But the rates of D-glucose uptake were 1.9-fold higher

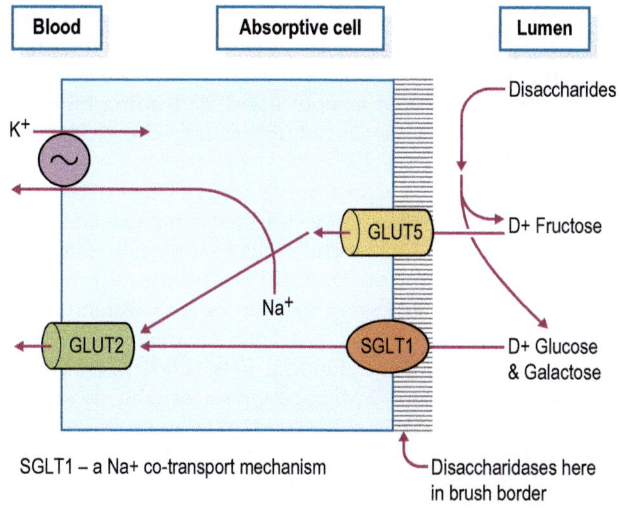

Figure 1.14 Mechanism of glucose absorption by the small intestine.

(215.5 ± 17.4 versus 115.9 ± 33.0 pmol/s/mg protein) in the jejunum and 3.7-fold higher in the ileum (139.5 ± 7.6 versus 38.4 ± 16.4 pmol/s/mg protein) than in horses fed pasture forage. The authors suggested that this was due an increase in the number of SGLT1 molecules. Using real time PCR, the increase in SGLT1 expression was confirmed not only in the ileum but also in the duodenum (Dyer et al 2009). The adaptation of SGLT1 expression to dietary change was slowly upregulated, with time. After one week of 60% hay, 40% grain feeding, there was no change in SGLT1 expression in the duodenum but a 2-fold increase in that in the ileum. Three weeks later on the same level of concentrate, SGLT1 expression in the duodenum was significantly increased to nearly twice the original level but that of ileal SGLT1 expression did not change. When the 40% hay, 60% grain diet was fed for a further month, duodenal SGLT1 expression was unchanged whereas there was a further increase in ileal SGLT1. This clearly demonstrated that not only the proximal but also and predominantly the distal small intestine have a capacity of enhancing SGLT1 expression (Dyer et al 2009).

In humans and a wide range of animal species, SGLT1 is upregulated by monosaccharides but not by starch. Two subunits of a sweet taste receptor 1 coupled to the α-subunit of the associated G-protein are required for upregulation of SGLT1 by luminal monosaccharides. The sweet taste receptor subunits as well as the associated G-protein are also expressed in the equine small intestine (Dyer et al 2009).

Regarding the slow upregulation of SGLT1, Dyer et al (2009) proposed that the lag period may be due to some other factors such as the time required for an α-amylase upregulation. In horses, amylase activity can be upregulated in response to increased dietary hydrolyzable carbohydrate intake. The mean activity of amylase within the jejunal chyme was reported to be 22.3 U/g wet weight (Kienzle et al 1994). The activity, however, was considerably higher when horses were fed grain diets (30.8 ± 15.4 U/g chime) for 24 h rather than maintained on an all-hay diet (15 ± 3.4 U/g). However, the increase was much smaller than in omnivorous species such as pigs or even in the carno-omnivorous dog. These results suggest that the primary rate limiting step in the increased glucose absorptive capacity of equine small intestine via SGLT1, is likely to be the inability of the horse to rapidly hydrolyze starch into glucose.

Glucose exits the enterocytes across the basolateral membrane by the Na^+-independent monosaccharide transporter, GLUT2 (Shirazi-Beechey 1995) (Fig. 1.14). Dyer et al demonstrated the absence of GLUT2 on the brush-border membrane. GLUT2 is expressed only on the basolateral membrane of intact villi of equine enterocytes. (Dyer et al 2009).

As for SGLT1, a similar pattern of increase in mRNA, protein abundance and glucose transport function was observed for the basolateral membrane glucose transporter, GLUT2, when horses received a grain concentrate (Dyer et al 2009). This indicates that there is a coordinated increase in the rate of glucose transport across the luminal and basolateral membrane of enterocytes resulting in enhanced transcellular transport of glucose from the lumen of the intestine into the blood.

It has been reported that fructose is well absorbed by horses (Bullimore et al 2000, Roberts 1975). It is transported across the luminal membrane of equine enterocytes by a Na+-independent facilitative transporter, equineGLUT5, which is insensitive to phlorizin and cytochalasin B. In horses maintained on a conventional, grass based diet, eGLUT5 protein is highly expressed on the brush-border membrane of duodenal and jejunal enterocytes, with lower levels in the ileal enterocytes. Furthermore, immunohistochemistry has shown that eGLUT5 protein is exclusively expressed on the brush-border membrane of the villus enterocytes and is not present in either the crypts or the enterocyte basolateral membrane (Merediz et al 2004).

Little is known in horses regarding the absorption of lactate but it is probable that similarly to what has been described recently in sheep, lactic acid is absorbed from the small intestine (Ding & Xu 2010) through active transporters. In mammals, lactate requires transporter proteins such as monocarboxylate transporters (MCTs) for absorption. MCT2 was suggested to be the main lactate transporter in mouse and pigs (Sepponen et al 2007, Teramae et al 2007).

Absorption of fat end-products

In humans, the mixed micelles formed with bile salts promote the permeation of lipids through the unstirred water layer to the enterocytes. LCFA are highly hydrophobic and they can only cross the aqueous diffusion barrier into mixed micelles which increase their aqueous concentration. Intestinal LCFA absorption starts with micellar dissociation: near the brush border, ionized LCFA are massively protonated due to the low pH microclimate which reduces their solubility into mixed micelles. Protonation induces the release of LCFA near the microvilli of absorptive cells which facilitates their subsequent cellular uptake mainly by diffusion. In humans again, three fatty acid-binding proteins (FABPs) have been isolated in the brush-border membrane of enterocytes. All of them are highly expressed in the jejunum and, to a lesser extent, in the ileum. Once within the enterocyte, LCFA and FACoA are reversibly bound to FABPs and acyl-CoA binding protein (ACBP), respectively. FACoA are rapidly re-esterified in TAG in the endoplasmic reticulum to form chylomicrons (Niot et al 2009). Currently due to lack of evidence in the horse, we can only assume that these same mechanisms are present.

Absorption of protein end-products

A net disappearance of nitrogen from the equine small intestine varying from 16% up to 58% indicates that nitrogen absorption can occur pre-cecally (Gibbs et al 1981, 1988, Glade 1983, Hintz et al 1971). The absorption appears to be primarily from the jejunum and ileum (Gibbs et al 1988, Glade 1983). The form of nitrogen absorbed from the equine small intestine has not been definitely stated but it is probably mainly amino acids, as in humans and most other mammals (Ganapathy et al 1994). It has been suggested that urea is absorbed per se from the equine small intestine and largely eliminated via the urine; thus, does not reach the microflora within the lower gut in sufficient amounts to be incorporated into protein and subsequently utilized by the host animal (Reitnour & Treece 1971).

In humans, it is known that di- and tripeptides plus free amino acids that result from hydrolyzation of dietary proteins by the brush-border peptidases are absorbed by the apical membrane of the enterocytes. Di- and tripeptides are transported via a H^+ driven transporter PEPT-1 into the cytoplasm and are then hydrolyzed by soluble cytoplasmic oligopeptidases into single amino acids, which move passively into portal blood down a concentration gradient (Dave et al 2004). In contrast, amino acids are transported by several distinct active transport systems into the enterocyte from which they are later liberated into portal blood. The amino acid transporters have been identified based on their ion (Na^+ and/or Cl^-) dependence and their profile of amino acids accepted (Dave et al 2004). Recently in horses, relative messenger RNA (mRNA) abundance of four Na^+ independent candidate AA transporter genes was measured. Data showed that abundance of cationic and neutral AA transporters was relatively uniform between the jejunum and the ileum (Woodward et al 2010).

Circulating and intraluminal amino acids can also be used by the intestinal epithelial cells as a source of metabolic fuel. In humans, glutamine is the principal fuel used by the small intestinal epithelial cells and its uptake far exceeds that of any other amino acid (Salloum et al 1993). This explains why most studies on amino acid absorption have been focused on that specific neutral amino acid. One group (Duckworth et al 1992) showed a marked capacity of the equine jejunum to extract glutamine and suggested that this uptake was likely higher than that of the large intestine. It occurs via two primary routes. The most important carrier is a high affinity sodium-dependent transporter. It is also transported by a sodium-independent system, although the contribution of this carrier to total uptake is considerably less than the sodium-independent route (Salloum et al 1993).

Absorption of minerals

It has long been stated that the absorption of calcium from the small intestine is vital as horses cannot absorb it from the large intestine (Stadermann et al 1992). That is questioned by recent work that has demonstrated the presence of receptors and transporters involved in the transcellular calcium transport at the level of the hindgut (Rourke et al 2010). In contrast to most domestic animals, horses can absorb a large proportion of the dietary calcium reaching up to 70% (Schryver et al 1970). The mechanisms involved have not been fully described but recent findings indicate that in horses, paracellular calcium transport may be more important than transcellular transport (Rourke et al 2010). Adaptation and fine regulation of the calcium demand is essentially driven by the transcellular calcium transport, which involves different receptors and transporters for the calcium entrance at the apical membrane channels, and crossing and exit of the cells. In the horse, the proximal small intestine is the main site for transcellular calcium transport. The transient receptor potential vanilloid member 6 (TRPV6) is the predominant apical membrane calcium channel in the small intestine (Breigdenbach et al 1998) with an expression approximately 4000-fold greater than the expression of the transient receptor potential vanilloid member 5 (TRPV5) (Rourke et al 2010). The calbindin D9k (CB9) is the main cytoplasmic calcium binding protein in the intestine (Breigdenbach et al 1998) with an expression in the duodenum and proximal jejunum 2 to 15-fold higher than in the distal jejunum, ileum, large intestine (Rourke et al 2010). The two basolateral transporters, the sodium calcium exchanger 1 (NCX1) and the plasma membrane calcium ATPase 1 (PMCA1) have an expression uniform throughout the intestine (Rourke et al 2010).

As for the vitamin D receptor (VDR), the mRNA expression was lowest in the small intestine compared to the large colon (Rourke et al 2010). These new data reinforce the fact that epithelial calcium transport in horses is not as dependent on vitamin D as in other species (Breigdenbach et al 1998, Rourke et al 2010).

In horses as in most mammalian species, inorganic phosphorus is probably absorbed at the duodenal and jejunal level. A putative phosphate-sodium carrier has not been identified yet from the brush border of enterocytes (Barlet et al 1995). Phosphorus absorption is modulated by many different factors such as other dietary constituents, quantity and type of phosphorus, and the age of the horse (NRC 2007). The majority of magnesium is absorbed in the small intestine in horses (Kapusniak et al 1988) and is modulated by other dietary constituents (NRC 2007).

Key Points

- Secretions into the duodenum are of intestinal, biliary and pancreatic sources. Pancreatic fluid volume is quite profuse with a pH of ~ 8.0, but the HCO_3^- concentration never attains levels seen in other species and digestive enzyme concentrations are relatively low. Within pancreatic tissue, lipase is the predominant enzyme, although amylase and proteolytic enzymes and pro-enzymes are also present.
- Oligosaccharides and residual α-dextrins initially produced by starch digestion by pancreatic endo-enzyme α-amylase are hydrolyzed by the brush border disaccharidases sucrase and maltase. Neutral and acid ß-galactosidase, which digest lactose, are also present in animals <4 years old.
- Transport mechanisms involved in glucose and fructose absorption are similar to those found in other species. Details concerning mechanisms of protein and fat assimilation in the horse are currently lacking.
- Diverse and numerous species of anaerobic and facultative aerobic bacteria are present, although no data are available about their nutritional involvement, if any, in carbohydrate, fat or protein digestion.
- The basic migrating motility complex (MMC) in the equine small intestine is qualitatively similar to that seen in other species, showing the three phases. Transit of contents is controlled by peristaltic and segmentation movements embedded within phase II. All of this is monitored and modulated by the ENS.

Cecum and colons

The equidae are among a group of herbivores, including elephants and rhinoceros, generally referred to as "hindgut fermenters". This group of animals has a highly developed large intestine designed to process and absorb ingested plant components that cannot be digested by the small intestine. Besides the large sacculated cecum, which can also be seen in other herbivores such as rabbits and guinea pigs, there is a vast compartmentalized great, or ascending, colon which has been anatomically divided into four sections: right ventral (RVC), left ventral (LVC), left dorsal (LDC) and right dorsal (RDC). In the adult 500 kg horse the average cecal volume is 33 liters and that of the great colon is 80 liters (Nickel et al 1979) which accounts for about 60% of the total GIT volume. Then there follows the short transverse colon and finally a well-delineated small colon wherein final desiccation of the digesta takes place and fecal balls are formed.

Histologically, the mucosa of the cecum and colon has prominent crypts of Lieberkuhn throughout that open directly into the lumen. There are no villi. As in the small intestine, however, the mucosal surface is composed primarily of columnar cells which have microvilli on their apical surface, although there are no digestive enzymes produced by these cells. Numerous goblet cells also line the crypts and there are single enteroendocrine cells within the basilar region of the crypts. There are no Paneth cells (Wille & Nakov 1999).

Secretion

As in the small intestine, active secretion within the large intestine is from the crypt intestinal cells and is primarily chloride driven. Under normal conditions, however, this activity, with respect to its effect on net water movement between lumen and plasma, is overshadowed by the osmotic effects of intracolonic fermentation and absorption of subsequent products (Argenzio et al 1974a, Clarke et al 1988, Clarke & Argenzio 1990a, b, Freeman et al 1997).

Digestive ecosystem and digestion/fermentation

In the large intestine, the host enzyme digestion has not been described and probably is negligible compared to the microbial digestion. The environmental parameters of the hindgut are favorable to a large density of strictly anaerobic microorganisms: the average pH values reported in the literature fluctuates around 7 with minimal pH values of 4.1 (Garner et al 1978) and 6.3 (Wolter et al 1978) and maximal values of 7.8 and 7.5 (Tisserand & Masson 1976) in the cecum and in the colon respectively. There are significant changes in the daily profile of the cecal and colonic pH. In both segments, the pH decreases rapidly during the first hours after feeding, reaching a minimal value of about a log less than the initial value 5 hours after the morning meal and staying at this low plateau for 2–4 hours. Then the pH increases progressively until the subsequent meal. The rate and extent of the pH drop differs depending on the diet: the decrease is more emphasized with a diet rich in concentrate than with a diet rich in forage. A recent study recording the pH at 1 minute intervals for nine hours detailed dynamics of the pH within the cecum: after oscillating around the initial value for 1.5 hours, the pH decreased and the minimal value was recorded six hours postprandially then it rose again (Brockner et al 2010).

Water content is between 88–97% and 76–85% in the cecum and colon, respectively (Goodson et al 1988, Hintz et al 1971, Wolter et al 1978). Water content decreases from the cecum to the distal colon (Hintz et al 1971, Sperber et al 1992, Varloud et al 2004) reaching 77–83% (Wolter et al 1980, Sperber et al 1992) due to water absorption through the intestinal wall. Electrolyte concentrations in the cecal contents are: Na^+ 122.0 ± 2.9, K^+ 13.2 ± 3.7, and Cl^- 28.6 ± 6.4 mmol/l, with an osmolality of 280.6 ± 15.2 mOsm/l. Electrolyte concentrations in large colon contents are: Na^+ 82.5 ± 11.4, K^+ 53.9 ± 8.1, and Cl^- 27.2 ± 5.2 mmol/l, with an osmolality of 295.0 ± 11.6 mOsm/l (Nicpoń et al 2000). The temperature of the hindgut contents is quite constant, being between 38–40°C (Philippeau, personal communication). As for redox potential, it was reported to average between - 488 mV (Da Veiga et al 2005) to- 212 mV (Philippeau et al 2009) in the right ventral colon.

Microorganisms

In 1911, Choukevitch observed large "ovals", bacilli and chains of cocci of up to 50 µm in size in the cecal contents of horses. Better microscopy and the development of strict anaerobic culture techniques (Hungate 1950) were decisive for improving our knowledge of intestinal microflora. Numerous bacteria, protozoa, anaerobic fungi, archaebacteria and recently phages have been isolated and described. However, it is evident that the majority of microorganisms within the equine large intestine have yet to be identified.

Concentrations of ciliate protozoa vary from 10^2 to 10^5 cells/ml of intestinal content (Goodson et al 1988, Kern et al 1973, Moore & Dehority 1993). Their distribution and their counts fluctuate depending on the different regions of the hindgut: the left dorsal colon presents the highest concentrations (Adam 1951, Moore & Dehority 1993); the microfauna are compartment-specific with a clear separation at the pelvic flexure (Moore & Dehority 1993). About six genera and fifty different species of protozoa have been described in the equine hindgut (Hsiung 1930).

In the cecal contents, the concentration of fungal zoospores varies from 10 to 10^4 ml^{-1} depending on the technique used (Dupuy-Julliand 1996, Orpin et al 1981). The majority of the fungal strains isolated from the cecum belonged to the genus *Piromyces* and four species have been identified.

The bacterial community represents the major part of the hindgut microbial biomass and was identified with molecular tools (Daly & Shirazi-Beechey 2003). It is dominated by the Firmicutes phylum (72%) followed by the Bacteroidetes (20%). The bacterial diversity is greater in the ventral colon than in the cecum (Daly & Stewart 2001, Daly & Shirazi-Beechey 2003). Interestingly, despite some variations due to experimental conditions, enumerations determined simultaneously in the cecal and the colonic contents showed that, in general, the microbial density tends to be higher in the colon than in the cecum (Julliand et al 2001, Kern et al 1974, Medina et al 2002a). A comparative study confirmed that the average total anaerobe concentrations were lowest in the cecum compared to the other digestive sections of the hindgut (de Fombelle et al 2003). All these data indicate that the function of the cecal ecosystem probably differs from that of the colon.

Since the digestion of cellulose and other plant fibrous material is essential in the nutrition of the horse, the fiber degrading bacteria play a major role. Nevertheless, their concentrations are low in the cecum, between 10^4 and 10^7 per ml of content and represented a small percentage of the total anaerobe count in horses (between 0.04% and 9%) (de Fombelle et al 2003, Julliand et al 1999, 2001, Kern et al 1973, Medina et al 2002a). *Ruminococcus flavefaciens* and *Fibrobacter succinogenes* have been identified as the predominating cellulolytic bacteria in the equine hindgut (Daly et al 2001, 2003, Julliand et al 1999). It was hypothesized that the cecum was probably the most propitious for cellulolysis because the proportion of cellulolytics among total anaerobes appeared to be greater in there than in the lower parts of the hindgut (de Fombelle et al 2003). However, a recent study found that cecal samples had significantly lower *R. flavefaciens* and *F. succinogenes* concentrations than those from the ventral and dorsal colons (Hastie et al 2008).

Glycolytic and amylolytic bacterial concentrations vary from 10^3 cfu/g (Nicpoń et al 2000) to 10^6 cfu/ml of cecal contents (de Fombelle et al 2003, Julliand et al 2001, Medina et al 2002a) and are mainly composed of streptococci, lactobacilli, and enterococci. (Bailey et al 2003, Al Jassim et al 2005). When enumerations were determined simultaneously within the cecal and the colonic contents, average concentrations of streptococci and lactobacilli were higher in the colon, approximating 10^7 cfu/ml^{-1} (de Fombelle 2003, Julliand 2001, Medina 2003). Hastie et al confirmed that *Streptoccus bovis* was more numerous in the luminal contents of the ventral colon and dorsal colon than in the cecum (Hastie et al 2008).

Concentrations of lactate-utilizing bacteria average 10^7 cfu/ml in the cecal and colonic contents (de Fombelle et al 2003, Julliand et al 2001, Medina et al 2002a) but tend to be generally higher in the colon than in the cecum. It appears that soluble carbohydrates and undigested starch that flow very quickly through the cecum and enter the colon, have a limited impact on the cecal microflora but stimulate the colonic microflora (Da Veiga et al 2005, de Fombelle et al 2001, 2003). The major lactate utilizing bacteria were identified as *Megasphaera* sp. and *Veillonella* sp. (Baruc et al 1983, Maczulak & Dawson 1985).

The average concentration of proteolytic bacteria was estimated around 10^7 cfu/ml of cecal contents (Kern et al 1973, Mackie & Wilkins 1988, Maczulak & Dawson 1985, Reitnour & Mitchell 1979). Mackie and Wilkins (1988) showed a higher number of proteolytic bacteria in the cecum than in the colon.

Digestion

Dietary carbohydrate utilization

Fiber degradation

Unlike the prececal segments, the hindgut shows an intense fibrolytic activity, as indicated by the high concentrations of VFA within the contents, averaging 58 mmol/l in the cecum and 80 mmol/l in the colon (de Fombelle et al 2003, Hintz et al 1971, Wolter et al 1980). In all segments the main VFAs produced are: acetate (74.9 vs 74.8% of the total), propionate (18.0 vs 16.9%), and butyrate (6.0 vs 6.3%) in the cecum and colon respectively (de Fombelle et al 2003).

The fibrolytic activity in the hindgut is probably mainly related to fungi and bacteria as protozoa do not seem to play an important role in cellulolysis (Moore & Dehority 1993). It starts with the adhesion of the microbial population to particles. A large bacterial population has been shown to be attached to grass cell walls in the cecum of the horse (Bonhomme-Florentin 1985). Fiber is broken down by enzymes excreted by the bacteria and fungi attached to particles and, to a lesser extent, by the free bacteria. The xylanasic activity, which represents the first step of the hemicellulose degradation, is greater than the carboxymethylcellulasic activity which corresponds to the first step of cellulose degradation (Jouany et al 2009). Accordingly, the β-D-glucosidase activity which represents the next step of the cellulose degradation is much greater than that of α-L-arabinosidase activity which represents the next step of the hemicellulose degradation. Interestingly, both carboxymethylcellulasic and xylanasic activities were higher in the colon than in the cecum (Jouany et al 2009).

The monomeric sugars produced are then hydrolyzed in bacterial cells, through the Embden–Meyerhoff pathway and lead to the formation of pyruvate and subsequently to the other VFA's and gases, namely CO_2, H_2 and CH_4 (Stewart & Bryant 1988). When horses are fed forage-based diets, cell wall degradation produces very little lactate.

Starch degradation

Recently, starch degrading activity in the hindgut was studied by estimating the amylolytic activity (primarily associated with the microbial population adhering to particles rather than the free microbes). The amylolytic activity was found to be similar between the cecum and the right ventral colon (Jouany et al 2009). The monomeric sugars produced are then hydrolyzed in bacterial cells leading mainly to lactate production. The average total lactate concentration ranges from 1.2 (Wolter et al 1980) to 4.6 mmol/l (Medina et al 2002a) in the cecum and 0.5 (Wolter et al 1980) to 4.9 mmol/l (Julliand et al 2001) in the colon (Table 1-5, Fig. 1.15).

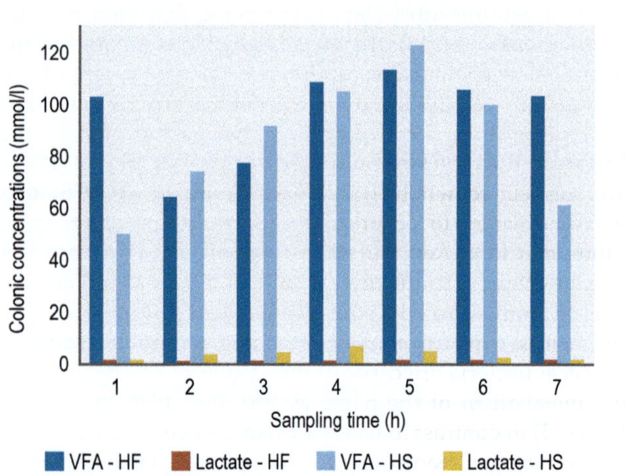

Figure 1.15 Post-prandial kinetics of L-lactate and total VFA in the colonic content depending on the diet (high fiber = HF or high starch = HS).

Table 1-5 Total Volatile Fatty Acid (VFA) Concentration in The Different Segments of The Small intestinal Content Depending on The Diet at Various Hours Post-Feeding

Diet		VFA concentration (mmol/l)			Reference
		2	5	8	
Complete pelleted feed	D		10.8		Wolter et al 1980
Complete semi expanded feed	D		12.8		Wolter et al 1980
Hay	D			10.7	Kleffken 1993
Hay	D		18.6		Kleffken 1993
Hay + cereals	D			3.9	Kleffken 1993
Hay + concentrate	D		23.4		Kleffken 1993
Oats	J		7.5		Kleffken 1993
Rolled oats	J		8.7		Kleffken 1993
Oats	J		16.9		Illenseer 1994
Corn	J		5.7		Kleffken 1993
Ground corn	J		4.3		Kleffken 1993
Hay + oats	J		4.6		Illenseer 1994
Hay	J			26.1	Kleffken 1993
Hay	J		15.1		Kleffken 1993
Hay + cereals	J			4.0	Kleffken 1993
Hay + concentrate	J		13.5		Kleffken 1993
Oats – pelleted feed	I		37.9		Kleffken 1993
Corn – pelleted feed	I		39.1		Kleffken 1993
Hay	I	6.6			Kern et al 1974
Hay	I			16.7	Kleffken 1993
Hay	I		8.2		Kleffken 1993
Hay + cereals	I			10.3	Kleffken 1993
Hay + concentrate	I		30.3		Kleffken 1993

D = duodenum. J = Jejunum. I = Ileum.

Dietary fat utilization

Lipolytic activity attributed to protozoa and bacteria has been demonstrated in vitro within cecal contents. In particular, the ciliate protozoa were shown to contribute actively to triglyceride hydrolysis (Bonhomme-Florentin 1976).

Dietary protein utilization

With respect to whole tract apparent nitrogen digestion, 40–70% appears to occur in the post-ileal compartments (Gibbs et al 1988, Reitnour & Salsbury 1972). Many bacteria of cecal origin can utilize gelatin, casein, peptones, amino acids or ammonia as the sole nitrogen source, but only very few bacteria can utilize urea (Baruc et al 1983). This suggests that cecal bacteria are capable of contributing to the amino-acid metabolism of the horse (Baruc et al 1983, Maczulak et al 1985) in contrast to urea that may not be used as a non-protein nitrogen feed source. However, little is known concerning the extent to which these microflora utilize dietary protein and non-protein nitrogen to contribute to the amino-acid pool in the horse.

Motility

All of the functions described above are dependent upon normal cecocolonic motility. If contents move too rapidly, optimal digestive (fermentative) activity and water absorption are reduced; if they move too slowly, impaction may result. Our knowledge of the myoelectrical and mechanical aspects of equine cecocolonic motility and how they are involved in the orderly movement of ingesta along the large intestinal lumen is still quite rudimentary. With respect to the cecum, myoelectrical and intra-luminal pressure studies suggest that contractile activity directed towards emptying begins in the apex (Ross et al 1986, 1989, 1990). An elegant radio-contrast study done in ponies indicates that this becomes a progressively defined ring of contraction as it approaches the cecal base, trapping ingesta and some gas within the region of the base referred to as the *cupola*. Coinciding with the arrival of this ring of contraction, the ileocecal area itself relaxes so that the ingesta from the cupola spills through the junction and into the RVC. Then this

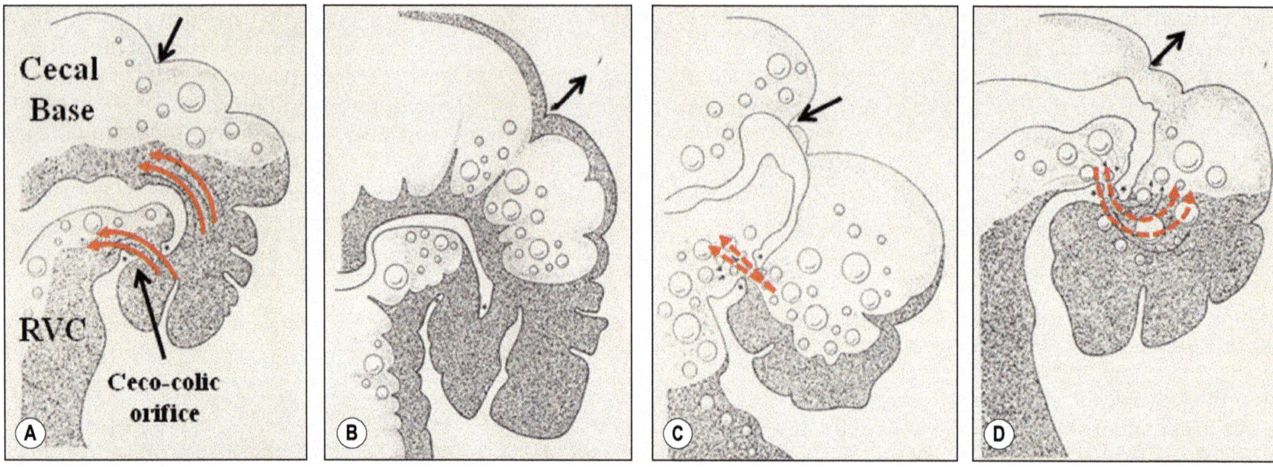

Figure 1.16 This series of drawings depicts a sequence of movements at the base of the cecum to transfer ingesta and gas between the cecum and the right ventral colon (RVC). These drawings were derived from cinefluoroscopic studies done in a pony whereby a barium (Ba) solution was injected into the cecum via a previously implanted cannula. In these drawings, the Ba-suffused digesta is shaded and gas is indicated by bubbles. **A)** The very terminal part of the cecal base, in which lies the cecocolic orifice, is called the *cupola*. In this panel, a contraction indicated by the black arrow is occurring at the junction between the cupola and the cecal base proper. This results in the simultaneous movement of digesta through the cecocolic orifice into the RVC and back into the cecal base (solid red arrows). **B)** As the cupola is now relaxing and drawing gas from the cecal base, the cecocolic orifice remains very open but there is little movement of either gas or digesta through it. **C)** The cupola is now contracting strongly and is pushing the gas drawn into it through the cecocolic orifice into the RVC (dashed red arrows). **D)** The cupola is relaxing once again and drawing some gas back from the RVC while the cecocolic orifice itself remains submerged in digesta.
Adapted from Dyce et al 1976.

contraction ring dissipates at the ileocecal junction there is some reflux of a small amount of ingesta from the RVC back into the cupola, but the net effect is movement of ingesta aborally (Dyce et al 1976) (Fig. 1.16). This activity repeats itself every 2–4 minutes, with the ileocecal orifice remaining open for 20–40 seconds during the cycle (Malbert & Roger 1989). As in other parts of the GI tract, feeding practices influence this activity. For instance, one study showed that horses fed ad libitum had a much more rapid cecal evacuation of a liquid marker than after they had been fasted for 12 hours (Vigroux et al 1975). Evacuation is also increased by pentagastrin and decreased by CCK (Malbert & Roger 1989). Lester et al found that the $T_{1/2}$ for emptying of a solid phase radio-labeled marker from the cecum of ponies was longer than that of a liquid phase marker (Lester et al 1998).

Myoelectrical events along the whole cecal body orientated towards the apex have also been described (Ross et al 1986, 1989, 1990). Undoubtedly, the associated motility is involved in circulating the contents throughout this large blind organ, but specific details of how this happens remain to be determined. It appears that turnover of contents within the cecum is relatively fast which represents less than 15% of the transit time through the equine GIT (Miyaji et al 2008).

With respect to the four large colon sections (RVC, LVC, LDC, RDC) there are some basic myoelectrical patterns that exist throughout and these are most clearly seen when the animal has been fasted for some hours. One of the most prominent of these patterns involves distinct, aborally migrating defined clusters of long spike bursts (LSB), which are indicative of contraction, that occur 10–20 minute intervals with cluster duration of 5–8 minutes and a propagation rate of 0.5–1.0 cm/min. These have been referred to as "slow migrating complexes" (SMC) (Merritt et al 1995). Dispersed between these distinct events is random LSB activity of up to 6 seconds each in duration that rapidly propagates in either an orad or aborad orientation (Fig. 1.17). All of the

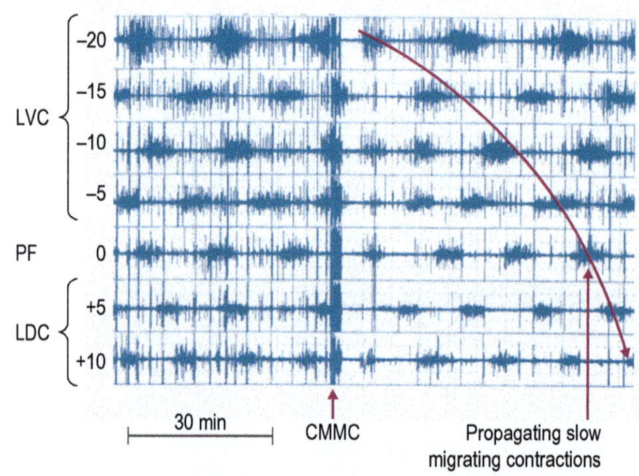

Figure 1.17 A myoelectrical recording of the large colon of a conscious horse, from which feed has been withheld for 12 hours, via 7 electrodes implanted at 5 cm intervals in the region of the pelvic flexure. Three types of action potential (spike burst) activity are prominent: (1) defined clusters of long spike bursts (LSB), designated as *slow migrating contractions (SMC)*, that occur at 10–20 minute intervals with cluster duration of 8–12 minutes and propagate aborally at a rate of 0.5–1.0 cm/min; (2) intermittent LSB activity that occurs between the SMC's; (3) very intense, repetitive LSB activity, designated as a "colonic migrating myoelectrical complex" (CMMC), that lasts ~5 minutes, propagates rapidly (~3 cm/s) in an aboral direction, and is followed by a period of relative electrical quiescence that lasts 5–15 minutes.
Adapted from Merritt et al 1995.

above activity is periodically interrupted by a burst of very intense, repetitive LSB activity, designated as a "colonic migrating myoelectrical complex" (CMMC), that lasts 5–8 minutes, propagates rapidly (~3 cm/s) in an aboral direction and is followed by a period of relative electrical quiescence that lasts 5–15 minutes (Lester et al 1998, Merritt et al 1995). In the fed animal, the CMMCs are much less frequent and distinct but the random LSB activity is markedly increased (Merritt et al 1995). Furthermore, Sellers et al suggested that within the pelvic flexure (PF) region, which differentiates LVC from LDC and is essentially the central point of the large colon, there exists "pacemaker" of the motility of the large colon as a whole (Sellers et al 1979). This is of considerable interest clinically because a common site for digesta impaction is within the LVC just orad to the pelvic flexure. Whereas there is definitely a greater concentration of components of the ENS within the PF region in contrast to the rest of the large colon (Burns & Cummings 1993, Hudson et al 1999) myoelectrical recordings done over many hours have not been able to identify distinct "pacemaker" properties in that region (Merritt et al 1995).

A direct relationship between localized myoelectrical and contractile events has been demonstrated (Merritt et al 1995) but there is still much to be learned about the motility of the equine large colon, especially with respect to its effects on digesta transit. Sellers et al have described a rapidly propagating contraction moving through the PF from LVC to LDC and pushing a bolus of ingesta in front of it that could be the motile expression of a rapidly propagating LSB mentioned above (Sellers et al 1984a). The orally directed events, combined with those that seem to be isolated and not propagated in either direction, are thought to hold up digesta transit and promote fermentation and absorption by "mixing" movements, which would be extremely important for a hind gut fermenter.

Nothing is known about the particulars of small colon motility in the horse.

Results of an early study of transit rate of markers of different sizes through the GIT of ponies by Argenzio et al (1974a) suggested that the rate of particulate markers of very small size is similar to liquid, but larger particles appear to evoke a direct size-related decrease in rate. For instance, in one study in ponies only about 40% of an experimentally fed nondigestible 2 cm size marker had appeared in the feces after ten days post-feeding in contrast to >90% of a 2 mm size marker (Argenzio et al 1974a). The implication from this study is that the larger particles of digesta entering the great colon are held up so that maximum microbial digestion can occur, in the process of which the particle size is reduced. However, results of more recent studies using general particulate markers indicate that 100% of a given test meal will have been excreted in the feces by 60 hours post-feeding (Bertone et al 1989, Orton et al 1985, Pearson & Merritt 1991). And, a review of the subject in 2006 found that published values for mean retention time (MRT) for digesta passage through the equine GIT ranged from 18–60 hours, depending upon many factors, including type of food and marker used, with most of the variability most likely occurring within the large intestine (Rosenfeld & Austbo 2009, Van Weyenberg et al 2006). However, a more recent study, using rare earth markers fed at varying times before slaughter to collect GIT contents, found that, although there were variable transit rates through various sections of the large intestine, there were no significant differences between a hay or silage diet. Specifically, the average MRT in cecum, RVC, LVC, LDC, RDC and small colon was 2.9, 3.1, 5.9, 1.0, 4.0 and 4.0 hours, respectively, for both diets combined, with a total tract (stomach through small colon) MRT of 29.75 hours. Furthermore, the DM weight of digesta was significantly related to the MRT in the RVC, LVC, LDC and RDC but not in the cecum or small colon (Miyaji et al 2008). These observations sustain the notion that DM content plays a part in determining rate of digesta passage, particularly through the various portions of the ascending colon where a significant amount of plant fiber digestion occurs. Potential sites of holdup of transit, particularly if the digesta contains larger particles or is dryer than normal, are at the pelvic flexure and the transverse colon where the lumen diameter becomes markedly smaller than that of the preceding LVC and RDC respectively (Drogoul et al 2000).

Absorption

Absorption of volatile fatty acids and lactate

With an average pKa of 4.8, about 95% of the VFAs are in their ionized form within the cecum and colon where the pH is ~7.0. However, they must be in a non-ionic form, protonated with H^+, in order for them to be efficiently absorbed across the luminal mucosal membrane. This protonated form is rapidly absorbed by a concentration-dependent passive diffusion process, with absorption rates reaching 8 μmol/cm^2/h (Argenzio et al 1977). The rate of absorption is inversely proportional to molecular weight, with the absorption of acetate > propionate > butyrate > lactate. Passive absorption is, unexpectedly, nearly independent from luminal pH. This is attributed to the presence of a constant pH-microclimate at the epithelial surface (Argenzio et al 1974b).

Recent work has described VFA transport at the luminal membrane via a monocarboxylate/H^+ symporter (Shirazi Beechey 2008). This activates the absorption of Na^+ and Cl^- in exchange for H^+ and HCO_3^- respectively. H^+ that are provided protonate more VFA which, therefore, can cross the apical mucosal membrane by nonionic diffusion. Thus, the transport of the VFA from the lumen of the equine colon into the colonocytes occurs along with NaCl absorption and H_2CO_3 secretion. Water follows the net VFA absorption (see next part on blood volume) (Argenzio et al 1974b, Clarke & Argenzio 1990, Clarke et al 1990b, Shirazi-Beechey 2008) (Fig. 1.18).

The equine colonic monocarboxylate/H^+ symporter transport of VFA is inhibited by the monocarboxylate

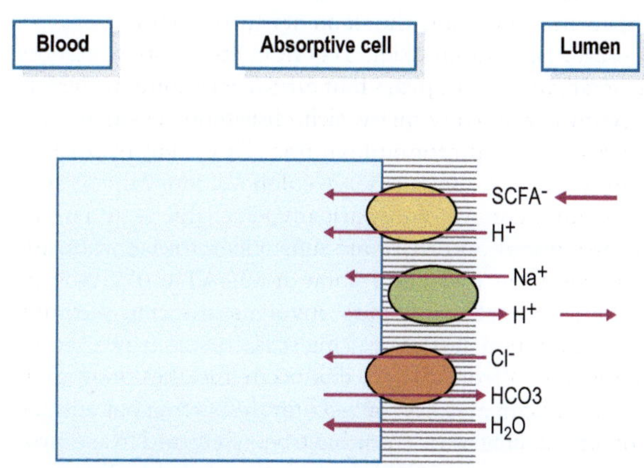

Figure 1.18 Mechanism of volatile short chain fatty acid (SCFA) absorption by the large intestinal mucosa via a monocarboxylase/H^+ symporter.

lactate. Lactic acid can enter the cell resulting in an intracellular acidification. This affects the expression of genes controlling apoptosis of the colonic epithelial cells thereby affecting colonic tissue homeostasis (Shirazi-Beechey 2008). In addition, alterations in the intracellular pH modulate the activity of the Na^+/H^+ antiporter and in turn influence salt, water and nutrient absorption. When horses receive high concentrate rations, lactate production increases, hindgut pH decreases, and the concentration and activity of fiber-degrading microorganisms decreases (Julliand et al 2001, Milinovich et al 2008).

Study of the transport of VFA across the colonic luminal membrane into colonocytes is complicated by the fact that substantial amounts, particularly butyrate, are metabolized within the epithelial cell itself. Currently, little is known about this in horses specifically.

Absorption of fat end-products

The mechanisms of fat absorption in the equine hindgut have not been studied yet.

Absorption of protein end-products

Horses can assimilate a large proportion of dietary nitrogen in the post-ileal compartments which explains how they can meet protein demand through hindgut fermentation (Gibbs et al 1988, Reitnour et al 1969, Reitnour & Salsbury 1972). In the small colon, most nitrogen is supplied by the conversion of the neutral detergent soluble fraction of the insoluble nitrogen-containing compounds to water soluble nitrogen-containing compounds (Glade 1983). Despite the significant role played by the hindgut in nitrogen absorption, little is known regarding the form of nitrogen absorbed in those segments. Different experiments conducted in vivo have shown evidence that horses can absorb ammonia and perhaps lysine, cystine and other essential amino acids of microbial origin as well from the cecum, although they did not provide direct information about AA transport by cecal or colonic mucosa (McMeniman et al 1987, Reitnour & Salsbury 1972, Slade et al 1971). But, subsequent in vitro studies showed that while radiolabeled L-alanine and cycloleucine were actively transported through the serosal (antiluminal) surface, there was no evidence for an active transport system on the mucosal (luminal) surface of the equine cecal mucosa. (Freeman et al 1989, Freeman & Donawick 1991) These data have not been confirmed in vivo.

Recently, candidate genes known to transport cationic and neutral AA across epithelial cells of other animal species were expressed in the equine large intestine. These transporters may facilitate the uptake and absorption of microbial and dietary-derived AA across the epithelium of the large intestine. The AA transporter b0,+AT which has a high affinity for cystine and cationic AA, was found uniformly all along the GIT. The distribution of b0,+AT in the cecum and colon appears to be unique to the horse and is relevant to its AA nutrition relying on microbial protein predominantly produced from dietary fiber fermentation occurring in post-ileal segments. AA transporter LAT-3 that has a high capacity and low affinity transporter for neutral AA, shows the greatest transcript in the large intestine probably contributing to maximizing absorption of neutral AA in those segments. The others underlined the fact that the observed differential mRNA abundances between segments and amongst the AA transporters studied translate into transporter protein levels or functional and phenotypic expression remains to be determined (Woodward et al 2010). Again, whether any of these transporters can actually move significant amounts of intact amino acids from lumen into blood still need to be determined.

Absorption of electrolytes and water

Calcium

In the equine hindgut, the mRNA expression of different proteins involved in transcellular *calcium* transport have been reported: the transient receptor potential vanilloid member 6 (TRPV6) and member 5 (TRPV5), the calbindin D9k (CB9) and D28k (CB28), the sodium calcium exchanger 1 (NCX1) and the plasma membrane calcium ATPase 1 (PMCA1). Their expression is much lower in the hindgut than in the small intestine except for the two basolateral transporters NCX1 and PMCA1 which are expressed uniformly throughout the intestine (Rourke et al 2010). The mRNA expression of the vitamin D receptor (VDR) is higher in the large colon (15–25-fold) than in the small intestine (Rourke et al 2010).

Sodium, chloride and water

The large intestine is a major water reservoir for hind gut fermenters. *When extrapolated to the surface area of the entire colon, net ion flux accounts for ±25% of net water flux* (Sneddon & Argenzio 1998). Thus, the fermentative process is of fundamental importance because the amount and composition of food ingested has a strong influence on both plasma and GIT water volume (Sneddon & Argenzio 1998). *As indicated above, along with the VFA absorption from the large colon there is also a net absorption of sodium, chloride and water from the lumen into the blood.* Thus, in the ascending (large) colon, the Na^+ absorption is primarily, though not exclusively, electroneutral, in exchange for H^+ which protonates the VFAs. In contrast, in the distal (small) colon Na^+ absorption is entirely electrogenic, is not coupled to SCFA absorption or acid/base adjustments, and is solely concerned with Na^+ and water conservation (Giddings et al 1974, Clarke et al 1992, Sneddon & Argenzio 1998, von Englehardt et al 1995). There is evidence that both of these mechanisms are up-regulated by aldosterone, although with the small colon responding more vigorously than the large (Clarke et al 1992). This has important implications regarding the effect of meal vs ad libitum food intake on the hydration of equine colonic contents. For instance, fermentation of a large single commercial hay/grain pelleted meal within the large intestine of ponies can cause up to 15% reduction in its plasma volume, which does not occur in those animals allowed to eat on a free choice basis (Clarke et al 1990a, b, Houpt et al 1988). This is because the production of VFAs within the large colon initially outstrips their absorption, thus pulling plasma water, by osmotic drag, into the colonic lumen. The resultant drop in plasma volume initiates renin-angiotensin, and then aldosterone release, promoting an enhanced Na^+, and thus water, absorption, particularly in the distal colon, over and above that which moves with VFA absorption (Clarke et al 1988, 1992). Theoretically, this could result in extra desiccation of colonic contents (Clarke et al 1990b).

Interestingly, Lopez et al (2004) did not observe a similar phenomenon in horses that were fed a grain meal and had free access to hay at all times, although they pointed out that they only collected their first blood samples at 5.5 hours after grain was offered while the dehydration effect reported by Clarke et al was seen within the first 3 hours of defined pelleted meal ingestion. Furthermore, Meyer has shown that with equal amounts of DM intake a high roughage diet resulted in increased amounts of water within the GIT of horses (Meyer 1996). *The question therefore arises – does strict meal feeding of horses, especially a meal which is easily fermentable, increase their chances of developing a colonic impaction?* The answer is still unknown.

In the final analysis, from the data presented by Argenzio et al, using ponies fed a commercial pelleted hay/grain meal, the greatest amount of the water expelled from the distal ileum through the ileocecal junction was absorbed, on a net basis, by the cecum, with a mean daily cecal turnover rate of 6.8 liters (Argenzio et al 1974a). The ventral colon absorbed the next greatest amount. The dorsal colon accumulated a small amount, resulting in a net colonic turnover rate of 3.3 liters/day. Finally, the small colon absorbed another 1.5 liters/day to form normal fecal balls. Thus, in this classic study, Argenzio et al. calculated that of the 19.5 liters of water that enters the large intestinal tract of a 160 kg pony each day, only about 1.5 liters leaves as fecal water. However, using a more direct measurement of flow in cecally and dorsal colonically cannulated ponies fed a chopped hay meal, Simmons and Ford reported considerably larger liquid turnover volumes of 54 and 49 liters/day in cecum and colon respectively (Simmons & Ford 1990). Clearly, this subject needs further attention.

Key Points

- The horse is a classic "hind gut fermenter", with both cecum and ascending (large) colon being involved. The normality of the fermentative process is highly dependent upon orderly delivery of contents into and through the system, maintenance of a strict anaerobic environment with limited fluctuations in pH, and rapid absorption of the fermentation by-products.
- Microbes involved in the fermentative process include various and numerous types of protozoa, fungi and bacteria working together to convert carbohydrate-based contents, primarily in the form of plant fiber, into volatile fatty acids (VFA). Some lactate may also be produced from any soluble carbohydrate entering the system.
- The VFAs are absorbed primarily by non-ionic diffusion or via a monocarboxylate/H^+ symporter within the luminal membrane that activates the absorption of Na^+ and Cl^- in exchange for H^+ and HCO_3^- secretion respectively. The H^+ provided protonate the VFA. Water passively follows the VFA and Na^+ absorption.
- Rate of production and absorption of organic acids within the large bowel mass has a profound influence on plasma volume via the osmotic effect of the acids on the direction of the transmucosal movement of water.
- Limited data presently available indicate that cecal and colonic motility is very complex and involves some specifically regional patterns of activity. Optimal digestive activity within and water absorption from the ceco-colon are highly dependent upon normal motor activity. Certain regions, such as the pelvic flexure in the large colon, contain a higher density of neurons involving various neurotransmitters, but the significance of this remains to be elucidated with respect to motor activity.

References

Adam, K.M.G., 1951. The quantity and distribution of the ciliate protozoa in the large intestine of the horse. Parasitology 41, 301–311.

Al Jassim, R.A.M., Scott, P.T., Trebbin, A.L., et al., 2005. The genetic diversity of lactic acid producing bacteria in the equine gastrointestinal tract. FEMS Microbiology Letter 248, 75–81.

Al Jassim, R.A.M., 2006. Supplementary feeding of horses with processed sorghum grains and oats. Animal Feed Science and Technology 125, 33–44.

Alexander, F., Davies, M.E., 1963. Production and fermentation of lactate by bacteria in the alimentary canal of the horse and pig. Journal of Comparative Pathology 73, 1–8.

Alexander, F., 1966. A study of parotid salivation in the horse. Journal of Physiology (London) 184, 646–656.

Alexander, F., Hickson, J.C.D., 1970. The salivary and pancreatic secretions of the horse. In: Phillipson, A.T. (Ed.), Physiology of Digestion and Metabolism in the Ruminant. Oriel Press, Newcastle upon Tyne, pp. 375–389.

Andrews, F.M., Jenkins, C.C., Blackford, J.T., et al., 1992. Effect of oral omeprazole on basal and pentagastrin-stimulated gastric secretion in young female horses. Equine Veterinary Journal 13, 80–83.

Andrews, F.M., Buchanan, B.R., Smith, S.H., et al., 2006. In vitro effects of hydrochloric acid and various concentrations of acetic, propionic, butyric, or valeric acids on bioelectric properties of equine gastric squamous mucosa. American Journal of Veterinary Research 67, 1873–1882.

Argenzio, R.A., Hintz, H.F., 1972. Effect of diet on glucose entry and oxidation rates in ponies. Journal of Nutrition 102, 879–892.

Argenzio, R.A., Lowe, J.E., Pickard, D.W., et al., 1974a. Digesta passage and water exchange in the equine large intestine. American Journal of Physiology 226, 1035–1042.

Argenzio, R.A., Southworth, M., Stevens, C.E., 1974b. Sites of organic acid production and absorption in the equine gastrointestinal tract. American Journal of Physiology 226, 1043–1050.

Argenzio, R.A., Stevens, C.E., 1975. Cyclic changes in ionic composition of digesta in the equine intestinal tract. American Journal of Physiology 228, 1224–1230.

Argenzio, R.A., Southworth, M., Lowe, J.E., et al., 1977. Interrelationship of Na, HCO_3 and volatile fatty-acid transport by equine large intestine. American Journal of Physiology 233, E469–E478.

Bailey, S.R., Baillon, M.L., Rycroft, A.N., et al., 2003. Identification of equine cecal bacteria producing amines in an in vitro model of carbohydrate overload. Applied Environmental Microbiology 69, 2087–2093.

Baker, S.J., Gerring, E.L., 1993. Technique for prolonged, minimally invasive monitoring of intragastric pH in ponies. American Journal of Veterinary Research 54, 1725–1734.

Barlet, J.P., Davicco, M.J., Coxam, V., 1995. Physiologie de l'absorption intestinale du phosphore chez l'animal. Reproduction and Nutritional Development 35, 475–489.

Baruc, C., Dawson, K., et al., 1983. The characterization and nitrogen metabolism of equine caecal bacteria. Proceedings 8th Equine Nutrition and Physiology Society Meeting, Lexington KY.

Bass, P., Code, C.F., Lambert, E.H., 1961. Motor and electrical activity of the duodenum. American Journal of Physiology 201, 287–291.

Berry, C.R., Merritt, A.M., Burrows, C.F., et al., 1986. Evaluation of the myoelectrical activity of the equine ileum infected with *Strongylus vulgaris* larvae. American Journal of Veterinary Research 47, 27–30.

Berthoud, H.R., 2006. Vagal and hormonal gut-brain communication: from satiation to satisfaction. Neurogastroenterology and Motility 20 (Suppl 1), 64–72.

Bertone, A.L., VanSoest, P.J., Johnson, D., et al., 1989. Large intestinal capacity, retention times, and turnover rates of particulate ingesta associated with extensive large-colon resection in horses. American Journal of Veterinary Research 50, 1621–1632.

Bonhomme-Florentin, 1976. Activité lipolytique des ciliés et des bactéries du caecum des equidés. Compte Rendu de l'Academie du Science Paris 282 (Série D), 1605–1608.

Bonhomme-Florentin, A., 1985. Attachement des ciliés du caecum du cheval aux fragments végétaux. Dégradation des chloroplastes. attachements des bactéries aux ciliés du caecum. Reproduction Nutrition Développement 25, 127–139.

Bonin, S.J., Clayton, H.M., Lanovaz, J.L, et al., 2007. Comparison of mandibular motion in horses chewing hay and pellets. Equine Veterinary Journal 39, 258–262.

Braun, T., Voland, P., Kunz, L., et al., 2007. Enterochromaffin cells of the human gut: Sensors for spices and odorants. Gastroenterology 132, 1890–1901.

Breigdenbach, A., Schlumbohm, C., Harmeyer, J., 1998. Peculiarities of vitamin D and of the calcium and phosphate homeostatic system in horses. Veterinary Research 29, 173–186.

Brockner, C., Austbo, D., Noesser, J.A., et al., 2010. The effect of sugar beet pulp on the caecal pH in Norwegian cold-blooded trotter horses. In: Ellis, A.D., Longland, A., Coenen, M, et al. (Eds.), The impact of nutrition on the health and welfare of horses. European Association for Animal Production publication N° 128, pp. 210–212.

Brown, M., Sonea, I., Nachreiner, R.F., et al., 1987. Serum immunoreactive gastrin activity in horses: Basal and postprandial values. Veterinary Research Communications 11, 497–501.

Bueno, L., Fioramonti, J., Ruckebusch, Y., 1975. Rate of flow of digesta and electrical activity of the small intestine of dogs and sheep. Journal of Physiology 249, 69–85.

Bullimore, S.R., Pagan, J.D., Harris, P.A., et al., 2000. Carbohydrate supplementation of horses during endurance exercise: comparison of fructose and glucose. Nutrition 130, 1760–1765.

Bullimore, S.R., Corfield, A.P., Hicks, S.J., et al., 2001. Surface mucus in the non-glandular region of the equine stomach. Research in Veterinary Science 70, 149–155.

Burns, G.A., Cummings, J.F., 1993. Neuropeptide distributions in the colon, cecum and jejunum of the horse. Anatomical Record 236, 341–350.

Burnstock, G., 2009. Purinergic cotransmission. Experimental Physiology 94, 20–24.

Camilleri, M., Malagelada, J.R., Brown, M.L., et al., 1985. Relation between antral motility and gastric emptying of solids and liquids in humans. American Journal of Physiology 249, G580–G585.

Campbell-Thompson, M.L., Merritt, A.M., 1987. Effect of ranitidine on gastric acid secretion in the young horse. American Journal of Veterinary Research 48, 1511–1515.

Campbell-Thompson, M.L., Merritt, A.M., 1990. Basal and pentagastrin-stimulated gastric secretion in young horses. American Journal of Physiology 259, R1259–R1266.

Campbell-Thompson, M.L., 1994. Secretagogue-induced [^{14}C]aminopyrine uptake in isolated equine parietal cells. American Journal of Veterinary Research 55, 132–137.

Cargile, J.L., Burrow, J.A., Kim, I., et al., 2004. Effect of dietary corn oil supplementation on equine gastric fluid acid, sodium, and prostaglandin E_2 content before and during pentagastrin infusion. Journal of Veterinary Internal Medicine 18, 545–549.

Carmalt, J.L., Allen, A.L., 2006. Effect of rostrocaudal mobility of the mandible on feed digestibility and fecal particle size in horses. Journal of the American Veterinary Medical Association 229, 1275–1278.

Ceccarelli, P., Pedini, V., Garguilo, A.M., 1995. Serotonin-containing cells in the horse gastrointestinal tract. Anatomia Histologia Embryologia 24, 97–99.

Cehak, A., Burmester, M., Geburek, F., et al., 2009. Electrophysiological characterization of electrolyte and nutrient transport across the small intestine in horses. Journal of Animal Physiology and Animal Nutrition (Berlin) 93, 287–294.

Chiocchetti, R., Bombardi, C., Mongardi-Fantaguzzi, C., et al., 2009. Intrinsic innervation of the horse ileum. Research in Veterinary Science 87, 177–185.

Choukevitch, J., 1911. Étude de la flore bactérienne du gros intestin de cheval. Annales de l'Institute Pasteur 25, 247–276 and 345–367.

Christensen, J., 1971. The controls of gastrointestinal movements: Some old and new views. New England Journal of Medicine 285, 85–98.

Clark, E.S., Morris, D.D., Whitlock, R.H., 1987. Esophageal manometry in horses, cows, and sheep during deglutition. American Journal of Veterinary Research 48, 547–551.

Clarke, L.L., Ganjam, V.K., Fichtenbaum, B., et al., 1988. Effect of feeding on renin-angiotensin-aldosterone system of the horse. American Journal of Physiology 254, R524–R530.

Clarke, L.L., Argenzio, R.A., 1990. NaCl transport across equine proximal colon and the effect of endogenous prostanoids. American Journal of Physiology 259, G62–G69.

Clarke, L.L., Argenzio, R.A., Roberts, M.C., 1990a. Effect of meal feeding on plasma volume and urinary electrolyte clearance in ponies. American Journal of Veterinary Research 51, 571–576.

Clarke, L.L., Roberts, M.C., Argenzio, R.A., 1990b. Feeding and digestive problems in horses: Physiological responses to a concentrated meal. Veterinary Clinics of North America: Equine Practice 6, 433–451.

Clarke, L.L., Roberts, M.C., Grubb, B.R., et al., 1992. Short-term effect of aldosterone on Na-Cl transport across equine colon. American Journal of Physiology 262, R939–R946.

Coenen, M., Probst, D., Gurer, C., et al., 1986. Studies on saliva production and composition in the horse. Journal of Animal Physiology and Animal Nutrition 56, 163.

Code, C.F., Marlett, J.A., 1974. The interdigestive myo-electric complex of the stomach and small bowel of dogs. Journal of Physiology 246, 289–309.

Cooke, H.J., 1986. Neurobiology of the intestinal mucosa. Gastroenterology 90, 1057–1081.

Crenon, I., Granon, S., Chapus, C., et al., 1994. Molecular cloning and expression of two horse pancreatic cDNA encoding colipase A and B. Biochimica Biophysica Acta 1213, 357–360.

Da Veiga, L., Chaucheyras-Durand, F., Julliand, V., 2005. Comparative study of colon and faeces microbial communities and activities in horses fed a high starch diet. Pferdeheilkunde 21, 45–46.

Dall'Aglio, C., Pascucci, L., Mercati, F, et al., 2009. Immunohistochemical identification and localization of orexin A and orexin type 2 receptor in the horse gastrointestinal tract. Research in Veterinary Science 86, 189–193.

Daly, K., Stewart, C.S., Flint, H.J., et al., 2001. Bacterial diversity within the equine large intestine as revealed by molecular analysis of cloned 16S rRNA genes. FEMS Microbiology Ecology 38, 141–151.

Daly, K., Shirazi-Beechey, S.P., 2003. Design and evaluation of group-specific oligonucleotide probes for quantitative analysis of intestinal ecosystems: their application to assessment of equine colonic microflora. FEMS Microbiology Ecology 44, 243–252.

Dave, M.H., Schultz, N., Zecevic, M., et al., 2004. Expression of heteromeric amino acid transporters along the murine intestine. Journal of Physiology 558, 597–610.

Delesalle, C., van Acker, N., Claes, P., et al., 2008. Contractile effects of 5-hydroxytryptamine (5-HT) in the equine jejunum circular muscle: functional and immunohistochemical identification of a 5-HT1A-like receptor. Equine Veterinary Journal 40, 313–320.

de Fombelle, A., Varloud, M., Goachet, A.G., et al., 2003. Characterisation of microbial and biochemical profile along the anatomic parts of the digestive tract of horses fed two distinct diets. Animal Science 77, 293–304.

de Fombelle, A., Veiga, L., Drogoul, C., et al., 2004. Effect of diet composition and feeding pattern on prececal digestibility of starches from diverse botanical origins measured with the mobile nylon bag technique in horses. Journal of Animal Science 82, 3625–3634.

Ding, Z., Xu, Y., 2010. Lactic acid is absorbed from the small intestine of sheep. Biomedical Research 31 (4), 239–249.

Domenghini, C., Radaelli, G., Arrighi, S., et al., 2004. Cholinergic, nitergic and peptidergic (Substance P- and CGRP utilizing) innervation of the horse intestine. A histochemical and immunohistochemical study. Histology Histopathology 19, 357–370.

Drogoul, C., Poncet, C., Tisserand, J.L., 2000. Feeding ground and pelleted hay rather than chopped hay to ponies: 1. consequences for in vivo digestibility and rate of passage of digesta. Animal Feed Science 87, 117–130.

Duckworth, D.H., Madison, J.B., Calderwood-Mays, M., et al., 1992. Arteriovenous differences for glutamine in the equine gastrointestinal tract. American Journal of Veterinary Research 53, 1864–1867.

Dulphy, J.P., Martin-Rosset, W., Dubroeucq, H., et al., 1997. Compared feeding patterns in ad libitum intake of dry forages by horses and sheep. Livestock Production Science 52, 49–56.

Dupuy-Julliand, V., 1996. Étude de l'écosystème cæcal des équidés: Aptitude à dégrader les polyosides pariétaux, - Caractérisation quantitative et qualitative des flores cellulolytiques bactériennes et fongiques dominantes. Thesis Food Sciences - Microbiology - ENSBANA, p. 121.

Dyce, K.M., Hartman, W., Aales, R.G.H., 1976. A cinefluoroscopic study of the caecal base of the horse. Research in Veterinary Science 20, 40–46.

Dyer, J., Fernandez-Castaño Merediz, E., Salmon, K.S.H., et al., SP, 2002. Molecular characterisation of carbohydrate digestion and absorption in equine small intestine. Equine Veterinary Journal 34, 349–358.

Dyer, J., Al-Rammahi, M., Waterfall, L., et al., 2009. Adaptive response of equine intestinal Na^+/glucose co-transporter (SGLT1) to an increase in dietary soluble carbohydrate. Pflugers Archives 458, 419–430.

Eckersall, P.D., 1984. Equine whole saliva - a sample system and biochemical analysis. Veterinary Record 115, 437–438.

Eckersall, P.D., Aitchison, T., Colquhoun, K.M., 1985. Equine whole saliva - variability of some major constituents. Equine Veterinary Journal 17, 391–393.

Ellis, A.D., Hill, J., 2005. Digestive Physiology of the Horse. In: Nutritional Physiology of the Horse. Nottingham University Press, Nottingham UK, pp. 7–41.

Elsden, S.R., Hitchcock, M.W.S., Marshall, R.A., et al., 1946. Volatile acid in the digesta of ruminants and other animals. Journal of Experimental Biology 22, 191–202.

Engelking, L.R., Anwer, M.S., Hofmann, A.F., 1989. Basal and bile salt-stimulated bile flow and biliary lipid excretion in ponies. American Journal of Veterinary Research 50, 578–582.

Feller, G., Bussy, O., Houssier, C., et al., 1996. Structural and functional aspects of chloride binding to *Alteromonas haloplanctis* α-amylase. Journal of Biological Chemistry 271, 23836–23841.

Fink, C., Tatar, M., Failing, K., et al., 2006. Serotonin-containing cells in the gastrointestinal tract of newborn foals and adult horses. Anatomy Histology and Embryology 35, 23–27.

Flemström, G., Isenberg, J.I., 2001. Gastroduodenal mucosal alkaline secretion and mucosal protection. News in Physiological Sciences 16, 23–28.

Freeman, D.E., Kleinzeller, A., Donawick, W.J., et al., 1989. In vitro transport of L-alanine by equine cecal mucosa. American Journal of Veterinary Research 50, 2138–2144.

Freeman, D.E., Donawick, W.J., 1991. In vitro transport of cycloleucine by equine cecal mucosa. American Journal of Veterinary Research 52, 539–542.

Freeman, D.E., Inoue, O.J., Eurell, T.E., 1997. Effects of flunixin meglumine on short circuit current in equine colonic mucosa in vitro. American Journal of Veterinary Research 58, 915–919.

Freeman, D.E., 2002. Dry matter content throughout the equine GIT and at sites of colonic impaction. In: Proceedings of the 7th International Equine Colic Research Symposium, Manchester, UK, p. 124.

Freytag, C., Seeger, J., Siegemund, T., et al., 2008. Immunohistochemical characterization and quantitative analysis of neurons in the myenteric plexus of the equine intestine. Brain Research 1244, 53–64.

Fujisawa, T., Itoh, K., Mitsuoka, T., 1993. *Lactobacilli* in the alimentary tract of horses. Bifidobacteria and Microflora 12, 87–90.

Furness, J.B., 2006. The Enteric Nervous System. Blackwell Publishing, Oxford.

Furness, J.B., 2008. The enteric nervous system: normal functions and enteric neuropathies. Neurogastroenterology and Motility 20 (Suppl. 1), 32–38.

Ganapathy, V., Brandsch, M., Leibach, F.H., 1994. Intestinal transport of amino acids and peptides. In: Johnson, L.R. (Ed.), Physiology of the Gastrointestinal Tract, third ed. Raven Press, NY, p. 1773.

Garner, H.E., Moore, J.N., Johnson, J.H., et al., 1978. Changes in the caecal flora. Equine Veterinary Journal 10, 249–252.

Gibbs, P.G., Potter, G., Kreider, J.L., et al., 1981. Partial and total tract protein digestion in ponies fed three forages. In: Proceedings of the Seventh Equine Nutrition and Physiology Symposium, Warrenton, VA.

Gibbs, P.G., Potter, G.D., Schelling, G.T., et al., 1988. Digestion of hay protein in different segments of the equine digestive tract. Journal of Animal Science 66, 400–406.

Giddings, R.F., Argenzio, R.A., Stevens, C.E., 1974. Sodium and chloride transport across the equine cecal mucosa. American Journal of Veterinary Research 35, 1511–1514.

Glade, M.J., 1983. Nitrogen partitioning along the equine digestive tract. Journal of Animal Science 54, 943–953.

Gonchar, M.V., Lavrenova, G.I., Rudenskaya, G.N., et al., 1984. Multiple forms of equine pepsin. Biokhimiya 49, 1026–1037.

Goodson, J., Tyznik, W.J., Cline, J.H., et al., 1988. Effects of an abrupt diet changes from hay to concentrate on microbial numbers and physical environment in the cecum of the pony. Applied and Environmental Microbiology 54, 1946–1950.

Goyal, R.K., Hirano, I., 1996. Mechanisms of disease - The enteric nervous system. New England Journal of Medicine 334, 1106–1115.

Goyal, R.K., Chadbury, A., 2008. Physiology of normal esophageal motility. Journal of Clinical Gastroenterology 42, 610–619.

Greet, T.R.C., 1982. Observations on the potential role of oesophageal radiography in the horse. Equine Veterinary Journal 14, 73–79.

Gronwall, R., Engelking, L.R., Anwer, M.S., et al., 1975. Bile secretion in ponies with biliary fistulas. American Journal of Veterinary Research 36, 653–654.

Hastie, P.M., Mitchell, K., Murray, J.A.D.M., 2008. Semi-quantitative analysis of *Ruminococcus flavefaciens, Fibrobacter succinogenes* and *Streptococcus bovis* in the equine large intestine using real-time polymerase chain reaction. British Journal of Nutrition 100, 561–568.

Healy, H.P., Siciliano, P.D., Lawrence, L.M., 1995. Effect of concentrate form on blood and gastric fluid variables in ponies. Journal of Equine Veterinary Science 15, 423–428.

Hersey, S.J., Sachs, G., 1995. Gastric acid secretion. Physiological Reviews 75, 155–189.

Hinder, R.A., Kelly, K.A., 1977. Canine gastric emptying of solids and liquids. American Journal of Physiology 233, E335–E340.

Hintz, H.F., Hogue, D.E., Walker, E.F., et al., 1971. Apparent digestion in various segments of the digestive tract of ponies fed diets with varying roughage grain ratios. Journal of Animal Science 32, 245–248.

Hirota, C.L., McKay, D.M., 2006. Cholinergic regulation of epithelial ion transport in the mammalian intestine. British Journal of Pharmacology 149, 463–479.

Holzer, P., 1998. Neural emergency system in the stomach. Gastroenterology 114, 823–839.

Holzer, P., Michi, T., Danzer, M., et al., 2001. Surveillance of the gastrointestinal mucosa by sensory neurons. Journal of Physiology and Pharmacology 52, 505–521.

Houpt, K.A., Perry, P.J., Hintz, H.F., et al., 1988. Effect of meal frequency on fluid balance and behavior of ponies. Physiology and Behavior 42, 401–407.

Houpt, K.A., 1998. Chapter 3: Biological rhythms and sleep. In: Domestic Animal Behavior for Veterinarians and Animal Scientists. Iowa State University Press, Ames IA, pp. 83–109.

Hsiung, T.S., 1930. A monograph on the protozoa of the large intestine of the horse. Iowa State College Journal of Science 4, 359–423.

Hudson, N.P.H., Pearson, G.T., Kitamura, N., et al., 1999. An immunohistochemical study of interstitial cells of Cajal (ICC) in the equine gastrointestinal tract. Research in Veterinary Science 66, 265–271.

Hudson, N.P.H., Mayhew, I.G., Pearson, G.T., 2001. In vitro microelectrode study of the electrical properties of smooth muscle in equine ileum. Veterinary Record 149, 707–711.

Hudson, N.P.H., Merritt, A.M., 2008. Equine gastrointestinal motility research: Where we are and where we need to go. Equine Veterinary Journal 40, 422–428.

Hungate, R.E., 1950. The anaerobic mesophilic cellulolytic bacteria. Bacteriological Reviews 14, 1–46.

Husted, L., Sanchez, L., Olsen, S.N., et al., 2008. Effect of paddock vs. stall housing on 24 hour gastric pH within the proximal and ventral equine stomach. Equine Veterinary Journal 40, 337–341.

Husted, L., Sanchez, L.C., Baptiste, K.E., et al., 2009. Effect of a feed/fast protocol on pH in the proximal equine stomach. Equine Veterinary Journal 41, 658–662.

Illenseer, M., 1994. Preileal digestibility of oat, potato and cassava diets in horses. Institut fur Tierernahrung, Tierarztliche Hochschule Hannover, Hanover, Germany.

Jansen, W.L., Van Oldruitenborgh-Oosterbaan, M.M., Cone, J.W., et al., 2007. High fat intake by ponies reduces both apparent digestibility of dietary cellulose and cellulose fermentation by faeces and isolated caecal and colonic contents. Animal Feed Science and Technology, 133, 298–308.

Johnsen, A.H., Sandin, A., Rourke, I.J., et al., 1998. Unique progastrin processing in equine G-cells suggests marginal tyrosyl sulfotransferase activity. European Journal of Biochemistry 255, 432–438.

Johnson, L.R., 2001. Digestion and absorption. In: Johnson, L.R. (Ed.), Gastrointestinal Physiology, sixth ed. CV Mosby, St Louis, pp. 119–141.

Jouany, J.-P., Broudiscou, L., Prins, R.A, et al., 1995. Metabolisme et nutrition de la population microbienne du rumen. In: Nutrition des Ruminants Domestiques. INRA, Pari, France, pp. 350–381.

Jouany, J.P., Medina, B., Bertin, G., et al., 2009. Effect of live yeast culture supplementation on hindgut microbial communities and their polysaccharidase and glycoside hydrolase activities in horses fed a high-fiber or high-starch diet. Journal of Animal Science 87, 2844–2852.

Julliand, V., de Vaux, A., Millet, L., et al., 1999. Identification of Ruminococcus flavefaciens as the predominant cellulolytic bacterial species of the equine cecum. Applied Environmental Microbiology 65, 3738–3741.

Julliand, V., de Fombelle, A., Drogoul, C., et al., 2001. Feeding and microbial disorders in horses: 3-Effects of three hay:grain ratios on microbial profile and activities. Journal of Equine Veterinary Science 21, 543–546.

Kapusniak, L.J., Greene, L.W., Potter, G.D., 1988. Calcium, magnesium and phosphorus absorption from the small and large intestine of ponies fed elevated amounts of aluminium. Equine Veterinary Science 8, 305–309.

Kelly, K.A., Code, C.F., Elveback, L.R., 1969. Patterns of canine gastric electrical activity. American Journal of Physiology 217, 461–470.

Kern, D.L., Slyter, L.L., Weaver, J.M., et al., 1973. Pony cecum vs. steer rumen: the effect of oats and hay on the microbial ecosystem. Journal of Animal Science 37, 463–469.

Kern, D.L., Slyter, L.L., Leffel, E.C., et al., 1974. Ponies vs. steers: microbial and chemical characteristics of intestinal ingesta. Journal of Animal Science 38, 559–564.

Khittoo, G., Vermette, L., Nappert, G., et al., 1991. Isolation of a major form of pepsinogen from gastric mucosa of horses. American Journal of Veterinary Research 52, 713–717.

Kidd, M., Tang, L.H., Miu, K., et al., 1996. Autoregulation of enterochromaffin-like cell histamine secretion via the histamine 3 receptor subtype. Yale Journal of Biological Medicine 69, 9–19.

Kienzle, E., Radicke, S., 1993. Effect of diet on maltase, sucrase and lactase in the small intestinal mucosa of the horse. Journal of Animal Physiology and Animal Nutrition 70, 97–103.

Kienzle, E., Radicke, S., Landes, E., et al., 1994. Activity of amylase in the gastrointestinal tract of the horse. Journal of Animal Physiology and Animal Nutrition 72, 234–241.

Kienzle, E., Pohlenz, J., Radicke, S., 1997. Morphology of starch digestion in the horse. Journal of Veterinary Medicine 44, 207–221.

Kitamura, N., Yamada, J., Calingasan, N.Y, et al., 1984. Immunocytochemical distribution of endocrine cells in the gastrointestinal tract of the horse. Equine Veterinary Journal 16, 103–107.

Kitchen, D.L., Merritt, A.M., Burrow, J.A., 1998. Histamine-induced gastric acid secretion in horses. American Journal of Veterinary Research 59, 1303–1306.

Kitchen, D.L., Burrow, J.A., Hartless, C.S., et al., 2000. Effect of pyloric blockade and infusion of histamine or pentagastrin on gastric secretion in horses. American Journal of Veterinary Research 61, 1133–1139.

Kleffken, D., 1993. Preileal digestibility of grain starch (barley/maize) depending on processing, roughage supply and amylase supplement in horses. Institut fur Tierernahrung, Tierarztliche Hochschule, Hannover, Germany.

Kolb, E., 1975. Physiologie de la digestion et de l'absorption. Physiologie des Animaux Domestiques, Vigot Frères, Paris, pp. 206–334.

Kollarczik, B., Enders, C., Friedrich, M., 1992. Effect of diet composition on microbial spectrum in the jejunum of horses. 1. Europäische Konferenz über die Ernährung des Pferdes-Physiologie und Pathologie des Verdauungskanals-Konsequenzen für die Ernährung, Pferdeheilkunde, Hannover, pp. 49–54.

Kotze, S.H., Van Aswegan, G., 1990. An immunohistochemical study of various peptide-containing endocrine cells and neurones at the equine ileocecal junction. Onderstepoort Journal of Veterinary research 57, 13–17.

Kunze, W.A.A., Furness, J.B., 1999. The enteric nervous system and regulation of intestinal motility. Annual Review of Physiology 61, 117–142.

Kwiatek, M.A., Menne, D., Steingoetter, A., et al., 2009. Effect of meal volume and calorie load on postprandial gastric function and emptying: studies under physiological conditions by combined fiber-optic pressure measurement and MRI. American Journal of Physiology 297, G894–G901.

Lengsfeld, H., Beaumier-Gallon, G., Chahinian, H., et al., 2004. Physiology of gastro-intestinal lipolysis and therapeutical use of lipases and digestive lipase inhibitors. In: Müller, G., Petry, S. (Eds.), Lipases and Phospholipases in Drug Development. Wiley-VCH Verlag GmbH & Co., pp. 195–229.

Lester, G.D., Merritt, A.M., Neuwirth, L., et al., 1998. Myoelectric activity of the ileum, cecum, and right ventral colon, and cecal emptying of radiolabeled markers in clinically normal ponies. American Journal of Veterinary Research 59, 313–319.

Lindner, A., Marx, S., Gansen, S., et al., 1999. Saliva collection and relationship between lactate concentration in blood and saliva of exercising horses.

16th Equine Nutrition and Physiology Symposium, Raleigh, North Carolina.

Liddle, R.A., 1995. Regulation of cholecystokinin secretion by intraluminal releasing factors. American Journal of Physiology 269, G319–327.

Lippold, B.S., Hildebrand, J., Straub, R., 2004. Tegaserod (HTF919) stimulates gut motility in normal horses. Equine Veterinary Journal 36, 622–627.

Lohmann, K., Roussel, A.J., Cohen, N.D., et al., 2000. Comparison of nuclear scintigraphy and aceomenophen absorption as a means of studying gastric emptying in horses. American Journal of Veterinary Research 61, 310–315.

Lopez, M.A.F., White, N.A., Crisman, M.V., et al., 2004. Effects of feeding large amounts of grain on colonic contents and feces of horses. American Journal of Veterinary Research 65, 687–694.

Lorenzo-Figueras, M., Merritt, A.M., 2002. Effects of exercise on gastric volume and pH in the proximal portion of the stomach of horses. American Journal of Veterinary Research 63, 1481–1487.

Lorenzo-Figueras, M., Merritt, A.M., 2006. Role of cholecystokinin in the gastric motor response to a meal in horses. American Journal of Veterinary Research 67, 1998–2005.

Lorenzo-Figueras, M., Preston, T., Ott, E.A., et al., 2005. Meal-induced gastric relaxation and emptying in horses after ingestion of high-fat versus high carbohydrate diets. American Journal of Veterinary Research 66, 897–905.

Lorenzo-Figueras, M., Morisset, S.M., Morisset, J., et al., 2007. Digestive enzyme concentrations and activities in healthy pancreatic tissue of horses. American Journal of Veterinary Research 68, 1070–1072.

Lundgren, O., 2004. Interface between the intestinal environment and the nervous system. Gut 53 (Suppl II), ii16–ii18.

Lybbert, T., Gibbs, P., Cohen, N., et al., 2007. Feeding alfalfa hay to exercising horses reduces the severity of gastric squamous mucosal ulceration. AAEP Proceedings 53, 525–526.

Lynn, A., Cochrane, M.P., 1997. An evaluation of confocal microscopy for the study of starch granule enzymic digestion. Starch 49, 106–111.

MacAllister, C.G., Morgan, S.J., Borne, A.T., et al., 1993. Comparison of adverse effects of phenylbutazone, flunixin meglumine, and ketoprofen in horses. Journal of the American Veterinary Medical Association 202, 71–77.

MacKay, R.J., French, T.W., Nguyen, H.T., et al., 1983. Effects of large doses of phenylbutazone administration to horses. American Journal of Veterinary Research 44, 774–780.

Mackie, R.I., Wilkins, C.A., 1988. Enumeration of anaerobic bacterial microflora of the equine gastrointestinal tract. Applied Environmental Microbiology 54, 2155–2160.

Maczulak, A.E., Dawson, K.A., Dawson, J.P., 1985. Nitrogen utilisation in bacterial isolates from the equine cæcum. Applied Environmental Microbiology 50, 1439–1443.

Madara, J.L., Trier, J.S., 1994. The functional morphology of the mucosa of the small intestine. In: Johnson, L.R. (Ed.), Physiology of the Gastrointestinal Tract. Raven Press, New York, p. 1577.

Malbert, C.H., Ruckebusch, Y., 1989. Vagal influences on the phasic and tonic components of the motility of the ovine stomach and gastroduodenal area. Gastrointestinal Motility 1, 15–20.

Malbert, C.H., Roger, T., 1989. Visualisation par échotomographie de la jonction caecocolique chez le poney – réponses pharmacologiques. Revue de Médicine Vétérinaire 140, 857–862.

Malone, E.D., Kannan, M.S., Brown, D.R., et al., 1999. Adrenergic, cholinergic, and nonadrenergic-noncholinergic intrinsic innervation of the jejunum in horses. American Journal of Veterinary Research 60, 898–904.

Malone, E.D., Kannan, M.S., Brown, D.R., 2000. Evaluation of substance P as a neurotransmitter in equine jejunum. American Journal of Veterinary Research 61, 1178–1184.

McCarthy, D.M., 2010. Adverse effects of proton pump inhibitor drugs. Current Opinion in Gastroenterology 26, 624–631.

McMeniman, N.P., Elliott, R., Groenendyk, S., et al., 1987. Synthesis and absorption of cysteine from the hindgut of the horse. Equine Veterinary Journal 19, 192–198.

Medina, B., 2003. Effets de la culture de levures vivantes Yea Sacc1026 (CBS 493.94) en function de deux ratios luzerne/orge dans un aliment complet granulé sur fonctionnement de l'ecosystème intestinal du cheval. Thesis presented to Department of Food Science – Animal Nutrition, University of Bourgogne.

Medina, B., Girard, I.D., Jacotot, E., et al., 2002a. Effect of a preparation of Saccharomyces cerevisiae on microbial profiles and fermentation patterns in the large intestine of horses fed a high fiber or a high starch diet. Journal of Animal Science 80, 2600–2609.

Medina, B., Drogoul, C., Julliand, V., 2002b. Pratique alimenataire et transit digestif. In: Nationaux, L.H. (Ed.), 28eme Journée de la Recherche Equine. INRA, Paris, pp. 91–102.

Merediz, E., Dyer, J., Salmon, K.S.H., et al., 2004. Molecular characterisation of fructose transport in equine small intestine Equine Veterinary Journal 36, 532–538.

Merritt A.M., Campbell-Thompson, M.L., Lowrey, S., 1989. Effect of xylazine treatment on equine proximal gastrointestinal tract myoelectrical activity. American Journal of Veterinary Research 50, 945–949.

Merritt, A.M., 1999. Normal equine gastroduodenal secretion and motility. Equine Veterinary Journal Suppl 29, 7–13.

Merritt, A.M., 2003. The equine stomach: a personal perspective. Proceedings of the 49th Annual AAEP Convention 49, 75–102.

Merritt, A.M., Panzer, R.B., Lester, G.D., et al., 1995. Equine pelvic flexure myoelectrical activity during fed and fasted states. American Journal of Physiology 269, G262–G268.

Merritt, A.M., Burrow, J.A., Horbal, M.J., et al., 1996. Effect of omeprazole on sodium and potassium output in pentagastrin-stimulated equine gastric contents. American Journal of Veterinary Research 57, 1640–1644.

Merritt, A.M., Burrow, J.A., Hartless, C.S., 1998. Effect of xylazine, butorphanol, and a combination of xylazine and butorphanol on equine duodenal motility. American Journal of Veterinary Research 59, 619–623.

Merritt, A.M., Sanchez, L., Burrow, J.A., et al., 2003. Effect of GastroGard™ and three compounded oral omeprazole preparations on 24 h intragastric pH in gastrically cannulated mature horses. Equine Veterinary Journal 35, 691–695.

Meschter, C.L., Gilbert, M., Krook, L., et al., 1990. The effects of phenylbutazone on the morphology and prostaglandin concentrations of the pyloric mucosa of the equine stomach. Veterinary Pathology 27, 244–253.

Metayer, N., Lhôte, M., Bahr, A., et al., 2004. Meal size and starch content affect gastric emptying in horses. Equine Veterinary Journal 36, 436–440.

Meyer, H., 1996. Influence of feed intake and composition, feed and water restriction and exercise on gastrointestinal fill in horses. Part 2. Equine Practice 18, 20–24.

Meyer, H., Ahiswede, L., Pferdekamp, M., 1980. Experiments on gastric contents and emptying in the horse. Deutsche Tierärztlichle Wochenschrift 87, 43–47.

Meyer, H., Coenen, M., Gurer, C., 1985. Investigations of saliva production and chewing in horses fed various feeds. Proceedings of the Equine Nutrition and Physiology Society, East Lansing MI, pp. 38–41.

Meyer, H., Coenen, M., Prost, D., 1986. Digestive physiology of the horse. 14 Feed insalivation and passage in the equine upper intestinal tract. Journal of Animal Physiology and Animal Nutrition 56, 171–183.

Meyer, H., Radicke, S., Kienzle, E., et al., 1993. Investigations on preileal digestion of oats, corn, and barley starch in relation to grain processing. Proceedings of the Equine Nutrition and Physiology Society, Gainesville FL, pp. 92–97.

Meyer, T.K., 2009. The larynx for neurologists. The Neurologist 15, 313–318.

Milinovich, G.J., Burrell, P.C., Pollitt, C.C., et al., 2008. Microbial ecology of the equine hindgut during oligofructose-induced laminitis. ISME Journal 11, 1089–1100.

Milligan, M., Beard, W., Kukanich, B., et al., S, 2007. The effect of lidocaine on postoperative jejunal motility in normal horses. Veterinary Surgery 36, 214–220.

Minami, H., McCallum, R.W., 1984. The physiology and pathophysiology of gastric emptying in humans. Gastroenterology 86, 1592–1610.

Miyaji, M., Ueda, K., Nakatsuji, H., et al., 2008. Mean retention time of digesta in the different segments of the equine hindgut. Animal Science Journal 79, 89–96.

Modlin, I.M., Tang, L.H., 1996. The gastric enterochromaffin-like cell: An enigmatic cellular link. Gastroenterology 111, 783–810.

Moeller, B.A., McCall, C.A., Silverman, S.J., 2008. Estimation of saliva production in crib-biting and normal horses. Journal of Equine Veterinary Science 28, 85–90.

Moore, B. (1898). Chemistry of the digestive processes. *Schafer's Textbook of Physiology. Vol. 1*, 312, New York.

Moore, B.E., Dehority, B.A., 1993. Effects of diet and hindgut defaunation on diet digestibility and microbial concentrations in the cecum and colon of the horse. Journal of Animal Science 71, 3350–3358.

Moreau, H., Gargouri, Y., Lecat, D., et al., 1988. Screening of lipases in several mammals. Biochimicha et Biophysica Acta 959, 247–252.

Morris, V.K., Kaihilahti, L., Girvan, M., et al., 2002. Chemical composition of digesta and microbial diversity in the fore stomach of the horse. 53rd Annual Meeting of the European Association for Animal Production, Le Caire, Egypte.

Morrissey, N.K., Bellenger, C.R., Baird, A.W., 2008. Bradykinin stimulates prostaglandin E2 production and cyclooxygenase activity in equine nonglandular and glandular gastric mucosa in vitro. Equine Veterinary Journal, 2008 40, 332–336.

Morton, A.J., Grosche, A., Rötting, A.K., et al., 2008a. Expression of cyclooxygenase-1 and -2 in the left dorsal colon after different durations of ischemia and reperfusion in horses. American Journal of Veterinary Research 70, 1536–1544.

Morton, A.J., Grosche, A., Freeman, D.E., 2008b. Characterisation of cyclooxygenase 1 and cyclooxygenase 2 expression in the gastrointestinal tract of horses. In; Proceedings of the 9th International Equine Colic Research Symposium. Liverpool, UK, 15–18 June 2008. pp. 144–145.

Murray, M.J., Schusser, G.F., 1993. Application of gastric pH-metry in horses: measurement of 24 hour gastric pH in horses fed, fasted and treated with ranitidine. Equine Veterinary Journal 25, 417–421.

Nadeau, J.A., Andrews, F.M., Mathew, A.G., et al., 2000. Evaluation of diet as a cause of gastric ulcers in horses. American Journal of Veterinary Research 61, 784–790.

Nadeau, J.A., Andrews, F.M., Patton, C.S., et al., 2003. Effects of hydrochloric, valeric, and other volatile fatty acids on pathogenesis of ulcers in the nonglandular portion of the stomach of horses. Ameriacn Journal of Veterinary Research 64, 413–417.

National Research Council, 2007. Minerals. In: Nutrient requirements of horses, 6th rev ed. National Research Council of the National Academies Press, Washington DC, pp. 69–108.
Nickel, R., Schummer, A., Seiferle, E., 1979. The Viscera of Domestic Animals, 2nd rev edn by Schummer A, Nickel R, Sack WO. Springer-Verlag, New York, pp. 180–198.
Nicpoń, J., Czerw, P., Zawadzki, W., 2000. Research of pathomechanism and therapy of colitis X. Electronic Journal of Polish Agricultural Universities, Veterinary Medicine, Volume 3, Issue 2.
Nieto, J.E., Snyder, J.R., Kollias-Baker, C., et al., 2000. In vitro effects of 5-hydroxytryptamine and cisapride on the circular smooth muscle of the jejunum of horses. American Journal of Veterinary Research 61, 1561–1566.
Niot, I., Poirier, H., Thi Thu Trang, T., et al., 2009. Intestinal absorption of long-chain fatty acids: Evidence and uncertainties. Lipid Research 48, 101–115.
Olowo-okorun, M.O., 1975. Gastrin activity along the gastrointestinal tracts of some ruminants and the donkey. General and Comparative Endocrinology 27, 111–114.
Orpin, C.G., 1981. Isolation of cellulolytic phycomycete fungi from the caecum of the horse. Journal of General Microbiology 123, 287–296.
Orsini, J.A., Dreyfuss, D.J., Vecchione, J., et al., 1991. Effects of histamine type-2 receptor antagonist (BMY-25368) on gastric secretion in horses. American Journal of Veterinary Research 52, 108–110.
Orton, R.K., Hume, I.D., Leng, R.A., 1985. Effects of exercise and level of dietary protein on digestive function in horses. Equine Veterinary Journal 17, 386–390.
Pearson, G.T., 1994. Structural organization and neuropeptide distributions in the equine enteric nervous system: an immunohistochemical study using whole-mount preparations from the small intestine. Cell Tissue Research 276, 523–534.
Pearson, R.A., Merritt, J.B., 1991. Intake, digestion and gastrointestinal transit time in resting donkeys and ponies and exercised donkeys given ad libitum hay and straw diets. Equine Veterinary Journal 23, 339–343.
Peretich, A.L., Abbott, L.L., Andrews, F.M., et al., 2009. Age-dependent regulation of sodium-potassium adenosinetriphosphatase and sodium-hydrogen exchanger mRNAs in equine nonglandular mucosa. American Journal of Veterinary Research 70, 1124–1128.
Peskar, B.M., Maricic, N., 1998. Role of prostaglandins in gastroprotection. Digestive Diseases and Sciences 43, 23S–29S.
Peskar, B.M., 2001a. Neural aspects of prostaglandin involvement in gastric mucosal defense. Journal of Physiology and Pharmacology 52, 555–568.
Peskar, B.M., 2001b. Role of cyclooxygenase isoforms in gastric mucosal defence. Journal of Physiology Paris 95, 3–9.
Pfeiffer, C.J., Dabareiner, R.M., 1992. Ultrastructure of Brunner's glands in the horse. Journal of Submicroscopic Cytology and Pathology 24, 581–588.
Philippeau, C., Faubladier, C., Goachet, AG., et al., 2009. Is there an impact of feeding concentrate before or after forage on colonic pH and redox potential in horses? Proccedings of the Equine Nutrition and Training Conference, Madrid, Spain.
Prause, A.S., Stoffel, M.H., Portier, C.J., et al., 2009. Expression and function of 5-HT_7 receptors in smooth muscle preparations from equine duodenum, ileum and pelvic flexure. Research in Veterinary Science 87, 292–299.
Rakestraw, P.C., Snyder, J.R., Woliner, M.J., et al., 1996. Involvement of nitric oxide in inhibitory neuromuscular transmission in equine jejunum. American Journal of Veterinary Research 57, 1206–1213.
Ralston, S.L., Foster, D.L., Divers, T, et al., 2001. Effect of dental correction on feed digestibility in horses. Equine Veterinary Journal 3, 390–393.
Reitnour, C.M., Baker, J.P., Mitchell, G.E., et al., 1969. Amino acids in equine cecal contents, cecal bacteria and serum. Journal of Nutrition 100, 349–354.
Reitnour, C.M., Treece, J.M., 1971. Relationship of nitrogen source to certain blood components and nitrogen balance in the equine. Journal of Animal Science 32, 487–490.
Reitnour, C.M., Salsbury, R.L., 1972. Digestion and utilization of cecally infused protein by the equine. Journal of Animal Science 35, 1190–1193.
Reitnour, C.M., Mitchell, G.E., 1979. Anaerobic proteolytic bacteria in caecal contents of ponies. Journal of Agricultural Sciences Cambridge 92, 507–509.
Respondek, F., Goachet, A.G., Rudeaux, F., et al., 2007. Effects of short-chain fructo-oligosaccharides on the microbial and biochemical profile of different segments of the gastro-intestinal tract in horses. Pferdeheilkunde 23, 146–150.
Ringger, N.C., Lester, G.D., Neuwirth, L., et al., 1996. Effect of bethanechol or erythromycin on gastric emptying in horses. American Journal of Veterinary Research 57, 1771–1775.
Roberts, M.C., Kidder, D.E., Hill, F.W.G., 1973. Small intestinal beta-galactosidase activity in the horse. Gut 14, 535–540.
Roberts, M.C., 1974. Amylase activity in the small intestine of the horse. Research in Veterinary Science 17, 400–401.
Roberts, M.C., 1975. Carbohydrate digestion and absorption in the equine small intestine. Journal of the South African Veterinary Association 46, 19–27.
Roberts, M.C., Hill, F.W.G., Kidder, D.E., 1974. The development and distribution of small intestinal disaccharidases in the horse. Research in Veterinary Science 17, 42–48.
Rosenfeld, I., Austbo, D., 2009. Effect of type of grain and feed processing on gastrointestinal retention times in horses. Journal of Animal Science 87, 3991–3996.
Ross, M.W., Donawick, W.J., Sellers, A.F., et al., 1986. Normal motility of the cecum and right ventral colon in ponies. American Journal of Veterinary Research 47, 1756–1762.
Ross, M.W., Rutkowski, J.A., Cullen, K.K., 1989. Myoelectrical activity of the cecum and right ventral colon in female ponies. American Journal of Veterinary Research 50, 374–379.
Ross, M.W., Cullen, K.K., Rutkowski, J.A., 1990. Myoelectric activity of the ileum, cecum, and right ventral colon in ponies during interdigestive, nonfeeding, and digestive periods. American Journal of Veterinary Research 51, 561–566.
Rourke, K.M., Coe, S., Kohn, C.W, et al., 2010. Cloning, comparative sequence analysis and mRNA expression of calcium-transporting genes in horses. General and Comparative Endocrinology 167, 6–10.
Ruckebusch, Y., 1973. Les particularités motrices du jéjuno-iléon chez le cheval. Extraits des Cahiers de Médecine Vétérinaire 42, 128–143.
Ruckebusch, Y., 1977. Elektromyographische analyse der dünndarmmotorik bei haustieren. Zentralblatt fur Veterinardezin A 24, 1–12.
Ruckebusch, Y., Bueno, L., 1976. The effect of feeding on the motility of the stomach and small intestine in the pig. British Journal of Nutrition 35, 397–405.
Ruckebusch, Y., Bueno, L., Fioramonti, F., 1981. La Mécanique Digestive chez les Mammifères. Masson, Paris, p. 35.
Stick, J.A., Derksen, F.J., McNitt, D.L., et al., 1983. Equine esophageal pressure profile. American Journal of Veterinary Research 44, 272–275.
Ruppin, H., 1985. Current aspects of intestinal motility and transport. Klinische Wochenschrift 63, 679–688.
Rutkowski, J.A., Ross, M.W., Cullen, K., 1998. Effects of xylazine and/or butorphanol or neostimine on myoelectrical activity of the cecum and right ventral colon in female ponies. American Journal of Veterinary Research 50, 1096–1101.
Sandin, A., Girma, K., Sjöholm, A., et al., 1998. Effects of differently composed feeds and physical stress on plasma gastrin concentration in horses. Acta Veterinaria Scandavania 39, 265–272.
Sangiah, S., McAllister, C.C., Amouzadeh, H.R., 1988. Effect of cimetidine and ranitidine on basal gastric pH, free and total acid contents in horses. Research in Veterinary Science 45, 291–295.
Sasaki, N., Yoshihara, T., 1998. The effect of motilin on the regulation mechanism of intestinal motility in conscious horses. Journal of Veterinary Medical Science 61, 167–170.
Sasaki, N., Yoshihara, T., Hara, S., 2000. Difference in the motile reactivity of jejunum, cecum, and right ventral colon to xylazine and metdetomidine in conscious horses. Journal of Equine Science 11, 63–68.
Sayegh, A.I., Anderson, N.V., Harding, J.W., et al., 1999. Purification of two equine pepsinogens by use of high-performance liquid chromatography. American Journal of Veterinary Research 60, 114–118.
Scheibner, J., Trendelenburg, A.U., Hein, L., 2002. Alpha 2-adrenoceptors in the enteric nervous system: a study in alpha 2A-adrenoceptor-deficient mice. British Journal of Pharmacology 135, 697–704.
Schemann, M., Mazzuoli, G., 2010. Multifunctional mechanosensitive neurons in the enteric nervous system. Autonomic Neuroscience 153, 21–25.
Schryver, H.F., Craig, P.H., Hintz, H.F., 1970. Calcium metabolism in ponies fed varying levels of calcium. Journal of Nutrition 100, 955–964.
Schubert, M.L., Peura, D.A., 2008. Control of gastric acid secretion in health and disease. Gastroenterology 134, 1842–1860.
Schwizer, W., Steingötter, A., Fox, M., et al., 2002. Non-invasive measurement of gastric accommodation in humans. Gut 51 (Suppl. 1), i59–i62.
Sellers, A.F., Lowe, J.E., Brondum, J., 1979. Motor events in equine large colon. American Journal of Physiology 237, E457–E464.
Sellers, A.F., Lowe, J.E., Rendano, V.T., 1984a. Equine colonic motility: Interactions among wall motion, propulsion, and fluid flow. American Journal of Veterinary Research 45, 357–360.
Sellers, A.F., Lowe, J.E., Cummings, J.F., 1984b. Trials of serotonin, substance P and α_2 -adrenergic receptor effects on the equine large colon. Cornell Veterinarian 75, 319–323.
Sepponen, K., Ruusunen, M., Pakkanen, J.A, et al., 2007. Expression of CD147 and monocarboxylate transporters MCT1, MCT2 and MCT4 in porcine small intestine and colon. Journal of Veterinary Medical Science 69, 599–604.
Shirazi-Beechey, S.P., 1995. Molecular biology of intestinal glucose transport. Nutrition Research Revue 8, 27–41.
Shirazy-Beechey, S.P., 2008. Molecular insights into dietary induced colic in the horse. Equine Veterinary Journal 40, 414–421.
Simmons, A., Ford, J.H., 1990. Liquid flow and capacity of the caecum and colon of the horse. Research in Veterinary Science 48, 265–266.
Sisson, S., Grossman, J.D., 1959. The Anatomy of Domestic Animals, fourth ed. W.B. Saunders Co., Philadelphia, pp. 406–407.
Slade, L.M., Bishop, R., Morris, J.G., et al., 1971. Digestion and absorption of 15N-labelled microbial protein in the large intestine of the horse. British Veterinary Journal 127, 11–13.
Slocombe, R.F., Todhunter, R.J., Stick, J.A., 1982. Quantitatative ultrastructural anatomy of esophagus in different regions in the horse: Effects of alternate methods of tissue processing. American Journal of Veterinary Research 43, 1137–1142.

Sneddon, J.C., Argenzio, R.A., 1998. Feeding strategy and water homeostasis in equids: the role of the hindgut. Journal of Arid Environments 38, 493–509.

Sojka, J.E., Weiss, J.S., Samuels, M.L., et al., 1992. Effect of the somatostatin analogue octreotide on gastric fluid pH in ponies. American Journal of Veterinary Research 53, 1818–1821.

Solinger, N., Sonea, I.M., 2008. Distribution of the neurokinin-1 receptor in equine intestinal smooth muscle. Equine Veterinary Journal 40, 321–325.

Sperber, I., Björnhag, G., Holtenius, K., 1992. A separation mechanism and fluid flow in the large intestine of the equine. 1- Europaische Konferenz über die Ernarhung des Pferdes, Pferdeheilkunde, Hannover, pp. 29–32.

Stadermann, B., Nehring, T., Meyer, H., 1992. Calcium and magnesium absorption with roughage or mixed feed. Pferderheilkunde 1, 77–80.

Stick, J.A., Robinson, N.E., Krehbiel, J.D., 1981. Acid-base and electrolyte alterations associated with salivary loss in the pony. American Journal of Veterinary Research 42, 733–737.

Stewart, C.E., Bryant, M.P., 1988. In: Hobson, P.N. (Ed.), The Rumen Microbial Ecosystem. Elsevier Applied Science, London, pp. 21–75.

Sutton, D.G., Bahr, A., Preston, T., et al., 2003. Validation of the ^{13}C-octanoic acid breath test for measurement of equine gastric emptying rate of solids using radioscintigraphy. Equine Veterinary Journal 35, 27–33.

Tack, J., 2000. The physiology and the pathophysiology of the gastric accommodation reflex in man. Verh K Acad Geneesk Belg 62, 183–207.

Teramae, H., Yoshikawa, T., Inoue, R., et al., 2007. The cellular expression of SMCT2 and its comparison with other transporters for monocarboxylates in the mouse digestive tract. Veterinary Journal 174, 122–128.

Tester, R.F., Karkalas, J., Qi, X., 2004. Starch structure and digestibility enzyme-substrate relationship. World's Poultry Science Journal 60, 186–195.

Treacy, P.J., Jamieson, G.G., Dent, J., 1990. Pyloric motor function during emptying of a liquid meal from the stomach in the conscious pig. Journal of Physiology 422, 523–538.

Tisserand, J.L., Masson, C., 1976. Effet de différents régimes sur l'activité biochimique dans le gros intestin du poney. 2e Réunion Annuelle de la Féderation. Européan Zootechnologie, Zürich, 23–26 août.

Van Weyenberg, S., Sales, J., Janssens, G.P.J., 2006. Passage rate of digesta through the equine gastrointestinal tract: A review. Livestock Science 99, 3–12.

Vanden Berghe, P., Janssen, P., Kindt, S., et al., 2009. Contribution of different triggers to the gastric accommodation reflex in humans. American Journal of Physiology 297, G902–G906.

Varloud, M., de Fombelle, A., Goachet, A.G., et al., 2004. Partial and total apparent digestibility of dietary carbohydrates in horses as affected by the diet. Animal Science 79, 61–72.

Varloud, M., 2006. Activité amylolytique des secretions salivaires. In: Implication des microorganismes de l'estomac dans la digestion de l'amidon par le cheval. Thesis presented to the National Agricultural Institute of Paris-Grignon, pp. 62–68.

Varloud, M., Roussel, A., Boisot, P., et al., 2006. A technique for the collection and the study of biochemical and microbial characteristics of postprandial gastric contents from conscious horses. Animal Feed Science and Technology 133, 259–274.

Varloud, M., Fonty, G., Roussel, A., et al., 2007. Postprandial kinetics of some biotic and abiotic characteristics of the gastric ecosystem of horses fed a pelleted concentrate meal. Journal of Animal Science 85, 2508–2516.

Venkatasubramanian, J., Ao, M., Rao, M.C., 2010. Ion transport in the small intestine. Current Opinion in Gastroenterology 26, 123–128.

Vigroux, P., Candau, M., Ruckebusch, Y., 1975. Motricité caecale et transit caeco-colique chez le cheval. Compte Rendu du Société de Biologie (Paris) 169, 1617–1621.

Von Engelhardt, W., Rösel, E., Rechemmer, G., 1995. Comparative views of electrophysiological parameters of large intestinal segments in pig, sheep, pony, guinea pig and rat. Deutsch Tierarztl Wochenschr 102, 157–159.

Vuyyuru, L., Schubert, M.L., Harrington, L., et al., 1995. Dual inhibitory pathways link antral somatostatin and histamine secretion in human, dog and rat stomach. Gastroenterology 109, 1566–1574.

Widenhouse, T.V., Lester, G.D., Merritt, A.M., 2002. Effect of hydrochloric acid, pepsin, or taurocholate on bioelectrical properties of gastric squamous mucosa in horses. American Journal of Veterinary Research 63, 744–749.

Windmueller, H.G., Spaeth, A.E., 1974. Uptake and metabolism of plasma glutamine by the small intestine. Journal of Biological Chemistry 25, 5070–5079.

Wille, K.H., Nakov, C., 1999. Functional morphology of the large intestinal mucosa of horses (*Equus przewalskii f. caballus*) with special regard to the epithelium. Anatomia Histologia Embryologia 28, 355–365.

Wolter, G., Gouy, D., Durix, A., et al., 1978. Digestibilité et activité biochimique intracaecale chez le poney recevant un même aliment complet présenté sous forme granulée, expansée ou semi-expansée. Annales de Zootechnie 27, 47–60.

Wolter, R., Chaabouni, A., 1979. Étude de la digestion de l'amidon chez le cheval par analyse du contenu digestif après abattage. Revue de Médecine Vétérinaire 130, 1345–1357.

Wolter, R., Nouwakpo, F., Durix, A., 1980. Étude comparative de la digestion d'un aliment complet chez le poney et le lapin. Reproduction Nutrition Développement 20, 1723–1730.

Wood, J.D., Galligan, J.J., 2004. Function of opioids in the enteric nervous system. Neurogastroenterology and Motility 16 (Suppl. 2), 17–28.

Woodward, A.D., Holcombe, S.J., Steibel, J.P., et al., 2010. Cationic and neutral amino acid transporter transcript abundances are differentially expressed in the equine intestinal tract. Journal of Animal Science 88, 1028–1033.

Wyse, C.A., Murphy, D.M., Preston, T., et al., 2001. The C-13-octanoic acid breath test for detection of effects of meal composition on the rate of solid-phase gastric emptying in ponies. Research in Veterinary Science 71, 81–83.

Young, D.W., Smythe, G.B., 1990. Molecular forms of gastrin in antral mucosa of the horse. Domestic Animal Endocrinology 7, 55–62.

Yuki, N., Shimazaki, T., Kushiro, A., et al., 2000. Colonization of the stratified squamous epithelium of the nonsecreting area of horse stomach by lactobacilli. Applied and Environmental Microbiology 66, 5030–5034.

2

Endocrine and metabolic physiology

Raymond J. Geor

As a nonruminant herbivore, the horse is adapted to survive on high roughage diets with a substantial proportion of daily energy requirements being met by the absorption of volatile fatty acids (VFA) produced by microbial fermentation of dietary fiber in the hindgut. However, the horse is also able to digest and absorb other energy substrates (particularly glucose and triglycerides) from the small intestine. Therefore, energy metabolism in the horse fed a roughage only diet is likely to be similar to that in ruminants but more akin to that in monogastric species when they are provided starch-based, low fiber feeds (e.g. corn) or oil-based concentrate feeds that are digested (primarily) in the foregut.

The goal of this chapter is to provide an overview of endocrine and metabolic physiology in horses as a basis for subsequent chapters in this book. The primary topics covered include the neuroendocrine regulation of appetite and energy balance; the role of major hormones in the regulation of energy substrate metabolism; an overview of macronutrient (energy substrate) metabolism; and the storage of energy substrates in key organs, emphasizing the effects of insulin in skeletal muscle and adipose tissue. Emphasis is also given to the effects of diet and feeding on carbohydrate metabolism in horses; this subject has been of considerable interest in recent years given: (1) the possible links between glucose/insulin responses and risk of adverse outcomes such as laminitis; and (2) the importance of muscle glycogen metabolism to athletic performance coupled with the fact that the post-exercise rate of muscle glycogen replenishment is very slow in the horse in comparison to other mammalian species.

Neuroendocrine regulation of appetite and energy balance

The central nervous system (CNS) modulates energy balance by regulating feed intake and energy expenditure in response to hormonal, neuronal and nutrient signals (Schwartz et al 2000; Fig. 2.1). In humans and other mammals, regulatory processes within the arcuate nucleus of the hypothalamus control feed intake and energy expenditure. Agouti-related peptide/neuropeptide Y (AgRP/NPY) neurons stimulate appetite (*orexigenic* hormones) and decrease metabolism, while proopiomelanocortin (POMC) neurons release α-melanocyte-stimulating hormone (α-MSH), a neurotransmitter that inhibits food intake (Schwartz et al 2000). A large number of hormones secreted by other tissues in particular the gut and adipose tissue as well as various nutrient signals, interact with these hypothalamic neurons to modulate appetite and metabolic rate. For example, peptide $YY_{3\text{-}36}$, a hormone secreted by the gut in direct proportion to the caloric content of a meal, decreases the activity of AgRP/NPY neurons and consequently suppresses appetite and food intake in rodent species (Murphy & Bloom 2006).

Very little information is available regarding the neuroendocrine control of energy balance in horses, although some data has emerged in recent years with respect to the hormones known to contribute to the control of appetite and energy homeostasis in other animals (e.g., leptin, adiponectin and ghrelin). The following sections briefly describe the functions of these key hormones and summarize the available equine data. Earlier work that investigated the effect of nutrient signals on feeding behavior in horses is also discussed. A more complete discussion on the more general factors affecting feed intake is presented in Chapter 3.

Leptin

Leptin is an adipocyte-derived hormone product of the *ob* gene that provides information to the brain (arcuate nucleus of the hypothalamus) regarding the availability of body fat stores, promoting satiety and reduction in food intake when energy balance is positive or fat stores are plentiful (Spiegelman & Flier 2001). Both AgRP/NPY and POMC neurons in the arcuate nucleus express leptin and insulin receptors, and the direct administration of either hormone into the brain of rodents reduces food intake (Schwartz et al 2000). The appetite suppressant effect of leptin is in part mediated by an increased expression of melanocortins, such as α-MSH, that induce satiety (see below). Leptin stimulates metabolism and energy expenditure by several mechanisms; it activates the sympathetic system in brown adipose tissue and increases the expression of uncoupling protein-1 and uncoupling protein-3 in skeletal muscle (Giacobino, 2002). Leptin also stimulates triglyceride and fatty acid metabolism by increasing lipolysis and fatty acid oxidation.

Leptin is secreted by adipocytes in proportion to their fat content, and therefore is an important signal to the brain

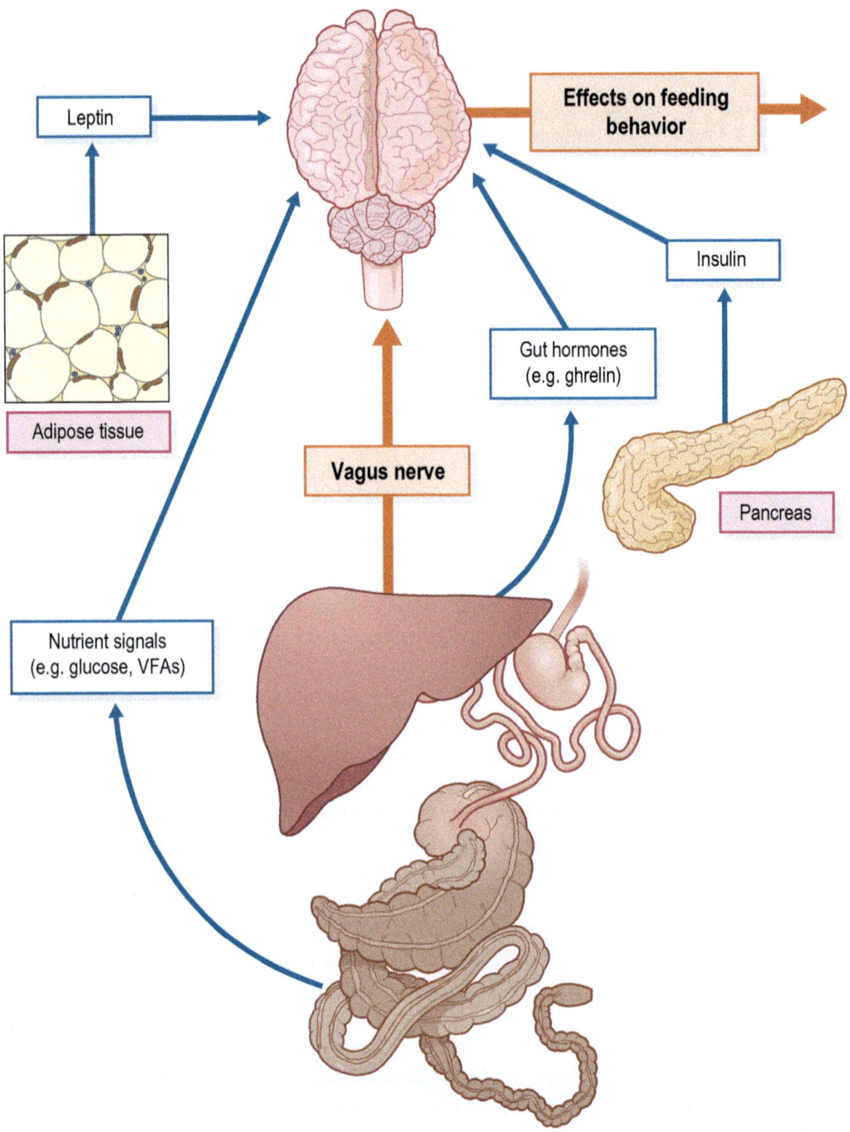

Figure 2.1 A general overview of the factors involved in the regulation of appetite and energy balance in humans and other mammals. VFAs = volatile fatty acids

regarding long-term energy stores. This importance is highlighted by the profound obesity that develops in animals with deletion of either the leptin protein or its receptor (Morton et al 2003). Increased fat stores and the resulting increased leptin secretion suppress appetite and increase metabolism (Schwartz et al 2000) but this feedback mechanism may fail beyond a certain level of adiposity. Indeed, obesity is associated with a marked increase in circulating leptin suggesting the development of leptin resistance (Considine et al 1996).

Studies in horses have shown a positive association between circulating leptin concentrations and BCS (Buff et al 2002, Carter et al 2009). Some studies, however, have shown a wide range of serum/plasma leptin concentrations in horses with similar apparent adiposity (Gentry et al 2002), suggesting that factors other than adipose tissue mass affect leptin production and secretion. Higher plasma leptin concentrations were reported in fed horses compared with fasted horses, with higher values in the afternoon than the morning being found only in the fed horses (Buff et al 2006). Plasma leptin concentration decreases in response to short-term feed restriction (McManus & Fitzgerald 2000, Van Weyenberg et al 2008) and increases following meal feeding (Cartmill et al 2005). The insulin increase associated with meal feeding appears to drive the postprandial increase in plasma leptin (Cartmill et al 2005). Dexamethasone administration has also been shown to be a potent stimulator of leptin secretion in horses, whereas physiological elevation of cortisol concentrations following adrenocorticotropic hormone (ACTH) administration produced only minor increases in leptin (Cartmill et al 2005). Leptin has seasonal variations in young and old mares, with plasma leptin levels increasing in the summer and decreasing in the winter, in correlation with body weight and fat mass (McManus & Fitzgerald 2000). Taken together, these observations suggest that leptin contributes to energy homeostasis in horses but its role in appetite regulation remains to be determined.

Insulin and glucose

Insulin crosses the blood–brain barrier and its receptors are found throughout the brain, with high concentrations observed in the arcuate nucleus of rodents (Bruning et al 2000). The intraventricular administration of insulin decreases feed intake in rats, partly due to an associated decrease in hypothalamic NPY and an increase in POMC expression (Sisley & Sandoval 2011). Glucose sensing in the brain also contributes to the regulation of feed intake, although the weight of evidence suggests that glucose availability is permissive to anorectic signals rather than glucose *per se* playing a primary role (Sisley & Sandoval, 2011). Ralston and Baile (1982a,b) investigated the effects of oral and intravenous glucose loads on feeding behavior in ponies. The intragastric administration of glucose (300 g) delayed the onset of feeding by ~113 min, with normal feeding behavior evident once the glucose-treated animals started to eat. This glucose effect on feeding was dose-related, with a shorter delay (latency) until the onset of feeding being observed after administration of 100 or 200 g glucose (Ralston & Baile, 1982b). On the other hand, IV glucose loads (0.2 or 1.0 g/kg BW) that induced marked hyperglycemia and hyperinsulinemia did not delay the onset of feeding but tended to prolong the interval between the first and second meal, suggesting an effect on satiety (Ralston & Baile 1982a). Further research is needed to clarify the effect of glucose and insulin signals on feeding behavior in horses.

Other nutrient signals

Ralston and Baile (1983) also compared the effects of intragastric corn oil (133 g) or mineral oil (133 g) on feeding behavior in ponies. Corn oil did not alter the onset of feeding or the size or duration of the first meal relative to control values. However, as observed with IV glucose administration, corn oil prolonged the first inter-meal interval and feed intake between 3 and 18 h post oil administration was 50% lower relative to the mineral oil (control) treatment (Ralston & Baile 1983). The mechanism(s) of this response was not investigated although in other species it is recognized that increased long-chain free fatty acids suppress food intake (at least in healthy, nonobese individuals) (Sisley & Sandoval 2011).

In ruminants, the infusion of volatile fatty acids (VFAs) into the rumen depresses feed intake. With the exception of propionate, however, this outcome seems to be due to the resultant increase in osmolality of rumen constituents vs. signaling by VFAs to central nervous system appetite centers because the injection of local anesthetics into the rumen eliminates the effects of acetate and butyrate infusions on feed intake (Faverdin 1999). In humans too, there is some evidence that propionate mediates satiety (Arora et al 2011). One study in ponies demonstrated that the intracecal infusion of 0.4 mmol propionate/kg BW increased feed intake by 7.5% relative to control values, while acetate (1.0 and 1.25 mmol/kg BW) and higher doses of propionate (0.75 mmol/kg BW) decreased feed intake by substantially prolonging the first inter-meal interval (Ralston et al 1983). Ralston and colleagues suggested that oropharyngeal stimuli have a dominant role in the short-term control of feed intake of ponies, whereas nutrient cues (e.g., glucose, VFAs) may be important in the regulation of meal frequency and long-term energy balance.

Ghrelin

Ghrelin is secreted by the hypothalamus and, in particular, P/D1 cells of the stomach. In humans, plasma ghrelin concentrations increase during the preprandial period and the magnitude of the increase is correlated with hunger scores (Cummings et al 2004). Intravenous infusion of ghrelin induces hunger and food intake in people (Korner et al 2009). For this reason, ghrelin is sometimes referred to as the "hunger hormone". In addition, to its orexigenic effect in humans, ghrelin stimulates gastrointestinal motility, gastric acid secretion and pancreatic exocrine secretion, all of which increase in anticipation of meals (Delzenne et al 2010). In horses, plasma ghrelin decreases in response to oral and intravenous glucose administration (Gordon & McKeever 2006). Feed intake and plasma ghrelin concentrations were higher in horses subjected to interval exercise vs. the control (no exercise) condition (Gordon et al 2006). These observations suggest that plasma ghrelin responds to nutritional signals and may play a role in appetite regulation in horses.

Melanocortins

The appetite suppressant effect of leptin is in part mediated by increased expression of melanocortin peptides, such as α-MSH and ACTH. In rats, under physiological conditions, there is evidence that both α-MSH and ACTH inhibit food intake by signaling through melanocortin-4 receptors that are located in several areas of the hypothalamus (Schulz et al 2010). Horses, similar to other species including sheep, demonstrate a seasonal rhythm in circulating concentrations of α-MSH and ACTH, with higher concentrations in the fall (autumn) than in winter and spring (Lincoln et al 2001, McFarlane et al 2011). In nondomesticated horses adapted to temperate climates, there are several other physiological adaptations that are entrained to photoperiod, including a decrease in appetite and metabolic rate as winter approaches (Fuller et al 2001). It is possible that the increases in α-MSH and ACTH contribute to this decrease in appetite in the fall.

Key Points – Neuroendocrine control of appetite and energy balance

- The central nervous system modulates energy balance by regulating feed intake and energy expenditure in response to hormonal, neuronal and nutrient signals.
- In horses, nutrient cues (e.g. increases in circulating glucose, insulin and volatile fatty acids) may modify aspects of feeding behavior in the short-term.
- The seasonal rhythm in circulating concentrations of α-MSH (melanocyte stimulating hormone) and ACTH (adrenocorticotrophic hormone) may contribute to longer-term regulation of feed intake and energy balance.

Endocrine regulation of metabolism

Hormones of the endocrine pancreas

The endocrine functions of the pancreas are mediated by cells of the islets of Langerhans (Fig. 2.2) that play a central role in systemic fuel homeostasis via secretion of hormones that directly influence the metabolic pathways involved in the uptake, deposition and utilization of fuel substrates. The two most important hormones in this context are insulin (synthesized and secreted by beta-cells) and glucagon (released by alpha-cells); a third major cell type (delta-cells) produces somatostatin, a hormone that suppresses insulin

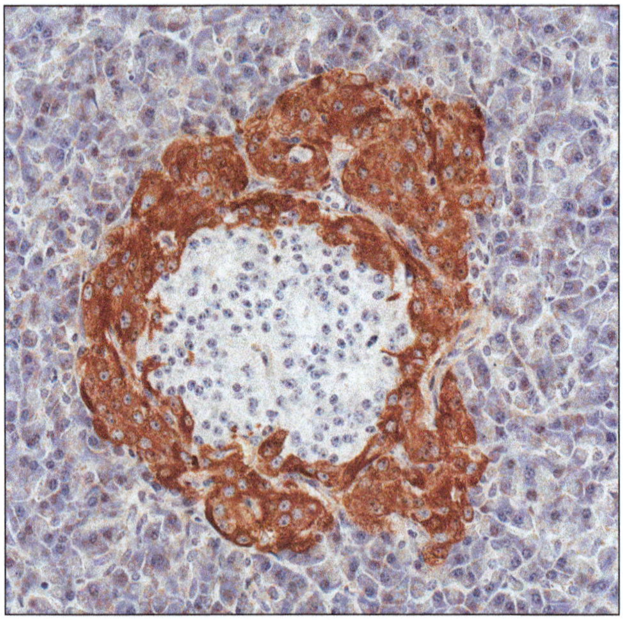

Figure 2.2 Photomicrograph of a section of equine pancreas stained with an anti-insulin antibody and demonstrating an islet of Langerhans. The peripheral distribution of insulin staining indicates that beta-cells are mainly in the periphery of the islet (×20 magnification).

Table 2-1 General Anabolic Effects of Insulin on Carbohydrate, Lipid and Protein Metabolism in Mammalian Species

Carbohydrate metabolism
Increased rate of glucose transport across the cell membrane in muscle cells and adipocytes
Stimulation of glycolysis in muscle and adipose tissue via activation of hexokinase and phosphofructokinase activity
Stimulation of glycogen synthesis in liver, adipose tissue and muscle
Inhibition of glycogenolysis and gluconeogenesis in liver; inhibition of glycogenolysis in muscle
Lipid metabolism
Decrease in the rate of lipolysis in adipose tissue, which results in a decrease in plasma or serum nonesterified fatty acids
Stimulates fatty acid and triacylglycerol synthesis in tissues
Increases the uptake of triglyceride from the blood into adipose tissue and muscle via activation of the enzyme lipoprotein lipase
Decreases the rate of fatty acid oxidation in muscle and liver
Increases cholesterol synthesis and very low density lipoprotein formation in liver
Protein metabolism
Increases the rate of transport of some amino acids (e.g. branched-chain) into tissues
Increases the rate of protein synthesis in muscle, adipose tissue, liver and other tissues
Decreases the rate of protein degradation in muscle
Decreases the rate of urea formation

Schmidt & Hickey 2009, Dimitriadis et al 2011.

secretion, intestinal blood flow and nutrient uptake. Immunohistochemical studies have identified all three cell types in equine pancreatic islets (Furuoka et al 1989).

In general, insulin and glucagon are secreted in a reciprocal manner in response to changes in the plasma concentrations of glucose and other metabolites. Insulin secretion occurs postprandially and favors the uptake of glucose and fatty acids in skeletal muscle, liver and adipose tissue. In the post-absorptive state, insulin secretion is reduced and glucagon secretion is enhanced, which results in stimulation of catabolic processes including the mobilization of glucose and fatty acids (Moore et al 2003). The actions of insulin and glucagon ensure that blood glucose concentrations are maintained within a fairly narrow range.

Insulin

Insulin is a pleiotropic hormone with numerous effects at the cellular, tissue, and whole-body level - indeed, it is now recognized that every organ in the body is a target for insulin action (Wilcox 2005). Insulin is primarily known for its role in carbohydrate metabolism, including the stimulation of glucose uptake and glycogen synthesis in skeletal muscle as well as suppression of glucose production (inhibition of glycogenolysis and gluconeogenesis) from the liver. Other metabolic effects of insulin include stimulation of triglyceride synthesis, inhibition of the release of free fatty acids from adipose tissue, and stimulation of the incorporation of amino acids into proteins (Wilcox 2005) (Table 2-1). Insulin also promotes cell division and growth through its mitogenic effects.

Insulin secretion

Insulin is a dipeptide containing A and B chains linked by disulfide bridges. Synthesis within beta-cells begins with the formation of preproinsulin, which is comprised of a signal peptide, the B chain, the connecting peptide (C-peptide) and the A chain (Wilcox 2005). Removal of the signal peptide in the endoplasmic reticulum forms proinsulin which is transported to the Golgi apparatus and then incorporated into soluble, zinc-containing hexamers (Wilcox 2005). Within secretory granules proteolytic removal of C-peptide from proinsulin yields insulin; this process allows a conformational change in the carboxy terminal of the B-chain of the insulin molecule that facilitates interaction with the insulin receptor (Wahren et al 2000). Insulin and C-peptide are co-secreted in equimolar amounts when mature granules release their contents into the portal circulation (Wilcox 2005). The effects of exogenous somatostatin, glucose infusion and insulin resistance on serum C-peptide concentrations in the horse have been described (Tóth et al 2010). Endogenous C-peptide secretion was markedly suppressed by somatostatin, while the C-peptide-to-insulin ratio decreased during an intravenous glucose tolerance test (300 mg dextrose/kg BW) from 3.60 ± 1.95 before injection to 1.03 ± 0.18 at 20 min after dextrose administration. The latter observation suggests that relative insulin clearance decreases as insulin secretion increases in response to dextrose administration. Median C-peptide and insulin concentrations were 1.5- and 9.5-fold higher, respectively, in insulin resistant horses when compared to healthy control animals (Tóth et al 2010). This perhaps reflects both increased insulin secretion and decreased insulin clearance in insulin resistant animals (Tóth et al 2010). The liver is the primary site of insulin clearance with up to two-thirds of the insulin secreted into the portal vein removed by first-pass hepatic metabolism (Wilcox 2005).

Glucose is the primary stimulus for insulin secretion, although other macronutrients (e.g., amino acids, lipids, and volatile fatty acids), hormones (e.g., glucagon-like peptide-1 [GLP-1] and somatostatin), humoral factors and neural input may modify the insulin secretory response (Pørksen et al 2002, Wilcox 2005 - see Table 2-2). In horses, a linear relationship between intravenous (IV) glucose dose and apparent insulin secretory response has been observed (Tóth et al 2009; Fig. 2.3). In humans and rats, a biphasic pattern to insulin secretion is observed in response to a sustained increase in plasma glucose concentration. There is a rapid increase in secretion that lasts only a few minutes and results in a well-defined peak in insulin concentrations, followed by a nadir and then a longer secondary phase of increased secretion that requires the augmenting action of glucose (Henquin et al 2002, Seino et al 2011). The first phase of secretion reflects rapid release of insulin from granules close to the cell membrane of beta-cells (*readily releasable pool*), while mobilization of the *reserve pool* of granules as well as newly synthesized insulin accounts for the second phase (Seino et al 2011). Some (Giraudet et al 1994, Tóth et al 2009) but not all (Dühlmeier et al 2001) studies in horses have reported that insulin secretion appears to occur as a single phase rather than as a biphasic response.

Pancreatic beta-cells are responsive to amino acids, including arginine, leucine and alanine (Wilcox 2005). The insulinotropic effect of arginine involves direct depolarization of the beta-cell plasma membrane (Sener et al 2000), whereas leucine-induced insulin secretion involves allosteric activation of glutamate dehydrogenase and an increase in adenosine triphosphate (ATP) production that leads to membrane depolarization (Heissig et al 2005). Arginine administration induces an insulin secretory response in fetal and neonatal foals (Fowden et al 2012) as well as mature horses (Sticker et al 2001). Leucine potentiates the insulin response to oral glucose administration in horses (Urschel et al 2010, Bröjer et al 2012). Both at rest and after a 60 min bout of exercise, the coadministration of glucose (1 g/kg BW) and leucine (0.3 g/kg BW) resulted in a greater than twofold increase in the area under the plasma insulin

Table 2-2 Nutrient, Hormonal and Neural Mediators of Insulin Secretion in Mammals

Stimulus	Nutrient	Hormone	Neural
Stimulatory	Glucose* Amino acids (arginine, leucine)*	Growth hormone Glucagon GLP-1 GIP Secretin Cholecystokinin Gastrin VIP Gastrin releasing peptide	β-adrenergic Vagal (parasympathetic)
Inhibitory		Glucocorticosteroids Somatostatin* Epinephrine Norepinephrine Galanin Neuropeptide Y Calcitonin gene-related peptide Prostaglandin E	α-adrenergic

Asterisk indicates that direct evidence exists in horses.
GLP-1, glucagon-like peptide-1; GIP, glucose-dependent insulinotropic polypeptide; VIP, vasoactive intestinal peptide.

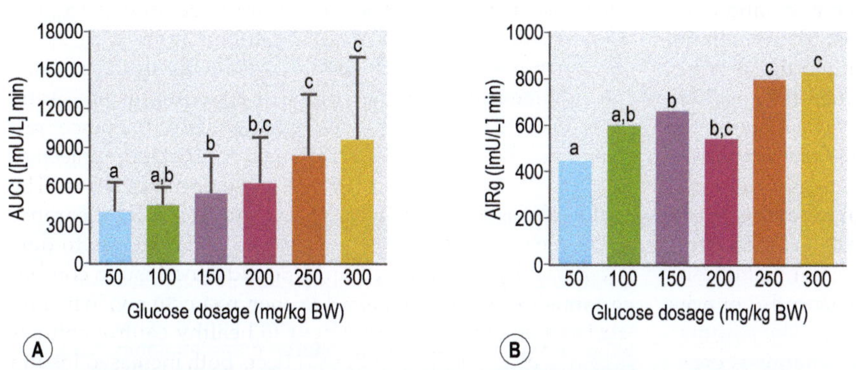

Figure 2.3 Serum insulin responses in 6 mixed-breed mares (aged 6–13 years) in response to 6 different dextrose dosages administered IV. **A)** Values (mean ± s.d.) for the area under the insulin vs. time curve (AUCi). **B)** Median values for the acute insulin response to glucose (AIRg), which is the area under the insulin curve during the first 10 min after dextrose injection. Values with different superscript letters differ significantly ($P < 0.05$).
Data taken from Tóth, F., Frank, N., Elliott, S.B., et al. 2009. Optimisation of the frequently sampled intravenous glucose tolerance test to reduce urinary glucose spilling in horses. Equine Veterinary Journal 41, 844–851.

response curve when compared to the administration of glucose (1 g/kg BW) alone (Urschel et al 2010). The addition of lower amounts of leucine (0.05, 0.1 or 0.2 g/kg BW) to a base feed, however, did not alter insulinemic responses in Quarter Horse yearlings (Etz et al 2011). Neither aspartic or glutamic acid nor *N*-methyl-D,L-aspartate affected insulin secretion in mature horses (Sticker et al 2001). The IV administration of butyrate but not acetate or propionate (all at 3.5 mmol/kg BW) elicited a modest insulin response in ponies (Argenzio & Hintz 1971); these responses are different to those reported for ruminants where IV propionate, butyrate and valerate are more potent stimulators of insulin secretion than glucose (Horino et al 1968).

The presence of nutrients in the gastrointestinal tract stimulates the secretion of hormones that augment glucose-induced insulin secretion (Kazakos 2011). In humans, it is well recognized that an oral glucose load results in a greater insulin response than that of an isoglycemic intravenous glucose infusion; this response is known as the *incretin effect* (Kazakos 2011, Irwin & Prentice 2011). This difference in insulin response is primarily attributed to the gastrointestinal peptides glucose-dependent insulinotropic polypeptide (GIP) and glucagon-like peptide-1 (GLP-1) – the so-called *incretin hormones*. In humans and other monogastric species, GIP is synthesized in enteroendocrine K cells in the proximal small intestine, whereas GLP-1 is synthesized in enteroendocrine L cells in the distal ileum and colon (Irwin & Prentice 2011). As much as two-thirds of the insulin secreted in response to meal ingestion in humans is due to the insulinotropic action of GIP and GLP-1 (Kazakos 2011). The extent to which these hormones contribute to insulin secretion in response to glucose administration or feed ingestion in horses is not known. Active GLP-1 concentrations have been measured in horses, with no change observed after weight gain in animals with histories of obesity and insulin resistance (Chameroy et al 2011). Dühlmeier et al (2001) observed a significant increase in plasma immunoreactive GIP in ponies and horses in response to oral but not IV glucose administration. These authors also reported a greater insulin response after oral when compared to IV glucose administration but an incretin effect could not be confirmed due to a fivefold difference in glucose dose (oral > IV; Dühlmeier et al 2001).

Age and physiologic state affect insulin secretory responses in horses. Several studies have characterized beta-cell function in foals during fetal development and the 10-day period postpartum (Forhead et al 2004, Fowden et al 2005, Holdstock et al 2004, 2012). Glucose administration had no effect on fetal insulin secretion between 175 and 230 days of gestation. However, insulin secretory responses to glucose increased in magnitude between 260 and 300 days of gestation, with a further increment in response late in gestation that coincided with the prepartum rise in circulating cortisol concentrations (Fowden et al 2005). Two hours after birth, the insulin response to glucose administration was low when compared to late gestation or days 5–7 of age (Holdstock et al 2004, Fowden et al 2005, 2012). The authors hypothesized that elevated circulating catecholamines contributed to the suppressed insulin secretory response at 2 h of age (Fowden et al 2012). Overall, pancreatic beta-cell response to glucose or arginine is little changed between days 2 and 10 postpartum (Holdstock et al 2004). However, the induction of parturition 24–48 h before full term as well as adverse conditions in utero results in an apparent increase in beta-cell sensitivity to glucose (Forhead et al 2004, Holdstock et al 2012). Induced foals had a 2–3-fold higher beta-cell response to exogenous glucose and arginine when compared to spontaneously delivered foals; these responses in the induced foals were associated with hypercortisolemia and the authors speculated that the increased insulin secretion may have been due to a cortisol-induced insulin resistance (Holdstock et al 2012). Neonatal pony foals that were overgrown in utero by transfer of pony embryos into Thoroughbred mares also demonstrated an increased beta-cell response to glucose (Forhead et al 2004), perhaps due to enhanced beta-cell growth during fetal development (Allen et al 2002).

Further alterations in pancreatic beta-cell response during preweaning foal development have been less well studied. Smyth et al (1993) reported higher post-feeding serum insulin concentrations in 3-month-old Arabian and Thoroughbred foals when compared to responses measured at 1 day, 1 week and 1 month of age. However, interpretation of these responses was confounded by differences in meal composition. In addition, the extent to which changes in insulin response reflected actual changes in beta-cell response vs. a compensatory response to decreased tissue insulin sensitivity was not determined. In this context, George et al (2009) reported a substantial decrease in insulin sensitivity in Thoroughbred foals between 5 and 160 days of age (George et al 2009; Fig. 2.4).

An upregulation of beta-cell function has been reported during pregnancy in humans and rodents (Sorenson & Brelje 1997) and similar changes have been proposed to occur during pregnancy in mares although specific measures are lacking (Fowden et al 1980). George et al (2011) observed higher acute insulin response to glucose (AIRg) but also lower insulin sensitivity (SI) in pregnant when compared to non-pregnant Thoroughbred mares. Therefore, the higher apparent insulin secretory response could, at least in

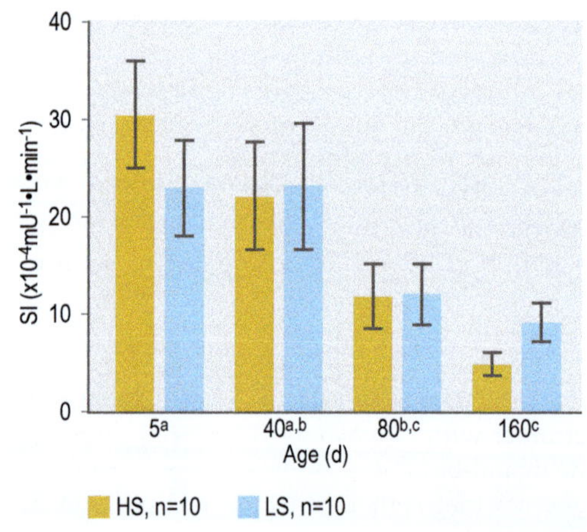

Figure 2.4 Minimal model insulin sensitivity (SI) derived from a frequently sampled intravenous glucose tolerance test performed in 20 Thoroughbred foals at 5, 40, 80 and 160 days of age. Foals were born to mares supplemented with either a high (HS) or low (LS) starch complementary feed. Different superscripts among the x-axis labels indicate significant differences ($P < 0.05$) between ages from repeated measures ANOVA.

Data redrawn with permission from George, L.A., Staniar, W.B., Treiber, K.H., et al. 2009. Insulin sensitivity and glucose dynamics during pre-weaning foal development and in response to maternal diet composition. Domestic Animal Endocrinology 37, 23–29.

part, have been compensation for reduced tissue insulin sensitivity.

In humans, glucose tolerance progressively declines with age due to decreases both in tissue insulin sensitivity and beta-cell responsiveness (Chang & Halter 2003). In horses, insulin response to oral or IV glucose administration was higher in old (mean age 27 years) when compared to middle-aged (15 years) and young (7 years) Standardbred mares (Malinowski et al 2002); however, it could not be determined whether this greater insulin response was due to increased insulin secretion, decreased insulin clearance, or both.

Insulin secretion is suppressed during exercise (Wasserman et al 1995). In horses, a decrease in serum insulin concentration was observed at exercise intensities greater than 50% of maximum aerobic capacity (VO_{2max}; McKeever 2002). There is a reciprocal increase in serum glucagon concentration and the rise in glucagon and fall in insulin, in part, mediate the increase in hepatic glycogenolysis during exercise. Exercise-induced increases in sympathetic drive and catecholamine release are thought to contribute to changes in insulin and glucagon secretion in the horse (Geor et al 2000a,b).

Insulin responses to feed deprivation and feeding

Consistent with observations in other species, feed withholding or restriction in horses results in a number of changes in plasma metabolite and hormone concentrations that reflect a shift to catabolic metabolism, including reduced insulin concentrations (Sticker et al 1995, 1996; also see Chapter 29). Several studies in horses have reported serum or plasma insulin responses to feeding (for example, Vervuert et al 2009a,b, Borgia et al 2011). However, it must be emphasized that to date few (if any) of these studies have employed specific measures of insulin secretory response, making it difficult to determine the relative contribution of insulin secretion vs. tissue insulin sensitivity to the overall insulin response. In general, the pattern of insulin secretion will depend on the relative proportions of various nutrients, the physical form of the feed, and the effects of several factors that may influence nutrient absorption and the stimulation of insulin release (e.g. rate of gastric emptying, intestinal motility, release of incretin hormones and neural input). See Chapter 8 as well as a subsequent section in this chapter (*Overview of Macronutrient Metabolism*) for further discussion on glycemic and insulinemic responses to feeding.

Mechanisms of insulin action

Insulin mediates its actions by binding to the insulin receptor, a heterotetramer with two extracellular alpha subunits that contain the ligand-binding domain and two transmembrane beta subunits that contain intrinsic tyrosine kinase activity. The insulin receptor has substantial structural homology with the insulin-like growth factor-1 receptor, which is also a member of the receptor tyrosine kinase super family (Nakae et al 2001). The binding of insulin to its receptor initiates a cascade of signaling events that result in mediation of insulin's metabolic, vascular and mitogenic effects (Fig. 2.5, also see *Storage of Energy Substrates in Skeletal Muscle and Adipose Tissue*). These signaling events have been characterized primarily in rodent and human skeletal muscle with very little investigation in horse tissue. The insulin

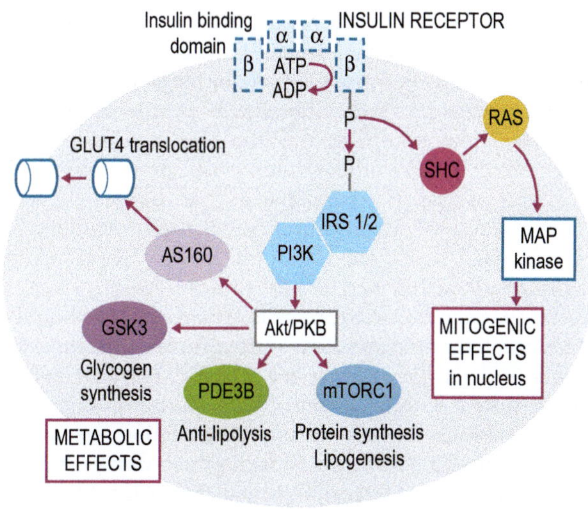

Figure 2.5 Highly simplified schematic of the insulin signaling pathways that mediate insulin's metabolic and mitogenic effects. Selected components have been partially characterized in equine skeletal muscle and adipose tissue – see text [AKT/PKB, protein kinase B; AS160, Akt substrate of 160 kDa; GSK3, glycogen synthase kinase 3; IRS1/2, insulin receptor substrate 1/2; MAP kinase; mitogen-activated protein kinase; MTORC1, mammalian target of rapamycin complex 1/2; PDE3B, phosphodiesterase 3B; PI3K, phosphatidylinositol 3-kinase; RAS, rat sarcoma GTPase protein subfamily; SHC, Src-homology-2-containing protein].

receptor has been detected in skeletal muscle as well as adipose and vascular tissues of the horse by use of Western immunoblot, PCR and immunohistochemical techniques (Annandale et al 2004, Asplin et al 2011, Burns et al 2011). In addition, at least three glucose transport proteins have been recognized in skeletal muscle and adipose tissue (GLUT1, GLUT4, GLUT12) and the effects of exercise and insulin stimulation on the phosphorylation of selected components of the insulin signaling cascade (e.g. Akt, glycogen synthase kinase-3, AS160) have been assessed in these tissues (McCutcheon et al 2006, Waller et al 2011a,b).

Key Points – Insulin

- As an anabolic hormone, insulin stimulates the tissue uptake and storage of glucose, fatty acids and amino acids.
- As in other mammals, glucose is the primary stimulus for insulin secretion in the horse. The amino acids arginine and leucine also stimulate insulin secretion but, unlike ruminants, an increase in circulating volatile fatty acids does not elicit a major secretory response.
- The *incretin effect*, wherein an oral glucose load results in a greater insulin response compared to an isoglycemic IV glucose infusion, is mediated by the gastrointestinal peptides glucose-dependent insulinotropic polypeptide (GIP) and glucagon-like peptide-1 (GLP-1).
- Insulin secretory responses in horses are affected by age and physiologic state (including pregnancy and exercise).

Glucagon

Glucagon is a primary regulator of hepatic glucose production; in the liver a rise in circulating glucagon results in increased glycogenolysis and decreased glucose uptake, the net result being an increase in hepatic glucose output (Ramnanam et al 2011). Glucagon secretion is regulated by glucose – hypoglycemia and hyperglycemia increase and decrease, respectively, hormone release from pancreatic alpha-cells. The glucagon action to stimulate hepatic glucose output is a critical component of the counter-regulatory response to hypoglycemia. Glucagon also protects against a fall in blood glucose during exercise. The exercise-induced increase in the uptake of blood-borne glucose (primarily by contracting muscle) is accompanied by an increase in both hepatic glycogenolysis and gluconeogenesis, mediated in part by a rise in glucagon and a fall in circulating insulin (Wasserman et al 1989).

In comparison to insulin, there is little information on the dynamics of glucagon secretion and action in the horse, with the bulk of available data coming from studies in fetal and neonatal foals (see Fowden et al 2012). Glucagon concentrations in fetal foals increase during late gestation, reaching a peak at birth and then decline during a 10-day post natal period (Fowden et al 2012, Holdstock et al 2012). Moderate fluctuations in blood glucose concentration do not appear to influence circulating glucagon concentrations in neonatal foals. The IV administration of arginine induces an increase in plasma glucagon in fetal and neonatal foals, with higher secretory responses being reported in foals induced to deliver 24–48 h before term, compared to foals born spontaneously (Holdstock et al 2012). The glucagon response to arginine administration increases during the 10-day period postpartum. It has been suggested that glucagon functions as a stress hormone in the perinatal period, with a primary role in stimulation of gluconeogenesis (Fowden et al 2012).

An increase in circulating glucagon has been observed in horses during and after exercise, the magnitude of which is proportional to exercise intensity (Hall et al 1982, Geor et al 2000a, 2002). The induction of β-blockade (propranolol, 0.22 mg/kg BW IV) suppressed the exercise-associated rise in plasma glucagon concentrations in horses (Geor et al 2000a), suggesting the involvement of sympathetic mechanisms in glucagon secretion during exercise. Exercise training was associated with a decrease in the plasma glucagon response to exercise performed at the same absolute workload before and after 6 weeks of conditioning (Geor et al 2002).

Other pancreatic hormones

Several other pancreatic hormones may contribute to the regulation of energy metabolism, including pancreatic polypeptide and somatostatin. There are no published data on concentrations of somatostatin in horses. However, consistent with its well known effect on pancreatic function in other species, recent studies in the horse have demonstrated suppression of insulin secretion in response to the administration of synthetic somatostatin (Tóth et al 2010, Geor et al 2010).

Adrenal hormones

The adrenal glands have two different structures: the medulla and the cortex. The adrenal medulla is a specialized part of the sympathetic nervous system that secretes catecholamines (epinephrine, norepinephrine). The adrenal cortex contains three zones: the zona glomerulosa, which produces mineralocorticoids (aldosterone); the zona fasciculata, which produces glucocorticoids (cortisol); and the zona reticularis, which synthesizes gonadocorticoids (androgens, estrogens).

Catecholamines

The catecholamines play a major role in the regulation of cardiovascular function and carbohydrate/fat metabolism, especially during "flight and fright" responses (stressful stimuli) as well as during exercise. In these circumstances, there is local release of norepinephrine from sympathetic nerve endings and systemic release of epinephrine and norepinephrine from the adrenal medulla. There are two groups of catecholamine (adrenergic) receptors: α- and β-adrenergic receptors, which are further divided into α1-, α2-, β1- and β2-adrenergic receptors. In horses, most information on the dynamics of plasma catecholamines has come from exercise studies. At low-to-moderate intensity exercise (<50–60% of VO_{2max}), there is minimal change in plasma catecholamine concentrations when compared to resting values. At higher exercise intensities, however, there is a curvilinear increase in catecholamines that is correlated with the change in plasma lactate concentrations (Gonzalez et al 1998; Nagata et al 1999).

Norepinephrine and epinephrine stimulate the mobilization of lipid and glucose stores. In adipose tissue, the catecholamines increase the activity of hormone sensitive lipase thereby stimulating lipolysis. Adrenergic control of lipolysis in adipocytes from subcutaneous adipose tissue of horses and ponies is dependent upon differential activation of β2-subtype (stimulatory) and α2-subtype (inhibitory) adrenergic receptors (Carrington et al 2003). In rats and ruminants, there is considerable variation in the lipolytic response to catecholamines between adipocytes from different fat depots (McNamara 1991, McNamara & Murray 2001); however, there have been no published equine studies on this aspect. Neither lipolytic responses to β-adrenergic agonists nor the expression of β2-adrenergic receptor mRNA was altered by early lactation in ponies (Carrington et al 2003), whereas lipolytic sensitivity is increased in the adipose tissue of cows during early lactation (McNamara 1991). The administration of the β-adrenergic antagonist propranolol (0.22 mg/kg BW IV) suppressed plasma non-esterified fatty acids (NEFA) concentrations at rest and during graded exercise in horses (Geor et al 2000a). Conversely, the administration of epinephrine resulted in a marked increase in plasma NEFA (Geor et al 2000b). Taken together, these data confirm the role of β-adrenergic mechanisms in lipolysis and systemic supply of NEFA in the horse (see Chapter 30 for further discussion on mechanisms controlling lipid mobilization).

Epinephrine participates in the regulation of glucose uptake into muscle as well as glycogenolysis in muscle, especially during exercise. Exogenous administration of epinephrine markedly decreases whole-body glucose disposal during exercise in man (Watts & Hargreaves 2002) and horses (Geor et al 2000b), suggesting that adrenergic stimulation impairs glucose uptake into muscle. Epinephrine also stimulates glycogenolysis in muscle (Geor et al 2000b) although studies in adrenalectomized human subjects have shown that glycogenolysis can occur in the absence of epinephrine (Kjaer et al 2000). In dog and man, epinephrine does not appear to mediate the increase in hepatic glucose production during low and moderate intensity exercise but may contribute during prolonged or heavy exercise when circulating epinephrine is very high (Wasserman 1995). The effect of epinephrine on hepatic glucose output in horses is not known.

Glucocorticoids

Cortisol is the major glucocorticoid secreted by the adrenal glands although smaller quantities of cortisone, corticosterone and deoxycorticosterone are produced. Cortisol secretion in horses shows a diurnal pattern with lowest values at night and highest values in the morning (6:00–10:00 a.m.; Thornton 1985). There is no published research on the effects of endogenous glucocorticoids on metabolism in horses; however, a number of studies have examined the effects of exogenous glucocorticoids (Freestone et al 1991, French et al 2000, Tiley et al 2007, Haffner et al 2009).

The glucocorticoids are catabolic hormones that stimulate substrate mobilization by enhancing gluconeogenesis, lipolysis and proteolysis. As one of the counter-regulatory hormones, cortisol acts to maintain plasma glucose concentrations by mobilizing substrates for hepatic gluconeogenesis (e.g., glycerol, amino acids) and by decreasing glucose utilization via antagonism of insulin-mediated glucose uptake (McMahon et al 1988). The parenteral administration of glucocorticoids to healthy horses induces moderate hyperglycemia (French et al 2000, Tiley et al 2007) as well as increases in plasma NEFA (French et al 2000) and serum triglyceride concentrations (French et al 2000). Hyperinsulinemia and decreased whole-body insulin sensitivity has been reported after single or repeated administration of glucocorticoids to horses (French et al 2000, Tiley et al 2007, Haffner et al 2009), although in one report the short-term administration of hydrocortisone apparently resulted in an increase in insulin sensitivity (de Graaf-Roelfsema et al 2005).

Somatotropic axis

The somatotropic axis, which consists of somatotropin (growth hormone, GH), insulin-like growth factors (IGF-I and -II) and their associated carrier proteins, plus GH and IGF receptors, plays a key role in the regulation of growth and metabolism. GH is synthesized in the anterior lobe of the pituitary, with its secretion under a dual control by two hypothalamic peptides – the GH releasing hormone (GHRH) which stimulates secretion, and somatostatin which is inhibitory. GH stimulates growth and development in young animals and, in animals of all ages, is regarded as the primary anabolic hormone during stress and fasting (Renaville et al 2002). GH exerts many of its somatotropic actions via IGF-I and IGF-II which are released from target tissues (e.g., liver) in response to GH (Renaville et al 2002). GH is one of the glucose counter-regulatory hormones (along with glucagon, epinephrine, and cortisol), reflecting its role in defending against hypoglycemia.

In general, nutritional status plays a major role in regulating the circulating concentrations of GH, IGF-I and binding proteins, as well as the number of cell membrane receptors. Elevated plasma GH concentrations are observed in growing cattle during prolonged fasting and in dairy cows during the first week of lactation, while GH concentrations are little changed in response to short-term (<24 h) feed restriction (Møller & Jørgensen 2009). In obese pony mares adapted to *ad libitum* feeding, 48-h of feed withholding resulted in increased pulse frequency, pulse amplitude and mean plasma concentrations of GH when compared to mares in the fed state (Buff et al 2007). Refeeding resulted in a rapid decrease in plasma GH concentrations. On the other hand, there was no effect of short-term (24 h) feed removal on GH in horses adapted to meal feeding (DePew et al 1994a, Sticker et al 1995), suggesting that feed deprivation exerts a stronger effect on GH secretion in horses and ponies that are fed *ad libitum*. A study of Welsh Mountain pony mares during winter and spring over 3 consecutive years examined the effects of longer term nutritional status on plasma GH and IGF-1 concentrations (Salazar-Ortiz et al 2011). Feed restriction (50% of energy requirements) or feeding management that mimicked the seasonal availability of pasture resulted in elevated GH when compared to the "well-fed" treatment, whereas plasma IGF-I was higher in the well-fed when compared to feed restricted groups. In this study, there was no correlation between plasma IGF-1 and GH concentrations but a significant correlation between IGF-1 and insulin was observed, raising the possibility that insulin stimulates IGF-1 secretion in the horse (Salazar-Ortiz et al 2011).

In other mammals, the most prominent metabolic effect of GH is a marked increase in lipolysis and fat oxidation (Renaville et al 2002). Thus, during prolonged feed withholding and other catabolic states, GH stimulates the release and oxidation of FFA which enables a reduction in glucose and amino acid oxidation and the preservation of glycogen reserves as well as lean body mass. The impact of GH on preservation of lean body mass in catabolic states is evidenced by the impact of GH deficiency during fasting, wherein amino acid oxidation, urea production rate, and muscle protein breakdown are all ~50% higher when compared to the values in non-GH deficient animals (Møller & Jørgensen 2009). GH antagonizes the hepatic and peripheral effects of insulin on glucose metabolism via mechanisms involving the concomitant increase in fatty acid flux and oxidation. Indeed, the anti-insulin effect of GH contributes to the relative insulin resistance that develops during fasting and inflammatory states. The administration of recombinant equine GH to healthy horses (20 µg/kg BW for 11 to 15 days) resulted in a significant 22% decrease in insulin sensitivity, as measured during a euglycemic–hyperinsulinemic clamp, when compared to horses treated with saline solution (de Graaf-Roelfsema et al 2005).

Key Points – Glucose counter-regulatory hormones

- Glucagon, the catecholamines (norepinephrine, epinephrine), cortisol, and growth hormone are collectively termed *glucose counter-regulatory hormones* because they oppose insulin action on glucose metabolism. In the face of hypoglycemia, these hormones stimulate hepatic glucose output and decrease glucose uptake into peripheral tissues.
- The catecholamines and, to a lesser extent, cortisol and growth hormone, also stimulate the mobilization and utilization of fatty acids.
- The action of growth hormone on lipid metabolism is critical to the preservation of lean body mass during prolonged feed withholding and other catabolic states.

Thyroid hormones

Thyroid hormone secretion is stimulated by thyroid-stimulating hormone (TSH) from the anterior pituitary gland, which itself is regulated by hypothalamic thyrotropin-releasing hormone (TRH). TSH exerts trophic effects on the thyroid glands including stimulation of follicular cell growth and activity, iodide uptake, and the synthesis of triiodothyronine (T_3) and thyroxine (T_4). The thyroid gland releases a much greater quantity of T_4 than T_3, and the majority of T_3 is derived from deiodination of T_4 in the peripheral tissues by type 1 and type 2 deiodinases, which are selenoproteins (Brehaus 2011). Therefore, T_4 is the major precursor for T_3 which is the more metabolically active of the two hormones. Major actions of the thyroid hormones include the stimulation of basal metabolic rate (oxygen consumption) and heat production, ionotropic and chronotropic effects in the heart, regulation of the expression of β-adrenergic receptors in multiple tissues, and fetal growth (especially brain development and skeletal maturation). The effects of the thyroid hormones on oxygen consumption and heat production are due in part to stimulation of Na^+-K^+-ATPase in most tissues.

Hypothyroidism is apparently rare in horses and few clinical abnormalities have been detected in mature horses subjected to bilateral thyroidectomy (Lowe et al 1974, Frank et al 2003, 2004). Plasma triglycerides, very low-density lipoproteins and low-density lipoproteins were higher in horses following thyroidectomy (Frank et al 1999) but adaptations to a higher fat diet (7.3% crude fat), including increases in post-heparin lipoprotein lipase and hepatic lipase activities, were not affected by thyroidectomy (Frank et al 2004). Decreased resting heart rate, cardiac output, respiratory rate and rectal temperature have also been observed after thyroidectomy, likely reflecting the effect of thyroid hormone deficiency on metabolic rate and β-adrenergic receptor expression (Vischer et al 1999). In young growing horses, however, thyroidectomy resulted in several abnormalities including decreased growth rate, delayed physeal closure, coarse hair coat, and lethargy (Lowe et al 1974). The thyroid hormones are essential for normal organ development and growth and it is therefore not surprising that deficiency results in more obvious clinical problems in foals when compared to mature horses.

Serum thyroid hormone concentrations are two- to threefold higher in neonatal foals when compared to the values in mature animals; concentrations gradually decrease to adult levels over the first 2–3 months of life (Irvine et al 1975, Chen & Riley 1981). Nutritional status, exercise and possibly season also influence serum thyroid hormone concentrations in horses but there is little information regarding mechanisms underlying these variations. Increases in serum T_3 and T_4 are observed with meal feeding in horses (Sticker et al 1996, Powell et al 2000). These responses are blunted in horses fed an energy-restricted diet (Powell et al 2000). However, neither short-term (45 h) feed deprivation (Sticker et al 1995a) nor the feeding of energy or protein restricted diets (50–70% of requirements; Sticker et al 1996, Powell et al 2000) altered basal serum T_4 and T_3 concentrations. In contrast, a rapid decrease in circulating thyroid hormone concentrations has been reported with dietary restriction in rats (Schalch & Cree 1985) and cattle (Blum et al 1985).

In weanling horses, the ingestion of a diet providing 130% of energy and protein requirements was associated with a more rapid and higher magnitude increase in serum T_3 when compared to a diet providing 100% of requirements. Serum T_4 concentrations decreased in response to feeding, and it was suggested that the meal-associated rise in insulin concentration accelerated the conversion of T_4 to T_3 (Glade & Reimers 1985). In a subsequent study, the intragastric administration of sucrose but not casein to weanling horses resulted in an increase in serum T_3 and T_4 concentrations, suggesting that the digestion of soluble carbohydrate (sucrose) but not protein triggers thyroid hormone responses in horses (Glade & Luba, 1987). These authors hypothesized that pronounced thyroid hormone responses to the feeding of high-starch or high-sugar diets to growing horses may increase risk of osteochondrosis and other development orthopedic disorders. However, subsequent studies have not found a link between diet composition, thyroid hormones and incidence of orthopedic problems in growing horses (e.g., Ott et al 2005). Also see Chapter 32.

In Quarter Horse mares maintained under constant energy balance, TSH secretion was greater in summer compared to winter, whereas mean T_4 concentrations were slightly greater in winter than in summer (Buff et al 2007). In contrast, seasonal variation in serum T_4 concentrations was not apparent in a small group of mixed-breed horses maintained under similar management conditions over a 1-year period (Place et al 2010).

In general, serum T_3 and T_4 increase in proportion to the intensity and duration of exercise in horses (Gonzalez et al 1998). In endurance horses, no change or only a transient decrease in plasma free T_4, free T_3, T_3 and T_4 was observed after rides between 40 and 56 km, whereas a more marked decrease was reported with longer rides (160 km; Graves et al 2006).

Overview of macronutrient metabolism

A large number of studies have examined aspects of nutrient metabolism in relation to diet composition, meal size, etc., and a comprehensive review of this literature is beyond the scope of this chapter. It should be recognized that little information is available on the mechanisms regulating nutrient metabolism in the horse. The following discussion provides an overview of macronutrient (carbohydrate, fat and protein) metabolism in relation to feeding state; where appropriate, information from work in other mammalian species is included to highlight important concepts.

Glucose and insulin responses

When horses ingest meals containing starch and/or sugar (e.g., cereal grains or a sweet feed that contains grains and molasses), there are post-feeding increases in blood glucose and insulin concentrations. The magnitude of the glycemic and insulinemic responses will depend on several factors, including size of meal, starch and sugar content, pre-cecal starch digestibility, and the rate of ingestion (Harris & Geor 2009). When starch of high prececal digestibility was provided in a compound feed, at levels between 0.3 g and 2.0 g starch/kg BW, serum glucose concentrations increased to reach a peak between 90 and 120 min post-feeding with a return to baseline concentrations by 4–7 hours. Serum insulin concentrations increased to reach a peak between 90 and 180 min post-feeding and similarly returned to baseline values by 4–7 hours (Vervuert et al 2009a; Fig. 2.6). In general, the magnitude of these responses increased as a

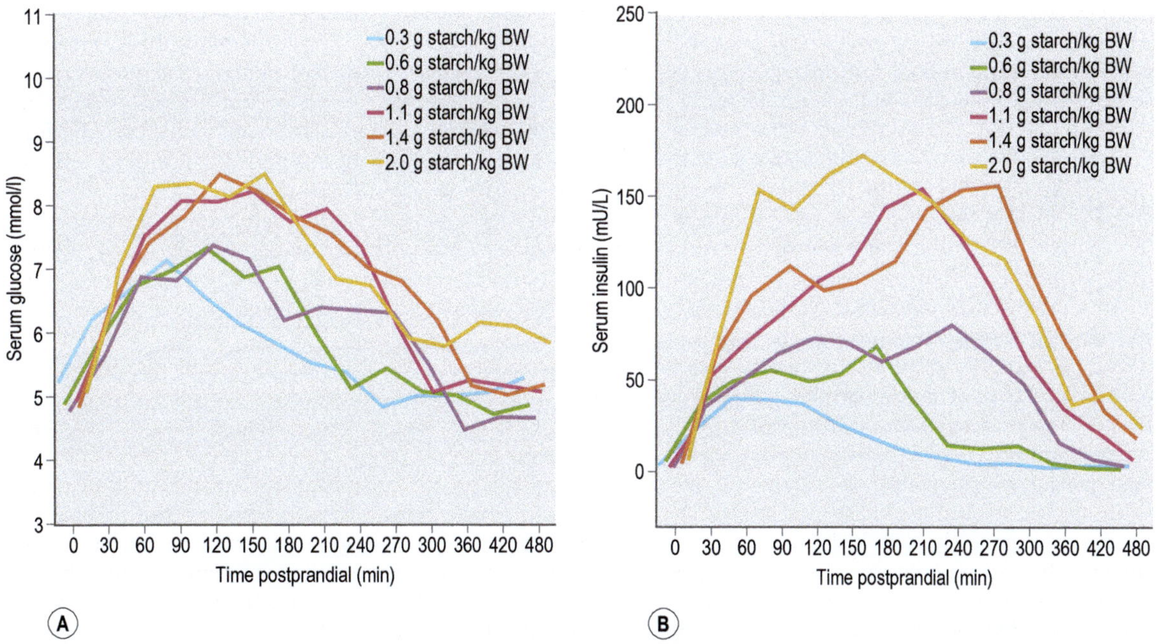

Figure 2.6 Mean serum glucose A) and insulin B) concentrations in four horses fed different amounts of starch in a compound feed. In general, glycemic and insulinemic responses were higher when 1.1–2 g starch/kg BW was fed compared to 0.3–0.8 g starch/kg BW. *From Vervuert, I., Voigt, K., Hollands, T., et al. 2009. Effect of feeding increasing quantities of starch on glycaemic and insulinaemic responses in healthy horses. The Veterinary Journal 182, 67–72. Reprinted with permission.*

function of starch dose but the relationship was not linear. The authors of this study recommended that starch intake be limited to no more than 1.1 g/kg BW (meal size 0.3 kg/100 kg BW when compound feeds and cereals contains 30–40% starch are fed) based on the moderate glycemic (increase from ~5 mmol/l to ~7 mmol/l) and insulinemic (from ~5 to ~50 μU/ml) responses observed at starch intakes below this threshold (Vervuert et al 2009a).

Glycemic and insulinemic responses are much smaller when horses consume roughage (e.g., preserved forage) when compared to grain-based feeds, although moderate increases in serum insulin concentrations have been observed after ingestion of hay with relatively high nonstructural carbohydrate (NSC) content (Borgia et al 2011). In horses fed "high" NSC (17.1% DM) Italian rye (*Lolium multiforum*) hay at 0.5% BW, serum insulin concentration increased from a mean of ~4 μU/ml to a peak of ~50 μU/ml between 60 and 120 min post-feeding, whereas there were minimal changes in serum insulin after ingestion of the same quantity of medium (10.6% NSC) and low (4.4% NSC) NSC content hay (Borgia et al 2011; Fig. 2.7). The results of this study lend support to the recommendation that laminitis-prone horses or ponies be fed hay with NSC content <10–12% to avoid post-feeding increases in circulating insulin concentrations that may increase risk of laminitis episodes. Interestingly, the addition of purified soluble (pectin) or insoluble (lignocelluloses) fiber to a meal of cracked corn did not affect postprandial glucose and insulin responses when compared to a meal of cracked corn alone (each treatment provided a starch intake of 2 g/kg BW; Vervuert et al 2009b). Similarly, the addition of alfalfa (crude fiber intake of 0.5 g/kg BW) before, mixed with, or after a meal of oats (2 g starch/kg BW) did not significantly alter glycemic and insulinemic responses; in this study, breath hydrogen production was lower when alfalfa was fed before or with the oats, perhaps reflecting improved starch hydrolysis in the small intestine along with reduced bacterial fermentation (Vervuert et al 2009c). As well, the addition of short-chop (<2 cm in length) alfalfa (Lucerne) chaff to a sweet meal did not alter glycemic response (Harris et al 2005). These findings contrasted with the results of earlier studies that demonstrated decreased glycemic responses when long fiber hay was fed before or mixed with a starch-based meal (Radicke et al 1994, Pagan & Harris 1999).

Glycemic and insulinemic responses to feeding may be modulated by the effects of meals consumed in the prior few hours. Gordon and McKeever (2005) fed Standardbred mares identical grain-based meals at 0730 and 1530 h, and observed significantly smaller increases in plasma insulin concentrations in response to the afternoon feeding (Fig. 2.8). This "second meal effect", characterized by enhanced glucose tolerance when successive glucose loads are ingested within a relatively short time span, is well described in humans (Wolever et al 1988). The colonic fermentation of indigestible carbohydrates in the first meal is thought to contribute to the second-meal effect in humans via a reduction in circulating NEFA that enhances glucose disposal (Brighenti et al 2006). The differential response between morning and afternoon meals, as reported by Gordon and McKeever (2005), may be in part due to the inhibitory effect of higher morning cortisol concentrations on insulin-mediated glucose utilization.

There is no information in horses on the disposition of the glucose load absorbed as a result of the pre-cecal digestion of starches and simple sugars. In humans and dogs, between one-quarter and one-third of an oral glucose load is taken up by the splanchnic tissues and liver, with about 10% of the glucose load extracted by the liver on first pass and the remainder removed from circulation on subsequent

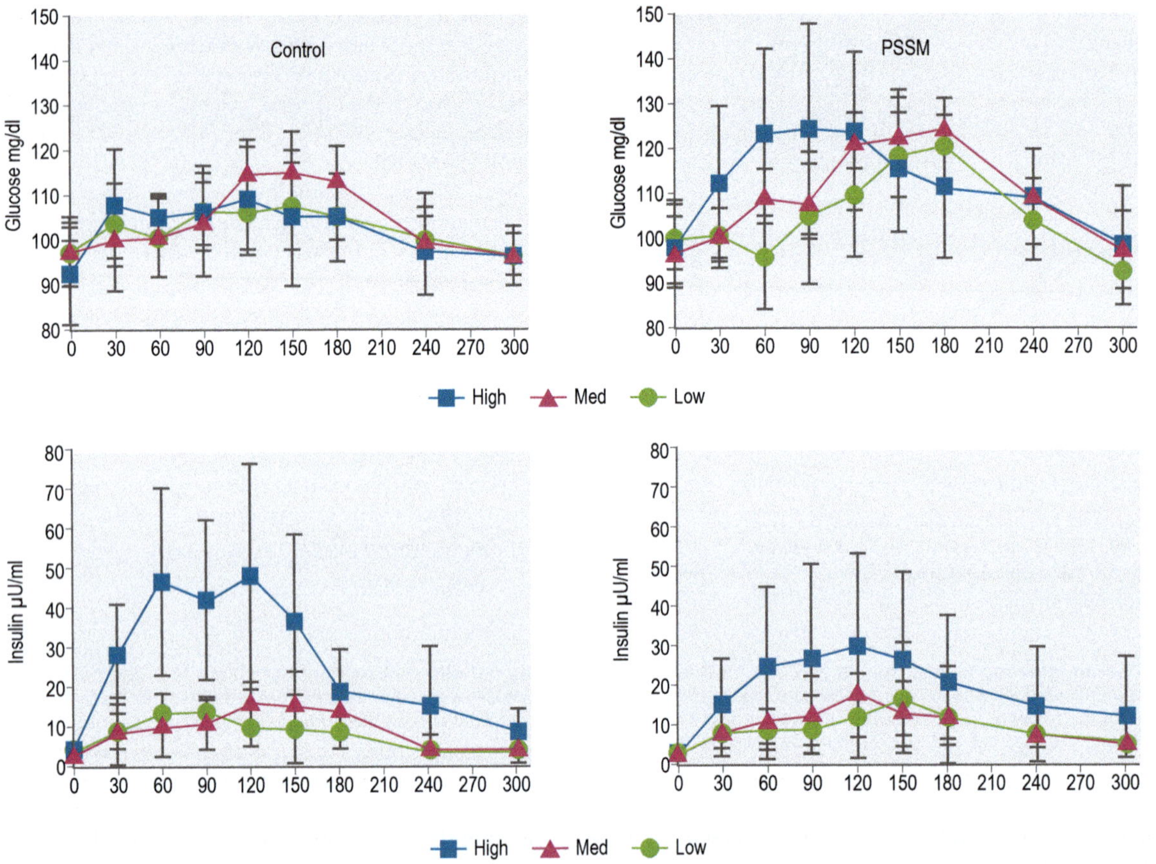

Figure 2.7 Mean ± SD post-prandial glucose and insulin concentrations for polysaccharide storage myopathy-affected and control horses fed high (HC = 17.1% DM; blue square), medium (MC = 10.6% DM, pink triangle) and low (LC = 4.4% DM, green circles) non-structural carbohydrate hay. Insulinemic response for control horses was significantly higher on HC than either MC or LC. Polysaccharide storage myopathy horses had a higher glycemic and lower insulinemic response than control horses on the HC but not the MC or LC hay.

Redrawn with permission from Borgia, et al. 2011. Journal of Animal Physiology and Animal Nutrition 95 (6), 798–807.

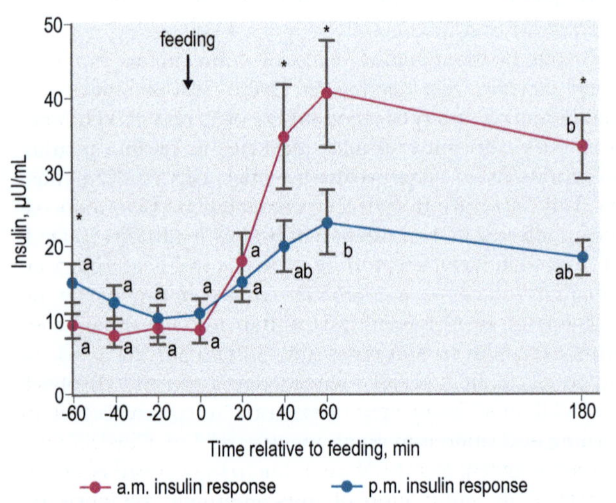

Figure 2.8 Man (± standard error of the mean) plasma insulin concentrations before and after ingestion of grain-based meals in the morning (pink symbols) and in the afternoon (blue symbols). Time 0 = time of feeding. Means within each group that do not have the same letter differ ($P < 0.05$). Asterisks indicate that means differ between a.m. and p.m. samples ($P < 0.05$).

Redrawn with permission from Gordon, M.E., McKeever, K.H., 2005. Diurnal variationof ghrelin, leptin, and adiponectin in Standardbred mares. Journal of Animal Science 83, 2365–2371.

passes (Dardevet et al 2002a). The liver takes up two to three times as much glucose following oral glucose ingestion as compared to uptake under similar hyperglycemic and hyperinsulinemic conditions induced by intravenous glucose infusion (Moore et al 2003). Approximately 35–45% of an oral glucose load is taken up by insulin-sensitive tissues (skeletal muscle and adipose tissue) and the remaining 25–30% is utilized by non-insulin-dependent tissues (e.g., red blood cells, central nervous system; Meyer et al

Key Points – Glucose and insulin responses to meal feeding

- Several factors affect the magnitude of glycemic and insulinemic responses to meal feeding, including meal size, starch and simple sugar content, the prececal digestibility of the starch, and the rate of feed intake.
- The addition of soluble or insoluble fibers to a grain-based meal or the mixing of moderate quantities of short chopped roughage (e.g., chaff) does not substantially alter postprandial glycemic and insulinemic responses.
- Glycemic and insulinemic responses to grain-based meals are lower in the afternoon when compared to the morning. Diurnal variation in cortisol concentrations may contribute to this differential response.

2002, Moore et al 2003; Dardevet et al 2002a). A similar partitioning of glucose disposal occurs after ingestion of a mixed meal in humans (Woerle et al 2003) but as noted above there is no information in the horse. The mechanisms of glucose utilization in insulin-sensitive tissues are discussed below (see Storage of energy substrates in skeletal muscle and adipose tissue).

Amino acid and protein metabolism

Basal (i.e., in the postabsorptive state in meal fed horses) plasma amino acid concentrations change little from day to day in mature horses at maintenance and do not show diurnal variation (Johnson & Hart 1974, Hackl et al 2006). Plasma concentrations also are fairly stable during short-term (≤24 h) feed withholding but increase during longer periods of fasting, likely reflecting catabolism of tissue proteins with utilization of amino acids for ATP synthesis or gluconeogenesis (Johnson & Hart, 1974, Russell et al 1986). Plasma concentrations of free amino acids increase following meal ingestion in horses (Johnson and Hart 1974, Russell et al 1986, Urschel et al 2011). The extent of these increases is dependent on the size and composition of the feed; in general peak concentrations occur 2–5 h post-feeding and then decrease toward basal values over a 4–8 h period (Russell et al 1986). In man and dog, it is well established that the splanchnic tissues extract a substantial proportion of the dietary amino acid load (Ferrannini et al 1988), with 20 to 96% of enterally administered amino acids utilized by the splanchnic bed (Mathews et al 1993). Several of the non-essential (dispensable) amino acids (e.g., glutamate and aspartate) are extensively oxidized by enterocytes of the small intestine with minimal entry of these amino acids into the portal circulation (Wu 2009). In addition, 30–50% of the essential (indispensable) amino acids may be subjected to first pass splanchnic extraction and metabolism (including urea synthesis) within enterocytes (Wu 2009). As a consequence, the nature and extent of postprandial increases in peripheral blood amino acid concentrations will not mirror the amino acid composition of the ingested feed.

After ingestion of low-protein pelleted feed (crude protein 8.1% DM; size of meal not provided) in mixed-breed geldings, concentrations of essential amino acids increased to 132% of basal values at 2 h post-feeding while nonessential amino acids increased to a lesser extent but remained elevated for a longer duration (Johnson & Hart 1974). In contrast, the ingestion of a high-protein feed (33.2% CP; lysine 1.63%; leucine 2.11% DM basis) at ~3.8 g/kg BW (as-fed basis) elicited a more substantial rise in the plasma concentrations of essential and non-essential amino acids; for example, plasma lysine increased from a mean baseline value of 124 μmol/l to 282 μmol/l at 80 min post-feeding while plasma leucine increased from 123 μmol/l to a peak of 188 μmol/l at 40 min post-feeding (Urschel et al 2011). The administration of a single dose of leucine alone (0.3 g/kg BW) resulted in an 8–10-fold increase in plasma leucine concentration and was accompanied by a decrease in all essential amino acids, especially the other branched-chain amino acids isoleucine and valine (Urschel et al 2010). Similarly, in growing Quarter Horses the addition of leucine (0.05, 0.1, or 0.2 g/kg BW) to a morning meal resulted in significant decreases in the plasma concentrations of valine and isoleucine between 120 and 420 minutes post-feeding (Etz et al 2011). In humans, there also is evidence that a marked rise in leucine is associated with decreases in isoleucine and valine concentrations (Eriksson et al 1981), perhaps due to the activation of the enzyme α-keto acid dehydrogenase that increases catabolism of all branched-chain amino acids (Aftring et al 1986).

The amino acid quality of the feed as well as the speed and site of protein digestion are also likely to influence post-feeding plasma amino acid responses. In horses fed a similar amount of CP (~850 g/day) from grass hay only or hay plus grain (HG), the post-feeding increase in the concentrations of several amino acids (e.g. methionine, leucine, isoleucine, and lysine) occurred more quickly and was of greater magnitude in HG when compared to the hay only treatment (Graham-Thiers & Bowen 2011). The authors concluded that the earlier rise in plasma amino acid concentrations in the post-feeding period reflected increased foregut digestibility as well as superior amino acid quality of the HG ration (Graham-Thiers & Bowen 2011).

Protein synthesis

Feeding is associated with an increase in whole-body protein synthesis and a decrease in proteolysis in man and dog (Rennie et al 1982, Volpi et al 1996). This pattern is reversed during the postabsorptive state such that whole-body protein mass remains fairly constant from day to day. These changes in protein metabolism are mediated primarily by feeding-induced increases in plasma concentrations of amino acids and insulin (Dardevet et al 2002a). Although skeletal muscle is a primary site of protein synthesis in the fed state, organs of the splanchnic bed (gut and liver) account for up to 25% of whole-body protein synthesis in humans (Barle et al 1997). Up to 40–50% of the protein synthesized in the liver is exported, much of it as albumin; in humans it has been suggested that the conversion of dietary amino acids to albumin provides a means of storing protein with breakdown of albumin providing essential amino acids for protein synthesis during periods of nutrient deprivation (De Feo & Lucidi 2002).

Within cells, signaling via the mammalian target of rapamycin (mTOR), a serine/threonine protein kinase, is a major mechanism for regulation of protein synthesis (Kimball 2007, Yang et al 2008). In skeletal muscle, signaling via amino acids or insulin causes an increase in mTOR phosphorylation, which in turn increases the phosphorylation of two targets key in the initiation of protein synthesis: eukaryotic initiation factor 4E binding protein 1 (4E-BP1) and ribosomal protein S6 kinase 1 (S6K1). These events result in the initiation of protein synthesis and possibly inhibition of autophagy, which is a major mechanism for the entry of proteins into the lysosome where they undergo hydrolysis (Wu 2009). Insulin phosphorylates mTOR in an Akt (protein kinase B)-dependent manner, whereas amino acids activate mTOR via mechanisms not involving Akt (Kimball 2007). In neonates, the stimulation of muscle protein synthesis by insulin and amino acids is independent (Davis et al 2002), whereas in mature mammals amino acids and insulin interact in promoting postprandial protein synthesis, and both factors appear to be important for maximal activation via mTOR (Bolster et al 2004). Aging in rats and human subjects is associated with a decline in the postprandial anabolic response of skeletal muscle, although supplementation with leucine or a mixture of essential amino acids can restore the muscle protein synthetic response (Dardevet et al 2002b, Timmerman & Volpi 2008).

Researchers are beginning to examine mechanisms that regulate protein synthesis in the skeletal muscle of horses. Urschel et al (2011) examined the effect of refeeding following an 18-h period of feed withholding on the phosphorylation of translation initiation factors in the skeletal muscle of mature Thoroughbred horses. In a crossover design, horses either continued to have feed withheld or were fed 2 g/kg BW of a 33% CP feed at time 0 and 30 min, and a biopsy sample of middle gluteal muscle was taken at 90 min. Plasma glucose, insulin and amino acid concentrations at the time of biopsy were markedly higher in the postprandial when compared to the postabsorptive state, and refeeding resulted in increased phosphorylation of 4E-BP1 and S6K1 in muscle independent of changes in the phosphorylation of Akt at Ser^{473}. These findings suggested that feeding stimulates protein synthesis in skeletal muscle of horses and that the postprandial rise in amino acids is the primary driver of this response (Urschel et al 2011). Stable isotope tracer techniques have also been used to examine the effects of amino acid supplementation on whole-body protein synthesis and breakdown in horses (Urschel et al 2012). In mature Arabian geldings provided a base diet containing the maintenance CP requirement, supplementation with equimolar amounts of glutamate (55 mg/kg BW/day), leucine (49 mg/kg BW/day) or lysine (55 mg/kg BW/day) resulted in increased plasma concentrations of the respective amino acids but did not alter non-oxidative phenylalanine disposal or phenylalanine release from protein breakdown. These findings indicated that leucine or lysine supplementation of horses provided a diet containing adequate CP with an appropriate amino acid profile does not alter net whole-body protein synthesis or breakdown (Urschel et al 2012). Further application of these newer methods will allow researchers to examine the regulation of whole-body and muscle protein synthesis in horses, studying for example the effects of age, diet, feeding strategy, and exercise.

Hepatic nitrogen metabolism

The liver plays a central role in the regulation of nitrogen-containing substrates in relation to body requirements for amino acids and glucose (i.e., use of amino acid precursors in gluconeogenesis) as well as the need to remove excess nitrogen (urea synthesis). There is a number of inter-organ amino acid carbon and nitrogen (N) cycles that shuttle carbon and N from peripheral tissues and portal-drained viscera to the liver for glucose and urea synthesis. The liver efficiently removes ammonia produced by bacterial fermentation within the gastrointestinal tract or from metabolism of amino acids, with the incorporation of N into urea. In ruminants, each of the N atoms of urea is supplied by balanced inputs of mitochondrial ammonia and cytosolic aspartate (Lobley et al 1995). A substantial proportion of N intake is absorbed into the portal vein as ammonia (as high as 65% in ruminants). Ammonia absorption and liver urea synthesis in ruminants are highly correlated with N intake, whereas amino acid absorption into the portal circulation is poorly correlated with urea synthesis (Reynolds & Maltby 1994).

Quantitative data on N handling in the equine liver or splanchnic tissues are not available but there are published data on the effects of diet and feeding state on serum or plasma urea N concentrations, a very crude indicator of amino acid catabolism and urea synthesis. In mares and stallions provided a 14.3% CP (as DM) feed after a 19-h period of feed withholding, there was an approximately 15% increase in urea N concentrations during the first 2 h post feeding (DePew et al 1994ab). The extent to which this rise in urea N reflected increased urea production vs. a feeding-associated decrease in plasma volume could not be determined. Restriction of dietary energy and/or protein impacts serum urea N concentrations. Sticker et al (1995b) fed mares Bermudagrass hay and a corn/cottonseed hull-based feed formulated to provide either 100% (control) or 50% (restricted) of the energy and(or) protein requirements for maintenance. Energy restriction increased urea N concentrations by ~19%, whereas protein restriction was associated with an ~19% reduction in plasma urea N; these effects of energy and protein restriction were evident within 24 h of initiating dietary treatments and were maintained throughout the 4-week dietary period (Sticker et al 1995b). The elevated plasma urea N concentrations during energy restriction likely reflect increased use of protein (amino acids) for ATP synthesis, whereas the reduced plasma urea N during protein restriction can be attributed to conservation of protein and an associated decrease in urea synthesis. The opposite is observed when horses are provided a diet that greatly exceeds CP requirements; horses fed diets with 12.9% or 18.5% CP for 2 weeks had serum urea N concentrations of ~12.5 and ~19 mg/100 ml, respectively (Miller & Lawrence 1988).

Key Points – Amino acid and protein metabolism

- Plasma free amino acid concentrations increase following meal ingestion but the nature and extent of these increases do not mirror the amino acid composition of the ingested feed due to the effects of splanchnic tissue amino acid metabolism.
- In skeletal muscle, signalling via the mammalian target of rapamycin (mTOR) is a major mechanism for the regulation of protein synthesis.
- Postprandial increases in insulin and amino acids stimulate protein synthesis in skeletal muscle via activation of mTOR.

Volatile fatty acids (VFA)

Acetate, butyrate and propionate are the primary volatile or short-chain fatty acids produced by bacterial fermentation within the gastrointestinal tract. In horses maintained on an all-roughage diet, the molar percentage of VFA in cecal or colonic fluid is approximately 74% acetate, 17% propionate, 6% butyrate and 3–4% other VFAs (isobutyrate, valerate, and isovalerate; Hintz et al 1971; also see Chapter A-1). With hay and grain/concentrate rations, the percentage of acetate decreases in concert with an increase in the proportion of propionate (Hintz et al 1971). There is little information on the portal flux of VFA in horses, nor data on the metabolic fate of absorbed VFAs. In ruminants, the net portal flux of acetate, propionate and butyrate represented 50%, 50% and 8%, respectively, of their production in the rumen (Bergman & Wolff 1971). Approximately 50% of the acetate and virtually all of the absorbed propionate and butyrate are metabolized by the total splanchnic bed (i.e., liver and portal vein-drained viscera; Reynolds & Maltby 1994). Much of the butyrate is utilized by enterocytes. In the liver, propionate is a substrate for gluconeogenesis and butyrate is converted to β-hydroxybutyrate, both of which are important sources of oxidizable carbon for peripheral tissues (Bergman 1990). In ruminants, the net flux of acetate across the liver is small with approximately equal rates of uptake and release. Acetate is a major substrate for fat synthesis (including milk fat synthesis) as well as an important substrate for immediate oxidation in peripheral tissues (Bergman 1990). In sheep, the liver, gut and muscle utilized, respectively, 17, 25, and 54% of total acetate flux (Pethick et al 1981).

It is assumed that the VFAs are a primary source of energy for horses, particularly for animals provided a forage-only ration. As in ruminants, propionate is a gluconeogenic precursor; the infusion of propionate into fasted ponies resulted in an increase in plasma glucose concentration (Argenzio & Hintz 1970) while in ponies fed a high-roughage diet, it was estimated that propionate from the large intestine accounted for up to 60% of endogenous glucose production (Ford & Simmons 1985, Simmons & Ford 1991). Plasma acetate concentrations in horses are affected by diet. For example, plasma acetate concentration was approximately 50% higher in lactating mares fed a 95% hay/5% concentrate diet (acetate ~1.6 mmol/l) when compared to a 50% hay/50% concentrate diet (~1.0 mmol/l; Doreau et al 1992). Acetate is likely a major fuel substrate in peripheral tissues of the horse. Nutrient uptake by the hindlimb was investigated by use of the arteriovenous difference technique in Thoroughbred horses fed to maintenance a diet of 100% roughage vs. 52% oat grain and 48% roughage (Pethick et al 1993). Approximately 40% of arterial acetate was extracted by the hindlimb, with no effect of diet. However, consistent with findings in other studies, plasma acetate concentrations were higher in hay fed when compared to grain-hay fed horses. Consequently, the estimated contribution by acetate to oxidation in the hindlimb was higher in horses fed roughage (~32% of total oxidation) when compared to grain-roughage (~21% of total) (Pethick et al 1993).

An *ex vivo* study of mesenteric and subcutaneous (neck crest) adipose tissue depots showed that acetate rather than glucose is the primary source of carbon for lipogenesis in horses (Suagee et al 2010). In addition, mesenteric adipose tissue had greater lipogenic activity than the subcutaneous adipose depot. Interestingly, liver tissue showed very little incorporation of carbon into fatty acids (from glucose or acetate), suggesting a low hepatic lipogenic capacity in horses compared to other species (Suagee et al 2010).

Key Points – Volatile fatty acid metabolism

- The volatile or short-chain fatty acids, acetate, propionate and butyrate are primary sources of energy for horses; particularly animals provided a forage-only ration.
- Propionate is an important gluconeogenic precursor; perhaps accounting for as much as 60% of endogenous glucose production in horses fed a high-roughage diet.
- Acetate is the preferred substrate for fat synthesis in the adipose tissue of horses and is a major fuel source for peripheral tissues including muscle.

Lipid metabolism

Descriptive data are available regarding lipid metabolism in horses after feeding or in response to feed withholding (Sticker et al 1995a, Frank et al 2002) but little is known about the fate of dietary fat in the postabsorptive state. Plasma or serum concentrations of NEFA and, to a lesser extent, triglycerides decrease after consumption of feeds that elicit a rise in circulating insulin, presumably due to the inhibitory effect of insulin on adipose tissue lipolysis as well as hepatic triglyceride production and secretion (Suagee et al 2011b). Insulin also increases the mRNA abundance of fatty acid transporters and lipoprotein lipase in equine skeletal muscle (Suagee et al 2011a), suggesting that insulin stimulates NEFA and triglyceride clearance from plasma. Interestingly, the post-feeding suppression of plasma NEFA was reduced in lean, healthy horses fed a high glycemic diet for 90 days, potentially indicating that insulin-induced suppression of adipose tissue lipolysis was reduced by adaptation to this starch-rich ration (Suagee et al 2011b).

Feed withholding induces marked increases in circulating NEFA and triglyceride concentrations. In one study, a 36-h period of feed withholding resulted in a 16-fold increase in serum NEFA and about a 2-fold increase in the concentrations of very low density lipoproteins (Frank et al 2002). Adaptation to dietary fat is associated with alterations in blood lipids; specifically, higher total cholesterol and lower triglyceride concentrations have been observed in horses fed higher fat (oil) diets (e.g., Orme et al 1997, Geelen et al 2001). In addition, an increase in dietary fat intake is associated with higher hepatic lipase and lipoprotein lipase activities (Orme et al 1997, Geelen et al 2001, Frank et al 2004). Further information concerning the effects of dietary fat on lipid metabolism in horses is described in Chapter 7.

Storage of energy substrates in skeletal muscle and adipose tissue

As in other mammals, the primary forms of stored energy in the horse are liver and muscle glycogen plus the triglycerides stored in adipose tissue as well as within muscle cells. These substrates are the main fuel sources available for ATP synthesis in skeletal muscle during exercise, with the relative proportion of substrates oxidized dependent on a number of factors, e.g., training state, the intensity and duration of exercise, and dietary adaptation (see Rivero & Piercy 2004 and Votion et al 2008 for a more comprehensive discussion on the energetics of exercise in horses). Equine skeletal muscle has a high capacity to store glycogen, with typical values of around 550–650 mmol/kg dry muscle (dm) in trained horses (or approximately 3500–4000 g for a 450–500-kg horse) as compared to human muscle in which resting glycogen stores are around 300–400 mmol/kg dm (Bergstrom et al 1972, Pösö et al 2008). In sedentary animals, liver glycogen content is more labile when compared to that in skeletal muscle, reflecting the dynamics of storage and utilization in relation to feeding state. Total liver glycogen content in mature horses likely ranges between 100 and 200 g depending on feeding state. Body fat stores are the largest energy substrate reserve; the vast majority of triglyceride is stored within subcutaneous and visceral adipose tissue depots with smaller amounts (perhaps no more than 1–2% of total TG stores) within muscle fibers (intramuscular triglycerides, IMTG). Given the limited carbohydrate reserves (glycogen), these fat depots are a very important fuel source for ATP synthesis in skeletal muscle, especially during endurance exercise. Reported values for IMTG in horses have varied markedly, ranging between <10 and 60 mmol/kg dm (Essén-Gustavsson 2008). The content of IMTG is two- to threefold higher in oxidative type I fibers, which also exhibit a greater capacity for fat oxidation. Additionally, IMTG content is higher in endurance horses than in Standardbred trotters and Thoroughbred racehorses (Essén-Gustavsson 2008), suggesting adaptations for greater use of fat during endurance exercise.

Glucose uptake into muscle (and adipose tissue)

Insulin stimulates transport of glucose into muscle and adipose tissue. Indeed, in humans, dogs and rodents skeletal muscle accounts for 80% of insulin-stimulated glucose disposal in peripheral tissues (Biddinger & Kahn 2006, Wasserman 2009). In general, there are three control points in glucose uptake: the rate that glucose is delivered to cells, the rate of transport into cells, and the rate that glucose is phosphorylated within the cell (Wasserman 2009). Movement of glucose from blood to the interstitium is determined by tissue blood flow, capillary recruitment and endothelial cell permeability to glucose. Insulin increases blood flow to muscle and adipose tissue by increasing vasodilation and capillary recruitment (Steinberg & Baron 2002). The effects of insulin on blood flow are mediated by an increase in endothelium-derived nitric oxide. Studies in humans and animals have demonstrated that the effect of insulin on blood flow, and thus the vascular delivery of glucose, is tightly coupled to insulin's effects on glucose uptake and metabolism (Dimitriadis et al 2011). The specific effects of insulin on blood flow have not be examined in horses; however, marked hyperinsulinemia in healthy horses (serum insulin concentration of ~1000 mU/l) was associated with development of prominent pulse amplitude in the digital arteries and an ~2°C increase in temperature of the hoof wall, changes indicative of an increase in distal limb blood flow (de Laat et al 2010).

Membrane glucose transport is the major barrier to cellular uptake, and occurs by facilitated diffusion through glucose transporter proteins (GLUTs). At least seven GLUT isoforms have been identified in the muscle and adipose tissue of man but the predominant isoforms are GLUT1 and GLUT4 (Stuart et al 2006). In skeletal muscle, GLUT4 is responsible for the majority of basal and insulin-stimulated glucose uptake. The translocation of GLUT4 from an intracellular pool to the cell surface is required for active transport; translocation is mediated by both insulin- and, in muscle, contraction-dependent mechanisms (Wasserman 2009). GLUT12 also is expressed in muscle and may participate in insulin-mediated glucose uptake (Stuart et al 2009).

Several studies have examined the expression and function of GLUT4 in equine skeletal muscle. GLUT4 is expressed in a fiber type-selective manner, with highest expression in the cytosol of type IIB (IIX) fibers observed in the vastus lateralis muscle of warmblood horses (van Dam et al 2004). Short- and longer-term exercise training as well strenuous, glycogen-depleting exercise over a 3-day period resulted in increased GLUT4 protein and mRNA content in skeletal muscle (McCutcheon et al 2002, Lacombe et al 2003, Stewart-Hunt et al 2006), whereas single bouts of exercise did not affect skeletal muscle GLUT4 protein content (McCutcheon et al 2002, Pratt et al 2007). These findings are similar to those observed in humans and other mammals (Jensen & Richter 2012). An increase in carbohydrate availability (and circulating insulin concentrations) via grain feeding or the IV administration of glucose also does not appear to affect middle gluteal muscle GLUT4 content in horses (Lacombe et al 2003).

There is some evidence to suggest that glucose transport into muscle is less sensitive to the effects of insulin in horses when compared to other species. In the semitendinosus muscle of Shetland ponies, even supraphysiological insulin concentrations resulted in minimal increase in GLUT4 translocation or glucose transport (Duehlmeier et al 2010). Similarly, GLUT4 translocation in middle gluteal muscle of Quarter horses was not enhanced by *in vitro* stimulation with insulin (Waller et al 2011a). The lack of increase in GLUT4 translocation in response to insulin stimulation may, in part, explain the lower whole-body insulin sensitivity in horses when compared to man and other species (Hoffman et al 2003). It has also been proposed that the high resting muscle glycogen concentration in horse muscle may be inhibitory to GLUT4 translocation via negative feedback (Waller et al 2011a), as has been reported in rodents (Fisher et al 2002). These observations are also relevant to the slow rate of post exercise muscle glycogen synthesis in horses (see below).

The capacity for glucose phosphorylation (i.e. formation of gluose-6-phosphate [G6P]) is determined by the amount of hexokinase (HK), HK compartmentalization within the cell, and the concentration of HK inhibitors (such as G6P). Phosphorylation of glucose is irreversible in adipocytes and muscle; i.e., this reaction traps glucose in the cell. Insulin increases HK activity in skeletal muscle and also enhances the binding of HK to mitochondria thereby increasing access to ATP, a substrate in the reaction that it catalyses (Wasserman 2009). In horses, hyperinsulinemia (insulin ~300 mU/l) resulted in an ~50% increase in HK activity in the middle gluteal muscle of Standardbred horses (Stewart-Hunt et al 2006). Insulin also increases the rate of glycolysis via stimulation of 6-phosphofructokinase (Dimitriadis et al 2011). Thus, when glycogen stores in muscle are replete, the glucose taken up is converted to lactate or completely oxidized in order to maintain glucose utilization and blood glucose homeostasis. Lactate produced in muscle or adipose tissue is taken up by the liver and used for glycogen synthesis (the *indirect pathway* of glycogen synthesis; Consoli et al 1992) or converted to glucose (the Cori cycle).

Glycogen synthesis

As above, once in the cell glucose (as G6P) can be directed to glycolysis or glycogenosis. For the latter, G6P is converted to glucose-1-phosphate and then incorporated into a glycogen molecule in a series of reactions (Fig. 2.9). Glycogen in human and equine skeletal muscle exists in two forms: *macroglycogen* (MG) and *proglycogen* (PG) (Adamo & Graham 1998, Bröjer et al 2002a,b). Both forms contain glycogenin, a

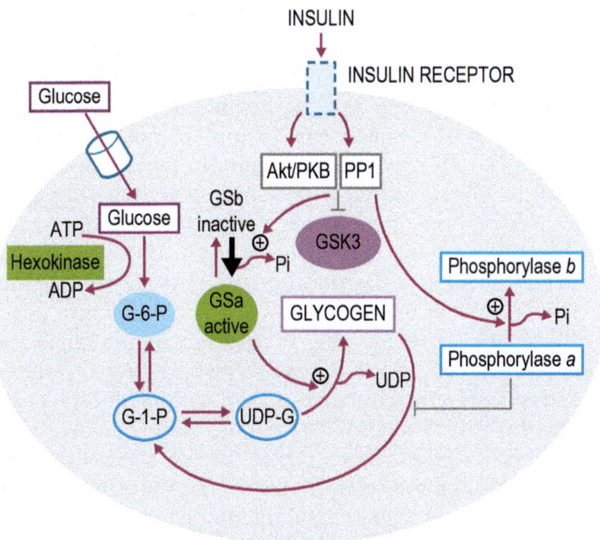

Figure 2.9 Simplified schematic of the biochemical pathway for the synthesis of glycogen in skeletal muscle under conditions of increased circulating glucose and insulin. Glucose entering the cell is phosphorylated to form glucose-6-phosphate (G-6-P) in a reaction catalyzed by hexokinase. Glycogen synthase catalyzes the addition of glucosyl units from UDP-glucose (UDP-G) to the glycogen polymer. GS is regulated by the concentrations of glycogen (autoregulation) and G-6-P, as well as insulin. Stimulation of GS by insulin involves activation of Akt (protein kinase B, PKB) that, in turn, leads to deactivation of glycogen synthase kinase 3 (GSK3). Deactivation of GSK3 enables conversion of GS from its inactive (GSb) to active form (GSa). Protein phosphatase 1 (PP1) also regulates glycogen synthetic activity via dephosphorylation reactions that activate GS and deactivate glycogen phosphorylase, thereby inhibiting glycogenolysis (⊕ = stimulates; ⊗ = inhibits)

protein primer for glycogen synthesis, and branching chains of glucose residues linked by α-1,4-glycosidic (primary polymerization) and α-1,6-glycosidic (branchpoints) bonds. As the name implies, MG is substantially larger (molecular weight ~10 000 000 daltons) than proglycogen (MW ~400 000 daltons). The physiologic importance of PG vs. MG with respect to muscle energetics remains to be determined.

Glycogen synthase (GS) is the "rate-limiting" enzyme in glycogen synthesis; GS is allosterically activated by increased cellular G6P and also by dephosphorylation reactions that are affected by insulin and exercise (Jensen & Richter 2012). In man, rodents, and horses, GS activity is also increased by low cellular glycogen content such that the rate of synthesis is inversely proportional to glycogen content (so-called *glycogen autoregulation;* Bergstrom et al 1972, Nielsen et al 2001, Lacombe et al 2004). Insulin also strongly inhibits the enzyme glycogen phosphorylase and, at physiological insulin concentrations, it has been argued that insulin stimulation of glycogen synthesis is more due to its inhibition of phosphorylase activity than stimulation of GS (Dimitriadis et al 2011). See below for further discussion on muscle glycogen synthesis in horses.

Lipid storage in skeletal muscle and adipose tissue

Very little is known regarding mechanisms regulating lipid (triglyceride) storage in adipose tissue and skeletal muscle of horses. Within muscle cells, triglycerides are stored as lipid droplets that are in close proximity to mitochondria. The uptake of fatty acids into skeletal muscle and adipose tissue is not yet fully understood. Recent studies in man and rodents have demonstrated the involvement of a protein-mediated transport mechanism, and a number of fatty acid transporters have been identified including fatty acid translocase (FAT)/CD36, plasma membrane-bound fatty acid binding protein (FABPpm), and the tissue-specific fatty acid transport protein (FATP) family (FATP 1–6) (Glatz et al 2010). The uptake of fatty acids into skeletal muscle depends on both NEFA concentrations in the blood and the regulation of these transporters (Glatz et al 2010). The exact proportion each of these transporters contributes to fatty acid uptake is not clear, but FAT/CD36 is thought to be a predominant transporter in muscle. Muscle contraction, insulin, leptin and AMP-activated protein kinase (AMPK) all rapidly induce translocation of FAT/CD36 from intracellular depots to the sarcolemma and increase fatty acid uptake (Zhang et al 2010). FAT/CD36 has been identified in the vastus lateralis muscle of warmblood horses (van Dam et al 2004) but as yet there is no information on the function or regulation of this transport protein in equine skeletal muscle.

In human and rodent tissue, NEFAs that are transported into the cytosol are esterified to long chain acyl CoA by fatty acyl CoA synthase. Under resting conditions, some of the long chain acyl CoAs enter mitochondria for β-oxidation but the majority (~60%) are esterified into TG (Shaw et al 2010). The activity of glycerol-3-phosphate acyltransferase (GPAT) is rate-limiting in the synthesis of TG (Wendel et al 2009). In mice, insulin stimulates TG synthesis via the PI3 kinase pathway (Dyck et al 2001). In humans, type I muscle fibers have the highest rate of IMTG synthesis at rest and also demonstrate higher content of GPAT and other enzymes involved in TG synthesis when compared to type II fibers (Shaw et al 2010).

In humans, exercise training is generally associated with an increase in IMTG content (Shaw et al 2010). Similarly, a modest increase in IMTG content has been observed after physical conditioning in horses (Essén-Gustavsson 2008). Few studies have examined whether diet (e.g., increased dietary fat/oil) influences IMTG content in horses; however, increases in lipoprotein lipase activity with fat adaptation point to increased capacity for uptake of fatty acids into muscle (see Chapter 7).

Within adipose tissue, the processes of fat storage and mobilization are regulated in a highly coordinated manner. In humans, adipose tissue is thought to play a central role in buffering the flux of fatty acids in circulation during the postprandial period, analogous to the buffering of blood glucose concentrations and flux by the liver and skeletal muscle post-feeding (Frayn 2002). In the postprandial state, adipose tissue increases the rate of TG clearance from circulation via an increase in the activity of lipoprotein lipase. Conversely, during fasting there is increased release of NEFA from adipose tissue via an increase in the activity of hormone-sensitive lipase, which catalyzes breakdown of stored TG (Frayn 1994). In humans and other mammals, insulin activates lipoprotein lipase and inhibits hormone-sensitive lipase (Dimitriadis et al 2011); to date there is no published information on the effect of insulin on the activity of these enzymes in the horse.

Key Points – Substrate storage in skeletal muscle and adipose tissue

- Equine skeletal muscle has high capacity to store glycogen, with highest content in glycolytic, fast twitch (type II) fibers.
- As in other mammals, insulin is thought to be the primary mediator of glucose transport into equine skeletal muscle and adipose tissue.
- The insulin-sensitive glucose transporter protein (GLUT4) has been identified in equine skeletal muscle and adipose tissue. Exercise training, but not a single bout of exercise or a short-term increase in carbohydrate availability, increases the expression of GLUT4 in equine skeletal muscle.
- Lipoprotein lipase (LPL) in adipose tissue and muscle mediates clearance of triglycerides, with liberation of fatty acids for tissue uptake. In other mammals, insulin activates LPL thereby facilitating blood triglyceride clearance in the postprandial state. The effect of insulin on LPL in the horse is unknown but adaptation to higher fat (oil) diets is associated with increased LPL activity.
- Fatty acid transport proteins, including the fatty acid translocase (FAT)/CD36, regulate the uptake of fatty acids into skeletal muscle and adipose tissue. FAT/CD36 has been identified in equine skeletal muscle and subcutaneous adipose tissue.

Insulin sensitivity and resistance

The association between insulin resistance (IR), obesity and risk for laminitis (see Chapter 27) has generated considerable interest in factors regulating insulin sensitivity in horses, including the effects of diet and exercise. The term *insulin sensitivity* is most often used in reference to insulin-mediated glucose disposal, and can be defined as the ability of insulin to enhance blood glucose disappearance (Bergman et al 1985). *Insulin resistance* (IR), on the other hand, represents a state in which the normal concentration of insulin fails to orchestrate a normal biological response, again usually in reference to insulin-mediated glucose disposal (Kahn 1978). Despite extensive study in humans and animal models, the molecular pathogenesis of IR remains incompletely understood.

Assessment of insulin sensitivity

A number of specific (direct) and nonspecific (indirect) methods have been used to assess insulin sensitivity *in vivo*. In humans, the euglycemic-hyperinsulinemic clamp (EHC) is regarded as the gold standard method for measurement of insulin sensitivity (Muniyappa et al 2008). In this procedure, the plasma insulin concentration is increased by a primed, constant-rate infusion of insulin while blood glucose is held steady ("clamped") at basal levels by a variable-rate infusion of glucose (dextrose) solution. The rate of glucose infusion averaged over the last 30–60 min of the procedure corresponds to whole-body glucose uptake and is a direct measure of whole-body insulin sensitivity (with the assumptions that hepatic glucose output is completely suppressed and that most of the glucose uptake is occurring in muscle and adipose tissues). Minimal model analysis of an insulin-modified frequently-sampled intravenous glucose tolerance test (FSIGTT) is another commonly used method to assess the effect of insulin on glucose homeostasis (Bergman et al 1985). In this procedure, a bolus of glucose is administered IV at Time = 0 min and then a dose of insulin is given IV at Time = 20 min after glucose administration. A two-compartment model is applied to plasma/serum glucose and insulin values obtained during a 180- or 240-min sampling period, providing model estimates of insulin sensitivity (SI) and glucose-mediated glucose disposal (Sg; also termed *glucose effectiveness*). In addition, the acute insulin response to glucose (AIRg) is calculated from the area under the insulin vs. time curve between Time = 0 and 10 min. A recent study examined the effect of glucose dosage (50 to 300 mg/kg BW) on urinary glucose spillover during the FSIGTT (Tóth et al 2009) in horses; based on the findings of this study the administration of 100 mg/kg BW dextrose followed by 20 mU/kg BW regular insulin 20 min later is recommended for use in horses.

Both the EHC and FSIGTT methods have been used in equine studies (see Kronfeld et al 2005 and Firshman & Valberg 2007 for comprehensive reviews). The clinical/field application of both methods is limited due to the time, labor input and expense required. Nonetheless, these methods are useful in experimental studies for which insulin sensitivity is an important outcome measure, bearing in mind that the within animal repeatability of the EHC and minimal model-FSIGTT is relatively poor and this can limit the ability to detect treatment effects. Figure 2.10 shows the rate of glucose infusion required to maintain euglycemia in Standardbred horses that underwent the EHC procedure before and after a 7-day period of exercise training that resulted in an ~12% increase in VO_{2max} (Stewart-Hunt et al 2006). After training, a significantly greater rate of glucose infusion was observed during the last 30 min of the EHC, indicating an increase in whole-body insulin sensitivity. Table 2-3 contains minimal model data from horses and ponies in a variety of physiological states and in response to dietary or exercise interventions.

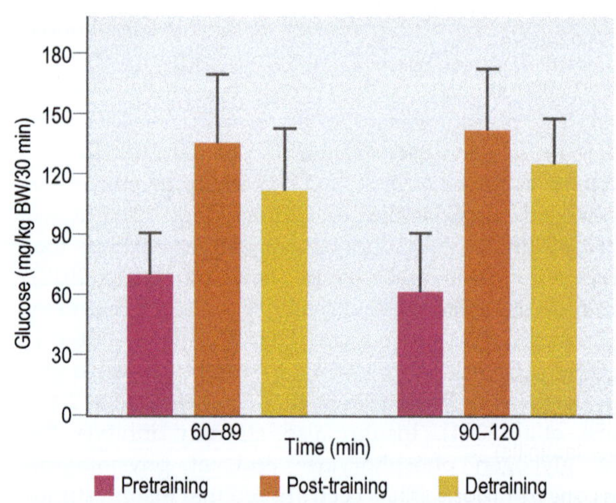

Figure 2.10 Mean (± standard error) rate of glucose infusion required to maintain euglycemia during the 30 min periods of a 2-h euglycemic–hyperinsulinemic clamp in 6 Standardbred horses before (Pretraining) and after (Post-Training) 7 consecutive days of treadmill exercise training, and after a further 5 days of stall rest (Detraining). Insulin infusion (3 μU insulin/kg BW/min) induced hyperinsulinemia that reached a plateau serum concentration of ~250 mU/l at 60 min and was maintained until the end of the clamp. Values with different superscript letters differ significantly ($P < 0.05$, repeated measures ANOVA). Note the more than twofold increase in glucose infusion rate post-training (i.e., increase insulin sensitivity to whole-body glucose disposal) that was maintained after 5 days of inactivity.

Table 2-3 Literature Values for Minimal Model Insulin Sensitivity (SI), Glucose Effectiveness (Sg) and Acute Insulin Response to Glucose (AIRg) in Different Horse Breeds and Ponies as Well as in Different Physiologic and Pathophysiologic States

Breed (physiologic state)	Number of animals	Insulin sensitivity (SI, $\times 10^{-4}$ l/min/mU)	Glucose effectiveness (Sg, min^{-1})	Acute insulin response to glucose (AIRg) ($[mU/l]min^{-1}$)	Reference
Thoroughbred mares (sedentary, open, at pasture)	35	3.19 ± 0.35	2.04 ± 0.24	245 ± 59	Unpublished data
Thoroughbred mares (6–7 months of pregnancy, at pasture)	22	1.34 ± 0.45	2.08 ± 0.18	595 ± 295	George et al 2011[a]
Thoroughbred mares (open, at pasture)	10	3.55 ± 0.57	3.05 ± 0.62	278 ± 151	George et al 2011[a]
Thoroughbred foals (5 days of age)	20	25.4 ± 9.4	3.62 ± 0.10	115 ± 24	George et al 2009[2]
Thoroughbred foals (40 days of age)	20	21.4 ± 10.5	4.24 ± 0.45	127 ± 29	George et al 2009[b]
Thoroughbred foals (80 days of age)	20	12.3 ± 3.8	2.5 ± 0.27	132 ± 34	George et al 2009[b]
Thoroughbred foals (160 days of age)	20	6.7 ± 0.32	2.23 ± 0.19	151 ± 28	George et al 2009[b]
Standardbred mares (sedentary, open)	14	1.68 ± 0.25	2.40 ± 0.33	149 ± 29	Stewart-Hunt et al 2006[c]
Standardbred mares (after 6 weeks exercise training)	14	2.56 ± 0.27	2.50 ± 0.25	179 ± 38	Stewart-Hunt et al 2006[c]
Arabian geldings (moderate BCS ~5–6)	13	2.07 ± 1.76	1.07 ± 0.52	206 ± 88	Carter et al 2009[d]
Arabian geldings (obese, BCS 8–9)	12	0.65 ± 0.54	1.08 ± 0.43	535 ± 174	Carter et al 2010[4]
Arabian geldings (exercised trained, adapted to SS feed)	6	2.32 ± 0.31	1.80 ± 0.27	404 ± 122	Treiber et al 2006b[e]
Arabian geldings (adapted to SS feed, tested during exercise)	6	14.2 ± 4.3	3.05 ± 0.95	155 ± 46	Treiber et al 2006b[e]
Arabian geldings (exercised trained, adapted to FF feed)	6	2.47± 0.26	1.85 ± 0.22	360 ± 110	Treiber et al 2006b[e]
Arabian geldings (adapted to FF feed, tested during exercise)	6	22.4 ± 6.7	3.65 ± 0.88	195 ± 48	Treiber et al 2006b[e]
Ponies (obese, insulin resistant)	6	0.32 ± 0.31	0.95 ± 0.25	841 ± 557	Tinworth et al 2011
Ponies (previously laminitic)	7	0.22 ± 0.18	2.39 ± 0.33	879 ± 274	Treiber et al 2007[f]
Ponies (never laminitic)	7	0.49 ± 0.14	2.05 ± 0.28	492 ± 167	Treiber et al 2007[f]

Unless otherwise indicated, the frequently sampled intravenous glucose tolerance test (FSIGTT) involved the administration of an IV glucose dose (300 mg/kg) at Time = 0 min, followed by insulin (20 mU/kg BW) at Time = 20 min. The data are means and standard errors unless otherwise indicated.

[a]George et al. 2011: Minimal model data were obtained from 10 non-pregnant mares at the same time that testing was performed in the 22 pregnant mares. All mares were kept at pasture and provided supplemental hay and a balancer supplement.

[b]George et al. 2009: Glucose and insulin dynamics with minimal model analysis were evaluated in 20 Thoroughbred foals at 5, 40, 80 and 160 days of age. Foals were born to mares that were fed either a starch-sugar (SS, n=10) or fat-fiber (FF, n=10) during the last trimester of gestation. Insulin dose for the FSIGT was 10 mU/kg BW. All mares were fed the FF during lactation. With the exception of Sg at Day 40 (FF foals > SS foals), there were no significant differences between the groups and the combined data are presented here. Note the decrease in values for SI between Day 5 and Day 160.

[c]Stewart-Hunt et al. 2006: The same animals were assessed in the sedentary state and after 6 weeks of treadmill exercise training. During the training phase, horses were fed either a starch-sugar (sweet feed) or a high-fat feed. As there was no difference between diet treatments, the combined data are presented.

[d]Carter et al. 2009, 2010 (data from both studies are means ± SD). The same horses were used in both studies. Initial values (moderate body condition) were obtained before the start of a weight gain feeding protocol. Data in the obese state were obtained approximately 8 months after completion of diet-induced weight gain; the horses had maintained overweight/obese condition during the interim and were fed a hay only diet. Note the lower SI and higher AIRg values in the obese state.

[e]Treiber et al. 2006b: The horses were maintained at pasture and fed a fat-fiber feed (FF, n=6) or a starch-sugar feed (SS, n=6) that provided ~30% of digestible energy requirements for 8 weeks while undergoing a program of regular exercise training on a treadmill. FSIGTT's with minimal model analysis were then applied at rest and during a 150 min low intensity exercise test. In both FSIGTT's, an IV glucose dose (600 mg/kg) was given at Time = 0 min, followed by insulin (0.01 iu/kg BW) at Time = 20 min).

[f]Treiber et al. 2007: FSIGTTs were applied to 7 ponies with a history of laminitis and 7 ponies of similar body condition without a history of laminitis.

A number of other testing procedures, measurements and calculations have been applied for assessment of insulin sensitivity in horse, including:

- A single "fasting" blood sample to determine blood glucose and insulin concentrations.
- "Proxy" measurements of insulin sensitivity and insulin secretory response derived from single sample measurements of glucose and/or insulin concentrations.
- Oral glucose tolerance test (oral administration of 1 g glucose/kg BW with blood samples obtained at regular intervals over a 5–6 hour period post-dosing for measurement of glucose and insulin concentrations).
- Oral sugar test (administration of 15 ml Light Karo™ Syrup per 100 kg BW with blood samples collected at 0 and 75 min of dosing or at 75 min only).
- Standard intravenous glucose tolerance test (IV administration of 0.3–0.5 g glucose/kg BW and measurement of glucose and insulin concentrations at regular intervals over a 3–4 h period).
- Combined glucose-insulin test (CGIT; the combined IV administration of 150 mg glucose/kg BW followed immediately by 0.10 U/kg BW regular insulin, with measurement of blood glucose concentrations at 10–15 min intervals for 90 min).
- An insulin tolerance test (IV administration of insulin with evaluation of glucose concentrations over time).

Single sample measurements are a convenient and cost-effective choice for clinical applications and/or use in the study of large populations. In horses and ponies, the most commonly used proxies have been RISQI (insulin$^{-0.5}$), QUICKI (1/(log[fasting insulin] + log[fasting glucose])) and MIRG (modified insulin-to-glucose ratio: $800 - 0.3 \times [\text{insulin} - 50]^2)/[\text{glucose} - 30]$). RISQI and QUICKI are estimates of insulin sensitivity while the MIRG is an estimate of insulin secretory response (or pancreatic beta-cell responsiveness; Treiber et al 2005a). Separate studies have shown that these proxies can distinguish between groups of laminitis-prone and control ponies (Treiber et al 2006a, Borer et al 2012), with lower RISQI and higher MIRG in laminitis-prone ponies that appear to have an insulin resistant phenotype. These proxies, however, do not accurately predict predisposition to laminitis in individual animals (Borer et al 2012). Seasonal variation in the proxy measurements of insulin sensitivity and insulin secretory response also has been observed (Borer et al 2012).

All of the methods listed above provide valuable information regarding the glucose-insulin system, and most have been used successfully in horses to assess changes in glucose and insulin dynamics in response to interventions such as exercise, diet and drug administration. However, it should be recognized that only the EHC and possibly also the minimal model method provide a direct measurement of insulin sensitivity. See Chapter 27 for further discussion on insulin sensitivity testing.

Key Points – Insulin sensitivity and resistance

- *Insulin sensitivity*, a term most commonly used in reference to insulin-mediated glucose disposal, is defined as the ability of insulin to increase blood glucose disappearance.
- *Insulin resistance (IR)* represents a state in which the normal concentration of insulin fails to orchestrate a normal biological response, usually in reference to insulin-mediated glucose disposal.
- The euglycemic–hyperinsulinemic clamp and minimal model analysis of an intravenous glucose tolerance test provide specific measures of whole-body insulin sensitivity; the clinical application of these methods is limited due to the time, labour input and expense required.
- Nonspecific measures of insulin sensitivity include proxy measures derived from single sample measurements of glucose and insulin, as well as dynamic assessment of the glucose and insulin system in response to oral or intravenous glucose loads.
- All measures of insulin sensitivity exhibit considerable within-animal variability, which can limit their utility in research and clinical settings.

Factors affecting insulin sensitivity in horses

A number of innate and environmental factors affect insulin sensitivity. This section briefly describes research findings in horses and ponies, with the discussion mostly restricted to studies that have applied specific (i.e., EHC or minimal model analysis) rather than nonspecific measures of insulin sensitivity.

Age, breed, and physiological state

Minimal model estimates of SI are quite high in neonatal Thoroughbred foals with a gradual decline in insulin sensitivity toward adult values over the first 5 months of life (Fig. 2.4; George et al 2009). High insulin sensitivity in the neonatal period may reflect adaptations to a milk-based diet that enable efficient disposition of the glucose load derived from digestion of lactose. At the other end of the age spectrum, there is evidence that advanced age is associated with low insulin sensitivity relative to young, mature horses (Liburt et al 2011). In a cross-sectional study of Thoroughbred mares, age was negatively correlated with insulin sensitivity measured by use of the EHC (Vick et al 2007). Studies in humans and other mammals have also reported age-related insulin resistance, with genetics, lifestyle (including diet and exercise), inflammation, and alterations in body composition (increased adipose, decreased lean tissue mass) all thought to be contributing factors (Vick et al 2007).

Few studies have examined for breed differences in insulin sensitivity (see Table 2-3). Ponies have considerably lower insulin sensitivity when compared to some horse breeds, as assessed by the minimal model (ponies vs. Thoroughbred and Arab horses; Treiber et al 2006a) or EHC (ponies vs. warmblood horses; Rijnen & van der Kolk 2003). Comparing data across studies that employed the EHC method (that achieved a similar degree of hyperinsulinemia), it appears that healthy Standardbred horses have higher insulin sensitivity when compared to Belgian horses and Quarter Horses, while the rate of glucose infusion needed to maintain steady-state blood glucose during hyperinsulinemia was approximately twofold higher in healthy Belgian horses compared to Quarter Horses (Pratt et al 2006, Annandale et al 2004, Firshman et al 2008). Further research is needed to examine breed differences in insulin sensitivity.

George et al (2011) reported lower minimal model SI and higher AIRg in pregnant (~7–8 months of gestation) when compared to non-pregnant mares kept at pasture. Advancing pregnancy in humans and other animal species is also characterized by a decrease in insulin sensitivity and an increase in insulin response to glucose. During late gestation, these adaptations are thought to enable the redirection of glucose away from maternal tissues to meet the nutritional demands of the rapidly growing fetus (Fowden & Forhead 2009).

Diet composition

There are conflicting data regarding the effects of diet composition on insulin sensitivity in horses. Initial studies reported that the feeding of a starch and sugar-based (sweet feed) complementary feed (along with forage) was associated with a decrease in minimal model- (Hoffman et al 2003, Treiber et al 2005b) or EHC-derived (Pratt et al 2006) measures of insulin sensitivity when compared to the feeding of forage alone or a diet of forage and a fat/fiber-based complementary feed. Down-regulation of insulin receptor and/or post-receptor signaling in response to postprandial hyperinsulinemia has been proposed as the mechanism underlying the effect of starch and sugar-based feeds on insulin sensitivity (Pratt et al 2006) but evidence is lacking. This apparent effect of dietary starch and sugar on insulin sensitivity was not apparent in horses undertaking regular physical conditioning (Pratt et al 2006, Treiber et al 2006b). Other studies have reported either no effect of higher starch and sugar diets on insulin sensitivity or improvement in insulin-mediated glucose disposal after adaptation to such diets. Minimal model insulin sensitivity in overweight, insulin resistant ponies did not differ when they were fed either was a base hay plus rice bran diet (NSC intake 1104 g/day) or the base diet to which glucose was added at 1.5 g/kg BW (NSC intake 1351 g/day) (Tinworth et al 2011). Pagan et al (2011) recently reported a higher rate of glucose clearance during an IV glucose tolerance test in healthy, nonobese horses adapted to a diet containing 20.3% non-structural carbohydrates (grass hay plus 2.3 kg whole oats; 31% of DE from NSC) compared to an isocaloric diet of forage alone. Finally, minimal model insulin sensitivity was evaluated in growing Quarter Horse foals at weaning and at 1 and 2 years of age under two dietary treatments: sweet feed (16% CP, 29.4% starch, 10.6% sugar, 5% fat) or a higher fat, lower starch feed (15.5% CP, 16.6% starch, 10.0% sugar, 9.5% fat). At 2 years of age, there was a trend ($P = 0.058$) for higher insulin sensitivity in horses fed the sweet feed compared to the higher fat, lower starch feed (Gordan et al 2011).

Similarly, there is a divergence of findings regarding the effects of dietary oil on insulin sensitivity and glucose tolerance. Using a switch-back design, Hoffman et al (2003) observed that Thoroughbred geldings adapted to a diet of ~60% forage (pasture) and ~40% fat and fiber feed (13.3% fat, DM basis) for 8 weeks had higher minimal model SI compared to a forage and starch/sugar feed diet treatment. A more recent study of healthy, aged Thoroughbred horses compared isocaloric diets of grass hay supplemented with either: (1) fiber (5.6 kg of additional hay); (2) alfalfa (3.1 kg alfalfa pellet); (3) carbohydrate (2.3 kg whole oats); or (4) fat (~500 g soybean oil with 1.3 kg alfalfa cubes); each supplement provided ~7.5 Mcal DE/day with ~11 Mcal/day from grass hay. The main finding was that oil supplementation was associated with a delayed insulin response and slower glucose clearance during an IV glucose tolerance test when compared to the other diet treatments (Pagan et al 2011). The horses in the Hoffman et al (2003) study received ~15% of daily DE intake from fat (oil), compared to ~30% of DE from fat in the Pagan et al (2011) study; thus it is difficult to directly compare these studies. Currently, it is not possible to draw firm conclusions regarding the effects of dietary energy source on insulin sensitivity in horses and further research is warranted (the effects of dietary fat on insulin sensitivity is also discussed in Chapter 7).

Exercise and physical conditioning

There is substantial evidence in man and rodents that a single bout of exercise results in an increase in insulin sensitivity to glucose uptake, measured by use of EHC or minimal model techniques (Cartee et al 1989, Wojtaszewski et al 2002, Bordenave et al 2008). This increased sensitivity to glucose transport into muscle persists for up to 24–36 h after exercise and is associated with increased recruitment of GLUT4 molecules to the plasma membrane. The mechanism behind the exercise effect on insulin sensitivity has not been determined. The proximal components in the insulin signaling cascade are unchanged by prior exercise (Wojtaszewski et al 2002) although current evidence indicates that contraction-mediated activation of the protein AS160 and p38 MAPK may play a central role in enhanced mobilization of GLUT4 to the plasma membrane after exercise (Treebak et al 2009). In fit Standardbred horses, no increase in insulin sensitivity was detected 0.5, 4 and 24 h after a single bout of exercise that reduced muscle glycogen content by ~30% from pre-exercise values (Pratt et al 2007), whereas an ~60% increase in insulin-mediated glucose uptake was observed when a hyperglycemic clamp was administered 30 min after completion of 45 min of exercise at 45% of VO_{2max} (Geor et al 2010). Differences in study design, especially the degree of hyperinsulinemia, may explain the discrepancies between studies.

Physical conditioning also enhances whole-body insulin sensitivity in association with adaptations in skeletal muscle that enhance glucose uptake, including increased protein expression of GLUT4 and insulin receptor substrate-1 (Goodyear & Kahn 1998). In horses, seven consecutive days of light (15–20 min in a round pen; Powell et al 2002) or moderate intensity (Stewart-Hunt et al 2006) resulted in an increase in insulin sensitivity measured by EHC. In the study by Stewart-Hunt et al (2006), the enhancement in insulin sensitivity was accompanied by weight loss and increases in skeletal muscle HK activity and GLUT4 protein expression; these changes persisted after 5 days of inactivity. The effects of longer term training on insulin sensitivity have been more variable. Treiber et al (2006b) found that the feeding of a fat and fiber based diet to Arabian horses during a 4-month period of training was associated with higher insulin sensitivity in comparison to a starch- and sugar-based diet when minimal model parameters were measured during low-intensity exercise at the end of conditioning. Consistent with other studies, "resting" minimal model SI values were higher after training. A longer period of exercise training (15 weeks) in young (mean age 7 years) and old (mean age 22 years) Standardbred mares also resulted in an increase in minimal model SI as well as glucose effectiveness

(Sg); the magnitude of the training-induced increase was greater in the young mares (Liburt et al 2011). In contrast, 8 weeks of mostly low intensity physical conditioning in overweight, insulin resistant geldings that were not subjected to dietary restriction did not alter minimal model SI or AIRg (Carter et al 2010). On balance, however, it appears that physical conditioning improves insulin sensitivity in horses but, as in other species, the magnitude of response is affected by the duration and intensity of training.

Insulin resistance in horses

Insulin resistance may be involved in the pathogenesis of several equine conditions, including the equine metabolic syndrome, laminitis, pituitary pars intermedia dysfunction (PPID), and hyperlipemia (see Chapters 27, 28, and 30). Although several studies have reported differences in insulin sensitivity between e.g. ponies with and without a history of recurrent laminitis, currently there is no clear-cut clinical definition of IR in horses and ponies and there has been very little study of the pathogenesis of IR in equids. It is evident from research in several species that IR is not a single entity and must be defined in terms of a specific action of insulin as well as the tissue or tissues involved (Biddinger & Kahn 2006). With respect to insulin's effects on glucose metabolism, IR may occur in the liver (hepatic IR) and/or in peripheral tissues (adipose tissue and skeletal muscle). Hepatic IR is associated with a reduced ability of insulin to suppress gluconeogenesis and glycogenolysis, whereas peripheral IR reflects defects in the insulin signaling cascade in insulin-sensitive tissues. Another manifestation of IR is reduced ability to inhibit lipolysis in adipose tissue, which contributes to the development of dyslipidemias in obesity and type 2 diabetes (Biddinger & Kahn 2006).

One research group (Waller et al 2011a, b) have compared selected measures of insulin-mediated glucose metabolism in skeletal muscle and adipose tissue from horses classified as insulin sensitive or insulin resistant based on minimal model analysis. In samples of skeletal muscle, IR was associated with reduced cell-surface expression of GLUT4 as measured by an exofacial bis-mannose photolabeling method. In addition, *in vitro* stimulation with insulin in both groups failed to enhance cell-surface GLUT4 expression. Total protein content of GLUT4 and GLUT12 as well as total or phosphorylated AS160 did not differ between the insulin sensitive and resistant groups (Waller et al 2011a). In adipose tissues from the same horses, Waller et al (2011b) observed lower total GLUT4 content in the omental fat of insulin resistant compared to insulin sensitive horses, but no difference between groups was seen in subcutaneous fat or other visceral depots. In addition, cell-surface GLUT4 in all fat depots was lower in insulin resistant compared to insulin-sensitive horses. Taken together, this preliminary work indicates that IR in horses is associated with altered cellular distribution of GLUT4 in muscle and adipose tissues. This reduction in cell-surface GLUT4 content could explain reduced insulin-mediated glucose transport (Waller et al 2011a). The application of techniques used in the studies by Waller et al (2011a, b) should facilitate further research on the pathophysiology of IR in horses and ponies.

Key Points – Factors affecting insulin sensitivity

- Age, physiologic state and breed affect insulin sensitivity of equids
  - Insulin sensitivity is high in neonates, with a decline to adult values by weaning
  - Horse > 20 years of age have lower insulin sensitivity compared to younger, mature horses
  - Insulin sensitivity is lower in ponies than some horse breeds; further work is needed to examine differences among horse breeds
  - Regular physical activity (exercise training) increases insulin sensitivity of healthy horses
  - Obese horses and ponies have lower insulin sensitivity when compared to lean and moderately conditioned animals
- There are conflicting data on the effect of diet composition (in particular, the relative proportion of energy sources) on insulin sensitivity in horses.

Skeletal muscle glycogen metabolism

The increased demand for energy (ATP) to sustain muscle contraction during exercise is matched by the increased utilization of energy substrates. The primary fuel sources within muscle are ATP, phosphocreatine (PCr), glycogen and TG, while the primary extramuscular fuel sources are blood-borne glucose (from hepatic glycogen and gluconeogenesis) and NEFA (from adipose TG stores). There are 3 immediately available energy sources in skeletal muscle: ATP, PCr and adenylate kinase (myokinase). These phosphagens have very low capacity with respect to providing fuel for contraction, and energy from glycolytic and oxidative metabolism is needed to sustain all but very brief (<20–30 s) periods of exercise (Brooks 2012). Muscle glycogen is the primary energy source for anaerobic glycolysis and oxidative phosphorylation during intense exercise in horses, and also is an important fuel during prolonged, lower intensity exercise. Indeed, experimental studies have suggested that most of the energy for exercise at intensities above 50% VO_{2max} is derived from carbohydrates (muscle glycogen, blood glucose, and lactate; Geor et al 2000a – see Fig. 2.11).

The depletion of muscle glycogen reserves can contribute to skeletal muscle fatigue and poor performance in high-intensity as well as endurance exercise in horses. Depletion of muscle glycogen stores has been associated with fatigue in horses during endurance racing (Snow et al 1981). Time to exhaustion in horses running at 6–7 mph was decreased by 35% when pre-exercise muscle glycogen content was 70% lower than in control horses (Topliff et al 1985), while anaerobic work capacity in horses during a sprint treadmill exercise test was decreased by approximately 28% when muscle glycogen content was 60–70% lower relative to a control treatment (Lacombe et al 2001).

A notable feature of skeletal muscle glycogen metabolism in horses is the slow rate of replenishment after glycogen-depleting exercise. As a result, horses that are exercised frequently (on a single day or on consecutive days) may have low muscle glycogen stores at the start of subsequent exercise bouts, which may impair physical performance. For these reasons, a considerable body of research has focused on potential nutritional strategies for enhancement of muscle glycogen replenishment after glycogen-depleting exercise. This section briefly reviews muscle glycogen utilization and resynthesis in the horse, and discusses the effect of nutrition and feeding management on muscle glycogen storage.

Glycogen depletion with exercise

The rate and extent of muscle glycogen depletion during exercise depends upon the intensity, duration and frequency of exercise (Pösö et al 2008; Fig. 2.12). With short duration, high intensity exercise (e.g., 1600-m of galloping by Thoroughbreds or trotting/pacing by Standardbred horses), muscle glycogen concentrations decrease by 30–35% (Harris et al 1987). Four repeat gallops over 620 m depleted muscle glycogen concentrations by ~40% (Snow et al 1985), while a 60% decrease in muscle glycogen content was observed in horses that completed the speed and endurance test (day 2) of a 3-day event (Hodgson et al 1984). Glycogen concentrations in middle gluteal muscle were decreased by as much as 75% after 100 to 160 km endurance rides, with evidence of complete depletion in a large number of individual fibres on histochemical examination (Snow et al 1981, Hodgson et al 1984, 1985). Similarly, complete depletion of the glycogen stores in individual fibres is observed with high-intensity exercise, with loss first occurring in the glycolytic, low oxidative type IIA and IIX fibers (that have higher resting glycogen content than oxidative type I fibers; Valberg 1985, White & Snow 1987). During maximal treadmill exercise, PG and MG contribute equally to glycogenolysis (Bröjer et al 2002b), whereas MG is used to a greater extent than PG during endurance exercise (Essén-Gustavsson et al 2002).

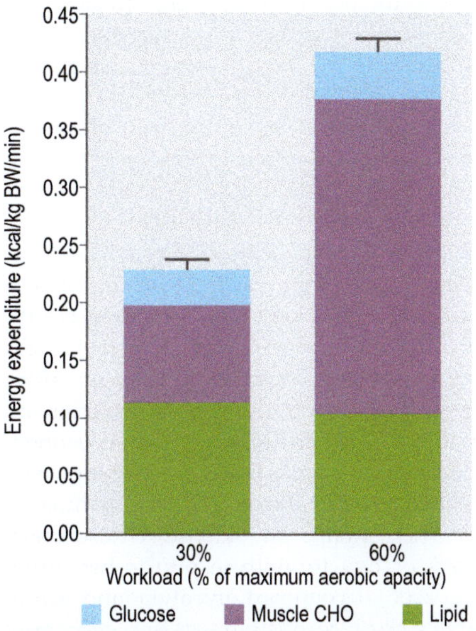

Figure 2.11 Contribution of energy from different substrate sources in six fit horses during treadmill running at a speed that elicited 30% and 60% of maximum aerobic capacity. Combined use of isotopic tracers and indirect calorimetry techniques enabled quantitative estimation of the contributions by fat (Lipid), blood-borne glucose (Glucose), and intramuscular carbohydrates (glycogen and lactate; Muscle CHO). Note that the increased energy expenditure associated with the higher intensity exercise was almost entirely met by use of muscle glycogen.
Data from Geor, R.J. 1999. The effects of glucose supply and sympathoadrenal mechanisms on glucose kinetics and substrate utilization in horses during sustained exercise. PhD dissertation, The Ohio State University.

Physical conditioning results in an increase in resting muscle glycogen concentrations in horses (Hodgson et al 1985, Essen-Gustavsson et al 1989, Foreman et al 1990), in part due to a training-associated increase in muscle oxidative capacity that results in a reduced rate of glycogenolysis during submaximal exercise. Nonetheless, 1600 m training gallops in Thoroughbred racehorses decreased glycogen concentrations by ~25% (from ~640 mmol/kg dm to ~460 mmol/kg dm), with at least 48 h required for restoration of glycogen reserves despite consumption of a conventional hay and grain ration (Snow et al 1991). As well, persistently low muscle glycogen concentrations were observed in Standardbred horses in race training (Essen-Gustavsson et al 1989).

Post-exercise muscle glycogen synthesis

Post-exercise replenishment of muscle glycogen is two- to threefold slower in horses than in man and other mammals (Waller & Lindinger 2010). During the first 24 hours post-exercise, very little repletion occurs under conventional feeding conditions and full recovery after exhausting exercise may take up to 3 days. In humans, muscle glycogen

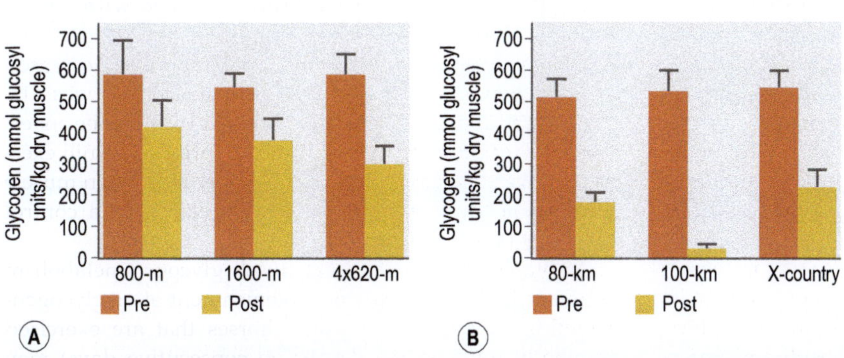

Figure 2.12 The effect of maximal (A) and endurance (B) exercise on muscle glycogen concentration in horses. Intense (galloping) exercise in Thoroughbred horses over distances of 800–1600 m results in an ~30–35% decrease in glycogen concentration; with a larger decrease evident in horses that completed 4 sprints over a distance of 620 m A). A more substantial glycogen depletion occurs during endurance racing or a speed-and-endurance test of a 3-day event B).
Data taken from several publications: Snow et al 1981, 1985, Harris et al 1987, Hodgson et al 1984.

synthesis following glycogen-depleting exercise follows two phases (Jentjens & Jeukendrup 2003). Initially, there is a period of rapid synthesis that functions independent of external factors such as insulin and last about 30–60 minutes. Exercise-induced translocation of glucose transport protein-4 (GLUT-4) to the sarcolemmal membrane, with increased permeability of the muscle membrane to glucose, is a key determinant of this rapid phase of glycogen re-synthesis. The second phase of re-synthesis is slower and lasts several hours. Systemic glucose availability, insulin stimulation of glucose uptake into muscle, and the activity of GS (the "rate-limiting" enzyme in glycogen synthesis) interact to control the rate of glycogen synthesis during this phase (Jentjens & Jeukendrup 2003). Another important component of this slower phase is a post exercise enhancement in skeletal muscle insulin sensitivity to glucose transport, an effect that persists for as long as glycogen stores remain below resting concentrations (Cartee et al 1989).

Several factors may account for the comparatively slow rate of muscle glycogen re-synthesis in horses (Waller & Lindinger 2010). In humans, an up to sixfold increase in muscle GS activity has been observed after glycogen-depleting exercise (Bergstrom et al 1972). GS activity is further increased in response to carbohydrate feedings or intravenous insulin administration (Bergstrom et al 1972). Skeletal muscle GS activity in horses is much lower when compared to humans (Geor et al 2006, Pratt et al 2007), only increases to a modest extent following exercise that depletes glycogen by 40–50% (Geor et al 2006), and no further increase in post exercise GS activity is observed in response to hyperinsulinemia (Pratt et al 2007) or following starch-rich meals (Lacombe et al 2004). Additionally, a post-exercise enhancement in insulin-stimulated glucose disposal (insulin sensitivity) does not occur in horses (Pratt et al 2007). Taken together, these observations suggest that glucose transport into muscle and the activity of GS restrain glycogen re-synthesis in horse skeletal muscle and, at least in part, may explain why nutritional strategies that emphasize hyperinsulinemia and increased glucose availability provide only a modest enhancement in the rate of muscle glycogen resynthesis (see below).

Diet and muscle glycogen storage

Several different feeding strategies for enhancement of the post exercise rate of muscle glycogen synthesis have been evaluated in horses, with a primary focus on carbohydrate feedings (glucose, glucose polymers or starch-rich meals) largely because these approaches have proven successful in human athletes (Waller & Lindinger 2010). However, it is now evident that feeding (or administering) glucose or starch in amounts comparable to that used with success in humans does not substantially (if at all) alter muscle glycogen recovery in horses (Table 2-4). For example, oral administration of a glucose polymer (3 g/kg BW) within 60 min of the completion of glycogen-depleting exercise or 1 g glucose/kg BW given at 0, 2, and 4 h post exercise (Geor et al 2006), did not alter the rate of muscle glycogen resynthesis in Standardbred horses. Provision of a 80% grain (corn, oats, and barley mix):20% hay diet modestly increased glycogen recovery over a 72-h period when compared to hay only or 50% grain:50% hay diets (Lacombe et al 2004). Feeding two meals of cracked corn at 0 and 4 h after glycogen-depleting exercise (2.2 kg corn/meal, total digestible energy intake of ~15 Mcal) enhanced systemic glucose supply (threefold increase in whole body glucose kinetics) but minimally enhanced muscle glycogen replenishment at 24 h post exercise when compared to feed withholding or isocaloric feedings of hay (grass and alfalfa hay mix) (Jose-Cunilleras et al 2006). In contrast, intravenous administration of glucose (3 g/kg BW over 6 hours or 6 g/kg BW over 12 h, or about 0.5 g/kg BW/h) was demonstrated to increase muscle glycogen recovery by 24 h post exercise (Davie et al 1995, Lacombe et al 2001, Geor et al 2006). It was hypothesized that the very large glycemic and/or insulinemic response to intravenous glucose contributed to the

Table 2-4 Comparison of Muscle Glycogen Synthesis Rates after Carbohydrate Administration in Horse and Man (Following Exercise that Depleted Muscle Glycogen by ~50–70%)

Species	Post exercise dietary protocol	Glycogen resynthesis rate (mmol kg bwt/h)	Reference
Horse	Oral: 0–3 h post exercise i) high CHO (grain-corn, oats barley; 2.3 g starch/kg BW) ii) mixed CHO (hay, grain; 1.5 g starch/kg BW) iii) low CHO (hay; 0.1 g starch/kg BW)	 i) 12 ii) 8 iii) 8	Lacombe et al (2004)
Horse	Oral: 0–4 h post exercise i) high CHO (corn; 2.7 g starch/kg BW) ii) low CHO (hay; 0.4 g starch/kg BW) iii) no feed	 i) 15 ii) 15 iii) 14	Jose-Cunilleras et al (2006)
Man	Oral: 0–4 h post exercise i) high CHO (5 g glucose/kg BW)	 i) 40	Jentjens et al (2001)
Horse	i.v. infusion: 0–6 h post exercise i) glucose (3 g/kg BW)	 i) 21	Geor et al (2006)
Man	i.v. infusion: 0–4 h post exercise i) glucose (1 kg)	 i) 85	Bergstrom and Hultman (1967)

Reprinted with permission from Waller, A.P., Lindinger, M.I. 2010. Nutritional aspects of post exercise skeletal muscle glycogen synthesis in horses: A comparative review. Equine Veterinary Journal 42, 274–281.

enhanced glycogen recovery under these conditions (Geor et al 2006).

The observation that glucose feedings or diets rich in hydrolysable carbohydrates (starch) are not beneficial for muscle glycogen recovery has prompted research into alternative strategies, including the addition of amino acids to glucose feedings, short-chain (volatile) fatty acid supplementation, and provision of a hypotonic electrolyte solution. Studies in humans have shown that the addition of protein hydrolysates or certain amino acids to carbohydrate/glucose feedings can enhance insulinemic response and glycogen replenishment when compared to carbohydrate alone (Ivy et al 2002). For example, the addition of whey protein or leucine to post exercise carbohydrate meals (0.8 g CHO/kg BW/h) augmented the insulin response and accelerated muscle glycogen recovery when compared to carbohydrate alone (Van Loon et al 2000). Leucine is an insulin secretatog and, in rodent studies, has been demonstrated to increase muscle glucose uptake; both mechanisms may promote muscle glycogenesis when leucine is fed along with glucose. It should be noted that protein or amino acid supplementation does not augment glycogenesis in humans when larger amounts of carbohydrate are consumed during recovery (~1.2 g CHO/kg BW/h) which is considered the optimal dosage for enhancement of glycogen re-synthesis) (Jentjens et al 2001).

In horses, the addition of 0.1 g/kg BW (Pösö & Hyyppä 1999) or 0.3 g/kg BW (Urschel et al 2010) leucine to a glucose dose was shown to substantially increase post-exercise plasma insulin responses when compared to glucose alone. However, the administration of leucine (0.1 g/kg BW at 0 and 4 h post exercise) in concert with glucose (1.0 g/kg BW at 0, and 4 h after exercise) did not alter post exercise glycogen replenishment in Standardbred horses (Bröjer et al 2012). Whereas amino acid supplementation may not enhance early post-exercise glycogen recovery, recent work has suggested that protein nutrition can affect muscle glycogen content. Specifically, the muscle glycogen concentration of Standardbred trotters fed a forage-only diet with 16.6% crude protein (CP) was higher (~630 mmol/kg dry weight [dw]) when compared to a forage diet providing 12.5% CP (~550 mmol/kg dw), and there also was a trend for faster post exercise glycogen recovery in horses fed the higher protein diet (Essén-Gustavsson et al 2010). The 16.6% CP hay also had greater NSC content and this difference may have contributed to the higher muscle glycogen concentration in this treatment. Nonetheless, further work is warranted to explore the effects of protein nutrition on muscle glycogen metabolism in horses.

Low availability of lipid metabolites during the post exercise recovery period may limit muscle glycogenesis by redirecting glucose away from glycogen synthesis to support immediate energy needs through the tricarboxylic acid (TCA) cycle (Hyyppä et al 1997), i.e., available glucose is partitioned to oxidation rather than storage. Therefore, post-exercise feeding strategies that directly or indirectly (e.g., via production of VFA by microbial fermentation) increase the availability of alternative substrates for the TCA cycle (such as acetate) could support glycogen synthesis. The ingestion of a glucose/acetate solution increased glycogen replenishment and GS activity in rats after exercise when compared to glucose alone (Fushimi et al 2002). In this context, Waller et al (2009a) reported that the administration of a sodium acetate-electrolyte solution (containing 500 g sodium acetate, 250 ml acetic acid, 32 g KCl, and 300 g glucose in 8 liters of water) modestly enhanced the early rate (measured at 4 h) of muscle glycogen synthesis in horses after glycogen-depleting exercise. The authors suggested that the administered acetate was rapidly taken up by skeletal muscle, converted to acetyl-CoA and acetylcarnitine and, in turn, metabolized to CO_2 and water via the TCA cycle. Presumably, synthesis of ATP by this mechanism would allow the partitioning of glucose into storage (glycogenesis) rather than oxidative pathways. The acetate–acetic acid mixture, however, appeared to depress appetite and may have elicited gastrointestinal discomfort, and therefore such a treatment cannot be recommended for use in the field pending further investigations of different acetate formulations.

The inclusion of oils in diets for athletic horses is widespread and there has been interest in the effects of higher oil diets on muscle glycogen storage in horses. Although early studies suggested that fat/oil supplementation was associated with higher "resting" muscle glycogen concentrations (Meyers et al 1989), more recent studies have reported no effect of oil supplementation on muscle glycogen stores (Eaton et al 1995, Hyyppä et al 1999). Few studies have examined the effects of oil supplemented diets on muscle glycogen replenishment in horses. In one study, the rate of post exercise muscle glycogen synthesis did not differ between horses fed a traditional hay/grain diet vs. a diet containing 5% fat (dry matter basis). However, the rate of glycogen re-synthesis was decreased in horses not adapted to the fat-supplemented diet (Hyyppä et al 1999). More recently, McCue et al (2009) reported that the administration of 217 ml of either corn or triheptanoin (a triglyceride containing fatty acid moieties with a chain length of seven carbons) 120 min before exercise did not influence post exercise glycogen repletion.

There is evidence that dehydration affects glycogen synthesis in muscle and liver. Within these tissues, glycogen is stored in a hydrated form associated with about 3 g water and 0.5 mmol K^+ per gram of glycogen, and adequate intracellular water and K^+ are required for glycogen synthesis. Indeed, studies in rodents have shown that cell shrinkage, as occurs with dehydration, impairs glycogen synthesis in skeletal muscle while cell swelling has the opposite effect (Low et al 1996). It is therefore possible that exercise-associated dehydration is one factor that constrains the post exercise rate of muscle glycogen re-synthesis in horses. To test this hypothesis, Waller et al (2009b) evaluated the effects of a hypotonic (~210 mOsmol/kg) electrolyte solution (12 g Na, 24 g Cl, 9 g K, 1 g Ca and Mg in 8 liters of water) on whole-body and muscle hydration state plus glycogen synthesis in horses after glycogen-depleting exercise. When compared to the control trial, the electrolyte treatment resulted in quicker restoration of hydration, evidenced by faster recovery of plasma protein concentration, maintenance of plasma osmolality and greater muscle intracellular fluid volume. Additionally, the electrolyte treatment enhanced the rate of muscle glycogen resynthesis; at 4 h and 24 h of recovery muscle glycogen was significantly higher than in the control treatment. Total water intake, including the 8 liters given via nasogastric intubation, was higher in the electrolyte treatment; at 24 h of recovery total water consumption in the electrolyte and control treatments was, respectively, 49.5 ± 4.2 and 34.8 ± 2.2 liters. Based on these findings, rehydration via administration of electrolyte solutions (and ensuring that horses have free access to fresh, palatable water) may be important in the context of muscle glycogen recovery.

Summary recommendations – diet and muscle glycogen

The need for nutritional strategies targeting rapid replenishment of muscle glycogen stores is dependent on the length and duration of the exercise session and on the timing of the next intense bout of exercise. A 1600-m Thoroughbred race may result in substantial muscle glycogen depletion but horses competing in such races are not likely to perform another hard training session or race for a few days. The timing and composition of post-exercise (post-race) feedings is therefore less critical with respect to replenishment of energy stores. Conversely, for other equine athletic disciplines such as show jumpers competing multiple times per day for several consecutive days, Standardbred racehorses running more than one heat in a single day, or 3-day eventers performing the stadium jumping test the day following the cross-country test, the timing and composition of postexercise feedings may be important.

Nutritional interventions with proven efficacy for enhancement of muscle glycogen recovery in humans and other species are not effective in horses, likely reflecting differences in physiology, in particular lower insulin sensitivity in horses vs. other mammals. Very high starch diets (e.g., grain at 70–80% of the as fed ration) have been shown to modestly increase the rate of muscle glycogen re-synthesis, but even then 48 hours or more are needed for complete replenishment. Concerns regarding the potentially adverse effects of high starch (grain), low forage diets, including increased risk of colic, gastric ulcer syndrome or laminitis, outweigh any benefit with respect to muscle glycogen recovery. In general, the composition of post-exercise meals should mirror the current base ration. The horse evolved as a hindgut fermenter, with fermentable carbohydrates from forage a primary source of energy in the form of volatile fatty acids. Accordingly, forage should be the *predominant* component of the diet, including horses engaged in elite level athletic competition. After training or competition exercise bouts, horses should initially be offered hay or other forage source. Fresh water should be offered as soon as possible after exercise and, especially in the hotter summer months, some salt (20–30 g NaCl) may be added to feedings or made available in a separate feed container.

Key Points – Skeletal muscle glycogen metabolism

- Muscle glycogen is an important source of energy during exercise, and depletion of muscle glycogen reserves can contribute to fatigue and poor exercise performance.
- Post-exercise replenishment of muscle glycogen is two- to threefold slower in horses than in man and other mammals, with up 48–72 h required for complete recovery following exercise that depletes glycogen by >50%. Factors that may contribute to the slow rate of muscle glycogen synthesis include:
  - A lack of post-exercise enhancement in insulin sensitivity to glucose disposal
  - Minimal effect of exercise or increased carbohydrate availability (hyperglycemia and hyperinsulinemia) on the activity of glycogen synthase
- Unlike humans, feeding strategies that enhance glucose availability and/or insulinemia in the post-exercise period have minimal to no effect on the rate of muscle glycogen replenishment
  - Intravenous but not oral glucose administration accelerates glycogen recovery
  - "Aggressive" grain feeding protocols do not alter glycogen recovery during the first 24 h post-exercise, although a modest enhancement has been observed at 48–72 h

References

Adamo, K.B., Graham, T.E., 1998. Comparison of traditional measurements with macroglycogen and proglycogen analysis of muscle glycogen. Journal of Applied Physiology 84, 908–913.

Aftring, R.P., Block, K.P., Buse, M.G., 1986. Leucine and isoleucine activate skeletal muscle branched-chain alpha-keto acid dehydrogenase *in vivo*. American Journal of Physiology Endocrinology and Metabolism 250, E599–E604.

Allen, W.R., Wilsher, S., Ousey, J.C., et al., 2002. The influence of maternal size on placental, fetal and postnatal growth in the horse: II. Endocrinology of pregnancy. Journal of Endocrinology 172, 237–246.

Annandale, E.J., Valberg, S.J., Mickelsen, J.R., et al., 2004. Insulin sensitivity and skeletal muscle glucose transport in horses with equine polysaccharide storage myopathy. Neuromuscular Disorders 14, 666–674.

Argenzio, R.A., Hintz, H.F., 1970. Glucose tolerance and effect of volatile fatty acids on plasma glucose concentrations in ponies. Journal of Animal Science 30, 514–518.

Argenzio, R.A., Hintz, H.F., 1971. Volatile fatty acid tolerance and effect of glucose and VFA on plasma insulin levels in ponies. Journal of Nutrition 101, 723–730.

Arora, T., Sharma, R., Frost, G., 2011. Propionate. Anti-obesity and satiety enhancing factor? Appetite 56, 511–515.

Asplin, K.E., Curlewis, J.D., McGowan, C.M., et al., 2011. Glucose transport in the equine hoof. Equine Veterinary Journal 43, 196–201.

Barle, H., Nyberg, B., Essen, P., et al., 1997. The synthesis rates of total liver protein and plasma albumin determined simultaneously *in vivo* in humans. Hepatology 25, 154–158.

Bergman, E.N., 1990. Energy contributions of volatile fatty acids from the gastrointestinal tract in various species. Physiological Reviews 70, 567–590.

Bergman, E.N., Wolff, J.E., 1971. Metabolism of volatile fatty acids by liver and portal-drained viscera in sheep. American Journal of Physiology 221, 586–592.

Bergman, R.N., Finegood, D.T., Ader, M., 1985. Assessment of insulin sensitivity *in vivo*. Endocrine Reviews 6, 45–86.

Bergstrom, J., Hultman, E., 1967. Synthesis of muscle glycogen in man after glucose and fructose infusion. Acta Medica Scandinavia 1982, 93–107.

Bergstrom, J., Hultman, E., Roch-Norlund, A.E., 1972. Muscle glycogen synthetase in normal subjects. Basal values, effect of glycogen depletion by exercise and a carbohydrate-rich diet following exercise. Scandinavian Journal of Clinical Laboratory Investigation 29, 231–236.

Biddinger, S.B., Kahn, C.R., 2006. From mice to men: insights into the insulin resistance syndromes. Annual Review of Physiology 68, 123–158.

Bolster, D.R., Jefferson, L.S., Kimball, S.R., 2004. Regulation of protein synthesis associated with skeletal muscle hypertrophy by insulin-, amino acid- and exercise-induced signaling. Proceedings of the Nutrition Society 63, 351–356.

Bordenave, S., Brandou, F., Manetta, J., et al., 2008. Effects of acute exercise on insulin sensitivity, glucose effectiveness and disposition index in type 2 diabetic patients. Diabetes and Metabolism 34, 250–257.

Borgia, L., Valberg, S., McCue, M., et al., 2011. Glycaemic and insulinaemic responses to feeding hay with different non-structural carbohydrate content in control and polysaccharide myopathy-affected horses. Journal of Animal Physiology and Animal Nutrition (Berlin) 95, 798–807.

Blum, J.W., Schnyder, P.L., Kunq, P.L., et al., 1985. Reduced and compensatory growth: Endocrine and metabolic changes during food restriction and refeeding in steers. Journal of Nutrition 115, 417–421.

Borer, K.E., Bailey, S.R., Menzies-Gow, N.J., et al., 2012. Use of proxy measurements of insulin sensitivity and insulin secretory response to distinguish between normal and previously laminitic ponies. Equine Veterinary Journal (in press, DOI: 10.111/j.2042-3306.2011.00475.x).

Brehaus, B.A., 2011. Disorders of the equine thyroid gland. Veterinary Clinics of North America Equine Practice 27, 115–128.

Brighenti, F., Benini, L., Del Rio, D., et al., 2006. Colonic fermentation of indigestible carbohydrates contributes to the second-meal effect. American Journal of Clinical Nutrition 83, 817–822.
Bröjer, J.T., Stämpfli, H.R., Graham, T.E., 2002. Analysis of proglycogen and macroglycogen content of muscle biopsy specimens obtained from horses. American Journal of Veterinary Research 63, 570–575.
Bröjer, J.T., Jonasson, R., Schuback, K., et al., 2002. Pro- and macroglycogenolysis in skeletal muscle during maximal treadmill exercise. Equine Veterinary Journal 34 (Suppl.), 205–208.
Bröjer, J.T., Nostell, K., Essen-Gustavsson, B., et al., 2012. Effects of repeated post-exercise supplementation with glucose and leucine on post-exercise glycogen storage and insulin response in horses. American Journal of Veterinary Research 73, 867–874.
Brooks, G.A., 2012. Bioenergetics of exercising humans. Comprehensive Physiology 2, 537–562.
Bruning, J.C., Gautam, D., Burks, D.J., et al., 2000. Role of brain insulin receptor in control of body weight and reproduction. Science 289, 2122–2125.
Buff, P.R., Dodds, A.C., Morrison, C.D., et al., 2002. Leptin in horses: tissue localization and relationship between peripheral concentrations of leptin and body condition. Journal of Animal Science 80, 2942–2948.
Buff, P.R., Spader, B.R., Morrison, C.D., et al., 2006. Endocrine responses in mares undergoing abrupt changes in nutritional management. Journal of Animal Science 84, 2700–2707.
Buff, P.R., Messer 4th, N.T., Cogswell, A.M., et al., 2007. Seasonal and pulsatile dynamics of thyrotropin and leptin in mares maintained under a constant energy balance. Domestic Animal Endocrinology 33, 430–436.
Burns, T.A., Watts, M.R., Geor, R.J., et al., 2011. Distribution of insulin receptor in the digital laminae of ponies fed a high-carbohydrate diet: An immunohistochemical study. In: Proceedings of the American College of Veterinary Internal Medicine Annual Forum. Denver, CO.
Cartee, G.D., Young, D.A., Sleeper, M., et al., 1989. Prolonged increase in insulin-stimulated glucose transport in muscle after exercise. American Journal of Physiology Endocrinology and Metabolism 256, E494–E499.
Carrington, E.F., Desautels, M., Naylor, J.M., 2003. β-adrenergic stimulated lipolysis in pony adipocytes is exclusively via a β2-subtype and is not affected by lactation. Comparative Biochemistry and Physiology Part A 136, 311–320.
Carter, R.A., Staniar, W.B., Cubitt, T.A., et al., 2009. Apparent adiposity assessed by standardized scoring systems and morphometric measurements in horses and ponies. Veterinary Journal 179, 204–210.
Carter, R.A., McCutcheon, L.J., Valle, E., et al., 2010. Effects of exercise training on adiposity, insulin sensitivity, and plasma hormone and lipid concentrations in overweight or obese, insulin-resistant horses. American Journal of Veterinary Research 71, 314–321.
Cartmill, J.A., Thompson, D.L., Storer, W.A., et al., 2005. Effect of dexamethasone, feeding time, and insulin infusion on leptin concentrations in stallions. Journal of Animal Science 83, 1875–1881.
Chameroy, K., Frank, N., Elliott, S., et al., 2011. Effects of weight gain on active glucagon-like peptide-1 concentrations in horses with histories of obesity and insulin resistance. In: Proceedings of the American College of Veterinary Internal Medicine Annual Forum. Denver, CO.
Chang, A.M., Halter, J.B., 2003. Aging and insulin secretion. American Journal of Physiology, Endocrinology and Metabolism 284, E7–E12.
Chen, C.L., Riley, A.M., 1981. Serum thyroxine and triiodothyronine concentrations in neonatal foals and mature horses. American Journal of Veterinary Research 42, 1415–1417.
Considine, R.V., Sinha, M.K., Heiman, M.L., et al., 1996. Serum immunoreactive-leptin concentration in normal-weight and obese humans. New England Journal of Medicine 334, 292–295.
Consoli, A., Nurjahan, N., Gerich, J., et al., 1992. Skeletal muscle is a major site of lactate uptake and release during hyperinsulinaemia. Metabolism 41, 176–179.
Cummings, D.E., Frayo, R.S., Marmonier, C., et al., 2004. Plasma ghrelin levels and hunger scores in humans initiating meals voluntarily without time- and food-related cues. American Journal of Physiology: Endocrinology and Metabolism 287, E297–E304.
Davie, A.J., Evans, D.L., Hodgson, D.R., 1995. Effects of intravenous dextrose infusion on muscle glycogen resynthesis after intense exercise. Equine Veterinary Journal 18 (Suppl), 195–198.
Davis, T.A., Fiorotto, M.L., Burrin, D.G., et al., 2002. Stimulation of protein synthesis by both insulin and amino acids is unique to skeletal muscle in neonatal pigs. American Journal of Physiology Endocrinology and Metabolism 282, E880–E890.
Dardevet, D., Moore, M.C., Remond, D., et al., 2002a. Regulation of hepatic metabolism by enteral delivery of nutrients. Nutrition Research Reviews 19, 161–173.
Dardevet, D., Stornet, C., Balage, G., et al., 2002b. Postprandial stimulation of muscle protein synthesis in old rats can be restored by a leucine-supplemented meal. Journal of Nutrition 132, 95–100.
De Feo, P., Lucidi, P., 2002. Liver protein synthesis in physiology and in disease states. Current Opinion in Clinical Nutrition and Metabolic Care 5, 47–50.
de Graaf-Roelfsema, E., Tharasanit, T., van Dam, K.G., et al., 2005. Effects of short- and long-term recombinant growth hormone and short-term hydrocortisone administration on tissue sensitivity to insulin in horses. American Journal of Veterinary Research 66, 1907–1913.
de Laat, M.A., McGowan, C.M., Sillence, M.N., et al., 2010. Equine laminitis: induced by 48 h hyperinsulinaemia in Standardbred horses. Equine Veterinary Journal 42, 124–131.
Delzenne, N., Blundell, J., Brouns, F., et al., 2010. Gastrointestinal targets of appetite regulation in humans. Obesity Reviews 11, 234–250.
DePew, C.L., Thompson Jr., D.L., Fernandez, J.M., et al., 1994a. Changes in concentrations of hormone, metabolites, and amino acids in plasma of adult horses relative to overnight feed deprivation followed by a pellet-hay meal at noon. Journal of Animal Science 72, 1530–1539.
DePew, C.L., Thompson Jr., D.L., Fernandez, J.M., et al., 1994b. Plasma concentrations of prolactin, glucose, insulin, urea nitrogen, and total amino acids in stallions after ingestion of feed or gastric administration of feed components. Journal of Animal Science 72, 2345–2353.
Dimitriadis, G., Mitrou, P., Lambadiari, V., et al., 2011. Insulin effects in muscle and adipose tissue. Diabetes Research and Clinical Practice 93S, S52–S59.
Doreau, M., Boulot, S., Bauchart, D., et al., 1992. Voluntary intake, milk production and plasma metabolites in nursing mares fed two different diets. Journal of Nutrition 122, 992–999.
Dühlmeier, R., Deegen, E., Fuhrmann, H., et al., 2001. Glucose-dependent insulinotropic polpeptide (GIP) and the enteroinsular axis in equines (*Equus caballus*). Comparative Biochemistry and Physiology A: Molecular and Integrative Physiology 129, 563–575.
Duehlmeier, R., Hacker, A., Widdel-Bigdely, A., et al., 2010. Insulin stimulates GLUT4 translocation in the semitendinosus muscle of Shetland ponies. Veterinary Journal 184, 176–181.
Dyck, D.J., Steinberg, G., Bonen, A., 2001. Insulin increases FA uptake and esterification but reduces lipid utilization in isolated contracting muscle. American Journal of Physiology Endocrinology and Metabolism 281, E600–E607.
Eaton, M.D., Hodgson, D.R., Evans, D.L., 1995. Effect of a diet containing supplementary fat on the capacity for high-intensity exercise. Equine Vet. J. Suppl. 18, 353–356.
Eriksson, S., Hagenfeldt, L., Wahren, J., 1981. A comparison of the effects of intravenous infusion of individual branched-chain amino acids on blood amino acid levels. Clinical Science 60, 95–100.
Essen-Gustavsson, B., McMiken, D., Karlstrom, K., et al., 1989. Muscular adaptation of horses during intensive training and detraining. Equine Veterinary Journal 21, 27–33.
Essén-Gustavsson, B., Jensen-Warren, M., 2002. Effect of an endurance race on muscle amino acids, pro- and macroglycogen and triglycerides. Equine Veterinary Journal 34 (Suppl.), 209–213.
Essén-Gustavsson, B., 2008. Triglyceride storage in the skeletal muscle. In: Saastamoinen, M.T., Martin-Rosset, W. (Eds.), Nutrition of the exercising horse. EAAP publication No. 125, Academic Publishers, Wageningen, pp. 31–42.
Essén-Gustavsson, B., Connysson, M., Jansson, A., 2010. Effects of crude protein intake from forage-only diets on muscle amino acids and glycogen levels in horses during training. Equine Veterinary Journal 42 (Suppl. 38), 341–346.
Etz, I.C., Lambert, N.M., Sylvester, J.T., et al., 2011. Supplemental leucine's influence on plasma glucose, insulin and amino acid responses in Quarter Horse yearlings. Journal of Equine Veterinary Science 31, 248–249.
Faverdin, P., 1999. The effect of nutrients on feed intake in ruminants. Proceedings of the Nutrition Society 58, 523–531.
Ferrannini, E., DeFronzo, R.A., Gusberg, R., et al., 1988. Splanchnic amino acid and glucose metabolism during amino acid infusion in dogs. Diabetes 37, 237–245.
Firshman, A.M., Valberg, S.J., 2007. Factors affecting clinical assessment of insulin sensitivity in horses. Equine Veterinary Journal 39, 567–575.
Firshman, A.M., Valberg, S.J., Baird, J.D., et al., 2008. Insulin sensitivity in Belgian horses with polysaccharide storage myopathy. American Journal of Veterinary Research 69, 818–823.
Fisher, J.S., Nolte, L.A., Kawanaka, K., et al, 2002. Glucose transport rate and glycogen synthase activity both limit skeletal muscle glycogen accumulation. American Journal of Physiology: Endocrinology and Metabolism 282, E1214–E1221.
Ford, E.J., Simmons, H.A., 1985. Gluconeogenesis from caecal propionate. British Journal of Nutrition 53, 55–60.
Foreman, J.H., Bayly, W.M., Allen, J.R., et al., 1990. Muscle responses of Thoroughbreds to conventional race training and detraining. American Journal of Veterinary Research 51, 909–913.
Forhead, A.J., Ousey, J.C., Allen, W.R., et al., 2004. Postnatal insulin secretion and sensitivity after manipulation of fetal growth by embryo transfer in the horse. Journal of Endocrinology 181, 459–467.
Fowden, A.L., Forhead, A.J., 2009. Endocrine regulation of feto-placental growth. Hormonal Research 72, 257–265.
Fowden, A.L., Barnes, R.J., Comline, R.S., et al., 1980. Pancreatic beta-cell function in the fetal foal and mare. Journal of Endocrinology 87, 293–301.
Fowden, A.L., Gardner, D.S., Ousey, J.C., et al., 2005. Maturation of pancreatic beta-cell function in the fetal horse during late gestation. Journal of Endocrinology 186, 467–473.

Fowden, A.L., Forhead, A.J., Ousey, J.C., 2012. Endocrine adaptations in the foal over the perinatal period. Equine Veterinary Journal 44 (Suppl. 41), 130–139.

French, K., Pollitt, C.C., Pass, M.A., et al., 2000. Pharmacokinetcs and metabolic effects of triamcinolone acetonide and their possible relationships to glucocorticoid-induced laminitis in horses. Journal of Veterinary Pharmacology and Therapeutics 23, 287–292.

Fuller, Z., Cox, J.E., Argo, C.M.C.G., 2001. Photoperiodic entrainment of seasonal changes in the appetite, feeding behavior, growth rate and pelage of pony colts. Animal Science 72, 65–74.

Furuoka, H., Ito, H., Hamada, M., et al., 1989. Immunocytochemical component of endocrine cells in pancreatic islets of horses. Nihon Juigaku Zasshi 51, 35–43.

Fushimi, T., Tayama, K., Fukaya, M., et al., 2002. The efficacy of acetic acid for glycogen repletion in rat skeletal muscle after exercise. International Journal of Sports Medicine 23, 218–222.

Frank, N., Sojka, J.E., Latour, M.A., 1999. Effect of hypothyroidism on blood lipid concentrations in horses. American Journal of Veterinary Research 60, 730–733.

Frank, N., Sojka, J.E., Latour, M.A., 2002. Effect of feed withholding on concentration and composition of plasma very low density lipoprotein and serum nonesterified fatty acids in horses. American Journal of Veterinary Research 63, 1018–1021.

Frank, N., Sojka, J.E., Patterson, B.W., et al., 2003. Effect of hypothyroidism on kinetics and metabolism of very-low-density lipoprotein in mares. American Journal of Veterinary Research 64, 1052–1058.

Frank, N., Sojka, J.E., Latour, M.A., et al., 2004. Effect of hypothyroidism on the blood lipid response to higher dietary fat intake in mares. Journal of Animal Science 82, 2640–2646.

Frayn, K.N., 2002. Adipose tissue as a buffer for daily lipid flux. Diabetologica 45, 1201–1210.

Freestone, J.F., Wolfsheimer, K.J., Ford, S.B., et al., 1991. Triglyceride, insulin, and cortisol responses of ponies to fasting and dexamethasone administration. Journal of Veterinary Internal Medicine 5, 15–22.

French, K., Pollitt, C.C., Pass, M.A., 2000. Pharmacokinetics and metabolic effects of triamcinolone acetonide and their possible relationships to glucocorticoid-induced laminitis in horses. Journal of Veterinary Pharmacology and Therapeutics 23, 287–292.

Geelen, S.N.J., Jansen, W.L., Sloet van Oldruitenborgh-Oosterbaan, M.M., et al., 2001. Fat feeding increases equine heparin-released lipoprotein lipase activity. Journal of Veterinary Internal Medicine 15, 478–481.

Geor, R.J., Hinchcliff, K.W., Sams, R.A., et al., 2000a. Beta-adrenergic blockade augments glucose utilization in horses during graded exercise. Journal of Applied Physiology 89, 1086–1098.

Geor, R.J., Hinchcliff, K.W., McCutcheon, L.J., et al., 2000b. Epinephrine inhibits exogenous glucose utilization in exercising horses. Journal of Applied Physiology 88, 1777–1790.

Geor, R.J., McCutcheon, L.J., Hinchcliff, K.W., et al., 2002. Training-induced alterations in glucose metabolism during moderate-intensity exercise. Equine Veterinary Journal Supplement 34, 22–28.

Geor, R.J., Larsen, L., Waterfall, H.L., Stewart-Hunt, L., McCutcheon, L.J., 2006. Route of carbohydrate administration affects early post exercise muscle glycogen storage in horses. Equine Veterinary Journal Supplement 36, 590–595.

Geor, R.J., Stewart-Hunt, L., McCutcheon, L.J., 2010. Effects of prior exercise on insulin-mediated and noninsulin-mediated glucose uptake in horses during a hyperglycemic clamp. Equine Veterinary Journal 42 (Suppl. 38), 129–134.

George, L.A., Staniar, W.B., Treiber, K.H., et al., 2009. Insulin sensitivity and glucose dynamics during pre-weaning foal development and in response to maternal diet composition. Domestic Animal Endocrinology 37, 23–29.

George, L.A., Staniar, W.B., Cubitt, T.A., et al., 2011. Evaluation of the effects of pregnancy on insulin sensitivity, secretion, and glucose dynamics in Thoroughbred mares. American Journal of Veterinary Research 72, 666–674.

Gentry, L.R., Thompson, D.L., Gentry, G.T., et al., 2002. The relationship between body condition, leptin, and reproductive and hormonal chracteristics of mares during the seasonal anovulatory period. Journal of Animal Science 80, 2695–2703.

Giacobino, J.P., 2002. Uncoupling proteins, lepti, and obesity: an updated review. Annals of the New York Academy of Sciences 967, 398–402.

Giraudet, A., Hinchcliff, K.W., Kohn, C.W., et al., 1994. Early insulin response to an intravenous glucose tolerance test in horses. American Journal of Veterinary Research 55, 379–381.

Glade, M.J., Luba, N.K., 1987. Serum triiodothyronine and thyroxine concentrations in weanling horses fed carbohydrate by direct gastric infusion. American Journal of Veterinary Research 48, 578–582.

Glade, M.J., Reimers, T.J., 1985. Effects of dietary energy supply on serum thyroxine, triiodothyronine and insulin concentrations in young horses. Journal of Endocrinology 104, 93–98.

Glatz, J.F., Luiken, J.J., Bonen, A., 2010. Membrane fatty acid transporters as regulators of lipid metabolism: implications for metabolic disease. Physiological Reviews 90, 367–417.

Goodyear, L.J., Kahn, B.B., 1998. Exercise, glucose transport, and insulin sensitivity. Annual Review of Medicine 49, 235–259.

Gonzalez, O., Gonzalez, E., Sanchez, C., et al., 1998. Effect of exercise on erythrocyte beta-adrenergic receptors and plasma concentrations of catecholamines and thyroid hormones in Thoroughbred horses. Equine Veterinary Journal 30, 72–78.

Gordon, M.E., McKeever, K.H., 2005. Diurnal variation of ghrelin, leptin, and adiponectin in Standardbred mares. Journal of Animal Science 83, 2365–2371.

Gordon, M.E., McKeever, K.H., 2006a. Oral and intravenous carbohydrate challenges decrease active ghrelin concentrations and alter hormones related to control of energy metabolism in horses. Journal of Animal Science 86, 1682–1690.

Gordon, M.E., McKeever, K.H., Bokman, S., et al., 2006b. Interval exercise alters feed intake as well as leptin and ghrelin concentrations in standardbred mares. Equine Veterinary Journal (Suppl 36), 596–605.

Gordon, M.E., Jerina, M.L., Raub, R.H., et al., 2011. Insulin sensitivity in growing horses fed a higher starch versus a higher fat diet for two years. Journal of Equine Veterinary Science 31, 277–278.

Graham-Thiers, P.M., Bowen, L.K., 2011. Effect of protein source on nitrogen balance and plasma amino acids in exercising horses. Journal of Animal Science 89, 729–735.

Graves, E.A., Schott 2nd, H.C., Marteniuk, J.V., et al., 2006. Thyroid hormone responses to endurance exercise. Equine Veterinary Journal 36 (Suppl), 32–36.

Hackl, S., van den Hoven, R., Zickl, M., et al., 2006. Individual differences and repeatability of post-prandial changes of plasma free amino acids in young horses. Journal of Veterinary Medicine A: Physiology, Pathology and Clinical Medicine 53, 439–444.

Haffner, J.C., Eiler, H., Hoffman, R.C., et al., 2009. Effect of a single dose of dexamethasone on glucose homeostasis in healthy horses by using the combined intravenous glucose and insulin test. Journal of Animal Science 87, 131–135.

Hall, G.M., Adrian, T.E., Bloom, S.R., et al., 1982. Changes in circulating gut hormones in the horse during long distance exercise. Equine Veterinary Journal 14, 209–212.

Harris, P.A., Sillence, M., Inglis, R., et al., 2005. Effect of short (<2 cm) Lucerne chaff addition on the intake rate and glycaemic response of a sweet feed. Pferdeheilkunde 21, 87–88.

Harris, P.A., Geor, R.J., 2009. Primer on dietary carbohydrates and utility of the glycemic index in equine nutrition. Veterinary Clinics of North America Equine Practice 25, 39–50.

Harris, R.C., Marlin, D.J., Snow, D.H., 1987. Metabolic response to maximal exercise of 800 and 2,000 m in the thoroughbred horse. Journal of Applied Physiology 63, 12–19.

Heissig, H., Urban, K.A., Hastedt, K., et al., 2005. Mechanism of the insulin-releasing action of alpha-ketoisocaproate and related alpha-keto acid anions. Molecular Pharmacology 68, 38–46.

Henquin, J.C., Ishiyama, N., Henquin, M., et al., 2002. Signals and pools underlying biphasic insulin secretion. Diabetes 51, S60-S67.

Hintz, H.F., Argenzio, R.A., Schryver, H.F., 1971. Digestion coefficients, blood glucose levels and molar percentage of volatile acids in intestinal fluid of ponies fed varying forage-grain ratios. Journal of Animal Science 33, 992–996.

Hodgson, D.R., Rose, R.J., Allen, J.R., et al., 1984. Glycogen depletion patterns in horses competing in day 2 of a three-day event. Cornell Veterinarian 75, 366–374.

Hodgson, D.R., Rose, R.J., Dimauor, J., et al., 1985. Effects of a submaximal treadmill training programme on histochemical properties, enzyme activities and glycogen utilization of skeletal muscle in the horse. Equine Veterinary Journal 17, 300–305.

Hoffman, R.M., Boston, R.C., Stefanovski, D., et al., 2003. Obesity and diet affect glucose dynamics and insulin sensitivity in Thoroughbred geldings. Journal of Animal Science 81, 2333–2342.

Holdstock, N.B., Allen, V.L., Bloomfield, M.R., et al., 2004. Development of insulin and proinsulin secretion in newborn pony foals. Journal of Endocrinology 181, 469–476.

Holdstock, N.B., Allen, V.L., Fowden, A.L., 2012. Pancreatic endocrine function in newborn pony foals after induced or spontaneous delivery at term. Equine Veterinary Journal 44 (Suppl. 41), 30–37.

Horino, M., Machlin, L.J., Hertelendy, F., et al., 1968. Effect of short-chain fatty acids on plasma insulin in ruminant and nonruminant species. Endocrinology 83, 118–128.

Hyyppä, S., Räsänen, L.A., Pösö, A.R., 1997. Resynthesis of glycogen in skeletal muscle from standardbred trotters after repeated bouts of exercise. American Journal of Veterinary Research 58, 162–166.

Hyyppä, S., Saastamoinen, M., Pösö, A.R., 1999. Effect of a post-exercise fat supplemented diet on muscle glycogen repletion. Equine Veterinary Journal Supplement 30, 493–498.

Irvine, C.H., Evans, M.J., 1975. Post-natal changes in total and free thyroxine and triiodothyronine in foal serum. Journal of Reproduction and Fertility 23 (Suppl), 709–715.

Irwin, D.M., Prentice, K.J., 2011. Incretin hormones and the expanding families of glucagon-like sequences and their receptors. Diabetes, Obesity and Metabolism 13 (Suppl. 1), 69–81.

Ivy, J.L., Goforth, H.W., Damon, B.M., et al., 2002. Early postexercise muscle glycogen recovery is enhanced with a carbohydrate-protein supplement. Journal of Applied Physiology 93, 1337–1344.

Jentjens, R., Jeukendrup, A., 2003. Determinants of post-exercise glycogen storage during short-term recovery. Sports Medicine 33, 117–144.

Jentjens, R., Van Loon, L.J., Mann, C.H., et al., 2001. Addition of protein and amino acids to carbohydrates does not enhance postexercise muscle glycogen synthesis. Journal of Applied Physiology 91, 839–846.

Jensen, T.E., Richter, E.A., 2012. Regulation of glucose and glycogen metabolism during and after exercise. Journal of Physiology 590 (5), 1069–1076.

Johnson, R.J., Hart, J.W., 1974. Influence of feeding and fasting on plasma free amino acids in the equine. Journal of Animal Science 38, 790–794.

Jose-Cunilleras, E., Hinchcliff, K.W., Lacombe, V.A., et al., 2006. Ingestion of starch-rich meals after exercise increases glucose kinetics but fails to enhance muscle glycogen replenishment in horses. Veterinary Journal 171, 468–477.

Kahn, C.R., 1978. Insulin resistance, insulin insensitivity, and insulin unresponsiveness: a necessary distinction. Metabolism 12 (Suppl. 2), 1893–1902.

Kazakos, K., 2011., Incretin effect: GLP-1, GIP and DPP4. Diabetes Research and Clinical Practice 93S, S32–S36. Journal of Endocrinology 2005;186:467–473.

Kimball, S.R., 2007. The role of nutrition in stimulating muscle protein accretion at the molecular level. Biochemical Society Transactions 35, 1298–1301.

Kjaer, M., Howlett, K., Langfort, J., et al., 2000. Adrenaline and glycogenolysis in skeletal muscle during exercise: a study in adrenalectomised humans. Journal of Physiology 528, 371–378.

Korner, J., Woods, S.C., Woodworth, K.A., 2009. Regulation of energy homeostasis and health consequences of obesity. American Journal of Medicine 122, S12–S18.

Kronfeld, D.S., Treiber, K.H., Geor, R.J., 2005. Comparison of nonspecific indications and quantitative methods for the assessment of insulin resistance in horses and ponies. Journal of the American Veterinary Medical Association 226, 712–719.

Lacombe, V.A., Hinchcliff, K.W., Geor, R.J., et al., 2001. Muscle glycogen depletion and subsequent replenishment affect anaerobic capacity of horses. Journal of Applied Physiology 91, 1782–1790.

Lacombe, V.A., Hinchcliff, K.W., Devor, S.T., 2003. Effects of exercise and glucose administration on content of insulin-sensitive glucose transporter in equine skeletal muscle. American Journal of Veterinary Research 64, 1500–1506.

Lacombe, V.A., Hinchcliff, K.W., Kohn, C.W., et al., 2004. Effects of feeding meals with various soluble carbohydrate content on muscle glycogen synthesis after exercise in horses. American Journal of Veterinary Research 65, 916–923.

Liburt, N.R., Fugaro, M.N., Wunderlich, E.K., et al., 2011. The effect of exercise training on insulin sensitivity and fat and muscle tissue cytokine profiles of old and young Standardbred mares. Journal of Equine Veterinary Science 31, 237–238.

Lincoln, G.A., Rhind, S.M., Pompolo, S., et al., 2001. Hypothalamic control of photperiod-induced cycles in food intake, body weight and metabolic hormones in rams. American Journal of Physiology Regulatory, Integrative and Comparative Physiology 281, R76–R90.

Lobley, G.E., Connell, A., Lomax, A., et al., 1995. Hepatic detoxification of ammonia in the ovine liver: possible consequences for amino acid metabolism. British Journal of Nutrition 73, 667–685.

Low, A.Y., Rennie, M.J., Taylor, P.M., 1996. Modulation of glycogen synthesis in rat skeletal muscle by changes in cell volume. J. Physiol. 495, 299–303.

Lowe, J.E., Baldwin, B.H., Foote, R.H., et al., 1974. Equine hypothyroidism: the long term effects of thyroidectomy on metabolism and growth in mares and stallions. Cornell Veterinarian 64, 276–295.

Malinowski, K., Betros, C.L., Flora, L., et al., 2002. Effect of training on age-related changes in plasma insulin and glucose. Equine Veterinary Journal 34 (Suppl.), 147–153.

Mathews, D.E., Marano, M.A., Campbell, R.G., 1993. Splanchnic bed utilization of leucine and phenylalanine in humans. American Journal of Physiology Endocrinology and Metabolism 264, E109–118.

McCue, M.E., Valberg, S.J., Pagan J.D., et al., 2009. Effect of triheptanoin on muscle metabolism during submaximal exercise in horses. American Journal of Veterinary Research 70, 1043–1052.

McCutcheon, L.J., Geor, R.J., Hinchcliff, K.W., 2002. Changes in skeletal muscle GLUT-4 content and muscle membrane glucose transport following 6 weeks of exercise training. Equine Veterinary Journal 34 (Suppl.), 199–204.

McCutcheon, L.J., Geor, R.J., Pratt, S.E., et al., 2006. Effects of prior exercise on components of insulin signaling in equine skeletal muscle. Equine Veterinary Journal 36 (Suppl.), 330–334.

McFarlane, D., Paradis, M.R., Zimmel, D., et al., 2011. The effect of geographic location, breed and pituitary dysfunction on seasonal adrenocorticotropin and α-melanocyte-stimulating hormone plasma concentrations in horses. Journal of Veterinary Internal Medicine 25, 872–881.

McKeever, K.H., 2002. The endocrine system and the challenge of exercise. Veterinary Clinics of North America Equine Practice 18, 321–353.

McMahon, M., Gerich, J., Rizza, R., 1988. Effects of glucocorticoids on carbohydrate metabolism. Diabetes Metabolism Reviews 4, 17–30.

McManus, C.J., Fitzgerald, B.P., 2000. Effects of a single day of feed restriction on changes in serum leptin, gonadotropins, prolactin, and metabolites in aged and young mares. Domestic Animal Endocrinology 19, 1–13.

McNamara, J.P., 1991. Regulation of adipose tissue metabolism in support of lactation. Journal of Dairy Science 74, 706–719.

McNamara, J.P., Murray, C.E., 2001. Sympathetic nervous system activity in adipose tissues during pregnancy and lactation in the rat. Journal of Dairy Science 84, 1382–1389.

Meyer, C., Dostou, J.M., Welle, S.L., et al., 2002. Role of human liver, kidney, and sketal muscle in postprandial glucose homeostasis. American Journal of Physiology Endocrinology and Metabolism 282, E419–E427.

Meyers, M.C., Potter, G.D., Evans, J.W., et al., 1989. Physiologic and metabolic responses of exercising horses to added dietary fat. Journal of Equine Veterinary Science 9, 218–223.

Miller, P.A., Lawrence, L.M., 1988. The effect of dietary protein level on exercising horses. Journal of Animal Science 66, 2185–2192.

Møller, N., Jørgensen, J.O., 2009. Effects of growth hormone on glucose, lipid, and protein metabolism in human subjects. Endocrine Reviews 30, 152–177.

Moore, M.C., Cherrington, A.D., Wasserman, D.H., 2003. Regulation of hepatic and peripheral glucose disposal. Best Practice & Research Clinical Endocrinology & Metabolism 17, 343–364.

Morton, G.J., Niswender, K.D., Rhodes, C.J., et al., 2003. Arcuate-specific leptin receptor gene therapy attenuates the obesity phenotype of Koletsky (fa(k)/fa(k)) rats. Endocrinology 144, 2016–2024.

Muniyappa, R., Lee, S., Chen, H., et al., 2008. Current approaches for assessing insulin sensitivity and resistance in vivo. American Journal of Physiology Endocrinology and Metabolism 294, E15–E26.

Murphy, K.G., Bloom, S.R., 2006. Gut hormones and the regulation of energy balance. Nature 444, 854–859.

Nagata, S., Takeda, F., Kurosawa, M., et al., 1999. Plasma adrenocorticotropin, cortisol and catecholamine responses to various exercises. Equine Veterinary Journal 30 (Suppl.), 570–574.

Nakae, J., Kido, Y., Accili, D., 2001. Distinct and overlapping functions of insulin and IGF-1 receptors. Endocrinology Reviews 22, 818–835.

Nielsen, J.N., Derave, W., Kristiansen, S., et al., 2001. Glycogen synthase localization and activity in rat skeletal muscle is strongly dependent on glycogen content. Journal of Physiology 531, 757–769.

Orme, C.E., Harris, R.C., Marlin, D.J., et al., 1997. Metabolic adaptations to a fat supplemented diet by the thoroughbred horse. British Journal of Nutrition 78, 443–458.

Ott, E.A., Brown, M.P., Roberts, G.D., et al., 2005. Influence of starch intake on growth and skeletal development of weanling horses. Journal of Animal Science 83, 1033–1043.

Pagan, J.D., Harris, P.A., 1999. The effects of timing and amount of forage and grain on exercise response in Thoroughbred horses. Equine Veterinary Journal 30 (Suppl.), 451–457.

Pagan, J.D., Waldridge, B.M., Lange, J., 2011. Moderate dietary carbohydrate improves glucose tolerance and high dietary fat impairs glucose tolerance in aged Thoroughbred geldings. Proceedings of the American Association of Equine Practitioners 57, 192 (abstract).

Pethick, D.W., Lindsay, D.B., Barker, P.J., et al., 1981. Acetate supply and utilization by the tissues of sheep in vivo. British Journal of Nutrition 46, 97–110.

Pethick, D.W., Rose, R.J., Bryden, W.L., et al., 1993. Nutrient utilisation by the hindlimb of thoroughbred horses at rest. Equine Veterinary Journal 25, 41–44.

Place, N.J., McGowan, C.M., Lamb, S.V., et al., 2010. Seasonal variation in serum concentrations of selected metabolic hormones in horses. Journal of Veterinary Internal Medicine 24, 650–654.

Pösö, A.R., Hyyppä, S., 1999. Metabolic and hormonal changes after exercise in relation to muscle glycogen concentrations. Equine Veterinary Journal 30 (Suppl.), 332–336.

Pösö, A.R., Hyyppä, S., Geor, R.J., 2008. Metabolic responses to exercise and training. In: Hinchcliff, K.W., Geor, R.J., Kaneps, A.J. (Eds.), Equine Exercise Physiology. Saunders Elsevier, Philadelphia, pp. 248–272.

Pørksen, N., 2002. The in vivo regulation of pulsatile insulin secretion. Diabetologica 45, 3–20.

Powell, D.M., Lawrence, L.M., Fitzgerald, B.P., et al., 2000. Effect of short-term feed restriction and calorie source on hormonal and metabolic responses in geldings receiving a small meal. Journal of Animal Science 78, 3107–3113.

Powell, D.M., Reedy, S.E., Sessions, D.R., et al., 2002. Effect of short-term exercise on insulin sensitivity in obese and lean mares. Equine Veterinary Journal 34 (Suppl.), 81–84.

Pratt, S.E., Geor, R.J., McCutcheon, L.J., 2006. Effects of dieary energy source and physical conditioning on insulin sensitivity and glucose tolerance in Standardbred horses. Equine Veterinary Journal 36 (Suppl.), 579–584.

Pratt, S.E., Geor, R.J., Spriet, L.L., et al., 2007. Time course of insulin sensitivity and skeletal muscle glycogen synthase activity after a single bout of exercise in horses. Journal of Applied Physiology 103, 1063–1069.

Radicke, S., Meyer, H., Kienzle, E., 1994. Über den Einfluß von Futterart und Fütterungszeitpunkt auf den Blutglucosespiegel bei Pferden. Pferdeheilkunde 10, 187–190.

Ralston, S.L., Baile, C.A., 1982a. Plasma glucose and insulin concentrations and feeding behaviour in ponies. Journal of Animal Science 54, 1132–1137.
Ralston, S.L., Baile, C.A., 1982b. Gastrointestinal stimuli in the control of feed intake in ponies. Journal of Animal Science 55, 243–253.
Ralston, S.L., Baile, C.A., 1983. Effects of intragastric loads of xylose, sodium chloride and corn oil on feeding behaviour of ponies. Journal of Animal Science 56, 302–308.
Ralston, S.L., Freeman, D.E., Baile, C.A., 1983. Volatile fatty acids and the role of the large intestine in the control of feed intake in ponies. Journal of Animal Science 57, 815–825.
Ramnanan, C.J., Edgerton, D.S., Kraft, G., et al., 2011. Physiologic action of glucagon on liver glucose metabolism. Diabetes, obesity and metabolism 13 (Suppl 1), 118–125.
Renaville, R., Hammadi, M., Portelle, D., 2002. Role of the somatotropic axis in the mammalian metabolism. Domestic Animal Endocrinology 23, 351–360.
Rennie, M.J., Edwards, R.H., Halliday, D., et al., 1982. Muscle protein synthesis measured by stable isotope techniques in man: the effects of feeding and fasting. Clinical Science (London) 63, 519–523.
Reynolds, C.K., Maltby, S.A., 1994. Regulation of nutrient partitioning by visceral tissues in ruminants. Journal of Nutrition 124, 1399S-1403S.
Rijnen, K.E., van der Kolk, J.H., 2003. Determination of reference range values indicative of glucose metabolism and insulin resistance by use of glucose clamp techniques in horses and ponies. American Journal of Veterinary Research 64, 1260–1264.
Rivero, J.L.L., Piercy, R.J., 2004. Muscle physiology: responses to exercise and training. In: Hinchcliff, K.W., Kaneps, A.J., Geor, R.J. (Eds.), Equine Sports Medicine and Surgery. Saunders, London, pp. 45–76.
Russell, M.A., Rodiek, A.V., Lawrence, L.M., 1986. Effect of meal schedules and fasting on selected plasma free amino acids in horses. Journal of Animal Science 63, 1428–1431.
Salazar-Ortiz, J., Camous, S., Briant, C., et al., 2011. Effects of nutritional cues on the duration of the winter anovulatory phase and on associated hormone levels in adult female Welsh pony horses (Equus caballus). Reproductive Biology and Endocrinology 9, 130.
Schalch, D.S., Cree, T.C., 1985. Protein utilization in growth: Effect of calorie deficiency on serum growth hormone, somatomedins, total thyroxine and triiodothyronine, free T_4 index, and total corticosterone. Endocrinology 117, 2307–2311.
Schmidt, S.L., Hickey, M.S., 2009. Regulation of insulin action by diet and exercise. Journal of Equine Veterinary Science 29, 274–284.
Schulz, C., Paulus, K., Lobmann, R., et al., 2010. Endogenous ACTH, not only α-melanocyte-stimulating hormone, reduces food intake mediated by hypothalamic mechanisms. American Journal of Physiology Endocrinology and Metabolism 298, E237–E244.
Schwartz, M.W., Woods, S.C., Porte Jr., D., et al., 2000. Central nervous system control of food intake. Nature 404, 661–671.
Seino, S., Shibasaki, T., Minami, K., 2011. Dynamics of insulin secretion and the clinical implications for obesity and diabetes. Journal of Clinical Investigation 121, 2118–2125.
Sener, A., Best, L.C., Yates, A.P., et al., 2000. Stimulus-secretion coupling of arginine-induced insulin release: comparison between the cationic amino acid and its methyl ester. Endocrine 13, 329–340.
Shaw, C.S., Clark, J., Wagenmakers, A.J.M., 2010. The effect of exercise and nutrition on intramuscular fat metabolism and insulin sensitivity. Annual Reviews in Nutrition 30, 13–34.
Simmons, H.A., Ford, E.J., 1991. Gluconeogenesis from propionate produced in the colon of the horse. British Veterinary Journal 147, 340–344.
Sisley, S., Sandoval, D., 2011. Hypothalamic control of energy and glucose metabolism. Review of Endocrine and Metabolic Disorders 12, 219–233.
Smyth, G.B., Young, D.W., Duran, S.H., 1993. Maturation of insulin and glucose responses to normal feeding in foals. Australian Veterinary Journal 70, 129–132.
Snow, D.H., Harris, R.C., 1991. Effects of daily exercise on muscle glycogen in the Thoroughbred racehorse. In: Persson, S.G.B., Lindholm, A., Jeffcott, L.B. (Eds.), Equine Exercise Physiology 3. ICEEP Publications, Davis, CA, pp. 299–304.
Snow, D.H., Baxter, P., Rose, R.J., 1981. Muscle fibre composition and glycogen depletion in horses competing in an endurance ride. Veterinary Record 108, 374–378.
Snow, D.H., Harris, R.C., Gash, S.P., 1985. Metabolic response of equine muscle to intermittent maximal exercise. Journal of Applied Physiology 58, 1689–1697.
Sorenson, R.L., Brelje, T.C., 1997. Adaptations of islets of Langerhans to pregnancy: beta-cell growth, enhanced insulin secretion and the role of lactogenic hormones. Hormone and Metabolic Research 29, 301–307.
Spiegelman, B.M., Flier, J.S., 2001. Obesity and its regulation of energy balance. Cell 104, 531–543.
Steinberg, H.O., Baron, A.D., 2002. Vascular function, insulin resistance and fatty acids. Diabetologica 45, 623–634.
Stewart-Hunt, L., Geor, R.J., McCutcheon, L.J., 2006. Effects of short-term training on insulin sensitivity and skeletal muscle glucose metabolism in standardbred horses. Equine Veterinary Journal 36 (Suppl.), 226–232.
Sticker, L.S., Thompson Jr., D.L., Bunting, L.D., et al., 1995a. Feed deprivation of mares: Plasma metabolite and hormonal concentrations and responses to exercise. Journal of Animal Science 73, 3696–3704.
Sticker, L.S., Thompson Jr., D.L., Bunting, L.D., et al., 1995b. Dietary protein and(or) energy restriction in mares: plasma glucose, insulin, nonesterified fatty acid, and urea nitrogen responses to feeding, glucose, and epinephrine. Journal of Animal Science 73, 136–144.
Sticker, L.S., Thompson Jr., D.L., Bunting, L.D., et al., 1996. Dietary protein and energy restriction in mares: Rapid changes in plasma metabolite and hormone concentrations during dietary alteration. Journal of Animal Science 74, 1326–1335.
Sticker, L.S., Thompson Jr., D.L., Gentry, L.R., 2001. Pituitary hormone and insulin responses to infusion of amino acids and *N*-methyl-d,l-aspartate in horses. Journal of Animal Science 79, 735–744.
Stuart, C.A., Yin, D., Howell, M.A., et al., 2006. Hexose transporter mRNAs for GLUT4, GLUT5 and GLUT4 predominate in human muscle. American Journal of Physiology Endocrinology and Metabolism 291, E1067–E1073.
Stuart, C.A., Howell, M.E., Zhang, Y., et al., 2009. Insulin-stimulated translocation of glucose transporter (GLUT) 12 parallels that of GLUT4 in normal muscle. Journal of Clinical Endocrinology and Metabolism 94, 3535–3542.
Suagee, J.K., Corl, B.A., Crisman, M.V., et al., 2010. *De novo* fatty acid synthesis and NADPH generation in equine adipose and liver tissue. Comparative Biochemistry and Physiology Part B 155, 322–326.
Suagee, J.K., Corl, B.A., Hulver, M.W., et al., 2011a. Effects of hyperinsulinaemia on glucose and lipid transporter expression in insulin-sensitive horses. Domestic Animal Endocrinology 40, 173–181.
Suagee, J.K., Corl, B.A., Swyers, K.L., et al., 2011b. A 90-day adaptation to a high glycaemic diet alters postprandial lipid metabolism in non-obese horses without affecting peripheral insulin sensitivity. Journal of Animal Physiology and Animal Nutrition (published online Nov 30, 2011). DOI:10.111/j.1439-0396.2011.01261.x.
Tiley, H.A., Geor, R.J., McCutcheon, L.J., 2007. Effects of dexamethasone on glucose dynamics and insulin sensitivity in healthy horses. American Journal of Veterinary Research 68, 753–759.
Timmerman, K.L., Volpi, E., 2008. Amino acid metabolism and regulatory effects in aging. Current Opinion in Clinical Nutrition and Metabolic Care 11, 45–49.
Tinworth, K.D., Raidal, S.L., Boston, R.C., et al., 2011. Effect of diet on insulin sensitivity in insulin-resistant ponies. Journal of Equine Veterinary Science 31, 258–259.
Thornton, J.R., 1985. Hormonal responses to exercise and training. Veterinary Clinics of North America Equine Practice 2, 477–496.
Topliff, D.R., Potter, G.D., Kreider, J.L., 1985. Diet manipulation, muscle glycogen metabolism and anaero.bic work performance in the equine. In: Proceedings of the 9th Equine Nutrition and Physiology Symposium. American Society of Animal Science, Champaign, IL, pp. 224–229.
Tóth, F., Frank, N., Elliott, S.B., et al., 2009. Optimisation of the frequently sampled intravenous glucose tolerance test to reduce urinary glucose spilling in horses. Equine Veterinary Journal 41, 844–851.
Tóth, F., Frank, N., Martin-Jimenez, T., et al., 2010. Measurement of C-peptide concentrations and responses to somatostatin, glucose infusion, and insulin resistance in horses. Equine Veterinary Journal 42, 149–155.
Treebak, J.T., Frosig, C., Pehmoller, C., et al., 2009. Potential role of TBC1D4 in enhanced post-exercise insulin action in human skeletal muscle. Diabetologica 52, 891–900.
Treiber, K.H., Kronfeld, D.S., Hess, T.M., et al., 2005a. Use of proxies and reference quintiles obtained from minimal model analysis for determination of insulin sensitivity and pancreatic beta-cell responsiveness in horses. American Journal of Veterinary Research 66, 2114–2121.
Treiber, K.H., Boston, R.C., Kronfeld, D.S., et al., 2005b. Insulin resistance and compensation in Thoroughbred weanlings adapted to high-glycemic diets. Journal of Animal Science 83, 2357–2364.
Treiber, K.H., Kronfeld, D.S., Geor, R.J., 2006a. Insulin resistance in equids: Possible role in laminitis. Journal of Nutrition 136, 2094S–2098S.
Treiber, K.H., Hess, T.M., Kronfeld, D.S., et al., 2006b. Glucose dynamics during exercise: dietary energy sources affect minimal model parameters in trained Arabian geldings during endurance exercise. Equine Veterinary Journal 36 (Suppl.), 631–636.
Treiber, K., Hess, T., Geor, R., et al., 2007. Insulin resistance and compensation in laminitis-predisposed ponies characterized by the Minimal Model. Pferheildekunde 23, 237–240.
Urschel, K.L., Geor, R.J., Waterfall, H.L., et al., 2010. Effects of leucine or whey protein addition to an oral glucose solution on serum insulin, plasma glucose and plasma amino acid responses in horses at rest and following exercise. Equine Veterinary Journal 42 (Suppl. 38), 347–354.
Urschel, K.L., Escobar, J., McCutcheon, L.J., et al., 2011. Effect of feeding a high-protein diet following an 18-hour period of feed withholding on mammalian target of rapamycin-dependent signaling in skeletal muscle of mature horses. American Journal of Veterinary Research 72, 248–255.
Urschel, K.L., Geor, R.J., Hanigan, M.D., et al., 2012. Amino acid supplementation does not alter whole-body phenylalanine kinetics in Arabian geldings. Journal of Nutrition 142, 461–469.

Valberg, S.J., 1985. Glycogen depletion patterns in the muscle of Standardbred trotters after exercise of varying intensities and durations. Equine Veterinary Journal 17, 439–444.

van Dam, K.G., van Breda, E., Schaart, G., et al., 2004. Investigation of the expression and localization of glucose transporter 4 and fatty acid translocase/CD36 in equine skeletal muscle. American Journal of Veterinary Research 65, 951–956.

Van Loon, L.J.C., Saris, W.H.M., Kruijshoop, M., et al., 2000. Maximizing postexercise muscle glycogen synthesis: carbohydrate supplementation and the application of amino acid or protein hydrolysate mixtures. American Journal of Clinical Nutrition 72, 106–111.

Van Weyenberg, S., Hesta, M., Buyse, J., et al., 2008. Short-term effects of energy changes on plasma leptin concentrations and glucose tolerance in healthy ponies. Veterinary Journal 178, 233–237.

Vervuert, I., Voigt, K., Hollands, T., et al., 2009a. Effect of feeding increasing quantities of starch on glycaemic and insulinaemic responses in healthy horses. Veterinary Journal 182, 67–72.

Vervuert, I., Klein, S., Coenen, M., 2009b. Effect of mixing dietary fibre (purified lignocelluloses or purified pectin) and a corn meal on glucose and insulin responses in healthy horses. Journal of Animal Physiology and Animal Nutrition (Berlin) 93, 331–338.

Vervuert, I., Voigt, K., Hollands, T., et al., 2009c. The effect of mixing and changing the order of feeding oats and chopped alfalfa to horses on: glycaemic and insulinaemic responses, and breath hydrogen and methane production. Journal of Animal Physiology and Animal Nutrition (Berlin) 93, 631–638.

Vick, M.M., Adams, A.A., Murphy, B.A., et al., 2007. Relationships among inflammatory cytokines, obesity and insulin sensitivity in the horse. Journal of Animal Science 85, 1144–1155.

Vischer, C.M., Foreman, J.H., Constable, P.D., et al., 1999. Hemodynamic effects of thyroidectomy in sedentary horses. American Journal of Veterinary Research 60, 14–21.

Volpi, E., Lucidi, P., Cruciani, G., et al., 1996. Contribution of amino acids and insulin to protein anabolism during meal absorption. Diabetes 45, 1245–1252.

Votion, D.M., Navet, R., Lacombe, V.A., et al., 2008. Muscle energetic in exercising horses. Equine and Comparative Exercise Physiology 4, 105–118.

Waller, A.P., Geor, R.J., Spriet, L.L., et al., 2009a. Oral acetate supplementation after prolonged moderate intensity exercise enhances early muscle glycogen resynthesis in horses. Experimental Physiology 94, 888–989.

Waller, A.P., Heigenhauser, G.J.F., Geor, R.J., et al., 2009b. Fluid and electrolyte supplementation after prolonged moderate-intensity exercise enhances muscle glycogen resynthesis in horses. Journal of Applied Physiology 106, 91–100.

Waller, A.P., Lindinger, M.I., 2010. Nutritional aspects of post exercise skeletal muscle glycogen synthesis in horses: A comparative review. Equine Veterinary Journal 42, 274–281.

Waller, A.P., Burns, T.A., Mudge, M.C., et al., 2011a. Insulin resistance selectively alters cell-surface glucose transporters but not their total protein expression in equine skeletal muscle. Journal of Veterinary Internal Medicine 25, 315–321.

Waller, A.P., Kohler, K., Burns, T.A., et al., 2011b. Naturally occurring compensated insulin resistance selectively alters glucose transporters in visceral and subcutaneous adipose tissues without change in AS160 activation. Biochimica et Biophysica Acta 1812, 1098–1103.

Wahren, J., Ekberg, K., Johansson, J., et al., 2000. Role of C-peptide in human physiology. American Journal of Physiology: Endocrinology and Metabolism 278, E759–E768.

Wasserman, D.H., 1995. Regulation of glucose fluxes during exercise in the postabsorptive state. Annual Review of Physiology 57, 191–218.

Wasserman, D.H., 2009. Four grams of glucose. American Journal of Physiology Endocrinology and Metabolism 296, E11–E21.

Wasserman, D.H., Spalding, J.A., Lacy, D.B., et al., 1989. Glucagon is a primary controller of hepatic glycogenolysis and gluconeogenesis during muscular work. American Journal of Physiology Endocrinology and Metabolism 257, E108–E117.

Watt, M.J., Hargreaves, M., 2002. Effect of epinephrine on glucose disposal during exercise in humans: role of muscle glycogen. American Journal of Physiology Endocrinology and Metabolism 283, E578–E583.

Wendel, A.A., Levin, T.M., Coleman, R.A., 2009. Glycerol-3-phosphate acyltransferases: rate limiting enzymes of triacylglycerol biosynthesis. Biochimica et Biophysica Acta 1791, 501–506.

Wilcox, G., 2005. Insulin and insulin resistance. Clinical Biochemistry Reviews 26, 19–39.

White, M.G., Snow, D.H., 1987. Quantitative histochemical study of glycogen depletion in the maximally exercised Thoroughbred. Equine Veterinary Journal 19, 67–69.

Woerle, H.J., Meyer, C., Dostou, J.M., et al., 2003. Pathways for glucose disposal after meal ingestion in humans. American Journal of Physiology Endocrinology and Metabolism 284, E716–E725.

Wojtaszewski, J.F.P., Nielsen, J.N., Richter, E.A., 2002. Invited review: effect of acute exercise on insulin signalling and action in humans. Journal of Applied Physiology 93, 384–392.

Wolever, T.M., Jenkins, D.J., Ocana, A.M., et al., 1988. Second-meal effect: Low glycemic index foods eaten at dinner improve subsequent breakfast glycemic response. American Journal of Clinical Nutrition 48, 1041–1047.

Wu, G., 2009. Amino acids: metabolism, functions, and nutrition. Amino Acids 37, 1–17.

Yang, X., Yang, C., Farberman, A., et al., 2008. The mammalian target of rapamycin-signaling pathway in regulating metabolism and growth. Journal of Animal Science 86, E36–E50.

Zhang, L., Keung, W., Samokhvalov, V., et al., 2010. Role of fatty acid uptake and fatty acid beta-oxidation in mediating insulin resistance in heart and skeletal muscle. Biochimica et Biophysica Acta 1801, 1–22.

3

Factors affecting feed intake

Derek Cuddeford

Knowledge of food intake is basic to the appropriate feeding of animals. Knowledge of daily nutrient requirements *per se* is of no value if the likely food intake of an animal is not known because the nutrients have to be "packaged" into a mass that the animal can consume within a 24 h period. Furthermore, underfeeding a horse in terms of feed mass, although not necessarily food nutrients, will mean that appetite will remain unsatisfied and, in the case of horses, this can lead to the development of undesirable stereotypic behaviors. Thus, it is essential to know the likely food intake of a horse or pony and also, to be aware of those factors that can moderate intake. Nowadays, obesity amongst the equid population is a problem of increasing significance and in order to limit or even control the intake of energy we must discover how to moderate this intake in a "welfare-friendly" fashion in order to maintain the health status of these animals. This chapter provides a summary of factors that are thought to influence intake (quality and quantity, palatability and appetite) as well as rate of intake. Hormonal regulation of feed intake is briefly discussed elsewhere (Chapter 2).

Quantitative intake

It is not known whether the controls of intake are the same for horses, ponies, different sexes, ages or breed types. However, we do know that breed size affects the rate of intake because of differences in the size of the harvesting (incisor arcade) and food processing features of the mouth (molar battery) that affect "handling time". This time increases linearly with bite size and the maximum processing rate increases with body size (Fleurance et al 2009). These authors suggested that smaller breeds are more constrained when bite size increases. Furthermore, they discovered a significant effect ($p<0.0001$) of the bite size × NDF interaction in ponies, which suggests that they are less well-adapted to dealing with high fiber feeds. It seems that when they encounter high fiber swards they limit their chewing activities rather than increasing their effort in handling.

Feedback mechanisms

Several feedback mechanisms appear to affect food intake by horses and these are detailed below.

Oropharyngeal monitoring

Ralston (1984) concluded that horses rely primarily on oropharyngeal and external stimuli to control the size and duration of an isolated meal. This conclusion was based on a study with ponies that were sham-fed but performed normal sequences of satiety behavior following a meal. However, only three ponies were used in the study and it is still possible that both metabolic and gastrointestinal inputs could moderate feeding behavior. The author considered that meal frequency is regulated by the presence and/or absorption of the products of digestion together with metabolic cues that may reflect body energy stores. However, the influence of the latter may be deemed weak in view of the fact that fat ponies tend to get fatter and remain fat. It is generally accepted (Cuddeford pers. observation) that equids are more sensitive to the feel, smell and taste of their food than are ruminants and thus, oropharyngeal monitoring must be more important in this species. This seems to be the case especially when offered clamp silage (Moore-Colyer & Longland 2000) or when fed straw. Dulphy et al (1997b) suggested that the organoleptic qualities of the latter may well limit its intake by horses.

Digestion end products

Ralston et al (1979) suggested a relationship between plasma glucose, subsequent meal size and rate of eating by ponies after a 3 h fast. After a 4 h fast, a control infusion of 2 liters of water had no effect on feeding behavior whereas an infusion of 2 liters of water containing 300 g of dissolved glucose decreased intakes of a pelleted diet 0 to 3 h post-treatment (Ralston & Baile 1982a). This probably represents a post-absorptive effect rather than a localized gastric response because of its duration. However, the tonicity of the glucose infusion solution could have affected fluid balance that, in itself could have had an effect. Ralston and Baile (1983) showed that reductions in intake occurred at times that would, in fact, reflect the postabsorptive state; 10 to 15 min for glucose and 4 to 6 h for cellulose. An intragastric infusion of 133 g of corn oil immediately after a 4 h fast, and before being given *ad libitum* access to a pelleted diet, did not affect consumption of the diet but did reduce subsequent intake by tripling the normal inter-meal interval. This could have resulted from metabolic feedback or a reduced rate of gastric emptying. Ralston and Baile (1982a) concluded that elevated levels of plasma glucose and insulin do not immediately generate satiety cues in ponies, although this view was based on glucose infusions via the jugular vein. Such an infusion would enable utilization of the metabolite and possibly, reduce effects at receptor sites. It is also probable that the glucose would have bypassed liver receptors as well. In this context it is worth noting that portal vein glucose sensors monitor glucose uptake from the gut and are involved in whole body glucose disposal, at least in rodents (Hevener et al 2001), dogs (Pagliassoti et al 1996) and pigs (Schmitt 1973). The signals generated affect the function of the liver and pancreas, tissues that are involved in glucose homeostasis (Burcelin et al 2001). Furthermore, signals enter the central nervous system to regulate functions such as feeding and satiety (Schmitt 1973). However, in the horse, it is hard to imagine that such an animal that has evolved essentially to ferment forage with the resultant evolution of volatile fatty acids (VFAs), will have a well-developed glucose sensing system in the portal vein.

Fermentation end products

Fermentation occurs throughout the horses' gastrointestinal tract (GIT) releasing VFAs such as acetic, propionic, and butyric acid. Most are produced in the large intestine and, following absorption, are available in the liver where they can be used as a source of energy or in fat storage. It is conceivable that, like glucose, they may have a role in appetite regulation. Intragastric infusion of acetate (0.75 mmol/kg LW) caused ponies to increase feed intake ($p<0.05$) by reducing the duration of the first inter-meal interval (Ralston et al 1983). Intravenous studies with short chain VFAs have not been undertaken and as a result, it is not known how circulating levels of these acids may affect voluntary dry matter intake (VDMI). Following a 4 h fast, above normal levels of acetate (1.0 and 1.25 mmol/kg LW) and propionate (0.75 mmol/kg LW) were introduced as a bolus into the cecum of ponies. VDMI was reduced in that the first inter-meal interval was prolonged (Ralston et al 1983). An intracecal infusion of 0.4 mol propionate per kg LW significantly ($p<0.05$) increased VDMI by 1.075 relative to control values. In contrast, an infusion of 1 mmol propionate per kg LW significantly ($p<0.01$) reduced by 0.22, the size of the first meal consumed without affecting subsequent feeding behaviors. Thus, there is some evidence to suggest local effects of VFAs within the GIT but the work was very limited. Furthermore, these animals were provided with complete pelleted diets that were fed *ad libitum* and consumed in 10/11 meals per day. However, the relevance of this type of research to the intake of an *ad libitum* forage-fed horse or pony is questionable.

Physical distention

The effect of gut fill on intake is equivocal. Intragastric infusions of kaolin had no significant effect on VDMI or feeding behavior of ponies when compared with control animals (Ralston & Baile 1982b). The authors suggested that stomach fill had no effect on intake although this ignores the fact that kaolin is inert and that it would not generate stimuli analogous to those produced by feed residues. Removal of 1.2 to 1.5 liters of cecal contents (equivalent to 0.22 of total cecal content of a 200 kg pony) also had no effect on subsequent feeding behavior of ponies (Ralston et al 1983). However, intra-gastric infusions of α-cellulose significantly ($p<0.05$) reduced total VDMI after 3 to 18 h post-infusion (Ralston & Baile, 1982b). Both of these results need to be interpreted with care because removal of a small amount of digesta is unlikely to have had much effect on intake and, in the case of α-cellulose, it could have had a "fill" effect, a metabolite effect or both. In fact, Ralston and Baile (1982a) suggested that intragastric loads of nutrients generate satiety cues in ponies that are not related to the volume or bulk of the treatment.

Neutral detergent fiber (NDF) apparent digestibility and NDF content of feed are not reliable predictors of VDMI ($r^2=0.266$) in horses (Cymbaluk 1990), suggesting that physical capacity of the large intestine is unlikely to limit feed intake. However, if fecal output were a determinant of VDMI then large intestinal capacity could have a role in controlling intake. The flow of digesta through the horse's GIT is slowed but it is not limited by particle size in the same way as it is in ruminants since there is no analogous structure to the reticulo-omasal orifice. Thus, digesta cannot be retained in the horse's GIT in the same way that it can in ruminants and therefore, there is less likelihood of "fill" negatively affecting intake.

The mean retention time (MRT) of feed residues in limit-fed ponies (17.5 g DM per kg LW/72 g DM per kg $W^{0.75}$) given lucerne silage alone, enzyme-treated silage or the same silage substituted with 0.30 DM sugar beet pulp (SBP) was not significantly different (Murray et al 2009). The excretion curves for hay and oats were very similar when fed to 500 kg cold-blooded Norwegian trotters and there seemed to be no difference in MRT between the hay and oats (Rosenfeld et al 2006). Furthermore, barley, maize, and wheat were ground, pelleted, extruded, or micronized to create a total of 12 processed grains and then fed in combination with hay to the same horses in order to measure gastrointestinal retention times (Rosenfeld & Austbø 2009). Processing appeared to affect passage rates and compartmental retention times, but did not affect the overall MRT. However, the authors seemed unclear as to which was the time-dependent compartment in the model used. The foregoing suggests that very different diets/feeds may have similar MRTs and thus, their respective intakes would be unlikely to be affected by feed residue residency times in the GIT.

Feed factors

Feed type

A horse may be fed a wide variety of different materials ranging in DM content from as low as 150 g/kg (almost akin to that of milk) to as high as 950 g/kg and furthermore, the cell wall content (NDF) can be as low as 100 and as high as 800 g/kg DM. This diversity in feed characteristics is likely to impact on the VDMI of these different feeds by horses.

Fresh forage

Archer (1973) was probably the first person to investigate the grass species preferences of horses and showed that the most palatable sward comprised a clover-rich mixture. Pasture varieties of perennial ryegrass were very palatable and as acceptable as timothy and cocksfoot. Tall fescue, crested dogs tail and wild white clover were other species found to be palatable for horses. Smith et al (2007) used the *n*-alkane technique to quantify the VDMI of horses grazing a clover-rich sward (dry herbage mass 1741 kg/ha, DM 230 g/kg, crude protein [CP] 101 g/kg DM, NDF 828 g/kg DM and acid detergent fiber [ADF] 691 g/kg DM), given no other feed. The estimated VDMI varied from animal to animal in the range 32 to 54 g/kg/day or from 150 to 254 g DM per kg $W^{0.75}$ measured over a 4-week period. Similar high intakes were estimated recently (Longland et al 2011a) in ponies (268±52 kg) based on LW change over a 6-week period at pasture (CP 129 g/kg DM, NDF 423 g/kg DM). The ponies averaged a daily gain of 0.96 kg and VDMI ranged from 0.029 to 0.049 LW. Edouard et al (2009) measured intakes up to only 152 g/kg $W^{0.75}$ but claimed to be the first to show that sward height affects patch selection and ingestive behavior in horses independently of variations in the nutritive value of forages. Daily VDMI averaged 21 g DM per kg LW per day (100 g/kg $W^{0.75}$) and varied between 14 and 32 g DM per kg LW per day (66 to 152 g/kg $W^{0.75}$) for individual horses; these differences were not significant. The horses selected vegetative patches of grass that they could ingest fastest and thus their feeding behavior accords with the predictions of optimal foraging models as proposed by Stephens and Krebs (1986) for large ruminant herbivores. It seems that horses have the ability to ingest large quantities of fresh herbage DM well in excess of need and that assumed by the National Research Council (2007) in their recommendations provided there is a high herbage mass. Furthermore, sward height rather than herbage quality seems to strongly influence selection. Clearly, estimates of the VDMI of fresh forage vary widely (66–254 g DM per kg $W^{0.75}$) and those horses that consume large quantities will become obese and thus prone to metabolic disease. The question remains as to why some horses are able to ingest so much more DM than others?

There is a paucity of information in relation to the VDMI of fresh forage by horses, but that which is available is detailed in Table 3-1. Dulphy et al (1997b) included data for 16 fresh forages (covering a range of NDF from 300 to 611 g/kg DM) and obtained a mean intake figure similar to that for grass hays whose NDF content varied from 495 to 709 g/kg DM. Published values for fresh forages obtained from the literature by Dulphy et al (1997b) varied between 90 and 117 g/kg, with a mean of 105 g DM per kg $W^{0.75}$, not that dissimilar from the data that they derived. As a result of these Institut National de la Recherche Agronomique (INRA) experiments, these authors suggested a probable fresh forage (grass) intake of 19–22 g DM per kg LW in the absence of a reliable means of predicting intake based on the classical parameters such as crude fiber (CF) and NDF as used for ruminants.

Forage intake work reported in New Zealand (Grace et al 2002a, b) with yearlings and lactating brood mares was based on fecal collection off the pasture and an *in vivo* assessment of pasture digestibility. The latter was done by cutting pasture and feeding it to confined horses in order to measure the apparent DM digestibility *in vivo*; VDMI by confined horses measured during a digestibility trial was lower than when grazing. The depression was 0.10–0.15 in stalled yearlings and 0.05–0.08 in corralled mares; both groups were offered about 0.30 excess herbage. This outcome illustrated the importance of grazing preference and its effect on VDMI (see earlier). The pasture intake by Australian stockhorse weanlings was measured differently by McMeniman (2000) in Australia using alkane markers but the results obtained (20–30 g DM per kg LW) were similar to those reported in New Zealand (~20 g DM per kg LW). Although the grass intakes by weanlings and yearlings in New Zealand met nutrient requirements, the intakes on the basis of $W^{0.75}$ were rather low.

Conserved forage

Hay Cymbaluk (1990) compared a number of Canadian grass hays, fed *ad libitum* to horses, together with long alfalfa hay and dehydrated alfalfa pellets and it appeared that horses voluntarily consumed more alfalfa hay than grass hay (see Table 3-2). It seems to be a consistent finding that

Table 3-1 Estimated Voluntary Dry Matter Intake (VDMI) of Fresh Forage

Horse type	Forage type	VDMI g/kg $W^{0.75}$ (range)	Reference
Mature (~500 kg)	Ryegrasses and lucerne	98 (77.4–123.0)	Chenost & Martin-Rosset 1985
	First cut pasture	87 (77–91)	Dulphy et al 1997b
	Second cut pasture	96 (78–123)	Dulphy et al 1997b
	Species-rich pasture	100 (66–152)	Edouard et al 2009
	Grass/clover sward	150–254[1]	Smith et al 2007
Camargue mares (~400 kg)	Semi-natural habitat of Camargue	144 (101–215)	Menard et al 2002
Mulassier Poitevin mares (674 kg)	Brackish grassland	172 (155–197)	Fleurance et al 2001
Lactating Camargue mares (~400 kg)	Semi-natural habitat of Camargue	155–188	Duncan 1992
Lactating T'bred mares (560 kg)	Perennial ryegrass/white clover pasture	118[2]	Grace et al 2002b
Weanlings[3] (300 kg)	Perennial ryegrass/white clover pasture	76[2]	Grace et al 2003
Yearlings[3] (350 kg)	Perennial ryegrass/white clover pasture	85[2]	Grace ND et al 2002a

[1]Mean not given, [2]no range given, [3]Thoroughbreds.

Table 3-2 Estimated Voluntary Dry Matter Intake (VDMI) of Hays

Horse type	Hay type	VDMI g/kg $W^{0.75}$	Reference
Yearlings	Alfalfa	134	LaCasha et al 1999
	Brome grass	123	
	Coastal Bermuda grass	92	
		111	Aiken et al 1989
Mature ponies	Grass	113	Hyslop et al 1998a
	Mature threshed grass	96	Hyslop et al 1998b
	Grass – early cut	89	Pearson et al 2006
	Grass – late cut	79	
Mature horses	Alfalfa (long)	122	Crozier et al 1997
		111	Dulphy et al 1997a
		92	
	Alfalfa hay (long)	114	Cymbaluk 1990
	Altai wild rye	81	
	Bluestem (big)	106	Reinowski & Coleman 2003
	Bluestem (Caucasian)	102	Crozier et al 1997
	Brome grass	114	Cymbaluk 1990
	Coastal Bermuda grass	96	Aiken et al 1989
	Crested wheatgrass	85	Cymbaluk 1990
	Eastern gamagrass	91	Reinowski & Coleman 2003
	Grass-regrowths	95–110	Dulphy et al 1997a
	Grass-early cut	104–115	
	Grass-normal cut	99–111	
	Grass-late cut	100–102	
	Indian grass	107	Reinowski & Coleman 2003
	Kentucky bluegrass	82	Cymbaluk 1990
	Oat	81	
	Reed Canary grass	99	
		74	Ordakowski-Burk et al 2006
	Timothy	141	Reinowski & Coleman 2003
		84	Ordakowski-Burk et al 2006

the intakes of legume hays are higher than that of grass hays and this may be for the reasons proposed by Minson (1990) to account for the higher intake of legumes by ruminants. He proposed that legumes had lower values for resistance to physical breakdown, percentage of cell wall, length-to-width ratios of fibers and energy required for mastication compared to grasses. In contrast, comparisons of the VDMI of chopped hays (legume and grass) by Arabian geldings (Crozier et al 1997) led to the conclusion that the higher intakes ($p<0.05$) of legume hay, compared to grass hays were a reflection of its significantly higher ($p<0.01$) dry matter digestibility (DMD). Overall, horses consume between 1.2 and 1.6 times more alfalfa hay than grass hay but the variation in intake between grass hays is not explainable although LaCasha (1999) has suggested that differences in cell wall composition may account for this variation between grass hays.

Ensiled forages The VDMI of ponies fed limited amounts (1.65 kg DM per 100 kg LW) of grass-derived products (haylage, big-bale silage and clamp silage) were significantly ($p<0.05$) different (Moore-Colyer & Longland 2000). The VDMI of clamp silage was less than 0.50 of that when the ponies were fed haylage, and hay VDMI was 0.80 of haylage VDMI. In view of the fact that the animals were limit-fed it would seem that intakes of the hay and clamp silage were probably limited by oropharyngeal factors such as palatability (for example silage fermentation characteristics including pH, VFA levels, DM, etc.) or, masticatory effort. Relative DM content of the hay, haylage, big-bale and clamp silage were 922, 676, 500 and 337 g/kg; the haylage was preferred against the high DM hay but the VDMI of the clamp silage was low. DM content seems irrelevant in relation to intake and physical distention/gut fill could not have limited intake of the clamp silage as the ponies consumed 2.93 kg/day more of the big-bale silage. Similar, but lower, intakes of big bale silage containing either long or short chopped grass have been reported (Morrow et al 1999). It appears that the type of forage ensiled has a major impact on its subsequent intake by horses. For example, Hale and Moore-Colyer (2001) measured the VDMIs of big-bales of grass or red clover silages and compared them with that of grass hay. Ponies consumed significantly ($p<0.05$) more red clover silage than hay, a finding in agreement with data presented in Table 3-2 that shows horses will eat more legume than grass-based forage; grass silage intakes were intermediate. The authors argued that maintenance of a constant bodyweight implied some degree of intake regulation although the short duration of the trial makes this conclusion uncertain. Low intakes of clamp grass silage (<0.50 of hay intake) by horses have been previously reported by others (McLean et al 1995). These low intakes were associated with significantly ($p<0.01$) longer MRT compared to a hay diet; 51.7 h compared with 36.8 h using either chromium-mordanted hay or C_{32} alkane markers (McLean 2001). Since physical regulation of intake appears to be unimportant in the horse, DM content of the forage *per se* cannot account for these measured differences although intake of maize silage has

Table 3-3 Estimated Voluntary Dry Matter Intake (VDMI) of Ensiled Forages

Horse type	Forage type	VDMI g/kg $W^{0.75}$	Reference
Ponies	Small bale grass haylage[a]	85–98	Bergero et al 2002
	Big-bale grass silage		Hale & Moore-Colyer 2001
	Big-bale red clover silage		
	Haylage[a]	79	Moore-Colyer & Longland 2000
	Big-bale grass silage	75	
	Clamp grass silage	39	
	Big-bale silage (long and short chop)	63	Morrow et al 1999
Horses	Clamp maize silage	56	Martin-Rosset et al 1987
		43[b]	Martin-Rosset & Dulphy 1987

[a]>500 g DM per kg, [b]40.6 is the value stated in the text of the paper.

Table 3-4 Estimated Voluntary Dry Matter Intake (VDMI) of High Temperature Dehydrated Forages

Horse type	Dehydrated product	VDMI g/kg $W^{0.75}$	Reference
Ponies	Grass (chopped)	110	Hyslop et al 1998a
	Alfalfa (chopped)	79	Hyslop & Calder 2001
	Alfalfa (chopped) + oil	78	
	Alfalfa (chopped)	155	Pearson et al 2001
		121	Pearson et al 2006
Horses	Alfalfa (pelleted)	98	Cymbaluk 1990

Table 3-5 Estimated Voluntary Dry Matter Intake (VDMI) of Straws

Horse type	Straw type	VDMI g/kg $W^{0.75}$	Reference
Ponies	Oat	95	Pearson et al 2001
	Barley	60	Pearson & Merritt 1991
	Barley	52	Pearson et al 2006
	Wheat	53	Tisserand et al 1991
Mature horses	Straws[a]	61	Dulphy et al 1997b
	Barley	43	Dulphy et al 1997a
		46	

[a]type not disclosed.

been shown to fall as dry matter content falls (Agabriel et al 1982). However, the nature of the conservation process is usually less good in low dry matter silages and the fermentation characteristics of clamp silage have long been known to affect the VDMI of ruminants (for example see McCullough 1966) and perhaps they also affect the VDMI of horses. *Ad libitum* feeding of maize silage to horses resulted in very low intakes (43 g DM per kg[1]$W^{0.75}$) and considerable refusals although conservation quality was considered satisfactory (Martin-Rosset & Dulphy 1987). This contrasted with *ad libitum* hay intakes in the same study of 99 g DM per kg$W^{0.75}$. Recently, Ragnarsson and Lindberg (2010) limit-fed Icelandic horses (363 kg) a big-bale haylage (0.9 timothy grass, 0.1 meadow grass, DM 679 g/kg) at the rate of 79 g DM per kg$W^{0.75}$ with 0.05 refusals in the first collection period and none thereafter; this accords with the VDMI haylage values shown in Table 3-3. It follows from the above that horses will have a high VDMI when fed high DM haylages.

Dehydrated products There is a large variation in the published intake values for high temperature artificially dehydrated forages (see Table 3-4). The alfalfa-based product used by the UK researchers had the same origin and yet, Pearson et al (2001, 2006) recorded much higher intakes and they suggested that this might be as a result of longer photoperiod during their trials. The parent material used for the UK product was young alfalfa and yet intakes of alfalfa hays (Table 3-1) were similar suggesting that stage of maturity of alfalfa has little impact on its intake by horses.

Cereal byproducts

Dulphy et al (1997a) measured the VDMI of barley straw by horses to be approximately half that of grass hays (see Table 3-5). Pearson and Merritt (1991) had previously reported a similar situation in resting donkeys; 81 and 37 g DM per kg $W^{0.75}$ per day respectively for hay and barley straw. However, the difference was not so great in resting ponies, 99 and 60 and surprisingly, the ponies appeared to be better able to compensate the poor quality of the forage offered. Pearson et al (2001) reported that the VDMI of oat straw by ponies was reduced by about 0.40 compared to when the ponies were fed *ad libitum* artificially dehydrated alfalfa. Similarly, Dulphy et al (1997b) reported a pooled intake value for undefined straws by adult light horses at maintenance that was rather lower than that reported for other dry forages. Thus, horses do not appear to be able to effectively compensate lower feed energy densities by eating more, although there is no evidence to support the view that intake is limited by the capacity of the GIT. Longer MRTs may inhibit intake although they may in themselves be a result of low intakes, furthermore, rate of elimination from the hindgut may have an impact on intake. Low intake of "cereal straw" may be influenced by its low palatability, a complex of organoleptic qualities including taste, structure, texture and smell. Surprisingly, results reported by Hyslop and Calder (2001) showed that the inclusion of approximately 0.50 oat straw in a short-chopped, dehydrated and molassed alfalfa diet had very little effect on total DMI, reducing it from 79 to 73 g DM per kg $W^{0.75}$. This confirmed the findings of Hansen et al (1992) who showed that an inclusion of 0.50 wheat straw in a chopped alfalfa hay diet had little effect on VDMI (79 vs. 76 g DM per kg $W^{0.75}$) in limit-fed (0.016 LW) horses although DMD was significantly ($p<0.01$) reduced from 0.49 to 0.36. It seems that cereal straws have a VDMI half that of grass hays but they do not seem to depress intake of legume hay when included at 0.50.

Dulphy et al (1997b) observed that VDMI was not influenced by forage CP content although the very low CP content of cereal straws could inhibit microbial fermentation in the hindgut. Hyslop et al (1997) showed that the hindgut microflora of the pony were similar to those in the rumen in terms of degrading feeds and Van Soest (1994) noted that diets containing <80 g CP per kg DM depress the VDMI by ruminants through the slow rate of fermentation in the rumen and thus, slow reduction in particle size. However, as noted above, digesta outflow from the hindgut of the horse is not limited in the same way as that from the rumen. An alternative explanation for low intakes of straw could be that the rate of comminution (food processing) falls as the quality of the diet declines (Forbes 1988) so a poorer quality diet, such as straw, takes longer to eat. In addition, longer inter-meal intervals are required and if time spent feeding is an important feedback mechanism in intake control, then it is understandable that horses have reduced intakes of straw. However, it has been shown recently (Fleurance et al 2009) that handling time (mouth processing) increased linearly with bite size but it was not affected by the fibrousness of swards. Furthermore these authors showed that smaller animals (ponies) would be more affected by sward fibrousness than larger horses. Their response was not to increase handling time in a proportionate manner and thus it was hypothesized that compensation would be achieved by increased digesta passage rate thus allowing for greater intakes. This in part is supported by some comparative work with donkeys and ponies (Pearson et al 2001) that were fed *ad libitum* oat straw. The ponies appeared to consume more DM with shorter retention times in the GIT and with lower apparent nutrient digestibilities compared to when fed alfalfa. The exceptionally high oat straw intake compared to other straws may also have been due to a seasonal effect.

Concentrated feed (compound/cereal)

Horses are rarely allowed *ad libitum* access to concentrated feed. One study was reported (Cuddeford & Hyslop 1996) in which ponies were offered a high-fiber feed (NDF 418, CP 166150 g/kg) and consumed between 76 and 137 (mean 104) g DM per kg $W^{0.75}$ which showed a great deal of variation in intake between ponies. A recent study (Henneke & Callaham 2009) investigated whether or not horses would self-regulate when given *ad libitum* access to a moderate energy-dense concentrate (C) and hay (H) in two trials. In a stall trial, total feed consumption began at 0.025 LW (0.01 C, 0.015 H), peaked at 0.0325 (0.025 C, 0.0075 H) and declined to 0.024 (0.021 C, 0.003 H) after a 21 day period. In a paddock-based trial, concentrate consumption peaked at 0.033 LW (22.45 kg/day) but eventually declined to 0.015 LW. Not surprisingly weight and condition score increased in both trials. Throughout these trials there was no evidence of colic or laminitis and the authors concluded that horses do have the ability to self-regulate the intake of both hay and concentrate after a suitable period of *ad libitum* feeding (~21 days) but some prefeeding, over a 2-5-week period, was necessary to allow the animals to adjust. There are insufficient data to allow firm decisions to be made about whether or not horses will self-regulate in the long-term and meet or exceed their needs. In the case of ponies, there is considerable risk in allowing them to "over eat" because of the concurrent risks of obesity and laminitis. However, it is clear that photoperiod (see below) affects the voluntary intake of *ad libitum* fed growing pony colts offered a complete pelleted diet (Fuller et al 2001). Long daylength resulted in increased intakes whilst short daylengths had the converse effect although responses were not immediate, taking 5 to 8 weeks to become evident.

Feed characteristics

In order to try to explain differences in VDMI of different feeds it is necessary to look in detail at the various characteristics of these feeds in order to identify those that might affect intake.

Fiber and protein content

A comparative study conducted in France (Dulphy et al 1997a) with mature horses showed very similar VDMIs for different hays. Alfalfa, regrowth grass, early cut, normal cut and late cut grass hays were fed in two trials. The authors concluded that because the horses consumed the different hays in practically the same amounts, it would be difficult to define precise criteria whereby it would be possible to predict likely intakes of dry forages by horses. Furthermore, the horses did not increase their intake as the energy concentration of the feed declined. Ponies offered *ad libitum* mature, threshed grass hay (Hyslop et al 1998c) were able to consume relatively large amounts of dry matter, even though this hay was of very poor quality (DMD, 0.30). These results supported the view of Dulphy et al (1997a) that there is a poor relationship between VDMI and the cell wall content of hays. A further experiment (Hyslop et al 1998a) showed that although the hay used was of poorer quality than the other forages fed to mature ponies, more was consumed. The difference in intake was non-significant but the difference in NDF digestibility was ($p<0.01$). Edouard et al (2008) have shown that forage digestibility declined as NDF increased and CP declined. NDF was a better predictor of DMD than CP for hays with a regression of DMD (%)=100.3−0.78×NDF (%) ($r^2=0.71$, $n=38$). These authors showed that the average VDMI of horses was unaffected by DMD or CP content but that VDMI appeared to decline slightly as NDF increased (DMI [150 g/kg LW]=24.91−0.12×NDF [%] [$r^2=0.10$, $n=45$]. An original discovery was that, by using mixed models that allowed for individual differences, as DMD declined, intake significantly increased. Similarly, as forage CP declined, VDMI increased. The authors concluded that most horses respond to a reduction in forage quality by increasing their VDMI as originally proposed by Janis (1976) but only until they reach a certain threshold as evidenced by the low VDMI of barley straw (0.5 that of grass hays, Dulphy et al 1997a).

Martin-Rosset and Dulphy (1987) and others (Pearson et al 2006) have suggested that variation in VDMI has little impact on the digestibility of the diet whereas other authors (Ott 1981, Cuddeford et al 1995) have shown a level of feeding effect. A study with Icelandic horses (Ragnarsson & Lindberg 2010) showed significant ($p<0.001$) differences between digestibility coefficients for DM, organic matter (OM), NDF and ADF measured at two levels of intake, 47 and 79 g DM per kg$W^{0.75}$. At first sight this contradicts the view of Martin-Rosset and Dulphy (1987) but examination of the French data showed that the CF digestibility of hay fed at 64 g DM per kg $W^{0.75}$ was 0.551, at 86 g DM per kg $W^{0.75}$ it was 0.487 and at 99 g DM per kg $W^{0.75}$ it was 0.498; clearly there is a level of feeding effect. Although these data do not decrement equally, CF digestibility was consistently lower above maintenance (M) feeding levels; at 1.4M it was 6.4 units lower and 5.3 units lower when fed *ad libitum*. Furthermore, the Icelandic work revealed substantial individual variation in terms of the horses' ability to digest fiber between feeding levels; NDF 0.012 to 0.102 (x=0.065) and ADF 0.004 to 0.109 (x=0.065). It should be no surprise that a limited intake of a quality feed will be associated with higher nutrient digestibility and a longer MRT; the refractory nature of straws, however, means that this scenario does not pertain to them.

A retrospective analysis of data obtained by the INRA and of values taken from published papers provided a data set for assessing VDMI of horses fed different dry forages (Dulphy et al 1997b). The pooled results for horses gave VDMIs for legumes (n=12), grasses (n=38) and regrowth grass hays (n=7) of 108, 93 and 98 g/kg $W^{0.75}$ respectively; the only significant ($p<0.05$) difference was between legume and grass hay. The authors concluded that voluntary intake of hay by horses was not influenced by either the CP, CF or NDF content of the forage. Multiple regression analysis yielded r^2 values between 0.11 and 0.13; in contrast, r^2 values for sheep calculated under similar conditions produced significant correlations of 0.78 to 0.84. Thus, it is impossible to reliably predict the intake of dry hays by horses based on forage analysis in contrast to ruminants, where effective equations have been derived and are based primarily on fiber content. Thus, Dulphy et al (1997b) have proposed that the voluntary intake of hays by housed, mature light horses will be in the range 19–22, 18–21 and 22–25 g/kg LW for grass, regrowth grass and alfalfa hays respectively. These values may be regarded as conservative estimates of VDMI by horses.

In contrast to the above, a review (Lawrence et al 2001) of published studies that reported both NDF and VDMI in mature horses fed long stem grass hays *ad libitum* concluded that there was a good relationship between the two parameters represented by:

$$\text{VDMI}\ (y) = 124.55 + 0.0155x^2 - 2.5742x \quad (r^2 = 0.67,\ p < 0.01)\ (x = \%\text{NDF},\ y = \text{g/kg LW per day}) \tag{1}$$

These authors tested the reliability of this equation in terms of predicting intake by feeding two orchard grass and two timothy hays to four mature equids (278–705 kg). Predicted daily intakes were not significantly different from actual intakes and in fact, the two were highly correlated (r^2=0.86, $p<0.001$). Incorporation of the experimental data into that derived from the literature (1) yielded:

$$\text{VDMI}\ (y) = 80.954 + 0.0073x^2 - 1.3677x \quad (r^2 = 0.50,\ p < 0.01,\ n = 21) \tag{2}$$

More recently, Reinowski and Coleman (2003) used equation (2) to predict likely *ad libitum* intakes of different grass hays (see Table 3-2) and then measured the actual intakes of the hays; the intakes met or exceeded those that were predicted. There was a strong correlation between actual DMI and the NDF content (%) of the hays fed:

$$\text{VDMI}\ (y) = 90.95 - 0.98x\ (r^2 = 0.68,\ p < 0.01,\ n = 16) \tag{3}$$

Dulphy et al (1997a) were able to show a negative relationship between VDMI and plant NDF content as follows:

$$\text{VDMI (g/kg LW)} = 53 - 0.0459 \times \text{NDF(\%)} \quad (r^2 = 0.23,\ n = 55,\ \text{NDF} = 30\text{–}83\%)$$

A weaker relationship was demonstrated by Mesochina (2000) over a wider range of forages:

$$\text{VDMI (g DM per kg } W^{0.75}) = 150.18 - 0.09 \times \text{NDF(\%)} \quad (r^2 = 0.23,\ n = 55,\ \text{NDF} = 30\text{–}83\%)$$

Both American and French workers have shown a relationship between NDF and VDMI but the strength of the association is variable and lacks the firm association measured in ruminants. NDF plays a role but where exactly in the digestive process? For example NDF can affect the processes of comminution, digestion in the small intestine and fermentation in the large intestine. Its precise role remains to be determined.

Replacing hay with concentrate reduced the ADF content of the ration by 0.19 but DDM of the hay and hay plus concentrate (H+C-70:30) diets remained the same at intakes of 84 and 92 g DM per kg $W^{0.75}$ respectively (Holland et al 1998). Although non-structural carbohydrate (NSC) digestibility was higher on the H+C diet, the NDF digestibility was reduced thereby explaining why DDM values were similar. Feces were approximately 0.02 drier from horses fed the H+C diet, probably because the diet contained less fiber (see below). Unfortunately, these horses were limit-fed so there was no opportunity to test if VDMI was affected. However, Turcott et al (2003) examined the effect of feeding diets containing different concentrate:forage ratios (70:30; 50:50; 30:70) and thus different NDF levels on the VDMI of Arabian and Quarter horse weanlings fed *ad libitum*. There were no differences at 5 and 8 months between the diets in terms of VDMI with animals consuming between 28 and 29 g DM kg^{-1} LW. Although the diets were digested to different extents this did not appear to affect intake confirming that sometimes NDF has little or no effect on intake.

Physical form

An early experiment (Haenlein et al 1966) demonstrated that three different physical forms of alfalfa hay (loose, wafered or pelleted) were consumed in different amounts. Whilst the three different forms were similar in chemical composition, they differed significantly in density and in mean particle size. Horses consumed 0.17 more wafers and 0.24 more pellets than loose hay. The CF of the pellets was significantly ($p<0.01$) less well digested than that of the loose hay presumably reflecting a more rapid rate of passage through the gut. Later work (Schurg et al 1978) involved feeding ryegrass straw to 500 kg horses either as long stem, pelleted, cubed or in a briquetted form. Respective VFIs were 5.5, 6.4, 6.0 and 5.9 kg/day; significantly ($p<0.01$) more of the compressed forms were eaten although DMD of the pelleted diet was significantly ($p<0.05$) depressed. Todd et al (1995) obtained similar results when feeding different forms of alfalfa to horses. When alfalfa-based forages were fed *ad libitum*, the range of VDMIs (g DM per kg $W^{0.75}$) reported in the literature were 75 to 122 for long hays (Haenlein et al 1966, Cymbaluk 1990, Crozier et al 1997, Dulphy et al 1997a,b), 88 to 139 for dried wafers, cubes or pellets (Haenlein et al 1966, Cymbaluk 1990, Todd et al 1995) and 100 to 155 for short-chopped, high temperature dried material (Pearson et al 2001). Altering the physical density of forage appears to encourage VDMI but those materials that were ground as part of the processing were less well-digested.

Thorne et al (2005) demonstrated that horses appeared to prefer short-chopped forages rather than the long form, possibly because they were bucket fed and horses did not have to expend effort pulling material from hay nets. Of the forages offered, molassed forms were preferred and molassed, chopped alfalfa was the most preferred. However, although the horses demonstrated preferences, all forages were sampled and foraging behavior was more frequent and longer in duration when offered multiple forages.

Water-holding capacity

The absence of a strong relationship in horses between food NDF content and intake that has been measured in ruminants may simply be due to the absence of a metering device in the horse that is analogous to their reticulo-omasal orifice. As an alternative to NDF, the horse may respond to the "bulkiness" of the food on offer. Kyriazakis and Emmans (1995) have proposed that in pigs, water-holding capacity (WHC) limited the intake of "bulky" foods rather than fiber content *per se*. Tsaras et al (1998) tested the proposal that WHC of a food was an adequate descriptor of its "bulk" and concluded that it accounted for the effects of different foods on VDMI of pigs. In contrast, CF, ADF and NDF of feeds were inadequate in this respect. In view of the fact that sugar beet pulp has been shown to depress VDMI in horses (Hyslop et al 1998b, Hyslop & Cuddeford 1999), perhaps the WHC of horse feeds should be assessed. Cuddeford et al (1992) showed that grass hay absorbed 4.4 times more water than short-chopped, high temperature dried alfalfa and that horses fed alfalfa produced drier feces. They explained this on the basis that the hay contained more hydrophilic hemicelluloses, and it is apparent from Table 3-2 that horses and ponies eat much more alfalfa than grass hay so could WHC explain higher alfalfa intakes? More recently (Spooner et al 2007) the effect of fiber type on hydration status has been measured in Arabian horses. This work was based on the fact that WHC varies between fiber sources and that a high WHC would be beneficial in terms of retaining body water for endurance horses. Certainly, body water content was affected differently according to the type of forage fed but it remains an open question as to whether or not VDMI can be influenced in this way.

Animal factors

1.3.1 Physiological status

Aiken et al (1989) fed Coastal Bermuda grass hay to both yearlings and mature geldings, and suggested that food intake was regulated by energy requirement, rather than by gut capacity. This was based on the fact that the yearlings, with higher nutrient need, consumed more DM *pro rata* than the mature horses; 0.025 versus 0.02 of body weight (see Table 3-2). This is in keeping with a view proposed by Frape et al (1982) that VDMI was proportionate to energy requirement rather than to gut volume. LaCasha et al (1999) also measured high intakes of alfalfa and brome grass hay (134 to 123 g/kg $W^{0.75}$) by yearlings although they recorded similar intakes for Coastal Bermuda Grass as Aiken and co-workers did for mature animals. Danish Warmblood colts were fed a total mixed ration (TMR) based on chopped forages (grass hay/silage, straw) and concentrate *ad libitum* and VDMIs were measured at 6, 9, 12, 18, 21 and 24 months of age (Søndergaard 2003) to be respectively 70, 75, 81, 93, 88 and 90 g/kg $^{.75}$. These intakes are lower than expected being all less than 0.02 of LW and perhaps show that young animals are less willing to consume high fiber diets (0.65 to 0.73 forage in TMR); barley straw inclusion at 0.23 to 0.36 could have also depressed intake. Furthermore, although the TMR was available *ad libitum*, residues of only 1 kg horse^{-1} were allowed so the opportunity for selection within the TMR was very limited perhaps contributing to the low intakes measured. Interestingly these animals were bedded on fresh straw daily so it is highly likely that they consumed some bedding although this was not recorded.

Boulot et al (1987) measured a 0.65 greater intake of forage by lactating mares (~530 kg) compared to those animals that were pregnant and this difference was confirmed recently (McCown et al 2011) when lactating mares (570–600 kg) consumed 0.33 more DM than pregnant mares ($p<0.05$). Others (Martin-Rosset et al 1990) fed a diet of 0.85 meadow hay and 0.15 concentrate *ad libitum* to dry, pregnant or lactating heavy horse (Comtois and Breton) breeds; their respective VDMIs were 117, 113 and 162 g/kg $^{.75}$. In the same study, light horse geldings consumed 100 g DM per kg $W^{0.75}$; this was significantly less ($p<0.02$) than that of the dry mares. This raises the question as to what is driving ingestive behavior. The most likely explanation is that it has a physiological basis and is thus probably mediated hormonally. The French experiment was repeated (Miraglia et al 2003) using the same animals and similar intakes were recorded at the same physiological state when fed the same diet. VDMIs for the heavy breeds were 104, 116 and 161 g/kg $W^{0.75}$ respectively; the value for the light horses was 98. The VDMIs of pregnant and lactating heavy breeds were significantly greater than that of light breeds. It is interesting to note that the intake of the dry heavy breed mares and light breed geldings in the most recent experiment was about the same. MRT was decreased (~0.33) at high intakes (lactating mares) and, as a result, nutrient digestibility was reduced; clearly, neither gut capacity nor rate of digestion was limiting VDMI in the lactating mares. However, pregnant mares had a MRT of only 21.7 h, similar to that of the lactating mares (21.4 h), indicating that, although their DMI of 116 was significantly less than that of the lactating mares (161 g/kg $W^{0.75}$), gut capacity was restricted. There is a limit to how much the abdominal cavity can expand during pregnancy and once this limit is reached, the growing conceptus will probably restrict gut capacity and thus feed MRT. However, some recent work (Winsco et al 2011) has shown that month of gestation does affect VDMI ($p<0.05$) regardless of whether fed forage alone or in combination with concentrate. Surprisingly, the Quarter horse mares (538–695 kg) consumed less during month 10 and more during the 11th month (0.0184 compared with 0.0219 LW) in contrast to other species where intake is reduced as pregnancy advances (e.g., ruminants; Forbes 1971). Of particular interest in this study was the fact that the forage-fed mares consumed 0.0225 LW whereas forage/grain-fed mares ate less DM (0.0179 LW, $p<0.01$) which perhaps suggests that the mare's VDMI was, in some way, proportionate to energy need (see below).

Energy requirements

There appears to be some sensitivity to energy intake since Laut et al (1985) showed that ponies ate larger meals more frequently when offered a standard pelleted diet of reduced energy density compared to when they were fed the undiluted pelleted diet. The ponies' response to changes in dietary energy density took between two and 14 days to stabilize, indicating a less precise mechanism than that shown to be present in other species (rats and monkeys) where compensation occurs in less than 24 h (Gibbs & Smith 1978). Others (Ralston & Baile 1982b, 1983) have shown that ponies were able to compensate intake of a pelleted diet that they were accustomed to accurately within a 24 h period when given additional intragastric inputs of energy in the form of glucose, corn oil or α-cellulose.

Given the opportunity, non-working horses and ponies will eat in excess of their energy needs and, as a result, become obese. Cuddeford and Hyslop (1996) showed in one particular study that, on average, housed ponies consumed in excess of three times their calculated digestible energy (DE) requirement, thereby indicating a complete failure to regulate their energy intake, at least in the short term. Hale and Moore-Colyer (2001) showed that the VDMI of red clover silage by ponies exceeded their maintenance requirements for energy and protein by 2.7 and 5.5 times respectively. Others (Hyslop et al 1998a, Pearson et al 2001) have confirmed this voluntary overconsumption during short-term Latin Square experiments. A grazing study over a period of several weeks (Smith et al 2007) estimated VDMIs of between 0.032 and 0.052 of mass and these high intakes were reflected in the mean daily change in mass of the horses that averaged +1.44 kg/day and varied from 1.0–3.7 kg/day. Clearly these horses, like so many that are offered excess feed, over consumed energy and, when allowed to continue this behavior, become obese.

Ralston (1992) abandoned an *ad libitum* experiment after 5 weeks because animals were becoming obese; however, with a little more time, intakes might have stabilized or reduced according to the opinion of others (Argo et al 2001) expressed below. In view of the fact that most Latin Square experiments utilize 21-day periods, intake data obtained from *ad libitum* feeding experiments under these circumstances could be of questionable validity. Evidence is provided above that physiological status (and thus energy requirement) can affect VDMI; higher requirements for energy appear to be able to drive higher intakes.

Seasonality

Photoperiod affects melatonin production and the latter has a very strong rhythm in horses (Piccione et al 2005) and may affect VDMI. Fuller et al (1998, 2001) have recorded higher energy intakes by ponies on "long days" than on "short days" at constant ambient temperatures. Dugdale et al (2010) showed that ponies fed *ad libitum* a chaff-based, complete diet ate more during the summer months (159 g DM per kg $W^{0.75}$) compared to the winter period (114 g DM per kg $W^{0.75}$) although this effect was confined to animals that were thin or in moderate body condition; the appetite of fat ponies was similar between seasons. Pearson et al (2001) suggested that the high intakes that they recorded for dehydrated alfalfa (155 g DM per kg $W^{0.75}$) and oat straw (95 g DM per kg $W^{0.75}$) compared to other published data was because their work was conducted throughout the summer months. In contrast, Dulphy et al (1997b) have suggested that horses do not seem to be sensitive to season and failed to take season into account when they conducted a retrospective analysis of data obtained from the literature and of that generated by INRA over the years (Chenost & Martin-Rosset 1985, Dulphy et al 1997a). More recently, a meta-analysis conducted by Edouard et al (2008) could not exclude any variability introduced by seasonality and its effect on variance in VDMI because diets fed to horses were not balanced across seasons. So far there are conflicting data about any effect of seasonality on VDMI although the indications and weight of evidence point to the fact that horses eat more during long photoperiods.

Individuality

Edouard et al (2008) suggested that horses are selected on traits that are not associated with feeding unlike ruminants, such as dairy cattle. This could be a reason why there is such a variance in their individual ability to consume food and digest it. These authors conducted a meta-analysis of 45 trials where intake and digestibility were measured in 21 saddle horses. They showed that at group level, intake declined slightly with increasing fiber content and there were no effects of CP or DMD on intake. However, at the individual level the coefficients of variation in intake were quite high; 0.09 for fresh forages, 0.13 for grass hays and 0.17 for alfalfa hays. Horses show different responses to changes in forage quality; some compensate for poor quality feed others do not, some horses eat well and others do not. Two horses that significantly ($p<0.05$) increased their DMI as digestibility declined could meet their energy and protein requirements even when fed the poorest quality forages. Some other individuals responded by decreasing intake as forage quality declined but in spite of this, they were still able to meet requirements. In general horses were able to compensate for reductions in forage quality by eating more as originally suggested by Janis (1976). Individuality in VDMI is reflected in differences in body condition and data obtained by Smith et al (2007) showed that individual grazing VDMI varied between 0.032 and 0.052 of mass. Knowledge of the impact that this individuality can have on results accounts for why Latin Square designs are so popular amongst scientists pursuing nutritional investigations. In practical situations knowledge about whether or not a horse will eat a lot or a little is very important. Unfortunately, we have scant information on this characteristic of horses.

Key Points – Quantitative intake

- Feedback mechanisms do not appear to play a major part in regulating VDMI
- The DMI of different feeds is very variable (37–254 g DM per kg $W^{0.75}$)
- Intake of fresh grass>lucerne>grass hay>grass silage>cereal straw
- There is a weak relationship between NDF and VDMI
- VDMI is affected by physiological status; lactation>pregnant/growing>non-pregnant/maintenance
- Energy need does not regulate VDMI in *ad libitum* fed horses/ponies at maintenance
- VDMI varies between season and individual

Qualitative intake

Horses select food based on its sensory properties and several attempts have been made (Goodwin et al 2004, 2005a, b) to assess the impact of flavors on food selection. The eight most readily consumed flavors were, in descending order of preference, fenugreek, banana, cherry, rosemary, cumin, carrot, peppermint and oregano. However, these were short-term studies and it is not clear that these flavors would have any long term impact. Furthermore, offering concentrates flavored with molasses, mint, herbs or garlic to horses failed to establish a flavor that was continuously preferred since horses switched between concentrates (Goodwin et al 2005b). The authors argued that providing sensory variety to stabled animals stimulated foraging behaviors.

Stabled horses were offered three diets varying in protein and fat content to try to assess whether or not horses would discriminate on the basis of nutrient content (Redgate et al 2007). Horses were adapted to an *ad libitum* diet medium in both fat (0.034) and protein (0.122) and then provided with a choice of two other diets (0.022 fat and 0.133 protein or 0.049 fat and 0.087 protein) together with the medium diet; two periods of self-selection were allowed. Initially the high fat/low protein diet was least preferred however, after a 4-day period of monadic feeding; in the second period of self-selection the intake of all of the diets was similar. Thus, it was discovered that initial diet preferences could be modified after exposure to other diets. Thus, there must be factors other than immediate sensory exposure that affect diet choice in the longer term.

Time allowed for feeding and, in particular, access to pasture can affect food selection. Smith (1999) showed that donkeys selected a more digestible diet when they had 23/24h access than when they had 8/24 h. Pearson et al (2001) showed that the DM digestibility was higher (0.43 vs 0.40) for oat straw when it was fed *ad libitum* (95 g DM per kg $W^{0.75}$) to ponies than when its intake was restricted (68 g DM per kg $W^{0.75}$); incidentally the difference was greater for donkeys, 0.50 vs 0.43 ($p<0.001$). It is probable that when fed *ad libitum*, ponies were able to select the more digestible components of the diet. Certainly, there is evidence in other species for this as for example in sheep (Savadogo et al 2000) and donkeys (Tisserand et al 1991). Grace et al (2002a, b) showed that DM digestibility was depressed by 0.10–0.15 in stalled yearlings and 0.05–0.08 in corralled mares compared to when they were grazing unlimited pasture although both groups were offered 0.30 excess herbage. Limiting the animal's ability to select was clearly affecting their qualitative intake and thus, their ability to utilize the nutrient resource. Other grazing studies (Gordon 1989, Naujeck et al 2005, Fleurance et al 2009) have suggested that ponies and horses will select different qualities of herbage when given the opportunity. The extent of the grazing resource and its diversity will affect the qualitative intake of both horses and ponies. Even stabled horses have been shown to exhibit foraging behaviors that mimic "patch foraging" as determined at pasture. It seems that stabled horses are motivated to move between locations if there is an opportunity to sample different forages (Goodwin et al 2007) and thus diversify their intake.

Cairns et al (2002) have shown that when horses were offered a choice test they appeared to select a higher energy diet. Konik ponies grazing natural vegetation selected about 0.52 of their diet based on the intake rate of digestible organic matter (DOMIR), a measure that is the product of bite size, bite rate and bite digestibility from the plants with the highest content of digestible organic matter (DOM) (van Wieren 1996). It seems clear that horses will select dietary components that will maximize their energy intake over time if given the opportunity.

Key Points – Qualitative intake

- Feed flavor can affect choice of feed
- Given the opportunity, horses will select the more digestible components of a diet and thus maximize nutrient/energy intakes

Rate of intake

The rate at which a horse eats its food is an important characteristic because it can significantly affect its well being. For example, rapid consumption of 12 mm pellets without adequate chewing and ensalivation can easily result in esophageal blockages (Frape 2010). Furthermore, inadequate comminution of food can increase the risk of acidosis when high starch diets are fed because particle size is not reduced sufficiently to enable satisfactory pre-ileal digestion (Meyer at al 1993). Thus, there are serious health issues associated with rate of intake of food and it is important to be aware of those factors that can modify it.

Physical form of forage

Grass can be presented to a horse in at least five forms; fresh, ensiled, artificially dehydrated, sun-cured or dried, ground and then pelleted. The rate at which dry matter is consumed will be lowest with the fresh grass and highest with the pellets because the concentration of DM (g DM per kg) in the latter will be about five times greater than it is in the grass (NRC 2007). Thus, the physical form of a feed is important because it affects the rate at which the horse can consume it and the quantity of fiber (for example g NDF per kg DM) *per se* is meaningless in this context. The rapid consumption of pelleted feed and the reduction in overall eating time is often associated with the development of abnormal behaviors such as wood chewing because normal eating behaviors cannot be satisfied (Haenlein et al 1966) and possibly also, the onset of diseases such as acidosis and laminitis (Frape, 2010).

Although the rate of consumption can be affected by modifying the physical form of forage with a resultant increase in VDMI, this is not always the case. For example, *ad libitum* provision of short-chop, dehydrated grass or traditional grass hay, both made from the same, second cut perennial ryegrass sward cut on the same day, resulted in similar intakes by ponies (Hyslop et al 1998a). However, Cuddeford et al (1992) measured marked differences in intake rates between precision chopped, high temperature dried alfalfa and long (33 cm) timothy hay that were fed to horses; the latter consumed 820 g DM per h of alfalfa and 1360 g DM per h of the hay. Earlier Gallagher et al (1984) had shown that chopping hay into a chaff form did not influence the digestibility of organic matter (OM) or ADF and Morrow et al (1999) measured no difference in nutrient digestibility or digesta passage rate when ponies were fed hay, either in long (18 cm) or short-chop (5.3 cm) form. These authors also showed that long and short-chop (29.3 and 6.8 cm respectively) forms of big bale silage did not differ in these respects. Forages produced for admixture with concentrates, compounds or cereals are normally sold as "chops" or "chaffs"; the nutrient digestibility and digesta passage rates for these materials should be the same as if the unprocessed forage were fed. Thus, the extent of physical treatment of forage will affect whether or not the rate of VDMI changes and whether digestibility parameters remain the same. Increasing the density of the forage can alter its rate of consumption by horses although altering its length appears to have little effect on total VDMI.

Physical form of concentrate

Argo et al (2001) compared the DE intakes of pony mares offered *ad libitum* access to the same complete diet in a pelleted or chaff form. Mean DE intakes of chaff and pellets increased ($p<0.01$) to attain maxima of 1.15 and 1.76 MJ/kg $W^{0.75}$ on days 25 and 26 respectively. During this period of time intakes of chaff-fed animals were only 0.73 ($p<0.001$) of pellet DE intake and during a second period (days 35 to 63), it was 0.79 ($p<0.01$). By the end of this second period, the digestibilities of measured parameters significantly declined ($p<0.001$) for both diets; GE: –0.16 and NDF: –0.28; chaff DE intake was reduced to 0.68 MJ/kg $W^{0.75}$. Ponies appear to eat more of a pelleted concentrate than when it is presented in a "muesli" format and thus the latter format is preferred where maximal intakes are not desired. Although condition score and average daily gain increased over the first 4 weeks of the study, growth and appetite returned to near maintenance values within 9 weeks. The authors concluded that nutritional characterization of *ad libitum* diets must account for physiological adaptation that in this case, took some 35 days.

A comparison of the rate of consumption of a meal based on steamed oat groats or rolled barley by horses resulted in a total time of 126±19 and 78±25 minutes for the oats and barley respectively (Jose-Cunilleras et al 2004). This clearly demonstrates that feed format greatly affects its intake rate by horses. Brøkner et al (2008) offered meals of whole oats, ground oats, muesli or 8 mm pellets to Icelandic horses and recorded the observed eating times (min/kg DM). They were respectively 25, 26, 30 and 17 min the latter two values being significantly ($p<0.001$) different from each other and from the other two values. It seems that the heterogeneity of the muesli required more jaw movements and thus contributed to the increased eating time. As expected, pelleted feed was consumed most rapidly agreeing with the findings of Argo et al (2002).

Hintz et al (1985) fed a grain mixture (0.36 oats, 0.34 maize, 0.20 soya, 0.06 molasses and 0.04 vitamin/mineral mix) in three different formats; unprocessed, pelleted (5 mm) and extruded (~5×10×10 mm). These diets weighed respectively 625, 580 and 330 g/l. Table 3-6 shows the outcome of this work and it is obvious that the less dense extruded food takes both horses and ponies significantly longer to eat. Coincidentally the digestibility of energy, DM and CP was highest when the extruded diet was fed although the rates of passage of the various diets were similar. It follows from the foregoing that pelleted feeds are always consumed more rapidly than coarse mixes/"sweet feeds", which in turn are eaten more quickly than extruded feeds. Thus, in order to minimize the incidence of gastrointestinal problems, pelleted feed should only be fed little and often.

Table 3-6 Rate of Intake (g/min) of Three Different Dietary Formats During the First 20 Minutes of a Meal (after Hintz et al 1985)

Animal type	Unprocessed	Pelleted	Extruded
Horses	97[a]	109[a]	67[b]
Ponies	60[a]	68[a]	45[b]

[a,b]values (mean of six animals) in the same row bearing unlike superscripts are significantly different ($p<0.01$).

Addition of chaff

It has been a long held tradition that, to slow down the rate of intake of concentrates/cereals during a meal, dried chopped forages or chaff should be mixed in with the feed. In fact, many concentrate feeds are now available with chaff already included as part of the formulation. Inclusion of 0.10, 0.20 or 0.30 straw, chopped into either 2.5 or 4 cm, in a concentrate pellet fed at between 1 and 1.2 kg that contained 0.10 chopped alfalfa (Ellis et al 2005) had no effect on rate of chewing but diets with straw added were consumed more slowly and the total number of chews per kg were significantly increased ($p<0.05$). Fiber length had no differential effect but the 0.30 straw addition increased the time taken to eat 1 kg of the concentrate from 7 to 16 min with an obvious increase in chewing time. The effect of separate addition of chaff was tested using a basal meal of oats (3 g/kg LW) to which was added longer (4 cm) or shorter ground (<2 cm) alfalfa chaff at five levels ranging from 0.07 to 0.375 of a mixed ration (Campbell et al 2005). Again, rate of food intake was unaffected by chaff length but declined as chaff addition increased with a maximal effect at an addition of 0.33. Horses, like many other species, vary their rate of feed consumption during a meal eating more quickly at the outset (see below). Thus, it is likely that the effect of chaff addition will depend on the size of the meal. Australian work failed to show that an overall inclusion of 26% (a 35% addition on top of the core ration) alfalfa chaff (<2 cm) in the ration significantly slowed the rate of consumption of either a sweet feed (Harris et al 2005a) or oats (Harris et al 2005b) when fed at 3 g/kg LW (~2 kg). Although intakes were reduced from respectively 77 and 58 g/min to 49 and 52 g/min for the sweet feed and oats but total time taken to eat the meal containing sweet feed was significantly increased. Of concern was the fact that the volume of the oat-based feed eaten per minute increased and this might adversely impact small intestinal starch digestion although there was no apparent effect on the glycemic response to the meal.

Meal size

Some work in Australia (Campbell et al 2006) has shown that neither meal size nor the inclusion of 0.10 molasses affected the rate at which a concentrate was consumed by Thoroughbred horses. Food intake was highest during the first 5 min (74 g/min) of the meal and then averaged

48 g min over the remaining 30 min; the decline in rate of intake was linear with respect to time. The study was extended to measure rate of intake in 34 Thoroughbreds, 30 Clydesdales and 9 Standardbred horses; individual rates varied between 28 and 125 g/min over a 10 min meal. As expected there was a linear relationship between body mass and intake rate reflecting the differences in oral processing ability. Rate of food intake was unaffected by sex, age or activity. However, at similar weights there were breed differences in eating rate–Clydesdales >Thoroughbreds>Standardbreds in terms of consumption rate. This probably has to do with mouth morphology and subsequent bite size.

Fresh forage

The relationship between the rate of grass VDMI by a grazing horse and the availability of herbage has not received detailed study. Naujeck and Hill (2003) showed that horses could recognize differences in grass height and that they increased bite dimensions with increasing grass height. To maximize rate of herbage intake horses should select from tall grasses but it is likely that the tall grasses will be of lower nutritive value so does the horse seek a balance between quantity and quality? Apparently not as evidenced by a recent investigation that was undertaken (Fleurance et al 2009) using natural swards whose biomass ranged from 82 to 513 g DM per m with heights from 3 to 63 cm (NDF: 530 to 680 g/kg DM) and offered to ponies (253 kg), saddle horses (602 kg) and heavy horses (953 kg). The mean maximum intake rates (±SE) calculated from measurements on the two highest sward biomass levels were for ponies 28.1 (1.6), saddle horses 59.5 (4.4) and heavy horses 85.1 (9.8) g DM per min. The relationship between bite size and sward biomass increased linearly over the range tested, but bite size increased faster for the large horses. As sward height increased bite size increased and, as a result, handling time per bite increased thereby lowering bite rate. The horses appeared to be relatively unaffected by differences in the plant fiber levels experienced although the ponies appeared to reduce their input into food processing at the higher fiber levels; the authors suggested that increases in rate of passage might compensate for reduced nutrient extraction per unit of food. The maximum processing rate of food significantly increased with body size which suggests that the intake rate of small horses was more limited when bite size increased than that of the larger horses. It is apparent that instantaneous intake rates scale to body size, the exact nature of this relationship (allometric, isometric, etc.) depends on the data set used. However, there is evidence that diet selection can be influenced by herbage quality since Gordon (1989) observed that ponies remained grazing short patches of better quality pasture rather than utilizing longer swards of inferior grasses. Similarly others (Naujeck et al 2005) have observed horses grazing short grass of lower bulk density rather than taller grass on perennial ryegrass swards so it seems that both sward height and herbage quality can influence diet selection. However, although horses in this study sampled their environment all of the time they returned to long patches of grass. Perhaps this was in order to optimize energy intake per bite per unit of time and thus to maximize their rate of intake. Grass height seemed to be the determining factor in selection rather than herbage allowance and enabled the highest rates of intake.

Horses (576 kg) grazing tall fescue pastures over an 8 h period averaged a VDMI of 0.166±0.015 kg DM per 100 kg LW per h, consuming 0.22±0.02 in the first 4 h and 0.11±0.02 kg DM per 100 kg LW per h in the second 4 h period (Dowler & Siciliano 2009). These rates of intake are much less than those recorded by Fleurance et al (2009) but similar to those measured by Duren et al (1989) in yearlings (374 kg) grazing a Cocksfoot-dominated pasture (0.160 kg DM per 100 kg LW per h) over a 3 h period. The higher rates of intake obtained in the French experiment were probably a consequence of the horses having been deprived of any food for 5 h before being offered sward trays in order to measure instantaneous intake rate. Thus, the information gathered using such protocols must be interpreted with care.

It is known that limiting access to pasture affects rate of intake and recently it has been shown (Longland et al 2011b) that the use of grazing muzzles can affect the rate of DMI on autumn pasture (sward height 8–15 cm). Without muzzles the ponies, on average, consumed 0.08 of their LW in a 3-h period (vs. 0.014 LW with muzzles). An experiment (Glunk & Siciliano 2011) that compared four different grazing time periods (24, 9, 6 and 3 h) also showed that the rate of DMI increased as the time allowed for grazing was reduced; 0.57, 1.12, 1.52 and 1.96 g DM per kg LW per h respectively. This type of compensatory intake may increase risk for those animals prone to laminitis. This effect could be compounded by giving limited access to grass after midday because Chavez et al (2011) have shown that horses eat more DM in the afternoon than in the morning over an 8-h period when the grass NSC content is at highest. Furthermore, Ince et al (2011) showed that restricting grazing to a 3-h period daily and allowing *ad libitum* access to haylage during 20 h in every 24 over 6 wks resulted in the ponies gradually increasing their rate of DMI at pasture. It was noteworthy that over the 6-week period overall VDMI remained fairly constant averaging 0.02 LW, allowing the ponies to gain, on average, 338 g/day. Pasture VDMI increased 1.86× from 0.049 in week 1 to 0.091 LW during the 3-h period in week 6. One can conclude from this that restricting pasture access becomes less effective, in terms of limiting grass intakes, as time progresses.

Individual feeds

Hill (2007) provides data on the short-term (10 min) intake (g DM per min) of various industrial by-products by young horses and pregnant mares, although animal weights were not given. Distillers' grains were consumed by the young horses at 46.8 (maize), 16.6 (barley), 53 (wheat) and by the mares respectively at 86.7, 70.2 and 93.3 g. In contrast, molassed SBP was eaten at 116.5 (young horses) and 161.4 (mares) g DM per min. The higher intakes by the mares would reflect bite size. Differences in palatability and fiber content would account for differences between feeds. However, short-term studies of this nature are of limited usefulness. Brøkner et al (2008) compared the rate of intake of unchopped barley straw, unchopped meadow hay, chopped and artificially dried alfalfa hay or chopped and artificially dried grass by Icelandic horses. The observed eating time (min/kg DM) for each feed was respectively 111, 70, 48 and 38; all values were significantly ($p<0.001$) different. The horses took 2.5 times longer to eat 1 kg straw DM compared to the same amount of dried grass. Others (Dulphy et al 1997a) measured a 0.48 greater mean eating time (min/kg NDF) for barley straw compared to hay whereas the difference measured in the Icelandic horses was only 0.17 greater. Brøkner et al (2008) showed that there were fewer jaw movements (293 per bout) and a slower chewing rate (86/min) when fed barley straw compared to dried grass (884 per bout, 91/min). These findings are commensurate with expectations based on the discussion above and the fact that straw VDMIs are generally lower than that of other roughages.

Key Points – Rate of intake

- Increasing the density of forage or concentrate increases its rate of intake
- Inclusion of 30% chaff in a meal will reduce the speed at which it is consumed
- Bite size controls the rate of intake
- The ease of comminution of a feed affects its rate of consumption
- Rates of VDMI increase when access to pasture is restricted.

Conclusions

Based on the information contained in the literature and reviewed above it is possible to determine appropriate VDMIs for horses in different situations, dependent on their specific requirements. Table 3-7 shows some of the likely VDMIs for a 500 kg horse based on the typical feeds that are used in the UK and on the horses' requirements for energy and protein.

Factors identified by others as affecting short-term (minute by minute) and long-term (24 h) feed intake of horses are sensory perceptions (olfactory, taste, temperature), metabolites and hormones (blood glucose and VFAs, insulin, growth hormones, sex hormones), digestive processes (meal size, fiber composition, feeding frequency, water intake, pH), and the physical state of the horses' body (peripheral energy stores) (National Research Council 2007).

It would appear that many of the data reported in the literature have been from short-term experiments using classical experimental designs (e.g., Latin squares) that do not allow sufficient time for physiological adaptation to enable true measures of intake. Furthermore, preference tests take a matter of a few days and can be affected by previous experience so care is needed in drawing inference from these studies.

The animal's daily rate of nutrient extraction from forages is a product of the animal's daily food intake and the digestibility of the ingested forage. The latter will depend to some extent on fiber content but also the rate of passage of forage through the GIT. The strategy adopted by hind-gut fermenters is to eat relatively more than ruminants (Janis 1976), especially of high fiber foods, because, without a selective delaying mechanism for large particles, digesta passes quickly through the fermentation zone (cecum and colon). Equids are capable of extracting more nutrients per day from *ad libitum* forage diets than bovids (Duncan et al 1990) although perhaps the daily energetic costs of the extra grazing (~6 h longer) outweigh the benefits. It is clear that the maximization of VDMI is critical to the adequate supply of nutrients to the horse. However, experiments that have measured straw intakes suggest that the model proposed for the horse does not always hold true. Ponies fed *ad libitum* artificially dehydrated lucerne or oat straw consumed respectively, 155 or 95 g DM per kg $W^{0.75}$ and when restricted to 0.70 of *ad libitum* intake, the equivalent figures were 70 or 68 g DM per kg $W^{0.75}$ (Pearson et al 2001). Ponies consumed less straw than lucerne and chromium-fiber MRTs were longer for the straw diets when compared to the respective lucerne diets. Was the longer MRT of oat straw a reflection of its lower intake, lower digestibility, and slower rate of emptying from the colon or lower CP content? Was the lower VDMI of oat straw relative to lucerne, a reflection of its higher NDF content (715 vs. 443 g/kg DM), lower OM digestibility (0.44 vs. 0.58), longer MRT of chromium-fiber (*ad libitum*, 31.5 vs. 21.3 h; restricted, 36.0 vs. 30.5 h), lower CP content (39 vs. 146 g/kg DM) or just greater fecal bulk? These questions remain to be answered.

There are many conundrums that arise following examination of the literature concerning VDMI by horses and ponies. For example the intake of alfalfa is greater than grass hay ("the legume effect"), which is greater than straw, but this is not a gut fill issue as there is less DM in the GIT of straw-fed animals. Of great interest in this context is that lactating mares have a much higher VDMI than pregnant mares although the rate of passage for feed residues is the same for both. Does this mean that abdominal space (reduced through growth of the conceptus) is limiting the capacity of the GIT such that residues can only remain for a limited time in the GIT of the pregnant mare? Intakes of clamp silages are less than big/small silages but this is not a DM content

Table 3-7 Likely Dry Matter Intakes of a 500 kg Horse at Maintenance, during Pregnancy, Lactating or in Hard Work Fed Typical UK Diets

Horse status	Requirements[1] (per kg $W^{0.75}$)		Dietary features (per kg DM)			DMI (g/kg $W^{0.75}$)	DMI (g/kg LW)
	Energy (MJ DE)	Protein (g CP)	Fiber (gNDF)	Energy (MJ DE)	Protein (g CP)		
Maintenance	0.66	6.0	660	8.0	75	80	17
Pregnant (month 11)	0.85	8.5	507	8.5	85	100	21
Lactating (month 2)	1.25	14.5	405	10.0	111	130	27
Hard work	1.37	9.5	303	10.5	73	130	27

[1]National Research Council (2007).

issue and the "legume effect" is apparent for both hays and silages. Intakes of grass, alfalfa and grass hay usually greatly exceed animal requirements-why and furthermore, what accounts for the large differences between individuals in terms of their VDMI? Level of feeding effect is complex. *Ad libitum* straw feeding results in higher DMD values presumably as a result of animal selection but, *ad libitum* feeding of higher quality forages can reduce MRT with a resultant reduction in DMD; limit feeding results in higher DMD values as a result of a longer MRT. Clearly, there can be a "trade off" between the amount of food processed and nutrient yield and the relative importance of these processes will depend on the animal's circumstances. There is an analogous problem when grazing. It appears that some horses select taller plants to maximize bite mass but tall plants will be mature and therefore of lower nutritive value. Should the horse select higher quality grass at a cost of reduced bite mass but rather, obtain a higher nutrient mass? Depending on the nature of the sward, herbage bite mass rather than grass height alone could be more important to maximize nutrient intake rather than VDMI alone.

References

Agabriel, J., Trillaud-Geyl, C., Martin-Rosset, W., et al., 1982. Utilisation de l'ensilage de mais par le poulain de boucherie. Bulletin Technical CRZV Theix, INRA 49, 5–13.

Aiken, G.E., Potter, G.D., Conrad, B.E., et al., 1989. Voluntary intake and digestion of Coastal Bermuda grass hay by yearling and mature horses. Equine Veterinary Science 9, 262–264.

Archer, M., 1973. The species preferences of grazing horses. Journal of the British Grassland Society 28, 123–128.

Argo, C.Mc.G., Fuller, Z., Cox, J.E., 2001. Digestible energy intakes, growth and feeding behaviour of pony mares offered *ad libitum* access to a complete diet in a pelleted or chaff-based form. Proceedings of the 17th Equine Nutrition and Physiology Society Symposium, Kentucky, USA, pp. 171–173.

Argo, C.Mc.G., Cox, J.E., Lockyer, C., et al., 2002. Adaptive changes in the appetite, growth and feeding behaviour of pony mares offered ad libitum access to a complete diet in either a pelleted or chaff-based form. Animal Science 74, 517–528.

Bergero, D., Peiretti, P.G., Cola, E., 2002. Intake and apparent digestibility of perennial ryegrass haylages fed to ponies either at maintenance or at work. Livestock Production Science 77, 325–329.

Boulot, S., Brun, J.P., Doreau, M., et al., 1987. Activités alimentaires et niveau d'ingestion chez la jument gestante et allaitante. Reproduction, nutrition, développment 27, 205–206.

Brøkner, C., Nørgaard, P., Hansen, H.H., 2008. Effect of feed type and essential oil product on equine chewing activity. Journal of Animal Physiology and Animal Nutrition 92, 621–630.

Burcelin, R., Da Costa, A., Drucker, D., et al., 2001. Glucose competence of the hepatoportal vein sensor requires the presence of an activated glucagon-like peptide-1 receptor. Diabetes 50, 1720. 1728.

Cairns, M.C., Cooper, J.J., Davidson, H.P.B., et al., 2002. Association in horses of orosensory characteristics of foods with their post-ingestive consequences. Animal Science 75, 257–265.

Campbell, T.E., Harris, P.A., Doughty, H.C., et al., 2005. Effect of chaff quantity and length on rate of intake in horses fed a concentrate diet. Asia Pacific Journal of Clinical Nutrition Supplement 14, S80.

Campbell, T.E., Harris, P.A., Doughty, H.C., et al., 2006. Factors that affect the rate of intake when horses are fed a concentrate diet. In: Proceedings of the Australian Equine Science Symposium 1, 34.

Chavez, S.J., Siciliano, P.D., Huntington, G.B., 2011. Horse intake estimation of AM versus PM grazing. Journal of Equine Veterinary Science 31, 296.

Chenost, M., Martin-Rosset, W., 1985. Comparaison entre especes (mouton, cheval, bovin) de la digestibilité et des quantités ingérées des fourrages verts. Annales de Zootechnie 34, 291–312.

Crozier, J.A., Allen, V.G., Jack, N.E., et al., 1997. Digestibility, apparent mineral absorption and voluntary intake by horses fed alfalfa, tall fescue and caucasian bluestem. Journal of Animal Science 75, 1651–1658.

Cuddeford, D., Hyslop, J.J., 1996. Intake and digestibility of a high fibre concentrate offered *ad libitum* to ponies and donkeys. Proceedings of the 47th Annual Meeting of the EAAP, Lillehammer, Norway, p. 296(a).

Cuddeford, D., Woodhead, A.D., Muirhead, R., 1992. A comparison between the nutritive value of short-cutting, high temperature-dried alfalfa and timothy hay for horses. Equine Veterinary Journal 24, 84–89.

Cuddeford, D., Pearson, R.A., Archibald, R.F., et al., 1995. Digestibility and gastro-intestinal transit time of diets containing different proportions of alfalfa and oat straw given to Thoroughbreds, Shetland ponies, Highland ponies and donkeys. Animal Science 61, 407–417.

Cymbaluk, N.F., 1990. Comparison of forage digestion by cattle and horses. Canadian Journal of Animal Science 70, 601–610.

Dowler, L.E., Siciliano, P.D., 2009. Prediction of hourly pasture dry matter intake in horses. Journal of Equine Veterinary Science 29, 354–355.

Dugdale, A.H.A., Curtis, G.C., Cripps, P., et al., 2010. Effect of dietary restriction on body condition, composition and welfare of overweight and obese pony mares. Equine Veterinary Journal 42 (7), 600–610.

Dulphy, J.P., Martin-Rosset, W., Dubroeucq, H., et al. 1997a. Compared feeding patterns in ad libitum intake of dry forages by horses and sheep. Livestock Production Science 52, 49–56.

Dulphy, J.P., Martin-Rosset, W., Dubroeucq, H., et al., 1997b. Evaluation of voluntary intake of forage trough-fed to light horses. Comparison with sheep. Factors of variation and prediction. Livestock Production Science 52, 97–104.

Duncan, P., 1992. Horses and grasses. The nutritional ecology of Equids and their impact on the Camargue. Springer-Verlag, New York.

Duncan, P., Foose, T.J., Gordon, I.J., et al., 1990. Comparative nutrient extraction from forages by grazing bovids and equids: a test of the nutritional model of equid/bovid competition and coexistence. Oecologia 84, 411–418.

Duren, S.E., Dougherty, C.T., Jackson, S.G., et al., 1989. Modification of ingestive behavior due to exercise in yearling horses grazing orchardgrass. Applied Animal Behaviour Science 22, 335–345.

Edouard, N., Fleurance, G., Martin-Rosset, W., et al., 2008. Voluntary intake and digestibility in horses: effect of forage quality with emphasis on individual variability. Animal 2, 1526–1533.

Edouard, N., Fleurance, G., Dumont, B., et al., 2009. Does sward height affect feeding patch choice and voluntary intake in horses? Applied Animal Behaviour Science 119, 219–228.

Ellis, A.D., Thomas, S., Arkell, K., et al., 2005. Adding chopped straw to concentrate feed: the effect of inclusion rate and particle length on intake behavior of horses. Pferdeheilkunde 21, 35–36.

Fleurance, G., Duncan, P., Mallevaud, B., 2001. Daily intake and the selection of feeding sites by horses in heterogeneous wet grasslands. Animal Research 50, 149–156.

Fleurance, G., Fritz, H., Duncan, P., et al., 2009. Instantaneous intake rate in horses of different body sizes: Influence of sward biomass and fibrousness. Applied Animal Behaviour Science 117, 84–92.

Forbes, J.M., 1971. The Regulation of Voluntary Feed Intake. Physiological changes affecting voluntary food intake in ruminants. Proceedings of the Nutrition Society 30, 135–142.

Forbes, J.M., 1988. Metabolic aspects of the regulation of voluntary food intake and appetite. In: Nutrition Research Reviews 1. Cambridge University Press, Cambridge.

Frape, D., 2010. Equine Nutrition and Feeding, fourth ed. Wiley-Blackwell Publishing Ltd, 9600 Garsington Road, Oxford, UK.

Frape, D.L., Tuck, M.G., Sutcliffe, N.H., et al., 1982. The use of inert markers in the measurement of the digestibility of cubed concentrate and of hay given in several proportions to the pony, horse and white rhinoceros (*Diceros simus*). Comparative Biochemistry and Physiology 72A, 77–83.

Fuller, Z., Cox, J.E., Argo, C.Mc.G., 1998. Photoperiodic entrainment of seasonal changes in appetite and growth in pony colts. Proceedings of the British Society of Animal Science 36, 131.

Fuller, Z., Cox, J.E., Argo, C.McG., 2001. Photoperiodic entrainment of seasonal changes in the appetite, feeding behaviour, growth rate and pelage of pony colts. Animal Science 72, 65–74.

Gallagher, J.R., Hintz, H., Schryver, H.F., 1984. A nutritional evaluation of chopped hay for equines. Animal Production in Australia 15, 349–352.

Gibbs, J., Smith, G.P., 1978. The gut and preabsorptive satiety. Acta-Hepato-Gastroenterology 25, 413–416.

Glunk, E.C., Siciliano, P.D., 2011. Effect of restricted grazing on dry matter intake rate. Journal of Equine Veterinary Science 31, 296–297.

Goodwin, D., Davidson, H.P.B., Harris, P., 2004. Flavour preferences in concentrate diets for stabled horses. In: Proceedings of the 38th International Congress of the International Society of Animal Ethology, Helsinki, Finland, pp. 47–48.

Goodwin, D., Davidson, H.P.B., Harris, P., 2005a. Sensory varieties in concentrate diets for stabled horses: effects on behaviour and selection. Applied Animal behaviour Science 90, 337–349.

Goodwin, D., Davidson, H.P.B., Harris, P., 2005b. Selection and acceptance of flavours in concentrate diets for stabled horses. Applied Animal Behaviour Science 95, 223–232.

Goodwin, D., Davidson, H.P.B., Harris, P., 2007. Responses of horses offered a choice between stables containing single or multiple forages. Veterinary Record 160, 548–551.

Gordon, I.J., 1989. Vegetation community selection by ungulates on the Isle of Rhum III. Determinants of vegetation community selection. Journal of Applied Ecology 26, 65–79.

Grace, N.D., Gee, E.K., Firth, E.C., et al., 2002a. Digestible energy intake, dry matter digestibility and mineral status of grazing New Zealand Thoroughbred yearlings. New Zealand Veterinary Journal 50, 63–69.

Grace, N.D., Shaw, H.L., Gee, E.K., et al., 2002b. Determination of the digestible energy intake and apparent absorption of macroelements in pasture-fed lactating Thoroughbred mares. New Zealand Veterinary Journal 50, 182–185.

Grace, N.D., Rogers, C.W., Firth, E.C., et al., 2003. Digestible energy intake, dry matter digestibility and effect of increased calcium intake on bone parameters of grazing Thoroughbred weanlings in New Zealand. New Zealand Veterinary Journal 51, 165–173.

Haenlein, G.F., Holdren, R.D., Yoon, Y.M., 1966. Comparative responses of horses and sheep to different physical forms of alfalfa. Journal of Animal Science 25, 740–743.

Hale, C.E., Moore-Colyer, M.J.S., 2001. Voluntary food intake and apparent digestibilities of hay, big-bale grass silage and red clover silage by ponies. In: Proceedings of the 17th Equine Nutrition and Physiology Society Symposium, Kentucky, USA, pp. 468–469.

Hansen, D.K., Webb, G.W., Webb, S.P., 1992. Digestibility of wheat straw or ammoniated wheat straw in equine diets. Journal of Equine Science 12, 223–226.

Harris, P.A., Sillence, M., Inglis, R., et al., 2005a. Effect of short (<2 cm) lucerne chaff on the intake rate and glycaemic response of sweet feed. Pferdeheilkunde 21, 87–88.

Harris, P.A., Sillence, M., Inglis, R., et al., 2005b. Effect of short lucerne chaff on the rate of intake and glycaemic response to oat meal. In: Proceedings of the 19th Equine Science Society Symposium, Tucson, USA, p. 151.152.

Henneke, D.E., Callaham, J.W., 2009. Ad libitum concentrate intake in horses. Journal of Equine Veterinary Science 29, 425–427.

Hevener, A.L., Bergman, R.N., Donovan, C.M., 2001. Hypoglycaemic detection does not occur in hepatic artery or liver: findings consistent with a portal vein glucosensor locus. Diabetes 50, 399–403.

Hill, J., 2007. Impacts of nutritional technology on feeds offered to horses: A review of effects of processing on voluntary intake, digesta characteristics and feed utilization. Animal Feed Science and Technology 138, 92–117.

Hintz, H.F., Scott, J., Soderholm, L.V., et al., 1985. Extruded feeds for horses. Proceedings of the 9th Equine Nutrition and Physiology Society Symposium, Lansing, Michigan, USA, pp. 174–176.

Holland, J.L., Kronfeld, D.S., Sklan, D., et al., 1998. Calculation of fecal kinetics in horses fed hay or hay and concentrate. Journal of Animal Science 76, 1937–1944.

Hyslop, J.J., Calder, S., 2001. Voluntary intake and apparent digestibility in ponies offered alfalfa based forages *ad libitum*. Proceedings of the British Society of Animal Science, p. 90.

Hyslop, J.J., Cuddeford, D., 1999. Soaked unmolassed sugar beet pulp as a partial forage replacer in equine diets when ponies are offered grass hay *ad libitum*. In: Proceedings of the British Society of Animal Science, p. 140.

Hyslop, J.J., Jessop, N.S., Stefansdottir, G.J., et al., 1997. Comparative degradation in situ of four concentrate feeds in the caecum of ponies and the rumen of steers. In: Proceedings of the 15th Equine Nutrition and Physiology Society Symposium. Fort Worth, Texas, USA, pp. 116–117.

Hyslop, J.J., Bayley, A., Tomlinson, A.L., et al., 1998a. Voluntary feed intake and apparent digestibility *in vivo* in ponies given *ad libitum* access to dehydrated grass or hay harvested from the same grass crop. Proceedings of the British Society of Animal Science, p. 131.

Hyslop, J.J., Roy, S., Cuddeford, D., 1998b. *Ad libitum* sugar beet pulp as the major fibre source in equine diets when ponies are offered a restricted amount of mature grass hay. Proceedings of the British Society of Animal Science, p. 132.

Hyslop, J.J., Tomlinson, A.L., Bayley, A., et al., 1998c. Voluntary feed intake and apparent digestibility *in vivo* in ponies offered a mature threshed grass hay *ad libitum*. Proceedings of the British Society of Animal Science, p. 130.

Ince, J., Longland, A.C., Newbold, J.C., et al., 2011. Changes in proportion of dry matter intakes by ponies with access to pasture and haylage for 3 and 20 hours per day respectively, for six weeks. Journal of Equine Veterinary Science 31, 283.

Janis, C., 1976. The evolutionary strategy of the equidae and the origins of rumen and cecal digestion. Evolution 30, 757–774.

Jose-Cunilleras, E., Taylor, L.E., Hinchcliff, K.W., 2004. Glycemic index of cracked corn, oat groats and rolled barley in horses. Journal of Animal Science 82, 2623–2629.

Kyriazakis, I., Emmans, G.C., 1995. The voluntary food intake of pigs given feeds based on wheat bran, dried citrus pulp and grass meal, in relation to measurements of food bulk. British Journal of Nutrition 73, 191–207.

LaCasha, P.A., Brady, H.A., Allen, V.G., et al., 1999. Voluntary intake, digestibility, and subsequent selection of Matua bromegrass, coastal bermudagrass, and alfalfa hays by yearling horses. Journal of Animal Science 77, 2766–2773.

Laut, J.E., Houpt, K.A., Hintz, H.F., et al., 1985. The effects of caloric dilution on meal patterns and feed intake in ponies. Physiology and Behaviour 35, 549–554.

Lawrence, A.C. St., Lawrence, L.M., Coleman, R.J., 2001. Using an empirical equation to predict voluntary intake of grass hays by mature equids. Proceedings of the 17th Equine Nutrition and Physiology Society Symposium, Kentucky, USA, pp. 99–100.

Longland, A.C., Ince, J., Harris, P.A., 2011a. Estimation of pasture intake by ponies from liveweight change during six weeks at pasture. Journal of Equine Veterinary Science 31, 275–276.

Longland, A.C., Barfoot, C., Harris, P.A., 2011b. The effect of wearing a grazing muzzle vs not wearing a grazing muzzle on pasture dry matter intake by ponies. Journal of Equine Veterinary Science 31, 282–283.

Martin-Rosset, W., Dulpy, J.P., 1987. Digestibility interactions between forages and concentrates in horses: influence of feeding level–comparison with sheep. Livestock Production Science 17, 263–276.

Martin-Rosset, W., Doreau, M., Boulot, S., et al., 1990. Influence of level of feeding and physiological state on diet digestibility in light and heavy breed horses. Livestock Production Science 25, 257–264.

Martin-Rosset, W., Doreau, M., Thivend, P., 1987. Digestion de régimes à base de foin ou d'ensilage de maïs chez le Cheval en croissance. Reproduction, Nutrition, Development 27, 291–292.

McCown, S., Brummer, M., Hayes, S., et al., 2011. Nutrient and dry matter intakes of broodmares fed high forage diets. Journal of Equine Veterinary Science 32, 264–265.

McCullough, M.E., 1966. The nutritive value of silage as influenced by silage fermentation and ration supplementation. Proceedings of the 10th International Grassland Conference, Helsinki, p. 581.

McLean, B.M.L., 2001. Estimating digesta passage rate of forage based diets in horses using N-alkanes. Proceedings of the 17th Equine Nutrition and Physiology Society Symposium, Kentucky, USA, pp. 192–194.

McLean, B.M.L., Afzalzadeh, A., Bates, L., et al., 1995. Voluntary intake, digestibility and rate of passage of a hay and a silage fed to horses and to cattle. Animal Science 60, 555.

McMeniman, N.P., 2000. Nutrition of grazing broodmares, their foals and young horses. RIRDC Publication No 00/28. Project No UQ-45A. Rural Industries Research and Development Corporation, Australia.

Menard, C., Duncan, P., Fleurance, G., et al., 2002. Comparative foraging and nutrition of horses and cattle in European wetlands. Journal of Applied Ecology 39, 120–133.

Mesochina, P., 2000. Niveau d'ingestion du cheval en croissance au pâturage: mise au point éthodologique et étude de quelques facteurs de variation. PhD. Institut National Agronomique Paris-Grignon, Paris, France.

Meyer, H., Radicke, S., Kienzle, E., et al., 1993. Investigations on preileal digestion of oats, corn and barley starch in relation to grain processing. Proceedings of the 13th Equine Nutrition and Physiology Society Symposium, Gainsville, Florida, USA, pp. 92–97.

Minson, D.J., 1990. Forage in Ruminant Nutrition, Academic Press, New York.

Miraglia, N., Poncet, C., Martin-Rosset, W., 2003. Effect of feeding level, physiological status and breed on the digesta passage of forage based diet in the horse. In: Proceedings of the 18th Equine Nutrition and Physiology Society Symposium, Michigan State University, East Lansing, USA, 4–7th June 2003, pp. 275–280.

Moore-Colyer, M.J.S., Longland, A.C., 2000. Intakes and *in vivo* apparent digestibilities of four types of conserved grass forage by ponies. Animal Science 71, 527–534.

Morrow, H.J., Moore-Colyer, M.J.S., Longland, A.C., 1999. The apparent digestibilities and rates of passage of two chop lengths of big bale silage and hay in ponies. Proceedings of the British Society of Animal Science, BSAS, P.O. Box 3, Penicuik, Midlothian, EH26 0RZ, UK, p. 142.

Murray, J.-A.M.D., Sanderson, R., Longland, A.C., et al., 2009. Assessment of mathematical models to describe the rate of passage of enzyme-treated or sugar beet pulp-substituted lucerne silage in equids. Animal Feed Science and Technology 154, 228–240.

National Research Council, 2007. Nutrient Requirements of Domestic Animals. Nutrient Requirements of Horses, fifth revised ed. National Academy of Sciences, Washington DC, USA.

Naujeck, A., Hill, J., 2003. The influence of sward height on bite dimensions of horses. Animal Science 77, 95–100.

Naujeck, A., Hill, J., Gibb, M.J., 2005. Influence of sward height on diet selection by horses. Applied Animal Behaviour Science 90, 49–63.

Ordakowski-Burk, A.L., Quinn, R.W., Shellem, T.A., et al., 2006. Voluntary intake and digestibility of reed canarygrass and timothy hay fed to horses. Journal of Animal Science 84, 3104–3109.

Ott, E.A., 1981. Influence of level of feeding on digestion efficiency of the horses. Proceedings of the 7th Equine Nutrition and Physiology Society Symposium, Virginia, USA, pp. 37–43.

Pagliassoti, M.J., Holste, L.C., Moore, M.C., et al., 1996. Comparison of the time courses of insulin and the portal signal on hepatic glucose and glycogen metabolism in the conscious dog. Journal of Clinical Investigation 97, 81–91.

Pearson, R.A., Merritt, J.B., 1991. Intake, digestion and gastrointestinal transit time in resting donkeys and ponies and exercised donkeys given *ad libitum* hay and straw. Equine Veterinary Journal 23, 339–343.

Pearson, R.A., Archibald, R.F., Muirhead, R.H., 2001. The effect of forage quality and level of feeding on digestibility and gastrointestinal transit time of oat straw and alfalfa given to ponies and donkeys. British Journal of Nutrition 85, 599–606.

Pearson, R.A., Archibald, R.F., Muirhead, R.H., 2006. A comparison of the effect of forage type and level of feeding on the digestibility and gastrointestinal mean retention time of dry forages given to cattle, sheep, ponies and donkeys. British Journal of Nutrition 95, 88–98.

Piccione, G., Caola, G., Refinetti, R., 2005. Temporal relationships of 21physiological variables in horse and sheep. Comparative Biochemistry and Physiology. Part A: Molecular and Integrative Physiology 142, 389–396.

Ragnarsson, S., Lindberg, J.E., 2010. Impact of level of feeding on digestibility of a haylage-only diet in Icelandic horses. Journal of Animal Physiology and Animal Nutrition (In press).

Ralston, S.L., 1984. Controls of feeding in horses. Journal of Animal Science 59, 1354–1361.

Ralston, S.L., 1992. Regulation of feed intake in the horse in relation to gastrointestinal disease. Pferdeheilkunde 15–18.

Ralston, S.L., Baile, C.A., 1982a. Plasma glucose and insulin concentrations and feeding behaviour in ponies. Journal of Animal Science 54, 1132–1137.

Ralston, S.L., Baile, C.A., 1982b. Gastrointestinal stimuli in the control of feed intake in ponies. Journal of Animal Science 55, 243–253.

Ralston, S.L., Baile, C.A., 1983. Effects of intragastric xylose, sodium chloride and corn oil on feeding behaviour of ponies. Journal of Animal Science 56, 302–308.

Ralston, S.L., Van den Broek, G., Baile, C.A., 1979. Feed intake patterns and associated blood glucose, free fatty acid and insulin changes in ponies. Journal of Animal Science 49, 838–845.

Ralston, S.L., Freeman, D.E., Baile, C.A., 1983. Volatile fatty acids and the role of the large intestine in the control of feed intake in ponies. Journal of Animal Science 57, 815–820.

Redgate, S.E., Hall, S., Cooper, J.J., et al., 2007. Dietary experience changes feeding preferences in the domestic horse. In: Proceedings of the 20th Equine Science Society Symposium. Maryland, USA, pp. 120–121.

Reinowski, A.R., Coleman, R., 2003. Voluntary intake of Big Bluestem, Eastern Gamagrass, Indian Grass and Timothy Grass hays by mature horses. In: Proceedings of the 18th Equine Nutrition and Physiology Society Symposium. Michigan State University, East Lansing, USA, 4–7 June, 2003, pp. 3–5.

Rosenfeld, I., Austbø, D., 2009. Effect of type of grain and feed processing on gastrointestinal retention times in horses. Journal of Animal Science 87, 3991–3996.

Rosenfeld, I., Austbø, D., Volden, H., 2006. Models for estimating digesta passage kinetics in the gastrointestinal tract of the horse. Journal of Animal Science 84, 3321–3328.

Savadogo, M., Zemmelink, G., Nianogo, A.J., 2000. Effect of selective consumption on voluntary intake and digestibility of sorghum (*Sorghum bicolor* L. Moench) stover, cowpea (*Vigna unguiculata* L. Walp.) and groundnut (*Arachis hypogaea* L.) haulms by sheep. Animal Feed Science and Technology 84, 265–277.

Schurg, W.A., Pulse, R.E., Holtan, D.W., et al., 1978. Use of various quantities and forms of ryegrass straw in horse diets. Journal of Animal Science 47, 1287–1291.

Schmitt, M., 1973. Influences of hepatic portal receptors on hypothalamic feeding and satiety centres. American Journal of Physiology 225, 1089–1095.

Smith, D.G., 1999. The impact of grazing time allowance on the dry matter intake and foraging behaviour of cattle and donkeys managed under traditional African grazing systems. PhD Thesis, University of Edinburgh.

Smith, D.G., Cuddeford, D., Mayes, R., Hollands, T., 2007. The dry matter intake of grazing horses. 46th Congress of the British Equine Veterinary Association 12th–15th September 2007, Edinburgh.

Søndergaard, E., 2003. PhD Thesis. Danish Institute of Agricultural Sciences, Department of Animal Health and Welfare, Tjele, Denmark.

Spooner, H.S., Nielsen, B.D., Harris, P.A., et al., 2007. Hydration status of horses during endurance exercise as affected by dietary fiber type. In: Proceedings of the 20th Equine Science Society Symposium. Maryland, USA, pp. 24–25.

Stephens, D.W., Krebs, J.R., 1986. Foraging Theory. Princeton University Press, Princeton, NJ, USA.

Thorne, J.B., Goodwin, D., Kennedy, M.J., et al., 2005. Foraging enrichment for individually housed horses: Practicality and effects on behavior. Applied Animal Behaviour Science 94, 149–164.

Tisserand, J.L., Faurie, F., Toure, M., 1991. A comparative study of donkey and pony digestive physiology. In: Fielding, D., Pearson, R.A. (Eds.), Donkeys, Mules and Horses in Tropical Agricultural Development. Centre for Tropical Veterinary Medicine, University of Edinburgh, pp. 67–72.

Todd, L., Sauer, W.C., Christopherson, R.J., et al., 1995. The effect of feeding different forms of alfalfa on nutrient digestibility and voluntary intake in mature horses. Journal of Animal Physiology and Animal Nutrition 73, 1–8.

Tsaras, L.N., Kyriazakis, I., Emmans, G.C., 1998. The prediction of the voluntary food intake of pigs on poor quality foods. Animal Science 66, 713–723.

Turcott, S.K., Nielsen, B.D., O'Connor, C., et al., 2003. The influence of various concentrate to roughage ratios on dietary intake and nutrient digestibilities of weanlings. In: Proceedings of the 18th Equine Nutrition and Physiology Society Symposium. Michigan State University, East Lansing, USA, 4–7 June 2003, pp. 1–2.

Van Soest, P.J., 1994. Nutritional Ecology of the Ruminant, second ed. Cornell University Press, Ithaca, NY.

Van Wieren, S.E., 1996. Do large herbivores select a diet that maximizes short-term energy intake rate? Forest Ecology and Management 88, 149–156.

Winsco, K.N., Wickersham, T.A., Hammer, C.J., et al., 2011. Effect of dietary energy manipulation on mares and their foals: Determination of voluntary dry matter intake of mares during late pregnancy using a dual marker system. Journal of Equine Veterinary Science 31, 265.

4

SECTION A Nutritional Foundations

Water

Nadia F. Cymbaluk

The desire for water is a basic motivating instinct for animals which is only exceeded by their need for air and the avoidance of severe pain. Water is a universal solvent therefore, "water is involved either directly or indirectly in virtually every physiologic process essential to life" (Raisbeck et al 2007). Water is critical to all biochemical reactions and thermoregulation. Water reserves in horses are more labile than energy reserves (body fat), which allows horses to tolerate feed deprivation for a longer period than a lack of water. Dehydration greater than 15% percent can be fatal for a horse (Carlson 1979). This is a fluid loss of about 95 liters for a 500 kg horse. Depending on environmental conditions and activity, fluid loss to this extent, as a result of obligatory fluid losses (Fig. 4.1), would be likely to take less than 7 days. Death due to starvation occurs after a body mass loss of about 50% (Stull, unpublished information). Depending on many factors (age, body condition, climate, activity), a weight loss of this magnitude for an average horse would likely take more than 90 days.

Body fluid compartments

Total body water accounts for 61–72% of the body weight (BW) of mature horses (Table 4-1: Julian et al 1956, Deavers et al 1973, Carlson et al 1979, Judson & Mooney 1983, Carlson 1987, Sneddon et al 1993, Forro et al 2000, Fielding et al 2004, 2007, 2008, Lindinger et al 2004, Waller & Lindinger 2005, Forro & Lindinger 2006) and has been estimated at 66–84% BW of foals varying with foal age or dilution method used (Oftedal et al 1983, Doreau et al 1986, Geerken et al 1988).

Total body water (TBW) is distributed within cells (intracellular) or outside of cells (extracellular). The intracellular fluid compartment (ICF) is estimated at 38–53% of body weight (BW) (Table 4-1). The extracellular fluid compartment (ECF) comprises fluid in blood, interstitial fluid (ISF), bone, connective tissue, and transcellular fluid. The ECF compartment has been estimated at 22–26% BW (Table 4-1; Andrews et al 1997, Fielding et al 2003, 2004, 2007, 2008, Waller et al 2008). Transcellular fluids are contained within epithelial-lined compartments such as the gut and urinary bladder. Depending on diet, the fluid sequestered by the horse's gastrointestinal content can account from 9 to 21% of equid weight (Robb et al 1972, Coenen & Meyer 1987, Gee et al 2003, Sneddon et al 2006) and has been speculated to be a fluid reservoir for the horse during physical activity and other brief periods when water is inaccessible (Sneddon & Argenzio 1998). The fluid holding capacity of the diet influences the water content in the equine gastrointestinal tract. Hay-fed horses had a total intestinal fluid capacity of 188 ml/kg BW which was 84% greater than horses fed a complete feed (102 ml/kg BW) (Coenen & Meyer 1987). Moreover, 77% of gut water in hay-fed horses was in the large bowel compared to 65% in horses fed complete feed. The large reservoir of gut fluid may explain why horses drink intermittently rather than sip continuously.

Total body water decreases linearly with age in horses and foals (Agrabriel et al 1984, Doreau et al 1986). The ECF of newborn foals is about 40% of BW but declines to 25% of body weight in adult horses (Table 4-1; Spensley et al 1987). Likewise, plasma volume in newborns is higher (9.6% BW) (Table 4-1) than in mature horses (4.7% BW) (Spensley et al 1987). These differences underscore why the approaches for fluid therapy in the foal must differ to that used for the mature horse.

Water balance

Water balance describes the homeostasis between water input and water output (Fig. 4.1). Water input occurs through drinking, water contained in feed, and water derived by metabolic processes. All horses lose fluid via four routes: fecal, urinary, respiratory, and cutaneous (sweat) losses. The latter two routes are called evaporative heat loss. Lactating mares have a fifth route of body fluid loss via milk secretion. The water balance equation for horses can be given as:

$$W_{balance} = (W_{feed} + W_{drink} + W_{metabolic}) - (W_{feces} + W_{urine} + W_{sweat} + W_{respiration})$$

W_{milk} is added to the equation for lactating mares. Two criteria are difficult to measure: metabolic water and water in respiration. Measuring cutaneous losses is difficult but not impossible. Although the water balance diagram (Fig. 4.1) implies a static relationship, the association between water intake and water output is dynamic.

Fluid output or loss

Fecal fluid loss

Feces are the main route of fluid loss in the mature, idle horse fed hay (Table 4-2) although diet, environment, physical activity and husbandry have a marked influence on absolute amounts of fluid lost by this route. Diet is one of the main determinants of intestinal, and therefore, fecal water content. Horses fed hay or silage (72–85% moisture) have

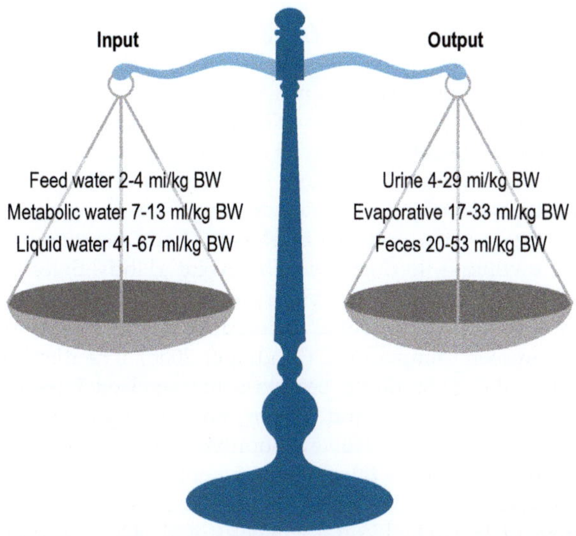

Figure 4.1 Elements of water balance in mature, idle horse.

wetter feces than horses fed hay diets with added grain (66% moisture) (Fonnesbeck 1968, Cymbaluk 1990a, Meyer 1995, Warren et al 1999, Zeyner et al 2004, Muhonen 2008). Absolute fecal fluid losses range from 16 to 38 mL/kg BW (Tasker, 1967c) (also see Table 4-1). Based on retrospective analysis of fecal moisture content of horses fed various hays (timothy, alfalfa-grass, oats, hay) plus limited grain mixes (less than 15%), fecal fluid output averaged 31.0 ± 4.9 ml/kg BW (range 19.6–52.7 ml/kg BW) (Cymbaluk unpublished data).

Fecal moisture content and total fecal water output were positively correlated to total DM intake and crude fiber content over a range of fecal moistures of 66 to 79% (Fonnesbeck 1968, Cymbaluk 1989). Water content of ingesta of horses unadapted to grain then acutely fed two high grain meals (4.55 kg/day) was approximately 5% lower than for horses fed an all hay diet free choice yet fecal water content did not differ significantly (Lopes 2002). Drier manure (less than 70%) was observed in horses fed high grain (greater than 50%), high glucose (15%), and high molasses beet pulp (26%) diets (Cymbaluk 1989, Olsman et al 2004). However, horses fed a high (12%) soluble fiber diet derived from beet pulp and alfalfa hay had a fecal moisture content (81.7%) 8% wetter than those fed a low (7%) soluble fiber diet of oats-orchardgrass–timothy hay as a result of a higher water:feed intake and adsorption of water to hydrophilic fiber (Warren et al 1999). Moreover, horses fed an all-hay diet maintained lower plasma protein concentration post-exercise than horses fed a limited hay-concentrate diet, which was inferred to represent conservation of plasma volume through greater movement of fluid from the gut (Danielsen et al 1995). For this reason, a higher dietary soluble fiber content has been speculated to have possible benefit during exercise when there is an increased water need. Although the pretreatment plasma volume of horses fed a high soluble fiber diet was higher, consuming a high or low soluble fiber diet

Table 4-1 Fluid Compartments of Adult Horses

Compartment	Volume (ml/kg BW)	Number of horses	Method of determination
Total body water	662 ± 55	149	Bioelectrical impedance, deuterium oxide, tritiated water
Extracellular fluid	241 ± 23	200	Sodium thiocyanate
Plasma volume	47 ± 9	255	Evans blue, ^{32}P, ^{51}Cr, ^{59}Fe
Gastrointestinal volume	147 ± 60	61	Post-mortem
Intracellular fluid	437 ± 66	61	Calculated

Table 4-2 Diet Effect on Water Intake, Fecal and Urinary Fluid Output of Idle Horses Kept in a Thermoneutral Environment (10°C, RH <75%)

Diet	Free + feed water intake	Fecal water	Urine	Ratio of imbibed water to		Feed:water ratio
		(ml/kg/day)		Fecal	Urine	
Timothy hay–15% grain	48.7	29.9	7.36	61.3	15.1	2.28
Oats hay	60.0	36.5	11.0	61.0	18.3	3.22
Timothy hay	50.0	30.3	9.5	60.6	19.0	2.50
Timothy hay – 15% (20% protein) pellet	51.9	28.9	8.2	55.6	15.8	2.65

Source: N.F. Cymbaluk, unpublished data.

had no effect on the plasma volume of horses after frusemide administration (Warren et al 1999). Similarly, no differences were observed in hydration status following a 60 km exercise test in horses fed a chopped grass hay compared to a grass hay : soluble fiber chop (Spooner et al 2009).

Intestinal disease that impairs water reabsorption by the gut increases fecal water loss. Horses with chronic diarrhea had a fecal output nearly fourfold greater (50.7 kg/day) than normal horses (12.04 kg/day) (Merritt 1975). The large fecal fluid loss by horses with chronic diarrhea was compensated for by a doubling of water intake (42 vs 24 liters/day). Likewise, horses with castor oil-induced diarrhea had fecal moistures of 90% or higher and lost twice the volume of fecal water (5.15 ml/kg BW/h) of normal horses (2.15 ml/kg BW/h) (Ecke et al 1998). For a 500-kg horse, these values equate to a daily fecal fluid loss of 61.8 liters/day during diarrhea compared to 25.8 liters/day in the normal horse. It is evident why horses with diarrhea become dehydrated if fluids are not replenished.

Urinary fluid loss

Body fluid homeostasis is controlled by the kidney. Although specific gravity (SG) alone has been used to classify urine concentration (Savage 2008), use of urine osmolality and urine SG provide a more accurate definition (Wilson 2007). Hyposthenuria describes urine with a SG less than 1.008 and an osmolality below 269 mOsm/kg (Wilson 2007). Isosthenuric urine is similar to plasma in concentration with an SG of 1.008–1.012 and osmolality between 260–300 mOsm/kg. Hypersthenuric urine has a SG greater than 1.012 with an osmolality greater than 300 mOsm/kg. Normal adults have hypersthenuric urine. Normal foals have hyposthenuric urine (Wilson 2007).

The obligatory loss of urine is the fluid required to eliminate various solutes via the kidney irrespective of fluid intake. Horses have an obligatory urine loss of about 5–6.3 ml/kg BW per day (Tasker 1967a) whereas "normal" urine volumes range from 6 to 29 ml/kg BW (Fonnesbeck 1968, Rumbaugh et al 1982, Freeman et al 1999). The average daily urine output for idle horses ($n = 340$) housed in a thermoneutral environment and fed a wide range of feeds was 8 ml/kg BW (range 4–18 ml/kg BW) (Cymbaluk, unpublished data). Variance in normal urine volume arises from differences in diet (composition and nutrient content), water or fluid availability, metabolic responses to ambient temperature, exercise load or gastrointestinal health (Tasker 1967b, c, Cymbaluk 1989, Knottenbelt 2000, Connysson et al 2006). Chronically diarrheic horses (4.15 liters/day) reduced urine output by 23% compared to normal horses (5.36 liters/day) (Merritt 1975). During and after heavy exercise, horses reduce urine output to conserve body fluid. Exercised Thoroughbred horses produced 1.4 liters less urine per day than idle horses perhaps to compensate for fluid losses in sweat (Pagan et al 1998). Yet, the impact of exercise on urine volume is unpredictable because fluid conservation is tied to sweat loss which depends on exercise intensity and the environmental conditions in which the exercise is performed.

Urine output in the horse varies quickly with changes in physiological and biochemical stimuli. Changes to the renal solute load created by protein, sodium, or potassium above the horse's requirements typically elevates urine volume. Urine flow rates quadrupled in donkeys fed alfalfa hay compared to a similar dry matter intake provided by a wheat straw diet because of an 8-fold higher nitrogen intake on the alfalfa diet (Izraely et al 1989). Because potassium homeostasis is regulated by the kidney, horses fed a high potassium diet (5.4 mmol K/kg BW) had a 26 to 30% higher urine output than horses fed a diet with 4.1 mmol K/kg BW (Jansson 1999, Jansson & Dahlborn 1999, Jansson et al 1999). Urinary output may be expected to increase when diets containing high-potassium feeds such as molasses (6.1% potassium) are fed to horses (NRC 2007). Although sodium is effectively conserved by the kidney, regulation of equine sodium homeostasis may be gastrointestinal rather than renal (Jansson & Dahlborn 1999). This is supported by data showing that ponies had similar urine volume when fed high (1–%) dietary salt (Schryver et al 1987).

Total evaporative fluid losses

Heat loss in horses occurs by water vaporization through respiration and/or sweating. At body temperature, 2.5 kJ or 578 calories of heat are removed during evaporation of 1 ml of water. Evaporative heat and, therefore, fluid loss, occurs by passive diffusion from skin and lungs whereas sweating is an active process, initiated by elevated body core temperatures, involving fluid secretion by sweat glands. Sweating occurs at thermoneutrality but increases greatly when core body temperatures increase in response to exercise or elevated ambient temperature (Lindinger 2008). The distribution of total evaporative heat loss in exercised horses is about 23% respiratory and 70% or more through sweating (Kingston et al 1997). Daily evaporative losses of idle Standardbred horses fed alfalfa hay and kept in thermoneutral (5–20°C) conditions were calculated at 10 liters/day with an average of 23 ml/kg BW (Groenendyk et al 1988). Standardbred horses kept in a climatic chamber had evaporative heat losses of 48 W/m^2 or about 20 ml/kg BW at thermoneutral temperatures (Morgan et al 1997).

Respiratory losses

Respiratory heat (fluid) loss by the idle horse varies with ambient temperature and humidity. In the exercised horse, fluid losses increase with length and duration of exercise. Respiratory fluid loss accounted for 19 to 30% of the total evaporative heat loss by exercised horses (Hodgson et al 1993, Kingston et al 1997). Thoroughbred horses exercised at 40, 65, and 90% of VO_{2max} for durations of 38, 15, 9 minutes, respectively, had estimated respiratory fluid losses of 2.1, 0.8 and 0.8 liters and concurrent sweat losses of 9, 9.2, and 6.9 liters, respectively (Hodgson et al 1993). Respiratory heat loss by Thoroughbred horses undergoing long duration exercise (202 min) at 40% VO_{2max} was estimated at 23% of evaporative heat loss (7.4 liters) with concomitant sweat losses of 22.7 liters (Kingston et al 1997). Heat acclimation occurs through increased sweating and respiration as discussed in more detail below (Geor et al 2000, McCutcheon & Geor 1999).

Sweat losses

Passive cutaneous evaporative loss by horses (average weight 429 kg) housed at temperatures between 5 to 20°C in a climatic chamber were estimated at about 8.5 liters per day (see above) (Morgan et al 1997) but in exercised horses, total fluid losses increase through sweat in proportion to exercise duration and intensity, environmental conditions, and climatic acclimation of the horse (McCutcheon & Geor 1998). Rates of fluid loss by horses doing low (40% VO_{2max}), moderate (65% VO_{2max}) and high (90% VO_{2max}) intensity treadmill work in an air-conditioned laboratory (21–23.5°C) were 0.61, 1.32 and 1.73 ml/kg BW/min (Hodgson et al 1993) Total body water losses attributed to sweating by cross-country event-horses ranged from 4.8 to 20.4 liters (2–6.1% of BW). (Ecker & Lindinger 1995). Body mass losses of 33.8 kg were obtained for 460-kg horses performing long-distance (45 km), low-intensity (40% VO_{2max}), activity on a treadmill (Kingston et al 1997).

Training, conditioning and temperature acclimation increase tolerance to high ambient temperatures. Training alone increases sweating rate of horses which is intensified as conditions of high humidity and high ambient temperatures are imposed (McCutcheon & Geor 1999). High ambient temperatures alone (>33–35°C) increased evaporative heat (fluid loss) by four- to five-fold in idle horses (Morgan et al 1997) and by 45–60% in exercising Standardbred and Thoroughbred horses relative to fluid loss at 20°C (Jansson 1999, McCutcheon et al 1995).

Sweating, in response to hot weather, requires time to become fully effective. Partial acclimation by horses to hot weather occurs within 2 weeks whether hot temperature exposure is intermittent or continuous but 3 weeks of exposure is required for full acclimation (Geor et al 2000, McCutcheon & Geor 1999). Acclimation to hot ambient temperatures does not confer resistance to dehydration.

Lactation losses

Milk output varies widely among individual mares, breeds, and over the lactation cycle (Doreau & Boulot 1989). Typically, primiparous mares produce less milk than multiparous mares irrespective of mare breed (Doreau et al 1991, Pool-Anderson et al 1994). Quarter horse mares produced 18–21 ml milk/kg BW daily (Gibbs et al 1982, Pool-Anderson et al 1994), Thoroughbred and Standardbred mares yielded 29 to 34 ml/kg BW per day (Oftedal et al 1983), primiparous and multiparous light and draft mares produced 24 to 27.5 ml milk/kg BW per day (Doreau et al 1991), Australian stock horses produced 37 ml/kg BW per day (Martin et al 1992), and Lusitano mares produced 23–30 ml/kg BW per day (Santos & Silvestre 2008). To offset lactational losses only, mares must increase water intake by 30 to 60% above maintenance.

Key Points – Water losses

- Feces are often the main route of fluid loss in idle horses but this depends on diet. Average daily fecal fluid output is about 31 ml/kg BW with a range between 20 to 53 ml/kg BW.
- Daily evaporative losses for horses average about 20 ml/kg BW (range 17–33 ml/kg BW) at thermoneutral conditions. Sweat fluid losses increase markedly with exercise, with further increments when exercise is conducted in hot conditions.
- Daily milk losses by mares range from 18 to 37 ml/kg BW under thermoneutral conditions. Water intake can be expected to increase by 30 to 60% to offset lactational losses alone. The metabolic requirements of lactation result in the consumption of at least 36% more feed during lactation than during pregnancy, thus water intake will increase proportionately to the increase in feed intake. Hot weather will further elevate water intake requirements.

Water intake

Water provision can be external (direct) or internal (indirect). External fluid supply is provided by liquid (free) water and feed water. Imbibed water generally supplies more than 80% of the water requirements of hay-fed horses whereas grazing horses obtain significant amounts of water from pasturage. Metabolic water is generated by tissue oxidation of protein, fats, and carbohydrates from feed and is estimated at 11–13% of daily water intake or 6.8–13 ml/kg BW (Groendyk et al 1988, Van den Berg et al 1998) and has been estimated at about 2.7 liters/day in a 500 kg horse (Carlson 1979).

Feed water

All horse feeds contain water. Basal feeds used in the stable such as hay, grain and processed feeds typically contain 10 to 15% moisture and so supply little fluid (1 to 2 liters/day) to the horse's water balance (Freeman et al 1999, Muhonen 2008). Haylage (32–45% moisture) and silage (55–64% moisture) can supply about 25% and 45% of the water needs of idle and worked horses resulting in a proportionate decrease in volume of liquid water consumed when these feeds are fed (Muhonen 2008). A vegetative perennial ryegrass pasture (80% moisture) in the amounts eaten by pregnant (68 kg) and barren mares (40 kg) provided 54.5 kg and 31 kg feed fluid, respectively (Marlow et al 1983), and nearly met the mares' water needs. Pasture moisture content declines over a growing season from more than 80% in the spring to less than 10% by late fall (McMillen et al 1943, Meissner & Paulsmeier 1995). This explains why equids drink infrequently (1.4 to 3.4 bouts/day) on lush pasture (Scheibe et al 1998) but drink more often as pastures senesce and when dry feeds are provided in stables (Sweeting et al 1985).

Liquid water

The total volume of water consumed by an idle horse is determined by its body weight. Therefore, an idle 1000-kg Percheron horse will typically drink more water than a 600-kg Quarter horse (Fig. 4.2). Adult horses fed hay to meet maintenance energy needs drink about 50 ml/kg BW daily. Daily free water intake by normal, idle horses fed alfalfa-timothy or alfalfa hay ad libitum was 51 to 56 ml/kg BW (Tasker 1967b, Sweeting et al 1985, Groenendyk et al 1988), stabled grass-fed Namib and Boerperd horses drank 41 to 48 ml water/kg BW (Sneddon et al 1993), stabled, mature ponies fed grass or alfalfa hay drank 50 to 55 ml/kg BW (Cymbaluk 1989), pregnant mares fed a grass hay-grain diet drank 45 to 59 ml water/kg BW (Freeman et al 1999).

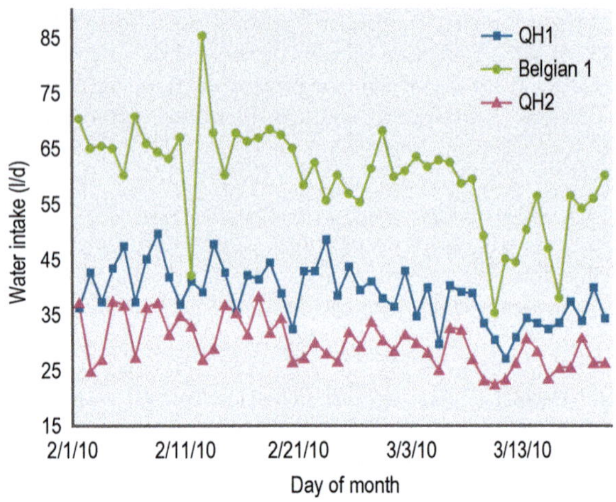

Figure 4.2 Daily absolute water intake of two Quarter Horse mares (QH1 wt 690 kg; QH2 wt 650 kg) and one Belgian mare (wt 880 kg) fed hay-concentrate diet to exceed nutrient requirements for pregnancy and housed at 10 to 15°C.

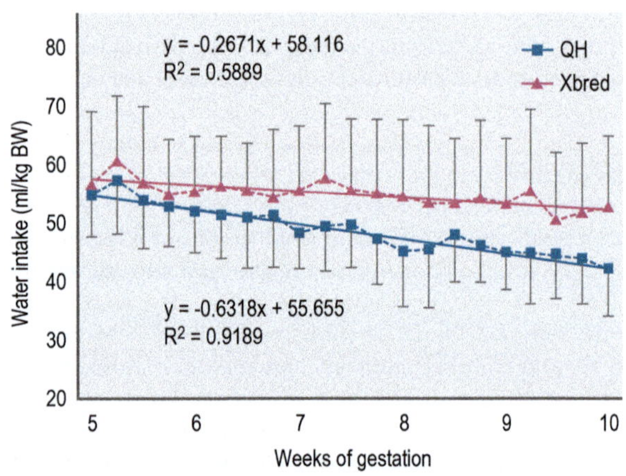

Figure 4.3 Water intake by 11 Quarter Horse mares and 11 Thoroughbred-draft cross mares from early to late gestation.

Horse breed may affect water intake but this factor has been inadequately tested. Thoroughbred horses and Highland ponies drank twofold more water per kg feed than donkeys or Shetland ponies (Cuddeford et al 1995). Draft-Thoroughbred cross mares (55.2 ± 11.5 ml/kg BW) fed the same diet drank 13% more water than Quarter horse mares (48.7 ± 7.75 ml/kg BW) (Cymbaluk, unpublished data) (Fig. 4.3) and donkeys drank 27% less water (51 ml/kg BW) than similarly housed and fed ponies (65 ml/kg BW) (Mueller & Houpt 1991).

Although daily maintenance water requirements are estimated at 50 ml/kg BW (range 41–67 ml/kg BW), individual horses of similar weight fed similar diets can drink very different amounts of water. Not only do individuals of similar breeds differ, an individual horse varies its water intake from day to day (Fig. 4.2) (Groenendyk et al 1988), likely because horses have a cyclic pattern of DM intake over time and may vary their intake of dietary ingredients (Jansson & Dahlborn 1999). Absolute water intake by pregnant mares varied 16 to 20% from the average (Freeman et al 1999) and by 21 to 25% in Standardbred horses (Nyman et al 2002). Daily water intake by individual Thoroughbred mares varied up to 75% (Smith et al 1996).

Diet effects on water intake

The total amount of feed eaten and its composition alters total water intake by the horse (Fonnesbeck 1968). Ponies drank 12 to 61% more water when fed all-hay diets than when fed mixed grain-hay diets (Cymbaluk 1989). Although Thoroughbred horses fed a hay-cube diet drank 26% more water than when fed a 40:60 grain:forage diet, water:feed ratios were similar (3.87 for all forage versus 3.66 for grain:forage; Pagan et al 1998). Thoroughbred horses fed diets with 50% grain drank significantly less ($p = 0.02$) water (17.4 liters) per day than those fed a 35% grain (22.4 liters water/day) and defecate less frequently ($p = 0.06$) (Freire et al 2009). Welsh ponies fed perennial ryegrass-timothy in a chopped, dehydrated form drank 23.8% more water than when the same forage was fed in the long form despite similarity in total DM intake (Hyslop 2003). Water:feed ratios for mature cross-bred ponies fed grass hay, alfalfa hay or high grain complete feed pellets were 3.2, 3.3 and 2.0, respectively (Cymbaluk 1989), and were 3.4, 3.3 and 2.6 for horses fed alfalfa-beet pulp, 77% orchardgrass-alfalfa-oats and forage-grain diets, respectively (Warren et al 1999). Ponies fed alfalfa and oat straw in ad libitum quantities had water:feed ratios of 4.4 and 3.8, respectively, but donkeys drank less water per kg DM than ponies when fed alfalfa (3.2 liters/kg) or oat straw (3.2 liters/kg) (Pearson et al 2001). The latter study also showed that water:feed ratios increased when horses were limit-fed at 70% of ad libitum feed intakes. The higher water intake by horses fed higher forage was attributed to a higher fiber intake of those diets. Adding grain to the diet reduces the total amount of feed and fiber eaten, which may explain the lower water intake by horses fed high grain diets.

Dietary composition

Doubling the salt intake in a compound feed from 50 to 100 mg/kg BW, increased water intake by 53% and increased urine output by 47% (Meyer et al 1987). Water intake in one study was linearly correlated to salt intake ($y = 36.5 + 0.22x$ where y = daily water intake in ml/kg BW and x = daily sodium intake in mg/kg BW) over a narrow range of intakes (Jansson & Dahlborn 1999). Others (Schryver et al 1987) have found no difference in water intake by ponies fed 1, 3, and 5% dietary salt.

Based on a limited range of protein intakes, water intake (WI, ml/kg BW) correlated linearly to nitrogen balance (N balance, mg/kg BW): N balance = 4.8339 WI − 54.696 (r^2 = 0.95) (Ragnarsson & Lindberg 2008). Similarly, Hyslop (2003) reported a linear relationship between water and protein intake for Welsh pony geldings of WI (liters/day) = 19.61 + 0.00838 CPI (g/day) based on the ad libitum intake of diets of two different protein concentrations. Daily water intake by Standardbred horses fed 291 g protein/100 kg BW from forage was 29% higher than by horses fed 200 g protein/100 kg BW also from forage (Connysson 2009). Yet in a recent study, we found that the longitudinal water intake by light and light-cross pregnant mares (31/group) fed either a 7 or 12% protein diet for a 20-week period did not differ ($p = 0.96$). Mares, weighing 603 kg, and eating 2.05 kg DM diet/100 kg BW drank 52.6 ml water/kg BW despite a difference in protein intake of 65% (Cymbaluk, unpublished data).

Temperature effects and water intake

Horses adapt to cold and hot ambient temperatures and changes in water intake are part of this adaptive process (Cymbaluk & Christison 1990, Geor et al 2000). Cold weather (below -8°C) reduced water intake by 6 to 14% by yearling horses with no concomitant reduction in feed intake (Cymbaluk 1990b). Water intakes increased from 23.4 liters/day at thermoneutrality (20°C, 45–50% RH) to 39.5 liters/day after 20 days of short-term exposure (4 h daily) to a hot, humid environment (33–35°C, 80–85% RH) (Geor et al 1996).

Water intake and pregnancy and lactation

Pregnancy does not appear to impose an increase in water needs beyond maintenance. Pregnant, stabled mares eating 2.2 kg DM hay-grain diet/100 kg BW drank 45–69 ml water/kg BW (Freeman et al 1999, Houpt et al 2000). Weight-scaled water intakes by mares declined during pregnancy without a reduction in feed intake (Fig. 4.3). Absolute water intake remained steady despite an increased BW with advancing gestation.

Few data have quantified water intakes by lactating mares but water intake is felt to increase significantly above maintenance and pregnancy needs as a result of fluid loss (milk) and the increased feed intake associated with lactation (Doreau et al 1992). Pregnant mares fed grass hay ad libitum and less than 0.5 kg/100 kg BW concentrate ate 2.2 kg DM/100 kg BW daily (Freeman et al 1999) compared to lactating draft mares, which ate 3 kg DM /100 kg BW of diets high in forage or concentrate (Doreau et al 1992). Based on these differences in feed intake, water intake by lactating mares would increase 40% solely to compensate for a higher feed intake with an added 20 to 30 ml/kg BW of fluid or water to compensate for milk loss. Total water intake by lactating mares housed at thermoneutrality could increase to 75–100 ml/kg BW or 150 to 200% above water intakes observed in pregnancy. However, lactating mares are typically fed diets with more grain than when they are pregnant which might mitigate the increase in water intake expected with lactation because of the lower water: feed ratio of grain.

Water intake by suckling foals

Daily fluid intake by foals at 11, 25, 39 days of age was estimated at 15.1, 14.2 and 16.6 kg/day or about 255, 188 and 182 ml/kg BW (Oftedal et al 1983), values roughly fourfold greater than for mature horses. Orphan foals drank 148 to 159 ml fluid/kg BW (water plus milk replacer) at 1 week old then decreased fluid intake to 102 to 108 ml/kg BW by 7 weeks old (Cymbaluk et al 1993). Nursing and orphan foals begin drinking supplemental water in addition to dam's milk or milk replacer at a relatively young age. Suckling 1-mo old foals drank 3.9 kg of water in addition to 17.4 kg milk and continued to increase water intake (5.5 kg/day) by 2-months old with no concurrent decrease in milk intake (Martin et al 1992).

Water or fluid intake in work or exercise

The impact of exercise on thermoregulation and fluid balance has recently been reviewed (Coenen 2005). Water needs of working or competitive horses are affected by a number of variables that influence sweat and respiratory fluid losses. The goal of fluid provision to exercised horses is to prevent dehydration and/or facilitate rehydration. Mild dehydration is described as a state of 5% total body fluid loss. In a 500-kg horse, whose total body water is about 350 liters, mild dehydration is a fluid loss of 17.5 liters whereas severely dehydrated horses have lost twice this amount. Not only is fluid lost, significant amounts of electrolytes are lost. Equine sweat is hypertonic to plasma (Lindinger 2008), while the dehydration created by sweating during vigorous exercise is hypotonic or isotonic. The plasma osmolality of horses with exercise-induced dehydration is insufficiently elevated to stimulate thirst (Waller et al 2008). Thus, providing only water, which has few electrolytes, to a horse in this physiological state will exacerbate plasma hypotonicity and further suppress the desire to drink. Strategies used for rehydration are discussed below.

Transportation

Transported horses exist in a temporary environment that can impose unique environmental, behavioral and dietary conditions. Horses transported for longer than 30 h without water became unfit for further transport whereas watered horses could tolerate an additional 2 h of transport (Friend 2000). Horses in transit consume water in response to thermal conditions, drinking more during hot temperatures and less during the cool periods of the day. During transport, both water and feed intake decrease, in amounts that are quite variable (Smith et al 1996). Light horses, accustomed to van transport, transported for 24 h during day time temperatures exceeding 30°C with humidity greater than 50%, lost 6% of body weight likely as fluid loss despite five stops to allow water consumption during the trip (Stull & Rodiek 2000). Weight losses of 3% were sustained in these horses for 24 h post-transport even though water was available ad libitum. Provision of water by bucket or trough should be considered for all transported horses and should be provided often (at least every 4 to 8 h) depending on weather conditions of the transport.

Drinking behavior of horses

True thirst or primary drinking results from a stimulus or desire caused by the need to replace fluid lost from intracellular and extracellular fluid reservoirs. Thirst is a response to changed plasma osmolality or blood volume, increased plasma sodium concentration or increased arterial blood pressure (Houpt & Yang 1995, Stricker & Sved 2000). Increases in plasma osmolality of 3% or less (about 8 mOsm) initiated drinking by horses (Sufit et al 1985, Jones et al 1989). Working horses in hot humid conditions that had high plasma osmolality (average 283 mOsm/kg) drank more frequently for longer drinking bouts and thus, had higher water intake than horses with lower plasma osmolality (Pritchard et al 2008). For idle horses, feed ingestion is the main reason for an increased plasma osmolality, which can increase by 3 to 5% within 1 h after feeding. Peri-prandial drinking (10 min before and 30 min after eating) is observed 75 to 89% of the time in horses fed ad libitum or four times daily (Sufit et al 1985, McDonnell et al 1999, Nyman & Dahlborn 2001). If watering stabled horses by hand, if water cannot be provided continuously, then water should be provided about the time of feeding.

Water drinking patterns of horses vary with husbandry (extensive or stabled), water availability and age of horse. Horses that have to walk a considerable distance drink less frequently than those which have water nearby. Water is consumed by horses in a circadian pattern associated with ambient temperature (Friend 2000). Horses receiving small forage meals (0.6 kg/h) appeared to drink more water at noon and 18:00 than at 15:00 (Jorgensen et al 2006) yet Quarter horse and Belgian mares consumed less water in the period from midnight to 9:00 which coincided with the absence of human activity in the barn and resting by the horses (Fig. 4.4; Cymbaluk, unpublished data).

A drinking bout is characterized by a long draught of water followed by short sips. Some horses take a drink of water, hold it in their mouths then either swallow or expel the water. Stabled horses whose feed is near the water source may dip their feed in the water causing soiling of the water bowl (McDonnell et al 1999). This behavior is likely a natural response to moisten dry hay to make it more palatable and easier to chew.

Normal drinking patterns for housed, mature horses is episodic occurring two to eight times per day for 10 to 60 s per episode irrespective of system of water delivery (McDonnell et al 1999). Stalled horses given water ad libitum from a large rectangular watering bowl drank 18 to 39 times daily for 13 to 26 s per drinking bout (McDonnell et al 1999). Horses provided with water by bucket, pressure-valve or float-valve water bowls drank 16 to 21 times daily with drinking bouts lasting 10 to 52 s per episode (Nyman & Dahlborn 2001) as did bucket-watered pony geldings whose drinking bouts lasted 12.2 to 24.2 s (Sweeting et al 1985). Drinking bouts by pastured mares lasted 23 ± 1.2 s (Crowell-Davis et al 1985) and transported horses drank for 11 to 28 s (Gibbs & Friend 2000). Horses drink more often (6–11 episodes) for the first 5 min post-exercise (Butudom et al 2004).

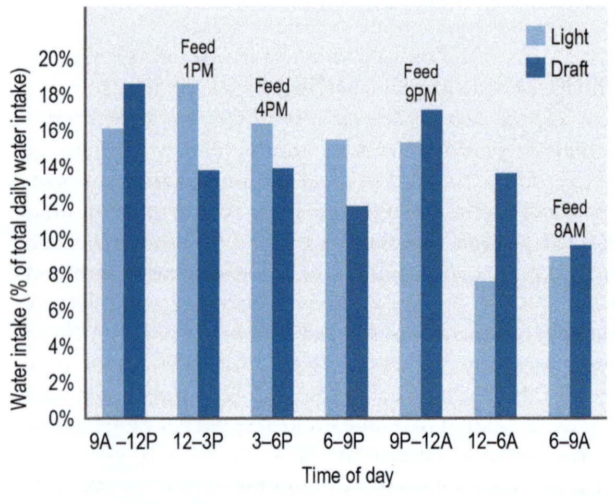

Figure 4.4 Water intake patterns of light and draft pregnant mares fed a 90:10 forage-grain diet housed in thermoneutral conditions. Data represents the average intake of 11 QH and 11 Belgian mares over 5 days. Grain was offered twice daily at 8:00 and 16:00; hay in ad libitum amounts was provided at each of the specified time periods.

The total time a horse spends drinking water every day is very short. Limit-fed ponies fed once or six times daily spent 0.4 to 0.6% (5 to 9 min) of their daily activity budget drinking water (Houpt et al 1988), whereas four limit-fed ponies fed twice daily spent 0.7 to 3.7% (10 to 53 min) drinking water (Sweeting et al 1985). Mares in early to mid gestation with ad libitum access to water drank for 6.2 min/day (McDonnell et al 1999) similar to mares given water intermittently by a float-water bowl (5.7 to 10.7 min/day) (Flannigan 2001). Standardbred geldings watered by bucket, float valve or pressure valve drank for 3 to 15 min/day (Nyman et al 2002). Longer daily drinking times (21 to 27 min/day) were reported for ponies fed and watered ad libitum (Sufit et al 1985), and by densely housed Arab mares with restricted feed access which spent 4.75% (68 min/day) drinking water (Benhajali et al 2008). In the latter study, the increased water intake was attributed to a lack of available feed.

Ambient temperatures affect the frequency of drinking and the amount consumed. Cold weather alone reduces water intake while hot ambient temperatures increase water intake. Pastured, lactating mares drank infrequently in cold weather (0–5°C) but as temperature increased so did drinking frequency which occurred every 1.8 h at temperatures of 30–35°C (Crowell-Davis et al 1985). The frequency of drinking by Hanoverian mares was reported to decrease as ambient temperatures declined (Niemann et al 2006). Drinking frequency by mares below 0°C was 1.32 ± 0.7, at 0 to 14 °C was 1.55 ± 0.97, at 15 to 24°C was 1.90 ± 1.22 and above 25°C was 2.5 ± 1.49.

Water temperature appears to influence total volume of water consumed only when ambient temperatures are cold. Pony stallions housed both outdoors and indoors at cool ambient temperatures drank 38 to 41% less icy water than warm water (19°C) (Kristula & McDonnell 1994). Yet, the converse effect, warm ambient temperature, did not hold. When the ponies were housed in a warm indoor environment conditions (15–29°C), they drank similar amounts of water whether warm (average 23°C) or icy (0–1°C) (McDonnell and Kristula 1996). Water intake by working horses and donkeys was unaffected when water temperatures ranged from 27 to 38°C (Pritchard et al 2006). Horses exercised on a treadmill at temperatures of 25°C when given physiological saline immediately post-exercise, preferred a lukewarm solution (20°C) to a cool (10°C) or warm solution (30°C) (Butudom et al 2004).

Key Points – Water intake

- The average daily water intake of an idle horse housed under thermoneutral conditions is about 50 ml/kg BW (range 41–67 ml/kg BW) but varies from day to day and from horse to horse.
- Horses drink more water when fed all-hay diets. The water:feed ratio for all-forage diets is about 3.2–4.4 and is about 2–2.6 for grain-based diets (more grain in the diet, less water consumed).
- Lactating mares need at least 75–100 ml fluid/kg BW or more depending on diet and temperatures above thermoneutrality.
- Suckling foals drink water, therefore water should be available in a water container (bowl, trough) at a height (75 to 90 cm) easily accessible by the foal.
- Horses fed dry feeds drink around the time of feeding and prefer cool to lukewarm water. Time spent drinking water per day is short usually about 5–6 min/day. Feed-deprived horses will spend more time drinking water.

Evaluating water supply and water intake

General evaluation of the water supply

Appraisal of the watering system is a critical part of the assessment of the adequacy of the dietary program of horses. The first step in evaluation of the water supply is assessment of water availability. Is the water supply freely available, and if not, how often is water provided and in what volume? In a recent epidemiologic study, the absence of water in the horse paddock was identified as another factor of many [diet availability, diet composition, confinement, training, pregnancy, age (Videla & Andrews, 2009)] that may increase risks of gastric ulceration in horses (Luthersson et al 2009). Based on survey data, a decrease in water consumption was a premonitory observation preceding colic in horses (Kaya et al 2009). The capacity of the water holding tanks or bowls should accommodate the needs of each individual horse whether it is alone or in a group (see below) under all weather extremes and feeding conditions (pasture, hay). Water quality should then be evaluated subjectively (color, smell, physical contamination, taste) and objectively (TDS, mineral, microbial properties) (see below).

Evaluation of water intake by individual horses

Mechanical measures

The most reliable way to assess water intake of a barn-housed horse fed dry feeds is to measure the volume of water consumed each day either using a graduated bucket (manual system) or by using an automatic watering bowl plumbed to an individual water meter (automatic watering system). Barn water meters can be used but do not provide information on individual horse water intakes. Errors in water flow can occur when water meters become plugged by sand, rust and other water contaminants. Spillage and water evaporation are generally unaccounted for in any watering system. Water records can be kept for each horse in the barn but as noted above daily variation should be expected.

Clinical measures

No single hydration test exists that is infallible in measuring the hydration status of horses for every type of clinical situation encountered. Body mass loss is considered a gold standard in measuring exercise induced fluid loss (Schott 2010) but may not be best measurement for chronically under-watered and underfed horses or those with chronic intestinal abnormalities. Multi-frequency bioelectrical impedance has been used to assess compartmental body water loss by exercising horses and may have future potential for measuring hydration status during transport, competition and clinical care (Waller & Lindinger 2006).

Water consumption is the best test of dehydration in working horses in a field situation (Pritchard et al 2008). Other, indirect, clinical measures have been used to assess adequacy of water intake and dehydration including fecal consistency, skin turgor ("tenting"), capillary refill time, and oral cavity moisture (Freeman et al 1999), but can be inaccurate (Pritchard et al 2006). Duration of the skin tent in dehydrated horses has been shown to vary from side to side, anatomical site used, coat moisture and age of the horse (Pritchard et al 2008). Young horses typically had shorter tent durations than older animals at similar states of hydration. Mucous membrane dryness also had limited usefulness as a diagnostic measure of dehydration. Evaluation of fecal moisture is an imprecise measure of water adequacy because many causes including intestinal, infectious, dietary composition (low or high protein) or management (rapid diet transitions) can temporarily alter fecal water content (Connysson 2009). Abrupt feed changes from moderate (13%) to high (17%) protein diets caused 5% changes in fecal moisture over the 24 h post-diet transition (Muhonen 2008).

Biochemical measures

Plasma osmolality has been used as a reference to assess dehydration but has limitations because of a circadian rhythm associated with drinking water and eating feed (Pritchard et al 2008). Other associated biochemical analyses that are used to predict hydration status, but also have limitations, are packed cell volume, total plasma proteins, serum electrolytes (sodium and chloride), urine SG and urine osmolality (Sufit et al 1985, Jones et al 1989, Freeman et al 1999, Friend 2000). Neither packed cell volume or total plasma proteins alone reflect the degree of dehydration in horses deprived of food and water (Carlson et al 1979). The ratio of packed cell volume to total plasma proteins may be the most accurate assessment of hydration status in horses with abdominal crises (Mueller & Moore 1998). Serum vasopressin and aldosterone responses have been used to evaluate horses with polydipsia or polyuria (Knottenbelt 2000).

Behavioral measures

Horses behave differently if they have partial or no access to water. The length of deprivation, the practices a horse is accustomed to, and whether the horse has access to feed during the deprivation influences the behavioral changes seen. Water-restricted horses spent less time eating and lipped their water buckets (Houpt et al 2000), whereas ponies water-deprived for 12 h, whinnied, stamped and pawed, and were generally anxious when water was present (Mueller & Houpt, 1991). Feeding activity gradual declines as water restriction is imposed (Houpt et al 2000). Horses continued to eat the grain portion of their diet but reduced hay intake by nearly half of that recorded with the "normal" non restricted diet, after 72 h of total water restriction (Sneddon et al 1993). In horses simultaneously deprived of feed and water, the physiological stimulus to thirst appears to be removed (Rumbaugh et al 1982) resulting in minimal behavioral changes (Tasker 1967b). Horses with only access to snow for nine days while being fed a grass silage diet, adapted to the absence of water by eating snow and showed no interest in water when offered (Mejdell et al 2005). Snow did not adversely influence water turnover rates or fluid balance in chronically cold exposed and limit-fed horses compared to similarly housed and fed horses given liquid water (Dieterich & Holleman 1973). Donkeys respond differently to water deprivation than ponies. Feed intake was reduced 13% in water-deprived donkeys compared to 32% by ponies under similar conditions (Mueller & Houpt 1991). Donkeys have water conservation strategies including high tolerance to body fluid loss (up to 30%) and thirst, reduced fecal dry matter content and evaporative losses, appetite retention, and the ability to rehydrate rapidly (Smith & Pearson 2005).

Water systems and maintenance

Choosing the best method to provide water to a horse depends on its housing. Horses on extensive pastures obtain their water from surface water (streams, dug-outs, lakes) or groundwater (wells) (see below). Stabled horses can be bucket watered or automatically watered. Water systems in stables are often taken for granted, but numerous interrelated factors affect water supply. Factors that influence automatic water systems are available water supply pressure and flow, manifold size, and the number of watering bowls or horses using the water supply. Intermittent provision of water by automatic or manual systems can supply water needs of horses (Freeman et al 1999, Nyman & Dahlborn 2001). Buckets are still commonly used in horse husbandry and are preferred by individual horses (Nyman & Dahlborn 2001) but may increase the risk of colic for horses compared to automatic watering systems which had a low risk of predisposing to colic (Kaya et al 2009). This contrasts to the survey data of Kaneene et al (1997) who indicated that buckets, automatic waterers and bulk tanks may be inadvisable for group housed horses because of a possible increased colic risk compared to other sources such as ponds. In the author's experience, automatic outdoor waterers with thermostat regulated cable heaters or use of automatic livestock float valves attached to large capacity holding tanks coupled with good feeding practices do not create a risk for colic in grouped horses.

Drinking frequency and total volume of water consumed are affected by water container and watering system. Lightly trained horses, adapted to both watering systems, drank 24 liters water daily when given by bucket but only 17 liters water from an automatic water bowl (Nyman et al 2002). Standardbred horses adapted to all watering systems pretrial, when offered water by bucket, pressure-valve or float-valve bowls showed a strong preference for drinking from buckets and drank more water from buckets (Nyman & Dahlborn 2001). When only a pressure-valve system was allowed, horses preferred water delivery at 8 l/min over 3 and 16 l/min (Nyman & Dahlborn 2001). Young horses, unfamiliar with automated water supply, preferred float-valve water bowls compared to push-valve water bowls and larger float-valve bowls to smaller volume bowls (Krawczel et al 2006). The authors concluded that the large float bowl was preferred for its openness, large volume of water retention and lower noise level during refilling. Native British ponies, naïve to artificial watering receptacles, on first exposure showed no preference for bucket, flowing water trough or automatic water bowl but after 4 days of exposure preferred the bucket over the flowing water trough and avoided the automatic water bowl (van de Weerd et al 2008).

The depth of the water bowl may influence how often the horse drinks and for how long. Horses watered from shallow, rectangular gravity-fed water containers (2.5 to 5 cm deep) appeared to sip rather than drink water (McDonnell et al 1999). Likewise, horses spent more time drinking from the pressure valve waterer but consumed less water compared to bucket or float water delivery systems (Nyman et al 2002). Water bowls and buckets require regular cleaning to prevent buildup of feed material and biofilm. Automatic watering systems must be checked daily in winter if temperatures fall below freezing to ensure a patent supply of water.

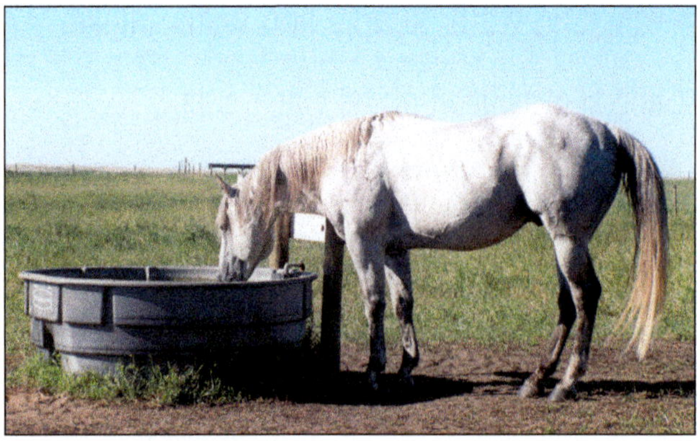

Figure 4.5 Stallion drinking from pasture water tank equipped with a stock float valve.

Watering systems for horses kept on extensive pastures or in paddocks differ to those needed in stables. Horses on pastures can obtain water from streams, dugouts, wells or hauled water. Few pastures have useable natural water sources and if using these sources, it is best to limit access, to reduce damage to riparian areas. Deep mud around natural water sources is a safety risk for animals especially for young foals. Frozen ponds and dugouts in winter also pose a risk of drowning for horses that fall through.

Galvanized steel, painted mild steel and plastic troughs can be selected depending on the volume needed, the pasture location and safety factors of the equipment (Fig. 4.5). Water troughs should be located so that most of the horses in the pasture can drink at the same time. This will minimize aggressive behavior and injury at the trough or tank. In pastures with stallions, the stallion will often determine the length of the drinking period so it is necessary to have a large trough that can be accessed quickly by the mares. Foals drink water on pasture but the height of the water receptacle, about 75–90 cm (30–36 in), is needed for them to drink comfortably.

Water can be pumped into a trough using gasoline or electric engines or by solar or water power. Troughs filled by gasoline pumps need to be filled daily depending on trough capacity. Troughs, that are filled daily, need to be sized according to an estimated daily water use by all horses in the pasture (at least 50 liters/day per animal). Daily filling of the water trough is a good opportunity to observe the health of the horse herd. Outdoor water troughs supplied by pressure systems can be regulated by a float value in the trough that allows refill as water is depleted.

Key Points – Evaluating water supply and intake

- The volume of water consumed by a horse is the best measure of water adequacy and horse hydration. Clinical and biochemical measures of hydration must be interpreted in context to the volume of water consumed by the horse.
- Water should be freely available for horses. The bucket, whose limitation is that water must be continuously replenished, is the preferred water container of horses.

Automatic water systems can provide a continuous clean water supply, but water intake by the horse is influenced by water receptacle and mechanism for dispensing water. Horses appear to prefer float valve over pressure valve systems and prefer large bowls to small bowls. Flow rate is critical in pressure valve systems and based on current data, horses prefer a flow rate of 8 l/min over 3 and 16 l/min.

Methods to maintain or increase water intake

The most common situations confronting clinicians and owners requiring improvement of water intake are: exercised horses with mild fluid losses (see above), horses moved to unfamiliar stabling and water supplies, transported and diarrheic horses. In the instance of the exercised horse, increasing intake of water or electrolyte solution is desired, whereas in the horse naïve to its surroundings, often there is a need to overcome disagreeable, new odors associated with the water source. Horses are very perceptive of odors and will reject most objectionable feeds and fluids. Odors in water can arise from sulfates, tannins, manure, rotting vegetation, algal, and microbial byproducts. Although these are suspected to affect water intake by horses, no quantitative data are available. Horses drank less feces-contaminated water (Friend 2000) but it is unclear whether odor, taste or the floating chunks of solid matter caused the horses to drink less. In the author's experience, the presence of sulfur-reducing bacteria at 200 CFU/ml in barn water resulted in total and enduring water rejection by four of four horses that were naïve to the water source. Sulfur-reducing bacteria in water create a "rotten egg" odor. Chemical remediation of the well with a commercial powdered acidifier and a hypochlorite oxidizer restored the palatability of the water source. Manganese, copper, iron, zinc, silver and aluminum cause water discoloration and the taste of the water (EPA 1992) but the impact of these cations on water intake by horses has not been identified.

Horses prefer sweet solutions to other tastes (Randall et al 1978, Danel & Merkies 2009). Horses provided with control or 1, 5, 10, 20 and 50 g sucrose/100 ml preferred solutions containing 1, 5 or 10 mg/100 ml but drank the highest volume of solution containing 10 g sucrose/100 ml (Danel & Merkies 2009). Foals provided with incrementally doubled sucrose concentrations ranging from 0.01 to 20 g/100 ml discriminated sweetness at 1.25 g/100 ml and showed moderate preferences for sucrose solutions up to 10 g sucrose/100 ml (Randall et al 1978). In both studies, individual horse preferences were observed. For example, one foal totally rejected solutions containing 10 and 20 g sucrose/100 ml (Randall et al 1978). Although the sugar sweetened water is palatable to horses, adverse side-effects of a high sugar intake need to be considered.

Foals tolerated a salty solution up to 0.63 g/100 ml (2331 mg sodium/l) but totally rejected solutions containing 1.25, 2.5 and 5 g salt/100 ml. Foals tolerated sour solutions containing 0.16 ml acetic acid/100 ml but rejected solutions with higher concentrations of acetic acid. Bitterness created by adding quinine caused rejection at concentrations of 20 mg quinine/100 ml (Randall et al 1978).

Anecdotally, it is claimed that horses can be enticed into drinking novel water by preconditioning them for 1–2 weeks before transportation to water flavored with apple cider vinegar, apple juice, Gatorade, Kool-aid and/or commercial flavorings and then using the flavoring to mask the taste of the novel water. Few studies have corroborated the effectiveness of flavorings to mask water tastes, but over a 2-day taste test, apple-flavored water was favored over clover-flavored water by Quarter horses mares following transportation (Mars et al 1992).

Liquid water can offset fluid loss for most horses partaking in light to mild recreational exercise. Horses doing intense physical work or exercise need more extensive intervention. Electrolytes in fluids must be used for rehydration of horses with exercise-induced dehydration. The calculation for replenishment is based on the amount of water and electrolytes required at maintenance plus the amount lost during work or exercise. In lightly worked horses, water alone is usually sufficient, but heavily-worked, mildly to moderately dehydrated horses will need not only fluid, but electrolyte, replacement. For example, Arabian and Arabian-type horses participating in a 50 or 100-mile endurance event, averaged BW losses of 15 ± 2.2®kg (maximum 28.2 kg) and 90% was attributed to sweat fluid losses (Schott et al 1997).

Various rehydration approaches have been studied with mixed outcomes. Isotonic electrolyte solution resulted in a more rapid return of plasma electrolyte and osmolality to normal than water or hypotonic electrolyte solutions (Sosa Leon et al 1995). Hypertonic oral electrolyte pastes, with or without glycerol, reduced but did not prevent the magnitude of weight (water) loss in horses post-exercise (Schott et al 1999). Hypertonic oral electrolyte solutions have also been reported to exacerbate gastric ulcers in mature horses when given once hourly for 8 h (Holbrook et al 2010). Water intake by frusemide-dehydrated horses was 30 to 35% higher when electrolyte pastes (potassium chloride, sodium chloride, and a mixture of potassium and sodium chloride) were used (Schott et al 2002). In a treadmill-simulated 60-km endurance ride conducted at 20°C and 40% relative humidity, horses drank notably less water (12.2 ± 1.7 liters) than horses given water with added electrolyte (23.5 ± 2.8 liters) or electrolyte in a glycerol solution (25.8 ± 2.2 liters) (Dusterdieck et al 1999). Other strategies that have been used for rehydration have been to provide oral rehydration solutions (electrolyte based) (Marlin et al 1998), electrolyte slurries pre- and mid-race and pastes (Schott et al 1997, 1999, Sampieri et al 2007) and hypotonic electrolyte solutions via nasogastric tube (Waller & Lindinger 2005, 2008, 2009). The impact of electrolyte supplementation is to stimulate drinking and to partially restore electrolyte imbalance.

A good electrolyte product should be a mixture of key electrolytes lost in sweat (sodium, potassium, chloride) that easily dissolves in water at room temperature with flavouring agents to increase palatability (Lindinger 2008). Training the horse to drink oral electrolyte solutions is another matter which typically involves adapting the horse to increasing proportions of electrolyte added to its drinking water. Depending on the type of exercise, electrolyte slurries and pastes may be given by dose syringe or nasogastric tube well in advance of exercise (30 min to 4 h), followed by mid-exercise dosing or at the end of exercise. Intravenous rehydration has been used in some instances but has been questioned by some clinicians unless dehydration is dire.

Water quality

Water quality refers to the characteristics of water which make it acceptable or unacceptable for animal use. Water standards are set by governmental agencies and differ by region, country and continent. Few controlled studies have been conducted on water quality for horses so most water quality criteria are based on studies done with other livestock. Upper limits and acceptable concentrations of cations and anions in water for horses are given in NRC (1974, 2007), but recently, Raisbeck et al (2007) have provided an updated review on the subject for wildlife and other species.

Surface and ground water are sources of water for horses. Surface water includes lakes, streams, and ponds located in pastures or premises. Ground water is obtained from wells. Both water sources are subject to contamination by livestock and agricultural activity (McDowell & Wilcock 2008). The chemical composition of the water depends on the bedrock and soil associated with the surface or well water. Surface water is felt to be more readily exposed to external contaminants such as smelters and agricultural applications contaminants (pesticide, fertilizer, animal feces), and human activity, but groundwater can ultimately be exposed to these same surface pollutants through percolation into underground water supplies. A comprehensive review of the pollutants and origin of the contamination of surface and groundwater used by humans has been published (Ritter et al 2002) and is applicable to water supplies used for horses. Horses themselves may be the contamination source of *Cryptosporidium* and *Giardia* into surface water (Sturdee et al 2003, Veronesi et al 2010). Increasingly, North American governmental water management policies recommend restricted access of livestock to surface water resources to reduce contamination of water downstream or into subterranean water sources.

Water composition is dynamic, changing by day with rainfall, and by season with snow melt, which is why water should be analyzed several times a year for an accurate picture of water quality. Spring run-off adds contaminants whereas summer droughts can exacerbate quality of surface water by concentrating contaminants. Commonly, water is tested every 6 months. Water analyses are conducted by local health or private commercial testing laboratories. Typical water analyses for livestock provide a limited array of chemical properties and seldom, physical properties.

Physical and chemical criteria of water

The physical properties of water include its turbidity, odor, color, and temperature. These criteria are readily perceptible but typically, water quality is defined in chemical terms. The most common indicator of water quality is the concentration of total dissolved solids (TDS), which is the total ionic content of the water but not its specific ionic composition. The term salinity is used interchangeably with TDS. Electrical conductivity (EC) measures the ionic activity of the solution by its ability to transmit current and is sometimes used to estimate TDS values. EC is not a suitable substitute for TDS values because the relationship between TDS and EC is non-linear. Australian and New Zealand (ANZEEC) livestock quality guidelines (2000) indicate that water with a TDS up to 4000 mg/l causes no ill-effects in horses and imply that horses are able to adapt to water containing TDS up to 6000 mg TDS/l water. The aesthetic objective for livestock water is below 1000 mg TDS/l but in practical situations in the Canadian Prairies, horses have thrived drinking water containing up to 3310 mg TDS/l water (Table 4-3). Threshold and limiting concentrations of salinity are estimated at 3000 and 7000 mg/l (Table 4-3).

Water pH indicates its acidity or alkalinity. Animals can consume water with pH values between 5 and 9 but the ideal range is 6.0 to 8.5 (Table 4-3). Water pH influences the dissolution of ions and can contribute to the precipitation or inactivation of antibiotics such as sulfonamides delivered through watering systems (Raisbeck et al 2007). Hardness principally measures the total cationic effect of calcium and magnesium in water. These cations are normally found in the horse's diet and in most situations, the calcium and

Table 4-3 Barn Water Analyses on 72 Equine Ranches and Suggested Component Thresholds

	Concentration on equine ranches[a]				Maximum tolerable levels[b]	
Component	Average	Min	Max	Mode	Threshold	Limiting concentration
TDS, mg/l	1112	350	3310	470	3000	7000
pH	7.80	7.12	8.62	7.72	6.0–8.5	5.5–9.0
Sulfate, mg/l	431	9	2330	9	<2000[Y]	3500
Nitrate plus nitrate, mg/l	3	0	30	0	100	400
Chloride, mg/l	96	9	1160	19	1500	3000
Sodium, mg/l	180	2	906	9	<1000[Y]	2000
Calcium, mg/l	119	5	403	165	500	1000
Magnesium, mg/l	55	2	164	24	250	500
Total coliforms (cfu/100 ml)	10	0	200	0	NA	NA

[a]Average of barn water samples taken on 72 equine ranches located in Manitoba, Saskatchewan (Canada) and North Dakota (USA). Groundwater (wells) water supply was used on 60 ranches; 12 ranches piped in water from surface sources (dugouts; lake). Well depths ranged from 3.1 to 108 m.
[b]Threshold and limiting concentrations based on NRC (1974, 2007); ANZECC (2000); CCME (2002), Raisbeck et al (2007) unless otherwise identified.
Based on research data (Cymbaluk, unpublished – see text).
NA = none available for horses.

magnesium in water do not add significant amounts to the dietary balance of the horse. High calcium content contributes to poor soaping properties of water and scaling of containers. Ion exchange water softeners can be used to remediate hard water and typically replace calcium ions with sodium. Unlike water calcium and magnesium, added water sodium can contribute significantly to the total sodium intake by the horse.

Sodium is a dominant cation in alkali and saline areas. The average water sodium concentration sampled from 72 horse ranches in Saskatchewan, Manitoba, and North Dakota was about 80 mg/l but some water sources exceeded 900 mg/l (Table 4-3). By extrapolation using an average water intake of 50 ml/kg BW and a dietary sodium requirement of 20 mg/kg BW (NRC 2007) a water sodium concentration of about 400 mg/l provides sufficient sodium to meet the daily sodium requirements of an idle 500-kg horse without adding salt to its diet. Of the 72 barn water samples tested (Table 4-3), 12 water samples (16.7%) exceeded this 400 mg/l threshold. Most of these samples were obtained from deep (30 m) wells. Sulfate was the associated anion in only 25% of the high sodium (>400 mg sodium/l) water samples. The presence of high sodium concentrations in the water supply requires critical evaluation of the total sodium intake by the horse obtained from supplemental sources. Commercial pelleted rations containing sodium would be inadvisable under these circumstances. In addition, if block or loose salt is the method used to provide trace mineral supplementation, alternative methods of provision will likely be needed.

High water sodium has been speculated to reduce water intake and potentially contribute to dehydration in horses, but this has not been confirmed with research data. Recently, our group compared the effect of providing high sodium water (1012 mg sodium/l as sodium chloride) relative to control water (2.3 mg/l) to eight horses over a 3-week period (Cymbaluk, unpublished observations). All horses showed an abrupt reduction in water intake the first day high sodium water was given but gradually water intake normalized. Over the study period, horses given high sodium water reduced their water intake by 13% with a concomitant 17% increase in urine volume. Two horses (25% of the group) reluctantly drank high salt water during the study. One horse drank 51% less water ($p < 0.05$), ate 25% less feed and lost weight over the 3-week study. However, water intake, appetite and weight gain returned to normal when the affected horses' water supply was reverted to low-salt water. None of the horses showed biochemical or clinical signs of dehydration. Voluntary salt intake was reduced, which is important in feeding systems where salt licks are the sole source of supplemental trace mineral.

Data confirming ideal or toxic concentrations of individual cations and anions in water used for horses are rare and moreover, these compounds are rarely analyzed by most laboratories that conduct water analyses. Inferential data are available in other sources (NRC 1974, 2007).

Nitrate

Water supplies in rural areas can receive nitrate contamination from agricultural sources such as livestock waste, manure and synthetic fertilizer application, and human activity such as waste disposal pits and leaking septic tanks (Katz & Bohlke 2000). Nitrate and nitrite in water was present in trace (0.1 mg/l) to moderate (29.9 mg/l) concentrations on 38 of 72 equine ranches tested (Table 4-3). The average nitrate plus nitrite concentrations on affected ranches was 2.65 ± 5.81 mg/l. Two water samples with nitrate concentrations of about 30 mg/l were obtained from shallow (<10 m) wells with a higher risk of fecal contamination.

Water analyses most often report nitrate as nitrate *and* nitrite concentrations or nitrate-nitrogen and nitrite-nitrogen concentrations. Nitrite is about 10 to 15 times more lethal than nitrate. Nitrite is the active ionic form which displaces oxygen on hemoglobin to form methemoglobin and nitrate is converted to nitrite by bacteria in the horse's cecum. Nonetheless, horses seem relatively tolerant to nitrate since hemoglobinemia due to nitrate poisoning is rarely reported (Oruc et al 2010). However, caution must prevail if using feeds and water containing high nitrate concentrations.

Nitrate and nitrite concentrations in water analyses are converted to their respective nitrogen values (nitrate-N and nitrite-N) by dividing by 4.43 and 3.29. The upper limit for nitrate-nitrogen in water for livestock is 100 mg/l and for nitrite-nitrogen at 10 mg/l (CCME 2002, NRC 1974). ANZEEC water guidelines use trigger values of 400 mg nitrate/l and 30 mg nitrite/l or about 90 mg/l nitrate-nitrogen and 9 mg/l nitrite-nitrogen (ANZECC 2000).

Sulfate

Water sulfate affects copper metabolism by ruminants but similar data is unavailable for horses. Upper limits of 1000 mg sulfate/l are used for cattle but tolerance level of water sulfate for horses remains unknown. To examine the short-term effect of high sulfate water on adult horses, our group compared effects of providing eight horses with high sulfate water (1992 mg/l from sodium sulfate) to normal water sulfate (29 mg/l) (Cymbaluk, unpublished observations). High sulfate water caused a 12% reduction in water intake over the 3-week period (Fig. 4.6) but this may have been caused by either a high sulfate or a high sodium effect (954 mg sodium/l), which had been previously shown to reduce water intake. The high sulfate water was astringent and bitter, which may have caused two horses (25% of the group) to drink less water than their cohorts and control horses. These horses reverted to normal when given low sulfate water. None of the horses showed clinical or biochemical dehydration. Copper utilization (70%) was unaffected by the high sulfate content of the water. On ranches where water supplies contained up to 2330 mg sulfate/l water (Table 4-3), water intake and health of the horses were normal. Nonetheless, precaution is required when high sulfate water is used. Sulfate toxicity was implicated in the deaths of horses consuming ten times this water sulfate concentration (Burgess et al 2010). Sudden death and/or profuse diarrhea in horses were observed following intake of extremely high water sulfate (greater than 22 500 mg/l) and high water salinity (greater than 36 800 mg/l) which resulted from evaporation of the surface water reservoir and inaccessibility to potable water (Burgess et al 2010).

Blue-green algae and coliform bacteria

Cyanophyceae (blue-green algae) are algal-like bacteria with photosynthetic capabilities that can contaminate surface water supplies mostly during warm summer months.

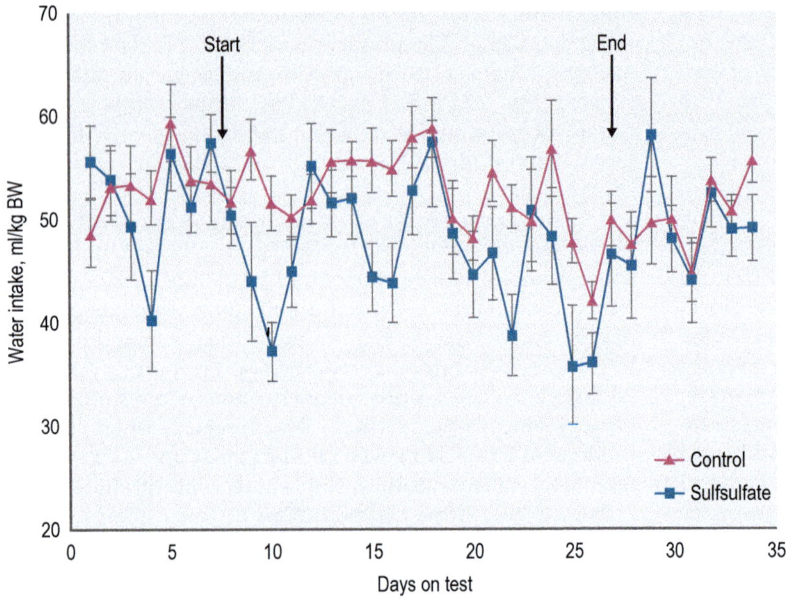

Figure 4.6 Water intake patterns of eight horses provided with control water (29 mg sulfsulfate/l) and eight horses given high sulfsulfate (1902 mg sulfsulfate/l) water derived from the addition of sodium sulfsulfate to control water.

The toxic component is microcystin, which gives the water a moldy, musty, grassy, or septic-tank odor. The proposed trigger value for microcystin-LR in water for horses is 2.3 μg/l or 11500 cells/ml but these recommendations are not based on studies using horses. Blue-green algal overgrowths on surface waters are treated with a registered copper sulfate product at the rate of 1 kg copper sulfate by weight per 2.1 million liters water (Government of Saskatchewan 2008).

Coliform bacteria were present in 100% of barn water on equine ranches (12 of 12 barns) with surface water supply and in 10% of barn water derived from wells (Table 4-3). The coliform population in contaminated wells averaged 39.8 ± 60.7 colony-forming units (cfu)/ml (range 2–200 cfu/ml water). One of the water supplies with the highest coliform count (165 cfu/ml) was piped from the water reservoir supplying the local town and community. All of the horses (greater than 1000) on ranches with coliform-contaminated water were clinically normal.

Tests for total coliform bacteria and total fecal coliforms in water determine the amount of fecal contamination of the water source. The threshold guideline for thermotolerant coliforms for livestock is given at 100 thermotolerant coliforms/100 ml (ANZECC 2000) whereas Canadian livestock water guidelines (CCME 2002) do not state a threshold number for coliforms because of the variable pathogenicity of enterobacteria. *Escherichia coli*, most commonly associated with enteric disease in humans, does not appear to affect horses similarly.

Summary

Horses require different volumes of water depending on many variables including their age, breed, weight, activity, health status, reproductive function, climate, and diet. As the preceding discussion has shown, normal horses have a wide range of water intakes and water outputs. Thus, it is unwise and potentially misleading to assume prescriptive recommendations for water intakes for various classes of horses are universally applicable.

The most common guideline given for watering horses is to provide fresh, clean water at all times. This recommendation ignores the observations (1) that an intermittent supply of water can be completely adequate for horses and (2) that water may appear to be fresh (flowing stream or obtained from a tap) and clean (not discolored, no floating creatures) and yet may contain toxic elements, or infectious bacteria and viruses that can cause clinical illness. The guideline should state: provide water chemically and microbially tested to be safe for horses in ad libitum or sufficient intermittent amounts to satisfy each individual horse's needs.

References

Agrabriel, J., Martin-Rosset, W., Robelin, J., 1984. Croissance et besoins du poulain. In: Jarrige, R., Martin-Rosset, W. (Eds.), Le Cheval. INRA, Paris, pp. 371–384.

Andrews, F.M., Nadeau, J.A., Saabye, L., et al., 1997. Measurement of total body water content in horses, using deuterium oxide dilution. Am J Vet Res 58, 1060–1064.

ANZECC (Australian and New Zealand Environment and Conservation Council, 2000. Livestock drinking water guidelines.) pp. 1–32 in Guidelines for Fresh and Marine Water Quality, vol. 3.

Benhajali, H., Richard-Yris, M.A., Leroux, M., et al., 2008. A note on the time budget and social behavior of densely housed horses. A case study in Arab breeding mares. Appl Anim Behav Sci 112, 196–200.

Burgess, B.A., Lohmann, K.L., Blakley, B.R., 2010. Excessive sulfate and poor water quality as a cause of sudden deaths and an outbreak of diarrhea in horses. Can Vet J 51, 277–282.

Butudom, P., Barnes, D.J., Davis, M.W., et al., 2004. Rehydration fluid temperature affects voluntary drinking in horses dehydrated by furosemide administration and endurance exercise. Vet J 167, 72–80.

Carlson, G.P., Rumbaugh, G.E., Harrold, D., 1979. Physiologic alterations in the horse produced by food and water deprivation during periods of high environmental temperatures. Am J Vet Res 40, 982–985.

Carlson, G.P., 1979. Fluid therapy in horses with acute diarrhea. Vet Clin North Am Equine Practice 1, 313–329.

Carlson, G.P., 1987. Hematology and body fluids in the equine athlete: A review. In: Gillespie, J.R., Robinson, N.E. (Eds.), 2nd Intern. Conf. Equine Exercise Physiology. ICEEP Publications, Davis, CA, pp. 393–425.

CCME (Canadian Council of Ministers of the Enviornment), 2002. (update). Canadian Environmental Guidelines for the Protection of Agricultural Water Uses. Chapter 5.

Coenen, M., Meyer, H., 1987. Water and electrolyte content of the equine gastrointestinal tract in dependence of the ration type. Proc Equine Nutr Physiol Symp 10, 531–536.

Coenen, M., 2005. Exercise and stress: impact on adaptive processes involving water and electrolytes. Livestock Prod Sci 92, 131–145.

Connysson, M., 2009. Fluid balance and metabolic response in athletic horses fed forage diets. Licentiate thesis Swedish Univ Agric Sci Uppsala 32.

Connysson, M., Muhonen, S., Lindberg, J.E., et al., 2006 Effects on exercise response, fluid and acid-base balance of protein intake from forage only diets in Standardbred horses. Equine Vet J 36 (Suppl), 648–653.

Crowell-Davis, S.L., Houpt, K.A., Carnevale, J., 1985. Feeding and drinking behavior of mares and foals with free access to pasture and water. J Anim Sci 60, 883–889.

Cuddeford, S., Pearson, R.A., Archibald, R.F., et al., 1995. Digestibility and gastro-intestinal transit time of diets containing different proportions of alfalfa and oat straw fed to Thoroughbreds, Shetland ponies, Highland ponies and donkeys. Anim Sci 61, 407–418.

Cymbaluk, N.F., 1989.Water balance of horses fed various diets. Equine Pract 11, 19–24.

Cymbaluk, N.F., 1990a. Comparison of forage digestion by cattle and horses. Can J Anim Sci 70, 601–610.

Cymbaluk, N.F., 1990b. Cold housing effects on growth and nutrient demand of young horses. J Anim Sci 68, 3152–3162.

Cymbaluk, N.F., Christison, G.I., 1990. Environmental effects on thermoregulation and nutrition of horses. Vet Clin North Am Equine Pract 6, 355–372.

Cymbaluk, N.F., Smart, M.E., Bristol, F., et al., 1993. Importance of milk replacer intake and composition in rearing orphan foals. Can Vet J 34, 479–486.

Danel, J., Merkies, K., 2009. Discrimination and selection by horses of sucrose solution. J Equine Vet Sci Abstracts 29, 384–385.

Danielsen, K., Lawrence, L.M., Siciliano, P., et al., 1995. Effect of diet on weight and plasma variables in endurance exercised horses. Equine Vet J Suppl 18, 372–377.

Deavers, S., Rosborough, J.P., Garner, H.E., et al., 1973. Blood volumes and total body water in the domestic pony. J Appl Physiol 34, 341–343.

Dieterich, R.A., Holleman, D.F., 1973. Hematology, biochemistry and physiology of environmentally stressed horses. Can J Zool 51, 867–873.

Doreau, M., Boulot, S., 1989. Recent knowledge on mare milk production: a review. Livestock Prod Sci 22, 213–235.

Doreau, M., Boulot, S., Martin-Rosset, W., et al., 1986. Relationship between nutrient intake, growth and body composition of the nursing foal. Reprod Nutr Develop 26, 683–690.

Doreau, M., Boulot, S., Martin-Rosset, W., 1991. Effect of parity and physiological state on intake, milk production and blood parameters in lactating mares differing in body size. Anim Prod 53, 111–118.

Doreau, M., Boulot, S., Bauchart, D., et al., 1992. Voluntary intake, milk production and plasma metabolites in nursing mares fed two different diets. J Nutr 122, 992–999.

Dusterdieck, K.F., Schott, H.C., Eberhart, S.W., et al., 1999. Electrolyte and glycerol supplementation improve water intake by horses performing a simulated 60 km endurance ride. Equine Vet J Suppl 30, 418–424.

Ecke, P., Hodgson, D.R., Rose, R.J., 1998. Induced diarrhoea in horses. Part I. Fluid and electrolyte balance. Vet J 155, 149–159.

Ecker, G.L., Lindinger, M.I., 1995. Water and ion losses during the cross-country phase of eventing. Equine Vet J Suppl. 20, 111–119.

Environmental Protection Agency (EPA), 1992. Secondary drinking water regulations: guidance for nuisance chemicals. EPA publication 810/K-92-001. EPA, Washington DC, p. 4.

Fielding, C.L., Magdesian, K.G., Elliott, D.A., et al., 2003. Pharmokinetics and clinical utility of sodium bromide (NaBr) as an estimator of extracellular fluid volume in horses. J Vet Intern Med 17, 213–217.

Fielding, C.L., Magdesian, K.G., Elliott, D.A., et al., 2004. Use of multifrequency bioelectrical impedance analysis for estimation of total body water and extracellular and intracellular fluid volumes in horses. Am J Vet Res 65, 320–326.

Fielding, C.L., Magdesian, K.G., Carlson, G.P., et al., 2007. Estimation of acute fluid shifts using bioelectrical impedance analysis in horses. J Vet Int Med 21, 176–183.

Fielding, C.L., Magdesian, K.G., Carlson, G.P., et al., 2008. Application of the sodium dilution principle to calculate extracellular fluid volume changes in horses during dehydration and rehydration. Am J Vet Res 69, 1506–1511.

Flannigan, G., 2001. Survey of stereotypies and time budgets of pregnant mares' urine (PMU) ranching industry production mares. MSc Univ Sask 118.

Fonnesbeck, P.V., 1968. Consumption and excretion of water by horses receiving all hay and hay-grain diets: J Anim Sci 27, 1350–1356.

Forro, M., Lindinger, M.I., 2006. Frusemide results in an extracellular to intracellular fluid shift in horses. Equine Vet J Suppl 36, 245–253.

Forro, M., Cieslar, S., Ecker, G.L., et al., 2000. Total body water and ECFV measured using bioelectric impedance analysis and indicator dilution in horses. J Appl Physiol 89, 663–671.

Freeman, D.A., Cymbaluk, N.F., Schott, H.C., et al., 1999. Clinical, biochemical and hygiene assessment of stabled horses provided continuous or intermittent access to drinking water. Am J Vet Res 60, 1445–1450.

Freire, R., Clegg, H.A., Buckley, P., et al., 2009. The effects of two different amounts of dietary grain on the digestibility of the diet and behaviour of intensively managed horses. Applied Anim Behavior Sci 117, 69–73.

Friend, T.H., 2000. Dehydration, stress and water consumption of horses during long-distance commercial transport. J Anim Sci 78, 2568–2580.

Gee, E.K., Fennessy, P.F., Morel, P.C., et al., 2003. Chemical body composition of 20 Thoroughbred foals at 160 days of age, and preliminary investigation of techniques used to predict body fatness. NZ Vet J 125–131.

Geerken, C., Doreau, M., Boulot, S., 1988. The use of urea as a marker of body water in the nursing foal. Reprod Nutr Develop 28, 257–263.

Geor, R.J., McCutcheon, L.J., Lindinger, M.I., 1996. Adaptations to daily exercise in hot and humid conditions in trained Thoroughbred horses. Equine Vet J Suppl 22, 63–68.

Geor, R.J., McCutcheon, L.J., Ecker, G.L., et al., 2000. Heat storage in horses during submaximal exercise before and after humid heat acclimation. J Appl Physiol 89, 2283–2293.

Gibbs, P.G., Potter, G.D., Blake, R.W., et al., 1982. Milk production of Quarter horse mares during 150 days of lactation. J Anim Sci 54, 496–499.

Gibbs, A.E., Friend, T.H., 2000. Effect of animal density and trough placement on drinking behavior and dehydration in slaughter horses. J Equine Vet Sci 20, 643–650.

Groenendyk, S., English, P.B., Abetz, I., 1988. External balance of water and electrolytes in the horse. Equine Vet J 20, 189–193.

Government of Saskatchewan, 2008. Blue-Green Algae-FAQs. http://www.agriculture.gov.sk.ca/Blue-Green_Algae_FAQs.

Hodgson, D.S., McCutcheon, L.J., Byrd, S.K., et al., 1993. Dissipation of metabolic heat during exercise. J Appl Physiol 74, 1161–1170.

Holbrook, T.C., Simmons, R.D., Paynton, M.E., et al., 2010. Effect of repeated oral administration of hypertonic electrolyte solution on equine gastric mucosa. Equine Vet J 37, 501–504.

Houpt, T.R., Yang, H., 1995. Water deprivation, plasma osmolality, blood volume and thirst in young pigs. Physiol Behav 57, 49–54.

Houpt, K.A., Perry, P.J., Hintz, H.F., et al., 1988. Effect of meal frequency on fluid balance and behavior of ponies. Physiol Behav 42, 401–407.

Houpt, K.A., Eggleston, K., Kunkle, K., et al., 2000. Effect of water restriction on equine behavior and physiology. Equine Vet J 32, 341–344.

Hyslop, J., 2003. Relationship between crude protein intake and water intake in forage based equine diets. Proc Brit Soc Anim Sci Emerging Equine Sci Conf 46–47.

Izraely, H., Chosniak, I., Stevens, C.E., et al., 1989. Factors determining the digestive efficiency of the domesticated donkey (*Equus asinus asinus*). Quart J Exp Physiol 74, 1–6.

Jansson, A., 1999. Sodium and potassium regulation with special reference to the athletic horse. Ph.D thesis. SwedUniv Agric Sci Uppsala.

Jansson, A., Dahlborn, K., 1999. Effects of feeding frequency and voluntary salt intake on fluid and electrolyte regulation in athletic horses. J App Physiol 86, 1610–1616.

Jansson, A., Lindholm, A., Lindberg, J.E., et al., 1999. Effects of potassium intake on potassium, sodium and fluid balance in exercising horses. Equine Vet J Suppl 30, 412–417.

Jones, N.L., Houpt, K.A., Houpt, T.R., 1989. Stimuli of thirst in donkeys (*Equus asinus*). Physiol Behav 46, 661–665.

Jorgensen, U.P., Raff, L., Norgaard, P., et al., 2006. Effects of forage type and time of feeding on water intake in horses. In: 57th Annual Meeting Eur. Assoc. Anim. Prod. Wageningen Academic Publishers, The Netherlands, p. 289 (Abstract).

Judson, G.J., Mooney, G.J., 1983. Body water and water turnover rate in Thoroughbred horses in training. In: Snow, D.H., Persson, S.G.B., Rose, R.J. (Eds.), Intern. Conf. Equine Exercise Physiology. Granta Editions, Cambridge UK, pp. 371–376.

Julian, L.M., Lawrence, J.H., Berlin, N.I., et al., 1956. Blood volume, body water and body fat of the horse. J Appl Physiol 8, 651–653.

Kaneene, J.B., Miller, R.A., Ross, W.A., et al., 1997. Risk factors for colic in the Michigan (USA) equine population. Prev Vet Med 20, 23–36.

Katz, B.G., Bohlke, J.K., 2000. Monthly variability and possible sources of nitrate in ground water beneath mixed agricultural land use, Suwanee and Lafayette counties, Florida. US Geological Survey, Water-Resources Investigations Report 00-4219, pp. 1–28.

Kaya, G., Sommerfeld-Stur, I., Iben, C., 2009. Risk factors of colic in horses in Austria. J Anim Physiol Anim Nutr 93, 339–349.

Kingston, J., Geor, R.J., McCutcheon, L.J., 1997. Use of dew-point hygrometry, direct sweat collection and measurements of body water losses to determine sweating rates in exercising horses. Am J Vet Res 58, 175–181.

Knottenbelt, D.C., 2000. Polyuria-polydipsia in the horse. Equine Vet Edu 12, 179–186.

Kristula, M.A., McDonnell, S.M., 1994. Drinking water temperature affects consumption of water during cold weather in ponies. Appl Anim Behav Sci 41, 155–160.

Krawczel, P.D., Friend, T.H., Johnson, R., 2006. A note on the preference of naïve horses for different water bowls. Appl Anim Behav Sci 100, 309–313.

Lindinger, M.I., McKeen, G., Ecker, G.L., 2004. Time course and magnitude of changes in total body water, extracellular fluid volume, intracellular fluid volume and plasma volume during submaximal exercise and recovery in horses. Equine Comp Exer Physiol 1, 131–139.

Lindinger, M.I., 2008. Sweating, dehydration and electrolyte supplementation: challenges for the performance horse. In: Proc 4th Eur. Equine Nutr. Health Congress. pp. 46–56. Available from www.ivis.org.

Lopes, M.A., 2002. Hydration of colonic ingesta and feces in horses fed large grain diets or treated with enteral fluid therapy, saline cathartics and

intravenous fluid therapy. PhD Thesis. Virginia Polytechnic Inst State Uni 147.
Luthersson, N., Nielsen, K.H., Harris, P., et al., 2009. Risk factors associated with equine gastric ulceration syndrome (EGUS) in 201 horses in Denmark. Equine Vet J 41, 625–630.
Marlin, D.J., Scott, C.M., Mills, P.C., et al., 1998. Rehydration following exercise: Effects of administration of water versus an isotonic oral rehydration solution (ORS). Vet J 156, 41–49.
Marlow, C.H., van Tonder, E.M., Hayward, F.C., et al., 1983. A report on the consumption , composition and nutritional adequacy of a mixture of lush green perennial ryegrass (Lolium perenne) and cocksfoot (Dactylis glomerata) fed ad libitum to Thoroughbred mares. J S Afr Vet Assoc 54, 155–157.
Mars, L.A., Kiesling, H.E., Ross, T.T., et al., 1992. Water acceptance and intake in horses under shipping stress. J Equine Vet Sci 12, 17–20.
Martin, R.G., McMeniman, N.P., Dowsett, K.F., 1992. Milk and water intakes of foals sucking grazing mares. Equine Vet J 24, 295–299.
McCutcheon, L.J., Geor, R.J., 1998. Sweating. Fluid and ion losses and replacement. Vet Clin North Amer Equine Pract 14, 75–95.
McCutcheon, L.J., Geor, R.J., 1999. Equine sweating responses to submaximal exercise during 21 days of heat acclimation. J Appl Physiol 87, 1843–1851.
McCutcheon, L.J., Geor, R.J., Hare, M.J., et al., 1995. Sweating rate and sweat composition during exercise and recovery in ambient heat and humidity. Equine Vet J Suppl 20, 153–157.
McDonnell, S.M., Freeman, D.A., Cymbaluk, N.F., et al., 1999. Behavior of stabled horses provided continuous or intermittent access to drinking water. Am J Vet Res 60, 1451–1456.
McDonnell, S.M., Kristula, M.A., 1996. No effect of drinking water temperature (ambient vs chilled) on consumption of water during hot summer weather in ponies. Appl Anim Behav Sci 49, 159–163.
McDowell, R.W., Wilcock, R.J., 2008. Water quality and the effects of different pastoral animals. NZ Vet J 56, 289–296.
McMillen, W.M., Williams, Q., Langham, W., 1943. Chemical composition, grazing value and vegetative changes in a typical plains pasture. J Anim Sci 2, 237–243.
Meissner, H.H., Paulsmeier, D.V., 1995. Plant compositional constituents affecting between plant and animal species prediction of forage intake. J Anim Sci 73, 2447–2457.
Mejdell, C.M., Simensen, E., Boe, K.E., 2005. Is snow a sufficient source of water for horses kept outdoors in winter? A case report. Acta vet Scand 46, 19–22.
Merritt, A.M., 1975. Chronic equine diarrhea - differential diagnosis and therapy. Proc Amer Assoc Eq Pract 21, 401–409.
Meyer, H., 1995. Influence of diet, exercise and water restrictions on the gut fill in horses. Proc Equine Nutr Physiol Symp 14, 90.
Meyer, H., Perez, H., Gonda, Y., et al., 1987. Postprandial renal and fecal water and electrolyte excretion in horses in relation to kind of feedstuffs, amount of sodium ingested and exercise. Proc Equine Nutr Physiol Symp 10, 67–72.
Morgan, K., Ehrlemark, A., Sallvik, K., 1997. Dissipation of heat from standing horses exposed to ambient temperature between -3 and 37°C. J Therm Biol 22, 177–186.
Mueller, P.J., Houpt, K.A., 1991. A comparison of the responses of donkeys (*Equus asinus*) and ponies (*Equus caballus*) to 36 hrs water deprivation. In: Fielding, D., Pearson, R.A. (Eds.), Donkeys, Mules and Horses in Tropical Agricultural Development. University of Edinburgh, Edinburgh, pp. 86–95.
Mueller, P.O., Moore, J.N., 1998. Gastrointestinal emergencies and other causes of colic. In: Orsini, J.A., Divers, T.J. (Eds.), Manual of Equine Emergencies. Treatment and Procedures. W.B. Saunders Co., Montreal, p. 160.
Muhonen, S., 2008. Metabolism and hindgut ecosystem in forage fed sedentary and athletic horses. PhD thesis. Uppsala, pp. 1–76.
NRC (National Research Council), 1974. Nutrients and Toxic Substances in Water for Livestock and Poultry. Washington, DC, p. 93.
NRC (National Research Council), 2007. Nutrient Requirements of Domestic Animals. No. 8. sixth revised ed. Nutrient Requirements of Horses. National Academy of Sciences, Washington, DC.
Niemann, B., Moors, E., Jockish, F.-J., et al., 2006. Drinking behavior of horses depending on the type of trough, concentrate feeding and climate condition. In: 57th Annu Meeting Eur. Assoc. Anim. Prod. Wageningen Academic Publishers, The Netherlands, p. 69 (Abstract).
Nyman, S., Dahlborn, K., 2001. Effects of water supply method and flow rate on drinking behavior and fluid balance in horses; Physiol Behav 73, 1–8.
Nyman, S., Jansson, A., Lindholm, A., et al., 2002. Water intake and fluid shifts in horses: effects of hydration status during two exercise tests. Equine Vet J Suppl 34, 133–142.
Oftedal, O.T., Hintz, H.T., Schryver, H.F., 1983. Lactation in the horse: milk composition and intake by foals. J Nutr 113, 2196–2206.
Olsman, A.F., Huurdeman, C.M., Jansen, W.L., et al., 2004. Macronutrient digestibility, nitrogen balance, plasma indicators of protein metabolism and mineral absorption in horses fed a ration rich in sugar beet pulp. J Anim Physiol Anim Nutr 88, 321–331.
Oruc, H.H., Akkoc, A., Uzunoglu, I., et al., 2010. Nitrate poisoning in horses associated with ingestion of forage and alfalfa. J Equine Vet Sci 30, 159–162.
Pagan, J.D., Harris, P., Brewster-Barnes, T., et al., 1998. Exercise affects digestibility and rate of passage of all-forage and mixed diets in Thoroughbred horses. J Nutr 128, 2704S–2708S.
Pearson, R.A., Archibald, R.F., Muirhead, R.H., 2001. The effect of forage quality and level of feeding on digestibility and gastrointestinal transit time of oat straw and alfalfa given to ponies and donkeys. Br J Nutr 85, 599–606.
Pool-Anderson, K., Raub, R.H., Warren, J.A., 1994. Maternal influences on growth and development of full-sibling foals. J Anim Sci 72, 1661–1666.
Pritchard, J.C., Barr, A.R., Whay, H.R., 2006. Validity of a behavioural measure of heat stress and a skin tent test for dehydration in working horses and donkeys. Equine Vet J 38, 433–438.
Pritchard, J.C., Burn, C.C., Barr, A.R., et al., 2008. Validity of indicators of dehydration in working horses: A longitudinal study of changes in skin tent duration, mucous membrane dryness and drinking behaviour. Equine Vet J 40, 558–564.
Ragnarsson, S., Lindberg, J.E., 2008. Nutritional value of timothy haylage in Icelandic horses. Livestock Sci. 113, 202–208.
Raisbeck, M.F., Riker, S.L., Tate, C.M., et al., 2007. Water quality for Wyoming Livestock and Wildlife. A Review of the Literature Pertaining to Health Effects of Inorganic Contaminants 94.
Randall, R.P., Schurg, W.A., Church, D.C., 1978. Responses of horses to sweet, salty, sour and bitter solutions. J Anim Sci 1978 47, 51–55.
Ritter, L., Solomon, K., Sibley, P., et al., 2002. Sources, pathways, and relative risks of contaminants in surface water and groundwater: A perspective prepared for the Walkerton inquiry. J Toxicol Environ Health Part A 65, 1–142.
Robb, J., Harper, R.B., Hintz, H.F., et al., 1972. Chemical composition and energy value of the body, fatty acid composition of adipose tissue, and liver and kidney size in the horse. Anim Prod 14, 25–34.
Rumbaugh, G.E., Carlson, G.P., Harrold, D., 1982. Urinary production in the healthy horse and in horses deprived of feed and water. Am J Vet Res 43, 735–737.
Sampieri, F., Schott, H.C., Hinchcliff, K.W., et al., 2007. Electrolyte supplementation for endurance horses: Effects on fluid losses and performance. Am Assoc Equine Pract 53, 82–85.
Santos, A.S., Silvestre, A.M., 2008. A study of Lusitano mare lactation curve with Wood's model. J Dairy Sci 91, 760–766.
Savage, C.J., 2008. Urinary clinical pathologic findings and glomerular filtration rate in the horse. Vet Clin North Am Equine Pract 24, 387–404.
Scheibe, K.M., Eichhorn, K., Kalz, B., et al., 1998. Water consumption and watering behavior of Przewalski horses (*Equus ferus przewalskii*) in a semireserve. Zoo Biol 17, 181–192.
Schott, H.C., 2010. Challenges of endurance exercise: hydration and electrolyte depletion. In: Proc. 17th Kentucky Equine Res. Nutr. Conf. Kentucky Equine Res, Versailles, KY, pp. 94–111.
Schott, H.C., McGlade, K.S., Molander, H.A., et al., 1997. Body weight, fluid, electrolyte, and hormonal changes in horses competing in 50- and 100-mile endurance rides. Am J Vet Res 58, 303–309.
Schott, H.C., Dusterdieck, K.F., Eberhart, S.W., et al., 1999. Effects of electrolyte and glycerol supplementation on recovery from endurance exercise. Equine Vet J Suppl 30, 384–393.
Schott, H.C., Axiak, S.M., Woody, K.A., et al., 2002. Effect of oral administration of electrolyte pastes on rehydration of horses. Am J Vet Res 63, 19–27.
Schryver, H.F., Parker, M.T., Daniluk, P.D., et al., 1987. Salt consumption and the effect of salt on mineral metabolism in horses. Cornell Vet 77, 122–131.
Smith, B.L., Jones, J.H., Hornof, W.J., et al., 1996. Effects of road transport on indices of stress in horses. Equine Vet J 28, 446–454.
Smith, D.G., Pearson, R.A., 2005. A review of the factors affecting the survival of donkeys in semi-arid regions of sub-saharan Africa. Tropical Anim Health Prod 37 (Suppl 1), 1–19.
Sneddon, J.C., van der Walt, J., Mitchell, G., 1993. Effect of dehydration on the volumes of body fluid compartments in horses. J Arid Environ 24, 397–408.
Sneddon, J.C., Argenzio, R.A., 1998. Feeding strategy and water homeostasis in equids: the role of the hindgut. J Arid Environ 38, 493–509.
Sneddon, J.C., Boomker, E., Howard, C.V., 2006. Mucosal surface area and fermentation activity in the hind gut of hydrated and chronically dehydrated working donkeys. J Anim Sci 84, 119–124.
Sosa Leon, L.A., Davie, A.J., Hodgson, D.R., et al., 1995. The effects of tonicity, glucose concentration and temperature of an oral rehydration solution on its absorption and elimination. Equine Vet J Suppl 20, 140–146.
Spensley, M.S., Carlson, G.P., Harrold, D., 1987. Plasma, red blood cell, total blood and extracellular fluid volumes in healthy horse foals during growth. Amer J Vet Res 48, 1703.
Spooner, H.S., Nielsen, B.D., Schott, H.C., et al., 2009. Evidence of the role of dietary fibre type on hydration status of horses performing endurance exercise. J Equine Vet Sci Abstracts 29, 367–368.
Stricker, E.M., Sved, A.F., 2000. Thirst. Nutrition 16, 821–826.

Stull, C.L., Rodiek, A.V., 2000. Physiological responses of horses to 24 hours of transportation using a commercial van during summer conditions. J Anim Sci 78, 1458–1466.
Sturdee, A.P., Bodley-Tickell, A.T., Archer, A., et al., 2003. Long-term study of Cryptosporidium prevalence on a lowland farm in the United Kingdom. Vet Parasitol 116, 97–113.
Sufit, E., Houpt, K.A., Sweeting, M., 1985. Physiological stimuli of thirst and drinking patterns in ponies. Equine Vet J 17, 12–16.
Sweeting, M.P., Houpt, C.E., Houpt, K.A., 1985. Social facilitation of feeding and time budgets in stabled horses. J Anim Sci 60, 369–374.
Tasker, J.B., 1967a. Fluid and electrolyte studies in the horse. III. Intake and output of water, sodium, and potassium. Cornell Vet 57, 649–657.
Tasker, J.B., 1967b. Fluid and electrolyte studies in the horse. IV. The effects of fasting and thirsting. Cornell Vet 57, 658–667.
Tasker, J.B., 1967c. Fluid and electrolyte studies in the horse. V. The effects of diarrhea. Cornell Vet 57, 668–677.
Van den Berg, J.S., Guthrie, A.J., Meintjes, R.A., et al., 1998. Water and electrolyte intake and output in conditioned Thoroughbred horses transported by road. Equine Vet J 30, 316–323.
Van de Weerd, H.A., Seaman, S., Wheeler, K., et al., 2008. Preference for artificial drinkers in British native ponies. In: 59th Annual Meeting Eur. Assoc. Anim. Prod. Wageningen Academic Publishers, Wageningen, the Netherlands, p. 219 (Abstract).
Veronesi, F., Passamonti, F., Caccio, S., et al., 2010. Epidemiological survey on equine Cryptosporidium and Giardia infections in Italy and Molecular Characterization of Isolates. Zoonoses Pub Health 57, 510–517.
Videla, R., Andrews, F.M., 2009. New perspectives in equine gastric ulcer syndrome. Vet Clinics of North Am Equine Practice 25, 283–301.
Waller, A., Lindinger, M.I., 2005. Time course and magnitude of fluid and electrolyte shifts during recovery from high-intensity exercise in Standardbred racehorses. Equine Comp. Exercise Physiol 2, 77–87.
Waller, A., Lindinger, M.I., 2006. Hydration of exercised Standardbred racehorses noninvasively using multi-frequency bioelectrical impedance analyis. Equine Vet J Suppl 36, 285–290.
Waller, A., Heigenhauser, G.J., Lindinger, M.I., 2008. Electrolyte supplementation after prolonged moderate-intensity exercise results in decreased plasma [TCO_2] in Standardbreds. Equine Comp Exer Physiol 4, 149–158.
Waller, A.P., Heigenhauser, G.J., Geor, R.J., et al., 2009. Fluid and electrolyte supplementation after prolonged moderate intensity exercise enhances muscle glycogen resynthesis in Standardbred horses. J Appl Physiol 106, 91–100.
Warren, L.K., Lawrence, L.M., Brewster-Barnes, T., et al., 1999. The effect of dietary fibre on hydration status after dehydration with frusemide. Equine Vet J Suppl 30, 508–513.
Wilson, M.E., 2007. Examination of the urinary tract in the horse. Vet Clin North Am Equine Pract 23, 563–575.
Zeyner, A. Geibler, C., Dittrich, A., 2004. Effects of hay intake and feeding sequence on variables in feces and fecal water (dry matter, pH value, organic acids, ammonia, buffering capacity) of horses. J Anim Physiol Anim Nutr 88, 7–19.

Energy systems and requirements

Andrea D. Ellis

Introduction

"The food is by no means ready to enter directly into the composition of the tissues of the body and add to its store of potential energy, but on the contrary, a very considerable amount of energy must be expended in the separation of the indigestible matters from the digestible and in the conversion of the latter into such forms as are suitable for the uses of the living cells in the body" (Armsby 1903).

Currently a variety of energy systems are available to calculate requirements for horses and to balance this with the provision of energy from feed. Each system has its strengths and weaknesses which has led to intensive and passionate discussion amongst scientists (Julliand & Martin-Rosset 2004). This chapter will give an overview of the main systems and discuss their practical application. The first section will try to provide a general understanding of the systems and their application and the second section will focus on more scientific details and an in depth discussion of systems. However, it is worth while to briefly reflect on why this area of nutrition science is so "exciting" and controversial.

On the one hand we have the very real, "live", actual energy requirements of an individual horse which are essential to maintain its bodyweight, biological function and ultimately to enable it to survive the various stages of life and environmental challenges. On the other hand we have the "abstract", paper based systems created by scientists/ nutritionists, in order to quantify, measure, calculate, estimate and predict these actual energy requirements and to quantify, measure, calculate, estimate and predict how they may be supplied by the feed. And all this is based on an abstract unit (Joule or Calorie). The original calorie was defined as the amount of energy required to heat 1 liter of water by 1°C – as determined by engineers when referring to steam engine technology. This "energy descriptor" is used by us in order to try and quantify the energy provided by organic nutrients (carbohydrates, fats, proteins) and converted metabolically into energy yielding compounds (glucose, fatty acids, volatile fatty acids, amino acids) which in turn are further metabolically catabolized into the key energy yielding unit adenosine triphosphate (ATP). This ATP is ultimately used to fuel maintenance of body systems, growth, production and movement. It is easy to see, therefore, why the energy requirements we estimate and subscribe to physiological functions cannot be "divorced" from the energy we estimate to be provided by feedstuffs.

Energy balance and defining energy units

Current energy systems (Table 5-1) try and predict the requirements of an individual animal (whether these are described in terms of GE, DE, ME, NE or any other unit), and match these against the supply from feed, i.e. match supply with demand and maintain the balance as illustrated in Fig. 5.1. Both supply and demand will depend on, and vary according to, a host of influencing factors which affect the digestive and metabolic processes (see Fig. 5.2). The energy value assigned can be obtained in several ways, each of which take into account different metabolic and digestive processes. This leads to a distinction between the energy units used. However, as long as the same energy unit (e.g., MJ digestible energy [DE] or MJ net energy [NE]) is used within a particular system a good balance can be obtained. A detailed discussion of the advantages and the disadvantages of each unit can be found at the end of this chapter.

Feed energy can be defined in terms of the gross energy of feed (GE = total heat that could be released = energy released through complete combustion of organic matter = relative to O_2 used); or the digestible energy of feed (DE = GE minus the fecal energy left after a feedstuff has passed through animal); or the metabolizable energy (ME = DE minus the energy lost in the gases and urine produced as a result of the feedstuff passing through the animal) or finally the net energy (NE = ME minus the associated heat increment lost through ingestion, digestion [fermentation] and metabolizing of food-substrates). This increment is represented by a coefficient (k) derived from estimating the efficiency at which ME is "converted" to NE (i.e., NE = ME × k, where k represents the efficiency in conversion of energy substrates to ATP).

In equine NE systems there is distinction made between energy for maintenance, production and/or work for requirements only, whereas ruminant systems distinguish between maintenance (m) and production (p) (i.e., k_m and k_p) only, but both for requirements and feed supply. Van Soest (1994) defined the net energy available from a feed for a given animal as being the *energy value realized in the form of product*. Such a product can be measured through the

Table 5-1 Energy Systems for Horses Currently in Use, Their Basis and Energy Units Used. The arrows predict the change in energy units that will occur (⟶) shortly (DLG 2011) and which may possibly occur (- - →) in the next few years.

System	Basis	Energy Unit	Country of use		
			DE	ME	(p)NE
NRC (2007)	DE	MCal DE	USA, GB, Australia, Canada, - - - →		
DLG (1994)	DE	MJ DE	Germany, Austria; ⟶	↓	
DLG (200?) in preparation	ME	MJ ME		Germany***	
INRA (1984)*	(p)NE	UFC			France, Spain, Portugal, Italy, Poland
CVB (2005)	(p)NE	EWpa			Netherlands, Belgium
SCAN Scandinavian** Systems based on CVB (1996) & INRA (1990) adaptations	(p)NE ME	UFC MJ ME FU		Sweden Finland	Denmark, Norway, Iceland

UFC = French Horse Feed Unit (NEfeed/NE of Barley; 1 kg DM Barley = 9.42 MJ NE = 1 UFC).
EWpa = Dutch Equine Feed Unit (NEfeed/NE of Oats; 1 kg DM Oats = 8.93 MJ NE = 1 EWpa).
FU = Feed Unit = 11.7 MJ ME (Finland).
*Described in detail by Vermorel and Martin-Rosset (1997)
**Described in Austbo (1996, 2004) and Jansson (2004)
***Described in Kienzle and Zeyner (2010), Coenen et al (2010a, b), Coenen (2011) pers.com, DLG 2011 – in preparation

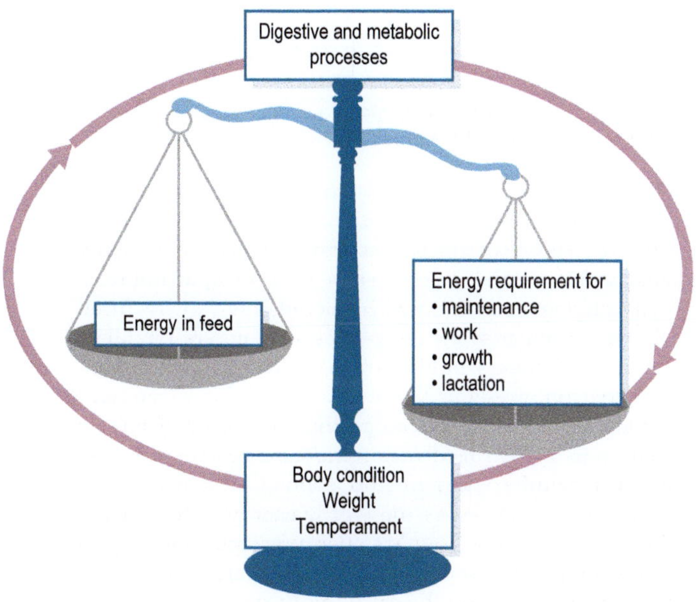

Figure 5.1 The "balance" that energy systems try to maintain.

energy "content" of animal tissue (growth in kg) or milk output but is much harder to define in terms of "work" or "horsepower". Current NE systems for horses therefore only determine the "product" at "maintenance" level with respect to food values – by estimating the end-substrates of food absorption which are then available for net use. With respect to requirements, the evaluation of the net energy used for work has been directly linked to oxygen consumption. This has resulted in the derivation of various equations which convert the ml of O_2 used above maintenance into energy values (Coenen 2005, Pagan et al 2005). In summary, Fig. 5.2 illustrates how the energy from feed and the energy required by the horse can be assessed. In terms of feed energy we move from left to right → of the pathway, starting with GE. Requirements, however, can only start to be measurable, using currently available techniques, at the ME and NE point and move from right to left ← up to the point of DE. The figure also highlights in gray boxes some of the major factors that influence the actual energy value that can be derived from feed and that is available to the horse.

The key factors at the feed or animal level which influence the actual energy value provided or required are shown in the gray boxes in Fig. 5.2. Herein lies the main problem and challenge – our energy systems are trying to fit a dynamic living process (energy metabolism, metabolic processes, multiple interactions) into a static list of values for supply and demand/requirement. The challenges are compounded as the methods we have currently at our disposal to measure these values at a given (static) point in time are often indirect and require additional calculations/estimations. Nevertheless, the ongoing process of gaining new knowledge and understanding of energy metabolism and supply has allowed us to optimize and continuously improve feeding systems and practices for production across different species, whether "production" is defined as athletic performance, growth, weight-gain, or lactation. In addition, it has given us vital understanding of the involvement of nutritional factors in maintaining health and wellbeing in the horse.

Key Points

- Feeding systems are a key towards understanding, quantifying and explaining digestive processes and energy metabolism
- Feed energy values are estimated from GE towards NE
- Energy requirements are estimated from NE and converted back to ME and DE.

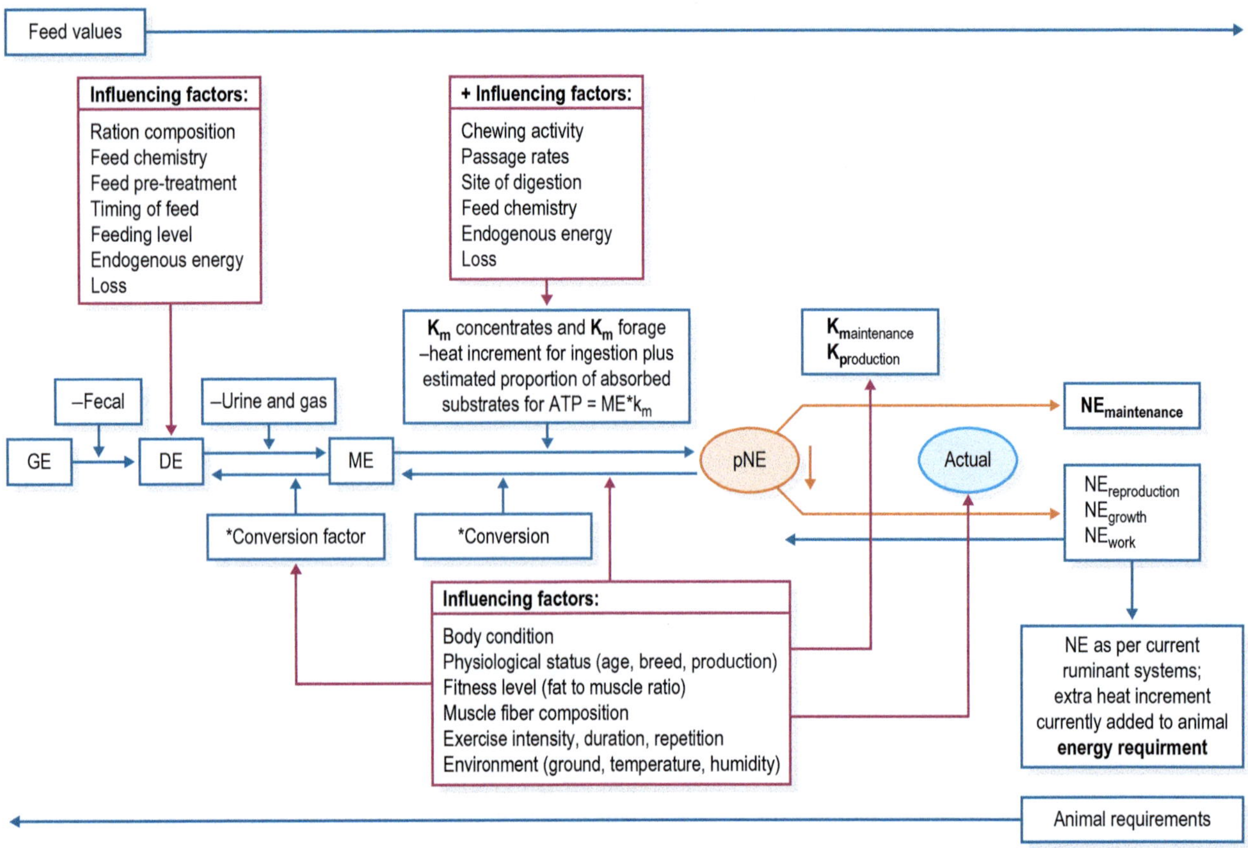

Figure 5.2 Schematic overview of reaching the energy unit assigned to feed (always starting with GE as the first measure point) and to requirements (always starting with NE (potential = pNE) as the first measure point for horses).
Adapted from Ellis 2002a.

Practical application of energy systems

In practice, the nutrition scientist can use the various formulas provided by each system to firstly calculate (a) feed values (Tables 5-2 and 5-3) and (b) energy requirements of horses (Tables 5-4, 5-5, and 5-6) and apply these to ration calculation and evaluation. They can then apply their knowledge of nutrient absorption and metabolic conversion in order to determine, as far as possible, the optimal chemical composition of the feed that should be provided for conversion into energy. This will vary according to the type and intensity of exercise and also needs to take into consideration the maintenance of good health and welfare.

The various equations can be used to derive table values, per system, which in turn can be applied to energy balance calculations (Table 5-3). This highlights that the values in the tables themselves *cannot be compared directly* as they are given in different units within a system.

The more applied nutritionist will tend to use tables, which give pre-estimated or measured values according to the type, lifestage and work of the horse, etc., rather than use the calculations. An example of how these summary calculations work for maintenance in a 500 kg horse, on medium quality grass hay is given in Table 5-4. *This highlights the fact that despite some differences in the theory behind each system and the units used the practical feed recommendations are fairly similar.* However, it is essential to understand that *systems and units cannot be "mixed" or easily converted* unless all the measures from that particular system are taken into account. This is one of the reasons why INRA (1984), Finland (Austbo 2004) and the Dutch system (CVB 1996) introduced a final conversion factor which moved them away from Mcal and MJ units, as the temptation to compare DE Mcal with NE or ME Mcal would be there for the less knowledgeable lay person.

Taking the approach of comparing the energy of a feed in relation to another feed within the same system can give some idea of differences in feed evaluation between the systems. Figure 5.3 shows the wet matter energy ratio of feeds either in relation to grass energy values or to barley energy values. It is important to note that this is "as fed"/wet matter/product and the calculations stated above have been used rather than in vivo table values.

As can be seen the energy values of forages in relation to that of grass, are fairly similar between all systems. However, differences occur with respect to the concentrate feed. This is due to the French NE system giving concentrates a higher value possibly due to the systems' equation's inclusion of sugar and starch when estimating energy content (Fig. 5.3A), whereas the NRC (DE) equation relates the energy value to the low ADF content. This is "mirrored" by the proportionally greater drop of energy values for forages in the NE system in relation to the barley value as compared to the other systems. Here the additional effect of the inclusion of a lower forage *k*-factor for energy derived from absorption of substrates in the hindgut can be seen (Fig. 5.3B). However, overall, the ratios show a similar order and relationship of feed values within the various systems. The

Table 5-2 Equations to Derive Feed Energy Values

USA, NRC (2007)	Germany, DLG (in preparation, 2011)	France, INRA (Vermorel & Martin-Rosset, 1997)
DE All table values according to formula (other formulas discussed in NRC 2007 but not used in the end)	ME Formulas only used in absence of in vivo digestibility coefficient	NE (pNE) In absence of in vivo dig. coefficient, regression formula from sheep dig. is used
Concentrates: DE (Mcal/kg DM) = 4.07 – 0.055 (%ADF) Forages: DE (Mcal/kg DM) = 2.118+0.01218 CP–0.00937ADF- 0.0383 (NDF-ADF) + 0.04718 EE + 0.02035 NFC – 0.0262 Ash Fats/oils: DE (Mcal/kg DM) = (–3.6 +0.211CP + **0.421**EE + 0.015 CF)/4.184 (Nutrients given in %/kg DM)	DLG (2011) (from Kienzle & Zeyner, 2010) ME(MJ/kg DM) = –3.54 + 0.0129 CP + 0.0420 EE – 0.0019 CF + 0.0185 NFE (Nutrients in g/kg DM) Derived from this and applied in the Dutch NET Energy system: k_{Conc} = (72,34 + 0.0119 × CF – 0.0081 × CP + 0,0112 × SS)/100 (CVB 1996) Derived from this and applied in the Dutch NET Energy system: k_{Forage}= (65,21 – 0,0178 × CF + 0.0181 × CP + 0,0452 × SS)/100 (CVB 1996) Derived from this: UFC/kg **OM** = 1.219 – 0.852ADF – 0.287 NDF – 0.857 ADL + 0.034 CP + 0.207 Starches (n = 35) r^2 = 0.98 RSD = 0.031	DE in MJ/kg DM = ED% * GE ED (%) = 0.034 + Δ + 0.9477 OMd (%) r^2 = 0.95 Δ = **–1.1** for forages Δ = **+1.1** for concentrates OMd horses from in vivo trials (majority of feedstuffs) OR Regression from OMd_{sheep} on 200 comparative studies (r^2 = 0.72–0.96) ME/DE (%) = 84.07 + 0.0165 CF – 0.0276 CP + 0.0184 CC for protein rich feed (>30% CP) ME/DE (%) = 94.36 – 0.0110 CF – 0.0275CP (Nutrients in g/kg DM) NE = ME × km km as per assumed energy (E) derived from end-products of digestion: Concentrate feed: km = 0.85 E_{GI} + 0.80 E_{LCFA} + 0.70 E_{AA} + (0.63 to 0.68) E_{VFA} Forages: km = 0.85 E_{GI} + 0.80 E_{LCFA} + 0.70 E_{AA} + (0.63 to 0.68) E_{VFA} minus 0.14(76.4 – E_{CH}) or minus 0.20_{CF} + 2.50

CP = crude protein, CC = cytoplasmic carbohydrates (INRA 1997) = starch + watersoluble carbohydrates; SS = starches and sugars); NFC = nonfibrous carbohydrates [NFC = 100 – %NDF – % CP – % Ash]; NFE = nitrogen free extractives (1000 – CP – CF – Ash-EE – in g DM); NDF = neutral detergent fiber; ADF = acid detergent fiber; ADL = acid detergent lignin; GI = glucose, LCFA – long chain fatty acids; VFA = volatile fatty acids; E_{CH} = *in vivo* energy cost of eating.

German (DLG) calculations make the smallest distinction between the metabolizable energy derived from oats and barley.

Maintenance

Table 5-4 highlights what happens when the hay values, as used in Fig 5.3, are linked to maintenance requirements according to each system. This provides a real practical example, as true comparison between the systems is only possible when both sides of the "balance" (intake and expenditure) are taken into account.

Although the descriptors of "low, average and high maintenance" from NRC (2007) cannot be completely equated to the three levels provided by INRA (1984) a similar relationship can be seen, with a slightly higher volume of hay needed by NRC to fulfil maintenance requirements for the more active animal and in the INRA system, for the Thoroughbred. The German system shows the highest differences in maintenance requirements according to type/breed of horse and details of the studies from which the data were used can be found in Kienzle et al (2010). In the end these requirements are "average" figures which should be considered as a mean with a range of ±10% depending on individual horse factors (body condition, temperament, breed, age, fitness level and worklevel), as well as environmental factors (temperature, humidity, social interaction, human requirement of body shape and temperament). There is no such thing as an "average" horse!

Table 5-3 Average Feed Energy Values Per kg Product (Wet Matter/as Fed) Listed according to the 3 Most Common Systems (Wet Matter Adjusted according to a Common DM Denominator So Using Same DM Values)

Feedstuff	DM	NRC (2007)	DLG (2011)	INRA (1984)
		DE (Mcal/kg)	ME (MJ/kg)	NE (UFC/kg)
Grass (ryegrass, summer)	20	0.47	1.65	0.13
Grass hay (medium quality)	84	1.90	6.20	0.49
Lucerne chop (heat dried)	84	2.16	6.40	0.52
Barley straw	91	1.52	4.31	0.42
Oats grain whole	88	3.13	11.01	0.88
Barley grain, rolled	88	3.45	11.62	1.01
Sugar beet pulp, unmolassed, dehydrated	91	2.40	8.20	0.71

Table 5-4 Equations from a Number of Systems to Calculate Maintenance Energy Requirements and example of how much hay (in kg WM) would fulfil Requirements of a 500 kg Horse at Maintenance

	Equation	Daily requirements 500 kg "mare/gelding"	= Daily intake of medium quality hay (kg)[1]	Experimental Basis
NRC 2007 Low[2] Average = low + 10% High = low + 20%	DE (kcal/day) 30.3 × BW (kg) 33.3 × BW (kg) 36.3 × BW (kg)	MJ DE/day 63.33 69.60 75.87	8.2 9.2 9.9	Cited in NRC (2007): Pagan and Hintz (1986) Wooden et al. (1970) Vermorel et al. (1997a,b)
DLG 2011 200–800 kg Pony Warmblood Warblood in training Thoroughbred Others	 ME(MJ/kg$^{0.75}$ BW) 0.40 0.52 0.58 0.64 0.4–0.5	 MJ ME/day 42 55 61 68 53	 6.4 8.4 9.8 10.3 8.0	Described by Kienzle and Zeyner (2010) & Kienzle et al. (2010) Vermorel et al. (1997a,b) Fingerling (1931–1939) Burlacu et al. (1993) Ragnarsson (2009) Kienzle et al. (2009)
INRA 1984 Cold-blood Ridinghorse Thoroughbred	Base 352 kJ/kg BW$^{0.75}$ or 0.038 UFC/kg BW$^{0.75}$ Mares/gelding Stallion +0% + 10% +5% + 15% +10% + 20%	UFC 4.0 UFC 4.2 UFC 4.4 UFC	8.2 8.6 9.0	Cited in: Vermorel & Martin-Rosset (1997) Voit (1901), Knox et al (1970) Zuntz & Hagemann(1898) Benedict (1938), Wooden et al (1970) Doreau et al (1988) Martin-Rosset (1990) Vermorel et al (1997a,b) Martin-Rosset & Vermorel (1991)

[1]Using energy values given by each system in the tables for a medium quality hay as per Table 5-5 above (NRC: Mcal/kg WM = 1.86 Mcal DE; DLG:5.6 MJ ME; INRA: 0.49 UFC).
[2]Low: Direct result from "stalled" horses in experiments, sedentary lifestyle; old horses (arthritic); stable rested; injured; small ponies; "good doers"; Average: normally moving around horses; walking in paddock; High: Highly strung; nervous; increased voluntary activity; young horses; stallions; "bad doers".

Pregnancy, lactation and growth

It is worth noting that with respect to pregnancy, lactation and growth all systems (see Table 5-5) start by calculating energy requirements from net energy for growth and lactation figures, using the energy accretion of the fetus during gestation, milk production, and average growth rates in kg/day. As these are based on net energy values they are then converted back to ME and DE as required according to system. The products themselves (kg growth and liters milk) are very tangible and measurable – unlike work output.

Work/exercise

When looking at the calculations and tables available for assessing work level it becomes clear that in practice these are very subjective or difficult to determine (see Table 5-6) and tend not to give clear guidance as to work level for individual horses. Trainers and riders therefore tend to ignore these systems unless there seems to be an obvious imbalance between energy expenditure and intake or other possibly nutrition related health problems. In the case of performance horses, professionals (veterinarian or

Table 5-5 Energy Requirements for Broodmares and Youngstock

System	Equation	Experimental basis
NRC 2007 Gestation <5 months gestation >5 months (PU = placental and uterine, G = gain)	DE (Mcal/day) As average maintenance (0.033BW) + (0.033 × 2 × (Fetal mass + PU mass) + [(0.03 × Fetal G × 9.4) + (0.2 × Fetal G × 5.6)]/0.6	PU data from 5 studies; Fetal gain data from Meyer & Ahlswende (1976) and Guissani et al (2005) For calculation of PU and Fetal G see NRC (2007)
Lactation <700 kg (high maint.) >700 kg (average maint.) Milk value 1 month = 0.0324, 2 month = 0.0299, 3 month = 0.0271 4 month = 0.0244	 (0.0363*BW) + (Milk production × 500)/600 (0.0333*BW) + (Milk production × 500)/600 Milk Prod = Milk Value × (month of lactation − 1) × BW	 Hoffmann et al (1998) Santos et al (2005) Martin et al (1992) Doreau et al (1992)
Foal Maintenance1–18 months (X = age in month) + Growth (ADG = average daily gain) ADG calculated (MBW = mature Bodyweight)	 $(56.5X^{-0.145}) \times BW$ + $(1.99 + 1.21X - (0.021X^2)) \times ADG$ MBW* (6.97 × Exp (−0.0772 × Age))/(30.4 × 100)	Ousey et al (1997) Cymbaluk et al. (1990) Based on mean values of 18 studies cited in NRC (2007) including various breeds: Morgan, Warmblood, Quarter horses, TB, Belgian, Arab, ponies
DLG 2011 (in preparation) Gestation For conceptus, d = day of gestation (d 240–340) Lactation (in preparation) d = day of lactation ($k_{lactation}$ = 0.6; conversion from NE to ME) Foal (in preparation)	MJ ME/kg Birthweight = 0.418 $0.000508848 \times e^{(0.0154d)}$ plus maintenance $\text{kJ ME/kg } BW^{0.82} = 141.3 \times d^{0.1727} \times e^{-0.00539d}/0.6$ plus maintenance in preparation	Presented in Coenen et al (2010a) Schmidt & Coenen (2010) Coenen et al (2010b)
INRA 1984* Gestation (For fetus: Y=%BW from Birthweight, a = chemical composition, GE, $k_{production}$ = 0.25; X = days of pregnancy) Lactation (GE = GE/kg milk, $k_{lactation}$ = 0.65) Milk yield/100 kg BW 1 month = 3 kg GE = 2.4 2–3 month = 2.5 kg GE = 2.09 4 month = 2 kg GE = 1.98 Foal a = maintenance requirements, bG = calorific value of daily gain 1.4 = allometry coefficient of adipose tissue in total BW	NE (MJ/day) = $(0.351 \text{ MJ/kg } BW^{75})$ + (Y × a × GE × km/kp) UFC/day = NE/9.42 $Y = -1.99 + 13.67 - 37.38X^2 + 45.51X^3 - 18.32$ NE (MJ/d) = $(0.351 \text{ MJ/kg } BW^{75})$ + (kg Milk × BW/100 × GE × km/kl) UFC/day = NE/9.42 NE (UFC/kg $BW^{0.75}$/day) $NE = a + bG^{1.4}$	Described in Martin-Rosset et al (2006a) Doreau et al (1991, 1992) Described in Martin-Rosset et al (2006b) Doreau & Boulot (1989) Doreau et al (1992) Described in Martin-Rosset & Ellis (2005)

nutritionist) may be called in to assess the diet and they may indeed use one of the energy systems to check if there are any obvious imbalances.

In Germany the practical table to evaluate work level can be seen below (GEH 1994, Table 5-7). This system is currently being revised and converted to ME, and bases energy requirements on oxygen consumption and average HR which in turn are linked to energy expenditure (Fig. 5.4).

The most practical advice and information is currently given by the French system, but even then it is still difficult for the practitioner to assign individual work programs to actual work level (Fig. 5.5).

In the UK and USA practitioners may use the new NRC (2007) System, where calculating energy requirements can now be done online: http://nrc88.nas.edu/nrh/. Here they will be asked to decide, without any further guidance, which level of maintenance is required (low, average or high) and which level of workload their horse does (light, medium, heavy, very heavy). The visitor to the website will probably not have the complete book at hand - but if they do - these are the guidelines given (Table 5-8):

In addition the NRC (2007) gives a table of percentage distribution of gaits within an hour for the first three work levels. Unfortunately a figure to depict this is not shown on the website or in the booklet for easy reference (Fig. 5.6). As was the case in the previous system (NRC, 1989), the individual equestrian sports have been assigned to various work levels but for the applied rider (scientific lay person)

Table 5-6 Summary of Various Levels of Calculations and Tables Used to Estimate Energy Requirements for Work per System

	NRC 2007	DLG 2011(in preparation)	INRA 1984
	DE	ME	NE
LEVEL 1 – Formula – Calculation	At this level NRC refers to a formula by Coenen (2005) based on O_2 consumption in relation to HR per minute: O_2 (ml/kg BW/min) = 0.0019 × $(HR)^{2.0653}$ Average HR per speed needs to be estimated from this–tables given and energy utilization factor for HR (beats/min) is used (kcal): 60 b/min = 24 90 b/min = 56 120 b/min = 99 150 b/min = 158 180 b/min = 230	The German system will be moving to ME energy expenditure (EE) based on the relationship between heart beats per minute and O_2 consumption allowing for estimation of anaerobic energy production at higher exercise levels (see Fig. 5.4) Energy expenditure (kJ/kg BW/ per minute exercise) = $0.566e^{-4} \times x^{1.9955} + 0.250e^{-6} \times e^{(0.073043x)}$ x = heartbeats/minute	Oxygen consumption VO_2 l/min = 3.78 + 0.0097 velocity (m/min) (Meixner 1981; based on 560 kg BW horse + 100 kg tack and rider) Linked to Energy Expenditure – thermal heat (NE kcal/min exercise) (Maintenance 1) Walk 1.2 Slow trot 2.5 Normal trot 10 Fast trot 15 Normal gallop 20 Fast gallop 40 Maximum velocity 60
LEVEL 2 – Simple Calculation Tables	Despite detailed description of the above Work energy values are then given as multiples of maintenance (*m*). Light = 1.2*m* Medium = 1.4*m* Heavy = 1.6*m* Very heavy = 1.9*m* Average time spent at various levels/hour are indicated (Table 5-8)	Users have the option to use a table which gives extra energy requirements per minute work per kg BW for: Walk: Slow, Fast Trot: Light, Medium Canter: Fast Collected, Medium Galop: Fast, Racing	Converted to exercise units of 1 hour (Fig. 5.5) with various % components of walk, trot, canter, jump and for school work (4 options) or open air work (4 options)
LEVEL 3 – Quick Reference Tables	Users have the option to get energy requirements from tables per day per type of horse per range of BW for work levels of: Light Medium Heavy Very Heavy	Users finally have the option to get energy requirements per day per range of BW for work levels of: Very light Light Medium Heavy Very heavy	Users finally have the option to get energy requirements per day per range of BW for work levels of: Very light Light Hack Moderate Intense

Table 5-7 Levels of Work in the German System (GEH 1994)

Work		Speed/ km/hour	kJ DE/kg weight*	kJ DE/kg Weight
Walk	Slow	3–3.5	1.2–1.8	7
	Fast	5–6	1.8	10
Trot	Light	12	2.3	27
	Medium	15	2.7	40
	Fast (collected canter	18	3.2	57
Gallop	Medium	21	3.9	81
	Fast	30	4–6	
	Racing	50–60	–40	

*Actual weight = horse and rider

as far as the author is concerned there is lots of scope for misinterpretation.

This brings the NRC (2007) system closer to European systems in providing practical guidance for horse trainers and riders. However, assessing the work level is still very ambiguous with the guidelines given. For heavy work just 1 hour speed work per week or 6–12 hours slow work per week are cited (Table 5-8). Both the French and Dutch systems give similar guidelines but at a slightly more detailed level.

In order to compare the three systems for a working horse, energy requirements for a 500 kg Gelding (Sports horse, average maintenance) plus 60 kg rider weight, in medium work (from Table 5-8 and Fig. 5.6 above), was calculated and balanced against the intake of 10 kg of hay (in units and values given per system, satisfying structural fiber requirements at 2% DM intake per day – total WM intake around 2.2% minimum). The remaining balance to achieve

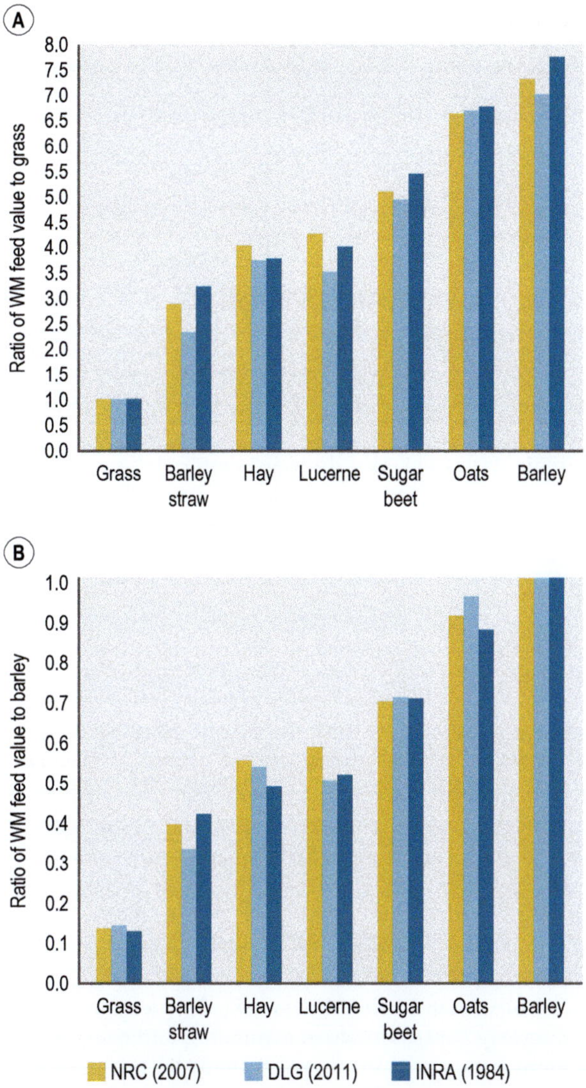

Figure 5.3 Relationship of table provided feed values/kg wet matter published within a system to each other: (A) in relationship to grass and (B) in relationship to barley values.

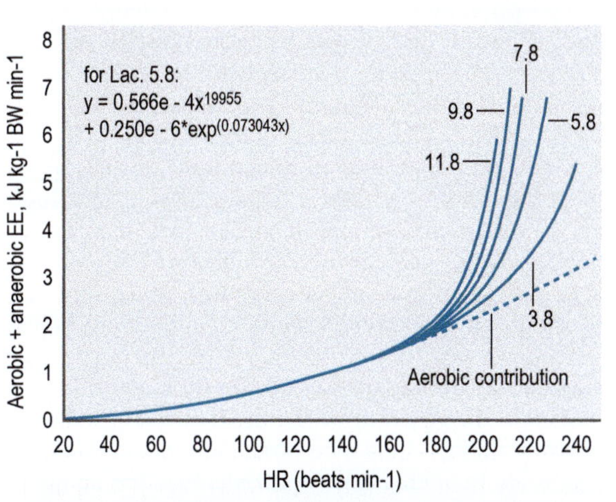

Figure 5.4 Relationship between heart beats per minute and aerobic/anaerobic energy expenditure (Coenen personal communication) (The duration, fitness level, muscle fibre composition/breed, slope and other environmental conditions will influence extent of anaerobic contribution – i.e., lactic acid production – Lac).

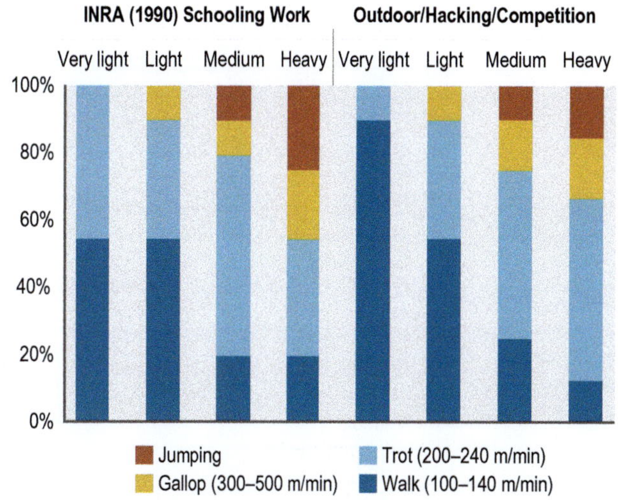

Figure 5.5 Estimated distribution of gaits during one hour of exercise per day for evaluation of work level.
Source: INRA 1990 – adapted from INRA 1990 (due to comments made by INRA).

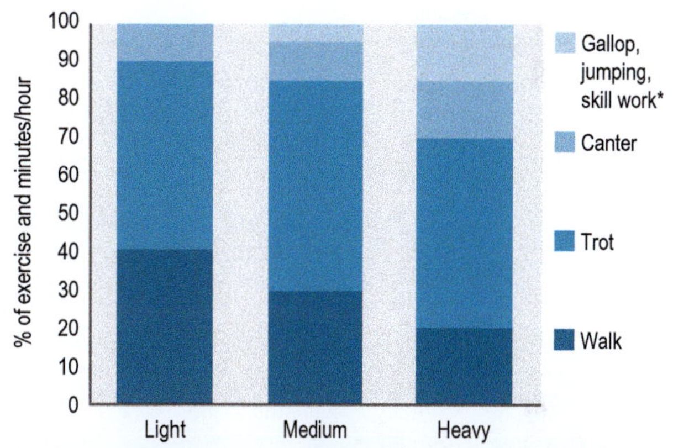

Figure 5.6 Illustration of average distribution of exercise within an hour at light medium and heavy work levels according to NRC (2007) * Other skill work not defined by NRC, possibly: Western, Ranch work, Polo.
Adapted from table in NRC (2007).

100% requirements has then been topped up with oats (Fig. 5.7).

Again – it can be seen that in the practical application of the systems (and when "average values" are taken = average oats and hay, average horse) there is fairly good accordance between the systems. How good this will fit with any individual horse is questionable and here the differences of "tabled" exercise descriptors will play an important role. The INRA system recommends slightly more, but when comparing exact definitions of medium work, this system's descriptor of medium work is probably slightly "harder" than the other two systems (less walk, more trot and jumping). The new German system is still in final development stages.

In practice some performance horse trainers and riders do now routinely use heart rate monitors, even GPS systems, to assess speed and distance covered, and also take regular lactate samples to assess fatigue tolerance (Naylor 2009). However, these measures are typically used to assess fitness level rather than energy requirements. Ultimately, in practice, energy balance is mainly assessed by maintenance or loss of body condition or according to traditional, at times misguided "thinking", of what is light, medium or heavy

Table 5-8 Work Level Descriptors according to NRC (2007)

	Sport	Hours/week	Mean heart rate
Light:	Recreational riding, Beginning of training programs, Show horses;	1–3 h/week	80 beats/ min
Medium:	School Horses, Recreational, Beginning of training/breaking, frequent Show horses, Polo, Ranch work	3–5 h/week	90 beats/ min
Heavy:	Ranch work, Polo, Show horses (frequent and strenuous), Low-Medium level eventing, Race training (middle stages)	4–5 h/week	110 beats/ min
Very Heavy:	Racing (Quater/ TB horse, Standardbred, Endurance) Elite 3-day event	6–12 h/week slow OR 1 h/ week speed work	110–150 beats/min

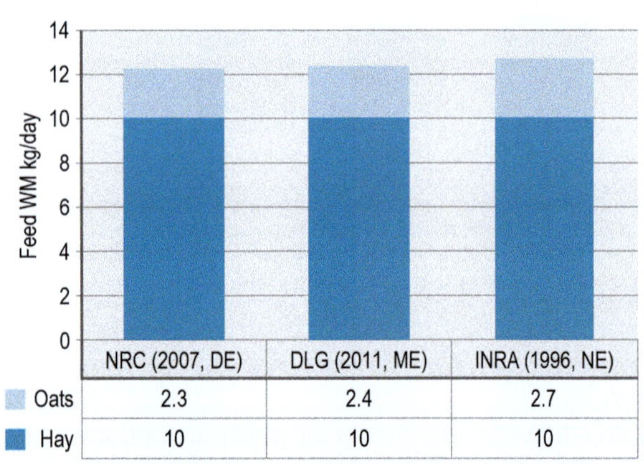

Figure 5.7 Feed requirements (kg WM) for a 500 kg Warmblood gelding (+60 kg rider) in medium work according to different systems.

work. Nevertheless the assessment and evaluation of energy requirements for work has led to increased knowledge on feed substrate use for conversion to work and thus optimizing performance. Research in this area will continue to deepen our understanding of exercise physiology.

The applied table values of all systems (Tables 5-6–5-8; Figs 5.5 and 5.6) become very insensitive to intensity, duration, repetition of exercise and additional effort (slope, temperature, humidity, fitness level, body condition) and therefore can at best only be very rough guides. There is scope for future development of a more detailed system for the end-user than the very simplistic table values given at the moment. This may help to keep a more direct link with the mathematical calculations which were originally used to estimate energy expenditure (Ellis 2008).

Key Points – Energy evaluation systems

- Always use same units/system for requirements and food values
- In practical application differences between systems diminish
- Correct work level assessment is key for practical rationing in working horses

Advantages and disadvantages of different systems

The energy values for feed and for requirements as utilized by each system are derived from a combination of in vivo measurements (direct or through extrapolation of key metabolic measures) and extrapolation from other species (through understanding and application of knowledge gained in these species) (NRC 2007, INRA 1990, DLG 1994, CVB 1996).

Terminology

An important note in respect of terminology: Disputes over terminology may distract from the true or potential advantages and disadvantages of the various systems. This is especially so with respect to the so called equine NE systems:

1. Units: The fact that the Dutch, Scandinavian and French systems use an additional conversion factor to avoid units of megaJoule or Calories is irrelevant to the discussion of the relative merits of each system – it is a pure factor of "naming" the energy units and is often incorrectly pointed out as a problem.
2. On the other hand using the term k_m does lead to unnecessary confusion when evaluating and comparing different systems, as in current systems for horses k (efficiency rate at which substrates are converted to ATP) is calculated according to feedstuffs (distinguishing between the k for concentrates and the k for forages) and is applied at the *potential* NE point (after nutrient absorption and ME loss but *prior to* partitioning for use in maintenance, work or production). In ruminant systems for feedstuffs and requirements, the k factor distinguishes between maintenance (k_m), work (k_w) and production (k_p) to assess the efficiency of substrate conversion to ATP (which changes depending on utilization). As Harris (1997) pointed out, the current "equine" $k_{maintenance}$ value is applied irrespective of maintenance, work and production status – so not truly a k_m factor. This highlights a key difference between the term k_m according to ruminant systems and k_m in the French and Dutch systems (INRA 1990, CVB 1996) and a change in "terminology" may be useful to avoid confusion. In the equine systems the reduced efficiency in substrate utilization is then potentially taken into consideration by increasing requirements when horses require energy above maintenance levels. This also occurs in ME and DE systems.
3. Finally, apart from possibly re-naming the k factor, the current equine NE systems should also highlight that their feed "NE" does not go as far as ruminant "NE" systems when assessing energy value of feed. One

suggestion could be to talk about *potential Net Energy (pNE) in feed.*

Derivation of the various energy values

Steps and calculations based on in vivo and direct knowledge are highlighted by green cards and green text (which represent verifiable measures/formulas based on regression from in vivo measurements). The estimated aspects which are based on less well substantiated values (e.g., some indirect physiological/biochemical factors) measured in vivo and in vitro are highlighted by the yellow cards. Finally, the disadvantages/unknown factors based on estimations from other species or pure in vitro results are given red cards and red text. This does not automatically mean that the information provided by these "red cards" does not bring us closer to "true" values, but at this point in time only educated estimates are possible. No doubt scientists will not all agree on the allocation and number of cards, for each system but clear logical arguments can be made based on the evidence at each point - this "card system" therefore needs to be seen as a basis for fruitful discussion and as an indicator of where future research should be targeted.

Figure 5.8 illustrates how, when matching up feed values and requirements of horses at each level along those points (in opposite directions), different issues may arise.

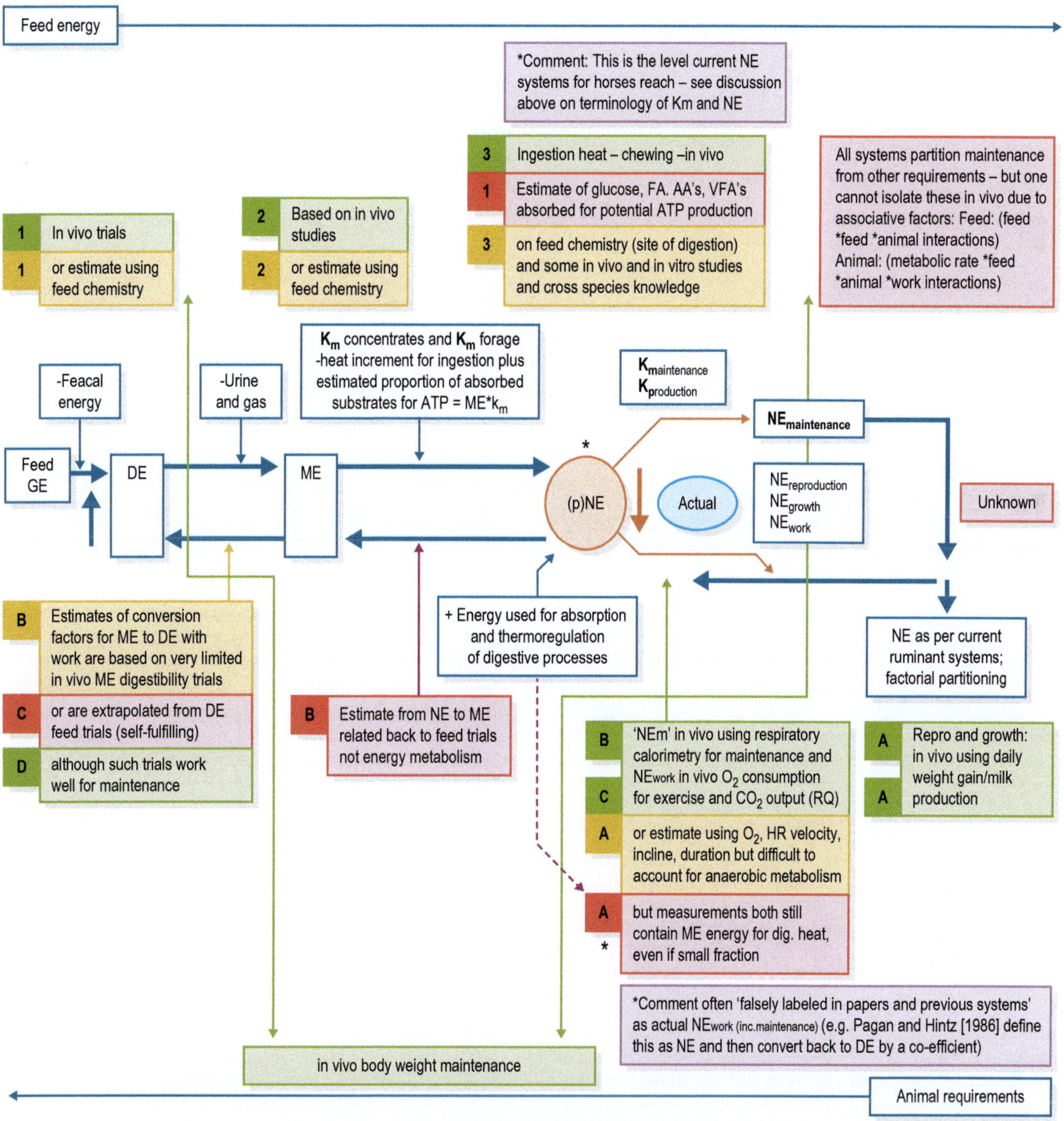

Figure 5.8 Schematic overview of calculations and estimations used to derive energy values (Cards: Values based on in vivo data [green], regressions and calculations from in vivo knowledge [yellow] or estimates from other species or in vitro values/ calculations [red]. For feed values cards are numbered numerically from left to right; for requirements cards are numbered alphabetically from right to left). Feed evaluation ends at (p) NE level and requirements end at DE level.

In Table 5-9 feed cards are added up from left to right starting from DE level and requirement cards from right to left, starting from potential NE level.

On both sides of the scales, and with each step of a system, advantages and disadvantages can be noted for calculation/estimation of feed energy and animal requirements. At this point in time we do not have enough knowledge to move to actual net energy partitioning for feed stuffs in particular but the current equine NE systems are not attempting to do this as yet. The discussion in Table 5-10 describes and evaluates the points summarized in Fig. 5.8 and Table 5-9.

Table 5-9 Number of Cards Accumulated by Systems

DE:	Feed:	1 1
	Requirements:	A B C D A B A B C
ME:	Feed:	1 2 1 2
	Requirements:	A B C A A B
(p)'NE':	Feed:	1 2 3 1 2 3 1
	Requirements:	A B C A A
End point of current systems		
		1 2 3 1 2 3 1 unknown
Actual NE:	Feed:	A B C A A

Conclusions

In summary the advantage of using the DE system lies with the ability to measure feed values relatively easily *in vivo* at maintenance, whereas the advantage of the NE system lies in the in vivo assessment of energy expenditure.

As can be seen from the above discussion most other arguments may apply to all the systems. Positives on the feed requirements side for one system may be counterbalanced by disadvantages on the feed evaluation side and vice versa. The process of increasing the accuracy of each system, as well as the discussion and integration of these systems into practical rationing has formed and still forms the basis of the nutrition scientists' quest for increased knowledge. Research into energy balance at various levels of work and body condition as well as physiological measures of the animal responses to various diets provide the basis for our improved understanding, such as the role different diets play in providing energy to horses working in different disciplines. This ultimately is translated to practical feeding recommendations.

Table 5-10 Advanced discussion on pros and cons of energy evaluation as per Figure 5.8

±	Discussion points for scientists	UNIT
Maintenance balance Plus	In practice the maintenance of bodyweight is the best way to asses that the diet is providing the required amount of energy. Indirect assessment of requirements seems to work extremely well in vivo at the maintenance level – by assessing feed units (whether determined as DE, ME or NE) required to maintain bodyweight. Equations which relate this energy requirement to the individual components of feed have been established from hundreds of digestibility trials using DE measures only and substantial data also exists from in vivo trials at the ME level. Similarly over 200 trial results using (p)NE feed values linked to BW maintenance have been carried out. These also supplied excellent information at the ME level. In addition, a number of trials have been linked directly to measures of (p)NE used through indirect calorimetry (O_2, RER, and limited caloric chamber work).	DE ME pNE
Exercise and production balance Plus	Direct in vivo assessment of the energy supplied from feed to maintain body condition in working, growing or breeding horses has been carried out – although to a lesser extent than for maintenance. All systems use this in vivo data and derived calculations (feed chemistry × conversion factors = estimated DE supply/ME supply) to make the association with requirements based on work/body-weight gain/ milk production or growth and even placental and foetal tissue accumulation.	DE ME pNE
Maintenance balance Minus	The energy required to maintain bodyweight and condition (the key indicator of energy balance) is influenced by various factors including breed, BW & size, body composition, age, growth, activity level (gender, temperament), environment, fitness level, exercise as well as the individual's digestive and metabolic efficiency. A number of studies have highlighted that the energy required at the maintenance level can vary up to ± 20% for horses of same bodyweight (e.g. Martin-Rosset 2008). Van Soest (1994) points out that a net energy maintenance requirement will always be somewhat inaccurate as heat production at low feeding levels will involve energy conservation, leading to unrealistically low maintenance levels. At a high feeding level, horses will store energy in adipose tissue, which requires different metabolic pathways than exercise would. Potter et al (1990) showed that horses fed on a fat-rich diet had a lower DE requirement for maintenance of constant bodyweight than horses fed on a control diet. Horses when exercised at two body conditions/weights had 30% greater amount of DE requirements to maintain a 8% higher bodyweight (Webb et al 1992) when fed on a very high sugar and starch diet (forage only 0.75% of BW).	ALL

Table 5-10 *Continued*

±	Discussion points for scientists	UNIT
Requirement and metabolism Minus Minus Minus/Plus Plus	Most feeding trials use mixed feed rations and in digestibility trials linking in vivo body weight maintenance to a feed value becomes a "self-fulfilling" prophecy – a circular calculation – and at the DE level takes least account of metabolic processes according to feed substrate availability. Factors such as diet composition (concentrate:forage ratio), type of feed, daily intake, meal volume and time of feeding in relation to exercise all can affect requirements in working horses. This is because the availability of one substrate affects the utilization of another. For example, due to a high glucose intake before exercise and consequent rising insulin, glucose uptake in the muscle is increased at the start of exercise, and peripheral glucose availability will be reduced (Febbraio et al 2000). Simultaneously increases in plasma insulin reduce lipolysis and fat availability, leading to utilization of muscle glycogen, reducing performance if exercise is sustained. Therefore, apart from type/composition of feed (e.g., addition of oil or replacement of carbohydrates with oil; effect of pre-treatment/processing on starch availability), the time of feeding for specific exercise (intensity and duration) can be vital for optimal substrate availability. At the ME level a little more differentiation is possible between feed and at NE level the *k*-factor allows for an estimate of metabolic efficiency according to feedstuff and substrates absorbed (see below).	ALL DE ME NE
Feed Factors Minus	Feed type and volume affect *in vivo* results even when horses are at similar body condition and fitness levels. The studies at ME level by Vermorel et al (1997a,b) which are the basis for both the French NE and the American DE system (NRC, 2007), highlight the differences in requirements due to changes in diet (Fig. 5.9). Note in particular the reduced daily ME requirement when feeding better quality hay with barley pellets (diet 5) versus the late cut poor quality hay (diet 1).	DE ME

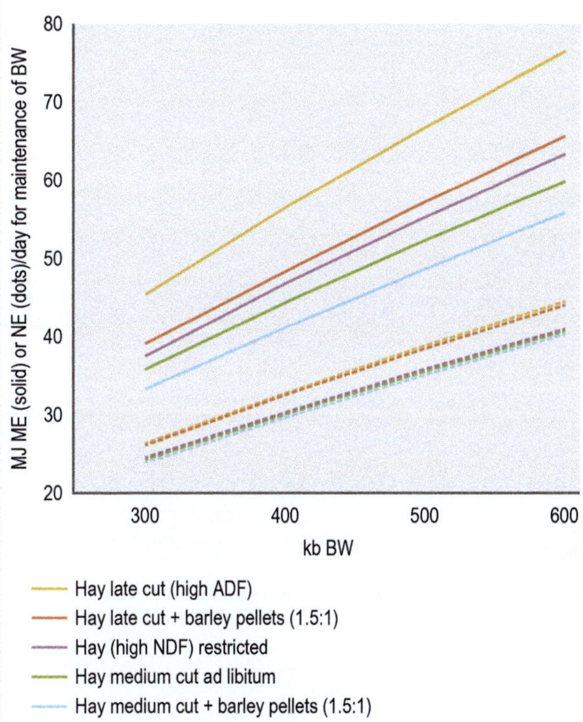

Figure 5.9 Solid lines: In vivo ME requirements of horses to maintain bodyweight (BW) (Original study: riding horses mean BW 475 kg; extrapolated according to MJ/kg $BW^{0.75}$). Dotted lines: Estimated NE requirements after conversion of ME to NE using *k*-factors derived according to chemical composition of feed (according to formula from CVB, 1996 described in Table 5-2 resulting in using the following conversion to NE = Late cut hay – 0.60*ME; Medium hay – 0.66*ME; Barley – 0.79*ME).
Adapted from Vermorel et al 1997a,b.

Table 5-10 *Continued*

±	Discussion points for scientists	UNIT
Feed factors Plus	When converting the in vivo results in the study illustrated in Fig. 5.9 to NE requirements (= dotted lines in Fig. 5.8), the large differences between the different feeds are significantly reduced. Such a conversion takes into account any differences in energy cost of chewing (Vernet et al 1995), digestibility and site of absorption and is the closest we can come to verifying NE of feed in vivo. The conversion from ME to NE, however, will always remain an educated estimate (estimated end products of digestion), based on in vitro work, evaluating energy metabolism at cellular level. The formula applied in the conversion used in Fig. 5.8 is based on the French estimations (of potential glucose, FA, AAs, VFAs absorbed) but has been adapted in the Dutch system in order to correlate with CP, CF and starches & sugars (which was tested though 19 in vivo ME trials : $r^2 = 0.96$; CVB 1996). In the Dutch system an additional k value for cereal byproducts, fats (animal or plant) and for sugar alone has been added, highlighting the scope for increasing the accuracy of determining the energy value of feed at the (p) NE level.	(p)NE
Feed composition Minus	However, the digestibility of a total ration is not equivalent to the weighted sum of individual components (due to associative effects, such as changes in: water holding properties, passage rates, bacterial population). Therefore when conducting *in vivo* studies with mixed diets, which maintain bodyweight balance, the allocation of energy provided by the individual feed becomes flawed for all systems. For example, Palmgren-Karlsson et al (2000) investigated the effect of oat inclusion rates of 0, 0.2, 0.4 and 0.6 to a hay diet, while feeding an isoenergetic diet (according to NRC 1989 DE). Results highlight the associative effect of feed components due to changes in passage rates, site of absorption and hindgut environment (Fig. 5.10). 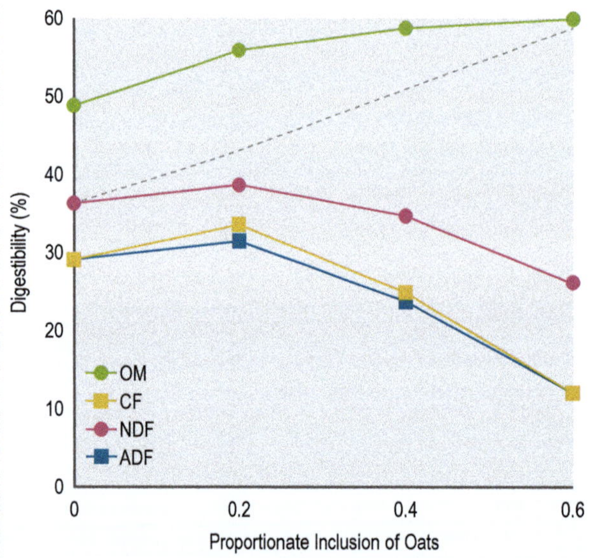 Figure 5.10 **Total ration nutrient digestibility (d) in horses fed different ratios of grass hay and whole oats.** The predicted total ration NDFd, assuming that predicted digestiblity in oats remains the same (i.e. no associate effect from oat inclusion) is shown by the dotted line. However, as oat inclusion increases fibre digestibility values decrease. OM – organic matter; CF – crude fiber; NDF – neutral detergent fiber; ADF – acid detergent fiber.) *Source: Ellis 2002a; adapted from Palmkren Karlsson et al 2000*	ALL

Table 5-10 *Continued*

±	Discussion points for scientists	UNIT
Chemical analysis Plus Plus	Fig. 5.10 also highlights the differences between assessing fiber fractions. When estimating the energy value of a feed according to chemical composition – the choice of indicators and chemical analysis methods play an important role. The NRC (2007) DE system distinguishes better between forages by using Van Soest's analysis (NDF, ADF but not ADL) than the German system which still focusses on CF from the Weende Analysis. The final regression formula used in the French system to calculate UFC includes the additional component : ADL (lignin) and more importantly includes a factor which takes into account the starch and sugar content of the feed (measured), whereas the NRC system refers to the calculated NFC (nonfibrous carbohydrates) value in its feed tables. In terms of affecting efficiency of the energy derived from a feed, lignin will be one of the most limiting factors, whereas knowledge of starches and sugars will allow for more accurate prediction of glucose absorbed. Both components play a key role in trying to predict interactions between feedstuffs. The latest recommendations of maximum starch levels in one meal (1 g/kg BW) in order to prevent an overspill into the hindgut are an applied example of this understanding (Julliand et al 2001, 2008).	DE (NRC) (p)NE
Requirement exercise Plus Minus	Measuring energy requirements in vivo during exercise by indirect energy expenditure (CO_2 out/O_2 in = respiratory exchange ratio (RER) at maintenance and respiratory quotient (RQ) during work) provides an indication of apparent net energy utilization by linking the CO_2/O_2 to the amount of ATP catabolized. The initial premise for this relationship at maintenance has been re-evaluated and described across species by Rolfe and Brown (1997) who concluded that 72% of mammalian oxygen consumption at base metabolism is linked to mitochondrial ATP synthesis. This, however, includes heat energy from maintenance and heat from O_2 utilization during metabolization of feed nutrients (ME). All systems are currently based on a measure of the NE required whether it be through O_2 consumption, RER ratio or more recently by HR linked to O_2 consumption (Fig. 5.11; Coenen, 2008). Coenen (2005) used data from 87 publications to evaluate the relationship between O_2 consumption and maximum volume of O_2 consumption (VO_{2max}). The effect of exercise and animal status (fitness level) on this base metabolism is less well established. In addition, there will once again be an associative effect and interaction between animal–diet–environment that will affect HR and VO_{2max}. In particular, in relation to estimating energy provision through anaerobic pathways limited data exists at this point. Coenen (2008) summarized from these that anaerobic energy expenditure can be measured as 1.03–1.8 J/s for each mmol of lactate produced (measured in average Lac/min). Currently estimating energy requirements for exercise in relation to VO_{2max} and/or RQ and subsequent correlations with HR (which if measured in vivo will take account of bodyweight, some account of fitness level and thus some account of metabolic rate) is the most accurate method to predict energy expenditure. More work in this area will help to clarify the effect of variations in exercise, animal status and of feed substrate supply for ATP production.	ALL

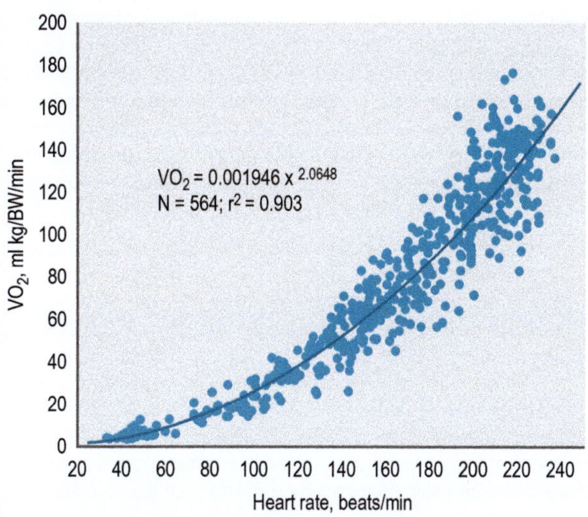

Figure 5.11 Oxygen consumption in dependence on heart rate.
Source: Coenen 2008.

Table 5-10 *Continued*

±	Discussion points for scientists	UNIT
Feed supply (ATP) and requirements Plus	Energy requirements as determined by in vivo trials using (p)NE feed energy go somewhat closer towards partitioning between substrate absorption according to diet composition. This is because they estimate the glucose, FA, AAs, VFAs absorbed for potential ATP production based on feed chemistry (site of digestion) and some cross species in vivo & in vitro studies. In the French system, glucose and lactate energy has been set at an average conversion of 85% net availability from glucose contents and an added 5% from cytoplasmic nitrogen free extract (cell wall carbohydrates digested enzymatically) for hays and dried grass, 8% for fresh grass, 10% for lucerne and 15% for concentrate feed. Energy derived from free fatty acids and amino acid supply has also been estimated, by applying current knowledge from *in vivo* research (Vermorel & Martin-Rosset 1997). An important aspect affecting the net energy derived from feed is the amount and composition of VFAs produced. Amount of VFAs was predicted by applying previous research results and linking them to digestibility of OM as shown below: VFA produced (g/kg DM feed) = (%DOM − %OM digested in SI) × 0.92 (DOM = digestible organic matter; SI = small intestine). Organic matter (OM) digested in the small intestine is based on a limited number of *in vivo* studies with horses which have an ileal or cecal canula inserted, and on extrapolation from measuring energy substrates in blood as well as knowledge of passage rates and other species. It remains a crude estimate but nevertheless allows for some basic distinction between feedstuffs. Knowledge in this area has increased considerably in the last few years (de Fombelle et al 2003, Julliand et al 2006, Vervuert et al 2004, 2007, 2009).	pNE
Requirement exercise Minus	Back conversion to estimated ME and then DE requirements from the NE requirements linked to net energy expenditure is currently difficult and based on indirect knowledge and estimation of energy efficiency (in turn often back linked to BW maintenance – so a "circular" reference). This has not been systematically explored possibly because in the animal "ME or DE" as a unit does not exist. The conversion factors often have been matched to DE or ME values derived from body weight maintenance trials and were not necessarily derived from within the same studies (Pagan & Hintz 1986: DE = NE/0.57) or to a limited number of BW balance trials of horses in work (Rose et al 1991, Anderson et al 1983, Hintz et al 1971). In a recent study Pagan et al (2005) attempted to link the NE measured through oxygen consumption to DE measured within the same trial and found a much lower efficiency of use of DE with a conversion of 28% efficiency for work (DE = NE/0.28). The implications of this highlight the weakness of attempting to convert requirements or "utilization" back to an abstract DE requirement value to match the very "measurable" and real DE value of feed.	DE ME
Requirement Minus	Challenges are added by the partitioning between efficiency of use of maintenance NE versus efficiency of use of work NE – adjustments to maintenance requirements in working horses are used in many systems to account for this. When it comes to using any energy value for horses above maintenance the biggest limiting factor is the attempt to partition maintenance from production energy both at a feed evaluation and at requirement level as the "line" between these is constantly shifting due to various factors (as illustrated in the gray boxes, Fig. 5.2) and this shift is nearly impossible to measure *in vivo* in horses. This applies to all levels (DE, ME and NE). All systems try to add work, growth and production requirements to maintenance requirements factorially. Perhaps the development of systems which do not build/add up maintenance and work but give total requirements according to status (body condition/fitness level and work level) is one way forward. On the other side of the "scales" it is perhaps just as difficult to accurately predict energy derived from concentrate feed when fed at various different combinations with roughage. Herein may lay a target for future research.	ALL
Requirement growth and lactation Plus Feed values and requirement growth and lactation Minus	Net energy as a result of "product" output – i.e. net weight gain (further subdivided by muscle, fat, bone tissue) or liters of milk produced can be applied directly in order to link with energy requirements as determined at any level (NE/DE, etc.). Hence, all systems use a basic maintenance level based on bodyweight (above discussion of advantages/disadvantages applies) and add additional requirement recommendations based on regression calculations from average daily weight gain (growth curves) in growing horses or body weight maintenance in lactating mares. Furthermore fetal growth data are applied for pregnant mares (Meyer & Ahlswende 1976). Although a direct net energy conversion of these "products" is most accurate, correlation to DE or ME requirements have been partially validated by a number of digestibility trials (see Table 5-5).	ALL

Table 5-10 *Continued*

±	Discussion points for scientists	UNIT
	Limitations across the board of all systems include the various animal factors as well as feed/environmental factors which may affect efficiency of energy conversion/utilization from feed and include: body composition, gender, breed differences, parity, feed sources and nutrient supply (especially amino acids), milk composition, suckling frequency (foal appetite), social interactions, weaning effects, season and temperature, age, % of adult BW reached at certain age (breed differences, speed of growth – given an exponential of growth curve, average daily gain) and exercise (housing). Current systems differ considerably in their incorporation of these factors into their calculations which could be the basis of an in depth discussion of the advantages or disadvantages of each system. However, these differences are not necessarily due to the energy scheme used (Martin-Rosset & Ellis 2005). Once again the debate over the distinction of maintenance requirements versus "production" should be highlighted here. In general, there is an assumption that the basal metabolic rate in relation to bodyweight for maintenance is higher in growing foals (Ott 2005). This assumption is reflected in the higher maintenance energy values for foals as seen in Table 5-5.	

Therefore, the practical application of this seemingly theoretical science is to devise feeding schedules for horses that meet their requirements while keeping them both healthy (in body and mind) as well as optimizing their performance.

References

Anderson, C.E., Potter, G.D., Kreider, J.L., et al., 1983. Digestible energy requirements for exercising horses. Journal of Animal Science 56, 91.

Argenzio, R.A., Hintz, H.F., 1971. Energy utilization in the horse. In: Cornell Nutrition Conference for Feed Manufacturers Proceedings. Cornell University, pp. 86–92.

Armsby, H.P., 1903. The principles of animal nutrition. Chapman & Hall, London.

Austbo, D., 1996. Energy and protein evaluation systems and nutrient recommendations for horses in.

Austbo, D., 2004. The Scandinavian adaptation of the French UFC system. In: Julliand, V., Martin Rosset, W. (Eds.), 2004, Nutrition of the Performance Horse. EAAP Publication No 111, Wageningen Academic Press, Wageningen, p. 69.

Barth, K.M., Williams, J.W., Brown, D.G., 1977. Digestible energy requirements of working and non-working ponies. Journal of Animal Science 44, 585–589.

Benedict, F.G., 1938. Vital energetics: a study on comparative basal metabolism. CanegieInst, Washington, pp. 503, 175–176. In: INRA 1984 Jarrige, R. Martin-Rosset, W. (Eds.), Le Cheval, Reproduction, Selection, Alimentation, exploitation, Institut National de la Recherche Argronomique, Paris.

Coenen, M., 2005. About the predictability of oxygen consumption and energy expenditure in the exercising horse, Proc 19th Meeting, Equine Science Society, Tuscon, AZ, pp123 adapted in: NRC 2007 Nutrient Requirements of Horses, sixth ed revised. National Academy Press, Washington DC.

Coenen, M., 2008. The suitability of heart rate in the prediction of oxygen consumption, energy expenditure and energy requirement for the exercising horses. In: Saastamoinen, M.T., Martin-Rosset, W. (Eds.), Nutrition of the exercising horse. EAAP Publication 125, Wageningen Academic Publishers, Wageningen, pp. 147–162.

Coenen, M., Kirchhof, S., Kienzle, E., et al., 2010a. A revision of the energy and nutrient requirements of mares: II Lactation. In: Ellis, A.D., Longland, A.C., Coenen, M. et al. (Eds.), (2010) The impact of nutrition on the health and welfare of horses. EAAP Publication No. 128, Wageningen Academic Publishers, Wageningen.

Coenen, M., Schmidt, St, Zeyner, A., et al., 2010b. A revision of the energy and nutrient requirements of mares: I. Gestation. In: Ellis, A.D., Longland, A.C., Coenen, M., et al. (Eds.), (2010) The impact of nutrition on the health and welfare of horses. EAAP Publication No. 128, Wageningen Academic Publishers, Wageningen.

CVB, 1996. Documentatierapport nr 15, Het definitieve VEP- en VREp-systeem the definitive Dutch Equine Energy and Protein System. CentraalVeevoederbureau, Lelystad.

CVB, 2005. The new energy-system for horses. Energie Waarde vor paarden, Centraal Veevoeder-Bureau, Lelystad, Netherlands.

Cymbaluk, N.F., Christison, G.I., Leach, D.H., 1990. Longitudinal growth analysis of horses following limited and ad libitum feeding. Equine Veterinary Journal 22, 198–204.

de Fombelle, A., Varloud, M., Goachet, A.G., et al., 2003. Characterization of the microbial and biochemical profile of the different segments of the digestive tract in horses given two distinct diets. Animal Science 77, 293–304.

DLG, 1994. Empfehlungen zur Energie und Nahrstoffversorgung der Pferde, Gesellschaft der Ernahrungsphysiologie der Haustiere. DLG Verlag, Frankfurt.

DLG, 2011. in preparation. M Coenen personal communication.

Doreau, M., Boulot, S., 1989. Recent Knowledge on Mare Milk Production. Livestock Production Science 22, 213–235.

Doreau, M., Martin-Rosset, W., Boulot, S., 1988. Energy requirements and the feeding of mares during lactation: a review. Livestock Production Science 20, 53–68.

Doreau, M., Boulot, S., Bauchart, D., et al., 1992. Voluntary intake, milk production and plasma metabolites in nursing mares fed two different diets. Journal of Nutrition 122, 992.

Doreau, M., Boulot, S., Chilliard, Y., 1993. Yield and composition of milk from lactating mares: effect of body condition at foaling. Journal of Dairy Research 60 (4), 457–466.

Ellis, A.D., 2002a. Energy assessment and standards in horses; Report 60 pages; Vpa-02-02-09. Research Institute for Applied Animal Husbandry, Animal Sciences Group, WUR, Lelystad, NL.

Ellis, A.D., 2002b. Energy sources and requirements for work, Internal report VPA-02-03. PraktijkonderzoekVeehouderij, Lelystad.

Ellis, A.D., 2008. Practical assessment of work levels in equines. In: Saastamoinen, M T., Martin-Rosset, W. (Eds.), Nutrition of the exercising horse. EAAP Publication 125, Wageningen Academic Publishers, Wageneingen, pp. 147–162.

Febbraio, M.A., Chiu, A., Angus, D.J., et al., 2000. Effects of carbohydrate ingestion before and during exercise on glucose kinetics and performance. Journal of Applied Physiology 89, 2220–2226.

GEH, 1994. Empfehlungen zur Energie und Nahrstoffversorgung der Pferde, Gesellschaft der Ernahrungsphysiologie der Haustiere, (Recommendation for energy and nutrient requirements of horses). DLG Verlag, Frankfurt.

Guissani, D.A., Forehead, A.J., Fowden, A.L., 2005. Development of cardiovascular function in the horse fetus. Journal of Physiology 565, 1019–1030.

Harris, P., 1997. Energy sources and requirements of the exercising horse. Annual Review of Nutrition 17, 185–210.

Hintz, H.F., Roberts, S.J., Sabin, S.W., 1971. Energy requirements of light horses for various activities. Journal of Animal Science 32, 100.

Hoffman, R. M., Kronfeld, D. S., Herblein, W.W., et al., 1998. Dietary carbohydrates and fat influence milk composition and fatty acid profile of mare's milk. Journal of Nutrition 18, 2708–2771S.

Hoffmann, L., Schiemann, W., Klippel, R., 1967. Untersuchungen über den Energieumsatz beim Pferd unter besonderer Berücksichtigung der horizontal Bewegung. Archiv Tierernährung 17, 441–449.

INRA, 1984. Le Cheval, Reproduction, Selection, Alimentation, Exploitation. In: Jarrige, R., Martin-Rosset, W. (Eds.), Institut National de la Recherche Agronomique, Paris.

INRA, 1990. In: Martin-Rosset, W. (Ed.), L'alimentation des chevaux. Institut National de la Recherche Agronomique, Paris.

Jansson, A., 2004. Utfodringsrekommendationer for hast (Feeding recommendations for horses). Sveriges Landbruksuniversitet SLU (Swedish Agricultural University, Sweden).

Julliand, V., de Fombelle, A., Drogoul, C., et al., 2001. Feeding and microbial disorders in horses: 3. Effects of three hay:grain rations on microbial profiles and activities. Journal of Equine Veterinary Science 21, 543–546.

Julliand, V., de Fombelle, A., Varloud, M., 2006. Starch digestion in horses: The impact of feed processing. Livestock Science 100, 44–52.

Julliand, V., Martin-Rosset, W., 2004. Nutrition of the performance horse. EAAP Publication No 111, Wageningen Academic Press, Wageningen, p. 69.

Julliand, V., Philippeau, C., Goachet, A.G., et al., 2008. Physiology of intake and digestion in equine animals. In: Miraglia, N., Martin-Rosset, W. (Eds.), Nutrition and feeding of the broodmare. EAAP Publication no. 120, Wageningen Academic Publishers, Wageningen, pp. 341–366.

Kienzle, E., Zeyner, A., 2010. Metabolizable energy for horses: development of a simple and flexible feed evaluation system. In: Ellis, A., Longland, A.C., Coenen, M., et al. (Eds.), The impact of nutrition on the health and welfare of horses. Metabolizable energy for horses: development of a simple and flexible feed evaluation system, Wageningen Academic Publishers, Wageningen, pp. 37–39.

Kienzle, E., Bertold, L., Zeyner, A., 2009. Effects of hay versus concentrate on urinary energy excretion in horses. Proceedings of Society of Nutrition and Physiology 18, 118.

Kienzle, E., Coenen, M., Zeyner, A., 2010. Der Erhaltungsbedarf von Pferden an umseztbaref Energie (Metabolisable Energy requirements for Maintenance) Übersicht. Tierernährung 38 (2010), 33–54.

Knox, K.L., Crownover, J.C., Wooden, G.R., 1970. Maintenance energy requirements for mature idle horse. In: Schurch, A., Wenk, C. (Eds.), Proceedings of the 7th Equine Nutrition and Physiology Symposium, Warenton, VA, pp. 186–19.

Martin, R.G., McMeniman, N.P., Dowsett, K.F., 1992. Milk and water intakes of foals sucking grazing mares. Equine Veterinary Journal 24, 295–299.

Martin-Rosset, W. (Ed.), 1990. L'alimentation des chevaux. Institut National de la Recherche Agronomique, Paris.

Martin-Rosset, W., 2008. Energy requirements and allowances of exercising horses. In: Saastamoinen, M.T., Martin-Rosset, W. (Eds.), Nutrition of the exercising horse. EAAP Publication 125, Wageningen Academic Publishers, Wageningen, pp. 103–138.

Martin-Rosset, W., Ellis, A.D., 2005. Evaluation of energy and protein requirements and recommended allowances in growing horses. In: Julliand, V., Martin-Rosset, W. (Eds.), The Growing Horse: Nutrition and Prevention of Growth Disorders, Second European Workshop on Equine Nutrition. ENESAD, Dijon, France, EAAP Publication No 114, Wageningen Academic Press, Wageningen, pp. 103–136.

Martin-Rosset, W., Vermorel, M., 1991. Maintenance energy requirements determined by indirect calorimetry and feeding trials in light horses. Equine Veterinary Science 11, 42–45.

Martin-Rosset, W., Austbo, D., Coenen, M., 2006b. Energy and protein requirements and recommended allowances in lactating mares. In: Miraglia, N., Martin-Rosset, W. (Eds.), Nutrition and feeding of the broodmare. EAAP Publication no. 120, Wageningen Academic Publishers, Wageningen, pp. 341–366.

Meixner, R., Hornicke, H., Ehrlein, H. J., 1981. Oxygen consumption, pulmonary ventilation and heart rate of riding horses during walk, trot and gallop. Biotelemetry 6.

Martin-Rosset, W., Vervuert, I., Austbo, D., 2006a. Energy and protein requirements and recommended allowances in pregnant mares. In: Miraglia, N., Martin-Rosset, W. (Eds.), Nutrition and feeding of the broodmare. EAAP Publication no. 120, Wageningen Academic Publishers, Wageningen, pp. 341–366.

Meyer, H., Ahlswende, L., 1976. Über das intrauterine Wachstum und die Korpuzusammenketzung von Fohlen sowie den Nahrstoffbedarf tragender. Stuten (On the intrauterine growth and bodycomposition of foals and nutrient requirements of mares) Übers Tiernarung 4, 263.

Naylor, J., 2009. Practical and controversial news on racehorse training. In: Lindner, A. (Ed.), 2009 Applied equine nutrition and training, Wageningen Academic Publishers. Wageningen, pp. 81–106.

NRC, 1989. Nutrient Requirements of Horses, fifth ed revised. National Academy of Sciences, Washington DC.

NRC, 2007. Nutrient Requirements of Horses, sixth ed revised. National Academy Press, Washington DC.

Ott, E.A., 2005. Energy and protein metabolism of normal growth. In: Julliand, V., Martin-Rosset, W. (Eds.), The Growing Horse: Nutrition and Prevention of Growth Disorders, Second European Workshop on Equine Nutrition. ENESAD, Dijon, France, EAAP Publication No 114, Wageningen Academic Press, Wageningen, pp. 91–102.

Ousey, J.C., Prandi, S., Zimmer, J., et al., 1997. Effects of various feeding regimens on the energy balance of equine neonates. American Journal of Veterinary Research 58, 1243.

Pagan, J.D., Cowley, G., Nash, D., et al., 2005. The efficiency of utilization of digestible energy during submaximal exercise. Proceedings of the 19th Equine Sci Symposium, Tuscon, Arizona, pp. 199–204.

Pagan, J.D., Hintz, H.F., 1986. Composition of milk from pony mares fed various levels of digestible energy. Cornell Vet 76, 139.

Palmgren-Karlsson, C.P., Lindberg, J.E., Rundgren, M., 2000. Associative effects on total tract digestibility in horses fed different ratios of grass hay and whole oats. Livestock Production Science 65, 143–153.

Potter, G.D., Webb SP Evans, J.W., Webb, G.W., 1990. Digestible energy requirements for work and maintenance of horses fed conventional and fat-supplemented diets. Journal of Equine Veterinary Science 10, 214–218.

Rolfe, F.F.S., Brown, G.C., 1997. Cellular energy utilization and molecular origin of standard metabolic rate in mammals. Physiology Review 77, 731–758.

Rose, R.J., Knight, P.K., Bryden, W.L., 1991. Energy use and cardiorespiratory responses to prolonged submaximal exercise. In: Persson, S.G.B., Lindholm, A., Jeffcott, L.B. (Eds.), Equine Exercise Physiology 3. ICEEP Publications, Davis, CA, p. 281.

Santos, A.S., Sousa, B.C., Leitao, L.C., et al., 2005. Yield and composition of milk from Lusitano lactating mares. Pferdeheilkunde 21 (Supplement), 115–116.

Schmidt, B., Coenen, M., 2010. Milk intake and foal growth - a review of literature. In: Ellis, A.D., Longland, A.C., Coenen, M., et al. (Eds.), The impact of nutrition on the health and welfare of horses. EAAP Publication No. 128, Wageningen Academic Publishers, Wageningen.

Van Soest, P.J., 1994. Nutritional ecology of the ruminant. Cornell University Press, London.

Vermorel, M., Martin-Rosset, W., 1997. Concepts, scientific bases, structure and validation of the French horse net energy system. UFC Livestock Production Science 47, 261–275.

Vermorel, M., Martin-Rosset, W., Vernet, J., 1997a. Energy utilisation of twelve forages or mixed diets for maintenance by sport horses. Livestock Production Sciences 47, 157–167.

Vermorel, M., Vernet, J., Martin-Rosset, W., 1997b. Digestive and energy utilisation of two diets by ponies and horses. Livestock Production Science 51, 13–19.

Vernet, J., Vermorel, M., Martin-Rosset, W., 1995. Energy cost of eating long hay, straw and pelleted food in sport horses. Animal Science 61, 581–588.

Vervuert, I., Bothe, C., Coenen, M., 2007. Glycaemic and insulinaemic responses to mechanical and thermal processed barley in horses. Journal of Animal Physiology and Animal Nutrition 91 (5–6), 263–268.

Vervuert, I., Voigt, K., Hollands, T., et al., 2009. Effect of feeding increasing quantities of starch on glycaemic and insulinaemic responses in healthy horses. Veterinary Journal 182 (1), 67–72.

Vervuert, I., Coenen, M., Bichman, M., 2004. Comparison of the effect of fructose and glucose supplementation on metabolic responses in resting and exercising horses. Journal of Veterinary Medicine A51, 171–177.

Voit, E., 1901. Über die Grösse des Energiebedarfs der Tiere im Hungerzustande. Zeitschrift der Biologie 41, 113. In: INRA 1984 Jarrige, R., Martin-Rosset, W. (Eds.), Le Cheval, Reproduction, Selection, Alimentation, Exploitation, Institut National de la Recherche Argronomique, Paris.

Webb, S.P., Potter, G.D., Evans, J.W., et al., 1992. Influence of body fat content on digestible energy requirements of exercising horses in temperate and hot environments. Equine Veterinary Science 10, 116–120.

Wooden, G. R., Knox, K., Wild, C.L., 1970. Energy metabolism of light horses. Journal of Animal Science 30, 544–548.

Zuntz, N., Hagemann, O., 1898. Untersuchungen über den Stoffwechsel des Pferdes bei Ruhe und Arbeit. Land Jahrb 27 (supp 3). In: INRA 1984 Jarrige, R., Martin-Rosset, W. (Eds.), Le Cheval, Reproduction, Selection, Alimentation, Exploitation, Instituut National de Agronomique, France.

6

Amino acids and protein

Kristine L. Urschel, Laurie M. Lawrence

Introduction

The word protein was derived from the Greek word *proteos*, meaning "of primary importance," and as such protein is a key nutrient that must be provided in the diets of horses of all ages. Protein is an organic macromolecule made up of chains of individual amino acids which are linked together by peptide bonds, and when protein is consumed in the diet, these bonds are broken down and individual amino acids can be absorbed for use in protein synthesis and metabolism. This chapter describes the structure and functions of protein and amino acids in the horse, and the mechanisms associated with amino acid digestion and absorption. Subsequent discussion focuses on the dietary sources of protein and amino acids, including the ever increasing number of commercially available amino acid supplements. Finally, protein and amino acid requirements are explained from a historical standpoint and in the context of horse's physiological state, the methods that can be used to assess requirements and dietary adequacy are explored, and the implications of both excess and deficient levels of intake are discussed. Areas where additional research is warranted are identified throughout the chapter.

Basic properties of proteins and amino acids

Chemical structure and classification

The general structure common to all amino acids is shown in Fig. 6.1. Each amino acid consists of an α-carbon that is attached to an amino group, a carboxylic acid group and a side chain group, which is unique to each amino acid. There are 21 different amino acids that are a part of mammalian proteins (Fig. 6.2), and these amino acids can be classified based on the chemical properties of the side chain group and on the basis of dietary essentiality.

A common method of classifying amino acids is based on whether or not the animal requires a preformed dietary source of the amino acid or whether the amino acid can be made through the animal's own metabolic processes in quantities sufficient enough to meet metabolic needs. Unlike bacteria, which have the metabolic pathways to synthesize all of the amino acids de novo, mammals only have the enzymatic ability to synthesize some amino acids. Amino acids that must be provided in the diet, because metabolic pathways for their synthesis do not exist or are insufficient to meet demands, are referred to as *indispensable* (essential) *amino acids*, and amino acids that the animal can make through its own metabolic pathways are termed *dispensable* (non-essential) *amino acids*. This classification system leaves a gray area for the amino acids where metabolic pathways are present, but under certain circumstances are unable to make sufficient quantities of the amino acids to meet metabolic requirements. These amino acids are termed *conditionally indispensable amino acids*. In mammals, there are nine amino acids that are classified as strictly indispensable amino acids: histidine, isoleucine, leucine, lysine, methionine, phenylalanine, threonine, tryptophan, and valine. Arginine is often included in this list because in many growing mammals the rate of its synthesis is insufficient to meet the animal's demands; however, with the exception of obligate carnivores, arginine appears to be made in adequate quantities in mature, healthy mammals, making a dietary source of this amino acid unnecessary (reviewed by Ball et al 2007). Arginine may also become an indispensable amino acid during illness or injury because of the roles that it plays in the immune system function and in the disposal of the excess nitrogenous wastes that are typical of a catabolic state. Other conditionally indispensable amino acids include: tyrosine, which can be synthesized from phenylalanine if sufficient phenylalanine is provided in the diet; cysteine, which can be synthesized from dietary methionine; glycine and proline, which may not be synthesized in sufficient quantities during growth; and glutamine which becomes essential in times of illness or physiological stress. The amino acids widely accepted as being dispensable among mammals are alanine, asparagine, aspartate, glutamate, and serine. Selenocysteine, a relatively "new" amino

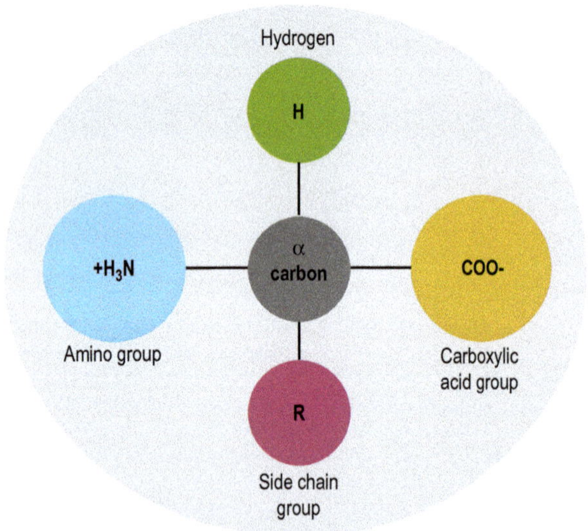

Figure 6.1 Basic structure of all α-amino acids.

acid discovery and a critical component in selenoproteins such as glutathione peroxidase, has not been officially classified on the basis of its dietary essentiality. However, because selenocysteine does not readily exist as a free amino acid and its synthesis occurs directly onto the tRNA molecule (Allmang et al 2009), this amino acid appears to be dispensable so long as adequate selenium is available.

Protein synthesis involves the transcription of the cell's genetic material, DNA, into RNA which is then translated into protein. During translation, the amino acids that are attached to the tRNA interact with the mRNA and adjacent amino acids are covalently joined together by peptide bonds (Fig. 6.3). These covalent peptide bonds are strong and once formed they can only be broken by enzymatic activity or by a combination of low pH and high heat. The amino acid sequence of each protein is unique and determines the three-dimensional structure and the specific function of the protein. For this reason, even a one amino acid substitution in a protein, can have major implications on the structure and subsequently the function of the protein.

Physiological roles of protein and amino acids in the body

Protein makes up ~15% of total body mass, with the muscle containing the largest portion of the body's protein. Some of the key functions of body proteins include providing structure (i.e., contractile proteins actin and myosin in the muscle, collagen, keratin), nutrient transport in the blood stream (i.e., hemoglobin, albumin), nutrient transport across cell membranes, regulation of metabolic function (i.e., enzymes, peptide hormones), as a component of the immune system (i.e., immunoglobins), and as a buffer to minimize fluctuations in body pH.

There are also several nitrogen-containing compounds that are synthesized from amino acids, but because they are formed through enzymatic reactions rather than through RNA transcription, they cannot be classified as proteins. These nitrogen-containing compounds have a variety of physiological functions. *Glutathione* (cysteine, glycine and glutamine) is an antioxidant that interacts with free-radicals and protects cells from oxidative damage. *Creatine* (arginine, glycine, and methionine) is involved in cellular energy metabolism, because when phosphorylated it can be used for the rapid generation of ATP. *Carnitine* (lysine, methionine) is necessary for the transport of fatty acids across the inner mitochondrial membrane for oxidation and ATP production. *Carnosine* (histidine and β-alanine) is present in very high concentrations in equine skeletal muscle fast twitch fibers (Sewell et al 1992), where it aids in buffering the lactic acid produced during glycolysis. The synthesis of the purine and pyrimidine bases, the molecular constituents of DNA and RNA, requires the nitrogen and/or carbon atoms from several amino acids: glutamine (purines/pyrimidines), aspartate (purines/pyrimidines), and glycine (purines).

Individual amino acids may also have important functions, independent of their role as a component of body protein. Arginine is a critical component of the urea cycle (necessary for nitrogen metabolism and excretion) and a precursor for nitric oxide (a potent vasodilator and involved in the immune response). Glycine is necessary for the synthesis of porphyrin, the oxygen-binding component of the hemoglobin molecule. Certain amino acids may be used extensively as a substrate for ATP production, such as the branched chain amino acids (BCAA; leucine, isoleucine, and valine) in the skeletal muscle, and glutamine in the gastrointestinal tract and immune cells. Alanine is formed in large amounts in skeletal muscle during exercise via the transamination of pyruvate, formed during glycolysis, with an α-keto acid, often one derived from muscle BCAA metabolism. In the liver, this alanine can then be converted back to glucose through the gluconeogenic pathway and is once again available to the muscle for use as a fuel. This cycling of alanine and glucose between the skeletal muscle and liver is known as the alanine cycle. There are several neurotransmitters and hormones that are derived from the amino acids serine (acetylcholine), tryptophan (serotonin) and tyrosine (epinephrine, norepinephrine, thyroid hormones, and melanin).

Considering all of the critical roles of proteins and amino acids in the horse, it is important to ensure that adequate amounts of protein and amino acids are provided in the diet. In order to provide dietary adequate protein and amino acids, it is necessary to have a thorough understanding of how protein is digested and absorbed, the different dietary sources of protein available to the horse, the protein and amino acid requirements for horses of various ages and physiological states, and how to assess whether or not appropriate levels of protein and amino acids are being fed.

Key Points

- Amino acids can be classified based on their chemical properties and on whether or not a dietary source must be provided
- Important functions of protein in the body include structural, enzymatic and hormonal roles, transport of nutrients across membranes and in the blood, and as a component of the immune system
- In addition to being a component of protein, certain amino acids have additional physiological roles

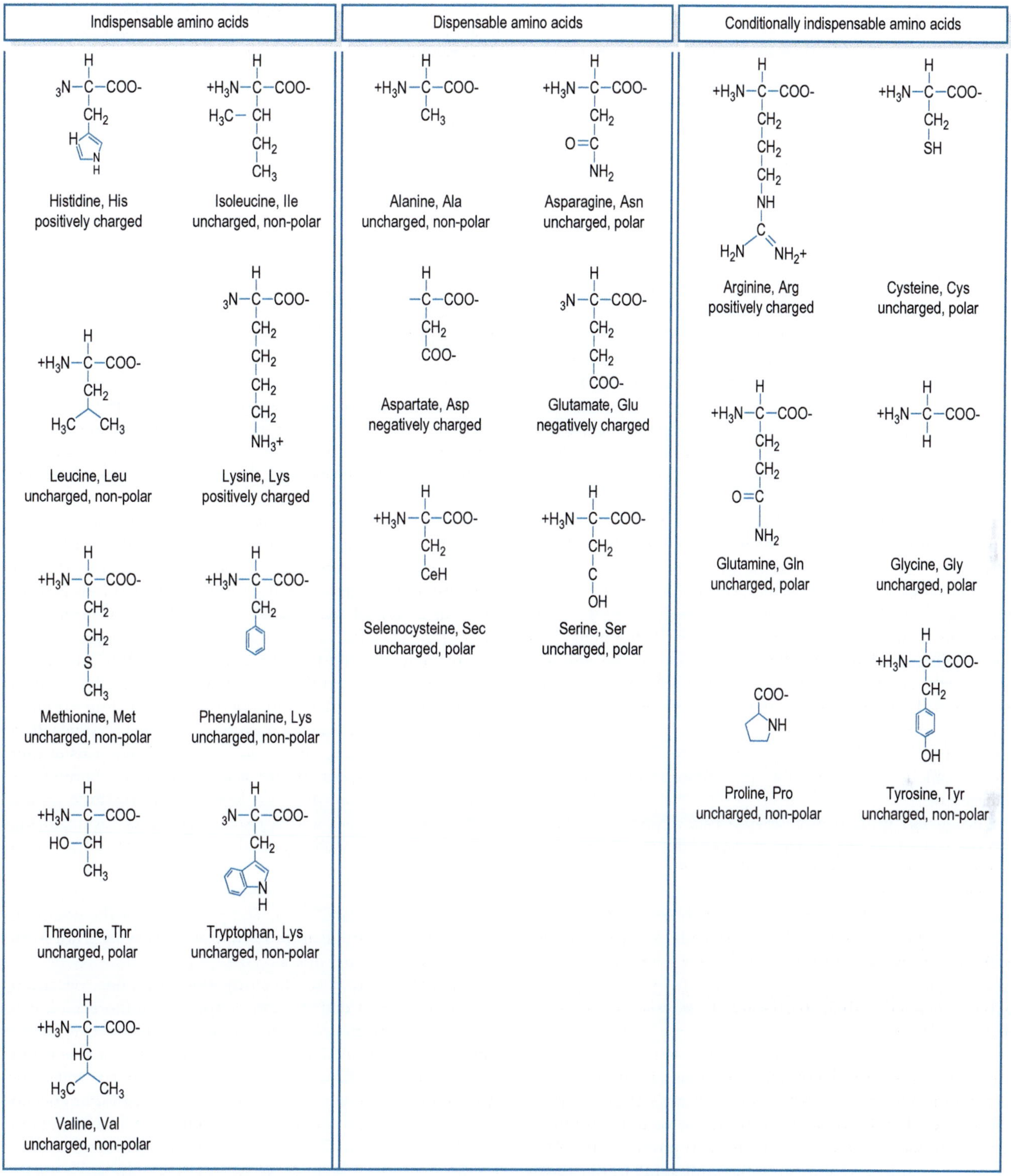

Figure 6.2 Structure and classification of the α-amino acids found in mammalian proteins. Although histidine is not shown with the additional proton and positive charge in this figure, the second nitrogen group is able to bind with hydrogen when pH drops, and in this way histidine acts as a buffer. For this reason, histidine is classified as a positively charged amino acid.

Protein and amino acid digestion and absorption

General overview of protein digestion

In order to be absorbed from the gastrointestinal lumen, dietary proteins must first be digested into individual amino acids and small peptides. The prececal processes involved in protein digestion in horses are essentially the same as in other monogastric species such as humans and pigs. Briefly, protein digestion begins in the stomach, with the release of hydrochloric acid and the zymogen (inactive enzyme) pepsinogen from the parietal and chief cells, respectively. The hydrochloric acid unwinds the three-dimensional protein structure, making the individual

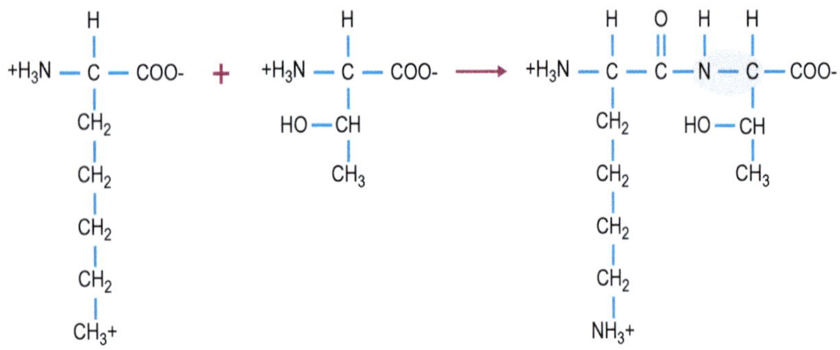

Figure 6.3 Peptide bond formation.

peptide bonds more assessable to the digestive enzymes. The hydrochloric acid also activates pepsinogen to pepsin, and the long peptide strands are cleaved into smaller chains. In the small intestine, the proteolytic enzymes secreted by the pancreas into the duodenum and the peptidases associated with the enterocyte brush border continue protein digestion. The pancreatic secretion contains several peptidase zymogens including trypsinogen, chymotrypsinogen, and procarboxypeptidases. Trypsinogen is activated to trypsin in the small intestinal lumen by enteropeptidase, secreted by duodenal enterocytes, and this trypsin activates the other pancreatic zymogens. The end products of pancreatic peptidase digestion are small oligopeptides, di- and tripeptide chains and free amino acids. The remainder of small intestinal protein digestion occurs at the enterocyte brush border membrane, by membrane-associated aminopeptidases and endopeptidases, primarily in the jejunum and ileum. The ultimate end products of the small intestinal protein digestion processes are the free amino acids, which are available for absorption into the enterocytes.

Undigested protein and unabsorbed amino acids pass into the large intestine, where, in other monogastrics, cecal peptidase activity is much lower than in the small intestinal segments (Bai 1993). There has been little research in horses about the microbial digestion of protein; however, microbial protein digestion in the rumen of cattle has been extensively studied and provides insight into the processes that may be occurring in the equine large intestine. In ruminants, proteases associated with the bacterial cell wall begin to degrade proteins into smaller peptide chains, which can then be absorbed by the bacteria, cleaved into individual amino acids and either used for microbial protein synthesis or further degraded to carbon skeletons and ammonia (Wallace 1996). In bacterial cells isolated from the cecal contents of horses, all species of bacteria could use partially digested protein as a nitrogen source, with smaller subsets of cecal bacteria also able to use ammonia and urea as sole nitrogen sources (Maczulak et al 1985). An important distinction must be made between the sites of microbial protein synthesis relative to the sites of protein digestion in ruminants versus monogastrics. In ruminants, the microbial protein is made proximal to the gastric and pancreatic secretions and therefore can be digested by the animal in a similar manner as dietary protein is digested in monogastrics. In horses, however, microbial protein synthesis occurs predominantly distal to the gastric and pancreatic secretions, and this has implications for both the digestion and absorption of these proteins.

Intestinal amino acid transport

In order to be absorbed from the intestinal lumen into the bloodstream, amino acids rely on specific transport proteins, often referred to as transport systems, to be transported across two sets of enterocyte plasma membranes: the apical (or luminal) membrane and the basolateral (serosal) membrane. In mammalian cells, many different amino acid transport systems have been identified and characterized on the basis of the chemical properties of the amino acids they transport, a requirement for metabolic energy, and whether they are sodium-dependent or independent (Broer 2008a). The expression of the various transport system proteins is membrane-specific, with some systems expressed on the apical membrane and others expressed on the basolateral membrane. Although the majority of the transport systems on the apical membrane transport amino acids into the enterocyte, the basolateral membrane has some systems that transport circulating amino acids into the enterocyte and others that transport amino acids out of the enterocyte. Glutamine, for example, is a key energy substrate in the gastrointestinal tract and is extensively taken up from the bloodstream by both jejunal and colonic enterocytes in horses (Duckworth et al 1992). There is also a well-characterized active transport system for di- and tri-peptides, PepT1 (Gilbert et al 2008a). The properties of the common mammalian intestinal amino acid transport system are summarized in Table 6-1 and Fig. 6.4.

Currently, only a single study exists that has measured the presence and distribution of specific amino acid transport systems in the equine intestine (Woodward et al 2009). This study examined the mRNA abundance of the genes corresponding to the apical membrane system $b^{0,+}$, the basolateral membrane system y^+ and for two genes that encode for the basolateral membrane system L. The $b^{0,+}$ system mRNA was similarly expressed in the jejunum, ileum, cecum and colon of mature horses, while the gene corresponding to the y^+ system was expressed to a greater extent in the small intestinal segments compared to the large intestinal segments (Woodward et al 2009). The mRNA abundance of the medium affinity L transport system was higher in the small intestine than in the large intestine; however, the abundance of mRNA corresponding to the lower affinity L system was higher in the cecum than in the jejunum (Woodward et al 2009). These findings provide a potential mechanism whereby amino acids synthesized by the large intestinal microbes could potentially be absorbed (for further discussion, see below), although additional research is necessary to characterize the distribution of other

Table 6-1 Systems Involved in Amino Acid Transport in the Mammalian Intestine

System name	Amino acids transported	Membrane localization	Na$^+$-dependent?
A	Gly, Pro, Ala, Ser, Gln, Asn, His, Met	Basolateral membrane	Yes
ASC	Ala, Ser, Cys, Thr, Gln	Apical membrane	Yes
B^0	Gly, Ala, Val, Leu, Ile, Met, Phe, Trp, Pro, Ser, Thr, Cys, Tyr, Asn, Gln	Apical membrane	Yes
$B^{0,+}$	Gly, Ala, Val, Leu, Ile, Met, Phe, Trp, Pro, Ser, Thr, Cys, Tyr, Asn, Gln, Arg, Lys, His	Apical membrane	Yes
$b^{0,+}$	Arg, Lys, cystine	Apical membrane	No
IMINO	Pro	Apical membrane	Yes
L	Gly, Ala, Val, Leu, Ile, Met, Phe, Trp, Ser, Thr, Cys, Tyr, Asn, Gln	Basolateral membrane	No
T	Phe, Trp, Tyr	Apical and basolateral membrane	No
X_{AG}	Asp, Glu	Apical membrane	Yes
y^+	Arg, Lys, His	Basolateral membrane	No
y^+L	Arg, Lys, His, Gln, Met, Leu	Basolateral membrane	Yes
PepT1	di- and tri-peptides	Apical membrane	Yes

Data from Broer 2008b, Closs et al 2004, Gilbert et al 2008b.

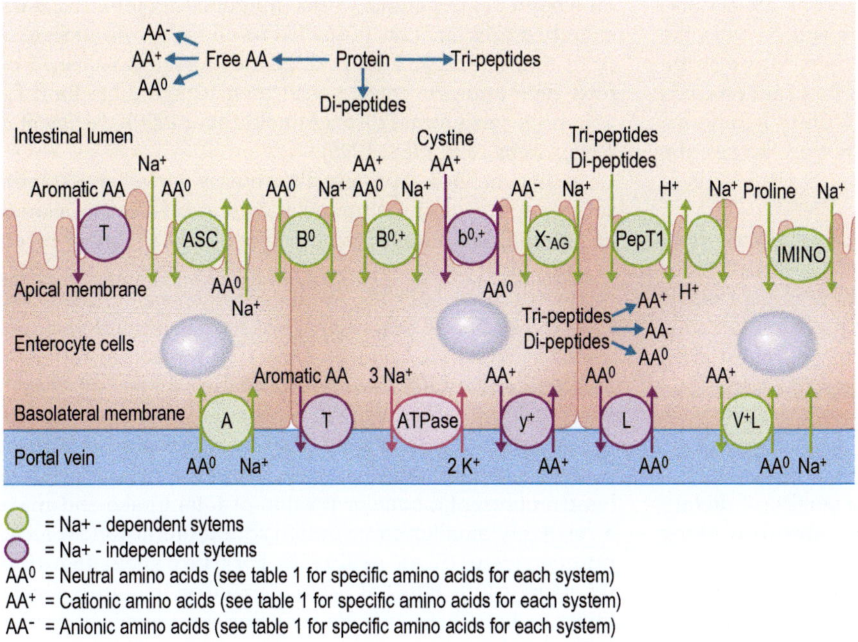

Figure 6.4 Transport systems involved with amino acid transport in the mammalian intestine.

amino acid transport systems along the equine intestinal mucosa.

The peptide transporter, PepT1, has also been identified throughout the small intestine of several domestic animals including cattle, pigs, sheep and chickens (Chen et al 1999) and in the cecum of chickens (Chen et al 1999; 2002), although at this time, PepT1 distribution has not been characterized in the equine intestinal mucosa. Incubation of the equine jejunal membrane with the dipeptide glycyl-L-glutamine, *in vitro*, resulted in an increase in current flow through the membrane, suggesting PepT1-like activity in the equine small intestine (Cehak et al 2009). However, in the rabbit, another hind-gut fermenter with a well-developed large intestine, PepT1 mRNA expression was not detectable in the cecum and was much lower in the colon than in the small intestinal segments (Freeman et al 1995), indicating only a limited capacity to absorb peptides in the large intestine.

Controversy exists about the extent to which amino acids can be absorbed from the large intestine of horses and over the last 40 years, a variety of studies have attempted to quantify the possible contribution of microbial amino acids to whole-body amino acid metabolism in horses. By infusing stable and radioactive isotope tracers into the cecum of horses, one study was able to detect the isotope label in the circulating indispensable amino acids (Slade et al 1971), whereas another study could not (Wysocki & Baker 1975). Orally administered isotopes also showed very minimal

(<10%) incorporation into circulating indispensable amino acids, and tissue and milk protein (McMeniman et al 1987, Schubert et al 1991), and because the isotope was fed, it is possible that some of these labeled amino acids were made by microbes proximal to the large intestine. The isotope data indicates that only a small portion of circulating and retained amino acids are synthesized by the large intestinal microbes, suggesting impairments in either the digestion or the absorption of microbially synthesized protein. The limitation in the absorption of microbial amino acids is further supported by the observation that the infusion of a large amount of lysine cecally does not result in the increase in portal vein plasma lysine concentrations that occurred when the lysine was administered gastrically (Wysocki & Baker 1975). Furthermore, the serum concentrations of several indispensable amino acids were significantly correlated to the dietary amino acid composition, but not to the amino acid composition of either cecal fluid or cecal microbes, indicating that the large intestine has only a minimal influence on whole-body amino acid status (Reitnour et al 1970).

The in vitro studies provide additional support that there is limited capacity to absorb amino acids across the apical membrane in both the cecal and colonic mucosa. At physiological concentrations, negligible amounts of lysine, histidine and arginine were able to cross the apical membrane in isolated colonic mucosa (Bochroder et al 1994), and although alanine and a leucine analog are able to cross the basolateral membrane of cecal mucosa, there was also no measurable apical membrane transport of these amino acids (Freeman et al 1989, Freeman & Donawick 1991). Ammonia, on the other hand, was readily transported across the mucosal membrane of the proximal colon (Bochroder et al 1994).

To summarize, despite the presence of some apical amino acid transport systems in the equine large intestine (Woodward et al 2009), it appears unlikely that the indispensable amino acids synthesized by microbes in the large intestine are absorbed to a large enough extent to make a substantial contribution to meeting the horse's amino acid needs.

Digestibility of dietary protein

The term protein digestibility refers to the portion of dietary protein that disappears, and is presumably absorbed, along the length of the gastrointestinal tract. A summary of the different types of digestibility that can be calculated is provided in Table 6-2. Digestibility can be defined as either total tract or prececal, depending on whether the undigested nitrogen is measured in the feces or ileal contents, respectively. Total tract protein digestibility is a measure of how much nitrogen is absorbed throughout the length of the intestine; however, it does not identify the location within the gastrointestinal tract of this digestion or the form (amino acids versus ammonia) that the nitrogen is absorbed in. Based on the discussion in the "Intestinal amino acid transport" section, it appears that the vast majority of amino acids are absorbed prior to the ileum and that most postcecal nitrogen absorption is likely to be largely as ammonia which is only available for protein synthesis if it is first incorporated into dispensable amino acids following absorption. Therefore, prececal protein digestibility (also referred to as ileal protein digestibility) may be a more reliable indicator of the amount of protein nitrogen that is absorbed in a form that is readily available for protein synthesis. Digestibility can also be classified as either true or apparent, depending on whether endogenous losses (microbial protein, enzymes, sloughed cells, etc.) are corrected for in the resulting fecal or cecal output (Table 6-2). Endogenous losses vary based on feed type and are greater with high forage diets than for primarily concentrate diets (Almeida et al 1999b, Farley et al 1995, Gibbs et al 1988, 1996).

Table 6-2 Calculation of Total Tract and Prececal Nitrogen Digestibility

Digestibility term[a]	Calculation
Apparent total tract nitrogen digestibility	Dietary nitrogen intake – fecal nitrogen output
Apparent prececal nitrogen digestibility	Dietary nitrogen intake – cecal nitrogen input
True total tract nitrogen digestibility	Dietary nitrogen intake – (fecal nitrogen output – endogenous nitrogen losses[b])
True pre-cecal nitrogen digestibility	Dietary nitrogen intake – (cecal nitrogen output – endogenous nitrogen losses[c])

[a]Protein is approximately 16% nitrogen, by weight. Therefore, nitrogen digestibility can be converted to crude protein digestibility by dividing by 0.16.
[b]Total tract endogenous nitrogen losses have been reported to range from 0.72–9.1 mg nitrogen/kg dry matter consumed (Almeida et al 1999b, Farley et al 1995, Gibbs et al 1988, 1996).
[c]Prececal endogenous nitrogen losses have been reported to range from 1.8 – 5.8 mg nitrogen/kg dry matter consumed (Almeida et al 1999b, Farley et al 1995, Gibbs et al 1988, 1996).

In mature horses, protein digestibility varies based on the protein source and the forage and concentrate composition of the diet, as summarized in Table 6-3. In the most recent version of the *Nutrient Requirements of Horses* (NRC 2007), total tract apparent nitrogen digestibility was estimated at 79% and pre-cecal apparent nitrogen digestibility was estimated at 51%. Based on the values summarized in Table 6-3, true and apparent prececal digestibility values are greater for cereal grains and oilseed meals than for forages. Apparent crude protein digestibility in horses increases with crude protein intake because as intake increases, the endogenous losses represent a smaller portion of total intake and make a relatively smaller contribution to total fecal (or prececal) nitrogen losses (Slade et al 1970). For true protein digestibility, there is little effect of protein intake on total tract digestibility, when there is a low to moderate level of protein intake and a constant protein source is used (Farley et al 1995). However, at high levels of protein intake, there may be a decline in both apparent and true pre-cecal digestibility (Farley et al 1995), likely due to limitations in the small intestinal digestive or absorptive capacity. Limited data exists regarding nitrogen digestibility in growing horses; however, in 3–7-month-old foals receiving a 70% concentrate diet, apparent total tract digestibility values of diets containing either milk protein or linseed (flax) meal ranged from ~35–45% (Hintz et al 1971), which is lower than similar high concentrate diets in mature horses (Table 6-3). In growing yearling horses, the apparent total tract digestibilities of 60% concentrate diets were ~80% (Antilley et al 2007), which are comparable to nitrogen digestibility estimates in mature horses (Table 6-3), suggesting that any limitations in nitrogen digestibility at ~6 months of age have been

Table 6-3 Estimates of Apparent and True Amino Acid Digestibilities of Feed Ingredients in Mature Horses

Ingredient/diet	Digestibility type	Apparent digestibility (%)	True digestibility (%)
Forages			
Coastal Bermuda grass hay	Prececal	9.6[a]	41[a]
	Total tract	57[a]	>100[a]
Alfalfa hay (15% CP)	Prececal	1.3[a]	27[a]
	Total tract	66[a]	>100[a]
Alfalfa hay (18.1% CP)	Prececal	21[a]	42[a]
	Total tract	74[a]	>100[a]
Cereal grains			
Corn	Prececal	48[b]	62[c]
	Total tract	98[b]	84[c]
Oats	Prececal	54[b]	68[c]
	Total tract	89[b]	75[c]
Barley	Prececal	ND	59[c]
	Total tract	ND	83[c]
Sorghum	Prececal	71[b]	ND
	Total tract	93[b]	ND
Protein feeds			
Soybean meal	Prececal	53[b]	ND
	Total tract	92[b]	ND
Cottonseed meal	Prececal	81[b]	ND
	Total tract	85[b]	ND
Forage and concentrate mixtures			
3:1 Coastal Bermuda grass to concentrate ratio	Prececal	39–56[b]	51–77[b]
	Total tract	83–88[2]	87–93[b]
2:1 Coastal Bermuda grass to concentrate ratio	Prececal	ND	ND
	Total tract	69–76[*,d]	83[d]
Complete pelleted diet (4.9% CP)	Prececal	37[e]	71[e]
	Total tract	63[e]	92[e]
Complete pelleted diet (9.5% CP)	Prececal	53[e]	71[e]
	Total tract	78[e]	94[e]
Complete pelleted diet (14% CP)	Prececal	60[e]	72[e]
	Total tract	86[e]	97[e]
Complete pelleted diet (16.5% CP)	Prececal	48[e]	58[e]
	Total tract	87[e]	97[e]
Oat hay/almond hulls + fish meal	Prececal	ND	ND
	Total tract	33–60[*,f]	80[f]
Oat hay/almond hulls + corn gluten meal	Prececal	ND	ND
	Total tract	36–59[*,f]	75[f]

*Apparent digestibility was linearly related to nitrogen intake, with increasing nitrogen intake resulting in increased apparent nitrogen digestibility.
Data from [a](Gibbs et al 1988); [b](Gibbs et al 1996); [c](Rosenfeld & Austbo 2009); [d](Freeman et al 1988); [e](Farley et al 1995); [f](Slade et al 1970).

overcome by 15 months of age. In the case of forage-based diets, ~⅔–¾ of the total tract true nitrogen digestion and absorption of nitrogen occurs in the large intestine (Table 6-3); whereas for grains more true nitrogen digestion and absorption occurred pre-cecally (> 70%) (Table 6-3).

Although prececal true protein digestibility values should give a reasonable estimate of protein absorbed in the form of amino acids, a better estimate would be to determine the prececal digestibility of each of the individual amino acids. In pigs, the true ileal digestibilities of the amino acids in many feed ingredients have been determined and individual amino acid requirements are provided on a true ileal digestible basis for pigs in a variety of physiological states (NRC 1998). There is very little research in horses that has quantified the prececal digestibilities of the individual amino acids and because of this lack of data it is not possible to estimate prececal digestibilities in the feed ingredients or to estimate the horse's requirements for prececally digestible amino acids. In growing foals receiving a diet with a 50:50 forage-to-concentrate ratio, the apparent digestibility of the amino acids increased with increasing crude protein intake (Almeida et al 1999a). Pre-cecal endogenous nitrogen losses

Table 6-4 Estimated Prececal Endogenous Losses and Total Digestibilities of Amino Acids in Growing Foals Receiving a Diet with a 50 : 50 Forage to Concentrate Ratio

Amino acid	Estimated endogenous losses (g/kg DM intake)	Prececal true digestibility (%)
Alanine	Value not given	41
Arginine	0.70	91
Aspartate	0.57	61
Cystine	0.86	86
Glutamate	Value not given	49
Glycine	0.45	56
Histidine	0.35	88
Isoleucine	Value not given	75
Leucine	0.45	72
Lysine	0.31	71
Methionine	0.15	81
Phenylalanine	0.27	100
Serine	1.00	85
Threonine	0.12	76
Tyrosine	Value not given	85
Valine	0.48	65

Data from Almeida et al 1999a.

(range: 0.12 to 1.00 mg/g dry matter consumed for threonine and serine respectively) and true pre-cecal digestibilities (range: ~30 to ~100% of intake for alanine and phenylalanine, respectively) were also calculated and are summarized in Table 6-4 (Almeida et al 1999b). These true prececal digestible amino acid values fall within the range of pre-cecal nitrogen digestion that have been reported (Table 6-3) and provide some indication of the extent to which dietary amino acids may be absorbed in the small intestine of horses. It is unknown how the pre-cecal digestibilities of the amino acids vary based on the feed ingredients used or the age/physiological state of the horse and additional research in this area is necessary.

Key Points

- Enzymatic protein digestion begins in the stomach and continues throughout the small intestine, with amino acids as the key end product. Microbial protein metabolism and digestion occurs in the large intestine, with ammonia as the major end product.
- Although luminal amino acid transport systems are present along the entire length of the intestine, it appears as though the majority of amino acid absorption occurs in the small intestine, whereas ammonia is the product absorbed from the large intestine. There is only minimal evidence to support the absorption of amino acids made by microbes in the large intestine.
- The majority of protein digestion from grains occurs prececally, whereas forage protein digestion occurs primarily postcecally.

Dietary sources of protein and amino acids

Milk

During the first few weeks of life, the foal obtains all or most of its dietary protein from milk. The protein concentration in fluid milk declines over the course of lactation. Colostrums may contain 10–19% crude protein on a fluid basis, but the protein concentration in milk is much lower (Martinez et al 1993, Ullrey et al 1966). During early lactation mare's milk usually contains 2–3% protein (Doreau et al 1992, Gibbs et al 1982, Glade 1991, Ullrey et al 1966). Between 2 and 4 months, the concentration of protein in fluid milk remains relatively constant at approximately 2% (Gibbs et al 1982, Ullrey et al 1966). In late lactation milk protein concentrations may be as low as 1.5 to 1.8% (Davison et al 1991, Mariani et al 2001).

Milk protein is considered a high quality protein source, because of its amino acid composition (Table 6-5) and its high digestibility. A classic study conducted by Hintz and coworkers (1971) demonstrated the importance of protein quality by comparing milk protein to linseed meal as the supplemental protein source in the diets of growing horses. Obviously milk is a source of high quality protein, but after the foal reaches 2–3 months of age most dietary protein will be derived from other sources.

Forages

Forages (hay, pasture, haylage, etc.) are important components of horse diets and can be excellent sources of protein and amino acids. However, forages can also be extremely variable in nutrient content.

Legumes that are used as forages for horses include alfalfa (lucerne), various types of clover, lespedeza, and varieties of peanut, pea, lupin, and soybean that have been selected for forage production. The crude protein concentration in common legume forages will usually exceed 14% on a dry matter basis.

Grasses are usually lower in crude protein than legumes. However, regular application of nitrogen-containing fertilizers to cool-season or warm-season grasses can increase the crude protein content. Well maintained cool-season pastures may contain 14 to 20% CP on a dry matter basis during the growing season (Harris 1997, Hoskin & Gee 2004, Lawrence et al 2006). Common cool season grasses that are used for horse hay or pasture include orchardgrass, Kentucky bluegrass, ryegrass, tall fescue and timothy. Warm-season grasses such as Bermuda grass and bahiagrass are also used for horses particularly in areas where winter temperatures are mild.

Stage of maturity at the time of harvest is one of the most important determinants of forage composition. Crude protein content of forages is highest when the plant is in a vegetative stage of growth and is lowest when the plant is in a late stage of maturity (Table 6-6). Stage of maturity also affects the neutral detergent fiber (NDF) and acid detergent fiber (ADF) in forage. Some of the protein in a forage may be associated with the NDF or ADF fraction, and the proportion of nitrogen found as acid detergent insoluble nitrogen (ADIN) increases with increasing forage maturity (Coblentz et al 1998, Elizalde et al 1999, Gonzalez et al 2001). It has

Table 6-5 Amino Acid Composition of Equine Skeletal Muscle and Mare's Milk

	Skeletal muscle		Mare's milk (~ 30 days lactation)	
Amino Acid	mg/g crude protein	% of lysine composition	mg/g total amino acids	% of lysine composition
Arginine	59	74	60	82
Histidine	46	58	22	30
Isoleucine	46	58	39	53
Leucine	77	97	93	127
Lysine	79	100	73	100
Methionine	24	30	22	30
Phenylalanine	41	52	43	59
Threonine	42	54	39	53
Tryptophan	7	9	ND	ND
Valine	49	61	47	64

Data from Badiani et al 1997, Davis et al 1994a, b. For both skeletal muscle and mare's milk, amino acid composition includes both free amino acids and amino acids contained in protein.

Table 6-6 Effect of Stage of Maturity on Crude Protein Content of Forages

	%CP
Alfalfa	
Pre-bud/bud	22–26
Early bloom	18–22
Midbloom	14–18
Full bloom	9–13
Cool season grasses	
Vegetative	16–20
Boot	12–16
Head	8–12
Warm season grasses	
Vegetative	16–18
Boot	6–8
Head	6–8

Adapted from Ball et al 2002.

been suggested that subtracting the amount of ADIN in a feed from total nitrogen can be used to estimate available dietary protein in horse feeds (NRC 2007).

Factors that influence the total protein concentration of forages will also affect the amino acid concentrations in the forage. In one study, the CP and lysine content of alfalfa hay harvested at three stages of maturity were 22% and 1.2%; 20.9% and 0.95%; and 16.9% CP and 0.64% lysine, respectively, on a dry matter basis (Garcia et al 1995). When the preceding lysine amino acid concentrations are expressed as a percentage of CP, it appears that with increasing stage of plant maturity, lysine decreases as a proportion of total protein, as well as a proportion of the dry matter. However, other researchers have not found a change in amino acid composition expressed as a percentage of CP in forages at different stages of maturity (Vanhatalo et al 2009).

Cereal grains and grain by-products

Cereal grains are incorporated into horse diets for energy, but they do provide protein and amino acids as well. The protein and amino acid composition of commonly used cereal grains are shown in Table 6-7. Within a type of grain, protein and amino concentrations are relatively consistent, and equations have been derived to estimate the amino acid composition of various feeds from their proximate components (NRC 1994). However some caution should be applied to this approach because there may be some differences among cultivars within a species and development of new cultivars has the potential to alter these characteristics. For example, to overcome low levels of lysine and methionine in typical corn varieties, higher lysine and higher methionine varieties have been developed. There are also differences in the protein characteristics of flint, dent, waxy, opaque and floury corn (Larson & Hoffman 2008). A new oat variety developed to have higher fat in the groat and lower lignin in the hull also has altered protein characteristics (Yu et al 2008). As new varieties of traditional cereal grains are used in horse rations, an understanding of their protein characteristics may be important. The crude protein in opaque and floury corn may have less zein than the crude protein in dent corn (Larson & Hoffman 2008). Zein is a type of prolamin protein that encapsulates starch. Higher levels of zein relative to the starch content may reduce the susceptibility of starch to digestion in ruminants (Larson & Hoffman 2008), and could be important in equine nutrition as well.

Both total tract and small intestinal protein digestion are generally greater for grains than for forages and there may be some differences between grain species in regard to the site or extent of protein digestion (Table 6-3). Limited information on small intestinal amino acid digestion by horses is available but reviews of relative digestibilities and bioavailabilities of amino acids in common swine and poultry feeds have been published (Lewis & Bayley 1995, NRC 1994, 1998).

Many byproducts of the grain processing industry are incorporated into horse feeds. Common examples include

Table 6-7 Amino Acid Composition of Feed Ingredients Commonly Used in Equine Diets

	Grass pasture	Legume pasture	Grass hay (mid-maturity)	Legume hay (mid-maturity)	Mixed grass/legume hay (mid-maturity)	Oats	Barley	Corn	Flax seed meal	Soybean meal	Rice bran
	Crude protein composition; % on a dry matter basis										
Crude protein	26.5	26.5	13.3	20.8	18.4	13.6	12.4	9.1	32.6	53.8	15.5
	Amino acid composition mg/g crude protein (% of lysine content)										
Arginine	43 (123)	52 (100)	39 (111)	51 (100)	42 (108)	68 (162)	51 (142)	46 (159)	88 (238)	73 (116)	78 (166)
Histidine	19 (54)	20 (38)	16 (46)	20 (39)	17 (44)	24 (57)	23 (64)	31 (107)	20 (54)	28 (44)	28 (60)
Isoleucine	34 (97)	43 (83)	33 (94)	42 (82)	36 (92)	38 (90)	35 (97)	33 (114)	46 (124)	46 (73)	34 (72)
Leucine	62 (177)	75 (144)	62 (177)	74 (145)	65 (167)	73 (174)	70 (194)	112 (386)	61 (165)	78 (124)	71 (151)
Lysine	35 (100)	52 (100)	35 (100)	51 (100)	39 (100)	42 (100)	36 (100)	29 (100)	37 (100)	63 (100)	47 (100)
Methionine	14 (40)	16 (31)	13 (37)	16 (31)	14 (36)	17 (40)	17 (47)	21 (72)	18 (49)	14 (22)	21 (45)
Phenylalanine	46 (131)	48 (92)	39 (111)	48 (94)	41 (105)	52 (124)	51 (142)	46 (159)	47 (127)	53 (84)	48 (102)
Threonine	36 (103)	44 (85)	36 (103)	44 (86)	38 (97)	35 (83)	34 (94)	36 (124)	38 (103)	40 (63)	39 (83)
Tryptophan	13 (37)	15 (29)	12 (34)	15 (29)	13 (33)	12 (29)	12 (33)	7 (24)	16 (43)	13 (21)	12 (26)
Valine	44 (126)	53 (102)	45 (129)	52 (102)	47 (121)	52 (124)	49 (136)	40 (138)	52 (141)	46 (73)	52 (111)

Data from NRC 2001, 2007.

wheat middlings and wheat bran, but corn gluten feed and rice bran are also considered in this category. In many cases the by-product feed has more crude protein than the parent grain. For example, corn grain has been reported to contain 8.3% CP whereas corn gluten feed contains 21.5% CP (as fed basis; NRC 1998).

As mentioned previously, cereal grains do not contain high quality protein. Consequently, grain by-products often contain moderate or low quality protein, even though they may be relatively high in CP. Therefore the amino acid content of by-product feeds should be considered when they are incorporated into horse feeds, especially if their inclusion reduces the use of ingredients with higher quality protein. Reference values for the amino acid composition of many by-product feeds have been published (NRC 1994, 1998, 2007); however, differences in milling procedures at individual plants may result in variation in protein and amino acid composition of these products. An alternative to using reference values for by-product feeds are prediction equations that have been developed to estimate amino acid composition from crude protein alone or in combination with other proximate components (NRC 1994, 1998).

Seed meals and other protein and amino acid supplements

When oil is extracted from the oil seeds of soybean, sunflower, canola, etc., the remaining seed meal is a high protein by-product that may be used in livestock feeds. Soybean meal is the most commonly used seed meal in horse feeds because it is widely available and it has a desirable amino acid profile. Raw soybeans contain several antinutritional factors that must be inactivated during the manufacturing process. When whole soybeans are incorporated into horse feeds they should be heated or extruded prior to feeding to inactivate the antinutritional factors. Although heat is essential for the production of useful soybean meal, too much heat can damage the protein and reduce amino acid availability. Amino acid availability may also be affected by soybean variety (Baker & Stein 2009). The protein content of commercially available soybean meal is often standardized at either 44% or 48% CP by the addition of soy hulls.

The protein and amino acid composition of many protein supplements have been well characterized (NRC 1994, 1998). The amino acid profile of soybean meal is generally superior to most other seed meals. Cottonseed meal, sunflower seed meal, safflower meal, peanut meal, canola meal and sesame meal are all comparatively low in lysine. Cottonseed meal and safflower meal are also low in sulfur-containing amino acids. When these protein sources are used it may be necessary to balance the amino acid profile using an amino acid supplement. Feed grade sources of several individual amino acids are available. Although amino acids can be synthesized in either the D or the L form, the amino acids that occur in plant and animal tissue are usually found as L-isomers. The ability of animals to use the D form of individual amino acids varies by amino acid and possibly by species or age of animal (Lewis & Baker 1995). The ability of horses to convert amino acids in the D form to the L form has not been investigated, although in other species the D-form of methionine can be converted to the L-form by the enzyme D-amino acid oxidase and is used as efficiently as the L-form in supporting growth (Baker & Boebel 1980, Chung & Baker 1992). However, supplements containing leucine, tryptophan, creatine, histidine, and β-alanine have also been manufactured for horses.

Key Points

- Common feed ingredients vary in protein quantity and quality
- Within a forage type, the most important factor affecting protein quantity is stage of maturity at the time of harvest
- Grain product feeds can also be variable with regards to protein quantity and quality

Supplementation of individual amino acids/ amino acid derivatives

Although most amino acids consumed by the horse come from forages and concentrates, there is an increasing number of supplements on the market that provide individual amino acids or combinations of amino acids. A brief summary of some of the commonly supplemented amino acids, their proposed mechanism of action in the horse and the results from any available research are provided below.

Branched chain amino acids (BCAA)

Because the BCAA (leucine, isoleucine and valine) are extensively oxidized for energy in the skeletal muscle, the supplementation of these amino acids has been suggested to have beneficial effects on athletic performance by sparing the use of dietary carbohydrates and glycogen (Harris & Harris 2005). At very low exercise intensities BCAA supplementation resulted in a reduction of plasma lactate concentrations (Glade 1989); however, in horses exercising at greater intensities, prolonged (4–5 weeks) BCAA supplementation (18–30 g/day) did not reduce plasma lactate concentrations or result in any improvements in athletic performance (Casini et al 2000, Stefanon et al 2000).

BCAA supplementation may also delay the onset of fatigue through the manipulation of mechanisms involved in the "central fatigue" hypothesis, which refers to a series of metabolic changes that occur during exercise that could result in an increase in tryptophan transport across the blood-brain barrier and increased serotonin synthesis. BCAA share a brain transport protein with tryptophan; therefore, if plasma BCAA concentrations decrease during exercise, the ratio of tryptophan to BCAA increases, relatively more tryptophan may be transported across the blood-brain barrier, leading to greater serotonin synthesis, which is proposed to result in fatigue. The role that supplemental BCAA may play in mediating the "central fatigue" response has not been investigated in horses. In endurance-trained humans, however, branched chain amino acid supplementation did reduce the brain uptake of tryptophan, but there was no corresponding improvement in time to exhaustion (van Hall et al 1995). The "central fatigue" hypothesis, and the possible role of BCAA in this mechanism, remains controversial.

Leucine is a potent activator of the mammalian target of rapamycin (mTOR) pathway, the pathway involved in the activation of muscle protein synthesis (Kimball 2007). In humans, providing a leucine-rich protein and carbohydrate supplement following resistance exercise increased rates of muscle protein synthesis compared to exercise stimuli alone due an increase in mTOR pathway activation (Dreyer et al 2008). In aging rats (Dardevet et al 2002) and humans (Rieu et al 2006), leucine supplementation increased post-feeding rates of muscle protein synthesis and may mitigate the loss of muscle mass that occurs with age. The role of BCAA in promoting muscle protein synthesis in horses of any age has not been investigated.

Methionine

Keratin, the major protein constituent of the hoof horn, is high in the sulfur amino acids methionine and cysteine; therefore, methionine is included in many equine hoof supplements. Although there is a lack of peer-reviewed research in horses, in cattle, methionine supplementation did result in increased rates of hoof growth during the spring and early summer (Clark & Rakes 1982) and in dry dairy cows (Smith et al 1999). However, the hooves of the cattle receiving the methionine supplement were not as hard as in receiving a control diet (Clark & Rakes 1982), and there was no improvement in the incidences of hoof horn disease (Laven & Livesey 2004). Although the benefits of dietary methionine supplementation on hoof growth and health remain unclear in cattle, because of the differences in gastrointestinal physiology and protein digestion in horses versus cattle, it is possible that dietary methionine supplementation may have different effects in horses and additional research is warranted.

Tryptophan

Tryptophan is included as an ingredient in many calming supplements (~0.8–13 mg/kg) because of its role as a serotonin precursor (Grimmett & Sillence 2005). Serotonin is a neurotransmitter and an elevation in serotonin levels in the brain has been associated with sedation, and reduced aggression and fear. An increase in circulating tryptophan concentrations, relative to the concentration of other amino acids, increases brain serotonin concentrations because more tryptophan is transported across the blood–brain barrier. Very low doses of supplemental oral tryptophan (>0.1 mg/kg) did not have a calming effect in horses subjected to isolation stress and actually appeared to increase excitability (Bagshaw et al 1994). Conversely, the oral supplementation of >300 mg/kg of tryptophan to ponies resulted in signs of respiratory distress and hemolysis (Paradis et al 1991) and an intravenous infusion of 100 mg/kg reduced endurance exercise capacity in mature mares, possibly by interfering with muscle glycogen utilization (Farris et al 1998). Oral feeding of 100 mg/kg of tryptophan, however, did not result in an early onset of fatigue when horses were pulling a 40 kg load on a treadmill at the walk and trot, and the authors speculated that even this high level of tryptophan intake was insufficient to increase brain serotonin levels (Vervuert et al 2005). In the studies that did evaluate the calming effect of tryptophan in horses receiving commercial tryptophan supplements (~13 mg/kg) and exposed to stimuli designed to elicit fear responses, the tryptophan-supplemented horses did not show any differences in any of the behavioral measures of fearfulness or in the heart rate parameters compared to untreated horses, despite elevated circulating tryptophan (Malmkvist & Christensen 2007, Noble et al 2008). At this time, there is no research to support the use of commercial calming supplements with tryptophan as the primary active ingredient.

Creatine

Phosphocreatine acts as phosphate donor to ADP to rapidly generate ATP, via the enzymatic reaction of creatine kinase.

$$\text{Creatine-P} + \text{ADP} \leftrightarrow \text{creatine} + \text{ATP}$$

Creatine is not present in plant material; therefore horses rely entirely on endogenous creatine synthesis by the kidney and liver. In the past 20 years, creatine supplementation in human athletes has received a great deal of attention because it has been shown to increase muscle creatine concentrations, muscle fiber area, strength and resistance to fatigue (reviewed by Kreider 2003), and appears to be related to improved performance in high-intensity or strength related athletic events (Kreider 2003). In humans, vegetarians are more responsive to creatine supplementation than those that regularly consume meat (Burke et al 2003); therefore, it seems plausible that horses may benefit from dietary creatine supplementation. However, equine studies using both short-term (50 g/day for ~7 days) (Schuback et al 2000) and longer-term (75 g/day for 30–90 days) (D'Angelis et al 2005) creatine monohydrate supplementation, showed no increases in either plasma or muscle creatine concentrations (Schuback et al 2000), no effect on muscle fiber cross-sectional area compared to a placebo group (D'Angelis et al 2005) and no improvements in either aerobic (D'Angelis et al 2005) or maximal (Schuback et al 2000) treadmill exercise performance. The discrepancy between the human and horse responses to creatine supplementation may be due to different intestinal absorption mechanisms resulting from horses having evolved as herbivores.

Carnitine

The majority of the body's carnitine is located in the skeletal muscle. Carnitine readily exchanges acyl groups with co-enzyme A, a key factor in the ATP production pathways, through the following reaction involving carnitine acyl/acetyltranferase enzymes:

$$\text{Carnitine} + \text{acyl-CoA} \leftrightarrow \text{acylcarnitine} + \text{coenzyme A}$$

The involvement of carnitine in this acyl exchange serves two key roles. First, long chain fatty acids must be in association with carnitine to be shuttled across the inner mitochondrial membrane for β-oxidation and ATP production. Second, the exchange of acetyl groups to carnitine prevents the accumulation of acetyl-CoA, which reduces the enzymatic activity of pyruvate dehydrogenase. A reduction in pyruvate dehydrogenase activity will limit the ability to produce ATP aerobically and will result in an increase in lactic acid production, eventually limiting anaerobic energy production and high intensity exercise performance. Carnitine is able to accept the acetyl groups from acetyl CoA, reducing the accumulation of acetyl-CoA and subsequently lactate, allowing for continued performance at relatively high exercise intensities. Only very low levels of carnitine are found in plant materials (Vaz & Wanders 2002); therefore as strict herbivores it is unlikely that horses consume large amounts of carnitine in their diets, although horses do have high muscle levels of carnitine compared to other species (Harris & Harris 2005). In practice, neither oral nor intravenous carnitine administration (>10 g/day for 56 and 28 days, respectively) in horses resulted in any increase in muscle carnitine levels, despite increases in plasma concentrations (Foster et al 1988, Harris et al 1995). In another study, however, there was a 50% increase in gluteal muscle carnitine levels in 2-year-old standardbred trotters following a 5-week conditioning program (Harmeyer et al 2001), although data from the unsupplemented horses undergoing the same conditioning program was not provided and therefore it is unclear whether the increase in muscle carnitine content was due to the supplementation or the conditioning program. In spite of the lack of consistent increase in muscle carnitine levels, there is some evidence that carnitine supplementation does increase VO_2 and/or reduce lactic acid production in both humans [summarized by (Brass 2000)] and horses [summarized by (Harris & Harris 2005)], although it is unclear how these effects are mediated in the apparent absence of increased muscle carnitine levels.

Key Points

- There are many commercially available supplements that are amino acids or amino acid derivatives
- The reasons for feeding amino acid supplements range from improved exercise performance to improved hoof health to calming an excitable horse
- At this time, there is little evidence to support the proposed effects of any of the commercially available amino acid supplements

Protein and amino acid requirements of horses

A variety of systems have been used to determine and express the protein requirements of horses. In its original publication addressing horse nutrition the NRC (1949) expressed the protein requirement of horses in pounds of digestible protein. In that publication, the daily protein allowance for maintenance was stated to be approximately four times the amount of nitrogen found in endogenous excretions. The requirements for medium work were approximately 45% greater than maintenance. The protein requirements for pregnant mares were developed from estimates of fetal and placental development and were about 45% higher than maintenance. The crude protein allowances above maintenance for lactating mares were calculated from a milk protein content of 2%, milk production of approximately 3% of BW and an efficiency of protein use of 50%. The allowances for growing horses were determined from maintenance and assumptions about rate of gain and composition of gain that were derived from calves. In this case, the efficiency of converting absorbed protein to gain was estimated at 50%. In order for users to determine actual feeding programs, the publication included the composition (including digestible protein) of more than 50 common horse feeds. In the most current publication the NRC (2007) still uses some of the original approaches to estimating requirements but crude protein and lysine have replaced digestible protein in the requirement tables.

The 1949 publication was named "Recommended Nutrient Allowances for Horses". In 1961, the NRC renamed the publication the "Nutrient Requirements of Horses" and expressed protein requirements in pounds of total protein as well as in pounds of digestible protein. Revisions of this document were published in 1966, 1971, 1978, 1989 and 2007. Requirements were expressed as both digestible protein and crude protein until the 5th revised edition was published in 1989 when the digestible protein recommendations were eliminated and an estimate of the daily lysine requirement was added. In the 50 years between the original publication and the current publication there have been relatively small changes in the protein recommendations for some types of horses. For example, the maintenance requirement was initially set at approximately 0.7 lb (0.32 kg) DP/day for a 1200 lb (545 kg) horse (NRC 1949). In 1978 the requirement was 0.31 kg DP/d and 0.68 kg CP/d (NRC 1978). In 2007, the maintenance requirement of a 545 kg horse was estimated at about 0.69 kg CP/day (NRC 2007) (Table 6-8). The requirements for a 1200 lb lactating mare were initially set at 2.3 lb (1.05 kg) DP/day. In 1978, the NRC estimates for the same mare were 0.92 kg DP/day and 1.48 kg CP/day. The 2007 NRC estimated the CP requirement of a 545 kg mare at 1.7 kg CP/day and 1.5 kg CP/day in the second and fourth months of lactation, respectively. Although the CP recommendations for some classes of horses have remained relatively constant, the emphasis on protein quality has resulted in some changes to the lysine requirements. For example, the lysine requirement of pregnant mares was previously estimated to be 3.5% of the crude protein requirement (NRC 1989); whereas the current daily lysine intake is estimated at 4.3% of the crude protein requirement (NRC 2007). A change in recommended lysine intake is most apparent for the lactating mare. The current recommendation of 92 g of lysine per day for a 545 kg mare in early lactation is almost 70% higher (NRC 2007) than the previous recommendation (NRC 1989). There were several factors that contributed to this increase, including a higher estimate of the amount of lysine needed for milk production and an increase in the amount of lysine needed by the mare maintenance. Many practical diets that are generally considered adequate for lactating mares do not provide the amount of lysine suggested by the NRC (2007); therefore it is possible that the current recommendations overestimate the lysine requirements of lactating mares.

Table 6-8 Crude Protein and Lysine Requirements of Horses with an Expected Mature Body Weight of 545 kg

	Crude protein (kg/day)	Lysine (g/day)
Maintenance (average)	0.69	30
Light work	0.76	33
Medium work	0.84	36
Heavy work	0.94	40
Very heavy work	1.1	47
Pregnant – 5 months	0.75	32
Pregnant – 8 months	0.83	36
Pregnant – 11 months	0.97	42
Lactation – 2 months	1.7	92
Lactation – 4 months	1.5	82
Growing – 6 months	0.74	32
Growing – 12 months	0.92	40

Data from NRC 2007.

While there has been good historical agreement on the protein requirements of broodmares and growing horses, there has been little agreement on the protein requirements of working horses. In 1949, it was suggested that working horses needed more protein than sedentary horses (NRC 1949). However, in 1961 and 1966 the protein requirements of 1200 lb (545 kg) working horses were estimated to be the same as sedentary horses (NRC 1961, 1966). In 1973, the requirements were increased to 0.6 kg DP/day and 1.1 kg CP/day (NRC 1973); justified by the desire to maintain a constant protein:calorie ratio in the diet. The authors of the fourth revised edition of the NRC (1978) were apparently unimpressed by this argument and once again reduced the protein requirements of working horses to the maintenance level (0.31 kg DP/day; 0.68 kg CP/day). In 1989, the protein:calorie ratio was reapplied and the crude protein requirements of 545 kg horses in moderate work were estimated to be 1.05 kg CP/day, which was about 50% greater than the needs of sedentary horses at the same body weight (NRC 1989). Experimental data from feeding experiments with exercising horses were used to establish the current recommendations, which are intermediate to the range of previous recommendations (0.84 kg CP for a 545 kg horse in moderate work). The lysine requirements of exercising horses are currently estimated to be 4.3% of the crude protein requirement (NRC 2007). In the previous recommendation, lysine comprised about 3.5% of the dietary crude protein; however, as mentioned previously, the recommended amount of crude protein was higher (NRC 1989). Consequently, the current recommendations for lysine intakes of exercising horses are similar to the previous estimates. The lysine intake for a 545 kg horse in moderate work was previously suggested to be about 37 g/day; whereas the current recommendation is 36 g/day.

Although CP and lysine are used to express the daily protein requirements of horses in the US, this system is not uniformly accepted across the world. Horse feeding standards in Japan use crude protein but in Germany requirements have been traditionally expressed as units of digestible crude protein (DCP). Researchers in France have developed feeding standards that express protein requirements as "Matieres Azotées Digestibles Cheval" (MADC) which is translated as horse digestible crude protein. However, the system accounts for more than just total tract protein digestibility of feeds. The French system is based on the assumptions that the amino acid composition of the feedstuff affects the value of the feed and that site of digestion affects the availability of amino acids in the feed. Therefore, MADC is similar to DCP for some feeds, such as concentrates and protein supplements. But for other feeds, such as mature forages, DCP overestimates the MADC because fewer amino acids in these feeds are available in the small intestine (Martin-Rosset 2001, Martin-Rosset & Ellis 2005). The MADC system has some advantage over the CP/lysine system employed in the US or a DCP system because it attempts to account for differences in the small intestinal availability of amino acids in various feeds. However, the system is more complicated and thus more difficult for some users to implement at the farm or stall level. In addition, to be accurate, information about the amino acid composition and amino acid digestibility of each feed must be available. As mentioned previously, there is considerable information about amino acid composition and digestibility of feeds that are used in swine and poultry production, but much less information exists about forages which often comprise the majority of the equine diet.

Feeding standards that include nutrient requirement tables should be used as a guide to formulating rations for horses. In practical application, recommended nutrient intakes must be adjusted to compensate for differences in environmental conditions, differences among feedstuffs and differences among individual horses. In depth discussion of the factors that influence the protein and amino acid requirements of specific classes of horses are covered in other chapters and will not be repeated here. However, the following section of this chapter will address various experimental approaches that have been used to determine protein and amino acid requirements in horses and other species. An understanding of the strengths and weaknesses of each method is necessary for the interpretation of the material included in the chapters addressing the nutrient requirements of specific groups of horses.

Key Points

- The National Research Council's recommendations for dietary protein intake are currently provided as crude protein and lysine requirements
- Although the American system for expressing protein requirements is on a crude protein basis, this is not a universal system. In Germany and France, alternate systems have been developed that attempt to account for protein digestibility and the sites of protein digestion
- Factors to consider when formulating rations for protein and lysine content include the requirements based on the physiological state of the horse, environmental factors and the characteristics of the feed ingredients used

Methods of assessing dietary protein/amino acid adequacy

The ability of a complete diet or an individual feed ingredient to provide adequate amounts of protein or, more specifically, each of the individual indispensable amino acids, can be assessed from two different standpoints: based on the amino acid composition of the feed ingredient relative to the amino acid requirements, or based on the physiological responses of animals receiving the specific diet(s)/ingredient(s). Some of the most commonly used methods of assessing dietary protein/amino acid adequacy are described below, along with their strengths and potential drawbacks, and when possible the previous use of these techniques in horses will be discussed.

Protein quality and amino acid scoring

Perhaps the easiest method of determining whether a particular diet or feed ingredient will adequately meet the needs of the horses is to compare the amino acid composition of the ingredient/diet to the amino acid composition of a reference protein, such as milk or muscle protein, in a process called amino acid scoring. The following equation is used to calculate the amino acid score for each indispensable amino acid:

$$\text{Amino acid score} = \frac{\text{Concentration of amino acid in the feed ingredient (mg/g CP)}}{\text{Concentration of amino acid in the reference protein (mg/g CP)}} \times 100\%$$

The amino acid provided in the lowest amount relative to the requirement is termed the *limiting amino acid*. In order for protein synthesis to occur, all amino acids must be present in a specific ratio. If even one amino acid is provided at a level less than what is required for protein synthesis, then the total amount of protein synthesis that can occur is limited to the level that can be supported based on the intake of the limiting amino acid. The barrel analogy (Fig. 6.5) is commonly used to illustrate the concept of the limiting amino acid: the barrel can only be filled as high as the shortest board just like protein synthesis can only occur up to the level supported by the limiting amino acid. In forage and cereal grain based diets fed to horses of a variety of ages, lysine is thought to be the first limiting amino acid (Breuer et al 1970, Graham et al 1994, Graham-Thiers & Kronfeld 2005b, Hintz et al 1971, Ott et al 1979, Potter & Huchton 1975), with threonine generally assumed to be the second limiting amino acid (Graham et al 1994, Graham-Thiers & Kronfeld 2005b, Staniar et al 2001). Although methionine is a limiting amino acid in legumes (i.e., soybean meal) (Iqbal et al 2010), methionine as a potentially limiting amino acid has received only minimal attention in horses (Breuer et al 1970, Glade & Luba 1987).

The *ideal protein concept* is frequently applied when formulating diets for poultry and swine. An "ideal" protein is one where the pattern of indispensable amino acids provided by the diet or feed ingredient closely resembles the pattern of the animal's requirements for these same amino acids. By closely matching the animal's intake of amino acids to the requirements, this ensures that none of the amino acids is limiting and minimizes the provision of excess dietary amino acids. For species where the indispensable amino acid requirements are well defined,

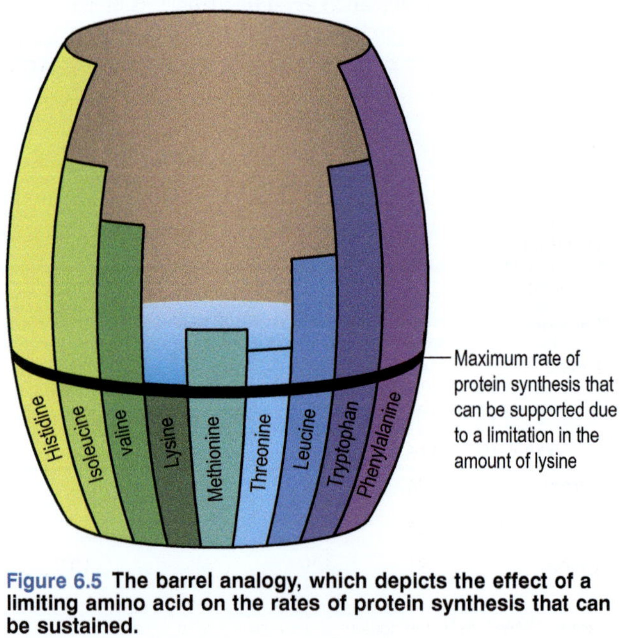

Figure 6.5 The barrel analogy, which depicts the effect of a limiting amino acid on the rates of protein synthesis that can be sustained.

the requirement for each amino is generally expressed as a percentage of the lysine requirement, and likewise the amount of each indispensable amino acid in the diet is also expressed as a percent of lysine intake. For horses, however, only the lysine requirement has been estimated (NRC 2007); therefore, in order to apply the ideal protein concept in assessing or formulating equine diets another reference amino acid profile must be used, such as that of skeletal muscle (Table 6-5).

The amino acid compositions of commonly used feeds in horse diets, expressed on both a percent of crude protein intake and as a percent of lysine intake, are provided in Table 6-7, and the amino acid scores for each amino acid, based on comparison to the skeletal muscle amino acid profile, are in Table 6-9. As expected, lysine is consistently one of the most limiting amino acid in equine feed ingredients, and in legumes methionine may also be limiting. Although histidine appears to be a limiting amino acid in several feed ingredients, histidine is not a limiting amino acid in any other monogastric species and a histidine deficiency has not been described in horses. Most likely, this is due to an overestimation of histidine in the skeletal muscle through the measurement of total muscle amino acid composition (Badiani et al 1997, Bryden 1991), which includes both free and protein bound amino acids. Muscle contains high amounts of the histidine containing dipeptide, carnosine (Sewell et al 1992), and this histidine would have been included in the published estimates of muscle histidine content, despite not being a part of protein.

Although an easy way to assess the quality of a dietary protein source, there are limitations to the amino acid scoring method. First, we do not have sufficient information to develop an "ideal protein" pattern for horses and using the amino acid composition of a single tissue such as skeletal muscle is not completely representative of the animal's whole-body needs. For example, although there is evidence to support that threonine is the second limiting amino acid for horses (Graham et al 1994), according to the amino acid scoring method using muscle amino acid composition as the reference profile (Table 6-9), threonine is not identified as one of the more limiting amino acids. A substantial amount of dietary threonine (up to 60%) (Bertolo et al 1998, Stoll et al 1998) is used by the gastrointestinal tract by other monogastrics for mucin synthesis (Law et al 2007, Nichols & Bertolo 2008), particularly when high fiber diets are fed (Myrie et al 2008). Therefore skeletal muscle threonine content likely underestimates total body threonine needs. Alternatives to skeletal muscle amino acid composition as the ideal amino acid profile are not readily available, although it has been suggested that the amino acid composition of mare's milk (Table 6-5) may be an appropriate amino acid profile for the growing or lactating horse (NRC 2007). We do not presently have requirements for any of the indispensable amino acids other than lysine in any age of horse, so it is not possible to design the reference protein profiles based on individual amino acid requirements. The amino acid scoring method also does not consider amino acid digestibility and metabolic availability and the amount of dietary amino acids absorbed by the horse and available for protein synthesis could vary quite dramatically from the actual amino acid composition. If individual amino acid requirements were known and amino acid digestibility/availability from a variety of feedstuffs were determined, then the use of the amino acid scoring method could be quite instructive when formulating rations.

In vivo methods to assess dietary protein and amino acid adequacy and requirements

The in vivo methods of assessing dietary amino acid adequacy are based on the physiological response of the horses

Table 6-9 Amino Acid Scores of Feed Ingredients Commonly Used in Equine Diets

	Grass pasture	Legume pasture	Grass hay (mid-maturity)	Legume hay (mid-maturity)	Mixed grass/legume hay (mid-maturity)	Oats	Barley	Corn	Flax seed meal	Soybean meal	Rice bran
	Amino acid score (% of muscle value)										
Arginine	73	89	66	88	72	117	87	79	151	125	133
Histidine	41	42	36	43	37	53	50	68	44	61	61
Isoleucine	74	94	72	92	77	82	76	72	101	99	75
Leucine	81	97	81	96	85	95	91	146	80	102	93
Lysine	44	65	44	64	49	53	46	36	46	79	59
Methionine	57	66	54	65	57	71	71	89	73	60	85
Phenylalanine	112	117	95	116	100	126	124	112	114	128	116
Threonine	84	104	85	104	90	82	81	84	89	94	91
Tryptophan	184	214	172	208	182	165	163	100	215	175	163
Valine	91	109	93	107	97	107	101	83	107	95	108

For each amino acid in each feed ingredient, the amino acid score was calculated by dividing the content of the amino acid in the feed ingredient (in mg/g protein; Table 6-4) by the content of the amino acid in the skeletal muscle (in mg/g protein; Table 6-6) and multiplying by 100%.

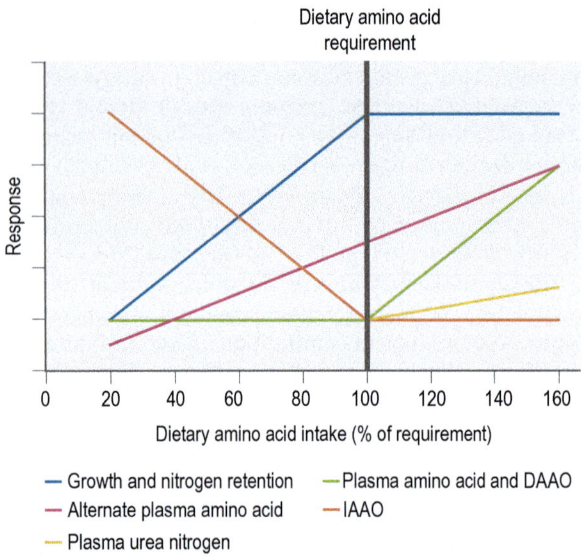

Figure 6.6 Expected patterns of response for the different criteria that can be used to assess the adequacy of dietary protein and amino acid intakes and measure requirements.

receiving a specific level of amino acid intake. There are three key patterns that can be observed in response to incremental increases in the intake of protein or an indispensable amino acid (Fig. 6.6) (Pencharz & Ball 2003). The level of intake where the slope of the response line changes is termed the "breakpoint" and represents the estimated amino acid/ protein requirement. The key methods that will be discussed are average daily gain, nitrogen retention, measurement of plasma metabolite concentrations and isotopic methods.

Average daily gain

Much of our knowledge about amino acid and protein nutrition in growing horses can be attributed to the measurement of average daily gain. When the intake of an indispensable amino acid of interest (or protein) increases from deficient to adequate, there is an incremental increase in average daily gain. Once the required amount is provided, further increases in the amino acid (protein) intake will not result in further increases in average daily gain (Fig. 6.6). This method is a relatively simple way to assess dietary amino acid (protein) adequacy and has been used to evaluate dietary protein quality and identify limiting amino acids in growing horse diets (Breuer et al 1970, Graham et al 1994, Hintz et al 1971, Ott et al 1979, 1981). However, this method can only be used to assess amino acid (protein) adequacy in growing horses. Additionally, in order to get an accurate assessment of growth rates, study periods need to be long (generally >100 days), making it impractical to study each subject at each level of dietary amino acid (protein) intake and therefore a large number of research subjects is necessary in order to detect significant differences in growth rate due to diet.

Nitrogen retention

The nitrogen retention method compares nitrogen intake to nitrogen losses and may also take into account "other miscellaneous nitrogen losses," which include nitrogen lost in sweat, as hair or in milk. The following equations are used in nitrogen retention calculations:

Nitrogen retained (g/kg/day) = Nitrogen intake (g/kg/day) − Nitrogen losses (g/kg/day)

Nitrogen losses (g/kg/day) = Nitrogen in feces + Nitrogen in urine + Other miscellaneous nitrogen losses

When nitrogen retention is plotted against nitrogen (amino acid) intake, nitrogen retention increases up to point where requirements are met and then additional increases in intake result in no further increases in nitrogen retention (Fig. 6.6). In adult mammals maintaining constant body weight, nitrogen retention should be zero, and this is termed *nitrogen balance*, and the level of intake where nitrogen balance is achieved is the amino acid (protein) requirement. For mature horses at maintenance, the sum of endogenous nitrogen losses in the feces, urine and through "other miscellaneous losses" should theoretically be equivalent to the dietary nitrogen requirement to obtain nitrogen balance. Fecal and urinary nitrogen excretion both increase linearly with protein intake (Olsman et al 2003), and using regression analysis of nitrogen excretion in response to nitrogen intake, endogenous losses can be estimated. While various calculations of endogenous renal nitrogen losses have yielded fairly consistent estimates of ~135 mg N/kg$^{0.75}$, estimates of endogenous fecal losses have been much more variable ranging from 27 to more than 100 mg N/kg$^{0.75}$, presumably due to imprecision in the measurements and the influence of other factors such as total dry matter intake and diet composition (Gibbs et al 1996, Meyer et al 1985, Olsman et al 2003). In one study that measured cutaneous nitrogen losses in horses, this value was estimated at 35 mg N/kg$^{0.75}$ (Meyer 1983). Based on these estimates, endogenous nitrogen losses could range from 197–270 mg N/kg$^{0.75}$ in a mature horse, meaning that amount of nitrogen would need to be digested and absorbed each day in order to attain nitrogen balance.

Growing horses, horses in athletic training that are building muscle and mid-to-late gestation horses should be actively accreting protein; therefore, when requirements are met, nitrogen losses will be less than nitrogen intake and horses will be in positive nitrogen balance (nitrogen retention > 0). When horses that are losing lean tissue, due to illness, weight loss or lactation they are said to be in negative nitrogen balance (nitrogen retention < 0).

The current dietary maintenance recommendations for dietary crude protein are also based on nitrogen retention techniques (NRC 2007). However, there are several criticisms of this method. Perhaps the largest concern is that it is extremely difficult to accurately quantify all nitrogen losses, particularly nitrogen lost as hair, skin and sweat. In previous nitrogen retention studies in horses (Antilley et al 2007, Freeman et al 1988, Hintz et al 1971, Hintz & Schryver 1972, Reitnour & Salsbury 1972, Slade et al 1970, Wall et al 1998), only nitrogen losses in urine and feces have been quantified, which underestimates total nitrogen losses and overestimates nitrogen retention. In horses, these miscellaneous losses could be an especially large concern as they would be expected to be highly variable between horses depending on the season, level of activity and individual horse characteristics and even more difficult to quantify that in humans or other species, although an estimate of 35 mg N/kg$^{0.75}$ for mature horses does exist (Meyer 1983). Nitrogen retention methodologies also require total fecal and urine collection which is not only labor intensive, but requires that horses are confined in relatively small areas, with little or no bedding, for the entire collection period (generally at least 4–5 days) (Antilley et al 2007). Because the urea pool takes several days to stabilize following changes in nitrogen (amino acid) intake (Rand et al 1976), generally at least 1 week is required to adapt to each new diet before urine and fecal collections can begin, making this technique impractical for studying requirements in rapidly growing animals, if each animal is to be studied on multiple levels of intake. Furthermore, a recent study in yearling fillies was unable to detect differences in nitrogen retention when the intake of each essential amino acids was reduced by ~ 25–35%, to a "deficient" level (Antilley et al 2007), suggesting that either the deficient diet was not actually deficient, that 6 animals per treatment was insufficient or that the nitrogen retention methodology they used was not an effective measure to assess the adequacy of amino acid intake in horses.

Plasma metabolite concentrations

Another method to measure to assess dietary amino acid (protein) adequacy is examining plasma metabolite concentrations, such as the concentration of plasma amino acids or urea. When the intake of an indispensable amino acid is below the requirement, it is predicted that the plasma concentration of that amino acid is low and constant, as incremental increases in the intake of that amino acid result in an increase in tissue uptake of that amino acid for use in protein synthesis, resulting in no net changes in plasma concentrations. Once the requirement for that amino acid is met, additional increases in dietary intake results in an accumulation of that amino acid in the plasma (Fig. 6.6). In reality, however, in many cases plasma amino acid concentrations vary directly with the amino acid content of the diet, and a breakpoint indicative of the requirement level may not be present (Fig. 6.6). A recent study attempted to determine dietary lysine requirements in mature horses using plasma lysine concentrations; however, only a very small number of subjects were used, and the "breakpoint" at the requirement level was not convincing as plasma amino acid concentrations appeared to increase in a linear manner with lysine intake (Ohta et al 2007).

For the plasma urea nitrogen response, when an indispensable amino acid ("test" amino acid) is provided below requirement, the use of the other indispensable amino acids will be limited by test amino acid intake and they will be catabolized, with the amino moiety is converted to urea for the excretion in the urine. As test amino acid intake becomes less limiting, more protein synthesis can occur and less urea is formed. Once test amino acid requirements are met, further increases in test amino acid intake result do not result in any additional protein synthesis and therefore the additional test amino acid is now in excess and must be catabolized, resulting in a slow increase in plasma urea nitrogen concentrations (Fig. 6.6). Plasma urea nitrogen concentrations have not been used to determine amino acid requirements in horses; however, they have shown that supplementing certain diets with lysine and threonine can improve dietary protein utilization and lower plasma urea nitrogen concentrations in growing (Graham et al 1994) and mature (Graham-Thiers & Kronfeld 2005b) horses.

These methods have the advantage that they are simple, less labor intensive than nitrogen retention techniques and require only a few blood samples following the adaptation period to the diet. However, they are not considered to be sensitive enough to stand alone in determining amino acid requirements (Pencharz & Ball 2003).

Isotopic methodologies

The "gold standard" methods for measuring protein and amino acid requirements in humans are the carbon oxidation techniques (World Health Organization 2007), where ^{13}C-labeled amino acid isotopes are infused and the appearance of the ^{13}C label in exhaled CO_2 is measured. There are two general categories of carbon oxidation methods: direct amino acid oxidation (DAAO), where the isotope is the same as the test amino acid, and indirect amino acid oxidation (IAAO), where an isotope of a different indispensable amino acid from the test amino acid, generally phenylalanine, is infused. Both methodologies are based on the ideal protein concept and the assumption that the carbon backbone of dietary indispensable amino acids that are provided in excess of what can be used for protein synthesis are oxidized to CO_2 (Pencharz & Ball 2003). For the DAAO, $^{13}CO_2$ formation increases once requirement is met, because the infused amino acid is now in excess of what can be used to support protein synthesis (Fig. 6.6) (Pencharz & Ball 2003). With the IAAO method, as test amino acid intake increases towards requirement, there is an increase in the amount of protein synthesis that can occur and incremental decreases in indicator amino acid oxidation and $^{13}CO_2$ appearance in the breath. Once the requirement is met, further increases in test amino acid intake do not result in any increase in the amount of protein synthesis and therefore indicator oxidation to $^{13}CO_2$ remains low and steady (Fig. 6.6) (Pencharz & Ball 2003). In other species, the DAAO and IAAO have been used extensively to measure individual indispensable amino acid requirements (Coleman et al 2003, Elango et al 2007, 2008, House et al 1998, Kriengsinyos et al 2002, 2004, Meredith et al 1986, Moehn et al 2004, Zello et al 1990, 1993), total protein requirements (Elango et al 2010, Humayun et al 2007a), determine limiting amino acids (Brunton et al 2007) and measure the metabolic availability of amino acids from different protein sources (Humayun et al 2007b, Moehn et al 2005).

These methods are extremely sensitive and typically only five to six subjects are required for an accurate estimate of the requirement (Pencharz & Ball 2003). In pigs and humans the adaptation period required prior to measurements has been shown to be extremely short, less than 2 days (Moehn et al 2004, Thorpe et al 1999), meaning that subjects only consume potentially deficient diets for a very short period of time. In theory, this would mean that an entire requirement study could be conducted in 3–4 weeks, a vast improvement over other methods. Finally, with the exception of the infusion and sampling procedures, subjects do not need to be confined as they do for the total urine and fecal collections needed for the nitrogen retention methodology. These methods are minimally invasive, as evidenced by the acceptance of these techniques for use in neonates and children (Bertolo et al 2003). At the present time, neither the DAAO nor IAAO methods have been used to measure amino acid (protein) requirements in horses; however, they show great promise in being applied to define indispensable amino acid requirements in horses of a variety of ages and physiological states.

Factorial method for determining protein and amino acid requirements

The current NRC protein recommendations for mature horses at maintenance are based on a meta-analysis of nitrogen retention data from several studies; however, due to insufficient research specifically examining the protein requirements during growth, gestation, lactation and during exercise, estimated requirements for these physiological states were calculated using a factorial approach. A factorial approach divides the total protein requirement into the maintenance and "production" components and also includes a correction factor for the efficiency of protein utilization and the digestibility of dietary protein. The production components include the protein content of average daily gain, fetal growth, milk production, and for muscle growth and sweat losses during growth, gestation (5 months to parturition), lactation and exercise, respectively (Table 6-10). The estimated efficiency of protein utilization is 50% during gestation, lactation and exercise. In the very young growing horse (less than 6 months old), the efficiency of protein use is also estimated at 50%, although this is reduced to 30% by 1 year of age. Dietary protein digestibility is estimated at 79% for all physiological states of horses. With the exception of lactation, where the dietary lysine requirement is based on the lysine content of milk in addition to the maintenance requirements, the lysine requirements for all "production" states are calculated in the same manner as the maintenance lysine requirement and is 4.3% of dietary crude protein requirement (NRC 2007).

Key Points

- Dietary protein quality can be assessed by comparing the amino acid profile of the feed ingredients to a profile that is representative of the horse's amino acid needs. However, at this time there is no universally recognized "ideal protein" profile in horses
- Protein and amino acid requirements can be determined by studying the physiological response (growth rate, nitrogen retention, plasma metabolite concentrations, isotope oxidation) to graded intakes of protein or amino acids and identifying the "breakpoint" in the response pattern
- Nitrogen retention measurements were used to estimate the protein requirements of horses at maintenance. For growth, lactation, gestation and during exercise, a factorial approach was used to calculate protein requirements

Signs of protein/amino acid deficiency and excess

Protein and amino acid deficiency

Horses do not technically have a metabolic requirement for crude protein, but rather requirements for each of the indispensable amino acids as well as enough amino acid nitrogen to synthesize the required dispensable amino acids. Therefore, protein deficiency can take one of two forms: inadequate amounts of one or more of the indispensable amino

Table 6-10 Factorial Approach to Estimating Protein Requirements in Horses in the 2007 Nutrient Requirements of Horses

Physiological state	Factorial calculation of the protein requirement
Growth	Maintenance protein requirement + Protein needs for growth[a] Example: A yearling with an estimated mature weight of 600 kg, a current weight of 385 kg and an average daily gain of 0.54 kg/day, of which 20% of the daily gain is protein deposited with an efficiency of 30% (assume 79% protein digestibility): = (1.44 g/kg/day × 385 kg) + [(540 g/day × 0.20)/(0.30 × 0.79)] = 1010 g protein/day
Gestation (5 months → parturition)	Maintenance protein requirement + Protein needs for fetal gains Example: A 500 kg mare pre-gestation, weighs 534 kg in her 9th month of gestation and has daily pregnancy-related gains of 0.41 kg/day, of which 20% of the daily gain is protein deposited with an efficiency of 50% (assume 79% protein digestibility): = (1.26 g/kg/day × 534 kg) + [(410 g/day × 0.20)/(0.50 × 0.79)] = 880 g protein/day
Lactation	Maintenance protein requirement + Protein needs for milk production Example: A 550 kg mare in her second month of lactation produces 18 kg of milk per day with a dietary crude protein requirement of 50 g/kg milk (milk is ~2% crude protein, with an efficiency of dietary protein use for milk production of 50% and estimated dietary protein digestibility of 79%): = (1.44 g/kg/day × 550 kg) + [18 kg × 50 g dietary protein/kg milk) = 1692 g protein/day
Exercise	Maintenance protein requirement + Protein needs for muscle growth + Protein needs to replace sweat losses[b] Example: A 600 kg competitive dressage horse in active training (heavy intensity workload) may deposit about 40 g of protein each day in muscle gains, with an efficiency of 30%. Sweat is produced at an estimated rate of 1% of body weight, with a protein content of 7.8 g protein/kg sweat, with an efficiency of dietary protein use for sweating of 50%. Estimated dietary protein digestibility is 79%: = (1.26 g/kg/day ×600 kg) + [(40 g/day)/(0.30 × 0.79)] + [(0.01 × 600 kg × 7.8®g/kg)/(0.50 × 0.79)] = 1043 g protein/day

[a]Protein needs for growth change throughout growth due to changes in average daily gain and declines in the efficiency of protein use for gain.
[b]Protein needs for muscle growth and to replace sweat losses will vary with the intensity of the exercise regime.

acids or inadequate total nitrogen intake that limits dispensable amino acid synthesis. Energy is typically the most limiting ingredient in the standard forage/grain diets that horses consume (NRC 2007); therefore, if adequate energy is consumed, generally enough total nitrogen is consumed to synthesize the dispensable amino acids. However, depending on the amino acid composition of diet ingredients, one or more of the indispensable amino acids may be limiting to protein synthesis (Graham-Thiers & Kronfeld 2005b).

Signs of dietary protein deficiency in horses are similar to the signs in other mammals: general non-thriftiness, depressed feed intake, weight loss, and poor hoof and hair coat quality (NRC 1989, 2007). These generic protein deficiency signs are all related to reductions in whole-body protein synthesis. If an indispensable amino acid is deficient in growing horses, this will be reflected by lower rates of average daily gain (Breuer et al 1970, Breuer & Golden 1971, Ott et al 1979, 1981), whereas a limiting amino acid during lactation could reduce milk protein and amino acid content and reduce rates of foal growth (Glade & Luba 1987). Other studies have also reported reduced milk production, increased weight loss in mares and reduced rates of foal growth if insufficient dietary protein is provided during lactation (summarized in the *Nutrient Requirements of Horses* (2007)). Because exercise training may increase lean mass and total nitrogen retention (Freeman et al 1988), athletic horses that do not consume enough indispensable amino acids or total nitrogen to maintain their increased muscle mass or replace nitrogen losses in sweat will begin to deplete the plasma amino acid pool (McKeever et al 1986) or lose muscle mass (Graham-Thiers & Kronfeld 2005b), resulting in increased nitrogen excretion.

Protein and amino acid excess

Dietary amino acids provided in excess of what can be utilized for protein synthesis and other metabolic functions cannot be stored, but must be catabolized to CO_2 and urea for excretion. With the exception of the BCAA, which are primarily catabolized in the skeletal muscle, the majority of protein catabolism and urea synthesis occurs in the liver. Urea synthesis is metabolically expensive, requiring ATP, meaning that, at least in theory, excess protein intake reduces growth efficiency due to the increased energy expenditure associated with nitrogen excretion. To illustrate, a horse consuming a commercial ration and forage at the rates recommended by the feed manufacturer may consume approximately twice the NRC recommendation (NRC 2007) for crude protein, which in a 600 kg horse would amount to ~2.5 g/kg/day. Based on regression equations that were developed in ponies to relate nitrogen intake to urea production (Prior et al 1974), this level of protein intake would be expected to result in ~400 g/day of urea production. If we account for the energy content of urea and the energy cost of making the urea, approximately 1 Mcal of energy would be associated with this urea production, which is 5% of the daily DE requirement of 20 Mcal/day for a 600 kg horse (NRC 2007). In support of these calculations, mature horses consuming a high protein diet with 15% greater metabolizable energy than the lower protein control diet did not gain any additional weight compared to the control horses, and the authors proposed that the increased dietary energy provided by the high protein diet was being consumed during the nitrogen excretion processes (Connysson et al 2006). Because urea is highly water soluble, excretion of urea also requires substantial amounts of water excretion (Meyer 1987); therefore adequate water intake is especially important when excess protein is fed. High levels of dietary protein intake resulted in reduced blood pH levels in horses both at rest (Graham-Thiers & Kronfeld 2005a) and following repeated sprints (Graham-Thiers et al 2001). Exercise already results in a decrease in blood pH due to lactic acid production (Roneus & Essen-Gustavsson 1997), and if muscle pH drops too low and acidosis develops, muscle fatigue will also occur (Spriet et al 1985). Therefore, a further reduction in blood pH due to excessive protein intake could, in theory, interfere with anaerobic energy production and exacerbate the onset of fatigue, although more rapid fatigue was not reported when the horses fed high protein diets underwent sprint exercise tests (Graham-Thiers et al 2001). In another study, high protein intake (18% crude protein) did not have an effect on heart rate, blood or muscle lactate levels, or muscle and liver glycogen utilization, compared to a control level of protein intake (9% crude protein) in post-absorptive horses performing sub-maximal exercise intensities (Miller-Graber et al 1991).

In healthy sedentary horses, under most circumstances there are few lasting health consequences of excess dietary amino acid intake; however, in horses with compromised liver or kidney function, excess amino acid intake may be extremely detrimental. During liver disease, ammonia produced by amino acid catabolism cannot be effectively metabolized to urea for excretion, resulting in high blood ammonia concentrations (Ralston 1990). In the case of renal failure, urea and other nitrogenous waste products accumulate in the blood, resulting in other signs such as reduced appetite (Jarvis 2009, Ralston 1990). For this reason, horses with known kidney and liver problems are generally fed low-protein diets, in order to reduce excess amino acids that need to be metabolized and excreted (Jarvis 2009, Ralston 1990). Furthermore, in cases of liver disease, inclusion of feed ingredients such as corn and beet pulp with a high BCAA to aromatic (tyrosine and phenylalanine) amino acid ratio are frequently advocated to prevent the accumulation of ammonia as well as aromatic amino acids in the blood (Jarvis 2009). It is important to note, however, that sustained excess protein intake has not been shown to actually cause kidney and/or liver disease.

Excess levels of intake of certain amino acids may interfere with the metabolism of other structurally related amino acids, in what is referred to as *amino acid antagonism* (Harper et al 1970). Specifically, the excess intake of one amino acid results in a deficiency in another amino acid, despite the fact that the intake of the antagonized amino acid(s) appears to be sufficient to meet the amino acid requirements. Amino acid antagonism has not been formally described in horses; however, in a recent study, a bolus nasogastric dose of leucine to adult horses following a period of either rest or exercise resulted in dramatic declines in plasma isoleucine and valine concentrations (Urschel et al 2010). This apparent antagonistic effect of leucine on the other BCAA in horses has important implications in cases where leucine may be supplemented, because if levels of isoleucine and valine drop to the point where they become limiting, then this would limit whole-body protein synthesis.

Perhaps one of the more overlooked consequences of excess dietary amino acid intake is the effects on the environment relating to high nitrogen excretion. Nitrogen excretion in both the urine and the feces increases with protein intake (Olsman et al 2003) and the excreted nitrogen can be volatized to ammonia and may leech into soils and groundwater, causing environmental acidification and eutrophication of waters [reviewed by (Rotz 2004)]. Ammonia emissions are a major cause of the unpleasant odors of animal housing areas, and are a health concern for workers (Mitloehner & Calvo 2008) and the animals (Drummond et al 1978). In pigs and cattle, reducing dietary crude protein, but still meeting all amino acid requirements, has no effect on animal performance but gives substantial decreases in nitrogen excretion and ammonia emissions (Frank et al 2002, Powers et al 2007). Studies in growing horses receiving low protein diets supplemented with free lysine and/or threonine found no deleterious effects in terms of growth (Graham et al 1994, Ott et al 1981, Staniar et al 2001) and better utilization of dietary protein as shown by reduced plasma urea concentrations and presumably reduced nitrogen excretion (Graham et al 1994). However, in order to implement lower protein diets in horses on a more widespread basis, the indispensable amino acid requirements must be known, in order to ensure that amino acid needs are met even with reduced total protein intake.

Key Points

- Protein deficiency is uncommon in horses fed typical diets that provide adequate dietary energy; however, depending on the protein quality of the diet, one or more individual amino acids may be deficient
- Signs of protein (amino acid) deficiency include weight loss, decreased feed intake, poor hoof and coat quality, decreased rates of gain in growing horses, and reduced milk production and lower rates of foal growth in lactating horses
- Feeding protein above the requirement levels offers no advantage to the horse, is metabolically expensive because excess nitrogen must be converted to urea for excretion and there are environmental consequences of high nitrogen excretion

Summary

Amino acids play many essential roles in the body as components of both protein and non-protein molecules. Prececal protein digestion and amino acid absorption in horses is believed to be similar to other monogastric species, with anywhere from ~30–80% of dietary protein being absorbed in the small intestine, depending on the specific feed ingredient. Although the abundant numbers of large intestinal microbes are able to use dietary amino acids to synthesize microbial protein, it is unknown how available this protein is to the horse for digestion and it does not appear that significant amounts of microbially derived amino acids can be absorbed in the large intestine. Horses receive their dietary amino acids from three key sources: forage, cereal grains, and seed meals. There are also many supplements currently being marketed for a variety of purposes that contain individual amino acids; however, at this time there is insufficient data to verify the majority of the supplement claims. In comparison to other species, relatively little is known about the individual indispensable amino acid requirements of horses, or how these change throughout the lifespan, and therefore protein requirements for horses are generally expressed on a crude protein basis. There are many avenues of future research that should be pursued in order to improve our understanding of protein and amino acid metabolism in horses.

References

Allmang, C., Wurth, L., Krol, A., 2009. The selenium to selenoprotein pathway in eukaryotes: more molecular partners than anticipated. Biochim Biophys Acta 1790, 1415–1423.

Almeida, F.Q., Valdares Filho, S.C., Donzele, J.L., et al., 1999a. Prececal digestibility of amino acids in diets for horses. Proceedings of the 16th Equine Nutrition and Physiology Symposium 274–279.

Almeida, F.Q., Valdares Filho, S.C., Queiroz, A.C., et al., 1999b. Endogenous nitrogen losses at the prececal, postileal, fecal, and urinary levels in horses. Proceedings of the 16th Equine Nutrition and Physiology Symposium 280–285.

Antilley, T.J., Potter, G.D., Gibbs, P.G., et al., 2007. Evaluating the technique of using nitrogen retention as a response criterion for amino acid studies in the horse. J Equine Vet Sci 27, 525–530.

Badiani, A., Nanni, N., Gatta, P.P., et al., 1997. Nutrient profile of horsemeat. J Food Comp Anal 10, 254–269.

Bagshaw, C.S., Ralston, S.L., Fisher, H., 1994. Behavioral and physiological effect of orally administered tryptophan on horses subjected to acute isolation stress. Appl Anim Behav Sci 40, 1–12.

Bai, J.P., 1993. Distribution of brush-border membrane peptidases along the intestine of rabbits and rats: implication for site-specific delivery of peptide drugs. J Drug Target 1, 231–236.

Baker, D.H., Boebel, K.P., 1980. Utilization of the D- and L-isomers of methionine and methionine hydroxy analogue as determined by chick bioassay. J Nutr 110, 959–964.

Baker, K.M., Stein, H.H., 2009. Amino acid digestibility and concentration of digestible and metabolizable energy in soybean meal produced from conventional, high-protein, or low-oligosaccharide varieties of soybeans and fed to growing pigs. J Anim Sci 87, 2282–2290.

Ball, D.M., Hoveland, C.S., Lacefield, G.D., 2002. Southern Forages. Potash and Phosphate. Inst and Foundation for Agronomic Res., Norcross GA.

Ball, R.O., Urschel, K.L., Pencharz, P.B., 2007. Nutritional consequences of interspecies differences in arginine and lysine metabolism. J Nutr 137, 1626S–1641S.

Bertolo, R.F., Brunton, J.A., Pencharz, P.B., et al., 2003. Arginine, ornithine, and proline interconversion is dependent on small intestinal metabolism in neonatal pigs. Am J Physiol Endocrinol Metab 284, E915–E922.

Bertolo, R.F., Chen, C.Z., Law, G., et al., 1998. Threonine requirement of neonatal piglets receiving total parenteral nutrition is considerably lower than that of piglets receiving an identical diet intragastrically. J Nutr 128, 1752–1759.

Bochroder, B., Schubert, R., Bodeker, D., 1994. Studies on the transport in vitro of lysine, histidine, arginine and ammonia across the mucosa of the equine colon. Equine Vet J 26, 131–133.

Brass, E.P., 2000. Supplemental carnitine and exercise. Am J Clin Nutr 72, 618S–623S.

Breuer, L.H., Golden, D.L., 1971. Lysine requirement of the immature equine. J Anim Sci 33, 227.

Breuer, L.H., Kasten, L.H., Word, J.D., 1970. Protein and amino acid utilization in the young horse. Proceedings of the 2nd Equine Nutrition Research Symposium 16–17.

Broer, S., 2008b. Amino acid transport across mammalian intestinal and renal epithelia. Physiol Rev 88, 249–286.

Broer, S., 2008a. Amino acid transport across mammalian intestinal and renal epithelia. Physiol Rev 88, 249–286.

Brunton, J.A., Shoveller, A.K., Pencharz, P.B., et al., 2007. The indicator amino acid oxidation method identified limiting amino acids in two parenteral nutrition solutions in neonatal piglets. J Nutr 137, 1253–1259.

Bryden, W.L., 1991. Amino acid requirements of horses estimated from tissue composition. Proc Nutr Soc Aust 16, 53.

Burke, D.G., Chilibeck, P.D., Parise, G., et al., 2003. Effect of creatine and weight training on muscle creatine and performance in vegetarians. Med Sci Sports Exerc 35, 1946–1955.

Casini, L., Gatta, D., Magni, L., et al., 2000. Effect of prolonged branched-chain amino acid supplementation on metabolic response to anaerobic exercise in standardbreds. J Equine Vet Sci 20, 120–123.

Cehak, A., Burmester, M., Geburek, F., et al., 2009. Electrophysiological characterization of electrolyte and nutrient transport across the small intestine in horses. J Anim Physiol Anim Nutr (Berl) 93, 287–294.

Chen, H., Wong, E.A., Webb, K.E., Jr., 1999. Tissue distribution of a peptide transporter mRNA in sheep, dairy cows, pigs, and chickens. J Anim Sci 77, 1277–1283.

Chen, H., Pan, Y., Wong, E.A., et al., 2002. Molecular cloning and functional expression of a chicken intestinal peptide transporter (cPepT1) in *Xenopus* oocytes and Chinese hamster ovary cells. J Nutr 132, 387–393.

Chung, T.K., Baker, D.H., 1992. Utilization of methionine isomers and analogs by the pig. Can J Anim Sci 72, 185–188.

Clark, A.K., Rakes, A.H., 1982. Effect of methionine hydroxy analog supplementation on dairy cattle hoof growth and composition. J Dairy Sci 65, 1493–1502.

Closs, E.I., Simon, A., Vekony, N., et al., 2004. Plasma membrane transporters for arginine. J Nutr 134, 2752S–2759S.

Coblentz, W.K., Fritz, J.O., Fick, W.H., et al., 1998. In situ dry matter, nitrogen, and fiber degradation of alfalfa, red clover, and eastern gamagrass at four maturities. J Dairy Sci 81, 150–161.

Coleman, R.A., Bertolo, R.F., Moehn, S., et al., 2003. Lysine requirements of pre-lay broiler breeder pullets: determination by indicator amino acid oxidation. J Nutr 133, 2826–2829.

Connysson, M., Muhonen, S., Lindberg, J.E., et al., 2006. Effects of exercise response, fluid and acid-base balance of protein intake from forage-only diets in Standardbred horses. Equine Vet J Suppl 36, 648–653.

D'Angelis, F.H., Ferraz, G.C., Boleli, I.C., et al., 2005. Aerobic training, but not creatine supplementation, alters the gluteus medius muscle. J Anim Sci 83, 579–585.

Dardevet, D., Sornet, C., Bayle, G., et al., 2002. Postprandial stimulation of muscle protein synthesis in old rats can be restored by a leucine-supplemented meal. J Nutr 132, 95–100.

Davis, T.A., Nguyen, H.V., Garcia-Bravo, R., et al., 1994a. Amino acid composition of human milk is not unique. J Nutr 124, 1126–1132.

Davis, T.A., Nguyen, H.V., Garcia-Bravo, R., et al., 1994b. Amino acid composition of the milk of some mammalian species changes with stage of lactation. Br J Nutr 72, 845–853.

Davison, K.E., Potter, G.D., Greene, L.W., et al., 1991. Lactation and reproductive performance of mares fed added dietary fat during late gestation and early lactation. J Equine Vet Sci 11, 111–115.

Doreau, M., Boulot, S., Bauchart, D., et al., 1992. Voluntary intake, milk production and plasma metabolites in nursing mares fed two different diets. J Nutr 122, 992–999.

Dreyer, H.C., Drummond, M.J., Pennings, B., et al., 2008. Leucine-enriched essential amino acid and carbohydrate ingestion following resistance exercise enhances mTOR signaling and protein synthesis in human muscle. Am J Physiol Endocrinol Metab 294, E392–E400.

Drummond, J.G., Curtis, S.E., Simon, J., 1978. Effects of atmospheric ammonia on pulmonary bacterial clearance in the young pig. Am J Vet Res 39, 211–212.

Duckworth, D.H., Madison, J.B., Calderwood-Mays, M., et al., 1992. Arteriovenous differences for glutamine in the equine gastrointestinal tract. Am J Vet Res 53, 1864–1867.

Elango, R., Ball, R.O., Pencharz, P.B., 2008. Indicator amino acid oxidation: concept and application. J Nutr 138, 243–246.

Elango, R., Humayun, M.A., Ball, R.O., et al., 2007. Lysine requirement of healthy school-age children determined by the indicator amino acid oxidation method. Am J Clin Nutr 86, 360–365.

Elango, R., Humayun, M.A., Ball, R.O., et al., 2010. Evidence that protein requirements have been significantly underestimated. Curr Opin Clin Nutr Metab Care 13, 52–57.

Elizalde, J.C., Merchen, N.R., Faulkner, D.B., 1999. Fractionation of fiber and crude protein in fresh forages during the spring growth. J Anim Sci 77, 476–484.

Farley, E.B., Potter, G.D., Gibbs, P.G., et al., 1995. Digestion of soybean meal protein in the equine small and large intestine at various levels of intake. J Equine Vet Sci 15, 391–397.

Farris, J.W., Hinchcliff, K.W., McKeever, K.H., et al., 1998. Effect of tryptophan and of glucose on exercise capacity of horses. J Appl Physiol 85, 807–816.

Foster, C.V., Harris, R.C., Snow, D.H., 1988. The effect of oral L-carnitine supplementation on the muscle and plasma concentrations in the Thoroughbred horse. Comp Biochem.Physiol A Comp Physiol 91, 827–835.

Frank, B., Persson, M., Gustafsson, G., 2002. Feeding dairy cows for decreased ammonia emission. Livestock Production Science 76, 171–179.

Freeman, D.E., Donawick, W.J., 1991. In vitro transport of cycloleucine by equine cecal mucosa. Am J Vet Res 52, 539–542.

Freeman, D.E., Kleinzeller, A., Donawick, W.J., et al., 1989. In vitro transport of L-alanine by equine cecal mucosa. Am J Vet Res 50, 2138–2144.

Freeman, D.W., Potter, G.D., Schelling, G.T., et al., 1988. Nitrogen metabolism in mature horses at varying levels of work. J Anim Sci 66, 407–412.

Freeman, T.C., Bentsen, B.S., Thwaites, D.T., et al., 1995. H^+/di-tripeptide transporter (PepT1) expression in the rabbit intestine. Pflugers Arch 430, 394–400.

Garcia, L., Perez-Alba, L., Alvarez, C., et al., 1995. Prediction of the nutritive value of Lucerne hay in diets for growing rabbits. Animal Feed Sci Tech 54, 33–44.

Gibbs, P.G., Potter, G.D., Blake, R.W., et al., 1982. Milk production of quarter horse mares during 150 days of lactation. J Anim Sci 54, 496–499.

Gibbs, P.G., Potter, G.D., Schelling, G.T., et al., 1988. Digestion of hay protein in different segments of the equine digestive tract. J Anim Sci 66, 400–406.

Gibbs, P.G., Potter, G.D., Schelling, G.T., et al., 1996. The significance of small vs large intestinal digestion of cereal grain and oilseed protein in the equine. Journal of Equine Veterinary Science 16, 60–65.

Gilbert, E.R., Wong, E.A., Webb, K.E., Jr., 2008a. Board-invited review: Peptide absorption and utilization: Implications for animal nutrition and health. J Anim Sci 86, 2135–2155.

Gilbert, E.R., Wong, E.A., Webb, K.E., Jr., 2008b. Board-invited review: Peptide absorption and utilization: Implications for animal nutrition and health. J Anim Sci 86, 2135–2155.

Glade, M., 1989. Effects of specific amino acid supplementation lactic acid production by horses exercised on a treadmill. 11th Conference of the Equine Nutrition and Physiology Symposium 244–248.

Glade, M.J., 1991. Dietary yeast culture supplementation of mares during late gestation and early lactation-effects on milk production, milk composition, weight gain and linear growth of nursing foals. J Equine Vet Sci 11, 89–95.

Glade, M.J., Luba, N.K., 1987. Benefits to foals of feeding soybean meal to lactating broodmares. Proceedings of the 10th Equine Nutrition and Physiology Symposium 593–597.

Gonzalez, J., Faria-Marmol, J., Rodriguez, C.A., et al., 2001. Effects of stage of harvest on the protein value of fresh lucerne for ruminants. Reprod Nutr Dev 41, 381–392.

Graham, P.M., Ott, E.A., Brendemuhl, J.H., et al., 1994. The effect of supplemental lysine and threonine on growth and development of yearling horses. J Anim Sci 72, 380–386.

Graham-Thiers, P.M., Kronfeld, D.S., 2005a. Dietary protein influences acid-base balance in sedentary horses. J Equine Vet Sci 25, 434–438.

Graham-Thiers, P.M., Kronfeld, D.S., 2005b. Amino acid supplementation improves muscle mass in aged and young horses. J Anim Sci 83, 2783–2788.

Graham-Thiers, P.M., Kronfeld, D.S., Kline, K.A., et al., 2001. Dietary protein restriction and fat supplementation diminish the acidogenic effect of exercise during repeated sprints in horses. J Nutr 131, 1959–1964.

Grimmett, A., Sillence, M.N., 2005. Calmatives for the excitable horse: a review of L-tryptophan. Vet.J 170, 24–32.

Harmeyer, J., Coenen, M., Verfuehrt, I., et al., 2001. Effect of L-carnitine (LC) supplementation during training on muscle carnitine and plasma biochemical values. Proceedings of the 2nd Equine Nutrition Research Symposium 282.

Harper, A.E., Benevenga, N.J., Wohlhueter, R.M., 1970. Effects of ingestion of disproportionate amounts of amino acids. Physiol Rev 50, 428–558.

Harris, P., 1997. Feeds and feeding in the United Kingdom, In: Current Therapy in Equine Medicine 4, Robinson, N.E. (Ed.), Saunders Co, Philadelphia, PA, pp. 698–704.

Harris, P.A., Harris, R.C., 2005. Ergogenic potential of nutritional strategies and substances in the horse. Livestock Prod Sci 92, 147–165.

Harris, R.C., Foster, C.V.L., Snow, D.H., 1995. Plasma carnitine concentration and uptake into muscle with oral and intravenous administration. Equine Vet J Suppl 18, 382–387.

Hintz, H.F., Schryver, H.F., Lowe, J.E., 1971. Comparison of a blend of milk products and linseed meal as protein supplements for young growing horses. J Anim Sci 33, 1274–1277.

Hintz, H.F., Schryver, H.F., 1972. Nitrogen utilization in ponies. J Anim Sci 34, 592–595.

Hoskin, S.O., Gee, E.K., 2004. Feeding value of pastures for horses. N Z Vet J 52, 332–341.

House, J.D., Pencharz, P.B., Ball, R.O., 1998. Lysine requirement of neonatal piglets receiving total parenteral nutrition as determined by oxidation of the indicator amino acid L-[1-14C]phenylalanine. Am J Clin Nutr 67, 67–73.

Humayun, M.A., Elango, R., Ball, R.O., et al., 2007a. Reevaluation of the protein requirement in young men with the indicator amino acid oxidation technique. Am J Clin Nutr 86, 995–1002.

Humayun, M.A., Elango, R., Moehn, S., et al., 2007b. Application of the indicator amino acid oxidation technique for the determination of metabolic availability of sulfur amino acids from casein versus soy protein isolate in adult men. J Nutr 137, 1874–1879.

Iqbal, A., Khalil, I.A., Ateeq, N., et al., 2010. Nutritional quality of important food legumes. Food Chem 97, 331–335.

Jarvis, N.G., 2009. Nutrition of the aged horse. Vet Clin North Am Equine Pract 25, 155–166, viii.

Kimball, S.R., 2007. The role of nutrition in stimulating muscle protein accretion at the molecular level. Biochem Soc Trans 35, 1298–1301.

Kreider, R.B., 2003. Effects of creatine supplementation on performance and training adaptations. Mol Cell Biochem 244, 89–94.

Kriengsinyos, W., Wykes, L.J., Ball, R.O., et al., 2002. Oral and intravenous tracer protocols of the indicator amino acid oxidation method provide the same estimate of the lysine requirement in healthy men. J Nutr 132, 2251–2257.

Kriengsinyos, W., Wykes, L.J., Goonewardene, L.A., et al., 2004. Phase of menstrual cycle affects lysine requirement in healthy women. Am J Physiol Endocrinol Metab 287, E489–E496.

Larson, J., Hoffman, P.C., 2008. Technical note: a method to quantify prolamin proteins in corn that are negatively related to starch digestibility in ruminants. J Dairy Sci 91, 4834–4839.

Laven, R.A., Livesey, C.T., 2004. The effect of housing and methionine intake on hoof horn hemorrhages in primiparous lactating Holstein cows. J Dairy Sci 87, 1015–1023.

Law, G.K., Bertolo, R.F., Adjiri-Awere, A., et al., 2007. Adequate oral threonine is critical for mucin production and gut function in neonatal piglets. Am J Physiol Gastrointest Liver Physiol 292, G1293–G1301.

Lawrence, L., Hayes, S., Allman, R., et al., 2006. Seasonal variation in cool season grasses. J Anim Sci 84 (Supplement 1), 331.

Lewis, A.J., Baker, D.H., 1995. Bioavailability of D-amino acids and DL-hydroxymethionine. In: Ammerman, C.B., Baker, D.H., Lewis, A.J. (Eds.), Bioavailability of nutrients for animals. Academic Press, San Diego, CA, pp. 67–82.

Lewis, A.J., Bayley, H.S., 1995. Amino acid bioavailability, In: Ammerman, C.B., Baker, D.H., Lewis, A.J. (Eds.), Bioavailability of nutrients for animals. Academic Press, San Diego, CA, pp. 35–65.

Maczulak, A.E., Dawson, K.A., Baker, J.P., 1985. Nitrogen utilization in bacterial isolates from the equine cecum. Appl Environ Microbiol 50, 1439–1443.

Malmkvist, J., Christensen, J.W., 2007. A note on the effects of a commercial tryptophan product on horse reactivity. Appl Anim Behav Sci 107, 361–366.

Mariani, P., Summer, A., Martuzzi, F., et al., 2001. Physicochemical properties, gross composition, energy value and nitrogen fractions of Haflinger nursing mare milk throughout 6 lactation months. Anim Res 50, 415–425.

Martin-Rosset, W., 2001. Feeding standards for energy and protein for horses in France. In: Pagan, J.D. (Ed.), Advances in Equine Nutrition - Volume 2. Kentucky Equine Research, Versailles KY, pp. 31–94.

Martin-Rosset, W., Ellis, A.D., 2005. Evaluation of energy and protein requirements and recommended allowances in growing horses, In: Julliand, V., Martin-Rosset, W. (Eds.), The Growing Horse: Nutrition, and Prevention of Growth Disorders (EAAP publication 114). Wageningen Academic Publishers, Wageningen Netherlands, pp. 103–135.

Martinez, T., Miller-Graber, P.A., Thompson, J., 1993. Taurine and selected free amino acids in colostrums and milk of mares with clinically normal foals. Proceedings of the 13th Equine Nutrition and Physiology Symposium 254–255.

McKeever, K.H., Schurg, W.A., Jarrett, S.H., et al., 1986. Resting concentrations of the plasma free amino acids in horses following chronic submaximal exercise training. J Equine Vet Sci 6, 87–92.

McMeniman, N.P., Elliott, R., Groenendyk, S., et al., 1987. Synthesis and absorption of cysteine from the hindgut of the horse. Equine Vet J 19, 192–194.

Meredith, C.N., Wen, Z.M., Bier, D.M., et al., 1986. Lysine kinetics at graded lysine intakes in young men. Am J Clin Nutr 43, 787–794.

Meyer, H., 1987. Nutrition of the Equine Athlete. In: Gillespie, J.R., Robinson, N.E. (Eds.), Equine Exercise Physiology 2. ICEEP Publications, Davis, CA, pp. 644–673.

Meyer, H., 1983. Protein metabolism and protein requirement in horses. Fourth Int.Symp.Protein Metabolism and Nutrition 343–364.

Meyer, H., von Stein, S., Schmidt, M., 1985. Investigations to determine endogenous faecal and renal N losses in horses. Proceedings of the 9th Equine Nutrition and Physiology Symposium 68–72.

Miller-Graber, P.A., Lawrence, L.M., Foreman, J.H., et al., 1991. Dietary protein level and energy metabolism during treadmill exercise in horses. J Nutr 121, 1462–1469.

Mitloehner, F.M., Calvo, M.S., 2008. Worker health and safety in concentrated animal feeding operations. J Agric Saf Health 14, 163–187.

Moehn, S., Bertolo, R.F., Pencharz, P.B., et al., 2004. Indicator amino acid oxidation responds rapidly to changes in lysine or protein intake in growing and adult pigs. J Nutr 134, 836–841.

Moehn, S., Bertolo, R.F., Pencharz, P.B., et al., 2005. Development of the indicator amino acid oxidation technique to determine the availability of amino acids from dietary protein in pigs. J Nutr 135, 2866–2870.

Myrie, S.B., Bertolo, R.F., Sauer, W.C., et al., 2008. Effect of common antinutritive factors and fibrous feedstuffs in pig diets on amino acid digestibilities with special emphasis on threonine. J Anim Sci 86, 609–619.

National Research Council, 1949. Recommended Nutrient Allowances for Horses. National Academy of Sciences publication, Washington DC.

National Research Council, 1961. Nutrient Requirements of Horses, first ed. National Academy of Sciences, Washington DC.

National Research Council, 1966. Nutrient Requirements of Horses, second ed. National Acedemy of Sciences, Washington DC.

National Research Council, 1973, Nutrient Requirements of Horses, third ed. National Academy of Sciences, Washington DC.

National Research Council, 1978, Nutrient Requirements of Horses, fourth ed. National Academy of Sciences, Washington DC.

National Research Council, 1989, Nutrient Requirements of Horses, fifth ed. National Academy Press, Washington DC.

National Research Council, 1994, Nutrient Requirements of Poultry, ninth ed. National Academy Press, Washington DC.

National Research Council, 1998, Nutrient Requirements of Swine, tenth ed. National Academy Press, Washington DC.

National Research Council, 2001, Nutrient Requirements of Dairy Cattle, seventh ed. National Academy Press, Washington DC.

National Research Council, 2007, Nutrient Requirements of Horses, sixth ed. National Academies Press, Washington DC.

Nichols, N.L., Bertolo, R.F., 2008. Luminal threonine concentration acutely affects intestinal mucosal protein and mucin synthesis in piglets. J Nutr 138, 1298–1303.

Noble, G.K., Brockwell, Y.M., Munn, K.J., et al., 2008. Effects of a commercial dose of L-tryptophan on plasma tryptophan concentrations and behaviour in horses. Equine Vet J 40, 51–56.

Ohta, Y., Yoshida, T., Ishibashi, T., 2007. Estimation of dietary lysine requirement using plasma amino acid concentrations in mature thoroughbreds. Anim Sci J 78, 41–46.

Olsman, A.F., Jansen, W.L., Sloet van Oldruitenborgh-Oosterbaan, M.M., et al., 2003. Assessment of the minimum protein requirement of adult ponies. J Anim Physiol Anim Nutr (Berl) 87, 205–212.

Ott, E.A., Asquith, R.L., Feaster, J.P., et al., 1979. Influence of protein level and quality on the growth and development of yearling foals. J Anim Sci 49, 620–628.

Ott, E.A., Asquith, R.L., Feaster, J.P. 1981. Lysine supplementation of diets for yearling horses. J Anim Sci 53, 1496–1503.

Paradis, M.R., Breeze, R.G., Bayly, W.M., et al., 1991. Acute hemolytic anemia after oral administration of L-tryptophan in ponies. Am J Vet Res 52, 742–747.

Pencharz, P.B., Ball, R.O., 2003. Different approaches to define individual amino acid requirements. Annu Rev Nutr 23, 101–116.

Potter, G.D., Huchton, J.D., 1975. Growth of yearling horses fed different sources of protein with supplemental lysine. Proceedings of the 4th Equine Nutrition and Physiology Symposium 19–10.

Powers, W.J., Zamzow, S.B., Kerr, B.J., 2007. Reduced crude protein effects on aerial emissions from swine. Appl Eng Agric 23, 539–546.

Prior, R.L., Hintz, H.F., Lowe, J.E., et al., 1974. Urea recycling and metabolism of ponies. J Anim Sci 38, 565–571.

Ralston, S.L., 1990. Clinical nutrition of adult horses. Vet Clin North Am Equine Pract 6, 339–354.

Rand, W.M., Young, V.R., Scrimshaw, N.S., 1976. Change of urinary nitrogen excretion in response to low-protein diets in adults. Am.J Clin.Nutr 29, 639–644.

Reitnour, C.M., Baker, J.P., Mitchell, G.E., Jr., et al., 1970. Amino acids in equine cecal contents, cecal bacteria and serum. J Nutr 100, 349–354.

Reitnour, C.M., Salsbury, R.L., 1972. Digestion and utilization of cecally infused protein by the equine. J Anim Sci 35, 1190–1193.

Rieu, I., Balage, M., Sornet, C., et al., 2006. Leucine supplementation improves muscle protein synthesis in elderly men independently of hyperaminoacidaemia. J Physiol 575, 305–315.

Roneus, N., Essen-Gustavsson, B., 1997. Skeletal muscle characteristics and metabolic response to exercise in young standardbreds. Am.J Vet Res 58, 167–170.

Rosenfeld, I., Austbo, D., 2009. Effect of type of grain and feed processing on gastrointestinal retention times in horses. J Anim Sci 87, 3991–3996.

Rotz, C.A., 2004. Management to reduce nitrogen losses in animal production. J Anim Sci 82 (E-Suppl), E119–E137.

Schuback, K., Essen-Gustavsson, B., Persson, S.G., 2000. Effect of creatine supplementation on muscle metabolic response to a maximal treadmill exercise test in Standardbred horses. Equine Vet J 32, 533–540.

Schubert, R., Zander, R., Gruhn, K., et al, 1991. First results on the incorporation and excretion of 15N from orally administered urea in lactating pony mares. Arch Tierernahr 41, 457–463.

Sewell, D.A., Harris, R.C., Marlin, D.J., et al., 1992. Estimation of the carnosine content of different fibre types in the middle gluteal muscle of the thoroughbred horse. J Physiol 455, 447–453.

Slade, L.M., Bishop, R., Morris, J.G., et al., 1971. Digestion and absorption of 15N-labelled microbial protein in the large intestine of the horse. Br Vet J 127, 11–13.

Slade, L.M., Robinson, D.W., Casey, K.E., 1970. Nitrogen metabolism in non-ruminant herbivores. I. The influence of nonprotein nitrogen and protein quality on the nitrogen retention of adult mares. J Anim Sci 30, 753–760.

Smith, M.B., Amos, H.E., Froetschel, M.A., 1999. Influence of ruminally undegraded protein and zinc methionine on milk production, hoof growth and composition, and selected plasma metabolites of high producing dairy cattle. The Professional Animal Scientist 15, 268–277.

Spriet, L.L., Matsos, C.G., Peters, S.J., et al., 1985. Effects of acidosis on rat muscle metabolism and performance during heavy exercise. Am.J Physiol 248, C337–C347.

Staniar, W.B., Kronfeld, D.S., Wilson, J.A., et al., 2001. Growth of thoroughbreds fed a low-protein supplement fortified with lysine and threonine. J Anim Sci 79, 2143–2151.

Stefanon, B., Bettini, C., Guggia, G., 2000. Administration of branched-chain amino acids to standardbred horses in training. J Equine Vet Sci 20, 115–119.

Stoll, B., Henry, J., Reeds, P.J., et al., 1998. Catabolism dominates the first-pass intestinal metabolism of dietary essential amino acids in milk protein-fed piglets. J Nutr 128, 606–614.

Thorpe, J.M., Roberts, S.A., Ball, R.O., et al., 1999. Prior protein intake may affect phenylalanine kinetics measured in healthy adult volunteers consuming 1 g protein. kg-1. d-1. J Nutr 129, 343–348.

Ullrey, D.E., Struthers, R.D., Hendricks, D.G., et al., 1966. Composition of mare's milk. J Anim Sci 25, 217–222.

Urschel, K.L., Geor, R.J., Waterfall, H.L., et al., 2010. Effects of leucine or whey protein addition to an oral glucose solution on plasma glucose, insulin and amino acid responses in horses at rest and following exercise. Equine Vet J 42 (Suppl 38), 347–354.

van Hall, G., Raaymakers, J.S., Saris, W.H., et al., 1995. Ingestion of branched-chain amino acids and tryptophan during sustained exercise in man: failure to affect performance. J Physiol 486 (Pt 3), 789–794.

Vanhatalo, A., Kuoppala, K., Ahvenjarvi, S., et al., 2009. Effects of feeding grass or red clover silage cut at two maturity stages in dairy cows. 1. Nitrogen metabolism and supply of amino acids. J Dairy Sci 92, 5620–5633.

Vaz, F.M., Wanders, R.J., 2002. Carnitine biosynthesis in mammals. Biochem J 361, 417–429.

Vervuert, I., Coenen, M., Watermulder, E., 2005. Metabolic responses to oral tryptophan supplementation before exercise in horses. J Anim Physiol Anim Nutr (Berl) 89, 140–145.

Wall, L.H., Potter, G.D., Gibbs, P.G., et al., 1998. Growth of yealing fillies fed alfalfa or soybean meal. J Equine Vet Sci 18, 266–269.

Wallace, R.J., 1996. Ruminal microbial metabolism of peptides and amino acids. J Nutr 126, 1326S–1334S.

Woodward, A.D., Holcombe, S.J., Steibel, J.P., et al., 2009. Cationic and neutral amino acid transporter transcript abundances are differentially expressed in the equine intestinal tract. J Anim Sci .

World Health Organization, 2007. Protein and Amino Acid Requirements in Human Nutrition. WHO Technical Report Series #935 WHO Press, Geneva.

Wysocki, A.A., Baker, J.P., 1975. Utilization of bacterial protein from the lower gut of the equine. Proceedings of the 4th Equine Nutrition and Physiology Symposium 21–43.

Yu, P., Rossnagel, B.G., Niu, Z., 2008. Protein value of a new genotype oat (CDC SO-I) for the NRC dairy model: Protein degradation balance and kinetics, protein fractions and total metabolizable protein supply. Can J Anim Sci 88, 507–513.

Zello, G.A., Pencharz, P.B., Ball, R.O., 1993. Dietary lysine requirement of young adult males determined by oxidation of L-[1-13C]phenylalanine. Am J Physiol 264, E677–E685.

Zello, G.A., Pencharz, P.B., Ball, R.O., 1990. Phenylalanine flux, oxidation, and conversion to tyrosine in humans studied with L-[1-13C]phenylalanine. Am J Physiol 259, E835–E843.

7

SECTION A Nutritional Foundations

Fat and fatty acids

Lori K. Warren, Kelly R. Vineyard

Historically fats and oils have been added to equine diets in relatively small quantities to improve the luster and shine of the hair coat, as well as to reduce dust, eliminate fines and aid in feed processing, such as pelleting. Although fat continues to be used today for some of the same reasons, recognition of the ability of horses to assimilate large amounts of dietary fat has encouraged inclusion of greater quantities in the diet. Fat's high energy density and efficiency of utilization have made it the "go-to" nutrient when additional calories are needed or as an alternative energy source to nonstructural carbohydrates (NSC). The characteristics and feeding potential of fat have inspired a great deal of research and led to the creation of high-fat feeds and supplements that are now widely available. Of late, there has been interest in the role that specific fatty acids (e.g., omega-3 and omega-6) play in various physiological functions. The purpose of this chapter is to summarize what is currently known about the horse's ability to utilize dietary fat and the benefits that potentially can be derived from fat-supplemented diets. The chapter concludes with some practical guidelines for including fat in the diet of horses.

Structural chemistry and nomenclature

Similar to other classes of nutrients, fats are chemically and structurally diverse. The structure of fat has direct bearing on its physical properties, as well as its biological behavior and activity. The naturally-occurring fats in forages and cereal grains exist as a mixture of simple lipids (di- and triacylglycerol, nonesterified fatty acids, waxes and sterols) and complex lipids (glycolipids, and phospholipids) (Hargin & Morrison 1980, Harwood 1996, Zhou et al 1999). By comparison, fats and oils added to equine diets consist mostly of triacylglycerols, which are also commonly referred to as triglycerides. Triacylglycerols consist of three fatty acids esterified to a 3-carbon glycerol molecule (Fig. 7.1). Each fatty acid is a hydrocarbon chain, which can vary in length from 2 to 28 carbons. However, the esterified fatty acids present in most feedstuffs are usually 12 to 22 carbons in length. Nonesterified fatty acids (NEFA) unbound from the glycerol backbone typically make up a very small portion of the fat. In fact, the presence of such "free" fatty acids in a feed or oil is used as an indicator of fat rancidity (oxidation).

Besides length, fatty acids can also differ in their degree of saturation or unsaturation (Figure 7.1). Fatty acids that contain no double bonds between carbon atoms are referred to as saturated fatty acids. Fatty acids with one or more double bonds are referred to as mono- or polyunsaturated fatty acids, respectively. Saturated fatty acids have a high melting point. Fat sources rich in saturated fatty acids, such as animal lard or tallow are solid at room temperature. In contrast, unsaturated fatty acids have a lower melting point, making the fat liquid (i.e., oil) or near liquid at room temperature. Most plant-based fats have relatively high unsaturated fatty acid content; notable exceptions are coconut oil and palm oil. In practice, the term "fat" is commonly used when referring to either solid fats or liquid oils. The usage of "fat" in this chapter will collectively represent the fatty acids, triacylglyercol and other complex lipid components in feeds and oils.

Each fatty acid has a carboxylic acid group at one end of the carbon chain and a methyl group at the other terminus. The carboxyl carbon is referred to as the delta (Δ) carbon, whereas the methyl carbon is the omega (ω or *n*) carbon (Fig. 7.1). Both of these landmarks have been used to reference the position of the double bond(s) in a fatty acid (i.e., the numbering of carbons in the chain can begin at either the Δ or ω carbon). The reference to the omega carbon is often favored when describing essential fatty acids. However, the international nomenclature system preferred by lipid biochemists references the position of double bonds from the delta terminus.

The length of a fatty acid, its degree of unsaturation, and the position of the double bonds within the fatty acid all dictate its biological function. As mentioned, there are numerous methods of nomenclature to identify each fatty acid based on these characteristics. In this chapter, the trivial name of the fatty acid (e.g., linoleic acid) and the shorthand numerical symbols are provided. The latter will consist of two numbers separated by a colon. The number to the left of the colon is the number of carbons in the fatty acid chain and the number to the right denotes the number of double bonds. Where appropriate, the specific omega family (e.g., *n*-3, *n*-6) that the fatty acid belongs to is also noted. For

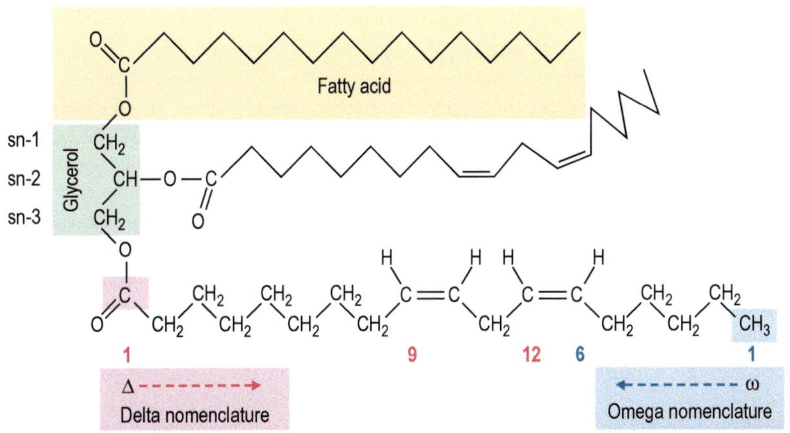

Figure 7.1 Example structure of a triacylglycerol composed of glycerol esterified to three fatty acids. This triacylglycerol has a 16-carbon saturated fatty acid (palmitic acid, 16:0) in the sn-1 position and two 18-carbon polyunsaturated fatty acids (linoleic acid, 18:2*n*-6) in the sn-2 and sn-3 positions. The numerical locations of the double bonds in reference to either the delta or omega terminal carbon have been highlighted in the third fatty acid.

example, the shorthand nomenclature for linoleic acid is 18:2*n*-6, indicating it is an 18-carbon fatty acid with two double bonds and is a member of the omega-6 family (Fig. 7.1). Although the nomenclature system presented herein is susceptible to some ambiguity, it remains the most widely used for identifying specific fatty acids in the scientific and popular literature. The reader is referred elsewhere for a more detailed tutorial on fatty acid nomenclature, including the more formal naming system recognized by the International Union of Pure and Applied Chemists and the International Union of Biochemistry (IUPAC-IUB 1976, Fahy et al 2005).

Key Points

- Dietary fats are chemically and structurally diverse, and may include triacylglycerol, phospholipids, glycolipids and other lipids.
- Plant sources of fat most often consumed by horses are generally rich in unsaturated fatty acids.
- The omega nomenclature system identifies the placement of double bonds from the methyl end of the fatty acid chain.

Fat digestion and absorption

Digestive physiology

Comprehensive study of the mechanisms of fat digestion and absorption in horses has not been performed. Although the basic process is likely similar in all animals, available research has found some aspects unique to equines. Thus, this section will describe the process of fat digestion that is presumed to be in place in horses, as well as highlight those aspects that are known to differ.

In general, digestion of fat consists of three phases: (1) mechanical disruption of large fat droplets into finely dispersed, emulsified particles; (2) enzymatic hydrolysis of lipid esters (i.e., triacylglycerol, phospholipids, and cholesterol esters); and (3) conversion of the water-insoluble products of lipolysis into a soluble form that can be readily absorbed. Mechanical disruption of fat begins in the oral cavity with chewing and continues in the stomach with physical churning. These processes emulsify dietary fat, resulting in the formation of small lipid droplets that provide a larger surface area for the attachment of enzymes and bile salts as the chyme flows through the small intestine.

Enzymatic digestion of fat begins in the stomach. In horses, the zymogen (chief) cells of the fundic mucosa are known to produce large amounts of gastric lipase that exhibits its peak activity at pH 4 (Moreau et al 1988). While it is presumed that gastric lipase initiates hydrolysis of triacylglycerols, the extent of fat lipolysis taking place in the equine stomach is unknown. In other species, the fatty acids released in the stomach are thought to be involved in priming the release of gastrointestinal hormones, which contribute to the emulsification of fat in the duodenum. Cholecystokinin is secreted from the duodenal mucosa in response to partially digested fats and proteins, and triggers the release of bile and pancreatic enzyme secretion. Additionally, the presence of gastric acid in the upper small intestine triggers the release of secretin, which in turn stimulates secretion of bicarbonate from the pancreas.

The products of digestion present in the lumen of the duodenum are one of many factors thought to regulate the rate of gastric emptying. For many species, it is generally believed that fat causes a greater inhibition of gastric emptying than carbohydrate (Meyer et al 1986); however, conflicting results have been reported for equids. Wyse et al (2001) fed ponies a small concentrate meal (0.4–0.6 g/kg BW) of oats and bran to which was added 0, 35 or 70 ml of soybean oil, resulting in meals containing approximately 0, 24 or 38% fat, respectively. Both fat-added meals resulted in a significant delay in gastric emptying compared to a meal without oil as measured by the ^{13}C-octanoic acid breath test. Using a similar technique, Geor et al (2001) found that the addition of corn oil (10%) to a sweet feed meal (2 g/kg BW) slowed gastric emptying in horses. Further, this effect was not influenced by the diet the horse was habituated to (with or without added fat), nor by a 4- or 8-week period of adaptation to a fat supplemented diet. By comparison, consumption of a high fat diet induces adaptation in humans, ultimately reversing the slowing effect of a fatty meal and enhancing gastric emptying (French et al 1995). Unfortunately, the specific role that fat plays in gastric emptying in horses is somewhat confounded in the studies of Wyse et al (2001) and Geor et al (2001), as control and fat-added test diets were not isocaloric. In other species, meal volume, caloric density, viscosity, and osmolality have also been shown to influence gastric motor function (Meyer et al 1986). A possible effect of viscosity was noted by Wyse et al (2001), where a delay in gastric emptying similar to that caused by the addition of soybean oil was observed when an indigestible oil (Olestra®) was added to the test meal. In contrast to these results, a series of studies performed by Lorenzo-Figueras et al (2005) demonstrated that small (0.5 g/kg BW) isocaloric meals high in carbohydrate or containing 8 or 12.3% fat had similar effects on gastric emptying (measured with the ^{13}C-octanoic acid breath test) and proximal gastric tone (measured with an intragastric barostat) in horses. Additional research is needed to clarify the effects of fat on gastric emptying in horses, as the mechanism may differ from other monogastrics that routinely consume greater amounts of dietary fat.

The proposed process of fat digestion and absorption in the small intestine is depicted in Fig. 7.2. As the acidic fat emulsion leaves the stomach and enters the duodenum, it is neutralized and modified by mixing with bile and pancreatic juice. The horse lacks a gall bladder to store bile, and instead bile is continuously secreted by the liver directly into the duodenum. Pancreatic fluid supplies bicarbonate to neutralize the acidic chyme as well as enzymes that cleave fatty acids from triacylglycerol, phospholipids and cholesterol esters. On a relative basis, the equine pancreas produces much more lipase than any other digestive enzyme (e.g., amylase, trypsin) and the activity of pancreatic lipase has been shown to be similar between adult horses, pigs and rats (Lorenzo-Figueras et al 2007). Pancreatic lipase catalyzes the hydrolysis of fatty acids from the outer positions (sn-1 and sn-3) of triacylglycerol, yielding two NEFA and one monoacylglycerol. The activity and efficiency of pancreatic lipase are enhanced by bile salts and pancreatic colipase. Bile salts accumulate on the surface of lipid droplets, increasing the surface area of the oil–water interface and permitting water-soluble lipase to be effective. Colipase ensures adsorption of lipase to the emulsified substrate by acting as an anchor.

The products resulting from lipid hydrolysis in the small intestine assemble into mixed micelles. Micelles contain a monolayer of bile acids, monoacylglycerol and lysophospholipids, which surround a core of NEFA, cholesterol and fat-soluble vitamins. Micelles deliver the lipids to the brush border of the small intestine and, because of their small size, are thought to pass readily into the unstirred water layer at the surface of the microvillus membrane where they release NEFA and monoacylglycerol. A protein-independent diffusion model and protein-dependent mechanisms have been proposed for the uptake and transport of fatty acids across the apical membrane of the enterocyte, although the relative contribution of each mechanism to fatty acid uptake is still unknown (Mansbach & Gorelick 2007). In humans, FAT/CD36 and FABPpm have been identified as fatty acid transport/binding proteins that are important for fatty acid uptake at the intestinal brush border (Mansback & Gorelick 2007, Iqbal & Hussain 2009).

Once inside the enterocyte, fatty acids are transported via cytosolic fatty acid transport/binding proteins to the endoplasmic reticulum where they are re-esterified to form triacylglycerol and phospholipids. The nucleotide sequence of one of these, intestinal fatty acid binding protein (I-FABP), has been characterized in the horse and was shown to share 87% identity with human I-FABP (Nieto et al 2005). In healthy horses, the I-FABP gene was found to be highly expressed in small intestinal mucosa with low expression

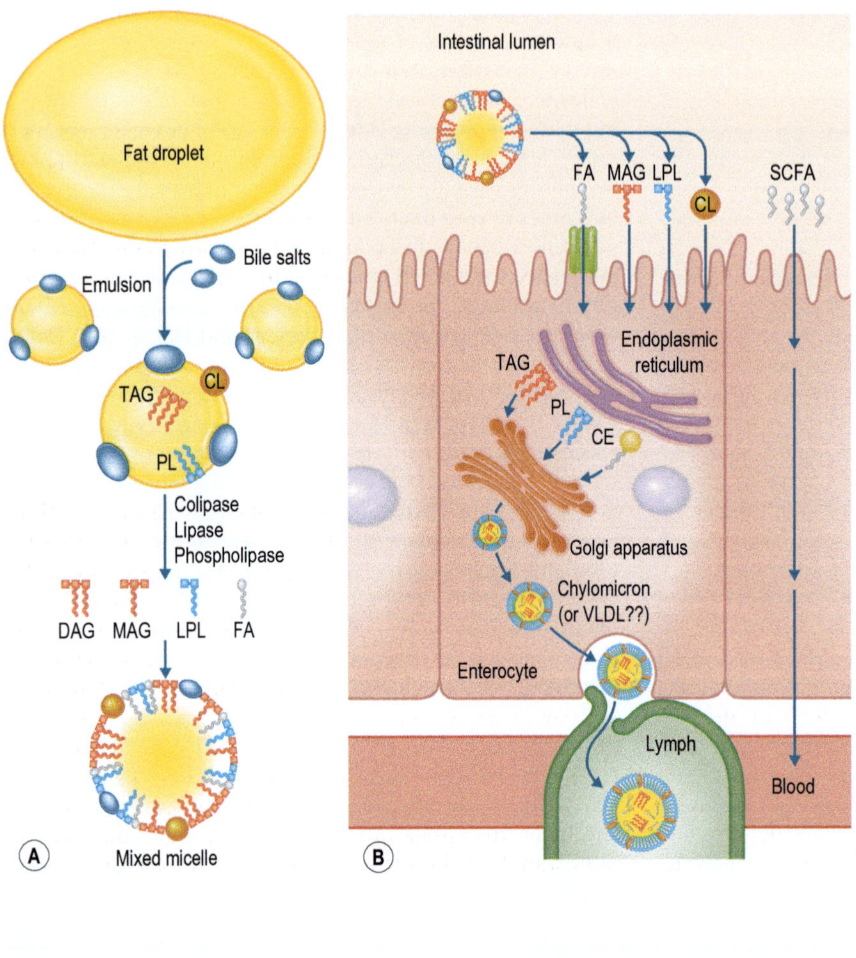

Figure 7.2 Illustration of fat digestion A) and absorption B) in the small intestine. CE = cholesterol ester; CL = cholesterol; DAG = diacylglycerol; FA = fatty acid; LPL = lysophospholipid; MAG = monoacylglycerol; PL = phospholipid; SCFA = short-chain fatty acid; TAG = triacylglycerol; VLDL = very low-density lipoprotein.

observed in the cecum and colon and virtually no expression in stomach mucosa (Nieto et al 2005).

For export into circulation, lipid products are repackaged within the enterocyte, creating a micellar particle with an outer monolayer of phospholipids, proteins and unesterified cholesterol, and a core of triacylglycerol, cholesteryl esters and fat-soluble vitamins. In most mammals, this enterocyte-derived lipoprotein is known as a chylomicron. However, it is unclear whether absorbed triacylglycerol is initially transported via chylomicrons in horses. A chylomicron-like lipoprotein has been identified in the non-fasting plasma of suckling foals, but not in mature horses or ponies maintained on forage and grain diets (see review by Watson et al 1993). Suckling foals were likely consuming more fat from mare milk compared to the mature horses evaluated. However, the fat content of the diet may not be the only factor influencing chylomicron formation as attempts to isolate this lipoprotein fraction from adult ponies following an acute oral fat load were unsuccessful (Watson et al 1993). In contrast, some investigators have reported very small concentrations of chylomicrons in the plasma of horses fed diets with or without added fat (e.g., Marchello et al 2000, van Dijk & Wensing 1989). However, the physical and chemical composition of the lipoprotein fractions were not described sufficiently in these studies to verify if these lipid fractions were in fact chylomicrons and not very low-density lipoproteins (VLDL). Although smaller and less dense, VLDLs are similar to chylomicrons in that they are triacylglycerol-rich. The lack of a chylomicron fraction in horses may reflect a mechanistic adaptation to relatively low fat, forage-based diets. In ruminants, dietary triacylglycerols are transported as modified VLDL when fed diets containing hay, silage and cereal grains, but chylomicrons are synthesized when large amounts of polyunsaturated fatty acids are infused into the small intestine (Byers & Schelling 1988). Even when present, ruminant chylomicrons are typically much smaller, lower in triacylglycerol, higher in phospholipids and less prevalent than described for humans (Byers & Schelling 1988). Differentiation of intestinally-derived chylomicrons (or modified VLDL) from liver-derived VLDL may prove difficult in the horse because the lipoprotein apo-B_{48}, secreted exclusively by the intestine in most mammals, is also secreted by the liver in horses (Greeve et al 1993). Although horses are capable of absorbing dietary fat (see the "Fat Digestibility" section), more study is needed to elucidate the process of triacylglycerol transport from the small intestine and how these mechanism(s) may be modified by diet.

The final phase of absorption involves the fusion of the triacylglycerol-rich lipoprotein (e.g., the chylomicron) with the basolateral membrane of the enterocyte and secretion into the extracellular space by exocytosis. This triacylglycerol-rich lipoprotein does not enter the plasma directly, but instead is excreted into the lacteals of the lymphatic system and eventually passes into circulation via the thoracic duct. Compared to the other products of absorption, dietary fats are unique in that they do not enter the hepatic portal vein and traverse the liver before entering systemic circulation. The exception are short- and medium-chained fatty acids (2 to 12 carbons), which are not re-esterified in the enterocyte and are instead rapidly absorbed into the capillary blood and transported to the liver bound to serum albumin.

The absorption of dietary fat takes place primarily in the distal duodenum and jejunum. Triacylglycerol-rich lipoproteins (e.g., chylomicrons, VLDL) transport absorbed fats and deliver them to the liver, adipose and other tissues. In man, the half-life of a triacylglycerol carried by a chylomicron released from an enterocyte is about 5 minutes, whereas the half-life of a whole chylomicron particle is approximately 13 to 14 minutes (Gurr et al 2002).

Similar to other nutrients, fats that are not digested and absorbed in the small intestine will pass into the hindgut. Based on the difference in ether extract between ileal contents and feces, Swinney et al (1995) reported that little to no fat disappearance occurred in the hindgut of miniature horses fed diets consisting of 35% forage and 65% concentrate that contained 5 to 25% added fat. This agrees with reports in ruminants, where loss of longer chain fatty acids from the rumen either by absorption across the ruminal epithelium or by catabolism to volatile fatty acids or carbon dioxide is minimal (Jenkins 1993). However, dietary fats that escape digestion in the equine small intestine have the potential to interfere with microbial fermentation in the hindgut. The amount of fat entering the hindgut has been shown to increase with increasing intake of soybean oil. Consumption of a concentrate diet with 0, 3.9 and 11% soybean oil resulted in 11, 20 and 99 g fat/kg DM of chyme entering the cecum, respectively (Coenen 1986). When the 11% fat-added concentrate was administered via nasogastric tube transit through the stomach and small intestine was accelerated, resulting in a larger quantity of fat entering the cecum (146 g/kg DM) and evident alterations to the microbiota (Coenen 1986). In ruminants, where the subject has been extensively studied, the negative impact of dietary fat on fiber digestion is believed to result from either the coating of feed particles or a direct toxic effect on rumen microorganisms (Hess et al 2008). The type of dietary fat is also relevant, whereby unsaturated fatty acids have been shown to have greater antimicrobial effects and promote greater inhibition of ruminal fermentation when compared to saturated fatty acids (Hess et al 2008). Presumably the same events would occur in the hindgut of horses, but further investigation on the effects of dietary fat on microbial fermentation using different fat sources and hay to grain ratios is warranted.

Fat digestibility

The digestibility of dietary fat is primarily affected by level of intake and type of lipid. The low levels of naturally-occurring fat in forages and cereal grains appears to be the most difficult for the horse to extract, with apparent digestibility of fat ranging from 5–57% in forages (Fonnesbeck et al 1967, Sturgeon et al 2000) and 55–76% in grains (Hintz & Schryver 1989). In contrast, diets supplemented with various sources of animal fat or vegetable oil have an apparent digestibility between 64% and 96% (Kane et al 1979, McCann et al 1987, Rich et al 1981, Swinney et al 1995, Bush et al 2001). After compiling data from five studies evaluating five basal diets (hay-grain mix, 23–37 g fat/kg DM) and 18 diets with added fat (76–233 g fat/kg DM), Kronfeld et al (2004) reported mean apparent digestibilities of 55% for forages, 81% for mixed diets including added fat, and 95% for added fats. Further modeling of this data indicated that the true digestibility of added fats was nearly 100% (Kronfeld et al 2004).

The reason for the differences in digestibility of naturally-occurring vs. supplemental fat sources is likely multifactorial. Animal fats and vegetable oils supplemented to equine diets are mostly in the form of freely available triacylglycerols. By comparison, fats in forages and grains are surrounded by plant cell wall components which may delay or prevent presentation to lipase in the small intestine. Modeling of data from several feeding trials led Kronfeld et al (2004) to suggest that enzymatic hydrolysis of fat might be slower as a consequence of the low fat intakes associated with forage and grains. In addition, although routinely used, ether extract methodology may not adequately characterize the types of lipid found in forages and cereal grains. Two-thirds of the lipid content in forage (Harwood 1996) and up to one-third in cereal grains (Hargin & Morrison 1980, Zhou et al 1999) is in the form of glycolipids and phospholipids that are incompletely extracted in ether. Similarly, forages contain waxes and other pigments that are extractable in ether but poorly digestible. Thus, if digestibility of fat in forages and cereal grains is based on ether extraction, the availability of naturally-occurring fat in forages and cereal grains might be underestimated as a significant portion of the lipid is not represented in the extract. The relatively small amount of fat, coupled with incomplete characterization of the lipid fractions digested, might also explain the wide variation in fat digestibility commonly observed with forages (see Fonnesbeck et al 1967).

Despite the fact that the digestive system of equids has evolved to process low-fat, high-fiber feeds, they appear quite capable of assimilating relatively large amounts of dietary fat (see reviews by Potter et al 1992, Kronfeld et al 2004, NRC 2007). Using data from a wide range of fat intakes (23–233 g/kg DM) Kronfeld et al (2004), demonstrated a linear relationship between fat intake (g/day) and fat absorbed (g/day), with an estimated daily endogenous loss of 0.22 g fat/kg BW. Additional modeling of these compiled data demonstrated that fat digestibility is maximized between 100 and 150 g/kg DM and sustained to at least 230 g/kg DM in horses adapted to fat-supplemented rations (Kronfeld et al 2004).

Few associative effects of dietary fat on the digestibility of other nutrients have been reported. In the studies compiled by Kronfeld et al (2004), the feeding of diets with up to 230 g fat/kg DM had no negative effects on the digestion of dry matter, crude protein, or fiber. The supplemental fat sources and the percent fat added to the total diet in Kronfeld's report included corn oil (5–20%), peanut oil (7.5–15%), tallow (7.5–15%), an animal–vegetable fat blend (7.5–15%), a blend of equal parts soy-lecithin and corn oil (10%), and a blend of equal parts soy-lecithin and soybean oil (10%). A similar lack of negative associative effects on nutrient digestibility have been reported by others with the addition of 5–15% corn oil (Kane et al 1979, Bush et al 2001, Lindberg & Karlsson 2001) and 8% linseed oil (Delobel et al 2008) to the concentrate portion of the diet. In contrast, a negative associative effect of soybean oil on crude fiber, neutral detergent fiber (NDF) and acid detergent fiber (ADF) digestion has been reported by Jansen et al (2000, 2001, 2002). In these studies soybean oil was added to the concentrate at a rate of 15–37%, resulting in 50–148 g fat/kg DM in the total diet. Other researchers have also found a negative effect on fiber digestion with fairly high levels of soybean oil inclusion in the concentrate portion of the diet (19–21%), but not lower levels (5–13%) (Godoi et al 2009, Morgado et al 2009). While reduced fiber intake associated with the feeding of high levels of soybean oil can possibly explain the reductions in fiber digestion observed by some (Godoi et al 2009, Morgado et al 2009), it does not explain the findings of Jansen et al (2000, 2001, 2002) who compared diets similar in energy and fiber by substituting corn starch and/or glucose for soybean oil. The mechanism by which soybean oil, but not other oils, might suppress fiber digestion is unknown. Higher fluxes of bile acids or fatty acids into the large intestine are not likely to be involved (Jansen et al 2007). A recent meta-analysis of 22 studies found that diets with added fat (15.5 to 217.5 g/kg DM) had no effect on digestion of crude protein or NDF but did result in a significant decrease in ADF digestibility (Sales & Homolka 2011). It is worth noting that this meta-analysis included the soybean oil supplementation studies of Jansen and coworkers. As ADF generally represents the least digestible fiber for the horse, the importance of this finding may have little practical relevance. To avoid potential negative effects on fiber digestion, the NRC (2007) recommended an upper limit of 0.7 g fat/kg BW (approximately 35 g/kg DM) when fat is supplemented in the form of soybean oil.

Only a small number of studies have evaluated the effect of fat supplementation on mineral absorption. In mature horses and ponies, absorption of calcium, phosphorus and magnesium appear to be largely unaffected by fat intakes of 80 to 98 g/kg DM (Davison et al 1991, McCann et al 1987, Meyer et al 1997). Although calcium absorption was not directly measured, growing horses fed a fat and fiber-based supplement (containing 11% corn oil) had lower radiographic bone density during the fall and winter months, but not the summer and spring months, compared to those fed an isocaloric supplement high in starch and sugar (Hoffman et al 1999). However, a follow-up study found no difference in radiographic bone density between weanlings provided fat and fiber when compared to starch and sugar-based feeds (Hoffman et al 2001). Given the potential for mineral availability to be decreased through the formation of fat-mineral soaps in the small intestine, additional study is needed to clarify the impact that high-fat diets have on the absorption of calcium and other minerals in growing horses.

The absorption of fat-soluble vitamins requires the presence of triacylglycerol and other fats in the small intestine. The impact of dietary fat on vitamin absorption has not been directly assessed in the horse. Kronfeld et al (2004) speculated that the lowered fat digestibility of traditional hay-grain diets may increase the risk of suboptimal vitamin A and E status. As evidence of this, ponies fed diets containing very low amounts of fat (0.05%) for 3 months were reported to have low plasma and tissue vitamin E concentrations, suggesting there may have been inadequate absorption of vitamin E (Sallmann et al 1991). The impact of dietary fat on vitamin absorption deserves further study, particularly as it may alter fat-soluble vitamin requirements in relation to dietary fat content.

Key Points

- The mechanics of fat digestion and absorption have received limited study in the horse.
- Dietary fat is principally digested and absorbed in the small intestine.
- Digestibility of fat from oils and other high fat feedstuffs is relatively high (85–100%).
- Inclusion of fat at up to at least 100 g/kg DM appears to have minimal impact on digestion of dry matter, crude protein, NDF or minerals.

Dietary sources of fat

Forages, cereal grains and most cereal by-products are naturally low in fat (i.e., <4% DM). Similarly, the use of highly efficient chemical methods to extract oils from oilseeds has resulted in oilseed meals (e.g., soybean meal) with relatively low fat content. There are, of course, some exceptions. For example, naked (hulless) oats and distillers grains may have 7–10% crude fat and oilseed meals generated from mechanical oil extraction may have up to 20% crude fat.

The fat content of equine diets can be augmented by a variety of fat-rich ingredients. The crude fat and fatty acid composition of feedstuffs commonly included in equine diets is provided in Table 7-1. Horses have been reported to accept a variety of plant oils added to their diet (depending on the processing method used for extraction), including canola, coconut, corn, cottonseed, flax (linseed), olive, palm, peanut, rice bran, safflower and soybean oils (Bush et al 2001, Delobel et al 2008, Duvaux-Ponter 2004, Frank et al 2004, Gatta et al 2005, Hallebeek & Beynen 2002, Holland et al 1998, Kronfeld et al 2004, Lindberg & Karlsson 2001, Meyer et al 1997).

Animal tallows and tallow-vegetable oil blends have also been used in horse rations (Holland et al 1998, McCann et al 1987, Rich et al 1981), although this practice is not as common today as it was 30 years ago and has been discouraged or prohibited in some countries based on perceived risk for transmission of bovine spongiform encephalopathy. In addition, palatability tests have generally indicated that horses have a preference for vegetable oils over animal fats (Bowman et al 1979, Holland et al 1998). More recently, interest in omega-3 fatty acids has led to the inclusion of marine fat sources in equine diets, including a variety of fish oils, seal blubber and algae to augment the omega-3 fatty acid content of the diet (Khol-Parisini et al 2007, King et al 2008, Vineyard et al 2010).

In addition to oils, which are essentially 100% crude fat, there are other feedstuffs that contain a relatively high percentage of DM (>20%) as crude fat; these include stabilized rice bran, heat-treated whole soybeans, flaxseed and sunflower seeds. Rice bran contains naturally high levels of phosphorus which can offset the ratio of calcium to phosphorus in the total diet. Because of this, some (but not all) companies have fortified their rice bran supplements with additional calcium to bring up the Ca : P ratio to more acceptable levels. Rice bran also contains an endogenous lipase that can be activated when the germ and bran are exposed to air. Unless deactivated by heat and moisture, the lipase can quickly hydrolyze the triacylglycerols and release fatty acids that are highly susceptible to oxidation. Modern mills stabilize rice bran after milling by passing the bran through an expander, a process which greatly reduces the potential for rancidity. Whole soybeans contain trypsin inhibitors that can interfere with protein digestion in monogastric animals; however, roasting or other processing methods that involve heating or toasting will generally inactivate this antinutritive factor.

Commercial concentrate rations with added fat typically include one or more of the oils or other high-fat feedstuffs described above. In general, products with a significant amount of added fat can be identified from the guaranteed analysis as having greater than or equal to 5% crude fat. Although horses can tolerate higher levels of fat in the diet, most fat-added concentrates available in the marketplace range from 5–14% crude fat. A variety of high fat supplements are also commercially available, the most common of which are stabilized rice bran and fat blends of varying composition and crude fat content. For horse owners, fat-added concentrates offer the advantage of convenience and also ensures that the feed is balanced with respect to other nutrients in the diet. In contrast, supplementing the basal ration with oil or other high fat feedstuffs can create nutrient imbalances that require additional fortification to correct, a practice that might negate any cost savings to the owner.

Key Points

- Forages and cereal grains that make up the bulk of most equine rations are generally low in fat (< 4% DM).
- Feedstuffs high in fat (20–100% DM) that can be added to equine rations include vegetable oils, marine oils, stabilized rice bran, flaxseed, and heat-treated soybeans among others.
- Horses have shown a preference for corn oil over other oils and vegetable oils over animal tallows and lards.
- Commercially available fat-added concentrates typically contain 5–14% crude fat.

Essential fatty acids

Linoleic acid (LA; 18:2*n*-6) and α-linolenic acid (ALA; 18:3*n*-3) are essential fatty acids (EFA) that must be supplied by the diet. Mammals lack the Δ12- and Δ15-desaturase enzymes necessary for desaturation of an 18-carbon fatty acid at the omega-3 (or Δ15) or omega-6 (or Δ12) positions. Therefore, LA and ALA cannot be synthesized in the body and are deemed "essential." By comparison, plants and algae contain ample amounts of the Δ12- and Δ15-desaturase enzymes and, as a result, LA and ALA are two of the most prevalent fatty acids found in plant tissues and oils.

An EFA deficiency has not been described for the horse, even in those consuming diets almost devoid of fat. Sallmann et al (1991) observed no clinical abnormalities in ponies fed very low fat diets containing 0.03% and 0.14% linoleic acid for 7 months. The absence of signs of deficiency in these ponies may have resulted from mobilization of body fat stores that could have met EFA needs during the prolonged period of low intake. In other species EFA deficiency is characterized by dry or scaly skin, dry coat, hair loss and decreased reproductive efficiency. The NRC (2007) has recommended a LA intake of 0.5% DM for horses although justification for this recommendation was not described. For a 500 kg horse with a DM intake of 2% BW,

Table 7-1 Average Crude Fat and Fatty Acid Composition (g/kg DM) of Feedstuffs Commonly Fed to Horses[a,b]

Feedstuff	Crude fat	SFA	MUFA	PUFA	Select omega-6 and omega-3 fatty acids					
					LA 18:2n-6	ALA 18:3*n*-3	AA 20:4*n*-6	EPA 20:5*n*-3	DPA 22:5*n*-3	DHA 22:6*n*-3
Forages										
Grass hay, cool-season	22.1	3.7	1.2	12.0	3.8	8.2	0	0	0	0
Grass hay, warm-season	20.0	5.3	0.6	8.2	3.6	4.6	0	0	0	0
Grass pasture, cool-season	25.0	4.0	1.5	13.8	4.5	9.3	0	0	0	0
Grass pasture, warm-season	24.4	6.3	0.7	15.0	3.9	11.1	0	0	0	0
Legume hay	25.5	5.2	0.8	11.8	3.9	7.9	0	0	0	0
Legume pasture	31.1	6.3	1.8	12.9	4.5	8.4	0	0	0	0
Concentrates										
Barley grain	23.0	4.8	3.0	11.1	10.0	1.1	0	0	0	0
Canola meal	54.0	4.3	27.4	16.9	12.1	3.5	0	0	0	0
Corn grain	47.4	6.7	12.5	21.6	21.0	0.7	0	0	0	0
Flax seed	421.6	36.6	75.3	287.3	59.0	228.1	0	0	0	0
Linseed (flax) meal	19.0	3.4	4.2	9.5	2.1	7.3	0	0	0	0
Oat grain	54.0	9.2	19.6	24.4	23.2	1.0	0	0	0	0
Rice bran	208.5	41.7	75.5	74.6	71.4	3.2	0	0	0	0
Soybean meal	16.0	3.1	2.7	7.2	5.9	1.0	0	0	0	0
Soybeans, whole roasted	216.2	31.3	47.8	122.1	107.6	14.4	0	0	0	0
Sunflower seeds	514.6	44.6	185.3	231.4	230.5	0.6	0	0	0	0
Wheat grain	24.7	4.5	3.4	9.8	9.8	0.5	0	0	0	0
Fats & oils										
Canola oil	1000	73.7	632.8	281.4	186.4	91.4	0	0	0	0
Coconut oil	1000	865.0	58.0	18.0	18.0	0	0	0	0	0
Corn oil	1000	129.5	275.8	546.8	532.3	11.6	0	0	0	0
Fish oil, Herring	1000	212.9	565.6	156.0	11.5	7.6	2.9	62.7	6.2	42.1
Fish oil, Menhaden	1000	304.3	266.9	342.0	21.5	14.9	11.7	131.7	49.2	85.6
Fish oil, Salmon	1000	198.7	290.4	403.2	15.4	10.6	6.8	130.2	29.9	182.3
Flaxseed (Linseed) oil	1000	94.0	202.0	660.0	127.0	533.0	0	0	0	0
Lard	1000	392.0	451.0	112.0	102.0	10.0	0	0	0	0
Olive oil	1000	138.1	729.6	105.2	97.6	7.6	0	0	0	0
Palm oil	1000	493.0	370.0	93.0	91.0	2.0	0	0	0	0
Peanut oil	1000	169.0	432.0	320.0	320.0	0	0	0	0	0
Rice bran oil	1000	197.0	393.0	350.0	334.0	16.0	0	0	0	0
Soybean oil	1000	156.5	227.8	577.4	504.2	67.9	0	0	0	0
Sunflower oil	1000	90.1	573.3	289.6	287.1	0.4	0	0	0	0
Tallow	1000	498.0	418.0	40.0	31.0	6.0	0	0	0	0

[a]SFA = saturated fatty acids; MUFA = monounsaturated fatty acids; PUFA = polyunsaturated fatty acids; LA = linoleic acid; ALA = α-linolenic acid; AA = arachidonic acid; EPA = eicosapentaenoic acid; DPA = docosapentaenoic acid; DHA = docosahexaenoic acid.
[b]Data from: Palmquist 1988, Boufaïed et al 2003, Warren & Kivipelto 2007a, b, USDA-ARS 2010.

the NRC recommendation would amount to a daily intake of 50 g of LA. Across a variety of other mammalian species, a minimum of 1% of total dietary energy intake as LA has been given as a general recommendation to prevent EFA deficiency (Gurr et al 2002). Extrapolating this to a 500-kg horse consuming 20 Mcal DE/day, and assuming a conservative estimate of 50% availability, the LA requirement is 45 g/day. Thus, the NRC (2007) recommendation for LA in horses appears to approximate the minimum intake guideline for other mammalian species. This requirement is likely to be met in horses consuming adequate quantities of good quality forage and is easily met by diets supplemented with fat, as most high-fat feedstuffs and oils are rich in LA (Table 7-1). Currently there are no guidelines for minimum daily ALA intake, although a horse consuming adequate amounts of fresh forage and/or good quality hay will likely receive ample amounts of ALA in the diet (Table 7-1). Supplementation with both LA and ALA should be considered in horses receiving poor quality or limited amounts of forage for prolonged periods of time. Because an ALA requirement has not been established for horses or other herbivores, provision of ALA in amounts resulting in a 5:1 to 10:1 ratio of LA:ALA might be considered adequate, as this has been recommended for other species (NRC 2005).

Key Points

- Linoleic acid (omega-6) and α-linolenic acid (omega-3) cannot be made by the horse and must be supplied by the diet.
- Essential fatty acid requirements have not been established for horses.
- Most equine diets will likely meet essential fatty acid needs unless poor quality rations are consumed for prolonged periods.

Omega-6 and omega-3 fatty acids

There has been a great deal of interest in the biological impact of different types of fatty acids supplied by various fat sources. In particular, omega-6 and omega-3 fatty acids have received attention for their roles in maintaining cell membrane fluidity and integrity, receptor and ion channel function, gene expression, neural and retinal development, and inflammation and immunity.

Both omega-6 and omega-3 fatty acids contribute to normal biological responses; however, the relative availability of omega-6 versus omega-3 fatty acids can influence the overall response. Linoleic acid (LA; 18:2*n*-6) is the "parent" omega-6 fatty acid and can be elongated and desaturated in the body to form the long-chain polyunsaturated fatty acids dihomo-γ-linolenic acid (DGLA; 20:3*n*-6) and arachidonic acid (AA; 20:4*n*-6) (Fig. 7.3). In the omega-3 family, α-linolenic acid (ALA; 18:3*n*-3) competes for the same elongase and desaturase enzymes to form eicosapentaenoic (EPA) and docosahexaenoic (DHA) acids. The initial step in this process catalyzed by Δ6-desaturase is thought to be rate-limiting, and studies in other species have indicated that there is a 1.5- to 3.0-fold higher Δ6-desaturase conversion rate for ALA compared with LA (Hussein et al 2005, Sprecher 2000, Sprecher et al 1995). The relative activities of

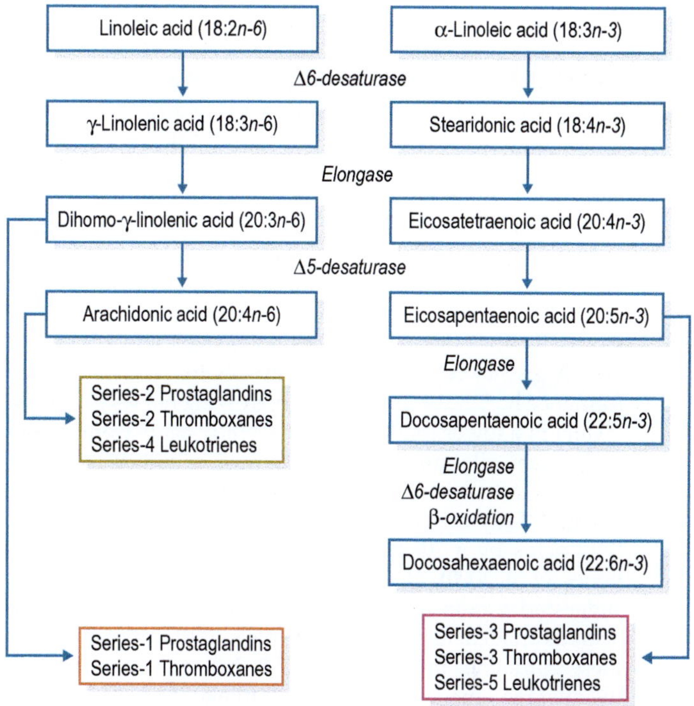

Figure 7.3 Elongation and desaturation of essential fatty acids and subsequent eicosanoid production.

Δ6- and Δ5-desaturase in horses have not been established. Nonetheless, horses appear to have the ability to synthesize the longer-chain polyunsaturated fatty acids from LA and ALA, as evidenced by the presence of AA, EPA and DHA in cell membranes despite not having consumed these fatty acids in the diet (Warren & Kivipelto 2008, Warren et al 2010).

In addition to competing for available enzymes, omega-3 and omega-6 fatty acids also compete for incorporation into cell membrane phospholipids. When greater quantities of EPA are present, it will be incorporated into cell membranes partially at the expense of AA (Calder 2006). The resulting changes in membrane fluidity and integrity, as well as cell receptor signaling and protein synthesis, can alter the biological response to trauma and infection. Furthermore, potent biological mediators known as eicosanoids are synthesized from the oxidation of EPA, DGLA and AA located in cell membranes. The eicosanoids, which include prostaglandins, leukotrienes and thromboxanes, mediate several events including inflammation, blood flow and pressure and blood clotting. DGLA and AA are precursors of the 1- and 2- prostaglandin and thromboxane series, whereas EPA serves as the precursor for the 3-series prostaglandins and thromboxanes and the 5-series leukotrienes (Fig. 7.3). In simplistic terms, eicosanoids derived from omega-6 fatty acids stimulate stronger pro-inflammatory responses, whereas those stemming from omega-3 fatty acids produce weaker inflammatory reactions. However, it is really the balance of the different eicosanoids produced that generates the final biological response. Because most cell membranes contain a greater concentration of AA than other 20-carbon fatty acids, AA is usually the principal precursor for eicosanoid synthesis (Calder & Grimble 2002).

Supplementation of omega-3 fatty acids

As an herbivore, the horse is adapted to a diet naturally high proportionally in omega-3 fatty acids. Forages, although low in total fat (2–4%), contain a significant portion of that fat (39–56%) as ALA (Boufaïed et al 2003, Warren & Kivipelto 2007a, b). In both fresh forage and hay, the proportion of ALA usually exceeds that of LA (Tables 7-1 and 7-2). In contrast, cereal grains, soybean meal, rice bran and most vegetable oils are enriched in the omega-6 fatty acid, LA. For example, corn oil and soybean oil contain over 50% LA, and the fat in rice bran contains approximately 35% LA (Table 7-1). A greater reliance on concentrates in the diets of performance horses, broodmares and growing horses generally results in a lower intake of omega-3 fatty acids from forage and, when oils are added to the diet, a higher intake of omega-6 fatty acids (Table 7-2). In humans, consumption of omega-6 fatty acids often greatly exceeds that of omega-3 fatty acids by a 20–25:1 margin (Calder & Grimble 2002, James et al 2000). Recent dietary recommendations have suggested a ratio of 5:1 to 10:1 of omega-6:omega-3 fatty acids as an ideal target for human diets (NRC 2005). Keeping these guidelines in mind, Table 7-2 shows a comparison of the average omega-6 and omega-3 intake from a variety of equine diets. According to the calculations and assumptions used in Table 7-2, most equine diets probably fall below the upper omega-6 to omega-3 ratio of 10:1, even with relatively high levels of omega-6 fatty acids provided from oil supplementation and using conservative estimates of fatty acid availability from forages in the small intestine. Such low omega-6:omega-3 ratios in equine diets compared to the typical human diet likely results from the potentially large contribution of ALA from forage. The ratio of omega-6 to omega-3 fatty acids is thought to be important because of the competitive nature of fatty acids and their different biological roles. However, there is also evidence that the absolute quantity of omega-3 or omega-6, more than the ratio, can influence conversion of precursor fatty acids to their longer chain derivatives, as well as the overall biological response (Goyens et al 2006). Much more work is needed in horses before an ideal omega-6:omega-3 ratio can be recommended, and to determine whether it is the ratio between these fatty acids or the amount consumed that has the biggest influence.

Table 7-2 Estimated Amounts of Omega-6 and Omega-3 Fatty Acids Available to a 500-kg Horse From Different Types of Diets[a,b]

Diet	Available omega-6 (g/day)	Available omega-3 (g/day)	Omega-6: omega-3 ratio
Pasture	25	75	0.3:1
Hay	35	60	0.6:1
Hay + Concentrate (4% crude fat)	50	25	2.0:1
Hay + Concentrate (6% crude fat)	135	30	4.5:1
Hay + Concentrate (10% crude fat)	275	35	7.8:1

[a]The estimates above were based on the following assumptions: a) 500-kg horse with a daily intake of 10 kg DM; b) hay + concentrate diets are based on total DM intake consisting of 50% hay and 50% as concentrate; c) concentrates are made up predominantly of cereal grains, grain byproducts and oil seed meals; d) corn oil, which is rich in omega-6, was used as the fat source for the concentrates with 6 and 10% crude fat; and e) 50% of the fatty acids in forages, 75% of the fatty acids in cereal grains, and 100% of the fatty acids in corn oil are available for absorption in the small intestine.
[b]Omega-6 and omega-3 fatty acids in example diets are predominantly in the form of linoleic acid and α-linolenic acid, respectively and are based on average fatty acid concentrations observed in commonly used feedstuffs (Warren et al 2007a, b, Vineyard et al 2010, Warren personal communication).

Given the potential anti-inflammatory and immunomodulatory activities ascribed to omega-3 fatty acids (Calder 2006), there has been interest in supplementing these fatty acids to the diets of horses. In addition to fresh grass and good quality hay, good sources of ALA in horse diets include flaxseed and flax (linseed) oil. The ALA content of canola and soybean oils tends to be higher than other vegetable oils, though still much outweighed by LA. Fish oil (e.g., menhaden, cod liver, salmon, herring) and algae supplements are sources rich in the long-chain omega-3 fatty acids EPA and DHA (Table 7-1). Marine-based oils are not without fault, however, as cod liver oil is known to be very high in vitamin A and some oils may be derived from fish contaminated with heavy metals such as copper or mercury, and organic pollutants such as PCBs or dioxins (Domingo et al 2007).

Flaxseed has been fed by horsemen for decades, most likely based on its anecdotal reputation for producing a shiny hair coat. Though generally well accepted by both horses and their owners, there remains some debate as to the ideal way to feed flaxseed. Feeding whole flaxseed is a safe and acceptable practice. Nonetheless, some insist that the flaxseed should be ground and/or stabilized in order to reap the full benefits. The practice of grinding flax may indeed be helpful, as grinding interrupts the hard outer seed coating, making the fat potentially more available for digestion in the small intestine. However, disruption of the seed coat also exposes the seed contents to air and therefore may hasten the oxidation and destruction of the fatty acids. Stabilization of ground flaxseed is intended to reduce the susceptibility of fatty acids to oxidation and is achieved by selection for mature and evenly colored seeds, the addition of natural and artificial antioxidants, or by employing further processing methods to protect the fat in the seed. Others claim that flaxseed must first be cooked before it can be fed to horses. Flaxseed contains cyanogenic glycosides that can interact with enzymes contained within the seed to release harmful cyanide (Oomah et al 1992). For this reason, some horsemen are compelled to boil flaxseed before feeding in order to volatilize and remove the cyanide. However, it is unlikely that harmful levels of cyanide are released with ingestion of flaxseed due to the ability of stomach acid to inactivate the enzymes contained within the seeds (O'Neill et al 2002). Whole flaxseed also contains more phosphorus (~0.65%) than calcium (~0.23%); thus if high quantities of flaxseed are fed, adjustments to the calcium:phosphorus ratio of the total diet may be necessary.

Feeding fish oil products to horses has sometimes been met with resistance due the unpleasant "fishy" odor, the increased expense, and limited availability compared to other oil sources. Some manufacturers of fish oil marketed specifically for horse consumption have been able to successfully reduce or even eliminate the "fishy" odor through further refining, as well as the addition of flavors and fragrances that horses (or their owners) find more acceptable. The popularity of feeding fish oil preparations to horses has grown in recent years and availability of these products has increased. Another way to supply EPA and DHA from fish oil is with a dry "encapsulated fish oil" pellet that contains approximately 23% fat. The encapsulation process is utilized to stabilize the fatty acids in the fish oil and to improve palatability. As an alternative to fish oil, algal-derived DHA supplements are also becoming more widely available for inclusion in equine rations.

Potential benefits of omega-3 fatty acid supplementation

The majority of omega-3 fatty acid supplementation research in horses has focused on inflammation. The results of early studies showed promising effects of linseed oil supplementation, including decreased monocyte procoagulant activity along with lowered thromboxane and tumor necrosis factor-α (TNF-α) production (Henry et al 1990, Morris et al 1991). More recently, horses supplemented with 3% fish oil had reduced prostaglandin E_2 (PGE_2) production by cells harvested from bronchoalveolar lavage fluid (BALF) when compared to horses supplemented with corn oil; however, delayed-type hypersensitivity skin test response, antibody response to vaccination, and TNF-α production by stimulated BALF cells were not different between diets (Hall et al 2004a, b). The effects of long-chain omega-3 fatty acids supplied as seal blubber to horses with recurrent airway obstruction revealed no improvements in several measures of pulmonary function and no improvement in clinical signs after 10 weeks of supplementation (Khol-Parisini et al 2007). Horses fed 10% corn oil had higher levels of the acute phase protein fibrinogen at rest and following exercise compared to those fed 10% soybean oil or a low-fat control diet (Wilson et al 2003).

Although in vitro and ex vivo methods of measuring immune function are important for gaining basic knowledge of how dietary omega-3 fatty acids can affect inflammatory processes, evaluation of in vivo response is essential for evaluation of clinical significance. Unfortunately, only a handful of equine studies have attempted to quantify the anti-inflammatory effects of omega-3 fatty acid supplementation using an in vivo model. In response to endotoxin administration, a longer whole blood recalcification and activated partial thromboplastin time, but no differences in inflammatory eicosanoid production, were observed when horses received a diet containing 8% linseed oil (Henry et al 1991). In a small cross-over study, six horses known to have Culicoides hypersensitivity had reduced lesion size after injection with Culicoides antigen when supplemented with 0.1% BW flaxseed compared to placebo (simply described as "bran") for 42 days (O'Neill et al 2002). In contrast to these findings, the level of pruritus or lesional surface area did not change in a study of 17 horses with Culicoides hypersensitivity after 6 weeks of supplementation with 200 mL linseed oil (Friberg et al 1999).

Supplementation with omega-3 fatty acids has also been touted to benefit horses with osteoarthritis. These claims are primarily based on findings from research performed in humans with rheumatoid arthritis that indicate fish oil supplementation may improve symptoms (Berbert et al 2005, Cleland et al 1988, Lau et al 1993). Studies in horses, however, are extremely limited and the results must be interpreted with caution, as the etiology of rheumatoid arthritis and degenerative osteoarthritis are very different. In one study, horses supplemented with encapsulated fish oil tended to have a longer trot stride suggestive of less pain than those receiving corn oil, but serum PGE_2 and TNF-α were not different between treatments (Woodward et al 2007). An experiment performed on equine synovial explants reported that treatment with ALA at high doses (300 μg/ml) increased ALA content of explant cell membranes and inhibited PGE_2 production after challenge with LPS (Munsterman et al 2005). However, it is unclear how the ALA dose used in this experiment relates to physiological levels of dietary ALA that could potentially reach the synovial fluid in vivo. Manhart et al (2009) supplemented arthritic horses with EPA and DHA for 90 days and reported a reduction in total leukocytes in synovial fluid in arthritic joints, decreased plasma PGE_2 concentration, and a trend for reduced fibrinogen concentrations compared to horses receiving no supplementation; however, force plate analysis indicated no effect of supplementation on gait abnormalities associated with the osteoarthritis. Although the authors concluded that omega-3 fatty acid supplementation would benefit horses with osteoarthritis, the inflammatory markers measured in this study were non-specific and there was no improvement in clinical signs. Collectively, these studies provide some useful preliminary data but they do not offer strong evidence that omega-3 fatty acids can attenuate arthritic inflammation in horses. More comprehensive investigation is needed to characterize the effects of omega-3 fatty acid supplementation on degenerative osteoarthritis in horses.

In a series of studies investigating the effects of fatty acid supplementation on aspects of innate and acquired immunity, lymphocyte proliferation and neutrophil function were not affected by omega-3 fatty acid supplementation (Vineyard et al 2007, 2008, 2010). Lymphocyte PGE_2 production was reduced and antibody response to vaccination was increased when either omega-3 (as fish oil) or omega-6 (as corn oil) fatty acids were supplied as part of a high fat (100 g/kg) feed (Vineyard et al 2008). Horses fed omega-3 fatty acids as fish oil or milled flaxseed also had an earlier increase in skin thickness after intradermal phytohemagglutinin injection compared to nonsupplemented controls (Vineyard et al 2010). Results from these studies suggest that both omega-6 and omega-3 fatty acids play a role in immune function of clinically normal horses. Further study is needed to identify the effects of feeding fat to horses with autoimmune or inflammatory diseases and the potential for increasing dietary omega-3 fatty acid intake to modulate the severity and/or progression of disease.

There has also been interest in supplementing omega-3 fatty acids to enhance reproductive function. In a cross-over design study with six stallions, an increase in daily sperm output and percentage of morphologically normal sperm were observed after 90 days of supplementation with a supplement containing fish oil that provided 29 g of DHA + EPA per day; however, omega-3 supplementation did not alter progressive motility in fresh, cooled or frozen semen (Harris et al 2005). In another cross-over design study with eight stallions, supplementation with 75 g of total omega-3 fatty acids per day (of which 20 g/day is estimated to be DHA + EPA) for 98 days did not improve characteristics of fresh semen, but did improve sperm motility after cooling and freezing (Brinsko et al 2005). Both of these studies noted that greater improvements in response to omega-3 supplementation were observed in stallions that produced semen with poor tolerance to cooling or cryopreservation. Further studies are needed on a larger number of stallions to confirm these findings and establish how consistently long-chain omega-3 fatty acid supplementation can improve semen viability. In addition, studies are needed in broodmares to evaluate potential influences of omega-3 fatty acids on fertility and maintenance of pregnancy.

Key Points

- Longer chain (>20 carbons) omega-3 and omega-6 fatty acids have important biological roles in the body.
- Horses have some ability to synthesize the longer-chain omega-3 and -6 fatty acids from essential fatty acid precursors.
- Forages, flaxseed, fish oils, and some algae are typically rich sources of omega-3 fatty acids, whereas cereal grains, vegetable oils, and rice bran are high in omega-6 fatty acids.
- Although research in other species has shown supplementation with omega-3 fatty acids can positively influence inflammation and immune function, studies in horses have shown mixed results.

Potential benefits of increasing fat intake

Research has demonstrated several potential benefits associated with the addition of fat to the equine diet. Research on the anti-inflammatory and immunomodulatory properties of omega-3 fatty acids were described in the previous section. This section will focus on the use of fat to increase the energy density of the diet, temper glycemic response, lessen excitable behavior, alter metabolism to favor utilization of fat, and the potential for dietary fat to reduce thermal load.

Increasing the energy density of the diet

One of the most common reasons for supplementing fat is to increase the energy density of the diet. From a gross energy standpoint, fats contain approximately 2.25 times the energy by weight as carbohydrates. Using data from several studies in which fat intake ranged from 23 to 233 g/kg DM, and with the assumption that fat has gross energy of 9.5 Mcal/kg, Kronfeld et al (2004) estimated mean DE values of 5.2, 7.7 and 9.0 Mcal/kg for ether extract in forages, mixed feeds including added fats and added fats, respectively.

Fat is also an efficient energy source. As might be expected when a fat source is added to an existing diet, Kane et al (1979) observed an increase in digestible and metabolizable energy and energy balance (an estimate of net energy) when either 50 or 96 g corn oil/kg DM was added to a basal diet of oats. When a similar amount of gross energy was provided by replacing some of the forage and cereal grains in the basal diet with 150 g/kg DM of corn oil, tallow or a vegetable oil-tallow blend, increases in digestible and metabolizable energy and energy balance were still apparent (McCann et al 1987). In both of these studies, the amount of energy lost as heat was similar between fat-added and non-fat added diets, although when evaluated as a proportion of DE heat production was lower in diets with added fat. Kane et al (1979) reported that the conversion of metabolizable energy to net energy was 85% in diets containing 29 to 123 g fat/kg DM; however, according to energy and heat production values reported by the author, this estimate seems very high. Using energy values from McCann et al (1987), the conversion of DE to net energy was approximately 26% in diets containing fat, whereas only 17% of DE remained to support energy-requiring processes in diets without added fat. If the energetics of just the fat sources used by McCann et al (1987) are evaluated, the efficiency of conversion of DE to net energy averaged 44%. Collectively, these results indicate the net energy available for growth, work or production could be increased if a portion of daily energy intake is provided as fat. However, it must be noted that the studies of Kane and McCann evaluated energy balance in mature ponies with maintenance-only requirements; the conversion to net energy for tissue accretion or milk production may be more or less efficient and deserves further study. In addition, while Kane et al (1979) observed an increase in the efficiency of energy utilization with increasing fat content in the diet, it would be useful to evaluate the level of dietary fat that may optimize this response. It can be concluded that oils and other high fat ingredients offer an efficient way to increase the overall caloric intake of the horse. Furthermore, such practices permit an increase in energy without drastically increasing DM intake, which may be useful for broodmares, hard-working performance horses, and thin horses that may already be at their upper limit of DM intake.

Alternative to starch as a dietary energy source

Recognition of the energy density of oils and other high-fat feedstuffs has made them a popular alternative energy source to cereal grains. Used in this manner, fat allows the replacement of calories normally provided by NSC, thereby reducing the digestive and metabolic risks associated with diets high in starch and sugar (Kronfeld & Harris 2003).

Modulation of glycemic and insulinemic responses

Replacement of starch and sugar with isocaloric amounts of fat and fiber in concentrates fed to horses has been shown to lower postprandial glycemic and insulinemic responses (Williams et al 2001, Zeyner et al 2006). Some studies have reported similar effects when 10% corn oil was top-dressed on grain-based feeds, which the authors attributed to fat-mediated alterations in gastric emptying (Geor et al 2001, Pagan et al 1999). In contrast, the addition of 0.2 ml/kg BW (~8%) soybean oil or fish oil to a meal of cracked corn had no effect on glycemic or insulinemic responses (Vervuert et al 2010). In addition, a nonisocaloric substitution of 8% linseed oil for barley in a concentrate feed had no effect on mean glucose response to a meal of concentrate but reduced mean serum insulin concentration by half (Fayt et al 2008). Discrepancies between studies may be due to differences in the amount of fat added to the meal, but could also be a result of differences in the starch and sugar content of the meal. For example, Vervuert et al (2010) combined oil with a meal that provided 2 g starch/kg BW, whereas the studies by Geor et al (2001) and Pagan et al (1999) provided 1.5 to

5 g of sweet feed per kg BW. Meal volume, rate of intake, and other dietary constituents may also alter glycemic and insulinemic responses. The type of fat also may impact insulin response. In humans and rodents, the replacement of saturated fats and *trans* fatty acids with monounsaturated or polyunsaturated fats has beneficial effects on insulin sensitivity (Risérus et al 2009). Further studies in horses are warranted to examine the effect of adding different quantities or types of fat to a high-NSC meal on postprandial glucose and insulin responses, particularly in view of current recommendations to add fat (or substitute NSC with fat) to rations for older or insulin resistant horses that have trouble maintaining body weight.

Behavior

Horse owners often comment that dietary fat alters behavior; specifically that horses are more tractable when receiving a ration with added fat. Holland et al (1996) reported that spontaneous activity and reactivity to pressure, loud noise and visual stimuli were reduced in horses fed diets containing 10% soy lecithin and corn oil. More recently, Nicol et al (2005) found that weanlings fed diets high in fat and fiber cantered less frequently and for a shorter duration, spent more time investigating, and took less time to complete a handling test compared to foals fed an isocaloric diet high in starch and sugar. Horses in dressage training had lower resting cortisol concentrations and a reduction in the intensity of their responses to a startle reaction test when fed a fat-added diet (11% DM) compared to an isocaloric diet higher in starch (Redondo et al 2009). Thus, there appears to be merit in the claims by horse owners that fat supplementation favorably alters behavior when used to replace some of the NSC in the diet (see Chapter 25).

Metabolic adaptations and responses to exercise

In horses adapted to high-fat diets, metabolic adaptations appear to favor the utilization of fat as an energy source. Supplementation with fat is generally characterized by an increase in plasma cholesterol and phospholipids and a reduction in plasma triacylglycerol (Frank et al 2004, Geelen et al 1999, Orme et al 1997). Lipoprotein lipase activity is increased with fat adaptation, indicating that skeletal muscle may have increased capacity for uptake of NEFA from circulating triacylglycerol (Geelen et al 1999, 2000, Orme et al 1997). As well, a lower respiratory exchange ratio during low to moderate intensity exercise has been observed in horses adapted to a high fat diet, suggesting that the capacity for oxidation of NEFA is increased with fat supplementation (Dunnett et al 2002, Pagan et al 2002). However, a similar response was not observed at higher workloads, suggesting a greater reliance on carbohydrate during more intensive exercise (Dunnett et al 2002). In two studies, the feeding of a diet supplying 25–30% of DE from fat resulted in a >30% reduction in the production and utilization of glucose during low intensity exercise (30–35% VO_{2max}), as measured by isotopic enrichment with [6-6-d_2]-glucose (Pagan et al 2002, Treiber et al. 2008). Collectively, these findings indicate an increase in the utilization of fat with a concomitant decrease in carbohydrate utilization in fat-adapted horses exercising at low to moderate intensity; however, substrate oxidation does not appear to be altered at higher exercise intensities (> 50–60% VO_{2max}). Although these results suggest fat supplementation may exert a glycogen-sparing effect, assessments of glycogen utilization during either submaximal or maximal exercise have shown no difference between high and low fat diets (Eaton et al 1995, Essen-Gustavsson et al 1991, Harkins et al 1992, Pagan et al 1987).

The metabolic response to fat supplementation is apparent after just 3 weeks of supplementation (Hughes et al 1995, Orme et al 1997). However, these effects are transient and dependent on the continued inclusion of fat in the diet, as the response is abolished within 5 weeks of withdrawal of fat supplementation (Orme et al 1997). The metabolic response to oil supplementation has also been reported to vary between horses, depending on their ability to utilize fat as a fuel source during exercise (Dunnett et al 2002).

Because dietary fat cannot be used as a substrate for glycogen synthesis, there has been some concern that high-fat diets would hamper glycogen repletion following exercise. Despite a reduction in NSC content to accommodate the addition of fat to the diet, some studies have reported an increase in resting muscle glycogen concentration in horses fed high fat diets (Harkins et al 1992, Meyers et al 1989, Oldham et al 1990). In contrast, several other researchers have reported no change or even a slight decrease in resting muscle glycogen when horses were fed comparable levels of fat (Eaton et al 1995, Hyyppa et al 1999, Geelen et al 2001, Orme et al 1997, Pagan et al 1987). Hyyppa et al (1999) reported that acute supplementation with 400 g rapeseed oil following moderate intensity exercise reduced the rate of glycogen repletion; however, this effect was abolished when horses were adapted to a diet containing 50 g fat/kg DM for 3 weeks.

Thermal load

Digestion and assimilation of nutrients as well as nutrient catabolism are not 100% efficient and, as a result, up to 80% of consumed gross energy may be lost as heat. This heat increases the body's thermal load and must be dissipated in order to maintain normal body temperature. Although energy balance studies in horses at rest have not demonstrated a lowered heat production with fat supplementation (Kane et al 1979, McCann et al 1987), such diets have been proposed to reduce the thermal load of horses during exercise (Kronfeld 1996). Using a theoretical model to compare the energetic efficiencies and heat production of three diets that provided varying proportions of fermentable carbohydrate, hydrolysable carbohydrate and fat, Kronfeld (1996) calculated that a hay, oat and corn oil diet (45:45:10% of intake) would result in approximately 2% less heat during moderate to heavy exercise and a 5% reduction (1.2 Mcal or 5 MJ) in total daily heat load compared to a diet of hay and oats (50:50). Although this calculated reduction in total heat load is small, it might be enough to benefit horses living and competing in hot and/or humid environments. However, it must be emphasized that these reductions in heat load are theoretical; thus, the real impact of a high fat diet on thermal load in vivo is unknown.

Athletic performance

Fat supplementation is often lauded for its ability to improve athletic performance, but research to support this claim is inconclusive. Studies have reported an increased time to fatigue during maximal exercise (Eaton et al 1995), faster times when performing repeated sprints (Meyers et al 1989, Oldham et al 1990, Scott et al 1992), and higher cutting scores indicative of greater work effort (Webb et al 1987) when horses were supplemented with greater than 12 to 15% of daily DE intake as fat. In contrast, an equal number of studies have reported no change in performance with similar levels of fat feeding (Topliff et al 1983, Pagan et al 1987, Essen-Gustavsson et al 1991, Hyyppa et al 1999). Mechanisms proposed for improved performance with fat supplementation have included increased stamina as a result of altered substrate use and a glycogen-sparing effect, improved power-to-weight ratio resulting from reduced DM intake and bowl ballast, and a reduction in acidemia and metabolic heat generated during exercise (Kronfeld 1996, Kronfeld et al 1998). However, many these mechanisms are theoretical and unproven while others have yet to be directly associated with the small improvements noted in performance. Ultimately, evidence that adaptation to fat affects exercise capacity is lacking.

Key Points

- The addition of fat to equine rations provides a means of increasing the energy density of the diet and/or replacing carbohydrates as a calorie source.
- Benefits ascribed to fat-added rations, such as modulation of glycemic/insulinemic responses and behavior, are likely related to the simultaneous reduction in NSC intake.
- Habituation to fat-added diets results in metabolic adaptations that favor the utilization of fat during low- to moderate-intensity exercise, but not high intensity exercise.
- Evidence that fat-added diets exert a glycogen-sparing effect, reduce thermal load, and in particular improve athletic performance is inconclusive.

Potential clinical applications of fat-added diets

Gastric ulceration syndrome

Feeding fat to reduce the incidence and severity of gastric ulceration in horses has been recommended but evidence of a beneficial effect in horses is lacking. In ponies, supplementation of a hay diet with corn oil (45 ml administered PO) for 5 weeks reduced gastric acid production and increased gastric fluid PGE_2 concentration when compared to a diet of hay alone (Cargile et al 2004). Although gastric ulceration was not assessed, the authors concluded that corn oil could potentially be helpful in reducing risk of ulceration associated with nonsteroidal anti-inflammatory drug administration. In another study, investigators fed 240 mL of corn oil, refined or crude rice bran oils, or water to horses for 6 weeks to identify effects on gastric ulceration (Frank et al 2005). Oils were added to a relatively high grain diet (estimated at 40:60 hay:grain) and fed for 5 weeks, followed by a 7-day intermittent feed deprivation (ulcer-inducing) protocol in which the same high grain diet was offered on alternating days. Neither of the rice bran oils nor corn oil prevented the formation of gastric ulcers or affected the severity of non-glandular mucosal ulceration (Frank et al 2005). It is possible that fat supplementation could help attenuate existing gastric ulcer severity if it permits total intake of NSC to be reduced (see Chapter 34). In conclusion, more research is needed to identify if vegetable oils have specific properties that may help protect gastric mucosal integrity.

Chronic exertional myopathies

The addition of fat to the diet can help in the management of horses afflicted with chronic exertional myopathies, including recurrent exertional rhabdomyolysis (RER) and Type 1 and 2 polysaccharide storage myopathy (PSSM). Thoroughbreds with RER had lower serum creatine kinase activity when fed a high fat, low starch diet (20% and 7% of DE, respectively) compared to an isocaloric diet high in starch (40% of DE) (McKenzie et al 2003). It has been suggested that replacing a portion of the NSC with fat may help assuage excitability or nervousness in horses with RER, which are believed to trigger episodes. For horses with RER, it has been recommended that at least 15% of DE requirements be supplied by fat, in combination with less than 20% of the total daily DE as starch (Valberg 2010). Several studies have demonstrated a reduction in clinical signs in horses with PSSM fed low starch (< 5% of DE), fat-added (≥12% of DE) diets compared to high starch diets (Firshman et al 2003, Ribeiro et al 2004). The benefit of a low starch, high fat diet for PSSM horses is believed to be the result of less glucose uptake by muscle and increased availability of fatty acids for use by muscle during exercise. The challenge in feeding horses with PSSM is providing enough calories to provide energy during exercise, yet preventing excessive weight gain. To further complicate matters, many PSSM horses are not in training and/or are overweight; thus, the additional calories supplied by dietary fat would simply result in unwanted weight gain. Because of the variation in training status and body condition of horses with PSSM, the need for fat supplementation can vary. Nonetheless, oils and other high fat feedstuffs can be used in lieu of ingredients rich in NSC when additional calories are required in the diet. However, it is worth noting that a recent study found that fats containing short-chain fatty acids (< 10 carbons) are ill-suited for reducing signs of PSSM compared to longer-chain fatty acids (>14 carbons) (Borgia et al 2010). Very few fat sources included in equine diets are naturally low in short chain fatty acids. Coconut oil has approximately 14% short chain fatty acids and thus might not be an ideal source of fat for horses with PSSM. The reader is referred to Chapter 31 for further information on feeding horses with PSSM and RER.

Insulin sensitivity

In humans and other species, a high fat diet (>38% daily caloric intake) that is mostly saturated fat has been associated with the development of insulin resistance (Risérus et al 2009). By comparison, "high fat" diets for horses supply less fat calories (10–20% of DE) and the plant oils and other high fat ingredients commonly added to equine diets generally contain an abundance of unsaturated fatty acids (Table 7-1). Currently, there is no evidence that this level of polyunsaturated fatty acid-rich oil supplementation results in insulin resistance in horses.

In humans, replacement of saturated fatty acids in the diet with mono- or polyunsaturated fatty acids often results in improvement in insulin sensitivity in both healthy and type II diabetic patients (Risérus et al 2009). Although omega-6 and omega-3 polyunsaturated fatty acids have been shown to directly impact membrane fluidity, insulin receptor binding/affinity, glucose transport, hepatic gluconeogenesis, and/or gene expression, their ability to improve insulin sensitivity in humans and other species appears to be mostly related to the concurrent reduction in saturated fat intake that accompanies the addition of polyunsaturated fatty acids to the diet (Fedor & Kelley 2009, Manco et al 2004, Risérus et al 2009). That is to say, supplementing an existing diet, particularly one already high in (saturated) fat with polyunsaturated fatty acids has not been shown to positively impact insulin responsiveness. The effect of different types of fatty acids on insulin sensitivity has not been as thoroughly examined in horses, but available evidence suggests that horses may respond similarly to other species. Although insulin sensitivity was not directly evaluated, glycemic and insulinemic responses were similar when horses were fed a meal of cracked corn with or without the addition of 8% soybean oil or fish oil (Vervuert et al 2010). Fayt et al (2008) reported a lower mean insulin concentration when linseed oil (8%) was substituted for some of the barley in a concentrate feed; however, this might be explained in part by a lower total intake of NSC when linseed oil was included.

Healthy adult and growing horses have been shown to have higher insulin sensitivity when consuming a concentrate rich in polyunsaturated fat and fiber compared to an isocaloric concentrate high in starch and sugar (Treiber et al 2005, Quinn et al 2008). Hoffman et al (2003) reported that insulin sensitivity was similar between pastured horses supplemented with hay or a concentrate rich in fat and fiber, yet insulin sensitivity was greater on these diets compared to a diet of pasture plus a concentrate rich in starch and sugar. Thus, the higher insulin sensitivity observed in horses supplemented with fat (and fiber) in these studies is more likely the result of a reduction in NSC than an increase in fat intake per se.

A comparison of fat-added vs. non-fat added diets in horses that have been diagnosed as insulin resistant or those confirmed to have equine metabolic syndrome or pituitary pars intermedia dysfunction has not been reported. Nonetheless, the use of fat supplements rich in unsaturated fatty acids are currently considered to be acceptable for use in the diets of horses who have insulin resistance when calorie-dense feedstuffs are needed to maintain adequate body condition.

Colic

The daily feeding of vegetable oil has been wrongly perceived as having the ability to "flush" or "lubricate" the gut, thereby preventing impaction or sand colic. Nasogastric administration of relatively large quantities of mineral oil is a common medical treatment for colic (Singer & Smith 2002) and is sometimes used prophylactically for evacuation of sand from the gastrointestinal tract (Hotwagner & Iben 2007). However, mineral oil differs from vegetable oils because it is a petroleum product that is not digested and cannot be absorbed. In contrast, vegetable oils included in the diet at common feeding rates are almost completely digested in the small intestine; thus, very little likely remains to "flush" the other contents through the gastrointestinal tract. Although feeding or administering large quantities of oil to horse that is not adapted to fat may cause loose, oily feces (Schumacher et al 1997), this outcome reflects digestive distress and should be avoided.

Key Points

- Dietary fat can serve as a useful calorie source for horses with special feeding needs.
- By replacing NSC as a calorie source, dietary fat has the potential to reduce risk of gastric ulcers, maintain insulin sensitivity, and reduce clinical signs of chronic exertional myopathies.
- There is no evidence that feeding vegetable oil will "lubricate" the gut or reduce colic risk.

Practical guidelines for feeding fat to horses

Various sources of fat have successfully been added to the diets of growing horses, broodmares, performance horses, older horses, and those with special needs (NRC 2007, Potter et al 1992). This section compares available options for adding fat to equine rations and provides guidelines on how to introduce oils and other high fat feeds to the diet.

Options for inclusion of dietary fat

Several options exist for adding fat to equine diets, ranging from the addition of a variety of vegetable oils or high-fat feedstuffs to an existing ration to the use of a commercial fat supplement or fat-added concentrate. The choice of a specific fat source or the method of fat inclusion will depend on the availability of the fat source or product, the horse's preference, the ease of incorporating the fat source into the feeding program, the owner's goal for feeding fat, and cost. Many owners find commercial fat-supplemented feeds to be a convenient means of including fat in their horse's diet. Such products also help to ensure the feed is balanced with respect to other nutrients in the diet. Most unfortified concentrates contain 2–4% crude fat, whereas "fat-added" feeds usually range from 5–14% crude fat. Fat fortification can raise the energy density of a concentrate by 10 to 50% (e.g., from 3.0 Mcal/kg to 4.5 Mcal/kg); thus commensurately less of a high-fat feed is needed to replace the quantity of a traditional concentrate. However, some commercial fat-added feeds contain additional fiber, which can neutralize the gain in energy density making it more similar to a traditional concentrate that is high in NSC.

Alternatively, horse owners may elect to top-dress oil on an existing ration. Preference tests have generally shown that horses prefer corn oil over other vegetable oils and vegetable oils over animal fats (Bowman et al 1979, Holland et al 1998) (Fig. 7.4). A standard measuring cup can hold 8 fl oz (250 ml) of water and 200 g (1.8 Mcal DE) of vegetable oil. One cup of oil is equivalent to approximately 10% of the maintenance DE requirement for a 500-kg horse. The DE of one cup of oil is equivalent to that provided in

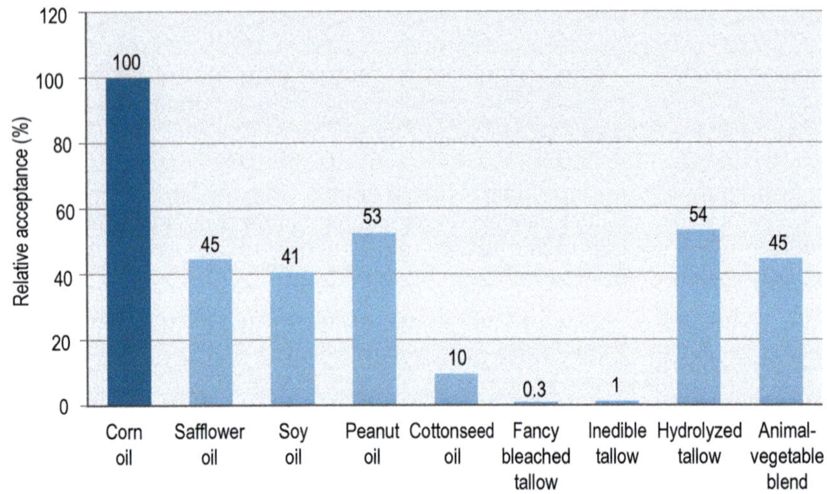

Figure 7.4 Relative acceptance of fats evaluated in palatability experiments compared to corn oil. *Data from* Holland et al (1998).

approximately 0.55 kg oats or rice bran and 0.50 kg corn. It should be cautioned that if oil is top-dressed on an existing ration, as opposed to using a fat-fortified feed, the diet may become unbalanced. It is especially important to evaluate the diets of growing horses and broodmares for nutrient deficiencies and imbalances that might be created by top-dressing oil. Oils provide calories, but they are devoid of protein and minerals. To a varying extent, oils also provide fat-soluble vitamins; however, many of the naturally-occurring tocopherols may be used in defense of lipid peroxidation during storage of the oil and are thus unavailable to aid in meeting the vitamin E requirements of the horse.

Amount of fat to include in the diet

The amount of fat to include in the diet will depend on the feeding goals. For example, it might only take a ½ cup (125 ml) of oil a day to add shine to a horse's hair coat, whereas 1 to 2 cups or more of oil per day for a 500-kg horse may be needed if the goal is to add a significant quantity of calories to the diet or to derive any potential performance benefits. Similarly, the specific feeding goal might dictate the type of fat that should be used. Table 7-3 summarizes the quantity, and in some cases the type, of dietary fat suggested or reported to be effective for a variety of desired outcomes. It should be noted that the quantities listed in Table 7-3 may not reflect the minimum level of fat needed to derive the specific benefit as this may not be established.

Inclusion of fat in the diets of performance horses is becoming commonplace. Anecdotally, some nutritionists recommend higher fat diets (8–10% DM intake, 20–25% of DE intake) for horses participating in more prolonged, submaximal activities, whereas lower fat intakes (5–6% DM intake, 10–15% of DE intake) are suggested for horses competing in racing or other high speed events (e.g., barrel racing). The philosophy behind such recommendations is rooted in the greater perceived need for carbohydrates as a substrate for muscle during maximal intensity, short-duration exercise. Fat supplementation does not appear to alter substrate oxidation in favor of the use of fat over carbohydrate at exercise intensities >50–60% VO_{2max} (Dunnett et al 2002). Thus, it's likely that diets for these horses should still contain a significant portion of hydrolysable carbohydrates to support higher intensity activities.

In contrast to the larger body of work evaluating fat supplemented diets for performance horses, little work has been carried out in broodmares and growing horses to establish ideal rates and types of dietary fat inclusion. While both groups would likely respond positively to fat as a calorie source, it is imperative that the diet as a whole remains balanced with regard to DE, protein, minerals and vitamins. Additional work is needed in young horses (especially those <1 year of age) to establish upper limits of fat inclusion (if it differs from mature horses), as well as verify the effects of high fat diets on absorption of calcium and other minerals crucial for bone development. Based on work at Virginia Tech, weanlings appear to do well when provided a feed with relatively low starch, high fiber and 10–15% crude fat, fed in a 1:1 to 1:2 ratio with forage (e.g., Hoffman et al 1999, 2001, Staniar et al 2007, Treiber et al 2005).

An adequate acclimatization period of up to 12 weeks may be required to reap the full benefits of fat supplementation, although some positive metabolic adaptations may be observed within 3–5 weeks of the introduction of fat into the diet (Dunnett et al 2002, Kronfeld & Harris 2003, Pagan et al 2002).

Upper limit of fat inclusion in equine diets

The upper limit of fat inclusion in equine diets has not been established for all sources of fat. Diets with up to 230 g fat/kg DM from added corn oil, peanut oil, tallow, and animal-vegetable fat blends appear to be acceptable to horses without negatively impacting digestion of other nutrients (Kronfeld et al 2004). In contrast, current information suggests that soybean oil should be limited to 0.7 g/kg BW/day (NRC 2007). Higher rates of fat inclusion may increase the risk for digestive disturbance, interfere with microbial fermentation of fiber in the hindgut, or reduce calcium absorption via formation of mineral-fat soaps. In addition, acceptance of high levels of dietary fat will likely vary between individual horses, based on palatability and texture preferences, as well as gastrointestinal tolerance. For example, some horses appear to dislike oils, but are more accepting of rice bran or flaxseed. Similarly, some horses will develop loose or greasy feces at lower levels of fat inclusion, while others will be able to consume relatively high quantities of fat with no apparent digestive problems. Although horses seem to tolerate relatively high levels of fat,

Table 7-3 Fat Source and Level of Inclusion in the Diet Shown to Produce Various Biological and Physiological Responses. Note That the Level of Inclusion Listed May Not Necessarily Represent the Minimum Amount Needed to Achieve the Desired Outcome

Biological or physiological response	Fat source used	Level of inclusion	Reference
Increase in plasma α-linolenic acid	Flaxseed	6 g ALA/100 kg BW	Stelzleni et al 2006
Increase in plasma eicosapentaenoic and decosahexaenoic acids	Fish oil (encapsulated)	2 g EPA+DHA/100 kg BW	King et al 2008
Skin improvement in response to Culicoides	Flaxseed	55 g ALA/100 kg BW	O'Neill et al 2002
Decrease in eicosanoid production	Fish oil (encapsulated)	7.2 g EPA+DPA+DHA/100 kg BW	Vineyard et al 2008
Decrease in eicosanoid production	Corn oil	43.2 g LA/100 kg BW	Vineyard et al 2008
Improved semen characteristics	Fish oil (encapsulated)[a]	3.1 g DHA/100 kg BW	Brinsko et al 2005
Reduced reactivity or excitability	Mix of soy lecithin and corn oil	200 g fat/100 kg BW	Holland et al 1996
Reduction in clinical signs of PSSM		≥ 13% of DE as fat[b]	Ribeiro et al 2004
Reduction in clinical signs of RER		15–25% of DE as fat[c]	McKenzie et al 2003
Decreased heat production during exercise	Vegetable oil	200 g oil/100 kg BW[d]	Kronfeld 1996
Metabolic adaptations to increase utilization of fat during exercise	Soybean oil	20% of DE as oil	Dunnett et al 2002

[a]25% DHA, 5% EPA.
[b]Paired with < 10% of DE from starch.
[c]Paired with < 20% of DE from starch.
[d]Based on theoretical calculations.

it is worth noting that in practice most rations are considerably lower than 230 g fat/kg DM, even with the use of so-called "high-fat" commercial feeds.

Introducing fat to the diet

Key to the success of any fat feeding program is gradual introduction of the oil or fat-added feed. Transition to high fat feeds or oils usually takes about 4 to 14 days in healthy horses. However, this will vary based on the quantity of fat fed and between individual horses. If top-dressing oil on an existing ration, a conservative approach is to start with ¼ cup (~60 ml) per meal and increase the amount by ¼ cup every 2-3 days until the desired 1 or 2 cups/day is reached in 2–3 weeks. Similarly, a fat-added feed or fat supplement should be introduced in small increments (~25% of the desired feeding rate) every 3 or 4 days. When initiating a fat feeding program, horses should be closely observed for signs of digestive upset and the rate of fat introduction adjusted accordingly. If the horse's feces are greasy, grayish in color, more abundant, or too loose, the introduction of fat may have been too rapid. These signs are usually preceded by sheen on well-formed fecal balls, a sign of some fat escaping digestion (Kronfeld et al 2004). In such cases, the amount of fat should be temporarily reduced until the feces return to normal, followed by reintroduction of fat at a slower rate.

Impact of fat-added diets on antioxidant requirements

Fatty acids, particularly unsaturated fatty acids, are prone to oxidation. As a result, it is often recommended that additional antioxidants be added to the diet. Unfortunately, there has been limited study on the impact of high fat diets on antioxidant requirements in horses. Vitamin E status was not negatively affected in horses fed diets with 64 g fat/kg DM (~20% of DE intake) from added soybean oil and 80 IU vitamin E/kg DM (Siciliano & Wood 1993). Vitamin E status was similarly unaffected in ponies fed a diet with 10% of DE intake from corn oil; however, plasma thiobarbituric acid reactive substances (TBARS) and breath pentane were elevated during exercise, especially in ponies with lower plasma vitamin E concentrations (McMeniman & Hintz 1992). Although TBARS and breath pentane are non-specific markers of oxidative stress, this finding indicates that additional vitamin E may be needed in the diet of horses with increased oxidative loads, even when including only moderate levels of fat. The level and type of endogenous tocopherols present in vegetable oils varies between different sources (Table 7-4), which may explain the discrepancy between these two studies. In addition, at least a portion of the naturally occurring tocopherols in oil may be used in defense of lipid peroxidation during storage and are thus unavailable to aid in meeting the vitamin E requirements of the horse. Functional and synergistic relationships between different antioxidant nutrients (e.g., selenium, vitamin C, carotenoids) and their level in the diet could further impact the need for additional supplementation; however, these relationships have not been investigated in the horse.

A general recommendation for the prevention of peroxidative damage is to provide a minimum of 100 IU of vitamin E per 100 ml of vegetable oil (Harris 1999, Stratton-Phelps et al 2003). This recommendation is based on research in rodents that concluded that 0.6 mg α-tocopherol equivalents per gram of linoleic acid was suitable for preventing excessive lipid peroxidation, and that some of the endogenous tocopherols in oil may be applied towards meeting this

Table 7-4 α- and γ-Tocopherol Content and Vitamin E Activity (as α-Tocopherol Equivalents) in Various Oils and Fats[a]

Fat source	α-tocopherol (mg/100 g)	γ-tocopherol (mg/100 g)	Vitamin E activity (mg/100 g)
Canola oil	21.0	4.2	21.5
Coconut oil	0.5	–[b]	0.7
Corn oil	11.2	60.2	19.8
Cottonseed oil	38.9	38.7	42.8
Olive oil	11.9	–	12.0
Palm oil	25.6	31.6	33.5
Peanut oil	13.0	21.4	15.2
Safflower oil	34.2	7.1	34.9
Soybean oil	7.5	79.7	17.1
Sunflower oil	48.7	5.1	49.2
Wheat germ oil	133.0	26.0	173.6
Cod liver oil	22.0	–	22.0
Herring oil	9.2	–	9.2
Menhaden fish oil	7.5	–	7.5
Lard	1.2	–	1.5
Tallow	2.7	–	2.7

[a]Data modified from Sheppard et al 1993.
[b]Dashes denote no value or trace.

additional tocopherol requirement (Valk & Hornstra 2000). Although research findings have been inconsistent, there is evidence in other species that supplementation with highly unsaturated fatty acids (e.g., EPA and DHA), even if coupled with lower total fat intakes, would require higher levels of vitamin E supplementation (Valk & Hornstra 2000). However, supplementation of yearling horses with high levels of EPA and DHA (6 g/100 kg BW) from encapsulated fish oil had no negative effects on plasma vitamin E or lipid-specific measures of peroxidative damage (e.g., lipid hydroperoxides, F2-isoprostanes) when diets contained adequate levels of vitamin E and a relatively low total fat content (4.2% DM) (White et al 2007). Further research on the impact of various fat sources on antioxidant requirements is needed, particularly in horses under increased oxidative stress (e.g., performance horses).

Product stability

Due to potential for oxidation, inclusion of fat in the concentrate can reduce the shelf life of the product compared to a non fat-added feed (e.g., by 1 to 2 weeks in hot and humid climates). Most feed manufacturers attempt to counteract the deterioration of fats by adding natural and/or artificial antioxidants to their products. Nonetheless, the risk of rancidity is still a concern if feeds are stocked for long periods in a warehouse or with distributors before being purchased or if owners fail to store products appropriately or utilize them in a timely manner. Fat with a high content of unsaturated fatty acids is particularly susceptible to oxidation, resulting in deterioration of fatty acids and the development of a number of components (e.g., hydroxyperoxides and aldehydes) which may have negative local and systemic effects on the horse if consumed. Rancid feeds should not be fed to horses.

Owners should regularly inspect fat-added feeds and supplements. Feeds that have gone rancid tend to have a sweet, alcohol-like smell and are generally, but not always unpalatable to horses. Fat-added feeds, supplements and oils should be stored in a cool, dry location and be purchased in quantities that can be fed in 2 to 4 weeks, depending on season and/or climate.

Potential contraindications for feeding fat to horses

Increasing the fat content of the diet can benefit many horses; however, there are a few scenarios in which this practice would be contraindicated. First and most obvious are horses or ponies that are already overweight or obese. Dietary fat is the most calorie-dense component that can be added to the diet; thus, adding fat to the diet of an animal that is overweight is not only unnecessary, it can contribute to diseases associated with obesity (e.g., insulin resistance) by promoting weight gain. Similarly, fat should not be added to the diet of ponies or horses prone to or experiencing hyperlipemia. Finally, added fat should not be a part of the initial refeeding program for starved or severely malnourished horses, as many of these horses have compromised gastrointestinal and organ function (Kronfeld 1993, Witham & Stull 1998).

Key Points

- Fat should be introduced into the diet gradually to avoid digestive problems.
- Be attentive to nutrient imbalances when top-dressing oil onto an existing ration.
- Commercial fat-added feeds are available and typically contain 5–14% crude fat.
- The level of fat to include in equine diets will depend on the feeding goals and desired outcome.
- Fat should not be added to equine diets indiscriminately and should be avoided in overweight horses.
- Inclusion of high levels of fat in the diet may precipitate a higher need for antioxidants such as vitamin E.

Conclusion

In today's equine industry, the inclusion of fat sources in horse rations has become commonplace even though this concept was considered fairly novel as little as 20 years ago. It could be argued that the widespread use of vegetable oils and the availability of fat-added rations, particularly those with higher fiber and lower starch, is perhaps the biggest change to horse feeding to occur in the last 20 or so years. Furthermore, this shift in feeding practice was driven by scientific research. Oils and other fat-rich feedstuffs offer a means to dramatically alter calorie intake in horses, not only in quantity but also in quality, enabling the formulation of safe and effective diets for healthy and special needs horses. Although great inroads have been made, there is still much to learn about how the horse utilizes fat, as well as the biological and physiological benefits that can be harnessed from different fat sources.

References

Berbert, A.A., Kondo, C.R., Almendra, C.L., et al., 2005. Supplementation of fish oil and olive oil in patients with rheumatoid arthritis. Nutrition 21, 131–136.

Borgia, L.A., Valberg, S.J., McCue, M.E., et al., 2010. Effect of dietary fats with odd or even numbers of carbon atoms on metabolic response and muscle damage with exercise in Quarter Horse-type horses with type 1 polysaccharide storage myopathy. Am J Vet Res 71, 326–336.

Boufaïed, H., Chouinard, P.Y., Tremblay, G.F., et al., 2003. Fatty acids in forages. I. Factors affecting concentrations. Can J Anim Sci 83, 501–511.

Bowman, V.A., Fontenot, J.P., Meacham, T.N., et al., 1979. Acceptability and digestibility of animal, vegetable and blended fats by equine. In: Proc 6th Equine Nutr Physiol Symp, College Station, TX. Equine Nutrition and Physiology Society, Savoy, IL, p. 74.

Brinsko, S.P., Varner, D.D., Love, C.C., et al., 2005. Effect of feeding a DHA-enriched nutraceutical on the quality of fresh, cooled and frozen stallion semen. Theriogenology 63, 1519–1527.

Bush, J.A., Freeman, D.E., Kline, K.H., et al., 2001. Dietary fat supplementation effects on in vitro nutrient disappearance and in vivo nutrient intake and total tract digestibility by horses. J Anim Sci 79, 232–239.

Byers, F.M., Schelling, G.T., 1988. Lipids in ruminant nutrition. The Ruminant Animal, Digestive Physiology and Nutrition. In: Church, D.C. (Ed.), Prospect Heights. Waveland Press, Inc, Illinois, pp. 298–312.

Calder, P.C., 2006. Polyunsaturated fatty acids and inflammation. Prostaglandins Leukotr Essent Fatty Acids 75, 197–202.

Calder, P.C., Grimble, R.F., 2002. Polyunsaturated fatty acids, inflammation and immunity. Eur J Clin Nutr 56 (suppl. 3), S14–S19.

Cargile, J.L., Burrow, J.A., Kim, I., et al., 2004. Effect of dietary corn oil supplementation on equine gastric fluid acid, sodium, and prostaglandin E2 content before and during pentagastrin infusion. J Vet Intern Med 8, 545–549.

Cleland, L.G., French, J.K., Betts, W.H., et al., 1998. Clinical and biochemical effects of dietary fish oil supplements in rheumatoid arthritis. J Rheumatol 15, 1471–1475.

Coenen, M., 1986. Verdaulichkeit und praecaecale passage einer suspendierfähigen diät in abhängigkeit von der applikationsform (spontane futteraufnahme bzw. Flüssig per sonde). J Anim Physiol Anim Nutr 56, 104–117.

Davison, K.E., Potter, G.D., Greene, L.W., et al., 1991. Lactation and reproductive performance of mares fed added dietary fat during late gestation and early lactation. J Equine Vet Sci 11, 111–115.

Delobel, A., Fabry, C., Schoonheere, N., et al., 2008. Linseed oil supplementation in diet for horses: Effects on palatability and digestibility. Livestock Sci 116, 15–21.

Domingo, J.L., Bocio, A., Falco, G., et al., 2007. Benefits and risks of fish consumption I. A quantitative analysis of the intake of omega-3 fatty acids and chemical contaminants. Toxicology 230, 219–226.

Dunnett, C.E., Marlin, D.J., Harris, R.C., 2002. Effect of dietary lipid on response to exercise: Relationship to metabolic adaptation. Equine Vet J 34 (Suppl), 75–80.

Duvaux-Ponter, C., Tournie, M., Detrimont, L., et al., 2004. Effect of a supplement rich in linolenic acid added to the diet of mares on fatty acid composition of mammary secretions and the acquisition of passive immunity in the foal. Anim Sci 78, 399–407.

Eaton, M.D., Hodgson, D.R., Evans, D.L., et al., 1995. Effect of a diet containing supplementary fat on the capacity for high intensity exercise. Equine Vet J 18 (Suppl), 353–356.

Essen-Gustavsson, B., Blomstrand, E., Karlstrom, K., et al., 1991. Influence of diet on substrate metabolism during exercise. In: Persson, S.G.B., Lindholm, A., Jeffcott, L.B. (Eds.), Equine Exercise Physiology 3. ICEEP Publications, Stockholm, Sweden, pp. 288–298.

Fahy, E., Subramaniam, S., Brown, H.A., et al., 2005. A comprehensive classification system for lipids. J Lipid Res 46, 839–861.

Fayt, J., Dotreppe, O., Hornick, J.L., et al., 2008. Spelt, an ancient cereal and first pressure linseed oil as ingredients of compound feedstuffs for modern horse feeding. J Anim Physiol Anim Nutr 92, 303–309.

Fedor, D., Kelley, D.S., 2009. Prevention of insulin resistance by n-3 polyunsaturated fatty acids. Curr Opin Clin Nutr Metab Care 12, 138–146.

Firshman, A.M., Valberg, S.J., Bender, J.B., et al., 2003. Epidemiologic characteristics and management of polysaccharide storage myopathy in Quarter Horses. Am J Vet Res 64, 1319–1327.

Frank, N., Sojka, J.E., Latour, M.A., 2004. Effect of hypothyroidism on the blood lipid response to higher dietary fat intake in mares. J Anim Sci 82, 2640–2646.

Frank, N., Andrews, F.M., Elliott, S.B., et al., 2005. Effects of dietary oils on the development of gastric ulcers in mares. Am J Vet Res 66, 2006–2011.

French, S.J., Murray, B., Rumsey, R.D., et al., 1995. Adaptation to high-fat diets: effects on eating behaviour and plasma cholecystokinin. Br J Nutr 73, 179–189.

Friberg, C.A., Logas, D., 1999. Treatment of culicoides hypersensitive horses with high-dose n-3 fatty acids: A double-blinded crossover study. Vet Derm 10, 117–122.

Fonnesbeck, P.V., Lydman, R.K., Vander Noot, G.W., et al., 1967. Digestibility of the proximate nutrients of forage by horses. J Anim Sci 26, 1039–1044.

Gatta, D., Casini, L., Liponi, G.B., et al., 2005. Effect of oils administration on diets digestibility and haematic fatty acids profile in exercising horses. Ital J Anim Sci 4 (Suppl 2), 415–417.

Geelen, S.N.J., Sloet van Oldruitenborgh-Oosterbaan, M.M., Beynen, A.C., 1999. Dietary fat supplementation and equine plasma lipid metabolism. Equine Vet J 30 (Suppl), 475–478.

Geelen, S.N.J., Jansen, W.L., Geelen, M.M., et al., 2000. Lipid metabolism in equines fed a fat-rich diet. Int J Vitam Nutr Res 70, 148–152.

Geelen, S.N.J., Blazquez, C., Geelen, M.J.H., et al., 2001. High fat intake lowers fatty acid synthesis and raises fatty acid oxidation in aerobic muscle in Shetland ponies. Br J Nutr 86, 31–36.

Geor, R.J., Harris, P.A., Hoekstra, K.E., et al., 2001. Effect of corn oil on solid-phase gastric emptying in horses. (Abstr.) Proc. 19th ACVIM. p. 853.

Godoi, F.N., Almeida, F.Q., Saliba, E.O.S., et al., 2009. Intake, digestive kinetics and nutrient digestibility in athletic horses fed diets with soybean oil. R Bras Zootec, online version, vol 38, doi: 10.1590/S1516-35982009001000011.

Goyens, P.L.L., Spiker, M.E., Zock, P.L., et al., 2006. Conversion of α-linolenic acid in humans is influenced by the absolute amounts of α-linolenic acid and linoleic acid in the diet and not by the ratio. Am J Clin Nutr 84, 44–53.

Greeve, J., Altkemper, I., Dieterich, J.H., et al., 1993. Apolipoprotein B mRNA editing in 12 different mammalian species: hepatic expression is reflected in low concentrations of apoB-containing plasma lipoproteins. J Lipid Res 34, 1367–1383.

Gurr, M.I., Harwood, J.L., Frayn, K.N., 2002. Lipid Biochemistry: an Introduction. fifth ed. Blackwell Science Ltd., Oxford, UK.

Hall, J.A., Van Saun, R.J., Tornquist, S.J., et al., 2004a. Effect of type of dietary polyunsaturated fatty acid supplement (corn oil or fish oil) on immune responses in healthy horses. J Vet Intern Med 18, 880–886.

Hall, J.A., Van Saun, R.J., Wander, R.C., 2004b. Dietary (n-3) fatty acids from menhaden fish oil alter plasma fatty acids and leukotriene b synthesis in healthy horses. J Vet Intern Med 18, 871–879.

Hallebeek, J.M., Beynen, A.C., 2002. The plasma level of triacylglycerols in horses fed high-fat diets containing either soybean oil or palm oil. J Anim Physiol Anim Nutr 86, 111–116.

Hargin, K.D., Morrison, W.R., 1980. The distribution of acyl lipids in the germ, aleurone, starch and non-starch endosperm of four wheat varieties. J Sci Food Agric 31, 877–888.

Harkins, J.D., Morris, G.S., Tulley, R.T., et al., 1992. Effect of added dietary fat on racing performance in Thoroughbred horses. J Equine Vet Sci 12, 123–129.

Harwood, J.L., 1996. Recent advances in the biosynthesis of plant fatty acids. Biochim Biophys Acta 1301, 7–56.

Harris, M.A., Baumgard, L.H., Arns, M.J., et al., 2005. Stallion spermatozoa membrane phospholipid dynamics following dietary n-3 supplementation. Anim Reprod Sci 89, 234–237.

Harris, P.A., 1999. Feeding and management advice for tying up. Proceedings of the BEVA Specialist meeting on Nutrition and Behaviour 100–104.

Hess, B.W., Moss, G.E., Rule, D.C., 2008. A decade of developments in the area of fat supplementation research with beef cattle and sheep. J Anim Sci 86 (E. Suppl.), E188–E204.

Henry, M.M., Moore, J.N., Feldman, E.B., et al., 1990. Effect of dietary alpha-linolenic acid on equine monocyte procoagulant activity and eicosanoid synthesis. Circ Shock 32, 173–188.

Henry, M.M., Moore, J.N., Fischer, J.K., 1991. Influence of an omega-3 fatty acid-enriched ration on in vivo responses of horses to endotoxin. Am J Vet Res 52, 523–527.

Hintz, H.F., Schryver, F.F., 1989. Digestibility of various sources of fat by horses. In: Proceedings of the Cornell Nutrition Conference for Feed Manufacturers. Syracuse, NY, pp. 44–48.

Hoffman, R.M., Lawrence, L.A., Kronfeld, D.S., et al., 1999. Dietary carbohydrates and fat influence radiographic bone mineral content of growing horses. J Anim Sci 77, 3330–3338.

Hoffman, R.M., Wilson, J.A., Lawrence, L.A., et al., 2001. Supplemental calcium does not influence radiographic bone mineral content of growing foals fed pasture and a fat and fiber supplement. In: Proceedings of Equine Nutrition and Physiology Society Symposium, Lexington, KY. Equine Nutrition and Physiology Society, Savoy, IL, pp. 122–123.

Hoffman, R.M., Boston, R.C., Stefanovski, D., et al., 2003. Obesity and diet affect glucose dynamics and insulin sensitivity in Thoroughbred geldings. J Anim Sci 81, 2333–2342.

Holland, J.L., Kronfeld, D.S., Meacham, T.N., 1996. Behavior of horses is affected by soy lecithin and corn oil in the diet. J Anim Sci 74, 1252–1255.

Holland, J.L., Kronfeld, D.S., Rich, G.A., 1998. Acceptance of fat and lecithin containing diets by horses. Appl Anim Behav Sci 56, 91–96.

Hotwagner, K., Iben, C., 2007. Evacuation of sand from the equine intestine with mineral oil, with and without psyllium. J Anim Physiol Anim Nutr 92, 86–91.

Hughes, S.J., Potter, G.D., Greene, L.W., et al., 1995. Adaptation of Thoroughbred horses in training to a fat supplemented diet. Equine Vet J 18 (Suppl), 349–352.

Hussein, N.E., Ah-Sing, P., Wilkinson, C., et al., 2005. Long-chain conversion of [^{13}C]linoleic acid and alpha-linolenic acid in response to marked changes in their dietary intake in men. J Lipid Res 46, 269–280.

Hyyppa, S., Saastamoinen, M., Poso, A.R., 1999. Effect of a post exercise fat-supplemented diet on muscle glycogen repletion. Equine Vet J 30 (Suppl), 493–498.

Iqbal, J., Hussain, M.M., 2009. Intestinal lipid absorption. Am J Physiol Endocrinol Metab 296, E1183–E1194.

IUPAC-IUB (International Union of Pure & Applied Chemistry-International Union of Biochemistry), 1976. The nomenclature of lipids. IUPAC-IUB Commission on Biochemical Nomenclature. J Lipid Res 19, 114–128.

James, M.J., Gibson, R.A., Cleland, L.G., 2000. Dietary polyunsaturated fatty acids and inflammatory mediator production. Am J Clin Nutr 71, 343S-348S.

Jansen, W.L., van der Kuilen, J., Geelen, S.N.J., et al., 2000. The effect of replacing nonstructural carbohydrates with soybean oil on the digestibility of fibre in trotting horses. Equine Vet J 32, 27–30.

Jansen, W.L., van der Kuilen, J., Geelen, S.N.J., et al., 2001. The apparent digestibility of fibre in trotters when dietary soybean oil is substituted for an iso-energetic amount of glucose. Arch Anim Nutr 54, 297–304.

Jansen, W.L., Geelen, S.N.J., van der Kuilen, J., et al., 2002. Dietary soybean oil depresses the apparent digestibility of fibre in trotters when substituted for an iso-energetic amount of corn starch or glucose. Equine Vet J 34, 302–305.

Jansen, W.L., Sloet van Oldruitenborgh-Oosterbaan, M.M., Cone, J.W., et al., 2007. Studies on the mechanism by which a high intake of soybean oil depresses the apparent digestibility of fibre in horses. Anim Feed Sci Tech 138, 298–308.

Jenkins, T.C., 1993. Lipid metabolism in the rumen. J Dairy Sci 76, 3851–3863.

Kane, E., Baker, J.P., Bull, L.S., 1979. Utilization of a corn oil supplemented diet by the pony. J Anim Sci 48, 1379–1384.

Khol-Parisini, A., van den Hoven, R., Leinker, S., et al., 2007. Effects of feeding sunflower oil or seal blubber oil to horses with recurrent airway obstruction. Can J Vet Res 71, 59–65.

King, S.S., Abughazaleh, A.A., Webel, S.K., et al., 2008. Circulating fatty acid profiles in response to three levels of dietary omega-3 fatty acid supplementation in horses. J Anim Sci 86, 1114–1123.

Kronfeld, D.S., 1993. Starvation and malnutrition: recognition and treatment. J Equine Vet Sci 13, 298–303.

Kronfeld, D.S., 1996. Dietary fat affects heat production and other variables of equine performance, under hot and humid conditions. Equine Vet J 22 (Suppl), 24–34.

Kronfeld, D.S., Harris, P.A., 2003. Equine grain-associated disorders. Comp Contin Educ Pract Vet 25, 974–983.

Kronfeld, D.S., Custalow, S.E., Ferrante, P.L., et al., 1998. Acid-base responses of fat-adapted horses: relevance to hard work in the heat. Appl Anim Behav 59, 61–72.

Kronfeld, D.S., Holland, J.L., Rich, G.A., et al., 2004. Fat digestibility in *Equus caballus* follows increasing first-order kinetics. J Anim Sci 82, 1773–1780.

Lau, C.S., Morley, K.D., Belch, J.J., 1993. Effects of fish oil supplementation on non-steroidal anti-inflammatory drug requirement in patients with mild rheumatoid arthritis - a double-blind placebo controlled study. Br J Rheumatol 32, 982–989.

Lindberg, J.E., Karlsson, C.P., 2001. Effect of partial replacement of oats with sugar beet pulp and maize oil on nutrient utilisation in horses. Equine Vet J 33, 585–590.

Lorenzo-Figueras, M., Preston, T., Ott, E.A., et al., 2005. Meal-induced gastric relaxation and emptying in horses after ingestion of high-fat versus high-carbohydrate diets. Am J Vet Res 66, 897–906.

Lorenzo-Figueras, M., Morisset, S.M., Morisset, J., et al., 2007. Digestive enzyme concentrations and activities in healthy pancreatic tissues of horses. Am J Vet Res 68, 1070–1072.

Manco, M., Calvani, M., Mingrone, G., 2004. Effects of dietary fatty acids on insulin sensitivity and secretion. Diabetes, Obesity and Metabolism 6, 402–413.

Manhart, D.R., Scott, B.D., Gibbs, P.G., et al., 2009. Markers of inflammation in arthritic horses fed omega-3 fatty acids. Prof Anim Sci 25, 155–160.

Mansbach, C.M., Gorelick, F., 2007. Development and physiological regulation of intestinal lipid absorption. II. Dietary lipid absorption, complex lipid synthesis, and the intracellular packing and secretion of chylomicrons. Am J Physiol Gastrointest Liver Physiol 293, G645–G650.

Marchello, E.V., Shurg, W.A., Marchello, J.A., et al., 2000. Changes in lipoprotein composition in horses fed a fat-supplemented diet. J Equine Vet Sci 20, 453–458.

McCann, J.S., Meacham, T.N., Fontenot, J.P., 1987. Energy utilization and blood traits of ponies fed fat-supplemented diets. J Anim Sci 65, 1019–1026.

McKenzie, E.C., Valberg, S.J., Godden, S.M., et al., 2003. Effect of dietary starch, fat, and bicarbonate content on exercise responses and serum creatine kinase activity in equine recurrent exertional rhabdomyolysis. J Vet Intern Med 17, 693–701.

McMeniman, N.P., Hintz, H.F., 1992. Effect of vitamin E status on lipid peroxidation in exercised horses. Equine Vet J 24, 482–484.

Meyer, H., Flothow, C., Radicke, S., 1997. Preileal digestibility of coconut fat and soybean oil in horses and their influence on metabolites of microbial origin of the proximal digestive tract. Arch Anim Nutr 50, 63–74.

Meyer, J.H., Mayer, E.A., Jehn, D., et al., 1986. Gastric processing and emptying of fat. Gastroenterology 90, 1176–1187.

Meyers, M.C., Potter, G.D., Evans, J.W., et al., 1989. Physiologic and metabolic response of exercising horses to added dietary fat. J Equine Vet Sci 9, 218–223.

Morgado, E.S., Almeida, F.Q., Godoi, F.N., et al., 2009. Carbohydrate digestion in horses fed diets composed by roughages or roughages supplemented with concentrate and/or soybean oil. Arquivo Brasileiro de Medicina Veterinaria e Zootecnia 61, 1112–1119.

Morris, D.D., Henry, M.M., Moore, J.N., et al., 1991. Effect of dietary alpha-linolenic acid on endotoxin-induced production of tumor necrosis factor by peritoneal macrophages in horses. Am J Vet Res 52, 528–532.

Moreau, H., Gargouri, Y., Lecat, D., et al., 1988. Screening of lipases in several mammals. Biochim Biophys Acta 959, 247–252.

Munsterman, A.S., Bertone, A.L., Zachos, T.A., et al., 2005. Effects of the omega-3 fatty acid, alpha-linolenic acid, on lipopolysaccharide-challenged synovial explants from horses. Am J Vet Res 66, 1503–1508.

Nicol, C., Badnell-Waters, A., Bice, R., et al., 2005. The effects of diet and weaning method on the behaviour of young horses. Appl Anim Behav Sci 95, 205–221.

Nieto, J.E., Aldridge, B.M., Beldomenico, P.M., et al., 2005. Characterization of equine intestinal fatty acid binding protein and its use in managing horses with colic. Am J Vet Res 66, 223–232.

NRC, 2005. Dietary reference intakes for energy, carbohydrate, fiber, fat, fatty acids, cholesterol, protein, and amino acids (macronutrients). The National Academies Press, Washington, DC.

NRC, 2007. Nutrient requirements of horses, sixth Rev ed. The National Academies Press, Washington, DC.

Oldham, S.L., Potter, G.D., Evans, J.W., et al., 1990. Storage and mobilization of muscle glycogen in exercising horses fed a fat-supplemented diet. J Equine Vet Sci 10, 353–359.

O'Neill, W., McKee, S., Clarke, A.F., 2002. Flaxseed (*Linum usitatissimum*) supplementation associated with reduced skin test lesional area in horses with culicoides hypersensitivity. Can J Vet Res 66, 272–277.

Oomah, B.D., Mazza, G., Kenaschuk, E.O., 1992. Cyanogenic compounds in flaxseed. J Agr Food Chem 40, 1346–1348.

Orme, C.E., Harris, R.C., Marlin, D.J., et al., 1997. Metabolic adaptation to a fat-supplemented diet by the Thoroughbred horse. Br J Nutr 97, 443–458.

Pagan, J.D., Essen-Gustavsson, B., Lindholm, A., et al., 1987. The effect of dietary energy source on exercise performance in Standardbred horses. In: Gillespie, J.R., Robinson, N.E. (Eds.), Equine Exercise Physiology 2. ICEEP Publications, Davis, CA, pp. 686–700.

Pagan, J.D., Harris, P.A., Kennedy, M.A.P., et al., 1999. Feed type and intake affects glycemic response in Thoroughbred horses. In: Proc 16th Equine Nutr Physiol Symp, Raleigh, NC. Equine Nutrition and Physiology Society, Savoy, IL, pp. 149–150.

Pagan, J.D., Geor, R.J., Harris, P.A., et al., 2002. Effects of fat adaptation on glucose kinetics and substrate oxidation during low intensity exercise. Equine Vet J 34 (Suppl), 33–38.

Palmquist, D.L., 1988. The feeding value of fats. In: Ørskov, E.R. (Ed.), World Animal Science. B. Disciplinary Approach. 4. Feed Science. Elsevier, Amsterdam, pp. 293–311.

Potter, G.D., Hughes, S.L., Julen, T.R., et al., 1992. A review of research on digestion and utilization of fat by the equine. Pferdeheilkunde: Sonderausgabe. 1. Europäische Konferenz über die Ernährung des Pferdes 119–123.

Quinn, R.W., Burk, A.O., Hartsock, T.G., et al., 2008. Insulin sensitivity in Thoroughbred geldings: effect of weight gain, diet, and exercise on insulin sensitivity in Thoroughbred geldings. J Equine Vet Sci 28, 728–738.

Redondo, A.J., Carranza, J., Trigo, P., 2009. Fat diet reduces stress and intensity of startle reaction in horses. Appl Anim Behav Sci 118, 69–75.

Ribeiro,, W.P., Valberg, S.J., Pagan, J.D., et al., 2004. The effect of varying dietary starch and fat content on serum creatine kinase activity and substrate availability in equine polysaccharide storage myopathy. J Vet Intern Med 18, 887–894.

Rich, G.A., Fontenot, J.P., Meacham, T.N., 1981. Digestibility of animal, vegetable and blended fats by equine. In: Proc 7th Equine Nutr Physiol Symp, Warrenton, VA. Equine Nutrition and Physiology Society, Savoy, IL, pp. 30–36.

Risérus, U., Willett, W.C., Hu, F.B., 2009. Dietary fats and prevention of type 2 diabetes. Prog Lipid Res 48, 44–51.

Sales, J., Homolka, P., 2011. A meta-analysis of the effects of supplemental dietary fat on protein and fibre digestibility in the horse. Livestock Sci 136, 55–63.

Sallmann, H.P., Kienzle, E., Fuhrmann, H., et al., 1991. Metabolic consequences of feeding ponies with marginal amounts of fat. In: Proc 12th Equine Nutr Physiol Symp, Calgary, Alberta. Equine Nutrition and Physiology Society, Savoy, IL, pp. 81–82.

Schumacher, J., DeGraves, F.J., Spano, J.S., 1997. Clinical and clinicopathologic effects of large doses of raw linseed oil as compared to mineral oil in healthy horses. J Vet Intern Med 11, 296–299.

Scott, B.D., Potter, G.D., Greene, L.W., et al., 1992. Efficacy of a fat-supplemented diet on muscle glycogen concentrations in exercising Thoroughbred horses maintained in varying body conditions. J Equine Vet Sci 12, 105–109.
Sheppard, A.J., Pennington, A.T., Welbrauch, J.L., 1993. Analysis and distribution of vitamin E in vegetable oils and foods. In: Packer, L., Fuchs, J. (Eds.), Vitamin E in Health and Disease. Marcel Dekker, Inc., New York, New York.
Siciliano, P.D., Wood, C.H., 1993. The effect of added dietary soybean oil on vitamin E status of the horse. J Anim Sci 71, 3399–3402.
Singer, E.R., Smith, M.A., 2002. Examination of the horse with colic: is it medical or surgical? Equine Vet Educ. 34, 87–96.
Sprecher, H., 2000. Metabolism of highly unsaturated n-3 and n-6 fatty acids. Biochim Biophys Acta 1486, 219–231.
Sprecher, H., Luthria, D.L., Mohammed, B.S., et al., 1995. Reevaluation of the pathways for the biosynthesis of polyunsaturated fatty acids. J Lipid Res 36, 2471–2477.
Staniar, W.B., Kronfeld, D.S., Akers, R.M., et al., 2007. Insulin-like growth factor I in growing Thoroughbreds. J Anim Physiol Anim Nutr 91, 390–399.
Stelzleni, E.L., Warren, L.K., Kivipelto, J., 2006. Effect of dietary n-3 fatty acid supplementation on plasma and milk composition and immune status of mares and foals. J Anim Sci 84 (Suppl. 1), 392–393.
Stratton-Phelps, M., Fascetti, A.J., Geor, R.J., 2003. Nutritional support in selected metabolic, hepatic, urinary, and musculoskeletal conditions. In: Robinson, N.E. (Ed.), Current Therapy in Equine Medicine 5. Elsevier Science, Philadelphia, PA, pp. 715–722.
Sturgeon, L.S., Baker, L.A., Pipkin, J.L., et al., 2000. The digestibility and mineral availability of matua, bermuda grass, and alfalfa hay in mature horses. J Equine Vet Sci 20, 45–48.
Swinney, D.L., Potter, G.D., Greene, L.W., et al., 1995. Digestion of fat in the equine small and large intestine. In: Proc 14th Equine Nutr Physiol Symp, Ontario, CA. Equine Nutrition and Physiology Society, Savoy, IL, pp. 30–35.
Topliff, D.R., Potter, G.D., Dutson, T.R., et al., 1983. Diet manipulation and muscle glycogen in the equine. In: Proc. 8th Equine Nutr Physiol Soc Symp, Lexington, KY. Equine Nutrition and Physiology Society, Savoy, IL, pp. 119–124.
Treiber, K.H., Boston, K.C., Kronfeld, D.S., et al., 2005. Insulin resistance and compensation in Thoroughbred weanlings adapted to high-glycemic meals. J Anim Sci 83, 2357–2364.
Treiber, K.H., Geor, R.J., Boston, R.C., et al., 2008. Dietary energy source affects glucose kinetics in trained Arabian geldings at rest and during endurance exercise. J Nutr 138, 964–970.
USDA-ARS (United States Department of Agriculture, Agricultural Research Service), 2010. USDA National Nutrient Database for Standard Reference, Release 23. Nutrient Data Laboratory. (http://www.ars.usda.gov/ba/bhnrc/ndl) accessed February 2011.
Valberg, S.J., 2010. Review of muscle diseases in sport horses. In: Proceedings of the Veterinary Sport Horse Symposium. Amer Assoc Equine Prac, Lexington, KY, pp. 107–120.
Valk, E.E., Hornstra, G., 2000. Relationship between vitamin E requirement and polyunsaturated fatty acid intake in man: a review. Int J Vitam Nutr Res 70, 31–42.
van Dijk, S., Wensing, T., 1989. Comparison of the lipoprotein pattern of the horse, the pony and the lactating and non-lactating cow obtained by a combination of an ultracentrifugation and a precipitation technique. Comp. Biochem. Physiol. B. 94, 735–738.
Vervuert, I., Klein, S., Coenen, M., 2010. Short-term effects of a moderate fish oil or soybean oil supplementation on postprandial glucose and insulin responses in healthy horses. Vet J 184, 162–166.
Vineyard, K.R., Warren, L.K., Kivipelto, J., 2007. Effect of fish oil supplementation on neutrophil function and antibody production in yearling horses. In: Proc 20th Equine Sci Soc Symp, Hunt Valley, MD. Equine Nutrition and Physiology Society, Savoy, IL, pp. 13–14.
Vineyard, K.R., Warren, L.K., Kivipelto, J., 2008. Effect of high fat diets and fat source on immune function in yearling horses. J Anim Sci 86 (E-suppl. 2), 376.
Vineyard, K.R., Warren, L.K., Kivipelto, J., 2010. Effect of dietary omega-3 fatty acid source on plasma and red blood cell membrane composition and immune function in yearling horses. J Anim Sci 88, 248–257.
Warren, L.K., Kivipelto, J., 2007a. Fatty acid content of grass and legume hays commonly fed to horses. J Anim Sci 85 (Suppl 1), 140–141.
Warren, L.K., Kivipelto., 2007b. Effect of season, forage maturity and grazing on the fatty acid composition of bahiagrass pasture. J Anim Sci 85 (Suppl 1), 141.
Warren, L.K., Kivipelto., 2008. Seasonal effects of diet on the omega-6 and omega-3 fatty acid composition of plasma and red blood cells in grazing horses. J Anim Sci 86 (E-Suppl. 2), 376.
Warren, L.K., Kivipelto, J., Gettinger, E., 2010. Evaluation of the capacity for maternal transfer and foal synthesis of long-chain polyunsaturated fatty acids. J Anim Sci 88 (E-Suppl. 2), 203.
Watson, T.D.G., Packard, C.J., Shepherd, J., 1993. Plasma lipid transport in the horse (Equus caballus). Comp. Biochem. Physiol. Part B Biochem. Mol. Biol. 106, 27–34.
Webb, S.P., Potter, G.D., Evans, J.W., 1987. Physiologic and metabolic response of race and cutting horses to added dietary fat. In: Proc 10th Equine Nutr Physiol Soc Symp, Fort Collins, CO. Equine Nutrition and Physiology Society, Savoy, IL, p. 115.
White, S., Warren, L.K., Vineyard, K.R., et al., 2007. Effect of dietary omega-3 fatty acid supplementation on vitamin E status and lipid peroxidation in growing horses. In: Proc. 20th Equine Science Society Symposium, Hunt Valley, MD, Equine Nutrition and Physiology Society, Savoy, IL, pp. 60–61.
Williams, C.A., Kronfeld, D.S., Staniar, W.B., et al., 2001. Plasma glucose and insulin responses of thoroughbred mares fed a meal high in starch and sugar or fat and fiber. J Anim Sci 79, 2196–2201.
Wilson, K.R., Potter, G.D., Michael, E.M., et al., 2003. Alteration in the inflammatory response in athletic horses fed diets containing omega-3 polyunsaturated fatty acids. In: Proc 18th Equine Nutr Physiol Symp, East Lansing, MI, Equine Nutrition and Physiology Society, Savoy, IL, pp. 20–23.
Witham, C.L., Stull, C.L., 1998. Metabolic responses of chronically starved horses to refeeding with three isoenergetic diets. J Am Vet Med Assoc 212, 691–696.
Woodward, A.D., Nielsen, B.D., O'Connor, C.I., et al., 2007. Supplementation of dietary long-chain polyunsaturated omega-3 fatty acids high in docosahexaenoic acid (DHA) increases plasma DHA concentration and may increase trot stride lengths in horses. Eq Comp Ex Physiol 4, 71–78.
Wyse,, C.A., Murphy, D.M., Preston, T., et al., 2001. The 13C-octanoic acid breath test for detection of effects of meal composition on the rate of solid-phase gastric emptying in ponies. Res Vet Sci 71, 81–83.
Zeyner, A.C., Hoffmeister, A., Einspanier, J., et al., 2006. Glycaemic and insulinaemic response of quarter horses to concentrates high in fat and low in soluble carbohydrates. Equine Vet J 36 (Suppl), 643–647.
Zhou, M., Robards, K., Glennie-Holmes, M., et al., 1999. Oat lipids. J Amer Oil Chem Soc 76, 159–169.

8 Carbohydrates

Rhonda M. Hoffman

The horse evolved primarily as a grazing and browsing, hind-gut fermenting herbivore with a wide range of forage carbohydrates - hydrolyzable to fermentable - as its main source of energy. Pastures provide the main habitat and nutrition for most horses, and the remaining stall-confined horses should have at least one-half of their dry matter intake supplied by conserved pasture. Horse owners supplement a diet of pasture and hay with energy-dense feedstuffs that often contain substantial quantities of cereal grains in order to meet energy demands of performance and to provide a carrier for micronutrients that are marginal or deficient in forages. Common experience has been supported by epidemiological and experimental studies that associate grain concentrates with several digestive and metabolic disorders, including colic (Clarke et al 1990, Tinker et al 1997, Hudson et al 2001), laminitis (Pass et al 1998, Hoffman et al 2007), gastric ulcers (Murray 1994), developmental orthopedic disease (Kronfeld et al 1990, Ralston 1996), insulin resistance (Hoffman et al 2003a, Treiber et al 2005) and polysaccharide storage myopathy (Valentine et al 2001, Ribeiro et al 2004). The abundant starch in grain concentrates has been implicated as the "culprit", leading to development and marketing of "low starch" concentrates for horses. Corresponding trends in human nutrition towards "low carb diets" have fed wide, consumer support for low starch feeds for horses, perhaps to excess.

While low starch complementary feeds ("concentrates") provide an alternative energy source that is critical for horses with a history of digestive and metabolic disorders that are sensitive to dietary starch load, these feeds are not a "one fits all" solution, as horses performing high intensity exercise may require some dietary starch in order to appropriately fuel performance. Horses have an opportunity for small intestinal metabolism of starch and simple carbohydrates to glucose, which is more metabolically efficient than hindgut fermentation of fibers to volatile fatty acids (Blaxter 1989, Kronfeld 1996). Compared to fatty acids, glucose (or its stored form glycogen) is aerobically metabolized nearly twice as fast to generate ATP for muscle contraction. As speed and exertion increase to the point of anaerobic work, glucose from glycogen is favored metabolically over fatty acids. Thus, in spite of the evidence that many horses perform well on high-forage, low-starch diets, some may not, and it should be noted that the critical lower limit of starch intake, especially for high intensity performance, is not known.

Carbohydrate nomenclature

From the perspective of plant physiology, carbohydrates may be divided into three general groups: simple sugars, polymeric storage molecules (e.g., starch, fructans), and structural polysaccharides (e.g., hemicelluloses, cellulose). From the perspective of equine digestive physiology, carbohydrates may be divided into two major groups: those that can be hydrolyzed to simple sugars in the small intestine, and those that cannot be digested by mammalian enzymes, but instead undergo bacterial fermentation to volatile fatty acids. Carbohydrates with α-1,4 glycosidic linkages are subject to enzymatic hydrolysis (although they may also be fermented), while β-1,4 linked molecules must be fermented. Specific descriptions of carbohydrates include the following descriptions and are noted in the scheme of carbohydrate fractions (Fig. 8.1).

Key Points

Carbohydrates may be divided into groups based on plant physiology: storage carbohydrates or structural carbohydrates, or equine digestive physiology: carbohydrates that are hydrolyzed and/or fermented.

Simple sugars include glucose, fructose and galactose, which are most often found as components of larger carbohydrate molecules. Free sugars do not occur in high concentrations in plants, but of those present, glucose and fructose are the dominating free sugars in forages.

Disaccharides include sucrose (glucose + fructose), commonly found in grass and legumes, maltose (glucose + glucose), which is produced as an intermediate in hydrolytic digestion of starch, and lactose (glucose + galactose), which is important for nursing foals.

Oligosaccharides. Some oligosaccharides are of note in equine nutrition, especially fructooligosaccharides, or fructans (see below) and the galactosylsucroses, also known as α-galactosides. The galactosylsucroses include raffinose,

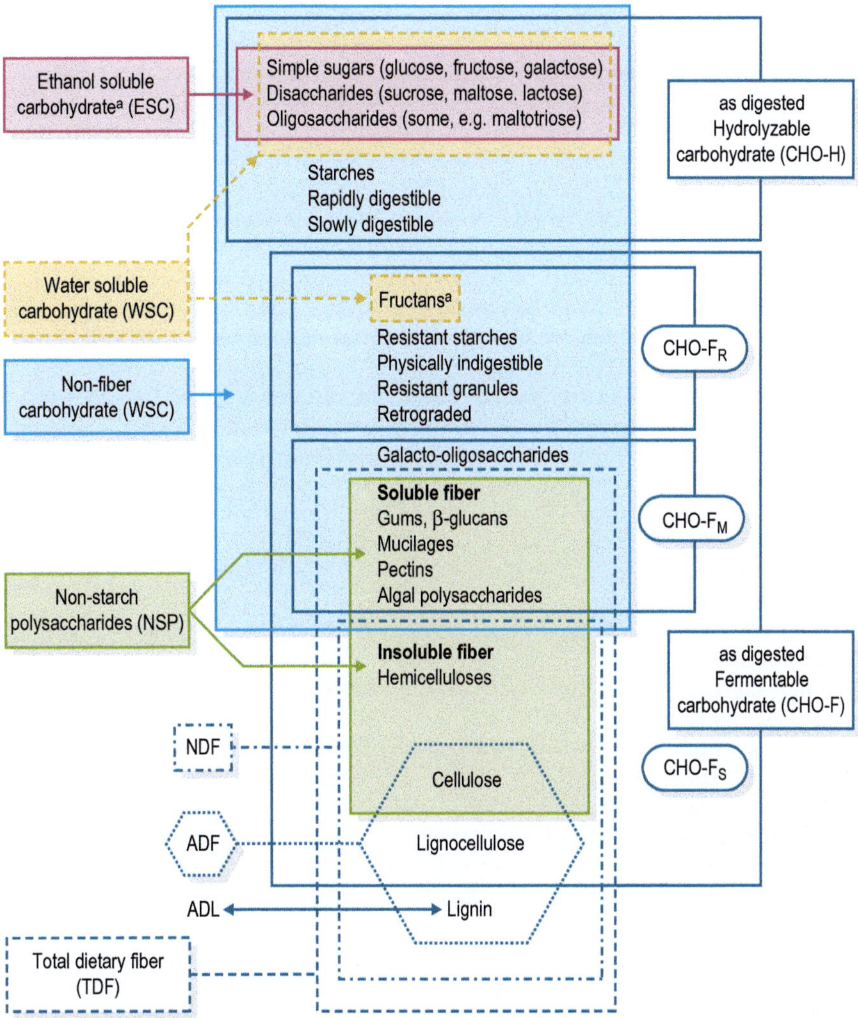

Figure 8.1 The scheme of carbohydrate fractions for the horse, as a comparison of proximate analysis fractions (left) with fractions as digested (right). Abbreviations: ADL, acid detergent lignin; ADF, acid detergent fiber; NDF, neutral detergent fiber; CHO-F_S, slowly fermentable carbohydrate (yielding mainly acetate and butyrate); CHO-F_M, moderately rapid fermentable carbohydrate (yielding mainly propionate and acetate), and CHO-F_R, rapidly fermentable carbohydrate (yielding mainly lactate). [a]Some low molecular weight fructans may be extracted in the ESC fraction. *Adapted and updated from Hoffman et al 2001.*

a trisaccharide with galactose + fructose + glucose, commonly found in sugar beet, molasses and cottonseed meal; stachyose, a tetrasaccharide with two galactose units + glucose + fructose, commonly found in legumes, especially soybean meal; and verbascose, a pentasaccharide with three galactose units + glucose + fructose, found in legumes. Horses are not known to produce the α-galactosidase enzyme required for small intestinal hydrolysis of these α-galactosides, but α-galactosidase is produced by fermentative microbes present in the hindgut.

Fructans, or oligo- and polyfructosyl sucrose polymers, contain a single sucrose starter molecule attached to a variable number of fructofuranose units (<10 = oligo; >10 = polyfructosyl); polymeric fructans may contain several thousand fructofuranose units. Depending on the polymerization, fructans may be considered either oligosaccharides or polysaccharides. Some fructans are linear with β-2,1 or β-2,6 glycosidic bonds, while others are branched, similar to starch. The two most common fructans in equine forages are *inulins*, generally linear with β-2,1 glycosidic bonds, and *levans*, linear with β-2,6 glycosidic bonds. A third type is *graminan*, a branched fructan containing both β-2,1 and β-2,6 glycosidic bonds, common in wheat and barley straw (Ritsema & Smeekens 2003). All are resistant to mammalian enzyme hydrolysis. Fructans are the main storage carbohydrate in cool season grasses and may comprise 5 to 40% of the dry matter in these grasses, depending on season and sunlight (Longland et al 1999, Cuddeford 2001, Harris & Geor 2009).

Starch is a polysaccharide containing glucose units linked by glycosidic bonds, including linear amylose with α-1,4 linkage and the branched amylopectin with α-1,6 linkages. Starch is produced in all plants but is the primary storage carbohydrate in grains, warm season grasses and legumes. Starch is subject to enzyme hydrolysis in the equine small intestine, but can be rapidly fermented. Like fructans, plant starch content is influenced by season and sunlight (McIntosh et al 2007a, b). *Resistant starch* is starch that is resistant to small intestinal enzyme hydrolysis, either due to physical or chemical structure.

Key Points

Fructans are of note in equine nutrition for three reasons:

- They are the storage carbohydrate in cool season grasses.
- They are resistant to hydrolysis in the equine small intestine and can be rapidly fermented in the hindgut.
- The putative association between fructan intake and risk of laminitis

Galactans are galactopolysaccharides found in hemicelluloses, sugar beet, soybean, as well as in gums and mucilages. Like galactosylsucroses, galactans are resistant to hydrolysis by mammalian enzymes and are considered to be soluble fibers.

Gums and *mucilages* are similar viscous galactopolysaccharides found in the woody parts of plants or in seed coatings. β-glucans are gums found in oats and barley, and are again resistant to mammalian enzyme hydrolysis. They are predominantly considered as soluble fibers.

Pectin is a structural polysaccharide that contains 1,4-linked α-D-galactosyluronic acid residues. They are found in most primary plant cell walls and the middle lamella where it helps bind cells together. Citrus pulp and sugar beet pulp are 30% pectin, apple pomace, 15%, and it is also found in potato, and pears, and frequently comprises about 2–5% of the DM in cereals and grasses. Pectins are fermented in the equine hindgut and are considered soluble fibers.

Hemicellulose includes several polysaccharides present in plant cell walls, most of which are polymers containing xylose, glucose, mannose, and arabinose, also known as xylans, glucomannans and arabinans. Most hemicelluloses are soluble in acid detergent and relatively easily and slowly fermented in the equine hindgut. It is generally approximated by concentrations of neutral detergent fiber (NDF) minus acid-digestible fiber (ADF) (see proximate analysis), and considered to represent insoluble fiber.

Cellulose is a polysaccharide containing as few as several hundred to over ten thousand glucose units linked by β-1,4 glycosidic bonds, which cannot be digested by small intestinal enzyme hydrolysis. An insoluble fiber, cellulose is the structural component of the cell walls of green plants and is fermented by cellulolytic bacteria in the equine hind gut.

Lignocellulose refers to polymers of hemicelluloses and cellulose that are bound' to lignin. They are difficult to ferment but may be degraded to varying degrees to cellulose and hemicelluloses by fungi and other microbes present in the equine hindgut.

Lignins are heterogeneous polyphenolic compounds found in lignocellulose, and as such are components of plant cell walls. Lignins are included in the proximate analysis of carbohydrates, and are therefore included here.

Sources of dietary carbohydrate and relevance to equine health

Forages

Forages contain nonstructural carbohydrates (sugars and starch) and structural carbohydrates (fructan, soluble and insoluble fibers, hemicelluloses, cellulose, and lignocellulose). During photosynthesis, green plants produce glucose and other simple sugars, with oxygen as a by-product, from water and atmospheric carbon dioxide in the presence of light:

$$6\,CO_2 + 12\,H_2O + \text{light energy} \rightarrow C_6H_{12}O_6 + 6\,O_2 + 6\,H_2O$$

When the production of sugars exceeds the energy requirements of the plant, they are converted to storage carbohydrates, most commonly starch or fructans. Cool season pasture grasses accumulate mainly fructans, while warm season grasses and legumes accumulate starch. The accumulation of storage carbohydrates in plants is affected by temperature, light intensity and plant growth rate (Longland et al 1999, Hoffman et al 2001; see Chapter 18). While plants that accumulate starch are limited to maximum storage when their chloroplasts are saturated, plants that accumulate fructans have no self-limiting mechanism, so high concentrations may accumulate.

Abrupt changes in fructan concentrations were observed from day to day in rapidly growing pastures and diurnally as plant composition changed from night to day or from shade to sunlight (Longland et al 1999, Longland & Byrd, 2006, McIntosh et al 2007a, b). Fructan concentrations usually rose during the morning, peaked in the afternoon, and declined to a low overnight until the early morning hours. Horses grazing in the afternoon, as compared to morning, may ingest between two to four times as much fructan (Longland et al 1999). See additional notes regarding fructans below and in Chapter 27.

Key Points

- Cool season pasture grasses accumulate fructans.
- Legumes and warm season grasses accumulate starch.
- Fructan and starch concentrations generally rise during the morning, peak in the afternoon, and decline to a low overnight.

Forages are the main component of equine diets, ranging from providing approximately 50% to 100% of the energy intake. There is currently no specific requirement for fiber (NRC 2007); rather, recommendations are made in order to avoid problems associated with under-provision of fiber, including colic (Clarke et al 1990, Tinker et al 1997), gastric ulcers (Murray 1994, see also Chapter 34), acidosis in the hindgut (Argenzio et al 1974, de Fombelle et al 2001, Medina et al 2002), and stereotypic behaviors such as cribbing (Gilham et al 1994). Plant fibers in horse nutrition are designated either by nomenclature (see above) or proximate analysis components (see below).

It has been generally assumed that voluntary forage intakes of horses sufficiently match their energy requirements; however, numerous studies indicate that intake of various forages and hay is highly variable and influenced by palatability, plant maturity, plant species and composition, time of day in which the hay was harvested (hence sugar/starch/fructan content), grazing patterns, interaction with other horses, and weather (Dulphy et al 1997a, b, MacKay et al 2003). Although NDF concentration has been highly correlated with voluntary intake of forages in cattle, voluntary dry matter intake in horses was not influenced by NDF of forages (Dulphy et al 1997b). See Chapter 3 for more information on factors affecting feed intake.

Key Points

Voluntary forage intake is highly variable in horses and influenced by palatability, plant maturity, plant species, time of day when hay was harvested, grazing patterns, interaction with other horses, and weather.

Grains and grain processing

It is common practice for horse owners to supplement forages with grain-based feeds in order to meet energy demands of performance and to provide a carrier for micronutrients required by horses. Although a wide variety of grains may be fed to horses, the most commonly used are oats, corn and barley. Oats and barley contain less starch and more fiber than corn (NRC 2007), but compared to corn and barley, oat starch appears to be more digestible in the small intestine (Radicke et al 1991, de Fombelle et al 2004).

Starch digestion is impeded when the physical form of the food limits contact with pancreatic amylase. This occurs if the starch is contained within whole grain or waxy seed coats, such as rice or corn, entrapped within rigid cell walls that hinder swelling and dispersion of the starch, such as soybeans, or if the starch is densely packed, which is more typical in human foods, such as pasta, than horse feeds. Such starch has been termed resistant starch by human nutritionists (Eerlingen et al 1993, Englyst et al 1996). Milling and grinding increased susceptibility to hydrolysis in vitro by breaking the seed coats and cell walls, as well as abrading the surface of starch granules at the microscopic level, which is smooth in its natural state (Gallant et al 1992). Preileal digestibility of starch was improved in horses when oats (slightly) or corn were ground, while rolling and breaking did not improve digestibility over that of whole grain (Kienzle et al 1992). Preileal digestibility of whole or crushed corn was 30%; grinding increased preileal digestibility to 51%, and popping increased preileal digestibility of corn to 90% (Meyer et al 1995). Similarly, the glycemic response, hence assumed preileal digestibility, was greatest to least, respectively, after equivalent meals of steam flaked, ground and cracked corn (Hoekstra et al 1999). In more recent studies, processing (whole, ground, steamed, micronized, steam-flaked and popped) had no effect on glycemic and insulinemic responses when using processed oats (Vervuert et al 2003) or corn (Vervuert et al 2004), but glycemic and insulinemic responses to barley feeding were influenced by processing method (Vervuert et al 2007).

Key Points

Starch may be resistant to small intestinal enzyme hydrolysis due to physical form, chemical structure, or when retrograded by excessive cooking. Resistant starch is rapidly fermented in the equine hindgut and may contribute to carbohydrate overload.

Key Points

Generally, processing of cereal grains increases digestibility.

Assessment of carbohydrates in feed

Proximate analysis

Standardized methods of proximate analysis (Van Soest 1963, Van Soest et al 1991) relate to plant anatomy and fit reasonably well with the digestive physiology of ruminants, but not as well with the digestive physiology of the horse. A comprehensive scheme was proposed in order to separate carbohydrates into groups for analysis appropriate for horses (Hoffman et al 2001). This scheme, which compares carbohydrate fractions obtained by current systems of analysis with fractions as digested by the horse, has been updated here (Fig. 8.1). The system of analysis for ruminant nutrition separates carbohydrates largely on the basis of plant anatomy into NDF, from plant cell walls, or nonstructural carbohydrate (NSC), mainly cell contents (Van Soest 1963, Van Soest et al 1991). NSC was traditionally calculated by difference, 100 - water - protein - fat - NDF, until a recent movement within academia and the industry to improve the definition of terms associated with the nonstructural or nonfiber carbohydrate portion of feeds. Laboratories now analyze NSC directly, and the calculated by difference fraction is now termed "non-fiber carbohydrate" (NFC) and assumed to contain carbohydrates not found in the NDF fraction of feeds and forages (Anon 2001).

NSC analysis currently refers to the portion of plant carbohydrates analyzed directly, either by extraction in water or ethanol, or by enzyme hydrolysis. Thus, the NSC fraction may be further annotated as water-soluble carbohydrates (WSC), ethanol-soluble carbohydrates (ESC), and starch. The WSC fraction includes simple sugars, disaccharides, oligosaccharides, and some polysaccharides, namely fructans (Smith, 1981, Van Soest 1994). The ESC fraction is a subset of WSC, including mainly sugars, glucose, fructose and sucrose, and low molecular weight fructans but not polymeric fructans. Even with the potential inclusion of low molecular weight fructans, the ESC fraction is the most practical method for estimating simple sugar content. Starch is analyzed by treating residues (previously subjected to extraction with ethanol) to acid or enzyme hydrolysis using α-amylase (Smith 1981, Hall et al 1989). Fructan may be analyzed directly by HPLC (Cairns & Pollock 1988) or colorimetrically (McCleary et al 1997), but the HPLC is rather costly for practical purposes, and the colorimetric method (Megazyme™) appears to substantially underestimate the fructan content of some forages, yielding widely variable results (Longland & Harris 2009). Estimating fructan by subtracting ESC from WSC is perhaps the most practical approach, but since ESC may contain low molecular weight fructans, this method can underestimate actual fructan content (Longland & Harris 2009).

Key Points

Nonstructural carbohydrate (NSC) is a measure of hydrolyzable carbohydrate, mainly sugar and starch. NSC may be specifically fractionalized as ethanol soluble carbohydrates (ESC, mainly sugars), starch, or water soluble carbohydrates (WSC, which includes sugars and fructan).

A system of carbohydrate analysis for human nutrition places greater emphasis on plant chemistry and includes non-starch polysaccharides (NSP) resistant to digestion by mammalian enzymes (Englyst et al 1982). Non-starch polysaccharides include soluble fibers (gums, β-glucans, mucilages, pectins) and insoluble fibers (hemicellulose and cellulose), but exclude lignin and lignocellulose, which have some significance in horse nutrition. Lignin and lignocellulose retard the rate of fermentation (Hall 1989) and are present in much larger proportions in horse feeds than in human diets. Additionally, lignocellulose may be degraded to cellulose by fungi and possibly other microbes present in the equine hindgut, so excluding this fraction may limit dietary assessment.

Neither the ruminant or human system fits well with the digestive physiology and intermediary metabolism of horses; however, the revised system that includes direct analysis of NSC, WSC and ESC is an improvement. Optimally, an analysis based on digestive, metabolic, and energetic efficiency of the animal, rather than plant properties, would include four main fractions useful in assessing diets for horses:

1. a hydrolyzed group (CHO-H) that yields sugars, mainly glucose for metabolism;
2. a rapidly fermented group (CHO-F_R) that yields primarily lactate and some propionate, which may be metabolized as 3- or 6-carbon units via glucose, but may cause hindgut dysfunction;
3. a moderately rapid fermented group (CHO-F_M) that yields primarily propionate as well as some acetate, which are metabolized largely as 3- or 6-carbon units, mainly via glucose, or 2-carbon unites via acetyl-CoA;
4. a slowly fermented group (CHO-F_S) that yields primarily acetate and butyrate, which are metabolized as 2- and 4-carbon units, largely via acetyl-CoA.

Until such an analysis is available, it may be practically approximated in terms of hydrolyzable carbohydrate (simple sugars + starch or practically ESC + starch), rapidly and moderately fermented carbohydrate (the difference between NFC and ESC + starch), and slowly fermented carbohydrate (approximated by NDF), as indicated in Fig. 8.1.

These approximations are based on limited data reported from in vivo studies (de Fombelle et al 2004, Moore-Colyer et al 2002, Longland et al 1997) but are limited by the NFC fraction, which is calculated by difference and accumulates laboratory errors. The NFC fraction contains hydrolyzable, rapidly and moderately fermentable portions, including sugars, starch and fructan as well as gums, mucilages, β-glucans, and pectins, which are not recovered by the NDF method. The NSC hydrolyzable fraction as analyzed directly is not equal to NFC, and accounts for about one-fifth of the NFC in hay, one-third of the NFC in pasture, one-half to two-thirds of the NFC in fiber-rich feeds, and the majority of the NFC in typical "sweet feed" grain-mixes for horses (Hoffman et al 2001). Old laboratory methods calculated NSC by difference using the same equation now used to calculate NFC. While it would be less confusing to drop the use of the by difference terminology altogether, some laboratories still employ the old method and equate NSC and NFC. Thus, care should be taken when interpreting laboratory reports. For example, the NFC method of calculating NSC (old laboratory method) estimates the hydrolyzable carbohydrate fraction of beet pulp around 32% DM, when it is actually closer to 11%.

Key Points

Non-fiber carbohydrate (NFC) is a fraction still used in some laboratories that provides little, if any, practical use in horse nutrition. NFC is calculated by difference, 100 – water – protein – fat – NDF, and generally includes hydrolyzable, rapidly and moderately fermentable carbohydrates that are not recovered by the NDF method.

Glycemic response and glycemic index

The glycemic response is a reflection of plasma glucose and insulin responses to a meal, an in vivo estimate, rather than a chemical analysis of the hydrolyzable carbohydrates in a feed. The glycemic index is a classification of feeds relative to their capacity to raise blood glucose, and is generally expressed as a percentage of the area under the curve response to a standard quantity of a test feed compared to that of a standardized reference: an oral glucose dose or white bread in human nutrition (Jenkins et al 1981, Englyst et al 1996). The glycemic index has been applied primarily in human nutrition for diabetics in order to formulate diets with a low glycemic impact (Wolever & Mehling 2002), but it has not been applied consistently in horse nutrition (Harris & Geor 2009). Meal-related responses of blood glucose and insulin to different diets in horses have been quantified in several reports (Stull & Rodiek 1988, Rodiek et al 1991, Williams et al 2001), but there has been a lack of standardization between laboratories regarding amounts of feed or NSC offered. Some fed equal weight meals (Hoffman et al 2009); some fed isocaloric meals (Rodiek & Stull 2007); some fed equivalent NSC meals (Jose-Cunilleras et al 2004), and some fed meals that increased in size or amount of NSC (Pagan et al 1999, Vervuert et al 2009b). Glycemic indices were quantified in a series of studies using whole oats as a standardized reference feed, with the calculated area under the curve for oats set to a standard value of 100. The range of feeds tested and their glycemic indices included (in ascending order of glycemic index) non-molassed beet pulp, 1; alfalfa hay, 26; timothy hay, 32; carrots, 51; oats, 100; barley, 101, and corn, 117 (Rodiek 2006). Similarly, other studies have compared ingestion of different feeds as either equal-weight or isocaloric meals and calculated glycemic index as a percentage of a standardized reference (oats, corn, or glucose via nasogastric tube). However, lack of standardization of methods, meal sizes, rates of intakes and reference feeds between studies has limited the applicable use of glycemic index in horses.

Additionally, while these studies provided meal-related blood glucose response, few assessed meal-related insulin response. Research regarding insulin resistance in horses (see below and Chapter 28), suggests that compared to blood glucose, insulin is a more important variable to consider.

Several factors may affect and confound glycemic response, including meal size and the relative amounts of hydrolyzable carbohydrates, oils and fiber within (isocaloric) meals (Métayer et al 2004, Pagan et al 1999, Stull & Rodiek 1988), processing (Vervuert et al 2007), rate of intake, digestibility and rate of absorption (Pagan et al 1999, Hoekstra et al 1999), and perhaps gastric emptying (Métayer et al 2004), thus contributing to high variability in repeated glycemic response testing (Kronfeld et al 2004, Harris & Geor 2009). Furthermore, common practice in the horse industry is to provide feeds formulated from a mixture of grains and grain products, plant protein products, fiber, fat, as well as vitamin and mineral supplements, rather than a single grain as commonly measured in a glycemic response test, and these mixtures themselves may affect glycemic response.

Key Points

Many factors affect glycemic responses, so there is high variability in repeated testing. Measurement of insulin rather than glucose dynamics may be more important in the horse.

Carbohydrate digestion and absorption

Carbohydrates may be hydrolyzed and/or fermented in horses, depending on the linkage of their sugar molecules: carbohydrates with α-1,4 linked molecules can be subject to enzymatic hydrolysis or may be fermented, while β-1,4 linked molecules must be fermented. Hydrolyzable carbohydrates include hexoses, disaccharides, some oligosaccharides, and starches not resistant to enzymatic hydrolysis. Fermentable carbohydrates include soluble fibers (e.g. gums, mucilages, pectins), some oligosaccharides and polysaccharides such as fructans, galactans and starches resistant to enzymatic hydrolysis, hemicellulose, cellulose, and lignocellulose.

Key Points

Carbohydrates may be hydrolyzed and/or fermented in horses, depending on the chemical linkage of their molecules.

Hydrolytic digestion

Enzymes secreted in the small intestine specific to carbohydrate hydrolysis include α-amylase, α-glucosidases (sucrase, glucoamylase, maltase), and β-galactosidase (lactase). Relatively little α-amylase is present in equine saliva, so limited hydrolysis occurs prior to arrival of carbohydrates in the stomach. In the stomach, gastric acid hydrolyzes carbohydrates to an extent, independent of enzymes. Limited microbial fermentation occurs in the stomach (see below), which may help initiate carbohydrate digestion but may also contribute to gastric distress, such as spasmodic colic, gas colic or ulcers (Murray & Grodinsky 1989, de Fombelle et al 2003).

Key Points

Hydrolyzable carbohydrates include simple sugars, disaccharides and starch. Hydrolysis of disaccharides and starch yields simple sugars for absorption.

In the small intestine, hydrolysis of carbohydrates is initiated primarily by pancreatic α-amylase. In the luminal phase, α-amylase cleaves α-1,4 linkages but not α-1,6 or terminal α-1,4 linkages of starch molecules. Amylopectinase cleaves α-1,6 linkages. The end products of the luminal phase are disaccharides and oligosaccharides such as maltotriose - no free sugars are yielded. Sucrase, lactase and maltase are expressed along the length of the equine small intestine at the brush border mucosal cells (Dyer et al 2002). Sucrase activity was higher in the duodenum and jejunum than the ileum, while maltase activity was similar in duodenum, jejunum, and ileum (Dyer et al 2002). Functional lactase was present in all portions of the small intestine of mature horses, higher in the duodenum and jejunum than the ileum. Although its activity was lower in mature than weaned horses, the presence of functional lactase suggests that mature horses can digest lactose (Dyer et al 2002). The action of these disaccharidases at the brush border mucosal cells completes hydrolysis to yield free sugars, glucose, galactose and fructose, providing relatively high energy yield. The activity of disaccharidases was shown to be unaffected by a diet rich in NSC compared to pasture alone (Dyer et al 2009).

Starch may be resistant to hydrolysis by physical entrapment, chemical structure, or by heating and retrogradation. Corn contains physically resistant starch, so its digestibility is improved with processing. Potato and manioc contain chemically resistant starch, with preileal digestibility of less than 10% (Meyer et al 1995).

Carbohydrate absorption

Two classes of glucose carrier proteins have been identified in mammalian cells (Shirazi-Beechey 1995): the high affinity, low capacity, Na^+/glucose cotransporter type I (SGLT1) and facilitative glucose transporters (GLUT). The SGLT1 is present on the intestinal luminal membrane and in kidney proximal tubule absorptive epithelial cells. It transports primarily D-glucose and D-galactose across the brush border membrane against the concentration gradient by active transport of Na^+ and the Na^+/K^+-ATPase (Dyer et al 2002). The sugars accumulate within the enterocytes and are transported down gradient into systemic circulation via GLUT (Joost & Thorens 2001). The major site of glucose absorption in horses is the proximal small intestine, with glucose transport highest in the duodenum, followed by jejunum and ileum (Dyer et al 2002).

The lag time between an abrupt change in dietary hydrolyzable carbohydrate and the appearance of enhanced SGLT1 was 12 to 24 h in mice (Ferraris & Diamond, 1993). Equine SGLT1 has 85% homology with mouse SGLT1 and 92% similarity at the amino acid level, and expression of SGLT1 is regulated at the level of mRNA abundance in the GI mucosa of horses (Dyer et al 2002). If a similar lag time for SGLT1 exists in horse, then in the event of an abrupt change in diet, sugar transport would be inadequate, thus exacerbating hydrolyzable carbohydrate overload to the hind gut. Recent work has shown that the SGLT1 protein and mRNA expression was twofold higher in the jejunum and three to fivefold higher in the ileum of horses that were adapted to a diet rich in NSC, compared to pasture alone (Dyer et al 2009). Additionally, changes in SGLT1 expression over time indicated an adaptation to an NSC-rich diet, compared to pasture only, when horses were adapted gradually over a two month period (Dyer et al 2009).

Genes encoding the GLUT proteins have been identified as GLUT 1–12, and are divided into three classes, based on structure and sequence similarities (James 1995, Joost & Thorens 2001). The class I transporters, GLUT 1–4 isoforms, facilitate glucose transport across the plasma membrane down gradient, either into or out of cells throughout the body. GLUT1 is expressed in endothelial cells within the brain, placenta, eye and testis; GLUT2 is found in liver, small intestine, kidney and pancreatic β-cells; GLUT3 is the primary glucose transporter in brain parenchymal cells, and GLUT4 is expressed primarily in tissues dependent on insulin signaling, including adipose tissue, skeletal and cardiac muscle. The class II transporter GLUT5 transports fructose and is expressed mainly in the small intestine but also in kidney, brain, muscle, adipose tissue, testes and sperm. Horses have the ability to absorb fructose in the small intestine (Bullimore et al 2000). Equine GLUT5 was expressed in enterocytes with greatest levels in the duodenum, followed by the jejunum and least in the ileum (Meredíz et al 2004). Other class II transporters, GLUT7, 9, 11, and class III transporters, GLUT6, 8, 10, 12, appear to have tissue and cell-specific expression similar to class I transporters (Joost & Thorens 2001).

Of these, GLUT4 is of interest in exercising horses. Repeated, strenuous, glycogen-depleting exercise and long-term exercise training increased GLUT4 content in skeletal muscle (McCutcheon et al 2002, Lacombe et al 2003, Jose-Cunilleras et al 2005). Dietary manipulation by feeding increased starch or i.v. administration of glucose, however, did not affect GLUT4 content (Lacombe et al 2003, Jose-Cunilleras et al 2005).

Fermentation

Fermentation occurs throughout the equine digestive tract, but predominantly in the hind gut. The concentrations of anaerobic, cellulolytic and lactic acid-utilizing bacteria, lactobacilli and streptococci have been determined in most sections of the equine gastrointestinal tract, with noted differences in microbial populations and fermentative products in different anatomical sections (Medina et al 2002, de Fombelle et al 2003, Al Jassim & Andrews 2009). Lactobacilli, streptococci, and lactate-utilizing bacteria were found throughout the GI tract, with highest populations in the stomach and small intestine, while cellulolytic bacteria populations were highest in the hindgut. Concentrations of total anaerobic bacteria were lowest in the cecum and highest in the stomach.

The presence of viable anaerobic bacteria as well as acetate, propionate, butyrate and lactate in the stomach suggests that some fermentation occurs. Highest fermentative activity occurs in the fundic region and favors lactic acid production – see Chapter 1 (Argenzio et al 1974, Kern et al 1974). Fermentative gases in breath exhalation indicate that microbial fermentation in the stomach and small intestine partially degrades starch and an inulin-type of fructan (Jerusalem artichoke), but not pectin and cellulose ((Zentek et al 1992, Moore-Colyer et al 2002, Coenen et al 2006). Based on breath hydrogen measures, it appears that adding chopped alfalfa to a meal of oats prolonged pre-cecal digestion of starch, although pre-cecal starch digestibility was not affected (Vervuert et al 2009a).

Key Points

Fermentable carbohydrates include fructans, starches resistant to enzymatic hydrolysis, soluble fibers, hemicellulose, cellulose and lignocellulose (plus any starch that escapes enzymatic hydrolysis). Fermentation produces volatile fatty acids, gas, heat and B-complex vitamins.

Carbohydrates fermented by intestinal microflora yield volatile fatty acids, mainly acetate, propionate, butyrate, and to a lesser extent, lactate and valerate (Hintz et al 1971, de Fombelle et al 2003). The efficiency of fermentation and relative proportions of volatile fatty acids produced are dependent on substrates, i.e. the proportions of dietary forage and concentrate (Longland et al 1997, de Fombelle et al 2001, 2003). Increasing proportions of grain favored production of propionate and lactate at the expense of acetate (Hintz et al 1971, Willard et al 1977, de Fombelle et al 2001). Feeding higher percentages of grain altered the microbial ecosystem throughout the equine GI tract, with the greatest changes in the stomach, and alterations significant enough in the cecum and colon to depress the efficiency of fiber utilization (de Fombelle et al 2001, 2003, Medina et al 2002). Rapid fermentation of starch favors proliferation of lactobacilli and production of lactate, which is poorly absorbed (Argenzio et al 1974, Garner et al 1978). Fermentation of soluble fibers such as pectin yields primarily acetate.

Management of nonstructural carbohydrate intake

While adequate hydrolyzable carbohydrate intake is required to provide glucose as needed to fuel work, overprovision may lead to obesity and exacerbate metabolic problems such as insulin resistance, polysaccharide storage myopathy and osteochrondrosis (Kronfeld et al 1990, De La Corte et al 1999, Hoffman et al 2003a). Over-provision of hydrolyzable carbohydrate may exceed the hydrolytic capacity of the small intestine resulting in their rapid fermentation in the hindgut. Rapidly fermentable carbohydrates (e.g., fructans, starch that exceeds the hydrolytic capacity of the SI, and resistant starches) are commonly thought to precipitate certain digestive and metabolic disorders in the horse, and overload may lead to hindgut acidosis, osmotic diarrhea, colic, and laminitis. Slow fermentation of insoluble fiber (mainly cellulosic) helps sustain healthy function of the large bowel. Volatile fatty acids produced from slowly fermentable fibers meet a large proportion of energy requirements.

Key Points

Efficiency of hindgut fermentation and volatile fatty acid production is dependent on proportions of dietary forage and other feeds. Increasing cereal grains over forage favors rapid fermentation, decreases efficiency of fiber utilization and alters the microbial ecosystem.

Hydrolysable carbohydrate overload

Simple sugars and starches are hydrolyzed in the equine small intestine up to the point at which the enzymatic capacity and/or absorptive capacity become overloaded, and the excess may be rapidly fermented in the hind gut. The critical capacity for starch overload to the hind gut varies depending on the amount and source of starch (Radicke et al 1991, Kienzle et al 1992, Potter et al 1992). Prececal digestion of corn starch increased from an intake of 1 g starch/kg BW/meal to peak at approximately 3.5 g/kg BW, then decreased at starch intakes above 4 g/kg BW, indicating significant overload (Potter et al 1992). Similarly, the presence of ileal starch remained at a plateau from intakes of 1 g starch/kg

BW to approximately 2.5 g/kg BW then increased exponentially at intakes above 2.5 g/kg BW per meal. Compared to oat starch, feeding corn starch resulted in lower cecal pH at levels of starch intake from 1 g/kg BW to 4 g/kg BW per meal, and differences in cecal pH between the corn and oat starch sources increased in proportion to starch intake (Radicke et al 1991). Cecal pH was suppressed with oat starch intakes of 2 g starch/kg BW/meal (Radicke et al 1991). Accumulation of lactic acid may overpower the buffering mechanism of the hind gut and lower pH, normally at 6.4 to 6.7 in grazing horses. A cecal pH of 6 was considered to represent subclinical acidosis (Radicke et al 1991). A pH less than 6 favors production of lactic acid (Garner et al 1978, Van Soest 1994) and was associated with clinical conditions such as osmotic diarrhea, overgrowth of undesired bacterial populations and lysis of desired bacterial populations, thus increasing the risk of endotoxemia and laminitis (Sprouse et al 1987, Bailey et al 2002). Recent work indicated that starch intake of <1 g/kg BW/meal reduced lactic acid producing bacteria and supported more stable microbial populations in the hindgut (Willing et al 2009). In general, horses fed diets containing high levels of nonstructural carbohydrates have a greater risk of colic (Shirazi-Beechey 2008). Slower gastric emptying was noted in horses fed small meals (3 g/kg BW/meal) with low (22%) starch, compared to horses fed small or large meals (7.5 g/kg BW/meal) with high (42%) starch (Métayer et al 2004). Thus, based on starch overload information to date, a commonly accepted recommendation is to limit starch intake regardless of the source, to <2 g/kg BW/meal in order to avoid overload and rapid hindgut fermentation (Julliand et al 2006).

Key Points

Limit starch intake to <2 g starch/kg BW/meal to avoid overload and rapid fermentation in the hindgut.

Key Points

Absorption of volatile fatty acids is integral to maintaining colonic pH above 6, as required for optimal populations of microbes.

- Forage-based diets high in fiber favor slow fermentation and production of acetate, butyrate and some propionate, all which are well absorbed.
- Rapid fermentation of starch favors production of lactate and other substances and may increase risk of diarrhea, colic, and laminitis.

Aside from excess hydrolyzable carbohydrates, other rapidly fermentable carbohydrates of note are fructans, which may comprise 5 to 40% of the dry matter in cool season grasses (Longland et al 1999, Cuddeford 2001). The β-2,1 and β-2,6 glycosidic bonds in fructan are not hydrolyzed in the mammalian small intestine but may be partially degraded by small intestinal microbes (Coenen et al 2006). Research studies have shown that a bolus dose (after a short adaptation phase) of fructans (oligofructose) at between 7.5 and 12.0 g/kg BW (the equivalent of approximately 3.75 to 6.25 kg for a 500-kg horses in a single meal) reliably induces laminitis in healthy horse (Pollitt et al 2003, van Eps & Pollitt, 2006) and in a recent study three out of eight horses given 5.0 g of oligofructose/kg BW developed laminitis (Kalck et al 2009). In vitro studies have demonstrated that inulin (one type of fructan) produced a more rapid fall in cecal pH than an equal amount of corn starch (Bailey et al 2002). Considering pasture intake and cool season pasture fructan concentrations, a horse grazing in the spring or summer potentially could ingest 5 kg or more of fructans per day (Longland et al 1999, Longland & Byrd 2006). Although the amount of fructan ingested while grazing can be as much as that used to clinically induce laminitis, it is relevant to consider that the gradual dose encountered over time during grazing likely has a far different impact than the entire dose in a single bolus during clinical induction of laminitis. In ponies, an increase in inulin intake (3 g/kg BW/day) was shown to affect fermentation fecal pH and fecal amine concentrations (Crawford et al 2007). Circadian and seasonal patterns in plasma glucose and insulin in grazing horses have been noted, however, to correspond with changes in pasture forage sugars, starches and fructan content (McIntosh et al 2007a, b). These changes during periods of pasture growth may increase the risk of laminitis by exacerbating insulin resistance in affected horses. Additional information may be found in the chapter on Laminitis.

Key Points

Circadian and seasonal patterns in plasma glucose and insulin in grazing horses correspond with pasture fluctuations in forage sugars, starches and fructan.

Insulin resistance

Insulin resistance has been generally defined as an abnormal metabolic state when normal concentrations of circulating insulin fail to elicit a normal physiologic response in target tissues (Kahn 1978). More specifically, cells in muscle, adipose tissue and liver that become insulin resistant require larger concentrations of circulating insulin to stimulate glucose uptake. Diets rich in simple sugars have been associated with insulin resistance in several animal and human studies (Storlien et al 2000, Bessesen 2001), and the common practice of feeding starch-rich cereal grains with high glycemic indices, often in over-provision, may promote insulin resistance in horses (Hoffman et al 2003a, Treiber et al 2005). Recently, decreasing insulin sensitivity and glucose tolerance was noted in pre-weaning foals born and raised for 160 days from mares fed during gestation a high starch diet and a high fat and fiber diet from when the foals were 5 days of age (George et al 2009).

Key Points

Insulin resistance in horses has been associated with obesity, laminitis, Cushing's disease, osteochondrosis, and equine metabolic syndrome.

Insulin resistance has been observed in obese (Hoffman et al 2003a, Frank et al 2006) and sedentary (Powell et al 2002) horses. Similar to humans, mares became insulin resistant during late pregnancy and recovered to normal sensitivity during early lactation (Hoffman et al 2003b, George et al 2007). Insulin resistance may be a risk factor in horses with hyperlipemia (Jeffcott & Field 1985, Jeffcott et al 1986), Cushing's disease (Garcia & Beech 1986, Johnson et al 2004), colic (Hudson et al 2001), and laminitis, especially chronic grass founder (Treiber et al 2006, Hoffman et al 2007, Frank 2009). Examination of weanling horses suggested an association between pronounced post-insulin responses and risk factor for osteochondrosis (Ralston 1996). Recent work suggests a genetic component in osteochondrosis that may play a role in abnormal insulin metabolism (Serteyn et al 2010). See Chapter 28 for additional discussion.

Managing intake

In human nutrition, the glycemic index provides a physiological classification of foods useful in developing nutritional programs for patients with insulin resistance or noninsulin-dependent diabetes. Lacking effective application of glycemic response and glycemic index data of horse feeds, the focus has been instead on restricting starch and simple sugar intake in horses. There is currently a trend in the horse feed industry to manufacture low or controlled starch feeds, with claims of reducing the risk of grain-associated metabolic disorders; however, lack of reports elucidating the effect of various starch intakes on relevant outcomes leaves questions regarding exact concentrations of dietary starch for horses that may be considered "low." Sufficient research supports limiting starch to no more than 2 g starch/kg BW/meal in order to avoid overload to the hind gut, but more research is needed to link minimum meal concentrations of starch for avoidance of other conditions that have been associated with dietary starch (e.g., gastric ulcer syndrome or equine metabolic syndrome). Recent work suggests that starch intake should be limited to <1 g starch/kg BW/meal in order to reduce risk of equine gastric ulcer syndrome (Luthersson et al 2009). An examination of glycemic and insulinemic responses to increasing starch intake of a mixed grain concentrate indicated that feeding <1.1 g starch/kg BW/meal resulted in lower glycemic and insulinemic responses, compared to meals up to 2 g starch/kg BW (Vervuert et al 2009b). A similar study in this laboratory examined glycemic responses to intakes of oat grain NSC (calculated as ESC + starch) ranging from 0.6 to 2.0 g/kg BW (Hoffman et al 2009). The glycemic response, calculated as the incremental area under the curve (AUC), plotted against NSC intake indicated a threshold of glycemic sensitivity (i.e. the inflection point, or knot) after which higher NSC intakes produced equally high AUC, at as little as 0.3 g NSC/kg BW/meal (Hoffman et al 2009).

While more work is needed in this area to determine recommended starch intake to reduce risks, a starting point for horse owners, feed manufacturers and veterinarians may be to limit starch intake to <1 g starch/kg BW/meal in horses, and perhaps <0.3 g starch/kg BW/meal in horses with documented metabolic disorders. Table 8-1 shows starch and ESC (sugar) composition of selected feed ingredients commonly fed to horses, and Table 8-2 shows starch and WSC (fructan and sugar) composition of forages commonly fed to horses. Table 8-3 indicates meal sizes of different cereal grains required to limit starch intakes to reduce

Table 8-1 Starch and Ethanol-Soluble Carbohydrates (DM Basis) of Feed Ingredients Commonly Fed to Horses

Feed	% Starch, mean	% Starch, range	% ESC[a], mean	% ESC, range
Corn	70.2	64.9–75.4	2.46	0.81–4.11
Wheat	62.1	54.7–69.4	2.05	0.90–3.19
Barley	54.9	46.3–63.5	2.29	0.98–3.59
Peas[b]	48.9	32.9–68.9	8.40	7.19–10.2
Oats	44.4	35.8–52.9	1.97	0.58–3.36
Wheat middlings	25.9	16.2–35.7	4.65	2.83–6.47
Wheat bran	21.9	15.0–28.8	5.10	2.82–7.39
Rice bran	22.2	8.49–35.9	5.46	1.79–9.13
Corn gluten meal	15.5	11.8–19.1	3.05	0.17–5.94
Distillers grains	5.42	1.22–9.62	6.31	4.03–8.59
Carrots	3.19	0–6.55	22.6	3.88–41.2
Linseed meal	2.85	0.30–5.39	5.21	3.15–7.27
Citrus pulp	2.08	0–6.18	22.3	12.2–32.3
Soybean meal	1.76	0.36–3.15	10.3	7.00–13.5
Soybean hulls	1.44	0.14–2.75	2.83	0.27–5.40
Sugar beet pulp (no molasses)	1.11	0–2.55	8.21	3.94–12.5
Molasses	0.94	0–2.32	37.8	23.3–52.2

[a]ESC, ethanol soluble carbohydrate, includes simple sugars, disaccharides and some oligosaccharides.
[b]Data include both smooth and wrinkled peas (Cerning-Beroard & Filiatre 1976, Gunawardena et al 2010, and Dairy One, a commercial website, http://www.dairyone.com). Compared to wrinkled peas, smooth peas are generally higher in starch and lower in ESC.
With the exception of peas, data taken from Equi-Analytical, a commercial website, accessed October 2010. http://www.equi-analytical.com

Table 8-2 Starch and Water-Soluble Carbohydrates (DM Basis) of Forages Commonly Fed to Horses

Forage	% Starch, mean	% Starch, range	% WSC[a], mean	% WSC, range
Mixed grass-legume pasture	2.59	0.73–4.45	11.1	6.47–15.8
Grass pasture	2.56	0.12–4.99	10.4	4.56–16.2
Legume[b] hay	1.90	0.92–2.88	9.15	7.32–11.0
Grass hay	2.26	0.83–3.69	10.9	6.5–15.3
Oat hay	5.14	1.66–8.63	16.8	9.06–24.6
Peanut hay	5.01	1.16–8.87	9.89	6.02–13.8
Soybean hay	5.13	2.70–7.57	9.85	6.60–13.1
Alfalfa cubes	1.71	0.55–2.87	8.26	6.34–10.2
Alfalfa pellets	2.76	0.27–5.24	7.47	5.54–9.40
Grass cubes	2.29	0.23–4.35	9.20	6.22–12.2
Straw	2.33	0–5.26	6.70	1.36–12.0

[a]WSC, water soluble carbohydrate, includes simple sugars, disaccharides, some oligosaccharides and fructans.
[b]Legume hay data references primarily alfalfa, also clover and lespedeza.
Data taken from Equi-Analytical, a commercial website, accessed October 2010. http://www.equi-analytical.com

Table 8-3 Maximum Intakes[a] per Meal of Common Types of Feeds and Cereal Grains Commonly Fed to Horses in Order to Avoid Starch Overload and Rapid Fermentation in the Hindgut, Reduce Risks of Conditions Associated with High Starch Intake, and Minimize Glycemic Impact in Metabolically Sensitive Horses

Feed	% Starch	Maximum intakes kg per meal		
		Target <2 g/kg BW/meal[b]	Target <1 g/kg BW/meal[c]	Target <0.3 g/kg BW/meal[d]
Traditional "high starch" sweet or pelleted feeds	50–65%	<1.5–2 kg	<0.75–1 kg	<0.4–0.6 kg
"Controlled starch" feed mixes	15–25%	<4–6.7 kg	<2–3.3 kg	<1.2–2 kg
"Low starch" feed mixes	10–12%	<8.3–10 kg	<4.2–5 kg	<2.5–3 kg
Corn	70%	<1.4 kg	<0.7 kg	<0.4 kg
Barley	56%	<1.8 kg	<0.9 kg	<0.5 kg
Oats	45%	<2.2 kg	<1.1 kg	<0.7 kg

[a]No consideration of factors other than starch concentration were given when calculating recommended maximum intakes. Other factors that may affect these recommended intakes include fat composition and physical form of the feed.
[b]Above all else, starch overload and rapid fermentation in the hindgut should be avoided by feeding <2 g starch/kg BW per meal.
[c]Reduce risk of conditions associated with high nonstructural carbohydrate intake by feeding <1 g starch/kg BW per meal.
[d]Manage starch intake in equids with a history of laminitis or other metabolic disorder, <0.3 g starch/kg BW per meal.
Calculated values are based on a 500 kg horse and consideration of starch concentrations only. Ranges of starch concentrations in mixes were compiled using advertised values of horse feeds from several commercial feed companies.

risk of hindgut overload and minimize glycemic impact and risk of disease. Since many factors impact glycemic response, care should be taken to consider qualities other than merely starch, such as fat (which potentially may slow gastric emptying and may moderate the glycemic response), intake time, and physical form of the feed.

Summary and overall recommendations

- Volatile fatty acid fermentation of fiber carbohydrates are a major source of energy. Dietary fiber can help to maintain integrity of the microbial population in the equine hindgut. Adequate and appropriate fiber provision may help to reduce risk of disorders such as colic, gastric ulcer syndrome, acidosis in the hindgut, and certain stereotypic behaviors.
- Excess intake of grain and other high-starch feeds may result in rapid hindgut fermentation and production of lactic acid and other substances which potentially contribute development of osmotic diarrhea, colic, and/or laminitis.
- To reduce risk of starch overload in the hindgut, limit starch intake to less than 2 g starch per kg BW per meal. A more severe restriction of dietary starch may be indicated in equidae at risk for gastric ulcer syndrome (<1 g starch per kg BW per meal) or with those documented metabolic disorders such as insulin resistance (<0.3 g starch per kg BW per meal).
- Over-provision of starch, sugars and/or fructan may promote or exacerbate several disorders, including obesity, insulin resistance, colic, laminitis, equine Cushing's disease, metabolic syndrome, osteochondrosis, and equine polysaccharide storage myopathy.

References

Al Jassim, R.A., Andrews, F.M., 2009. The bacterial community of the horse gastrointestinal tract and its relation to fermentative acidosis, laminitis, colic, and stomach ulcers. Vet Clin North Amer Equine Pract 25, 199–215.

Anon, 2001. NSC vs. NFC. In: Dairy One Forage Update. Dairy One Forage Lab, Ithaca, NY, USA, 24:4.

Argenzio, R.A., Southworth, M., Stevens, C.E., 1974. Sites of organic acid production and absorption in the equine gastrointestinal tract. Amer J Physiol 226, 1043–1050.

Bailey, S.R., Rycroft, A., Elliott, J., 2002. Production of amines in equine cecal contents in an *in vitro* model of carbohydrate overload. J Anim Sci 80, 2656–2662.

Bessesen, D.H., 2001. The role of carbohydrates in insulin resistance. J Nutr 131, 2782S–2786S.

Blaxter, K.L., 1989. Energy Metabolism in Animals and Man. Cambridge University Press, Cambridge, UK.

Bullimore, S.R., Pagan, J.D., Harris, P.A., et al., 2000. Carbohydrate supplementation of horses during endurance exercise: comparison of fructose and glucose. J Nutr 30, 1760–1765.

Cairns, A.J., Pollock, C.J., 1988. Fructan synthesis in excised leaves of *Lolium temulentum*: 1) chromatographic characterization of oligofructans and their labeling patterns following 14 CO_2 feeding. New Phytologist 109, 399–405.

Cerning-Beroard, J., Filiatre, A., 1976. A comparison of the carbohydrate composition of legume seeds: horsebeans, peas, and lupines. Cereal Chem 53, 968–978.

Clarke, L.L., Roberts, M.C., Argenzio, R.A., 1990. Feeding and digestive problems in horses. Vet Clin N Amer Equine Pract 6, 433–451.

Coenen, M., Mosseler, A., Vervuert, I., 2006. Fermentative gases in breath indicate that inulin and starch start to be degraded by microbial fermentation in the stomach and small intestine of the horse in contrast to pectin and cellulose. J Nutr (Suppl) 36, 2108S–2110S.

Crawford, C., Speulveda, M.F., Elliot, J., et al., 2007. Dietary fructan carbohydrate increases amine production in the equine large intestine: implications for pasture-associated laminitis. J Anim Sci 85, 2949–2958.

Cuddeford, D., 2001. Starch digestion in the horse. In: Pagan, J.D., Geor, R.J. (Eds.), Advances in Equine Nutrition II. Nottingham University Press, Loughborough, UK, pp. 95–103.

de Fombelle, A., Julliand, V., Drogoul, C., et al., 2001. Feeding and microbial disorders in horses: effects of an abrupt incorporation of two levels of barley in a hay diet on microbial profile and activities. J Equine Vet Sci 21, 439–445.

de Fombelle, A., Varloud, M., Goachet, A.G., et al., 2003. Characterization of the microbial and biochemical profile of the different segments of the digestive tract in horses given two distinct diets. Animal Science 77, 293–304.

de Fombelle, A., Veiga, L., Drogoul, C., et al., 2004. Effect of diet composition and feeding pattern on the prececal digestibility of starches from diverse botanical origins measured with the mobile nylon bag technique in horses. J Anim Sci 82, 3625–3634.

De La Corte, F.D., Valberg, S.J., MacLeay, J.M., et al., 1999. Glucose uptake in horses with polysaccharide storage myopathy. Amer J Vet Res 60, 458–462.

Dulphy, J.P., Martin-Rosset, W., Dubroeucq, H., et al., 1997a. Compared feeding patterns in ad libitum intake of dry forages by horses and sheep. Livest Prod Sci 52, 49–56.

Dulphy, J.P., Martin-Rosset, W., Dubroeucq, H., et al., 1997b. Evaluation of voluntary intake of forage trough-fed to light horses. Comparison with sheep. Livest Prod Sci 52, 97–104.

Dyer, J., Al-Rammahi, M., Waterfall, L., et al., 2009. Adaptive response of equine intestinal Na^+/glucose co-transporter (SGLT1) to an increase in dietary soluble carbohydrate. Pflugers Arch 458, 419–430.

Dyer, J., Fernandez-Castano Merediz, E., Salmon, K.S., et al., 2002. Molecular characterization of carbohydrate digestion and absorption in equine small intestine. Equine Vet J 34, 349–358.

Eerlingen, R.C., Cronbez, M., Delcour, J.A., 1993. Enzyme-resistant starch I: quantitative and qualitative influence of incubation time and temperature of autoclaved starch on resistant starch formation. Cereal Chem 70, 339–344.

Englyst, H.N., Veenstra, J., Hudson, G.J., 1996. Measurement of rapidly available glucose (RAG) in plant foods: a potential *in vitro* predictor of the glycaemic response. Br J Nutr 75, 327–337.

Englyst, H., Wiggins, H.S., Cummings, J.H., 1982. Determination of the non-starch polysaccharides in plant foods by gas-liquid chromatography of constituent sugars as alditol acetates. Analyst 107, 307–318.

Ferraris, R.P., Diamond, J.M., 1993. Crypt/villus site of substrate-dependent regulation of mouse intestinal glucose transporters. Proc Natl Acad Sci 90, 5868–5872.

Frank, N., 2009. Equine metabolic syndrome. J Equine Vet Sci 29, 259–267.

Frank, N., Elliot, S.B., Brandt, L.E., et al., 2006. Physical characteristics, blood hormone concentrations, and plasma lipid concentrations in obese horses with insulin resistance. J Amer Vet Med Assn 228, 1383–1390.

Gallant, D., Bouchet, J.B., Buléon, A., et al., 1992. Physical characteristics of starch granules and susceptibility to enzymatic digestion. Euro J Clin Nutr 46, S3–S16.

Garcia, M.C., Beech, J., 1986. Equine intravenous glucose tolerance test: glucose and insulin responses of healthy horses fed grain or hay and of horses with pituitary adenoma. Amer J Vet Res 47, 570–572.

Garner, H.E., Moore, J.N., Johnson, J.H., et al., 1978. Changes in the caecal flora associated with the onset of laminitis. Equine Vet J 10, 249–252.

George, L.A., Staniar, W.B., Cubitt, T.A., et al., 2007. Nutritional effects on insulin sensitivity and glucose dynamics in pregnant and non-pregnant mares. In: Proceedings 20th Equine Sci Soc. Hunt Valley, MD, USA, pp. 3–4.

George, L.A., Staniar, W.B., Treiber, K.H., et al., 2009. Insulin sensitivity and glucose dynamics during pre-weaning foal development and in response to maternal diet composition. Domest Anim Endocrinol 37, 23–29.

Gilham, S.B., Dodman, N.H., Shuster, L., et al., 1994. The effect of diet on cribbing behavious and plama beta-endorphin in horses. Appl Anim Behav Sci 41, 147–153.

Gunawardena, C.K., Zijlstra, R.T., Goonewardene, L.A., et al., 2010. Protein and starch concentrates of air-classified field pea and zero tannin faba bean for weaned pigs. J Anim Sci 88, 2627–2636.

Hall, J.M., 1989. A review of total dietary fiber methodology. Cereal Foods World 34, 526–528.

Harris, P., Geor, R.J., 2009. Primer on dietary carbohydrates and utility of the glycemic index in equine nutrition. Vet Clin Equine 25, 23–37.

Hintz, H.F., Argenzio, R.A., Schryver, H.F., 1971. Digestion coefficients, blood glucose levels and molar percentage of volatile acids in intestinal fluid of ponies fed varying forage-grain ratios. J Anim Sci 33, 992–995.

Hoekstra, K.E., Newman, K., Kennedy, M.A.P., et al., 1999. Effect of corn processing on glycemic response in horses. Proc 16th Equine Nutr Physiol Soc. Raleigh, NC, USA, pp. 144–148.

Hoffman, R.M., Wilson, J.A., Kronfeld, D.S., et al., 2001. Hydrolyzable carbohydrates in pasture, hay, and horse feeds: direct assay and seasonal variation. J Anim Sci 79, 500–506.

Hoffman, R.M., Boston, R.C., Stefanovski, D., et al., 2003a. Obesity and diet affect glucose dynamics and insulin sensitivity in Thoroughbred geldings. J Anim Sci 81, 2333–2342.

Hoffman, R.M., Kronfeld, D.S., Cooper, W.L., et al., 2003b. Glucose clearance in pregnant mares is affected by diet, pregnancy and lactation. J Anim Sci 81, 1764–1771.

Hoffman, R.M., Haffner, J.C., Eiler, H., et al., 2007. The role of insulin resistance in carbohydrate-sensitive versus stress-induced laminitis. In: Proceedings of the 20th Equine Science Soc. Hunt Valley, MD, USA, pp. 106–107.

Hoffman, R.M., Haffner, J.C., Crawford, C.A., et al., 2009. Nonstructural carbohydrate and glycemic response of feeds: how low is "low" starch? J Equine Vet Sci 29, 379–380.

Hudson, J.M., Cohen, N.D., Gibbs, P.G., et al., 2001. Feeding practices associated with colic in horses. J Amer Vet Med Assoc 219, 1419–1425.

James, D.E., 1995. The mammalian facilitative glucose transporter family. News Physiol Sci 10, 67–71.

Jeffcott, L.B., Field, J.R., 1985. Current concepts of hyperlipaemia in horses and ponies. Vet Record 116, 461–466.

Jeffcott, L.B., Field, J.R., McLean, J.G., et al., 1986. Glucose tolerance and insulin sensitivity in ponies and Standardbred horses. Equine Vet J 18, 97–101.

Jenkins, D.J.A., Thomas, D.M., Wolever, T.M.S., et al., 1981. Glycemic index in foods: a physiological basis for carbohydrate exchanges. Am J Clin Nutr 34, 362–366.

Johnson, P.J., Messer, N.T., Ganjam, V.K., 2004. Cushing's syndromes, insulin resistance and endocrinopathic laminitis. Equine Vet J 36, 194–198.

Joost, H.G., Thorens, B., 2001. The extended GLUT-family of sugar/polyol transport facilitators: nomenclature, sequence characteristics, and potential function of its novel members. Mol Membr Biol 18, 247–256.

Jose-Cunilleras, E., Taylor, L.E., Hinchcliff, K.W., 2004. Glycemic index of cracked corn, oat groats and rolled barley in horses. J Anim Sci 82, 2623–2629.

Jose-Cunilleras, E., Hayes, H.A., Toribio, R.E., et al., 2005. Expression of equine glucose transporter type 4 in skeletal muscle after glycogen depleting exercise. Am J Vet Res 66, 379–385.

Julliand, V., De Fombelle, A., Varloud, M., 2006. Starch digestion in horses: The impact of feed processing. Livestock Science 100, 44–52.

Kahn, C.R., 1978. Insulin resistance, insulin sensitivity, and insulin unresponsiveness: a necessary distinction. Metabolism 27, 1893–1902.

Kalck, K.A., Frank, N., Elliott, S.B., et al., 2009. Effects of a low- dose oligofructose treatment administered via nasogastric intubation on induction of laminitis and associated alterations in glucose and insulin dynamics in horses. Am J Vet Research 70 (5), 624–632.

Kern, D.L., Slyter, L.L., Leffel, E.C., et al. Ponies vs. steers: microbial and chemical characteristics of intestinal ingesta. J Anim Sci, 1974;38, 559–564.

Kienzle, E., Radicke, S., Wilke, S., 1992. Praeileale stärkeverdauung in abhängigkeit von stärkeart und -zubereitung. Pferdeheilkunde 1, 103–106.

Kronfeld, D.S., 1996. Dietary fat affects heat production and other variables of equine performance under hot and humid conditions. Equine Veterinary Journal Suppl 22 (Vol 11), 24–35.

Kronfeld, D.S., Rodiek, A.V., Stull, C.L., 2004. Glycemic index, glycemic load, and glycemic dietetics. J Equine Vet Sci 24, 399–404.
Kronfeld, D.S., Meachem, T.N., Donoghue, S., 1990. Dietary aspects of developmental orthopedic disease in young horses. Vet Clin N Amer Equine Pract 6, 451–466.
Lacombe, V.A., Hinchcliff, K.W., Devor, S.T., 2003. Effects of exercise and glucose administration on content of insulin-sensitive glucose transporter in equine skeletal muscle. Am J Vet Res 64, 1500–1506.
Longland, A.C., Byrd, B.M., 2006. Pasture nonstructural carbohydrates and equine laminitis. J Nutr (Suppl) 136, 2099S–2012S.
Longland, A.C., Harris, P.A., 2009. Comparison of a colorimetric and a high performance liquid chromatography method for the determination of fructan in pasture grasses for horses. J Equine Vet Sci 29, 376–377.
Longland, A.C., Moore-Colyer, M., Hyslop, J.J., et al., 1997. Comparison of the *in sacco* degradation of the non-starch polysaccharide and neutral detergent fibre fractions of four sources of dietary fibre by ponies. In: Proceedings of the 15th Equine Nutr Physiol Soc. Fort Worth, TX, USA, pp. 120–121.
Longland, A.C., Cairns, A.J., Humphreys, M.O., 1999. Seasonal and diurnal changes in fructan concentration in *Lolium perenne*: Implications for the grazing management of equines pre-disposed to laminitis. In: Proceedings of the 16th Equine Nutr Physiol Soc. Raleigh, NC, USA, pp. 258–259.
Luthersson, N., Nielsen, K.H., Harris, P., et al., 2009. Risk factors associated with equine gastric ulceration syndrome (EGUS) in 201 horses in Denmark. Equine Vet J 41, 625–630.
McCleary, B.V., Murphy, A., Mugford, D.C., 1997. Determination of oligofructans and fructan polysaccharides in foodstuffs by an enzymatic/spectrophotometric method. Collaborative study. J AOAC International 83, 356–360.
McCutcheon, L.J., Geor, R.J., Hinchcliff, K.W., 2002. Changes in skeletal muscle GLUT4 content and muscle membrane glucose transport following 6 weeks of exercise training. Equine Vet J Suppl 34, 199–204.
McIntosh, B., Kronfeld, D., Geor, R., et al., 2007a. Circadian and seasonal fluctuations of glucose and insulin concentrations in grazing horses. In: Proceedings of the 20th Equine Science Soc. Hunt Valley, MD, USA, pp. 100–101.
McIntosh, B., Kronfeld, D., Geor, R., et al., 2007b. Circadian and seasonal patterns in forage nonstructural carbohydrate content. In: Proceedings of the 20th Equine Science Soc. Hunt Valley, MD, USA, pp. 102–103.
MacKay, L.C., Mayland, H.F., MacKay, W.P., 2003. Horse preference for alfalfa-grass hay harvested in the afternoon or morning. In: Proceedings Western Section. Amer Soc Anim Sci 54, 193–195.
Medina, B., Girard, I.D., Jacotot, E., et al., 2002. Effect of a preparation of *Saccharomyces cervisiae* on microbial profiles and fermentation patterns in the large intestine of horses fed a high fiber or high starch diet. J Anim Sci 80, 2600–2609.
Métayer, N., Lhôte, M., Bahr, A., et al., 2004. Meal size and starch content affect gastric emptying in horses. Equine Vet J 36, 436–440.
Merediz, E.F., Dyer, J., Salmon, K.S., et al., 2004. Molecular characterisation of fructose transport in equine small intestine. Equine Vet J 36, 532–538.
Meyer, H., Radicke, S., Kienzle, E., et al., 1995. Investigations on preileal digestion of starch from grain, potato and manioc in horses. Zentralbl Veterinarmed A 42, 371–381.
Moore-Colyer, M.J.S., Hyslop, J.J., Longland, A.C., et al., 2002. The mobile bag technique as a method for determining the degradation of four botanically diverse fibrous feedstuffs in the small intestine and total digestive tract of ponies. Br J Nutr 88, 729–740.
Murray, M.J., 1994. Gastric ulcers in adult horses. Compend Contin Ed Pract 16, 792–797.
Murray, M.J., Grodinsky, C., 1989. Regional gastric pH measurement in horses and foals. Equine Vet J (Suppl 7), 73–76.
NRC, 2007. Nutrient Requirements of Horses (6th Ed.). National Academy Press, Washington, DC, USA.
Pagan, J.D., Harris, P.A., Kennedy, M.A.P., et al., 1999. Feed type and intake affects glycemic response in Thoroughbred horses. In: Proc 16th Equine Nutr Physiol Soc. Raleigh, NC, USA, pp. 149–150.
Pass, M.A., Pollitt, S., Pollitt, C.C., 1998. Decreased glucose metabolism causes separation of hoof lamellae *in vitro*: a trigger for laminitis? Equine Vet J 26, 133–138.
Pollitt, C.C., Kyaw-Tanner, M., French, K.R., et al., 2003. Equine laminitis. In: Proceedings Amer Assn Equine Pract. New Orleans, LA, USA, pp. 103–115.
Potter, G.D., Hughes, S.L., Julen, T.R., et al., 1992. A review of research on digestion and utilization of fat by the equine. Pferdeheilkunde 1, 119–123.
Powell, D.M., Reedy, S.E., Sessions, S.R., et al., 2002. Effect of short-term exercise training on insulin sensitivity in obese and lean mares. Equine Vet J Suppl 34, 81–84.
Radicke, S., Kienzle, E., Meyer, H., 1991. Preileal apparent digestibility of oats and corn starch and consequences for caecal metabolism. Proc 12th Equine Nutr Physiol Soc. Calgary, Canada, pp. 43–48.
Ralston, S.L., 1996. Hyperglycemia/hyperinsulinemia after feeding a meal of grain to young horses with osteochondritis dissecans (OCD) lesions. Pferdeheilkunde 12, 320–322.
Ribeiro, W., Valbery, S.J., Pagan, J.D., et al., 2004. The effect of varying dietary starch and fat content on creatine kinase activity and substrate availability in equine polysaccharide storage myopathy J Vet Intern Med 18 (6), 887–94.
Ritsema, T., Smeekens, S., 2003. Fructans: beneficial for plants and humans. Curr Opin Plant Biol 6, 223–230.
Rodiek, A., 2006. Glycemic index of practical horse feeds. Agri Res Instit Pub No 00-2-034-1B. California Agricultural Technology Institute, California State Univ, Fresno, CA, USA.
Rodiek, A., Bonvicin, S., Stull, C., et al., 1991. Glycemic and endocrine responses to corn or alfalfa fed prior to exercise. Equine Exercise Physiology 3, 323–330.
Rodiek, A.V., Stull, C.L., 2007. Glycemic index of ten common horse feeds. J Equine Vet Sci 27, 205–211.
Serteyn, D., Piquemal, D., Vanderheyden, L., et al., 2010. Gene expression profiling from leukocytes in horses affected by osteochondrosis. J Orthoped Res 28, 965–970.
Shirazi-Beechey, S.P., 1995. Molecular biology of intestinal glucose transport. Nutr Res Rev 8, 27–41.
Shirazi-Beechey, S.P., 2008. Molecular insights into dietary induced colic in the horse. Equine Vet J 40, 414–421.
Smith, D. 1981. Removing and analyzing total non-structural carbohydrates from plant tissues. Wisconsin Ag Exp Station Report No R2107, Madison, WI, USA.
Sprouse, R.F., Garner, H.E., Green, E.M., 1987. Plasma endotoxin levels in horses subjected to carbohydrate induced laminitis. Equine Vet J 9, 25–28.
Storlien, L.H., Higgins, J.A., Thomas, T.C., et al., 2000. Diet composition and insulin action in animal models. Br J Nutr 83, S85–S90.
Stull, C.L., Rodiek, A.V., 1988. Responses of blood glucose, insulin and cortisol concentrations to common equine diets. J Nutr 118, 206–213.
Tinker, M.K., White, N.A., Lessard, P., et al., 1997. Prospective study of equine colic risk factors. Equine Vet J 29, 454–458.
Treiber, K.H., Boston, R.C., Kronfeld, D.S., et al., 2005. Insulin resistance and compensation in Thoroughbred weanlings adapted to high-glycemic meals. J Anim Sci 83, 2357–2364.
Treiber, K.H., Kronfeld, D.S., Geor, R.J., 2006. Insulin resistance in equids: possible role in laminitis. J Nutr (Suppl) 136, 2094S–2098S.
Valentine, B.A., Van Saun, R.J., Thompson, K.N., et al., 2001. Role of dietary carbohydrate and fat in horses with equine polysaccharide storage myopathy. J Amer Vet Med Assoc 219, 1537–1544.
van Eps, A.W., Pollitt, C.C., 2006. Equine laminitis induced with oligofructose. Equine Vet J 3, 203–208.
Van Soest, P.J., 1963. The use of detergents in the analysis of fibrous feeds II. A rapid method for the determination of fiber and lignin. J Assoc Off Anal Chem 46, 829–835.
Van Soest, P.J., 1994. Nutritional Ecology of the Ruminant, second ed. Cornell University Press, Ithaca, NY, USA.
Van Soest, P.J., Robertson, J.B., Lewis, B.A., 1991. Methods for dietary fiber, neutral detergent fiber and nonstarch polysaccharides in relation to animal nutrition. J Dairy Sci 74, 3583–3597.
Vervuert, I., Coenen, M., Bothe, C., 2003. Effects of oat processing on the glycaemic and insulin responses in horses. J Anim Physiol Anim Nutr (Berl) 87, 96–104.
Vervuert, I., Coenen, M., Bothe, C., 2004. Effects of corn processing on the glycaemic and insulinaemic responses in horses. J Anim Physiol Anim Nutr (Berl) 88, 348–355.
Vervuert, I., Bothe, C., Coenen, M., 2007. Glycaemic and insulaemic responses to mechanical or thermal processed barley in horses. J Anim Physiol Anim Nutr (Berl) 91, 263–268.
Vervuert, I., Voigt, K., Hollands, T., et al., 2009a. The effect of mixing and changing the order of feeding oats and chopped alfalfa to horses on: glycaemic and insulinaemic responses, and breath hydrogen and methane production. J Anim Physiol Anim Nutr (Berl) 93, 631–638.
Vervuert, I., Voigt, K., Hollands, T., et al., 2009b. Effect of feeding increasing quantities of starch on glycemic and insulinaemic responses in healthy horses. Vet J 182, 67–72.
Willard, J.G., Willard, J.C., Wolfram, S.A., et al., 1977. Effect of diet on cecal pH and feeding behavior of horses. J Anim Sci 45, 87–93.
Williams, C.A., Kronfeld, D.S., Staniar, W.B., et al., 2001. Plasma glucose and insulin responses of Thoroughbred mares fed a meal high in starch and sugar or fat and fiber. J Anim Sci 79, 2196–2201.
Willing, B., Vörös, A., Roos, S., et al., 2009. Changes in faecal bacteria associated with concentrate and forage-only diets fed to horses in training. Equine Vet J 41, 908–914.
Wolever, T.M.S., Mehling, C., 2002. High-carbohydrate-low-glycemic index dietary advice improves glucose disposition index in subjects with impaired glucose tolerance. Br J Nutr 87, 477–487.
Zentek, J., Nyari, A., Meyer, H., 1992. Investigations on postprandial H_2- and CH_4-exhalation in the horse. Pferdeheilkunde 1, 64–66.

9

SECTION A Nutritional Foundations

Vitamins

Annette Zeyner, Patricia A Harris

Introduction

Vitamins can be described as organic compounds that are required in tiny amounts for essential vital functions (e.g., as cofactors for metabolic reactions or for the immune response) and are not degraded as sources of energy. By convention, the term "vitamin" does not include other nutrients, essential for life, such as minerals or selected amino acids. Vitamins are very heterogeneous, both in terms of their chemical composition and their metabolic function. They are generally classified according to their solubility: Vitamins A, D, E, and K are soluble in fats and lipophilic solvents, whereas vitamins of the B-complex and vitamin C are soluble in water. Many vitamins are represented by more than one chemical compound, which may vary considerably in biological potential.

The traditional view is that vitamins cannot be synthesized in sufficient quantities by more highly developed animals and therefore must be obtained from the diet. However, the validity of this statement depends on the vitamin and the species in question. As an example, vitamin D_3 can be formed, under exposure to UV light, from a precursor in the skin and is further activated in the liver and kidney (Schenk & Kolb 1982). Vitamin C can be synthesized in the liver of all mammals (Chattergee 1973) apart from guinea pigs, bats and one of the two major primate suborders (which includes human beings). Certain gut microbes are able to synthesize some vitamins (e.g., those of the B-complex) but the question remains, to what extent these vitamins can be absorbed from the gut and thus used by the host?

Certain provitamins exist (e.g., β-carotene and 7-dehydrocholesterol) that do not possess vitamin activity but which can be converted into active vitamins by the body. The ability of the body to store reserves of vitamins also varies. For example, while vitamin A stores in liver can last for 2–6 months and reserves of vitamin B_{12} can last for a year through enterohepatic cycling, reserves of thiamin may be sufficient for only 1–2 weeks (Saastamoinen & Harris 2008).

The vitamin contents in feeds and forage typically decrease during storage. As many horses do not have access to good quality, fresh green forage all year round, vitamin supplementation is often required to meet requirements. For this reason industrially produced vitamins are often added to horse diets in order to supplement the intake of natural vitamins. Although this practice is sound, it does create the potential for over supplementation and toxicity. In one survey of feeding practices in racing stables, vitamin A and D were often overdosed (up to more than 6 times above the requirement) while the vitamin E supply just met requirements (Meyer et al 1991). This means that when discussing appropriate vitamin provision one needs to cover not only the requirements on an individual basis but also the prevention of undesirable toxic effects, especially if multiple vitamin-containing supplements are fed.

General considerations regarding vitamin requirements

Derivation of requirement recommendations

Vitamin requirement figures are usually derived from factorial calculations or dose–response relationships. The predominantly functional nature of vitamins would seem to make the latter the method of choice. However, there are very few good quality, published data sets that can be used for deriving vitamin requirements of horses; response curves are often based on too few data and typically extrapolations from other species are made. In addition, several internal factors (e.g., animal age, amount of exercise and reproductive status) as well as external factors influence the amount of an individual vitamin needed for the particular metabolic or immunologic function in question, which complicates the characterization of a clear dose–response curve. External factors, such as the type and quality of the diet and the amount of access to sunlight, also need to be taken into account when considering an individual animal's requirements. This can be achieved by increasing or reducing the more general requirements in response to the individual circumstances e.g. due to the known importance of vitamin B_1 for carbohydrate metabolism (Bates 2001) it can be assumed that sport horses being exercised at a given level would need more vitamin B_1 when on a high-starch diet than when consuming a high-fat feed. *Vice versa,* it is likely that horses on a high-fat diet would benefit from a higher intake of vitamin E. Various health problems such as recurrent airway obstruction (RAO), nephropathy or gastrointestinal diseases can also modify the utilization of, and therefore the need for, several vitamins. However, this is not an issue that should be considered when formulating requirement figures, rather the health status should be taken into account when adapting the respective requirement figures for the individual circumstances.

Another question is to decide whether vitamins that can be formed through metabolism (such as vitamin C) or produced by gut microbes (vitamin K and vitamins of the B-complex) also need to be given via the feed. The extent of the absorption of vitamins derived from microbial production is largely unknown. The potential for vitamin synthesis is large given the size of the hindgut fermentation vat. However, the extent to which vitamins are absorbed from the caecum and large intestine is not known. Nonetheless, it is evident that horses can survive without additional oral intake of vitamin K or vitamins of the B-complex. It may be that these vitamins are produced in sufficient quantities by microbes in the terminal small intestine and absorbed there or that there is sufficient vitamin absorption from the hindgut (Schenk & Kolb 1982). However, it cannot be excluded that the status of those vitamins can be low under some circumstances of modern horse husbandry in the absence of dietary supplementation. It may also be that changes in the ration, strenuous exercise or other stressful conditions cause alterations of the microflora resulting in inadequate production of B-vitamins (Linerode 1967).

Experimental data from horse studies do not enable robust derivation of vitamin requirements that take into consideration all the major modifying factors. However, by using multiple smaller data sets with different response variables (e.g., serum kinetics after vitamin ingestion and minimal vitamin intake required to prevent critical conditions such as night blindness), requirements have been estimated for vitamins A, D, E, thiamin and riboflavin (NRC 2007). It should be noted that the absolute requirement for a given vitamin may differ depending on the test variable used. For vitamin K, most vitamins of the B-complex and vitamin C, experimental data do not allow development of definitive recommendations for dietary intakes. An exception is made for thiamin and, using less rigorous demands for scientific verification, also for riboflavin. Vitamin K, biotin and vitamin C are discussed in this chapter with respect to the interest in these vitamins; however, precise dietary requirements are not given for these vitamins. Because of a lack of scientifically-derived data in horses, the other B-vitamins are discussed only very briefly in this chapter.

Rationale

Vitamin requirements have mostly been derived from studies that have used horses of a medium body size. The practical use of such requirement figures when expressed per unit of body weight (BW) may work quite well when the weight range of the horses from the original studies covers the BW of the target animal. The problem is, however, the remarkably high BW variability of equines: ranging from less than 100 kg in miniature Shetland ponies to 1000 kg and more in Shire horses. The same problem occurs with dogs (NRC 2006). Extrapolating BW-based requirements to larger-sized animals may lead to an unrealistic overestimate. Based on such extrapolations, for example, a Shire horse would need a much higher nutrient density (per unit of energy) in the feed than a medium-sized horse in order to cover maintenance requirements but this does not fit with practical experience.

Maintenance energy requirement is an alternative to consider as the basis for vitamin requirements, but again this is not a viable option due to wide variation in energy needs. Depending on breed, training status and body composition, energy needs may range from 0.40 to 0.64 MJ of metabolizable energy per kg of metabolic BW ($BW^{0.75}$) with additional variance of ±10% associated with spontaneous activity and temperature regulation (Kienzle et al 2010). Taking a mean conversion rate of 83%, which may fit well for hay-based feeding rations supplemented with limited amounts of concentrates (Kienzle & Zeyner 2010), this would be equal to 0.48 to 0.77 MJ (~60% variation) of digestible energy per kg of $BW^{0.75}$. There is no evidence that vitamin requirements for healthy animals at maintenance vary by this amount.

Using maintenance DM intake as the basis for vitamin requirements is also not promising because either the DM intake is assumed to be ~2% of the BW (GfE 1994, NRC 2007), which preserves the problems that occur when BW is taken as the basis, or the DM intake is taken to be that which is needed to provide the maintenance energy requirement for that individual. The latter also can lead to confusion, e.g. there is no evidence that the vitamin requirement is significantly modified when obese horses are being fed a restricted diet with low energy intake.

Rucker (2007), however, suggests that the amount of specific substances (which are generally thought to be nutritionally essential or conditionally important) needed per day is similar among animal species (or in animal species with a considerably high variation in BW) when expressed per $BW^{0.75}$. Theoretical considerations on this subject were developed more than 60 years ago (Brody 1945, Lucky 1951). The rationale is that it is more likely for nutrients involved in biochemical reactions (e.g., as catalysts or cofactors) to be linked to basal metabolism (expressed as ¾ power of BW) rather than to absolute BW (Rucker & Storms 2002, Rucker & Steinberg 2002). For example, Grollmann & Lehninger (1957) described the potential synthesis of vitamin C from D-glucuronic acid, for which glucose and galactose serve as precursors. Vitamin C synthesis in vivo obviously cannot be greater than the amount of glucose and galactose shunted through the oxidative pathway which is essential for vitamin C synthesis (Grollmann & Lehninger 1957, Rucker et al 1980, Rucker & Steinberg 2002). When expressed relative to the $BW^{0.75}$, extrapolation from the available animal data yields values that are basically in keeping with the human requirement (Rucker 2007). Accordingly, it is suggested that in addition to basal daily energy utilization, allometric scaling based on $BW^{0.75}$ may be used to predict and compare basal nutrient requirements among widely varied species, as well as make comparative toxicological and other biological assessments and predictions (Rucker 2007).

Key Points

- Vitamin requirements for both maintenance and production/performance are best expressed as a function of metabolic body weight ($BM^{0.75}$).
- The NRC and many other reference books still use bodyweight as the basis for vitamin requirement recommendations; this approach results in unrealistic overestimates in larger-sized horses.

Life stage and life style

Maintenance vitamin requirements need to be adjusted for the additional needs associated with production, for example the transfer of vitamins to the fetus or into milk. Lack of data concerning the optimal quantity of vitamin in the target tissue and the transfer rate from the consumed vitamin to the respective product hampers use of the factorial method. For example, weighted means of 2077 and 128 international units (IU) of vitamin A (n=159) and D_3, (n=87), respectively, per kg of mare milk have been extracted from the literature (Coenen et al 2010). Such data may serve as a basis for calculations, but it is not known whether these numbers represent ideal milk vitamin content or just values found in certain management systems. Furthermore, while orally provided vitamin A may increase serum retinol to a certain extent (Sklan & Donoughue 1982) even very high intakes of vitamin A do not automatically result in significant enrichment in the mares' milk (Großer et al 1995).

Finally, the partial or additional requirements for any performance parameter are often more functionally founded (e.g., extra need for higher immune response) than product-related which also hinders the development of factorial derivations.

Fat-soluble vitamins

Vitamin A and β-carotene

Vitamin A belongs to the group of retinoids. However, the various retinoids and carotinoids which are precursors of vitamin A differ considerably in their biological activity. One international unit (IU) of vitamin A is equivalent to the biological activity of 0.300 µg all-*trans*-retinol, 0.334 µg of all-*trans*-retinyl acetate, 0.359 µg all-*trans*-retinyl propionate or 0.550 µg of all-*trans*-retinyl palmitate for example (Seehawer & Schliffka 2006).

Major biological functions

Vitamin A plays an important direct role in vision (Wald 1968). It helps to regulate cell differentiation by influencing gene expression (Solomons 2001) and to maintain epithelial surfaces as well as the innate and the adaptive immune response (Kolb 1995, Stephensen 2001). The last two functions represent the key importance of vitamin A in the defense against infection. However, the most crucial role vitamin A plays is in the reproduction process. Both deficiency and oversupply result in impairment of fertility and may cause severe teratogenic effects in mammals (for review see Schweigert 1998a, b). Retinoic acid exerts its effect in a similar manner to a steroid hormone *via* nuclear receptors. Thus, vitamin A has a key role in various endocrine regulatory systems, which explains the numerous effects of this vitamin, including its role as a morphogen in embryonic development.

Whether β-carotene has a vitamin A-independent essential biological function is not known. However, in contrast to vitamin A, β-carotene serves as an unique antioxidant and a highly efficient single oxygen quencher (Bendich 1989).

Sources

Vitamin A

Vitamin A is available only from feed supplements that contain this vitamin in the form of retinyl-esters such as retinyl-palmitate or retinyl-acetate. They are thought to be hydrolyzed to retinol in the small intestine and absorbed there (Schweigert 1998b). According to one study (Bjondahl & Virkki 1977), the absorption of vitamin A is more rapid with xylitol and polyol as a vehicle than if water is used. After absorption, the majority of the vitamin will be transported to the liver and stored there or distributed via the blood stream to target tissues. In the blood, retinol occurs in a protein-bound form. The release of vitamin A from the liver is assumed to occur in response to demand by peripheral tissues (Schweigert 1998a). Jarrett and Schurg (1987) described an increase in plasma concentrations of vitamin A four hours after intake. However, despite the fact that plasma concentrations of retinol and retinyl esters respond to oral intake (Sklan & Donohue 1982, Jarret & Schurg 1987), plasma or serum levels do not adequately reflect the overall vitamin A status of the horse because hepatic vitamin A stores maintain blood retinol homeostasis in the face of changing dietary supply (Bondy & Sklan 1984, Jarrett & Schurg 1987, Mäenpää et al 1988a, Saastamoinen & Juusela 1992, Greiwe-Crandell et al 1997). Meyer et al (1995) did not detect a plasma response to oral vitamin A but did observe increased liver retinol levels. Measurement of the serum retinol response after a period of depletion may provide a more sensitive indication of overall vitamin status (Greiwe-Crandell et al 1995, 1997).

β-carotene

Natural feedstuffs for horses do not contain vitamin A but contain varying amounts of carotenoids that act as provitamins. The most important of these vitamin A precursors is β-carotene. Apart from yellow corn (where not all the color comes from β-carotene) most complementary feeds or concentrates only contain negligible quantities of β-carotene. However, this provitamin can be found in large amounts in green grass and in decreasing quantities in artificially dried grass followed by grass silages and then hay (Table 9-1).

For horse rations, therefore, fresh grass and good-quality leafy hay are the most important natural sources of vitamin A (retinol) (Fonnesbeck & Symons 1967). Corn provides

Table 9-1 Guide to the Mean (min – max, in mg/kg of Air Dried Material) Levels of ß-Carotene and Vitamin E in Selected Types of Roughage (AWT 2001)

Roughage	β-carotene		Vitamin E	
	mean	range	mean	range
Grass	200	100–400	200	100–400
Grass silage	100	20–250	60	10–200
Grass hay	20	0–100	30	5–80
Alfalfa	50	100–500	20	50–300
Alfalfa hay	50	10–150	20	5–60
Maize silage[a]	20	0–50	15	5–40

[a]Entire plant.

only about 1/8th the amount of β-carotene when compared to green forage. Factors affecting the content of β-carotene in pasture include the plant species, climatic conditions, and stage of maturity. Ballet et al (2000) described mean values of about 278 vs. 59 mg of β-carotene per kg of DM in vegetative vs. mature grasses. The leaf-to-stem ratio is important because leaves have much higher levels of β-carotene. Carrots provide high concentrations of β-carotene but there are differences between varieties. In general, β-carotene content is positively associated with intensity of color. However, crop fertilization practices further influence the carotene content (Evers 1989). Beta-carotene may be absorbed intact and then converted to retinol or can be converted to retinol or retinyl-esters in the intestinal mucosa (Ullrey 1972, Bondy & Sklan 1984, Napoli 2000).

Bioavailability

In humans, ~90% of retinol is absorbed but only ~3% of carotenoids (Sate & Patel 2010). Similar to the other fat-soluble vitamins, retinol requires bile acids for emulsification and micelle formation in order to be absorbed into enterocytes. Within the cell, retinol is re-esterified and packaged into chylomicrons which then enter the lymphatic system. Retinol is primarily removed by the liver where it is stored within the hepatic stellate cell (Sate & Patel 2010). It is presumed that a similar process occurs in the horse, although the role of chylomicrons remains uncertain due to the controversy over their presence in adult horses (see Chapter 7).

The bioavailability of synthetic β-carotene in horses is another topic that has not been satisfactorily examined. Greiwe-Crandell et al (1997) suggested that retinyl-palmitate (72 000 IU vitamin A), but not a vitamin A equivalent water-dispersible-carotene preparation, given in two large doses per week was effective for improving the vitamin A status (in terms of serum retinol and relative dose response) of mares throughout a 20 month repletion period following 8 months of depletion. A similar water-dispersible preparation of β-carotene given in daily doses of 1.8 mg β-carotene/kg BW also failed to alter plasma β-carotene concentration (Watson et al 1996, Eitzer & Rapp 1985). Kienzle et al (2002) reported an increase in plasma β-carotene concentrations when either natural β-carotene or a synthetic beadlet preparation was fed at half the amount (0.8 mg β-carotene/kg BW) given by Watson et al (1996). However, different synthetic preparations of both vitamin A and β-carotene, such as beadlets, coated and spray-dried products, may differ in terms of their dispersion within aqueous solutions. It is therefore likely that the absorption of synthetic β-carotene depends on the preparation used, which means that the effects of one preparation may not be directly inferred from the results of another. Plant oils may facilitate the transfer of fat-soluble vitamins and pro-vitamins to micelles and, thus, enhance absorption rate.

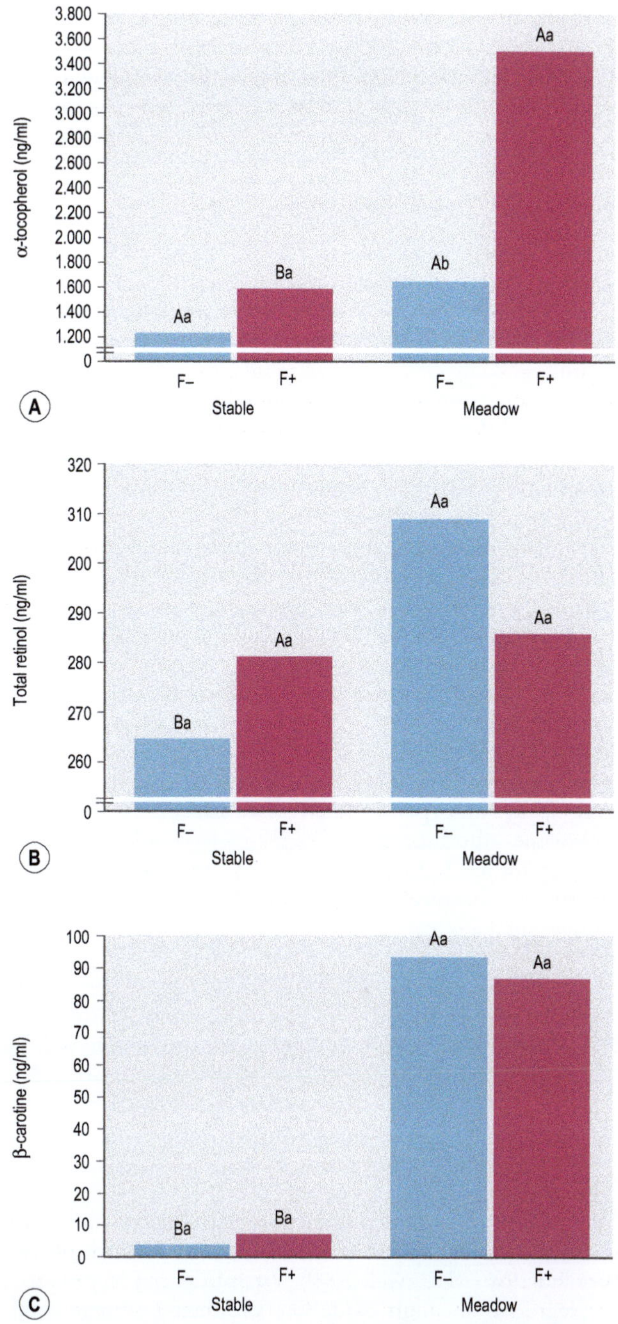

Figure 9.1 Concentrations of α-tocopherol A), total retinol B) and β-carotene C) in the blood serum of Warmblood-type horses (n=6) fed oats (F–) or a mixed feed providing 0.87 g of partly hardened soybean oil per kg of BW and day (F+) either in the stable feeding period (with hay as forage) or on pasture (with meadow grass as forage). All horses were given 69 000 IU vitamin A and 1725 mg vitamin E per day by a mineral-vitamin-supplement. ([ab] different small letters indicate with $p<0.05$ significant differences between means within "stable" or "meadow"; [AB] different large letters indicate with $p<0.05$ significant differences between F– or F+; ± pooled SD for α-tocopherol, total retinol and β-carotene: 108.6, 33.9 and 4.71; Zeyner et al 1995.)

Effect of concurrent oil administration

According to expectations, Zeyner et al (1995) found a substantially higher concentration of β-carotene in the blood serum of horses fed a diet of meadow grass vs. grass hay. Interestingly, the corresponding differences in serum retinol levels appeared to be affected by supplemental soybean oil (Fig. 9.1). Kienzle et al (2002) described an increase in serum β-carotene when sunflower oil was added (4.7% of the diet) to the diet. Zeyner et al (1995) did not find an effect of 0.33, 0.66, 1.00, and 1.33 g of soybean oil per kg of BW/day on plasma retinol but did show that serum β-carotene concentrations were significantly elevated with the highest oil feeding level. In contrast, feeding a concentrate with 15% partly hardened soybean oil did not have an effect on the serum concentration of retinol and ß-carotene when given together with hay or with meadow grass (Fig. 9.1). However, in the study by Zeyner et al (1995) β-carotene came from natural sources only, whereas Kienzle et al (2002) provided supplemental β-carotene as a synthetic beadlet preparation.

Conversion

Horses convert β-carotene to vitamin A rather inefficiently with an average conversion rate of about 33% (NRC 2007). Many factors such as age, activity, environmental conditions and vitamin A status may influence this conversion rate (Bondy & Sklan 1984). Studies in rats, for example, suggest higher conversion rates in pregnant than in growing animals (McDowell 1989). In mares, Schweigert & Gottwald (1999) found a marked increase in plasma levels of β-carotene (absolute values and in relation to the concurrently measured increase in vitamin A) between day 42 to day 2 antepartum. Possible reasons include an improved absorption of carotene and/or a reduced conversion into vitamin A, as well as a mobilization from tissue storages or a reduced uptake into tissues other than the mammary gland. However, the conversion rate from β-carotene to vitamin A seems to decrease when animals consume particularly large amounts of β-carotene (Ullrey 1972, Bondy & Sklan 1984, Solomons 2001). Although this has not been explicitly studied in horses it makes sense from a physiological point of view to avoid oversupply and possibly adverse effects. Furthermore, β-carotene utilization in horses seems to be affected by the type of forage fed, as indicated by more stable plasma vitamin A concentrations when alfalfa hay, which provides a lower intake of carotene, was fed (Fonnesbeck & Symons 1967).

Despite the fact that the suggested levels for conversion range between 300–555 IU of vitamin A per mg of β-carotene, it is generally assumed that 1 mg of the provitamin will be metabolized into 400 IU of vitamin A (NRC 1989, GfE 1994).

Stability

Vitamin A

The stability of vitamin A in the feed depends upon the formulation used and the methods of protection employed (Coelho 1996, McDowell 2000). Vitamin A can in principle be degraded through oxidation, prolonged storage, high temperatures during pelleting, catalytic effects of trace minerals as well as the peroxidizing effects of rancid fats (McDowell 2000). Although retinyl-acetate is susceptible to oxidation due to its five double bonds, synthetic sources of vitamin A are said to be more stable and thus less likely to be degraded during storage. Between 30 and 40% of the vitamin A present at mixing may be destroyed through the process of pelleting (McDowell 2000). Furthermore, the inclusion of trace minerals in premixes increases the risk of oxidation. The 2-month-stability of crosslinked vs. not crosslinked vitamin A within a prepared mixed feed was 90% vs. 65% (Seehawer & Schliffka 2006). Environmental conditions also are important. In one study, vitamin A was reduced to around 2% of the starting value when stored under high temperature and high humidity conditions over a period of 3 months compared to 88% under conditions of low temperature and low humidity (see McDowell 2000).

β-carotene

Carotenes appear to be one of the most difficult nutrients within forage to preserve (Fonnesbeck & Symons 1967; for review see Saastamoinen & Harris 2008). They may be destroyed by oxidation and this process is promoted by ultraviolet radiation and heat (Ballet et al 2000). In contrast to vitamin D, sun-cured hay has lower concentrations than fresh forage. It has been reported that the process of conserving forages can destroy around 80% of the β-carotene present and then biological oxidation continues at a rate of 6–7% per month during storage (McDowell 2000, Ballet et al 2000). Production of haylage leads to a loss of around 14% of the original β-carotene (Müller et al 2007) and further reductions occur during storage. Drying in the barn seems to preserve levels better, even though prolongation of the drying process may lead to similarly high losses (Ballet et al 2000). In addition, the loss of leaves also decreases the carotene content of hay. Certain legumes, particularly alfalfa and soybeans, contain the enzyme lipoxidase that unless quickly inactivated readily destroys much of the carotenes (McDowell 2000). Rapid dehydration can help preserve the carotene content of alfalfa (with 0–30% loss depending on residual moisture levels). In one study the β-carotene content of corn decreased to about 50% after 8 months of storage at 25°C and to 25% after 3 years (McDowell 2000).

Requirements

Limited evidence-based information exists regarding vitamin A nutrition of horses in different physiological states. Requirements figures are therefore poorly founded and can only be regarded as provisional.

Maintenance

The vitamin A requirement for maintenance derives from the intake needed to prevent night blindness plus an extra need to secure tissue storage (NRC 1989). Guilbert et al (1940) suggested, based on a depletion-repletion study with growing Percheron horses, a minimum intake of 17 to 22 IU vitamin A/kg BW/day to be necessary to prevent night blindness. The same group reported that about three times this amount (51 to 66 IU/kg BW/day) was needed for appropriate tissue storage in rats. Taking daily vitamin A intakes of horses without night blindness (22.9±5.1 IU/kg BW/day, n=10) from Guilbert et al (1940) and adding two standard deviations comes close to the vitamin A requirement for maintenance given by NRC (1989): 30 IU/kg BW. This is similar to the 150 IU/kg $BW^{0.75}$ recommended in Table 9-2.

Exercise

Precise recommendations for vitamin A nutrition of the performance horse are not available. Gastrointestinal tract permeability and resistance to infection may be affected by exercise and this could be a rationale for increasing the recommendations for Vitamin A in athletic horses given its role in helping to support mucosal integrity and the immune system. It has been suggested, for example, that vitamin A deficiency impairs innate immunity by impeding normal regeneration of mucosal barriers damaged by infection and by diminishing the function of neutrophils, macrophages and natural killer cells (Stephensen 2001). The NRC (2007) stayed with the recommendation that the requirement for

Table 9-2 Requirements (GEH) for the Daily Vitamin Supply for Horses of Different Physiological States (per kg of $BW^{0.75}$)

Vitamin		Maintenance	Work	Gestation	Lactation	Growth
A	[IE]	150	225	300	300	300
D	[IE]	30	30	30[a]/50[b]	50	70–110[c]
E[d]	[mg]	5[e]	5–10[f]	5–10[g]	5–10[g]	10
B_1	[mg]	0.3	0.3–0.6[h]	0.3	0.3	0.3
B_2	[mg]	0.2	0.2	0.2	0.2	0.2

[a]Till month 7 of gestation.
[b]From month 8 of gestation.
[c]In IU/kg $BW^{0.75}$: 0–6 month: 110, 7–12 month: 90, 13–18 month: 80, 19–24 month: 70 and 25–36 month: 50.
[d]Expressed as DL-α-tocopherol-acetate (1 mg = 1 IU).
[e]When a high-fat diet is given, which is unlikely under maintenance conditions the horse should receive 10 mg/kg $BW^{0.75}$/day.
[f]The higher quantity should be given when a high-fat diet is fed and in horses exercised more intensively. According to empirical experiences it is conceivable that horses susceptible to myopathy such as equine rhabdomyolysis syndrome (Harris 2005b) and particularly heavily exercised horse may profit from a significantly higher supply of around 20 mg/kg $BW^{0.75}$ per day.
[g]Under certain conditions (high infection pressure or overall critical health status) it may be beneficial to provide 10 mg of vitamin E/kg $BW^{0.75}$/day to mares in the last month of pregnancy and first month of lactation.
[h]Exercised horses with elevated carbohydrate metabolism should receive the higher quantity.

work lies somewhere between maintenance (30 IU/kg BW/day) and that for gestation and lactation (60 IU/kg BW/day): i.e., 45 IU/kg BW/day. Most recommendations in the literature vary between 45 and 90 IU/kg BW/day (NRC 2007, INRA 1990, GfE 1994). Transformed to metabolic body weight this corresponds to a daily vitamin A requirement for work of 225 IU/kg $BW^{0.75}$ (Table 9-2).

Pregnancy and lactation

Several studies reported seasonal variations in vitamin A status in broodmares (Mäenpäa et al 1988a, b, Greiwe-Crandell et al 1997). These variations may in part be due to changes in the diet i.e. access to pasture *vs.* feeding preserved forages (Fonnesbeck & Symons 1967, Greiwe-Crandell et al 1997). However, it has also been shown that the seasonal decline in the vitamin A status is more pronounced in pregnant than non-pregnant mares (Mäenpäa et al 1987, 1988a) indicating that vitamin A metabolism is higher during pregnancy. Furthermore, Stowe (1982) suggested that vitamin A utilization increases around parturition due to elevated secretion of the vitamin into colostrum. However, the seasonal decline in vitamin A status occurs in broodmares without (<0.8 IU vitamin A/kg BW/day) and with supplementation of vitamin A in the form of retinyl-palmitate (125 IU vitamin A/kg BW/day; Greiwe-Crandell et al 1997). Stowe (1967) suggested that oral or parenteral doses of a combination of vitamin A and vitamin E will improve reproductive state (e.g., more serviced heats and live foals). However, it should be noted that although vitamin A status of unsupplemented mares without access to pasture decreases, no negative effects due to this decline have been reported. To date there is no evidence suggesting that the vitamin A requirements for pregnant and lactating mares are different from those previously recommended by NRC (1989, 2007): 60 IU/kg BW/day), which is equal to 300 IU/kg $BW^{0.75}$ (Table 9-2).

Whether horses have a need for supplemental β-carotene independent from that of vitamin A is controversial (Enbergs & Klemt 1987, Schubert et al 1991) with most work in this area focused on the pregnant and lactating mare. Some reports indicated that supplemental β-carotene may benefit the fertility of broodmares (for review see Enbergs & Klemt 1987). However, the described endocrinological and clinical effects of supplemental beta-carotene could not be clearly distinguished from a possible impact of additional vitamin A. In an attempt to resolve this problem, Schubert et al (1991) fed two groups of 12 Shetland pony mares a semi-purified diet that was free of β-carotene. After one year of depletion, the mares received over a period of 4 years either 12000 IU (year 1 and 2) and 15000 IU (year 3 and 4) of vitamin A per day (control group) or 150 mg of β-carotene plus 10000 IU of vitamin A per day (year 1-4, treatment group). There was a tendency for the conception rate to be higher in the carotene-free group whereas embryo loss and abortion tended to be lower in the carotene-supplemented mares. The concentrations of progesterone, pregnant mare serum gonadotropin, thyroxine, and triiodthyronine in the blood were unaffected by the dietary treatment. However, total protein and several protein fractions (α- and β-globulin) in the mares' serum as well as the foals' birth weight (in % of the weight of the dam) and the weight gain till the 5th month of life were significantly higher in the carotene-supplemented group. Whether these outcomes would have been achieved by just providing more vitamin A supplementation remains unclear. These results do not support the opinion that supplemental β-carotene impacts fertility although there may be benefits to foal health. Enbergs & Klemt (1987) found that the duration of neonatal foal diarrhea was inversely correlated with serum β-carotene concentration of the mares. In contrast, Kuhl et al (2011) reported that supplementation of Warmblood broodmares at 1000 mg of β-carotene per day from 14 days before the expected date of foaling to 42 days after parturition did not affect the incidence of foal diarrhea. Carotene intake via the core diet, however, was not reported in this study.

Further work is needed to clarify the effect of pre- and postpartum diet on the foal's vitamin A status. One study showed that plasma β-carotene is highly correlated (r^2=0.9) with concentrations in the mare's colostrum (Schweigert & Gottwald 1999). Interestingly, levels of β-carotene in the colostrum were 65 times higher compared to milk collected later in lactation while concentrations of vitamins A and E were only 3 to 6 times higher. However, the addition of 20000 or 100000 IU vitamin A to a basal diet (hay, oats, and mineral supplement) of Haflinger mares did not change the vitamin A concentration of colostrum (Großer et al 1995).

Zeyner et al (2004) demonstrated a substantial decrease in serum concentrations of total retinol (from first sucking until 6 h after birth) and β-carotene (until 12 h after birth) in trotter mares whereas serum retinol in the foals increased over time (Fig. 9.2). Although the mares' β-carotene pool was apparently utilized, no corresponding increase in serum β-carotene of the foals was detected. In fact, serum β-carotene activity in the foals was below the limit of detection of the assay. One reason may be that mares' β-carotene pool was in part used to maintain their own serum retinol concentrations (Fig. 9.2). Alternatively, the serum concentrations of β-carotene in this study were particularly low, compared to other published data from mares around parturition (Schweigert & Gottwald 1999). This in turn was probably due to dietary deficiencies resulting from feeding hay that had been stored for a long period together with a mixed feed that was not fortified with β-carotene or vitamin A. This supports the need to provide pregnant mares with an adequate vitamin A intake throughout gestation - supplementation will become particularly important if the dam is kept inside and fed very mature forage during the final stages of gestation.

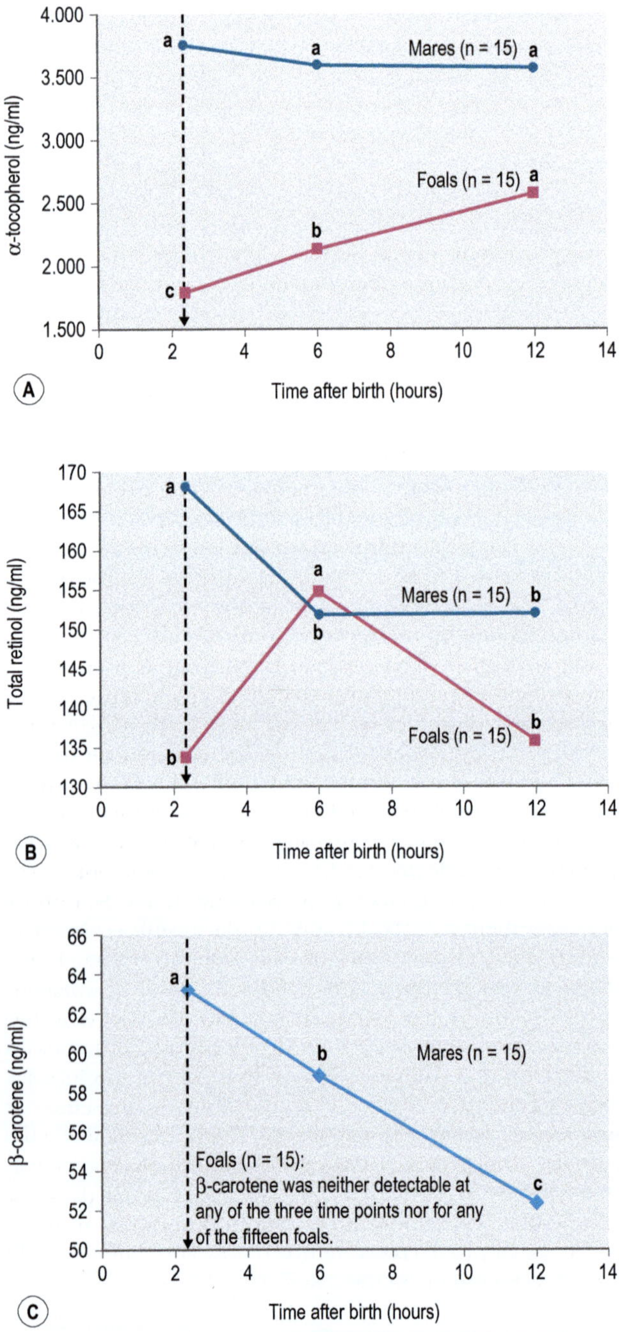

Figure 9.2 Concentrations of α-tocopherol (A), total retinol (B) and β-carotene (C) in the blood serum of trotter mares and their foals (n=15 each) immediately after first sucking (2.37±1.36 hours) and 6 and 12 hours after birth. ([abc] different small letters indicate with $p<0.05$ significant differences between means within mares or foals; ± pooled SD for α-tocopherol, total retinol and β-carotene: 203.0, 14.8, and 5.37 [mares only]; Zeyner et al 2004.)

In summary, additional supplementation of synthetic β-carotene around parturition may be beneficial under some circumstances but more research is required. Supplementation of the late pregnant and early lactating mare with 1 to 2 g of β-carotene/kg BW/day may support foal health and development. However, many questions remain regarding the possible mode of action, the most effective form (natural vs. synthetic β-carotene) and the optimal dosage.

Growth

Guilbert et al (1940) reported no apparent problems with growth in Percheron horses (119 to 444 days old) consuming 22.9±5.1 IU vitamin A/kg BW/day. Donoghue et al (1981), however, suggested from a study of 4- to 12-month-old ponies that a dose ranging from 60 to 200 IU/kg BW/day was necessary for optimal growth. Despite using younger horses (orphan foals), Stowe (1968) reported a minimum requirement of vitamin A that was substantially lower (9.5–11 IU/kg BW/day). For reasons of "security", however, the daily intake of vitamin A recommended by the NRC 2007 for growing horses lies at the lower limit of the range given by Donoghue et al (1981); i.e., 60 IU/kg BW. On a metabolic body weight basis the recommendation is 300 IU/kg $BW^{0.75}$ (Table 9-2).

Effects of deficiency and excess

Deficiency

In humans, vitamin A deficiency is most commonly seen with malnutrition or fat malabsorptive states (e.g., chronic liver disease; Sathe & Patel 2010). Based on data from several mammalian species, vitamin A deficiency may cause impaired growth resulting in developmental orthopedic disease (DOD), reduced protective function of epithelial cells, decreased efficiency of the immune system, disturbed maturation of spermatozoa, reduced storage of rhodopsin (which may cause night blindness), lowered secretion of glucocorticoids, and increased early embryonic mortality (Kolb 1995). The classical clinical sign of vitamin A deficiency is night blindness, which appeared when growing Percheron horses consumed 5 to 10 μg total carotene/kg BW/day (no more than 2 to 4 IU vitamin A/kg BW/day) for 265 to 627 days (Guilbert et al 1940). However, mares did not show any clinical signs even when they consumed hay with extremely low β-carotene (4 mg /kg of dry matter, DM) for 22 months (Greiwe-Crandell et al 1997). In orphan foals, signs of vitamin A deficiency were observed when feeding a semi-purified diet devoid of vitamin A activity (Stowe 1968). Impairments to growth and hematopoiesis may be the most sensitive indicators of deficiency (Donoghue et al 1981). Vitamin A is stored in the liver (McDowell 2000) and this reserve store may help to buffer a short-term deficiency in dietary intake. This means that serum retinol activity will not accurately indicate marginal vitamin A status. In contrast, the relative dose response (RDR) test is an indirect measure for liver vitamin A stores, potentially allowing a more precise description of vitamin A status (Greiwe-Crandell et al 1995). Overall, vitamin A deficiency is very rare in horses and only likely to occur under extreme conditions of deprivation (Frape 2000, NRC 2007).

Excess

Vitamin A toxicity may result in elevated bone fragility, hyperostosis, exfoliated epithelium, and teratogenesis (NRC 1987) as well as DOD in growing horses (Donoghue et al 1981, Kronfeld et al 1990). Doses of 160 IU/kg (Jarrett & Schurg, 1987) and 220 IU/kg BW (Saastamoinen & Juusela, 1992) have been fed for 9 months or more without harmful effects but also without beneficial effects. According to NRC (2007), the safe upper safe limit is 16 000 IU/kg dry matter (~360 IU/kg BW/day) although it was noted that this is most likely erroneous based on the absence of toxicity in horses consuming such amounts. Even though the intake of β-carotene from pasture could theoretically reach critically high levels if all the β-carotene was fully converted into vitamin A (with a conversion rate assumed to be 400 IU of vitamin A per 1 mg of β-carotene), toxic effects of β-carotene have not yet been reported in horses. This is thought to be due to a reduction in the conversion rate at high intakes.

Vitamin D

Vitamin D (calciferols) has two forms, vitamin D_2 (ergocalciferol) and vitamin D_3 (cholecalciferol). Despite not being chemically identical, both are derived from steroids. They are formed from their respective pro-vitamins following exposure to ultraviolet radiation (UV-B radiation wavelength 290–318 nm). Ergosterol, found in plant material, is the precursor of vitamin D_2. In the majority of domestic species, 7-dehydrocholesterol within the skin (which is synthesized through the animal's metabolism) serves as the precursor to vitamin D_3. In general, vitamin D_3 has higher potency than vitamin D_2 (Harrington & Page 1983) but there is species variation (Schenk & Kolb 1982). In humans, vitamin D from the skin (D_3) binds to D-binding protein in the blood and is transported to the liver. Following emulsification and micelle formation ~80% of ingested vitamin D_2 is absorbed by enterocytes in the duodenum and ileum, incorporated into chylomicrons and transported to the liver via the lymphatic system (Sathe & Patel 2010). To become biologically active, vitamin D must be activated via reactions in the liver (hydroxylated on carbon 25 forming calcidiol; 25-OH-D) and then in the kidney (synthesis of calcitriol via hydroxylated on carbon 1; 1,25-OH-D). The active form, 1,25-OH-D, should actually be classified as a hormone. In humans, vitamin D status appears to be best assessed by measuring calcidiol levels because with vitamin D deficiency, parathyroid hormone increases the renal production of calcitriol resulting in apparently normal concentrations (Sathe & Patel 2010).

In the majority of mammalian species, vitamin D plays a key role in regulation of calcium and phosphorus homeostasis, especially in bone. However, the importance of vitamin D is questionable in equines, not least because of the significantly low plasma levels of vitamin D activating products (Smith & Wright 1984, Mäenpää et al 1987, 1988b, Harmeyer et al 1992) and the absence of clear evidence of biological effects.

Major biological functions

In the majority of domestic species, vitamin D is suggested to be largely responsible for (1) stimulating the intestinal absorption of calcium, (2) the renal reabsorption of calcium and phosphorus (in the presence of the parathyroid hormone), (3) building up the bone matrix, and (4) the calcification of osteoblasts. The anabolic effect of vitamin D metabolites within bone results from a combination of (1) indirect suppression of bone resorption, (2) direct stimulation of osteoblastic matrix synthesis, and (3) osteoblastic bone formation (Bante et al 1996). This biological effect of vitamin D is linked to the presence of receptors, similar to those for steroid hormones, in different cells and tissues. This explains how vitamin D influences many other biological processes, including the growth and differentiation of epidermal cells, differentiation of cells of the hematopoietic system, immune modulation, in addition to the already mentioned influence on calcinogenesis (Kolb & Grün 1996).

Although Hintz et al (1973) reported that supplemental vitamin D promotes calcium and phosphorus resorption in horses, the actual impact of the vitamin on calcium metabolism in the horse seems to be rather low compared to other domestic animals (Harmeyer et al 1992). However, a particularly high protein level of a vitamin D-dependent receptor has been identified *ex vivo* in the duodenal wall of horses (Sprekeler et al 2011). This receptor is commonly known to be involved in an active, vitamin D-dependent transcellular pathway of Ca^{2+}. The mRNA level of this receptor did not change remarkably throughout the intestine. Using chamber studies revealed Ca^{2+} active absorption in the duodenum but not in the cecum and specific sites of the colon (Sprekeler et al 2011). Horses therefore appear to have the capacity for active Ca^{2+} transport but passive mechanisms may be dominant. Breidenbach et al (1998) concluded that vitamin D does not seem to play a key role in regulating the homeostasis of calcium and inorganic phosphorus in horses under normal circumstances. However, the situation is different when pharmacological doses of vitamin D_3 are given (Harmeyer & Schlumbohm 2004). Overall, it does appear that the metabolism and biologic functions of vitamin D in the horse differ in many respects from those of other mammalian species such as human beings, pigs or rats (Breidenbach et al 1998). For example, plasma levels of calcidiol (<10 nmol/l) and calcitriol (20–40 pmol/l) are very low even in healthy animals and would clearly be regarded as deficient in humans or pigs (Kaune & Harmeyer 1987, Harmeyer 1999, Sathe & Patel 2010). Furthermore, in vitro results indicate that, contrary to other species, equine kidney tissue does not synthesize the active form of vitamin D hormone from its precursor calcidiol (Harmeyer 1999). This area would benefit from further research.

Sources and bioavailability

In principle, there are three ways for horses to obtain vitamin D: (1) via direct exposure to sunlight; (2) through the intake of vitamin D_2 from desiccated plant material or yeasts following prior exposure to ultraviolet radiation; and (3) via supplemental vitamin D from complementary feeds and supplements.

How much vitamin D is formed in the skin (Webb & Holick 1988) depends on the duration and intensity of the sunlight and thus also on the geographical location as well as the season of the year (Nutrition Reviews 1989) and the type of housing management. Ultraviolet radiation tends to be low in the morning and during the winter season, due to the shorter daylight time. This is particularly true at latitudes above 50° which may be a problem when horses are trained in the morning and then housed for the remainder of the day (Saastamoinen & Harris 2008). It has been suggested that horses in such regions, especially in the winter season, may have a deficiency of vitamin D when not supplemented (Mäenpää et al 1987) as exemplified by seasonal changes in serum 25-OH-D. However, Saastamoinen & Juusela (1992) did not find such a seasonal variation nor an impact of dietary supplementation on serum levels.

In naturally preserved forages, some vitamin D_2 will be synthesized from ergosterol if the forage is exposed, after cutting, to sunlight during desiccation (McDonald et al 1988, McDowell 2000). Because of reduced exposure to ultraviolet radiation, artificially dried hay will contain much less vitamin D_2 than sun dried material (Ballet et al 2000: around 971 IU/kg DM when sun dried vs. 470 IU/kg DM when barn dried). As the highest quantity of vitamin D_2 is found in dried leaves, the leaf to stem ratio is another influencing factor. The range of vitamin D_2 content in selected forages from a study by Ballet et al (2000) is given in Table 9-3. As ergosterol is also present in other plant forms like fungi and yeasts, irradiated yeast can be used as a source of vitamin D_2.

Both forms (D_2 and D_3) are used in the formulation of commercial complementary feeds and mineral-vitamin premixes, although use of vitamin D_3 is most common. It has been suggested that vitamin D_2 and D_3 are absorbed at a similar rate from the gut, ~60–80% (Schenk & Kolb 1982). There is, however, a lack of studies explicitly addressing absorption rates in horses.

Stability

Inexpert mechanical handling of sun cured forages, especially hay, can lead to loss of leaf and thus of vitamin D. Furthermore, many other factors influence the stability of vitamin D in the feed including the presence of heavy metals, alkaline components, and exposure to light when O_2 is present (Schenk & Kolb 1982). McDowell (2000) described a loss of 10 to 30% when complementary mixed feeds, which included mineral-vitamin premixes, were stored for either 4 or 6 months at 22°C.

Requirements

Based on blood levels, vitamin D status is low compared to other animal species (Smith & Wright 1984, Mäenpää et al 1987, 1988b, Harmeyer et al 1992). Supplemental vitamin D has been reported to increase calcium and phosphorus absorption in horses (Hintz et al 1973). However, no study has clearly shown the need for additional vitamin D on top of that synthesized in the skin through exposure to sunlight when horses are maintained under typical field conditions, including some pasture turnout. In situations when horses need to be kept inside (because of illness for example) or when the exposure to sunlight is restricted for other reasons, there may be a rationale for supplementation with vitamin D. Again without scientific evidence, it also is proposed that other life stage/life styles may benefit from the added security of knowing the animal has been provided with a known level of vitamin D through the diet. This may also be true for pregnant and lactating mares, when horses grow rapidly, or when young-stock come into training at an early age, all of which may increase vitamin D requirements. To ensure an adequate intake, vitamin D requirements for horses of different age and performance are given (Table 9-1) which are close to the recommendations published by GfE (1994) and NRC (2007). The main difference between these recommendations is the reference to $BW^{0.75}$ instead of BW: 30 IE/kg $BW^{0.75}$ for maintenance and early gestation (until the 7th month), 50 IU/kg $BW^{0.75}$ for late gestation (from the 8th month when fetal development accelerates) and lactation. As already suggested by NRC (2007), it is also proposed here to provide relatively high quantities of vitamin D to very young growing horses with intensive bone development (110 IE/kg $BW^{0.75}$ until the 6th month of age) with a subsequent decrease in provision (70 IE/kg $BW^{0.75}$ at 19–20 months of age) as they become older.

Table 9-3 Guide to Typical Concentrations of Vitamin D_2 in Selected Forages (Ballet et al 2000)

Roughages	Vitamin D_2 (range, in IU/kg of DM)
Fresh green forages	31–1800
Dehydrated lucerne	176–617
Cattle silages	80–866
Hay	90–5560

Effects of deficiency and excess

Deficiency

Signs of vitamin D deficiency in domestic animals principally occur due to: (1) inadequate intake and low exposure to sunlight; (2) insufficient metabolic activation (e.g., with liver or kidney diseases); or (3) in conjunction with a critically low calcium or phosphorus status. Under such conditions, the absorption rate of calcium and phosphorus may be decreased and the activity of plasma alkaline phosphatase increased. In other domestic animals and human beings, reduced mineralization of the skeleton is the most important outcome of vitamin D deficiency, which in turn results in the replacement of stable bone tissue by osteoid with insufficient mechanical strength. Growing animals develop rickets whereas osteoporosis is the typical characteristic of severe vitamin D deficiency in adult animals. In horse, these problems are very seldom, if ever, reported (Harmeyer & Schlumbohn 2004). Growth and development were similar in pony foals fed a diet containing 1000 IU of vitamin D per day with no exposure to sunlight vs. a ration without vitamin D but having exposure to sunlight (Elshorafa et al 1979). The growth and development of ponies was adversely affected in a third group that received neither a dietary vitamin D supply nor exposure to sunlight. Even so, the externally visible bone deformities were not typical of rickets. Thus, no clear evidence currently exists for a need for dietary vitamin D in horses that receive exposure to sunlight. For this reason deficiency of vitamin D is not considered to be a major problem in the horse industry.

Nonetheless, commercial complementary feeds are normally enriched with either vitamin D_2 or D_3.

Excess

Oversupply of vitamin D may be an issue. Ergocalciferol cannot be stored to any great extent in the body of mammals but storage of cholecalciferol in the liver, kidney, adipose tissue and to a lesser extent protein-bound in the blood plasma is possible (Schenk & Kolb 1982). In horses, an extreme oversupply of vitamin D or the excessive intake of substances with similar biological activity is known to cause serious health problems, including calcinosis with multiple foci of calcification in soft tissues (myocardia, large arteries and coronary arteries, gastric mucosa, lung, kidney) (Rambeck et al 1979, Köhler 1981, Harrington 1982, Rambeck & Zucker 1982, Harrington & Page 1983, Grabner et al 1985, Weisweiler et al 1993) and possibly death (Hintz et al 1973). Soft tissue calcifications are typically fatal in the horse, especially nephrocalcinosis (Harmeyer & Schlumbohm 2004). Calcinosis can occur even though pharmacological doses of vitamin D_3 (10 000 IU/kg BW i.m. for 4 consecutive days) do not increase plasma calcitriol concentrations above 40 pmol/l (Harmeyer 1999). However, this level of vitamin D_3 administration led to a persistent increase in plasma Ca (although it remained within the normal range) and P (from 1.38 to 3.33 mmol/l) concentrations (Harmeyer et al 1994). There are conflicting results in the published literature as to the effects of high doses of vitamin D on plasma Ca concentration. No significant elevation in plasma Ca concentration was reported by McClure (1987) and Harrington & Page (1983), but an increase has been demonstrated in other studies (Muylle et al 1974, Papasteriades et al 1988). A pronounced increase in plasma P has been reported after high doses of both vitamin D_2 and D_3 (Harrington 1982, Harrington & Page 1983, McClure 1987), suggesting that both forms are potentially toxic in horses. These studies have demonstrated that extremely high vitamin D doses (between 10000 to 33000 IU/kg BW) can induce toxic effects but it is possible that lower doses over a longer time frame may also cause calcification of soft tissues. That may be the reason why the NRC (1987) gave an upper safe level of vitamin D of 44 IU/kg BW/day.

It is difficult to assess, both in terms of quantity and activity, the importance of substances present in calcinogenic plants like yellow oat grass (*Trisetum flavescens* L.), which contain vitamin D_3 (Rambeck et al 1979, Rambeck & Zucker 1982) as well as a water-soluble compound with a similar activity (Rambeck & Zucker 1982). These substances maintain their activity, at least in part, when the plant is desiccated.

In the event of vitamin D intoxication, it may help to restrict the intake of calcium and phosphorus immediately in an attempt to diminish soft tissue calcification (Harmeyer & Schlumbohn 2004). Harmeyer and Schlumbohn (2004) gave only 53% and 34% of the normally required Ca and P intake for 14 days after calcitriol challenge, and 88% and 34% of calcium and phosphorus afterwards (for an undisclosed period of time).

Vitamin E

Vitamin E is a collective term for all tocol and tocotrienol derivatives. These are fat-soluble substances which consist of a chromanol ring with different isoprenoid side chains which affect activity. The eight naturally occurring compounds with vitamin E activity include four tocopherols (α, β, γ, δ) that have a saturated side chain, and four tocotrienols (α, β, γ, δ) with a threefold unsaturated side chain. The designation as α, β, γ and δ forms relates to the placement of methyl groups on the chromanol ring (stereoisomery). The side chain of α-tocopherol contains three asymmetric carbons. This results in eight different stereoisomers. The naturally-occurring form has a *2R 4'R 8'R* configuration, commonly referred to as *RRR* (NRC 2007). Synthetic vitamin E forms represent a racemic mixture of the different stereoisomers, designated as *all-rac*-forms.

Major biological functions

The most prominent biological function of vitamin E is that of an antioxidant. Together with other substances (albumin, bilirubin, glutathione, uric acid) it represents the nonenzymatic defense system of the body. This works in conjunction with the various anti-oxidative enzymes, such as isoenzymes of the glutathione peroxidize family or superoxide dismutase. Vitamin E is the most important lipid-soluble antioxidant responsible for the integrity of biological structures such as cell membranes (Combs et al 1975). In situations of oxidative stress, vitamin E trapping of reactive oxygen species, including lipid peroxides, prevents free radical-induced damage (Harris & Dyson 1996). Vitamin C, as part of the water-soluble antioxidant system, is able to regenerate vitamin E through the acquisition of oxygen from the tocopherols' oxidized form. In addition, vitamin E promotes the syntheses of ubiquinone and thus is important in the respiratory chain (for overview see Kolb 1966). A lack of vitamin E also seems to cause disturbances in the metabolism of nucleic acids and signs of vitamin A deficiency may be attenuated if simultaneously high doses of vitamin E are given (Schenk & Kolb 1982). Furthermore, vitamin E is said be important with respect to function of the gonads and is therefore referred to as an anti-sterility vitamin (Domke et al 2004). Vitamin E also may be important in the regulation of cell proliferation and gene expression (Sathe & Patel 2010) and the development of humoral immune response (Baalsrud & Overnes, 1986).

Sources and bioavailability

Vitamin E may be provided either from natural feedstuffs or via synthetic sources within complementary feeds, premixes and supplements. In nature, tocopherols and tocotrienols are only synthesized by plants. The α, β, γ and δ configurations all have different biological activities (Lynch 1996a, b). *RRR*-α-tocopherol is considered to be the most active form (Table 9-4) and comprises around 90% of

Table 9-4 Biological Activity of Individual Forms of Vitamin E (in IU/mg; Brubacher & Weiser 1967)

Vitamin E	RRR-form	all-rac-form
α-tocopheryl acetate	1.36	1.00
α-tocopherol	1.49	1.10
β-tocopherol	0.40	0.30
γ-tocopherol	0.20	0.15
δ-tocopherol	0.016	0.012

the total vitamin E activity in plant material (Kolb 1966). The α-tocopherol transfer protein which is responsible for blood transport of vitamin E (in very low density lipoproteins) has highest affinity for natural α-tocopherol. γ-tocopherol, which is mainly found in soy products, shows lower activity. In humans, however, supplementation of α-tocopherol decreased concentrations of γ-tocopherol in blood and tissues whereas ingested γ-tocopherol increased both α- and γ-tocopherol (Jiang et al 2001). For this reason, it is currently being discussed whether a particular function of γ-tocopherol needs to be ascribed. Most synthetic vitamin E forms exhibit a considerably lower activity than their natural counterpart (Table 9-4) and also appear to have higher bioavailability (Gansen et al 1995). Pagan et al (2005) reported that natural forms of vitamin E (especially micellized forms) were superior in increasing plasma α-tocopherol levels in horses. On the contrary, Hakkarainen and Pehrson (1987) stated that there are no differences in the bioavailability of different vitamin E isomers. In addition, there was no difference in the availability of vitamin E from forages *vs.* grain sources. The highest concentrations of vitamin E are found in the adrenal and pituitary glands (Kolb 1966) but adipose tissue represents the largest body store (Roneus et al 1986).

High levels of vitamin E are found in wheat germs and vegetable oils, including wheat germ oil (Kivimäe & Carpena 1973). In wheat germ-, sunflower- and olive oil, *RRR*-α-tocopherol is the main form (wheat germ oil, up to 2435 mg total tocopherols/kg with 49% α-tocopherol; sunflower oil, 454–810 mg total tocopherols/kg with 86–99% α-tocopherol; olive oil, 46–224 mg total tocopherols/kg with 89–100% α-tocopherol). In soybean-, maize germ- and palm oil, γ-tocopherols represent the majority (Domke et al 2004). Another rich vitamin E source is dehydrated green feed (Kivimäe & Carpena 1973). On a DM basis, fresh forages and those harvested at an immature state can contain remarkably high concentrations of vitamin E (30–100 IU/kg DM; NRC 2007). However, the level of vitamin E in forages is very variable and depends upon the stage of growth and the time of harvesting, the genetic variety, processing and storage (Kivimäe & Carpena 1973). Levels in hays and haylages can be very low (personal observation). Vitamin E is typically low in cereal grains (20–30 IU/kg DM). As a consequence, the total tocopherol contents and proportion of α-tocopherol in mixed feeds will depend upon their composition.

Effect of concurrent oil administration

Tocopherols are soluble in fats and lipophilic solvents and, thus, their absorption may be increased with fat-enriched feeding (Siciliano & Wood 1993, Zeyner et al 1995, 1999). Providing increasing amounts of soybean oil (0, 0.33, 0.67, 1.00, 1.33 g/kg BW/day) to Warmblood-type horses receiving 1000 mg vitamin E per day through a mineral-vitamin-mix elevated the concentration of α-tocopherol in the blood serum (Zeyner et al 1995). However, the serum response seems to have an interaction with the basal feed, at least the forage type. In Warmblood-type horses supplemented with 1725 mg of vitamin E per day, serum tocopherol concentrations were only slightly higher when animals had free access to meadow grass vs. hay. When compared to a control diet (no added fat), the addition of 0.87 g/kg BW/day partly hardened soybean oil led to a small increase in serum tocopherol of horses fed oats plus hay and a larger increase when the animals were fed oats plus meadow grass (Zeyner et al 1995; Table 9-1).

Stability

Vitamin E is highly susceptible to oxidation processes. Every kind of processing causes some loss of vitamin E; milling, flaking, and shredding produce heavy losses and only the refining of oils results in relatively small losses (Kivimäe & Carpena 1973). Vitamin E decreases during harvesting and drying of hay, with further losses during storage. In alfalfa stored for 3 months at 33°C, vitamin E content decreased by 54–73% (Lynch 1996b). High moisture and temperature during storage exacerbate vitamin E losses (Kivimäe & Carpena 1973). However, it should also be noted that vitamin E is sensitive to oxidative damage even at low temperatures (Dju et al 1958). Because free vitamin E compounds are particular unstable, the more stable ester forms are typically used in feed supplements (Gassmann & Ulbricht 1979). *All-rac*-α-tocopheryl acetate (termed "synthetic vitamin E") and *RRR*-α-tocopheryl acetate (termed "natural vitamin E") forms are most commonly used.

Requirements

Maintenance

Vitamin E requirements for maintenance have been derived from studies with quite different aims and target outcomes. Stowe (1968) found that 0.233 mg/kg BW were required to maintain erythrocyte stability in vitamin E-deficient foals. In another study, 0.27 mg/kg BW was needed to maintain basal metabolism in horses at rest, but 1.4 to 4.4 mg/kg BW was considered necessary to maximize tissue stores (Roneus et al 1986). However, optimal tissue storage levels are unknown and the latter result should not be overvalued. Baalsrud and Overnes (1986) reported that 1 mg vitamin E/kg BW/day together with 5 mg selenium/day had the ability to enhance humoral immune function in mature horses, which was suggested to be essential to support resistance to influenza and tetanus. Another question is whether feeding supplemental fats and oils alters the need for vitamin E due to a greater need for antioxidants in the face of increased ingestion of unsaturated fatty acids. Studies in humans suggest that the requirement for vitamin E increases as a function of polyunsaturated fatty acid (PUFA) intake (Wardlaw 1999). From studies in other species, it has been concluded that the need for vitamin E per g of fatty acid is 0.6 mg of α-tocopherol for linoleic acid (C18:2*n*-6) and 3 mg of α-tocopherol for α-linolenic acid (C18:3*n*-3) and other omega-3 PUFA (cited according to Saastamoinen & Harris 2008). With the assumptions that: (1) no more than 1 g supplemental fat/kg BW/day be fed to horses for avoidance of detrimental effects associated with disturbed microbial fermentation in the hindgut and reduced fiber digestibility as well as possibly decreased production of B-vitamins (Zeyner 2002); and (2) all of the fat consists of PUFA, the extra requirement for vitamin E is 0.6 mg (all omega-6 PUFA) and 3 mg (all omega-3 PUFA) of vitamin E/kg BW/day. This is equal to 3 and 15 mg/kg $BW^{0.75}$/day. However, such a high intake of omega-3 PUFA is unrealistic because oils containing omega-3 PUFA do not have such high concentrations of these particular fatty acids. Additional vitamin E in the range of 1–1.5 mg/1 ml supplemented oil is a more realistic recommendation (Harris 2005b). Assuming the recommended maximal intake of supplemental fats and oils (Zeyner 2002), this would be equivalent to an extra need of 5–7 mg vitamin E/kg $BW^{0.75}$/day. However, under maintenance conditions where fat is oxidized rather slowly an extra supply of 5 mg vitamin E/kg $BW^{0.75}$/day should be enough.

Taking all of this information together it is recommended to provide horses under maintenance conditions a minimum of 5 mg of vitamin E per kg of $BW^{0.75}$/day (which is equal to 1 mg/kg BW for medium-sized horses) (Table 9-2). Horses on a fat-enriched ration should receive double this amount (i.e., 10 mg/kg $BW^{0.75}$/day, which is equal to 2 mg/kg BW for medium-sized horses; Table 9-2). Some nutritionists (P. Harris included) recommend this level of intake in all circumstances but substantive experimental evidence in support of this recommendation is currently lacking.

Exercise

Common recommendations for vitamin E intake by exercising horses range from 0.27 to 2 mg/kg BW/day, but as much as 4 mg/kg BW/day has been recommended for horses in intense training (INRA 1990, GfE 1994, Frape 2000, NRC 2007, P. Harris personal recommendation). Total intakes of 1.5 mg/kg BW/day (1 mg/kg BW/day as supplement) were not sufficient to maintain serum vitamin E levels of exercising horses during the winter season (Saastamoinen & Juusela 1993). Several studies have provided evidence that high intakes (1.5 to 5 mg vitamin E/kg BW/day) are necessary to maintain vitamin E status in exercising horses (Putnam 1986, Roneus et al 1986, Saastamoinen & Juusela 1993, Siciliano et al 1997). The concentration of vitamin E in blood serum, as well as liver, skeletal muscle and adipose tissue was used as an indicator of vitamin E status in these studies (Roneus et al 1986). Steiss et al (1994), however, stated, that the vitamin E status of horses is difficult to assess by means of serum α-tocopherol concentration because of its high short-term fluctuation. Schubert et al (1993) did not find a convincing effect of 200 mg supplemental vitamin E per day (to a core diet containing ~15 mg vitamin E/kg DM) on serum α-tocopherol in broodmares, foals or geldings over a 12-month period. Furthermore, calculating serum α-tocopherol concentrations in proportion to lipids (Stahe & Patel 2010) does not substantially reduce variability of measurements in horses (Craig et al 1989). Adipose tissue α-tocopherol concentrations also demonstrate high variability in horses (Steiss et al 1994).

With respect to dietary vitamin E and athletic performance, a 3-year study of 247 Thoroughbreds from 10 different yards reported superior race performance in horses that received 1000 mg of vitamin E per day (~2.5 mg/kg BW/day) vs. animals provided no supplement (with the core diet providing 0.2 mg vitamin E/kg BW/day) (Schubert & Heinrich 1988).

For athletic horses, it is necessary to distinguish between low and high intensity work. The maintenance vitamin E requirement (5 mg/kg $BW^{0.75}$/day; Table 9-2) is adequate for horses used in pleasure riding activities. When horses are exercised to a higher level or receive a high-fat diet, vitamin E intake should be twice maintenance (10 mg/kg $BW^{0.75}$/day), as recommended by GfE (1994) and NRC (2007). Horses in very intense training and those prone to recurrent myopathy (Harris 2005b) may benefit from higher vitamin E supply (~20 mg/kg $BW^{0.75}$/day).

Breeding, pregnancy and lactation

There is no evidence from literature that supplemental vitamin E supports fertility of stallions (Rich et al 1983) or mares. However, studies on this subject are scarce. Providing 100 mg vitamin E per day to barren mares did not affect reproduction (Stowe 1967). Furthermore, the supply of 46 mg vitamin E/day to foaling mares, where the base ration already covered the requirement (NRC 1978), did not influence re-breeding efficiency (Ott & Asquit 1981). Serum α-tocopherol decreased during gestation in mares fed a base ration consisting of preserved forage supplemental 200–400 mg vitamin E/day, but no negative health effects were observed (Mäenpäa et al 1988b). Vitamin E nutrition (up to 2000 mg/day) also does not appear to affect vitamin E concentrations in colostrum (Schubert et al 1993; Großer et al 1995). However, a doubling of vitamin E intake (from 80 mg/kg DM to 160 mg/kg DM) increased colostral immunoglobulin G (IgG) content as well as foal serum IgG concentration (Hoffman et al 1999). In mares fed according to German recommendations (GfE 1994), serum α-tocopherol concentrations remained constant during the first 12 hours after birth while the serum concentrations increased in the foals (Zeyner et al 2004, Fig. 9.2).

The current literature does not suggest a need to alter the vitamin E recommendation for broodmares from that given by NRC (1989). Thus, it can be recommended to provide 10 mg of vitamin E/kg $BW^{0.75}$/day (Table 9-2) to pregnant and lactating mares. This is similar to the NRC (1989) recommendation of 2 mg vitamin E/kg BW/day for medium-sized horses. Basing on the observed increase in IgG in the colostrum of mares and blood serum of foals when the mares received 160 vs. 80 mg vitamin E/kg DM (Hoffman et al 1999), it may be beneficial to provide a ration containing 20 mg of vitamin E/kg $BW^{0.75}$/day (160 mg vitamin E/kg DM assuming a dry matter intake of 2.5% BW) under some circumstances (e.g., on farms with high infection pressure). Nevertheless, more research is needed before this can be incorporated into general recommendations.

Growth

Apart from the study done by Stowe (1968) which described satisfactory erythrocyte stability in foals consuming 0.233 mg vitamin E/kg BW, there have been no published studies concerning the vitamin E requirement of growing horses. For reasons of security however, it seems to be appropriate to supply growing horses as much vitamin E as recommended for broodmares (10 mg/kg $BW^{0.75}$/day).

Effects of deficiency and excess

Deficiency

Clinical signs of vitamin E deficiency have been mainly studied in rats and food-producing animals. The following deficits were encountered in rats: degenerative changes in the testes, accumulation of stillbirths and increased number of nonviable fetuses (with normal ovarian function and cycle), necrosis and edema in the cerebellum, reduction of the size of the zona fasciculata in the anterior pituitary, disrupted steroid metabolism, and degenerative processes in the muscle (for review see Kolb 1966). Clinical expression of vitamin E deficiency is influenced by selenium status (e.g., liver dystrophy in pigs). In humans, most cases of vitamin E deficiency are secondary to fat malabsorption and may present with hemolytic anemia, muscle weakness or neurological deficits such as ataxia (Sathe & Patel 2010).

Perhaps more related to a deficiency of selenium (Lofstedt 1997) than of vitamin E (Schougaard et al 1972, Wilson et al 1976) is the so-called "white muscle disease" (WMD) or "nutritional muscle dystrophy" in foals, a disorder characterized by a noninflammatory degeneration of skeletal and cardiac muscle. The bright appearance (white color) of damaged muscle tissue gives the disease its name. In the majority of cases, foals are already affected at birth, and are often too weak to stand with weak or absent suckling reflex. However, WMD has been described in foals up to 11 months of age (Lofstedt 1997). The treatment involves administration of high doses of vitamin E and selenium. The vitamin E and selenium status of broodmares should be investigated to determine the need for dietary adjustments.

Whether vitamin E deficiency contributes to the development of myopathies in adult horses is controversial. Although "tying-up" has been associated with low serum concentrations of vitamin E (Watanabe et al 1982) there is no evidence of causation (Saastamoinen & Harris 2008). In one case report (Zentek 1991), 6 of 35 horses exhibited severe myopathy within a 3-week period. Vitamin E intake was very low (0.06 mg/kg BW/day) but dietary selenium also was inadequate and therefore it was not possible to ascribe the myopathy to pure vitamin E deficiency.

Vitamin E deficiency also may play a facilitating role in equine degenerative myeloencephalopathy (EDM; Liu et al 1983, Mayhew et al 1987, Harris & Mayhew 1998, Gandini et al 2004), although this hypothesis has been disputed (Dill et al 1989). This condition probably has a genetic background, affects horses aged up to two years, and is characterized by gait abnormalities and degenerative changes in the spinal cord and parts of the brain (Blythe et al 1991, Blythe & Craig 1991). From the clinical point of view, EDM cannot be distinguished from other forms of neuroaxonal dystrophy (NAD) where NAD is the generic term for neurodegenerative diseases characterized by dystrophy on neurons and axons and the formation of spheroids. In a study with Quarter Horses, which developed NAD on a pasture poor in vitamin E and selenium, the addition of vitamin E had no positive impact on already diseased animals (Aleman et al 2011). However, additional supplementation to mares did appear to decrease the incidence and severity of disease in the subsequent crop of foals.

Equine motor neuron disease (EMND) is associated with low vitamin E status (Hintz & Cymbaluk 1994, Divers 2005). Affected horses typically have very low serum α-tocopherol concentrations and the condition has been experimentally induced in horses after 18–22 months of continuous ingestion of a vitamin E-deficient diet. Clinical signs of EMND usually develop in horses older than 2 years of age and include an acute onset of trembling, almost constant shifting of weight in the rear legs when standing, prolonged recumbency, and muscle wasting (Divers 2005). The primary pathology of EMND is degeneration of somatic lower motor neurons (Divers 2005). For further information see Chapter 38.

Excess

In humans, vitamin E toxicity is rare. Interestingly, clinical signs of vitamin toxicity are similar as for deficiency and include fatigue plus altered coagulation, but they are not seen until a chronic intake of >1000 mg/day (Sathe & Patel 2010). In preterm infants necrotizing enterocolitis has been reported with the use of hyperosmolar oral vitamin E preparations. Data from other animals suggest coagulopathy and impaired bone mineralization can occur when diets with excessive vitamin E (above the upper safe limit of 1000 mg/kg DM; NRC 1987) are consumed. However, in horses no signs indicating vitamin E toxicosis have yet been reported even at the high intakes recommended for treatment of EMD and other conditions.

Vitamin K

General introduction and major biological functions

The term vitamin K represents a group of vitamins, which are all derived from naphthoquinone. They are involved in the post-translational synthesis of γ-carboxyglutamic acid (Gla), ultilizing the glutamic acid residues within certain precursor proteins (Ferland 2001). This results in the formation of vitamin K-dependent proteins, so called Gla-proteins. The Gla residues act as calcium binding groups in these proteins and are essential for their biological activity e.g. the ability to bind calcium (Ca^{2+}) is required for the activation of the seven vitamin K-dependent clotting factors in the coagulation cascade. Gla-proteins are also involved in vascular health, bone metabolism and sphingolipid metabolism in the brain (Dowd et al 1995, Vermeer et al 1996, 2004, Denisova & Booth 2005). The role of vitamin K in blood coagulation is perhaps best understood. In this process, vitamin K carboxylates glutamate-residues from preprothrombin and preliminary stages of the coagulation factors VII, IX, and X. The γ-carboxyglutamic acid residues bind calcium ions causing a local enrichment of precursors of clotting factors around phospholipid membranes in the area of an injured vessel.

Although vitamin K is thought to play an important role in bone health, results from studies on the effects of vitamin K supplementation in adult humans have been conflicting (Kalkwarf et al 2004, Bonjour et al 2009). In osteoblasts and osteocytes, vitamin K is part of an enzyme system which carboxylates glutamatic acid residues to form several key vitamin K-dependent proteins including osteocalcin, bone GLA protein, matrix Gla protein, protein S and periostin; osteocalcin is the most abundant (Shearer 1997). The γ-carboxyglutamic acid residues of osteocalcin attract calcium ions enabling them to be incorporated into the hydroxyapatite molecule. It has therefore been hypothesized that vitamin K is necessary for bone mineralization (Shearer 1997). Vitamin K deficiency results in an increase in undercarboxylated osteocalcin, a protein with low biological activity (Bugel 2003). Vitamin K also has been shown to increase osteoblastogenesis and decrease osteoclastogenesis, thereby increasing bone formation and decreasing bone resorption. Whether menaquinone 4 (MK-4) has a unique role independent to the recognized coenzyme function of vitamin K is currently unknown but levels in the brain suggest that it may be important for neural function (Okano et al 2008).

Sources and bioavailability

Natural vitamin K exists in two molecular forms: phylloquinone and the menaquinones (MKs). Phylloquinone (PK or vitamin K_1: 2-methyl-3-phytyl-1,4-naphtoquinone) is a single compound primarily found in plants in association with chlorophyll. The levels of PK vary in fresh cut grass and levels will decrease with UV radiation so that dried preserved forage can have markedly reduced levels (Biffin et al 2008). PK in plants may have low bioavailability due to its tight binding within chloroplasts; in a small pilot study of Thoroughbred yearlings kept at pasture it was observed that plasma vitamin K levels increased in response to supplementation (3 mg/day for 9 days; Biffin et al 2008).

There are at least 15 types of menaqinones referred to as menaquinone-*n* (MK-n), where *n* stands for the number of isoprenyl residues in the unsaturated side chain. The MK-n forms are collectively referred to as vitamin K_2 (2-methyl-1,4-naphtoquinones). The long chain menaquinones MK-7 to MK-9 are synthesized by bacteria and gut microflora in mammals or in certain fermented feeds (Schenk & Kolb 1982, Okano et al 2008, Bonjour et al 2009). Interestingly MK-4 does not appear to be produced in significant amounts by bacteria; instead, it appears to be synthesized from phylloquinone within the body (Okano et al 2008). Furthermore, a synthetic vitamin named menadione (vitamin K_3) exists which is used as a feed additive (the other synthetic types of Vitamin K: K_4 and K_5 are not fed to horses). It is thought that menadione is metabolized into MK-4, the active form (Okano et al 2008). The concentration of vitamin K is substantially higher in forages (3–22 mg/kg DM) than in cereal grains (0.2–0.4 mg/kg DM) (McDowell 1989, Siciliano et al 2000a).

The absorption of vitamin K from the intestine should in theory be enhanced by fine emulsification and micelle formation. However, the mechanisms of absorption in horses have not been elucidated, nor is it known if absorption is enhanced by feeding fats or oils. One pilot study in horses reported that a soluble vitamin K form was more effective than an oil-based preparation but full data were not provided and so firm conclusions cannot be reached (Biffin et al 2008). Menaquinones produced by gut microbes can be absorbed in humans and rodents, but the extent of absorption from the large intestine is not known with some suggestion that this process is inefficient (Groenen-Van Dooren et al 1995, Suttie 1995). Siciliano et al (2000b) described that vitamin K status in foals and weanlings (measured by undercarboxylated osteocalcin) increased with age. The age effect may be related to either higher forage intakes or more effective microbial production or both.

One small study from Japan looked at the plasma concentrations of vitamin K homologs in Thoroughbred horses either provided with 9 mg/day of menadione (vitamin K_3) vs. a nonsupplemented diet (Inoue et al 2009). The authors reported that menadione supplementation increased plasma MK-4 concentrations. MK-7 (from bacterial production) was not detected in the plasma of most of the horses whereas it was found in the plasma of lactating cows. It was suggested that bacterial synthesis of vitamin K_2 may not be significant in the horse (Inoue et al 2009).

In mammals, vitamin K_1 is stored primarily in the liver (Schenk & Kolb 1982) although cardiac tissue may have similar concentrations (Okano et al 2008). However, vitamin K_1 storage capacity is quite low because most is converted to the primary active form, 2-methyl-3(geranyl-geranyl)-napthochinone, which is rapidly degraded after being active. The products of degradation are primarily excreted in bile. There is, however, some conservation via vitamin K recycling.

Requirements

Dietary requirements have not been determined in horses. The absorption of vitamin K from feed and from menaquinones synthesized by the gut microbes, however, seems to be adequate for maintenance of vitamin K status if no antagonistic factors are present (e.g., the coumarin derivatives that inhibit the recycling of vitamin K). Whether increased amounts are required when there are disturbances to the gut microflora or in cases of chronic liver disease or fat malabsorption is currently unknown.

The fact that there are at least five GLA proteins in bone and cartilage that require vitamin K dependent modification for function does suggest that there is a need for an optimal supply of vitamin K for bone health throughout life. However, the level of optimal osteocalcin carboxylation is unknown even in humans. A recent meta-analysis suggested a strong association between vitamin K supplementation and reduced fracture incidence as well as mitigation of bone loss in osteoporosis (see Bonjour et al 2009), but often the doses used were very high (pharmacologic) rather than nutritional. There is no evidence that exercise loading (e.g., the initiation of exercise training in young horses) alters serum concentrations of undercarboxylated osteocalcin (Siciliano et al 2000a). Currently, there is insufficient data to make any recommendation with respect to vitamin K supplementation and bone health.

Vitamin K supplementation should be only used in the case of vitamin K deficiency and to treat specific blood coagulation problems, not with the aim to prevent exercise-induced pulmonary hemorrhage (Maxie et al 1992) or bone abnormalities.

Effects of deficiency and excess

Deficiency

Effects of vitamin K deficiency are mediated by the production of undercarboxylated Gla-proteins that lack biological activity. The most obvious effect of vitamin K deficiency is impaired blood coagulation (McDowell 1989). In humans, vitamin K deficiency is associated with diseases of the blood vessels and impaired bone health (Vermeer et al 2004). The latter may be related to undercarboxylated osteocalcin. In horses, however, serum undercarboxylated osteocalcin was neither correlated to medial radiographic bone density in foals and weanlings nor to exercise associated changes in bone mineral content or bone pathology (Siciliano et al 2000a, b).

Primary vitamin K deficiency has never been described in horses. Coumarin derivatives, such as dicoumarol and warfarin, however, may act as antagonists. One case has been described in which dicoumarin produced in moldy sweet clover impaired blood coagulation (McDonald 1980). This effect can also be observed after warfarin administration (0.8 mg/kg BW/day for 4–5 days; Byars et al 1986). It has been suggested that there may be an increased risk of coagulation defects with the ingestion of certain plants, if microbial fermentation in the terminal tract is severely depressed or if the liver function is seriously impaired (Harris 2005a).

In other species large doses of vitamin A (due to interference with vitamin K absorption) or vitamin E (inhibition of vitamin K-dependent carboxylase enzymes) have been associated with vitamin K antagonism (Both et al 2004). It is not known whether this antagonism occurs in the horse.

Excess

Studies in laboratory animals have shown that high doses of phylloquinone (25 g/kg BW; oral or parenteral) do not cause adverse health effects (Molitor & Robinson 1940) and the food and nutrition board reported no known toxicity for vitamin K_1 or K_2 (Food and Nutrition Board 2001). Dietary menaquinones and menadione also have low toxicity (NRC 2007). Intramuscular or intravenous administration of 1.8–8.3 mg/kg BW of menadione bisulfite to horses, however, caused renal colic, hematuria, azotemia and electrolyte abnormalities consistent with acute renal failure (Rebhun et al 1984). Findings at necropsy indicated renal tubular nephrosis. Studies in human neonates have indicated that phylloquinone injectables are safer than menadione injectables (American Academy of Pediatrics 1971). Menadione injection in infants can induce liver toxicity, jaundice and hemolytic anemia and is no longer used for treatment of vitamin K deficiency. Phylloquinone forms are also likely to be safer in other mammalian species.

Water-soluble vitamins

Vitamin B_1 (thiamin)

Thiamin in the form thiamine pyrophosphate is required by enzymes involved in the use of substrates (e.g. glucose) for ATP-synthesis (pyruvate dehydrogenase, α-ketoglutarate dehydrogenase) and in the pentose phosphate pathway (transketolase). Thus, the vitamin is highly involved in carbohydrate metabolism (Bates 2001) and is particularly important for nervous system function. The latter is indicated by its alternative name, "Aneurin" (Schenk & Kolb 1982). High concentrations of thiamin pyrophosphate can be found in the myocardium, the liver, the kidney and the brain.

Sources and bioavailability

Feedstuffs with significant levels of thiamin are cereal grains (~3–5 mg/kg), protein supplements (~6–11 mg/kg) and grain by-products (10–15 mg/kg) (McDowell 1989, McMeniman et al 1995). Highest concentrations can be found in brewers' and bakers' yeast (~150–160 mg/kg; McDowell 1989). The thiamin content in forages seems to be substantially lower (~0.1–4.5 mg/kg DM; Ballet et al 2000). There is a paucity of knowledge of vitamin B_1 content in silages. Thiamin hydrochloride and thiamin mononitrate are used as synthetic feed supplements.

Requirements

Investigations on the concentration of individual vitamins of the B-complex in the horse's gut provide evidence for microbial synthesis of thiamin, particularly in the anterior part of the large colon (Carroll et al 1949). Production and absorption or both, however, may be insufficient under some circumstances. This has been demonstrated in two 2-year-old Percheron horses that developed signs of thiamin deficiency (poor appetite, weight loss and ataxia) when consuming a semisynthetic ration containing 1.1 mg of thiamin per kg DM for 4 months (Carroll et al 1949). One horse died 3 weeks after the end of the feeding period and the other improved over a 4-month period when consuming 0.25 mg thiamin per kg $BW^{0.75}$/day. Other studies have reported positive effects of dietary vitamin B_1 on weight gain of weanling ponies (3.3 mg thiamin/kg DM; Jordan 1979) and the thiamin status of exercising horses as indicated by blood thiamin levels and post-exercise pyruvate dehydrogenase activity (4 or 28 mg vs. 2 mg thiamin/kg DM; Topliff et al 1981). From published literature, the NRC (1989, 2007) stated that horses should receive 0.06 mg thiamine/kg BW/d which is equivalent to 0.3 mg/kg $BW^{0.75}$/day (Table 9-2). For exercising horses this level of intake may not be adequate (Topliff et al 1981) and it can be recommended to double the supply (0.6 mg/kg $BW^{0.75}$/day; Table 9-2), particularly to support elevated carbohydrate metabolism. Based on current literature, there is no evidence to suggest a further differentiation of the recommendations according to life stages and performance of horses. Overall requirements, however, are normally met without supplementation when rations containing grains or cereal grain products are fed (McMeniman et al 1995).

Effects of deficiency and excess

Deficiency

In the rat, which relies primarily on oral intake, the thiamin content of most organs decreased significantly after 10 days of deficiency (McIlwain 1966). Clinical signs included decreased appetite, increased irritability, and a reduced heart rate. Chronic conditions of the digestive tract as well as diarrhea inhibit the absorption of thiamin (Schenk & Kolb 1982). Anorexia, bradycardia, muscle fasciculations, hyperesthesia, ataxia and convulsions have been described as signs of thiamin deficiency in horses (Carroll et al 1949, Roberts et al 1949, Cymbaluk et al 1978). However, thiamin deficiency seems to have no practical significance in horses fed typical diets in the absence of interfering ingredients (arsenic, mercury, phenol derivatives, thiaminases of microbial or plant origin, amprolium). Only by feeding a semipurified diet with only 1.1 mg thiamin per kg over a period of 16 weeks were signs of thiamin deficiency induced (Carroll et al 1949; for details see "Requirements"). Such signs may also be caused by the ingestion of interfering substances, e.g. thiaminases from marsh horsetail (*Pteridium aquilinum*), bracken fern (*Equisetum palustre*; Roberts et al 1949), or the coccidiostat amprolium (Cymbaluk et al 1978). However, ponies that ingested 5, 10, and 20% of their total dietary DM intake as dried marsh horsetail (0.128 mg palustrine/kg DM) developed no clinical signs (Hünsche et al 2010). Plasma thiamin concentrations (5.05–23.8 µg/l) also did not indicate depletion due to increased thiaminase activity. In the same study, ruminants (cows and sheep) developed moderately severe clinical signs of thiamin deficiency following the ingestion of similar quantities of marsh horsetail.

Excess

Thiamin toxicity has not been described in horses.

Vitamin B_2 (riboflavin)

Vitamin B_2 is called riboflavin because of the content of ribitol in the molecule and its yellow color. The other synonym "lactoflavin" derives from its high content in milk. The most important metabolic function of riboflavin may be as a precursor for the coenzymes flavin adenine mononucleotide (FAM) and flavin adenine dinucleotide (FAD). FAM and FAD are required for the formation of several enzymes involved in ATP synthesis, lipid metabolism, dehydration of amino acids and oxidation-reduction reactions (Schenk & Kolb 1982, Rivalin 2001).

Sources and bioavailability

FAM and FAD are the only riboflavin-containing substances in naturally occurring feedstuffs. Feed tables (NRC 1982) indicate that legumes are rich in riboflavin (13–17 mg/kg DM), followed by grass hays (7–10 mg/kg DM) and further by cereal grains with clearly lower contents (1.4–1.7 mg/kg DM). As feed additives, pure riboflavin and riboflavin preparations are in use. Further, riboflavin synthesized by gut microbes seems to be a remarkable source (Jones et al 1946, Carroll et al 1949, Linerode 1967). However, the hindgut is the part of the intestine with the highest microbial density and activity, but the small intestine is assumed to be the site of vitamin absorption.

Requirements

The NRC (1949) developed a riboflavin requirement for horses based on the work by Pearson et al (1944a, b). The authors calculated that a horse needs to ingest 2.2 mg riboflavin/kg DM to maintain body stores. The NRC (1989) revised this amount to 2 mg riboflavin/kg DM, which corresponds to 0.04 mg/kg BW, assuming a DM intake of 2% of BW. From today's perspective there is no serious justification for the assumption that horses have an oral need for riboflavin. However, for reasons of security the recommendation should provisionally be maintained. When converted to metabolic body weight the recommendation given by the NRC (1989) would correspond to 0.2 mg/kg $BW^{0.75}$/day (Table 9-2). This, however, should normally be fulfilled without supplementation by a normal ration (see "sources and bioavailability").

Effects of deficiency and excess

Deficiency

In species others than horses, deficiency of riboflavin leads to decreased activity of FMN- and FAD-dependent enzymes with reduced protein synthesis and growth as main consequences (Schenk & Kolb 1982). Clinical signs of riboflavin deficiency have not been described in horses, even after feeding a riboflavin-deficient diet (0.4 mg/kg DM; Carroll et al 1949). Carroll et al (1949) reported that the riboflavin concentration in the ingesta DM increased markedly during passage through the gastrointestinal tract with concentrations in the cecum and anterior small colon, respectively, 18- and 30-fold higher when compared to the DM of the feed. Riboflavin provision via microbial synthesis seems to be sufficient to compensate for low riboflavin intakes, although no data are available on absorption from the large intestine. This is supported by the finding that riboflavin supplementation to conventional oats or corn based diets did not change the activity of riboflavin-containing enzymes in exercising horses (McMeniman et al 1995).

Excess

Evidence for riboflavin toxicity exists only in rats where the oral LD_{50} was extremely high (10 g/kg BW; Schumacher et al 1965). Riboflavin toxicity is not likely to occur with typical horse feeding practices.

Biotin

Nearly all cell types take up biotin and convert it to carboxy biotin, which is a component of a wide group of diverse enzymes (pyruvate carboxylase, acetyl-CoA carboxylase, B-methylcrotonyl-CoA carboxylase, propionyl-CoA carboxylase and carbamylphosphate synthetase I and II). Due to the activity of these enzymes, biotin is involved in fatty acid synthesis, gluconeogenesis, amino acid metabolism and other metabolic pathways. The vitamin may also play an important role in gene expression and biotinylation of histones, which are required for cell proliferation and, thus, growth.

Sources and bioavailability

Biotin is derived from synthesis by gut microbes and dietary sources. With respect to microbial synthesis, Carroll et al (1949) showed an enrichment of the digesta DM biotin content during its passage through the intestinal tract with highest concentration in the anterior large colon (3.8 mg/kg DM vs. 0.01 and 0.1 mg/kg DM in the feed and small intestine, respectively). There is very little information on the biotin content of typical feedstuffs for horses. High concentrations have been reported in fresh alfalfa (~0.5 mg/kg DM), moderate concentrations in alfalfa hay (~ 0.2 mg/kg DM), oats (~0.1–0.4 mg/kg DM), barley (~0.1–0.2 mg/kg DM) and soybean meal (~0.2–0.5 mg/kg DM) and particularly low levels in maize (~0.1 mg/kg DM) (NRC 1982, McDowell 1989).

In natural feedstuffs, biotin occurs in a form bound to protein such as biocytin (δ-*N*-biotinyl-L-lysine). Bioavailability varies between feedstuffs (Schenk & Kolb 1982) and depends on the digestibility of the specific binding protein in the species in question (Baker 1995). A specific case is avidin, the alkaline biotin binding protein in raw egg white, which cannot be broken down by proteolytic digestive enzymes unless denatured by boiling (Schenk & Kolb 1982). Biotin availability has not been studied in horses, but in poultry and swine on a corn and soybean diet it is quite high (75–100% and 100%, respectively; Baker 1995).

Requirements

There is no evidence from the literature for a dietary biotin requirement above the quantity supplied by the gut microbes. Nevertheless, biotin supplementation may be beneficial in some horses with poor hoof quality. One reason for the helpful effect may be that biotin has a positive effect on the synthesis of intercellular glue (Geyer 2005). In vitro studies indicated that biotin supplementation increases cytokeratins, which are normally increased upon terminal differentiation of epidermal cells in vivo suggesting a direct stimulation of the differentiation of epidermal cells by biotin (Fritsche et al 1991). In a double-blind, placebo-controlled clinical trial with 42 Lipizzaner horses, the effect of 20 mg biotin per day on hoof growth and hoof horn quality was studied over a period of 19 months. The supplemented horses showed a small but significant improvement in hoof horn quality by nine months, which was also present at the end of the study and this was maintained over 2.5 further years of observation (with continued supplementation). In this study there was no effect of supplementation on horn wall growth (~0.25 mm/day with or without supplementation). The core diets being fed were not ideally balanced with respect to calcium and phosphorus and the zinc intake was marginal. In another study with 24 riding horses, beneficial effects were described when 15 mg of biotin were used rather than 7.5 mg, both being fed for 10 months (Josseck et al 1995, Zenker et al 1995). Measures of hoof wall quality did not differ between horses that received 3 mg biotin/100 kg BW/day or no supplement for 1 year (the horses entered the study with poor hoof horn quality; Philipp & Kienzle, 2008). In this study, 1 mg of zinc/kg BW/day (as zinc sulfate) was reported to have no effect on hoof wall quality in another group of horses. In summary, biotin supplementation may positively affect subjective measures of hoof quality in some horses but it does not seem to impact hoof growth rate. However, in ponies fed very high levels of biotin (0.12 mg/kg BW; equivalent to 60 mg for a 500-kg horse) hoof growth rate was 15% higher (0.19 mm/day) than in nonsupplemented ponies (0.16 mm/day) (Reilly et al 1998).

Studies have shown that the equine hoof wall takes approximately 9–12 months to grow from the coronary band to the weight-bearing surface. It is not surprising that research has also shown that in feeding trials, where supplemental biotin was added over a lengthy period of time (up to several years), it often took a long time before significant improvements were detected. One trial, which showed an improvement in hoof horn condition in those animals which received 5 mg of biotin /100–150 kg BW for 8–15 months, concluded that in cases of poor hoof quality, a reduction in the dose or a complete stopping of the biotin would tend to result in the deterioration of the hoof (Geyer & Schulze 1994). On this basis, it is often recommended that any supplemental biotin is fed for at least 6 to 9 months and if this results in an improvement in the hoof quality it may be advisable to provide such levels of supplemental biotin on a continual basis.

The amount of biotin recommended for horses with poor quality hoof horn is 3–4 mg/100 kg BW/day (i.e., 15–20 mg/day for a 500-kg horse), although higher intakes up to 30 mg have been suggested (NRC 2007). The daily amount can be given all at once or divided throughout the day. The question is, however, why biotin helps to improve poor hoof quality in some horses but does not in others. Kempson (1987) described two different types of defect using the hoof clippings from horses with brittle feet. The first showed a loss of structure in horn from the outermost layer of the hoof wall, which could apparently be helped by biotin supplementation. The second defect, which the author reported as being found in around 94% of cases, showed a marked loss of tubular structure in the inner layers of the hoof wall and was thought to be due to poor attachment of the horn cells. This type did not respond to biotin supplementation alone, but according to the author 95% of horses with such a defect responded to the addition of calcium (along with either biotin or protein). It is important to note that in the one case reported in detail in this paper, the additional calcium supplementation may just have corrected a calcium–phosphorus imbalance. This therefore does not suggest that additional calcium above that normally recommended will always be of value or necessary (and in some cases may not be advisable). Some types of hoof horn defects may not respond to biotin alone and may require other nutrients to be present in adequate levels. However, the supply of biotin required to improve hoof horn quality in particular horses lies clearly above normal dietary recommendations and cannot be described as a standard requirement.

Effects of deficiency and excess

Deficiency

Deficiency of biotin in other species results in poor quality of skin, coat and hoof or claw horn. Biotin deficiency may slow mitosis in the stratum basale meaning that the tips of the dermal papillae in the coronary region become more susceptible to physical damage, resulting in hemorrhage and bleeding into the horn (Kempson 2005). In pigs, experimentally induced biotin deficiency caused poor claw horn (Geyer 2005). As above, poor biotin status in horses may be one but not the only reason for reduced hoof quality.

Excess

The danger of an excess is not very high because surplus biotin is excreted in the urine. In rats, subcutaneous injection of extremely high doses (50 to 100 mg biotin/kg BW) caused fetal resorption (cited from NRC 2007). Poultry and pigs tolerate at least 10-fold the dietary biotin requirement without adverse signs (NRC 2007). In horses, detrimental effects of high biotin doses have not been described. Currently no recommended upper daily intake limit has been set for biotin, but as a guide horses should receive no more than 12 mg/100 kg BW/d.

Other B vitamins

There are few data available on requirements for the other B vitamins. Saastamoinen & Harris (2008) described the suggested requirement for folic acid: 0.55 mg/kg DM feed or 0.012 mg/kg BW for adult horses at rest and in light to moderate work, and 1.7 mg/kg DM or 0.043 mg/kg BW for those in intensive work. INRA (1990) recommends about 0.04 mg/kg BW. However more work is required to support these provisional recommendations. It should be noted that folic acid supplementation is not recommended (Toribio et al 1998) or should be carried out with caution in horses treated with dihydrofolate reductase inhibitors (for equine protozoal myelitis).

No deficiency of niacin has been reported in horses, two trials in exercising Thoroughbred horses showed that neither acute nor chronic (3 g/day) niacin supplementation appeared to affect exercise metabolism or niacin status (Parker et al 1997) and no dietary requirements have been established by the NRC. INRA (1990) recommended 0.40 mg/kg BW in intense work. There are no recommendations concerning the intake and need for pantothenic acid (B_5), pyridoxine (B_6), nor choline in the NRC 2007, but INRA (1990) suggested 0.16, 0.04, and 2.18 mg/kg BW/day for B_5, B_6 and choline, respectively. Again more work is needed before firm recommendations can be given.

Vitamin C

Vitamin C includes L-ascorbic acid and dehydro-L-ascorbic acid with equivalent biological activities. It represents a prominent part of the water-soluble antioxidant system. The most important physiologic effect is preventing radical attacks and regenerating other substances within the antioxidant system such as vitamin E (Johnston 2001). Vitamin C (ascorbic acid) is also required for the hydroxylation of proline and lysine to form hydroxyproline and hydroxylysine.

Sources and bioavailability

Like most other mammals, equines are able to synthesize vitamin C in the liver from glucose (Pearson et al 1943, Stillions et al 1971) with rates identified in horses to be approximately 72 g/day (Alawad et al 1994). Despite that, the concentration of ascorbic acid in the muscle and heart of horses appears to be low (Alawad et al 1994). Plasma concentrations in horses have been measured in a range between ~0.8–6.5 mg/l (Pearson et al 1943, Jaeschke & Keller 1978, Snow et al 1987, Snow & Frigg 1989, 1990, Zeyner & Lengwenat 1993, Hargreaves et al 2002, Marlin et al 2002, Williams et al 2004). Serum levels have been reported to be lower in the winter than in the summer (Rasbech & Koefoed-Johnsen, 1987, Snow et al 1987).

Plasma concentrations may be elevated after intake of supplemental vitamin C. Meyer et al (1996) did not find differences in the preileal absorption of ascorbic acid (10 mg/kg BW) whether provided in crystalline form or as polyphosphate. Other studies, however, indicate that the bioavailability of vitamin C depends on the source fed, with low absorption of crystalline and amorphous ascorbic acid but higher bioavailability with other sources (Errington et al 1942, Löscher et al 1984, Snow et al 1987, Snow & Frigg 1989, 1990, Zeyner & Lengwenat 1993, Deaton et al 2003; Table 9-5). Among the presently available products (e.g., crystalline and amorphous ascorbic acid, coated ascorbic acid, ascorbyl palmitate, ascorbyl phosphates such as calcium-ascorbyl-2-monophosphate, ascorbylsulfates like disodium-L-ascorbat-2-sulfat), ascorbyl palmitate seems to be most bioavailable in horses.

Stability

Robust data on the content and stability of vitamin C in typical feedstuffs for horses are not available. Supplemental vitamin C as part of premixes, however, is highly susceptible to destruction by several environmental factors, particularly if a protected form is not used (Coelho 1996). A number of vitamin C products have claims of improved stability during feed manufacture, including those composed of a mixture of the phosphate esters of L-ascorbic acid. Bioavailability of this latter form of vitamin C in horses appears to be slightly greater than ascorbic acid, but slightly reduced in comparison with ascorbyl palmitate (Deaton et al 2003).

Requirements

An important question is whether the body's own synthesis of vitamin C will be sufficient under stressful conditions or in horses with particular health problems when the hepatic synthesis of the vitamin may be decreased or the need for vitamin C is elevated. It has been reported that plasma concentrations of ascorbic acid are reduced in horses with poor performance, in the postoperative and post-traumatic state, with wound infections, epistaxis, strangles, influenza, fever, pneumonia, and recurrent airway obstruction (Jaeschke & Keller 1978, Kolb et al 1983, Jaeschke 1984, Rasbech & Koefoed-Johnsen 1987, Snow et al 1987, Deaton et al 2002, 2004a, b, 2005). Because it is known that supplemental vitamin C elevates the concentration of ascorbic acid in blood plasma (Errington et al 1942, Löscher et al 1984, Snow et al 1987, Snow & Frigg 1989, 1990, Zeyner & Lengwenat 1993, Deaton et al 2002) and bronchoalveolar lavage pulmonary epithelial lining fluid (Deaton et al 2002), it is conceivable that oral vitamin C can be helpful under such conditions. Kolb et al (1983) recommended 30 mg/kg BW of supplemental vitamin C (ascorbyl-2-triphosphate) under such conditions.

The effect of training and acute exercise on plasma ascorbic acid concentrations may be modified by several factors such as duration and intensity of the individual exercise bout, training status of the horse, and climatic conditions (Petersson et al 1991, McMeniman & Hintz 1992, White et al 2001, Hargreaves et al 2002, Marlin et al 2002, de Moffarts et al 2004). Despite this variability, high doses of supplemental vitamin C are widely used in exercised horses. The timing of vitamin C supplementation, however, may need to be chosen carefully because oral vitamin C has been reported to reduce cortisol secretion (Kolb et al 1983). In Standardbred trotters, plasma cortisol was significantly decreased following ingestion of different vitamin C

Table 9-5 Plasma Ascorbic Acid (AA, in mg/l) and Cortisol (CO, in ng/ml) Levels Following Oral Administration of 20 g Ascorbic Acid from Different Sources or a Placebo to Standardbred Trotters (n = 5; Zeyner & Lengwenat 1993)

	Time after feeding (hrs)									
	0		4		6		8		12	
	AA	*CO*	*AA*	*CO*	*AA*	*CO*	*AA*	*CO*	*AA*	*CO*
Acr	4.28	54.8	5.36	43.2	5.28	42.0	4.96	40.7	4.80	31.5
Apa	3.88	58.3	7.52	49.5	8.92	47.9	7.62	43.8	7.06	43.6
Aph	3.74	61.0	6.68	37.8	6.18	39.5	6.16	37.7	5.92	28.5
Alc	3.66	46.8	5.62	46.8	5.64	37.1	5.32	35.9	5.16	26.6
PL	3.90	55.9	4.34	54.4	4.08	40.8	3.98	39.7	4.54	28.0

Acr, crystalline ascorbic acid; Alc, lipid coated AA; Apa, ascorbyl palmitate; Aph, ascorbyl-2-monophosphate; PL, placebo.
Peak AA levels are underlined; significant (p<0.05) differences ([a, b, c, d]) for postprandial AA areas under the curves: Acr[c], Apa[a], Aph[b], Alc[c], PL[d].

products, but this reaction was similar to the placebo effect (Zeyner & Lengwenat 1993). The measured cortisol decrease may in fact be of circadian or general postprandial nature rather than specifically being induced by supplemental vitamin C.

Currently, there is no scientifically robust argument that supports recommending a regular oral supply of vitamin C to healthy horses. For animals that are housed for prolonged periods of time in environments which provide a challenge to respiratory system defenses additional vitamin C supplementation may be of value, but administration should not be abruptly stopped.

Effects of deficiency and excess

Deficiency

Classic signs of vitamin C deficiency have not been described in horses.

Excess

Daily doses of 20 g ascorbic acid/kg BW have been given for 8 months without any obvious negative effect (Snow et al 1987). Although there have been no reports of toxicity in horses, it should be taken into consideration that excessive ascorbic acid may act as metabolic acidifier (Wood et al 1990). It may also act as a pro-oxidant and cause gastrointestinal disturbance. In other species it is known that high oral doses may cause allergic reactions and decrease the body's own synthesis of the vitamin.

References

Alawad, A., Kolb, E., Leo, M., et al., 1994. Gehalt an Ascorbinsäure in 13 Geweben und Aktivität der L-Gulonolacton-Oxidase in der Leber von Pferden. Prakt Tierarzt 75, 40–47.

Aleman, M., Finno, C.J., Higgins, R.J., et al., 2011. Evaluation of epidemiological, clinical and pathological features of neuroaxonal dystrophy in Quarter Horses. J Am Vet Med Assoc 239, 823–833.

American Academy of Pediatrics, Committee of Nutrition, 1971. Vitamin K supplementation for infants receiving milk substitute infant formulas and for those with fat malabsorption. Pediatrics 48, 483–487.

AWT, 2001. Vitamine in der Tierernährung. Agrimedia, Bergen/Dumme.

Ballet, N., Robert, J.C., Williams, P.E.V., 2000. Vitamins in forages. In: Givens, D.I., Owen, E., Axford, R.F.E., et al (Eds.), Forage evaluation in ruminant nutrition. CABI publishing, pp. 399–432.

Baalsrud, K.J., Overnes, G., 1986. Influence of vitamin E and selenium supplement on antibody production in horses. Equine Vet J 18, 472–474.

Baker, D.H., 1995. Vitamin bioavailability. In: Ammermann, C.B., Baker, D.H., Lewis, A.J. (Eds.), Bioavailability of nutrients for animals: amino acids, minerals, vitamins. Academic Press, New York, p. 399.

Bante, U., Erben, R.G., Stangassinger, M., 1996. Tagungsband der 12. Tagung der DVG-Fachgruppe Physiologie und Biochemie: 'Warum wirkt die chronische Applikation von Vitamin-D-Metaboliten in vivo knochenanabol?' Hannover. 1996. 10–12 March, p. P49.

Bates, C.J., 2001. Thiamin. In: Bowman, B.E., Russel, R.M. (Eds.), Present knowledge in nutrition. Washington D.C.: ISLI Press, p. 184.

Bendich, A., 1989. Symposium conclusions: Biological actions of carotenoids. J Nutr 119, 135–139.

Biffin, J.R., Regtop, H.L., Talbot, A.M., 2008. Pasture content and availability of vitamin K in yearlings. Proc Aust Equine Sci Symp 2, 54.

Bjondahl, K., Virkki, M., 1977. Comparative studies on vitamin A utilization using three different base solutions (xylitol, polyol and water) in the ADE-vitamin solution. Nutr Rep Int 15, 519–527.

Blythe, L.L., Craig, A.M., 1997. Degenerative myeloencephalopathy. In: Robinson, N.E. (Ed.), Current therapy in equine medicine. Philadelphia: W.B. Saunders.

Blythe, L.L., Craig, A.M., Lassen, E.D., et al., 1991. Serially determined plasma alpha-tocopherol concentrations and results of the oral vitamin E absorption test in clinically normal horses and horses with degenerative myeloenephalopathy. Am J Vet Res 52, 908–911.

Bondy, A., Sklan, D., 1984. Vitamin A and carotene in animal nutrition. Progress in food and nutrition Sci 8, 165–191.

Bonjour, J.-P., Gueguen, L., Palacios, C., et al., 2009. Minerals and vitamins in bone health: The potential value of dietary enhancement. Br J Nutr 101, 1581–1596.

Both, S.L., Golly, I., Sacheck, J.M., et al., 2004. Effect of vitamin E supplementation on vitamin K status in adults with normal coagulation status. Am J Clin Nutr 80, 143–148.

Breidenbach, A., Schlumbohm, C., Harmeyer, J., 1998. Peculiarities of vitamin D and of the calcium and phosphorus homeostatic system in horses. Vet Res 29 (7), 173–186.

Brubacher, G., Weiser, H., 1967. Biologische Wirksamkeit von Tocopherol und von Antioxidantien. Wiss. Veröff. Deutsche Ges. Ernährung 16, 50–66.

Brody, S., 1945. Bioenergetics and growth. Reinhold, New York: NY.

Bugel, S., 2003. Vitamin K and bone health. Proc Nutr Soc 62, 839–843.

Byars, T.D., Greene, C.E., Kemp, D.T., 1986. Antidotal effect of vitamin-K-1 against warfarin-induced anticoagulation in horses. Am J Vet Res 47, 2309–2312.

Carroll, F.D., Goss, H., Howell, C.E., 1949. The synthesis of B vitamins in the horse. J Anim Sci 8, 290–299.

Chattergee, I.B., 1973. Evolution and the biosynthesis of ascorbic acid. Science 182, 1271–1273.

Coelho, M., 1996. Stability of vitamins affected by feed processing. Feedstuffs 68, 9–14.

Coenen, M., Kirchhof, S., Kienzle, E., et al., 2010. An update on basic data for the factorial calculation of energy and nutrient requirements in lactating mares., Rev Anim Nutr 38 (1), 91–121.

Combs, G.F., Noguchi, T., Scott, M.L., 1975. Mechanism of action of selenium and vitamin E in protection of biological membranes. Fed Proc 34, 2090–2995.

Craig, A.M., Blythe, L.L., Lassen, E.D., et al., 1989. Variations of serum vitamin E, cholesterol, and total serum lipid concentrations in horses during a 72-hour period. Am J Vet Res 50, 1527–1531.

Cymbaluk, N.F., Fretz, P.B., Loew, F.M., 1978. Amprolium-induced thiamine deficiency in horses: clinical features. Am J Vet Res 39, 255–261.

Deaton, C.M., Marlin, D.J., Roberts, C.A., et al., 2002. Antioxidant supplementation and pulmonary function at rest and exercise. Equine Vet J, Suppl. 34, 58–65.

Deaton, C.M., Marlin, D.J., Roberts, C.A., et al., 2003. Pulmonary bioavailability of ascorbic acid in an ascorbate-synthesising species, the horse. Free Radical Res 37, 461–467.

Deaton, C.M., Marlin, D.J., Smith, N., et al., 2004a. Antioxidant supplementation in horses affected by recurrent airway obstruction. J Nutr 134, 2065S-2067S.

Deaton, C.M., Marlin, D.J., Smith, N., et al., 2004b. Pulmonary epithelial lining fluid and plasma ascorbic acid concentrations in horses affected by recurrent airway obstruction. A J Vet Res 65, 80–87.

Deaton, C.M., Marlin, D.J., Smith, N., et al., 2005. Effect of acute airway inflammation on the pulmonary antioxidant status. Exp Lung Res 31, 653–670.

de Moffarts, B., Kirschvink, N., Art, T., et al., 2004. Impact of training and exercise intensity on blood antioxidant markers in healthy Standardbred horses. Equine Comp Exerc Physiol 1, 211–220.

Denisova, N.A., Booth, S.L., 2005. Vitamin K and sphingolipid metabolism: evidence to date. Nutr Rev 63, 111–121.

Dill, S.G., Kallfelz, F.A., de Lahunta, A., et al., 1989. Serum vitamin E and blood glutathione peroxidase values of horses with degenerative myeloencephalopathy. Am J Vet Res 50, 166–168.

Divers, T.J., 2005. Equine motor neuron disease. J Equine Vet Sci 25, 238–240.

Dju, M.Y., Filer, L.J., Mason, K.E., 1958. Effect of storage on tissue tocopherols. A J Clin Nutr 6, 61–64.

Domke, A., Großklaus, R., Niemann, B., et al., 2004, Verwendung von Vitaminen in Lebensmitteln – Toxikologische und ernährungsphysiologische Aspekte. In: BfR-Wissenschaft, 03/2004 (ed: Bundesinstitut für Risikobewertung). Pressestelle des BfR, Hausdruckerei des BfR, Berlin.

Donoghue, S., Kronfeld, D.S., Berkowitz, S.J., et al., 1981. Vitamin A nutrition of the equine: growth, serum biochemistry and hematology. J Nutr 111, 365–374.

Dowd, P., Ham, S.W., Naganathan, S., et al., 1995. The mechanism of action of vitamin K. Annu Rev Nutr 15, 419–440.

Eitzer, P., Rapp, H.J., 1985. Zur oralen Anwendung von synthetischem beta-Carotin bei Zuchtstuten. Prakt Tierarzt 66, 123–128.

Elshorafa, W.M., Feaster, J.P., Ott, E.A., et al., 1979. Effect of vitamin-D and sunlight on growth and bone-development of young ponies. J Anim Sci 48, 882–886.

Enbergs, H., Klemt, P.W., 1987. Der Einfluss von beta-Karotin auf Zyklus und Trächtigkeit der Stute sowie auf die Gesundheit der Fohlen. Prakt Tierarzt 68, 52–58.

Errington, B.J., Hodkiss, W.S., Jaynw, E.P., 1942. Ascorbic acid in certain body fluids of horses. Am J Vet Res 3, 242–247.

Evers, A.-M., 1989. Effects of different fertilization practices on the carotene content of carrot. J Agric Sci Finl 61, 7–14.

Ferland, G., 2001. Vitamin K. In: Bowman, B.A., Russel, R.A. (Eds.), Present knowledge in nutrition. Washington D.C.: ILSI Press.

Fonnesbeck, P.V., Symons, L.D., 1967. Utilization of the carotene of hay by horses. J Anim Sci 26, 1030–1038.

Food and Nutrition Board, 2001. Vitamin K. Dietary reference intakes for vitamin A, vitamin K, arsenic, boron, chromium, copper, iodine, iron, manganese, molybdenum, nickel, silicon, vanadium, and zinc. National Academy Press, Washington, D.C, pp. 162–196.

Frape, D., 2000. Equine nutrition and feeding, second ed. Blackwell Science, Oxford, p. 564.

Fritsche, A., Mathis, G.A., Althaus, F.R., 1991. Pharmacologic effects of biotin on epidermal cells [Pharmakologische Wirkungen von Biotin auf Epidermiszellen.] Schweizer Archiv für Tierheilkunde 133 (6), 277–283.

Gandini, G., Fatzer, R., Mariscoli, M., et al., 2004. Equine degenerative myeloencephalopathy in five Quarter horses: clinical and neuropathological findings. Equine Vet J 36, 83–85.

Gansen, S., Lindner, A., Wagener, A., 1995. Influence of a supplementation with natural and synthetic vitamin E on serum α-tocopherol content and V_4 of Thoroughbred horses. In: Proc. 14th Equine Nutr. Physiol. Symp., Ontario, CA. Equine Nutrition and Physiology Society, Savoy, IL, p. 68.

Gassmann, B., Ulbricht, G., 1979. Bases and consequences of the newly recommended daily intakes of vitamins for the population of the German Democratic Republic. Molec Nutr Food Res 23, 83–89.

Geyer, H., 2005. Nutritional management to keep the hoof healthy. In: Lindner, A. (Ed.), Applied equine nutrition, Proceedings of ENUCO. Wageningen: Academic Publishers, pp. 43–60.

Geyer, H., Schulze, J., 1994. The long term influence of biotin supplementation on hoof horn quality in horses. Schweizer Archiv Fur Thierheilkunde 136 (4) 137–149.

GfE, 1994. Energie- und Nährstoffbedarf landwirtschaftlicher Nutztiere. Nr. 2: Empfehlungen zur Energie und Nährstoffversorgung der Pferde (Hrsg.: Ausschuß für Bedarfsnormen der Gesellschaft für Ernährungsphysiologie der Haustiere). DLG-Verlag, Frankfurt (Main).

Grabner, A., Kraft, W., Essich, G., Hänichen, T., 1985. Enzootische Kalzinose beim Pferd. Tierärztl Praxis Suppl. 1, 84–93.

Greiwe-Crandell, K.M., Kronfeld, D.S., Gay, L.A., et al., 1995. Seasonal vitamin A depletion in grazing horses is assessed better by the relative dose response test than by serum retinol concentration. J Nutr 125, 2711–2716.

Greiwe-Crandell, K.M., Kronfeld, D.S., et al., 1997. Vitamin A repletion in thoroughbred mares with retinyl palmitate or beta-carotene. J Anim Sci 75, 2684–2690.

Groenen-Van Dooren, M.M.C.L., Ronden, J., Soute, B.A.M., et al., 1995. Bioavailability of phylloquinone and menaquinones after oral and colorectal administration in vitamin K-deficient rats. Biochem Pharmacol 50, 797–801.

Grollmann, A.P., Lehninger, A., 1957. Enzymatic synthesis of L-ascorbic acid in different animal species. Archives Biochem Biophysics 69, 458–467.

Großer, K., Schubert, R., Kluge, H., et al., 1995. Einfluß einer unterschiedlichen Vitamin-A- und -E-Versorgung auf den Gehalt dieser Vitamine in der Stutenmilch. In: Schubert, R., Flachowsky, G. (Eds.), Vitamine und Zusatzstoffe in der Ernährung von Mensch und Tier. Verlag Gbr. Franke KG, Gera, pp. 73–76.

Guilbert, H.R., Howell, C.E., Hart, G.H., 1940. Minimum vitamin A and carotene requirements of mammalian species. J Nutr 19, 91–103.

Hakkarainen, J., Pehrson, B., 1987. Vitamin E and polyunsaturated fatty acids in Swedish feedstuffs for cattle. Acta Agric Scand 37, 341–346.

Hargreaves, B.J., Kronfeld, D.S., Waldron, J.N., et al., 2002. Antioxidant status of horses during two 80-km endurance races. J Nutr 132, 1781S-1783S.

Harmeyer, J., 1999. Die Bedeutung von Vitamin D für die Regulation des Calcium- und Phosphathaushalts beim Pferd. In: Schubert, R., Flachowsky, G., Bitsch, R., et al (Eds.), Vitamine und Zusatzstoffe in der Ernährung von Mensch und Tier. Verlag Gbr. Franke KG, Gera, pp. 20–35.

Harmeyer, J., Schlumbohm, C., 2004. Effects of pharmacological doses of vitamin D3 on mineral balance and profiles of plasma vitamin D3 metabolites in horses. J Steroid Biochem Molec Biol 89–90, 595–600.

Harmeyer, J., Twehues, R.C., Schlumbohm, C., et al., 1992. The role of vitamin D on calcium metabolism in horses. In: 1. Europäische Konferenz über die Ernährung des Pferdes. Pferdeheilkunde, Sonderausgabe, pp. 81–85.

Harmeyer, J., Twehues, R.C., Schlumbohm, C., et al., 1994. Peculiarities of calcium and phosphate regulation in horses. In: Norman, A.W., Bouillon, R., Thomasset, M. (Eds.), Vitamin D, a Pluripotent Steroid Hormone: structural studies, molecular endocrinology and clinical applications, Walter de Gruyter, Berlin and New York, pp. 787–788.

Harrington, D.D., 1982. Acute vitamin-D_2 (ergocalsiferol) toxicosis in horses - case-report and experimental studies. J Am Vet Med Assoc 180, 867–873.

Harrington, D.D., Page, E.H., 1983. Acute vitamin D3 toxicosis in horses: Case reports and experimental studies of comparative toxicity of vitamins D2 and D3. J Am Vet Med Assoc 182, 1358–1369.

Harris, P., Dyson, S., 1996. Muscle disorders in the horse. Vet Pract 28, 6–8.

Harris, P.A., 2005a. Feeding and management advice for tying up/azoturia/ Monday Morning disease/equine rhabdomyolysis syndrome. In: Harris, P.A., Mair, T.S., Slater, J.D., Green, R.E. (Eds.), Equine Nutrition for All. Proc. 1st BEVA & WALTHAM Nutr. Symp. Harrogate, pp. 113–118.

Harris, P.A., 2005b. Feeding and management advice for tying up/azoturia/ Monday Morning disease/Equine Rhabdomyolysis Syndrome. In: Suomen Eläinlääkäriliiton luentokokoelma. Fennovet Ltd., Helsinki, pp. 184–192.

Harris, P.A., Mayhew, I.J., 1998. Musculoskeletal disease. In: Bayly, W., Reed, S. (Eds.), Equine Internal Medicine. Publisher: WB Saunders, pp. 371–427.

Hintz, H.F., Cymbaluk, N.F., 1994. Nutrition of the horse. Ann Rev Nutr 14, 243–267.

Hintz, H.F., Schryver, H.F., Lowe, J.E., et al., 1973. Effect of vitamin-D on Ca and P metabolism in ponies. J Anim Sci 37, 282.

Hoffman, R.M., Morgan, K.L., Lynch, M.P., et al., 1999. Dietary vitamin E supplemented in the periparturient period influences immunoglobulins in equine colostrum and passive transfer in foals. Proc. 16th Equine Nutr. Physiol. Symp. Raleigh, NC. Equine Nutrition and Physiology Society, Savoy, IL, p. 96.

Hünsche, K., Wolf, P., Lange, K., et al., 2010. Investigations on adverse effects of feeding tried marsh horsetail (Equisetum palustre) to ruminants and horses. Proc Soc Nutr Physiol 19, 132.

Inoue, Y., Ohba, Y., Kobayashi, Y., et al., 2009. Determination of plasma concentrations of vitamin K homologues in Thoroughbred horses. J Equine Vet Sci 29, 395–396.

INRA, 1990. L'Alimentaion des Chevaux. Martin-Rosset, W. (Ed.), INRA Publications, Paris.

Jaeschke, G., 1984. Influence of ascorbic acid on physical development and performance of racehorses. In: Wegger, I., Tagwerker, F.J., Moustgaard, J. (Eds.), Proc. Ascorbic Acid in Domestic Animals. Danish Agricultural Society, Copenhagen, pp. 139.

Jaeschke, G., Keller, H., 1978. Beitrag zum Ascorbinsäurestatus des Pferdes. 2. Mitteilung: Klinische Aspekte und Mangelsituationen. Berliner Münchener Tierärztl. Wochenschrift, 91, 375–379.

Jarrett, S.H., Schurg, W.A., 1987. Use of modified relative dose response test for determination vitamin A status in horses. Nutr Rep Int 35, 733–742.

Jiang, Q., Christensen, S., Shigenaga, M.K., et al., 2001. γ-Tocopherol, the major form of vitamin E in the US diet, deserves more attention. Am J Clin Nutr 74, 714–722.

Johnston, C., 2001. Vitamin C. In: Bowman, B.A., Russel, R.M. (Eds.), Present Knowledge in Nutrition. ILSI Press, Washington D.C.

Jones, T.C., Roby, T.O., Maurer, F.D., 1946. The relation of riboflavin to equine periodic ophthalmia. Am J Vet Res 7, 403–416.

Jordan, R.M., 1979. Effect of thiamin and vitamin A and D supplementation on growth of weanling ponies. In: Proc. 6th Equine Nutr. Physiol. Symp.: College Station, TX. Equine Science Society, Champaign, IL, p. 67.

Josseck, H., Zenker, W., Geyer, H., 1995. Hoof horn abnormalities in Lipizzaner horses and the effect of dietary biotin on macroscopic aspects of hoof horn quality. Equine Vet J 27, 175–182.

Kalkwarf, H.J., Khoury, J.C., Bean, J., et al., 2004. Vitamin K, bone turnover, and bone mass in girls. Am J Clin Nutr 80, 1075–1080.

Kaune, R., Harmeyer, J., 1987. Die quantitative Bestimmung von Vitamin D3 und seiner metaboliten im Plasma. Biol Chem Hoppe-Seyler 367 (11), 1135–1140.

Kempson, S.A., 1987. Scanning electron microscope observations of hoof horn from horses with brittle feet. Vet Rec 120, 568–570.

Kempson, S.A., 2005. Nutritional management of horses with hoof diseases. In: Applied equine nutrition. In: Lindner, A. (Ed.), Proceedings of ENUCO Wageningen Academic publishers. pp. P105–112.

Kienzle, E., Zeyner, A., 2010. The development of a metabolisable energy system for horses. J Anim Physiol Anim Nutr 94, e231–e240.

Kienzle, E., Coenen, M., Zeyner, A., 2010. Maintenance metabolisable energy requirements in horses. Rev Anim Nutr 38 (1), 33–54.

Kienzle, E., Kaden, C., Hoppe, P.P., et al., 2002. Serum response of ponies to β-carotene fed by grass meal or synthetic beadlet preparation with and without added dietary fat. J Nutr 132, 1774S–1775S.

Kivimäe, A., Carpena, C., 1973. 'The level of vitamin E content in some conventional feeding stuffs and the effects of genetic variety; harvesting; processing and storage.' Acta Culturae Scandinavica, Suppl. 19, 161–167.

Köhler, H., 1981. Zur Kalzinose in Österreich. IX. Kalzinose beim Pferd?' Zentralblatt für Veterinärmedizin Reihe A 28 (3), 187–200.

Kolb, E., 1966. Die ernährungsphysiologische Bedeutung der Vitamine und die wichtigsten Vitamin-Mangelerkrankungen bei Mensch und Tier. In: Hock, A. (Ed.), Vergleichende Ernährungslehre des Menschen und seiner Haustiere. VEB Gustav Fischer Verlag, Jena, pp. 687–804.

Kolb, E., 1995. Die Bedeutung des Vitamins A für das Immunsystem - Übersichtsreferat (The significance of vitamin A fort the immune system - a review). Berl Münch Tierärztl Wschr 108, 385–390.

Kolb, E., Grün, E., 1996. Die Bedeutung der D-Vitamine für das Immunsystem. Der praktische Tierarzt 1/1996, 11–15.

Kolb, E., Schneider, J., Prietz, G., et al., 1983. Der Gehalt an Askorbinsäure im Blutplasma von Pferden. Prakt Tierarzt 64, 720–725.

Kronfeld, D.S., Meacham, T.N., Donoghue, S., 1990. Dietary aspects of development orthopedic disease in young horses. In: Hintz, H.F. (Eds.), Vet. Clinics North Am. W.B. Saunders, Philadelphia.

Kuhl, J., Winterhoff, N., Wulf, M., et al., 2011. Changes in faecal bacteria and metabolic parameters in foals during the first six weeks of life. Veterinary Microbiology (doi: 10.1016/j.vetmic.2011.03.017).

Linerode, P.A., 1967. Studies on the synthesis and absorption of B-complex vitamins in the horse. Equine Pract 13, 283–314.

Liu, S.K., Dolensek, E.P., Adams, C.R., et al., 1983. Myelopathy and vitamin E deficiency in six Mongolian wild horses. J Am Vet Med Assoc 183, 1266–1268.

Löscher, W., Jaeschke, G., Keller, H., 1984. Pharmacokinetics of ascorbic acids in horses. Equine Vet J 16, 59–65.

Lofstedt, J., 1997. White muscle disease of foals. Vet Clin North Am, Equine Pract 13, 169–185.

Lucky, T., 1951. A single diet for all living organisms. Science 120, 396–398.

Lynch, G.L., 1996a. Vitamin E structure and bioavailability. In: Coelho, M.B. (Ed.), Vitamin E in animal nutrition and managelment. BASF, Mount Olive, NJ, p. 1.

Lynch, G.L., 1996b. Vitamin E structure and bioavailability. In: Coelho, M.B. (Ed.), Natural occurrence and content of vitamin E in feedstuffs. BASF, Mount Olive, NJ, p. 51.

Mäenpää, P.H., Lappeteläinen, R., Virkkunen, J., 1987. Serum retinol, 25-hydroxyvitamin D and tocopherol of racing trotters in Finland. Equine Vet J 19, 237–240.

Mäenpäa, P.H., Koskinen, T., Koskinen, E., 1988a. 'Serum profiles of vitamins A, E and D in mares and foals during different seasons'. J Anim Sci 66, 418–1423.

Mäenpäa, P.H., Pirhonen, A., Koskinen, E., 1988b. Vitamin A, E and D nutrition in mares and foals during the winter season: effect of feeding two different vitamin-mineral concentrates. J Anim Sci 66, 1424–1429.

Marlin, D.J., Fenn, K., Smith, N., et al., 2002. Changes in circulatory antioxidant status in horses during prolonged exercise. J Nutr 132, 1622S–1627S.

Maxie, G., van Dreumel, T., McMaster, D., 1992. Menadione (vitamin K3) toxicity in six horses. Can Vet J 33, 756–757.

Mayhew, I.G., Brown, C.M., Stowe, H.D., 1987. Equine degenerative myeloencephalopathy: a vitamin E deficiency that may be familial. J Vet Int Med 1, 45–50.

McClure, J.J., 1987. Vitamin D intoxication in a thoroughbred racehorse, compendium on continuing education for the practicing. Veterinarian 9 (5). 573–578.

McDonald, P., Edwards, R.A., Greenhalgh, J.F.D., 1988. Animal Nutrition, fourth ed. Pearson Education Ltd, Harlow.

McDonald, G.K., 1980. Moldy sweet clover poisoning in a horse. Can Vet J 21, 250–251.

McDowell, L.R., 1989. Vitamins in animal nutrition, first ed. Academic Press, New York.

McDowell, L.R., 2000. Vitamins in animal and human nutrition, second ed. Iowa State Press, Ames, p. 793.

McIlwain, H., 1966. Biochemistry and the central nervous system. Churchill Livingstone, London.

McMeniman, N.P., Hintz, H.F., 1992. Effect of vitamin E status on lipid peroxidation in exercised horses. Equine Vet J 24, 482–484.

McMeniman, N.P., Thornton, J.R., Dowsett, K.F., 1995. Effect of grain type and supplementation on performance of exercising horses. Equine Vet J, Suppl. 18, 367–371.

Meyer, H., Boos, A., Weisweiler, B., et al., 1995. Ein Beitrag zum Beta-Carotin und Vitamin-A-Stoffwechsel des Pferdes. Pferdeheilkunde 11, 259–262.

Meyer, H., Kienzle, E., Zmija, 1991. Fütterungspraxis in Trainingsställen von Galopp- und Trabrennpferden. Pferdeheilkunde 7, 365–370.

Meyer, H., Radicke, S., Völker, L., 1996. Ein Beitrag zur präilealen Vitamin-C-Absorption beim Pferd. Pferdeheilkunde 12, 851–852.

Molitor, H., Robinson, H.J., 1940. Oral and parenteral toxicity of vitamin K-1, Phthiocol and 2 methyl 1, 4, naphthoquinone. Proc Soc Exp Biol Med 43, 125–128.

Müller, C.E., Möller, J., Krogh Jensen, S., Uden, P., 2007. Tocopherol and carotenoid levels in baled silage and haylage in relation to horse requirements. Anim Feed Sci Technol 137, 182–197.

Muylle, E., Oyaert, W., De Roose, P., et al., 1974. Hypercalcaemia and mineralisation of non-osseous tissues in horses due to vitamin-D toxicity. Zbl Vet Med A 21 (8), 638–643.

Napoli, J.L., 2000. A gene knockout corroborates to the integral function of cellular retinol-binding protein in retinoid metabolism. Nutr Rev 58, 230–236.

NRC, 1949. Recommended nutrient allowances for horses. National Academy Press, Washington, D.C., USA.

NRC, 1978. Nutrient requirements of horses, fourth ed. National Academy Press, Washington, DC.

NRC, 1982. Nutritional data for United States and Canadian Feeds. National Academy Press, Washington, DC.

NRC, 1987. Vitamin tolerance of animals. National Academy Press, Washington, DC.

NRC, 1989. Nutrient requirements of horses, fifth ed. National Academy Press, Washington, D.C., USA.

NRC, 2006. Nutrient requirements of dogs and cats, third ed. National Academy Press, Washington, D.C., USA.

NRC, 2007. Nutrient requirements of horses, sixth ed. National Academy Press, Washington, D.C., USA.

Nutrition Reviews, 1989. Season, latitude, and ability of sunlight to promote synthesis of vitamin D_3 in skin. Nutr Rev 47, 252–253.

Okano, T., Shimomura, Y., Yamane, M., et al., 2008. Conversion oh phylloquinone (vitamin K_1) into menaquinone-4 (vitamin K_2) in mice. Two possible routes for menaquinone-4 accumulation in cerebra of mice. J Biol Chemistry 283, 11270–11279.

Ott, E.A., Asquit, R.L., 1981. Vitamin and mineral supplementation of foaling mares. In: Proc. 7th Equine Nutr. Physiol. Symp., Warrenton, VA. Equine Nutrition and Physiology Society, Savoy, IL, p. 44.

Parker, A.L., Lawrence, L.M., Rokuroda, S., et al., 1997. The effects of niacin supplementation on niacin status and exercise metabolism in horses. In: Proc. 15th Symp. Equine Nutr. Physiol. Soc., Worth, Texas. Equine Nutrition and Physiology Society, Savoy, IL, p. 19.

Pearson, P.B., Sheybani, M.K., Schmidt, H., 1943. The metabolism of ascorbic acid in the horse. J Anim Sci 2, 175–180.

Pearson, P.B., Sheybani, M.K., Schmidt, H., 1944a. Riboflavin in the nutrition of the horse. Arch Biochem 3, 467–474.

Pearson, P.B., Sheybani, M.K., Schmidt, H., 1944b. The B-vitamin requirements of the horse. J Anim Sci 3, 166–174.

Petersson, K.H., Hintz, H.F., Schryver, H.F., et al., 1991. The effect of vitamin E on membrane integrity during submaximal exercise. In: Persson, S.G.B., Lindholm, A., Jeffcott, L.B. (Eds.), Equine Exercise Physiol. 3. pp. 315–322.

Pagan, J.D., Kane, E., Nash, D., 2005. Form and source of tocopherol affects vitamin E status in Thoroughbred horses. Pferdeheilkunde 21, 101–102.

Papasteriades, S., Argioudes, S., Lentides, S., et al., 1988. Case of vitamin D intoxication in race horses. In: Proc 4th Hellenic Vet Congr Athens, Greece, pp. 131–136.

Philipp, M., Kienzle, E., 2008. A double blind placebo controlled field study on the effect of biotin or zinc on the state of poor hoof horn quality. In: Proc. 12th Congr. Europ. Soc. Vet. Comparative Nutr. Vienna, Austria, p. 19.

Putnam, M.E., 1986. The role of vitamins in nutrition of performance horses. Mod Vet Pract 1986, 121–124.

Rambeck, W., Oesterhelt, W., Vecchi, M., et al., 1979. Occurrence of cholecalciferol in the calcinogenic plant *Trisetum flavescens*. Biochemical and Biophysical Research Communications 87 (3), 743–749.

Rambeck, W., Zucker, H., 1982. Vitamin D-artige Aktivitäten in calcinogenen Pflanzen. Zentralblatt für Veterinärmedizin Reihe A 29 (4–5), 289–296.

Rasbech, N.O., Koefoed-Johnsen, H.H., 1987. Undersogelser over askorbinsyrestatus hos fulblodhesta I Danmark. Dansk Veterinärtidsskrift 70, 1121–1128.

Rebhun, W.C., Tennant, B.C., Dill, S.G., et al., 1984. Vitamin K3-induced renal toxicosis in the horse. J Am Vet Med Assoc 184, 1237–1239.

Reilly, J.D., Cottrell, D.F., Martin, R.J., et al., 1998. Effect of supplementary dietary biotin on hoof growth and hoof growth rate in ponies: a controlled trial. Equine Vet J Suppl. 26, 51–57.

Rivalin, R.S., 2001. Riboflavin. In: Bowmen, B.A., Russel, R.A. (Eds.), Present knowledge in nutrition. Washington D.C.: ILSI Press, p. 191.

Roberts, H.E., Evans, E.T., Evans, W.C., 1949. The production of bracken staggers in the horse and its treatment by B1 therapy. Vet Rec 61, 549.

Roneus, B.O., Hakkarainen, R.V.J., Lindholm, C.A., et al., 1986. Vitamin E requirements of adult Standardbred horses evaluated by tissue depletion and repletion. Equine Vet J 18, 50–58.

Rich, G.A., McGlothlin, D.E., Lewis, L.D., et al., 1983. Effect of vitamin E supplementation on stallion semen characteristics and sexual behavior. In: Proc. 8th Equine Nutr. Physiol. Symp. Lexington, KY. Equine Nutrition and Physiology Society, Savoy, IL, p. 85.

Rucker, R.B., 2007. Allometric scaling, metabolic body size and interspecies comparisons of basal nutritional requirements. J Anim Physiol Anim Nutr 91 (3–4), 148–156.

Rucker, R.B., Steinberg, F., 2002. Vitamin requirements: relationship to basal metabolic need and functions. J Biochem Molec Biol Educ 30, 86–89.

Rucker, R.B., Storms, D., 2002. Interspecies comparisons of micronutrient requirements: metabolic vs. absolute body size. J Nutr 132, 2999–3000.

Rucker, R.B., Dubick, M.A., Robinson, J., 1980. Hypothetical calculations of ascorbic acid synthesis based on estimates in vitro. Am J Clinical Nutr 33, 961–964.

Saastamoinen, M.T., Harris, P.A., 2008. Vitamin requirement and supplementation in athletic horses. In: Saastamoinen, M.T., Martin-Rosset, W. (Eds.), Nutrition of the exercising horse. EAAP publication no. 125. Wageningen Academic Publishers, Wageningen, pp. 233–266.

Saastamoinen, M.T., Juusela, J., 1992. Influence of dietary supplementation on serum vitamin A and D concentrations and their seasonal variation in horses. Agr Sci Finl 1, 477–482.

Saastamoinen, M.T., Juusela, J., 1993. Serum vitamin-E concentration of horses on different vitamin-E supplementation levels. Acta Agric Scand Section A - Anim Sci 43, 52–57.

Sate, M.N., Patel, A.S., 2010. Update in pediatrics: Focus on fat-soluble vitamins. Nutr Clin Pract 25, 340–346.

Schenk, M., Kolb, E., 1982. Grundriß der physiologischen Chemie. VEB Gustav Fischer Verlag, Jena.

Schougaard, H., Simesen, M.G., Basse, A., et al., 1972. Nutritional muscular-dystrophy (NMD) in foals. Nordisk Veterinaer Medicin 24, 67–84.

Schubert, R., Großer, K., Stötzner, L., et al., 1993. Untersuchungen zum Vitamin-E-Status von Pferden im Jahresverlauf. In: Flachowsky, G. & Schubert, R. (Eds.), Vitamine und weitere Zusatzstoffe bei Mensch und Tier. Friedrich-Schiller-Universität Jena, Jena (Germany), pp. 140–143.

Schubert, R., Heinrich, A., 1988. Die Wirkung von bedarfsüberschreitenden Dosen an Vitamin E auf die Leistung von Galopprennpferden. In: Schwark, H.J. (Eds.), Züchtung, Leistungsprüfung und Ernährung von Pferden. Karl-Marx-Universität Leipzig, pp. 612–617.
Schubert, R., Zimmermann, C., Börner, A., et al., 1991. Einfluss der Vitamin-A- und ß-Karotinversorgung auf Reproduktionsparameter sowie Hormon- und Proteinkonzentrationen im Serum von Ponystuten. In: Schubert, R., Flachowsky, G., Bitsch, R., Jahreis, G. (Eds.), Vitamine und weitere Zusatzstoffe bei Mensch und Tier. pp. 42–47.
Schumacher, M.F., Williams, M.A., Lyman, R.L., 1965. Effect of high intakes of thiamine, riboflavin, and pyridoxine on reproduction in rats and vitamin requirements of the offspring. J Nutr 86, 343–349.
Schweigert, F.J., 1998a. Vitamin A: Stoffwechsel, Genexpression und embryonale Entwicklung. Übers. Tierernährung 26, 1–24.
Schweigert, F.J., 1998b. Metabolism of carotinoids in mammals. Carotenoids 3, 249–284.
Schweigert, F.J., Gottwald, C., 1999. Effect of parturition on levels of vitamins A and E and of beta-carotene in plasma and milk of mares. Equine Vet J 31 (3), 319–323.
Seehawer, J., Schliffka, W., 2006. Vitamine. In: Futtermittelzusatzstoffe. Technologie und Anwendung. Agrimedia, Bergen/Dumme, pp. 181–204.
Shearer, M.J., 1997. The role of vitamin D and K in bone health and osteoporosis prevention. Proc Nutr Soc 56, 915–937.
Siciliano, P.D., Wood, C.H., 1993. The effect of added dietary soybean oil on vitamin E status of the horse. J Anim Sci 75, 1553–1560.
Siciliano, P.D., Parker, A.L., Lawrence, L.M., 1997. Effect of dietary vitamin E supplementation on the integrity of skeletal muscle in exercised horses. J Anim Sci 75, 1553–1560.
Siciliano, P.D., Kawcak, C.E., McIlwraith, C.W., 2000a. The effect of initiation of exercise training in young horses on vitamin K status. J Anim Sci 78, 2353–2358.
Siciliano, P.D., Warren, L.K., Lawrence, L.M., 2000b. Changes in vitamin K status of growing horses. J Equine Vet Sci 20, 726–729.
Sklan, D., Donoghue, S., 1982. Serum and intracellular retinol transport in the equine. Brit J Nutr 47, 273–280.
Smith, B.S.W., Wright, H., 1984. 25-hydroxyvitamin D concentrations in equine serum. Vet Rec 115, 579.
Snow, D.H., Frigg, M., 1989. Oral administration of different formulations of ascorbic acid to the horse. Equine Vet Sci 9, 30–33.
Snow, D.H., Frigg, M., 1990. Bioavailability of ascorbic acid in horses. J Vet Pharm Therapie 13, 393–403.
Snow, D.H., Gash, S.P., Cornelius, J., 1987. Oral administration of ascorbic acid to the horse. Equine Vet Sci 9, 30–33.
Solomons, N.W., 2001. Vitamin A and carotinoids. In: Bowman, B.A., Russell, R.M. (Eds.), Present knowledge in nutrition. ILSI Press, Washington D.C.
Sprekeler, N., Müller, T., Kowalewski, M.P., et al., 2011. Expression patterns of intestinal calcium transport factors and ex-vivo absorption of calcium in horses. BMC Vet Rec 7, 65–76.
Steiss, J.E., Traber, M.G., Williams, M.A., et al., 1994. Alpha tocopherol concentrations in clinically normal adult horses. Equine Vet J 26, 417–419.
Stillions, M.C., Teeter, S.M., Nelson, W.E., 1971. Ascorbic acid requirement of mature horses. J Anim Sci 32, 249–251.
Stephensen, C.B., 2001. Vitamin A, infection, and immune function. Annu Rev Nutr 21, 167–192.
Stowe, H.D., 1967. Reproductive performance of barren mares following vitamin A and E supplementation. In: Proc. 13th Am. Ass. Equine Pract. New Orleans, LA. American Association of Equine Practitioners, Lexington KY, p. 81.
Stowe, H.D., 1968. Experimental equine avitaminosis A and E. In: Proc. 14st Equine Nutr. Res. Soc. Lexington. University of Kentucky, Equine Science Society, Champaign, IL, p. 27.
Stowe, H.D., 1982. Vitamin A profiles of equine serum and milk. J Anim Sci 54, 76–81.
Suttie, J.W., 1995. The importance of menaquinones in human nutrition. Annu Rev Nutr 15, 399–417.
Topliff, D.R., Potter, G.D., Kreider, J.L., et al., 1981. Thiamin supplementation of exercising horses. In: Proc. 7th Equine Nutr. Physiol. Symp. Warrenton, VA. Equine Nutrition and Physiology Society, Savoy, IL, p. 167.
Toribio, R.E., Bain, F.T., Mrad, D.R., et al., 1998. Congenital defects in newborn foals of mares treated for equine protozoal myeloencephalitis during pregnancy. J Am Vet Med Assoc 212, 697–701.
Ullrey, D.E., 1972. Biological activity of fat-soluble vitamins: vitamin A and carotene. J Anim Sci 35, 648–657.
Vermeer, C., Gijsbers, B.L., Craciun, A.M., et al., 1996. Effects of vitamin K on bone mass and bone metabolism. J Nutr 126, S1187–S1191.
Vermeer, C., Shearer, M.J., Zittermann, A., et al., 2004. Beyond deficiency: potential benefits of increased intakes of vitamin K for bone and vascular health. Eur J Nutr 43, 325–335.
Wald, G., 1968. Molecular basis of visual excitation. Science 162, 230–239.
Wardlaw, G.M., 1999. Perspectives in nutrition, fourth ed. WBC Mc Graw-Hill, New York.
Watanabe, H., Yoshikazu, F., Ichikawa, F., et al., 1982. A high-performance liquid-chromatographic analysis of serum tocopherols in thoroughbred horses. Bull Equine Res Inst 19, 51–58.
Watson, E.D., Cuddeford, D., Burger, I., 1996. Failure of beta-carotene absorption negates any potential effect on ovarian function in mares. Equine Vet J 28, 233–236.
Weisweiler, B., Twehues, R., Kuczka, A., et al., 1993. Einfluß hoher Vitamin-D-Dosierungen auf Calcium-, Magnesium- und Phosphatstoffwechsel von Pferden, klinische und pathomorphologische Befunde. Pferdeheilkunde 6/1993, 343–352.
Webb, A.R., Holick, M.F., 1988. The role of sunlight in the cutaneous production of vitamin D_3. Ann Rev Nutr 8, 375–399.
White, A., Estrada, M., Walker, K., et al., 2001. Role of exercise and ascorbate on plasma antioxidant capacity in thoroughbred racehorses. Comp Biochem Physiol Av Mol Integr Physiol 128, 99–104.
Williams, C.A., Kronfeld, D.S., Hess, T.M., et al., 2004. Antioxidant supplementation and subsequent oxidative stress of horses during an 80-km endurance race. J Anim Sci 82, 588–574.
Wilson, T.M., Morrison, H.A., Palmer, N.C., et al., 1976. Myodegeneration and suspected selenium-vitamin-E deficiency in horses. J Am Vet Med Assoc 169, 213–217.
Wood, T., Weckman, T.J., Henry, P.A., et al., 1990. Equine urine pH: normal population distributions and methods of acidification. Equine Vet J 22, 118–121.
Zenker, W., Josseck, H., Geyer, H., 1995. Histological and physical assessment of poor hoof horn quality in Lipizzaner horses and a therapeutic trial with biotin and a placebo. Equine Vet J 27, 183–191.
Zentek, J., 1991. Myopathien in einem Reitpferdebestand. Tierärztl Praxis 19, 167–169.
Zeyner, A., 2002. Ernährungsphysiologische Wirkungen eines Austausches von stärkereichen Komponenten durch Sojaöl in der Reitpferdeernährung. Habilitation Thesis, Georg-August-Universität Göttingen.
Zeyner, A., Lengwenat, O., 1993. Untersuchungen zur Verfügbarkeit verschiedener oral verabreichter Askorbinsäureverbindungen beim Pferd. In: Flachowsky, G., Schubert, R. (Eds.), Vitamine und weitere Zusatzstoffe bei Mensch und Tier. Friedrich-Schiller-University, Jena, pp. 220–223.
Zeyner, A., Buchholz, I., Schweigert, F.J., 1995. Untersuchungen zum Einfluß von Fettgaben auf die Konzentration an beta-Carotin, Vitamin A und Vitamin E im Blutserum von Pferden. In: Schubert, R., Flachowsky, G. (Eds.), Vitamine und Zusatzstoffe in der Ernährung von Mensch und Tier. pp. 97–100.
Zeyner, A., Buchholz, I., Schweigert, F.J., 1999. Untersuchungen zum Einfluß von Fettgaben auf die Konzentration an beta-Carotin, Vitamin A und Vitamin E im Blutserum von Pferden. 2. Mitteilung: Sojaöl und Sojalecithin. In: Schubert, R., Flachowsky, G., Bitsch, R., Jahreis, G. (Eds.), Vitamine und Zusatzstoffe in der Ernährung von Mensch und Tier. pp. 358–361.
Zeyner, A., Vergos, A., Schmitz, M., et al., 2004. Studies on the metabolic situation of mares and their foals during an early period after birth. In: Juliand, V., Martin-Rosset, W. (Eds.), The growing horse: Nutrition and prevention of growth disorders. EAAP publication no. 114. Wageningen, The Netherlands: Wageningen Academic Publishers, pp. 237–238. (ISBN 9-0769-9862-0).

10

SECTION A Nutritional Foundations

Macro and trace elements in equine nutrition

Manfred Coenen

Overview

The elements discussed in this chapter (Table 10-1) are essential for animals as well as for most plants. The differentiation between macro- and trace elements is not linked to their chemical structure but simply reflects their essentiality and average required dietary concentration: ≥100 ppm = macro, <100 ppm = trace element. This approach is very helpful in practice and is linked to content of these elements in animal tissue.

The differences in the required amounts of macro vs. trace elements and the potential to induce negative effects in the animal when provided in excess form the foundation for the differing legislation which covers the various elements. In most countries, more detailed legal restrictions exist regarding the trace elements in comparison to the macro elements.

Inadequate intake is still a common event and can be associated with visible clinical signs. However, such occurrences are not typically due to a lack of available knowledge either with respect to *requirements* or the *availability* from mineral carriers but are usually due to poor application of this information or even lack of understanding. In addition, it is important to recognize that there is limited tolerance for high mineral intakes. Common reasons for oversupplementation, in particular with trace elements, include the selection of inappropriate mineral supplements or the unthinking usage of such supplements. The potential for adverse consequences to develop when mineral intake exceeds the upper safe margins is commonly underestimated; this practice does pose a high risk for negative effects on health and performance.

The adverse effects of mineral deficiencies or excesses on horse health are an important veterinary issue and can be divided into acute and chronic responses.

Acute responses: For some elements, effects may be seen within a relatively short time scale when the available amounts do not cover tissue requirements; hypocalcemia is a prominent example. In these circumstances, effects are typically linked to disturbances in the internal balance and distribution of an element even when the intake is not particularly low. Acute responses can also occur if the intake increases to toxic levels (e.g., Se toxicosis), in which cases the high intakes are typically mirrored by abnormal tissue concentrations.

Chronic derangements in mineral intake induce adaptations in the animal; however, even these adaptations can be overridden by critically low or high intakes that may induce nonspecific effects such as growth retardation. Certain tissues become depleted or enriched depending on the intake. The value of ration evaluation to support the development of a clinical diagnosis is commonly underestimated. There might be some difficulties in quantifying feed intake precisely but use of estimates for intake and typical mineral concentrations in the feeds can yield at least sufficient basic information to judge whether one needs further, potentially costly, ration analysis and evaluation or not.

Factors determining requirements

In theory, zero mineral intake, a situation that can occur under experimental conditions, results in a negative mineral balance due to continual mineral excretion, mainly via the feces, urine and skin. The required intake to compensate for these unavoidable losses, defined as endogenous losses, represents the maintenance requirement. Such data, with respect to horses, are available for all of the macrominerals apart from sulfur (S). Data analysis for the balance between intake and retention, based on a broad range of intakes, ideally yields a linear relationship: $y=a+bx$. The principle is presented in Fig. 10.1. The value for "a" represents the endogenous losses and "b" gives the rate of utilization; both parameters are specific for the individual elements.

The value of "a" '(endogenous loss) is influenced by the

1. physiological role of the element
2. dry matter intake (see below)
3. concentration of the mineral in various secretions as part of its role within tissues, e.g., bile secretion
4. capability of an organ to activate conservation mechanisms (e.g. renal reabsorption of sodium).

Dry matter intake (DMI) may impact mineral requirements by inducing an increase in mucosal cell apoptosis and cell regrowth. Additionally, most secretions in the gastrointestinal tract (GIT) are related to DMI (e.g., saliva).

The utilization of the element b, visualized by the slope of the regression line, is affected by the:

1. type/ chemical nature of the naturally occurring compound (e.g. $CaCO_2$ vs. Ca-phosphate)
2. digestibility of the feedstuff or supplement containing the element
3. distribution in tissues
4. physiological uptake by tissues.

Table 10-1 Macro- and Trace Elements with Nutritional Relevance

Element		When identified	Atomic mass	Occurrence		Toxicity[1]	Legal status[3]
				Earth crust*	Typical horse feeds[2]**(g/kg)		
Calcium	Ca	1808	40.08	3.68%	1–>15	+/+	available without legal restrictions as mineral compounds which are classified as a single feedstuff, like salt
Phosphorus	P	1669	30.97	0.12%	<1-5	++/++	
Magnesium	Mg	1808	24.31	2%	<1-5	+/+	
Sodium	Na	1807	22.99	2.27%	<1-5	+/++	
Potassium	K	1702	39.10	2.4%	5–35		
Chloride	Cl	1774	35.45	0.1 g/kg	<1–10	+/++	
Sulfur	S	1777	32.06	0.4 g/kg			
					mg/kg[2]		max.[3]
Copper	Cu	~5000BC	63.5	20 mg/kg	2–15	+/++	25
Zinc	Zn	16th C	65,38	70 mg/kg	5–60	+/+	150
Iron	Fe	~2000BC	55.85	4.7%	10->500	++/+	750
Manganese	Mn	1774	54.9	950 mg/kg	10–80	+/+	150
Selenium	Se	1817	78.96	0.09 mg/kg	<0.05–0.3	++/+++	0.5
Iodine	J	1811	126.9	0.2 mg/kg	0.03–0.1	++/++	4
Cobalt	Co	1735	58.9	18	0.05–2		2
Chromium	Cr	1897	52.0	126	0.03–0.8	+/+++	Not regulated

[1]Indication of the likelihood of toxicity to occur/ how serious or life-threatening such toxicity may be; likelihood: + very rare, experimentally has been produced, ++ may happen, +++ frequently seen; life-threatening if toxic doses are ingested:+ no, ++ possible +++ in most cases; note that the given range for the elements in typical horse feeds are far below toxic levels (see Table 10-4)
[2]per kg dry matter
[3]for the EU; legally defined upper limits for a complete diet and daily ration, respectively, referring to 88% dry matter.
*Merian et al 2004, Anke 2004; **Hohenheim 1976.

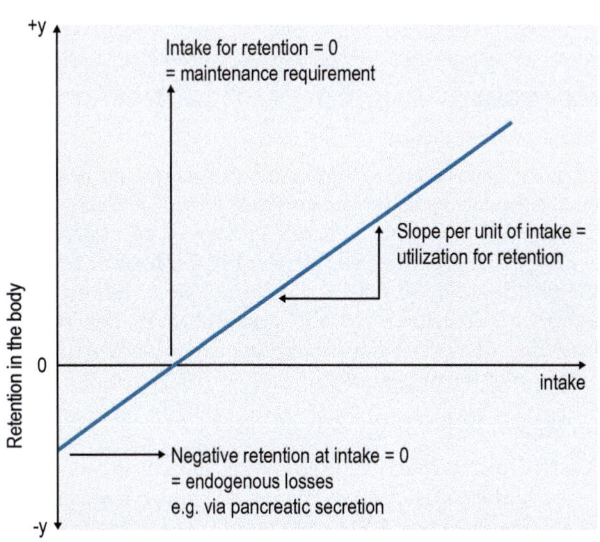

Figure 10.1 Principle of mineral balance trials with very low and high intake.

When considering the requirements for gestation, lactation, growth and exercise, mineral accretion in the respective "products" must be considered, i.e., in the pregnant uterus, in postnatal weight gain, milk, and sweat. As energy and mineral requirements do not change in parallel to the increase in these products, it is not possible to give a certain mineral:energy ratio as a guideline for feeding in practice. Commonly, recommendations are given in g or mg per kg body weight (BW), kg metabolic BW ($BW^{0.75}$) or per kg feed on a DM basis. However, the accuracy of latter as a target value for rations is low, due to the wide variability in possible DM-intakes (range of 15–>40 g DM/kg BW; see Chapter 3).

Trace element balance studies are very challenging and despite the high quality of some of the existing knowledge, requirements are less precisely defined than for the macroelements. Most data are based on dose-response studies in which the required intake for ensuring adequate tissue levels (blood or organ, e.g., muscle) is evaluated. Although it is not recommended to use the factorial approach to determine intake requirements for trace elements, it is possible to use their known concentrations in products such as milk to determine rough estimates based on such a factorial approach. This enables evaluation of the plausibility of requirement data.

In theory, there is no tissue that acts as a designated mineral sink (an exception is the liver for Cu) or a strategic reservoir when intake exceeds requirements. This is in contrast to the capacity of the body to store energy in adipose tissue. Even bone is not adapted to store Ca above that required for the optimal level of bone strength. However, bone can act as a buffer in case of a temporary shortage in exogenous Ca supply. Consequently, simple strategies are required for the organism to manage naturally occurring high intakes:

- limiting absorption (e.g., Fe) and increasing fecal excretion
- enforced renal excretion (e.g., Na)
- enforced excretion via milk (e.g., iodine).

Key Points

- Overconsumption of minerals induces an abnormal load in certain tissues and increases the risk of cell damage. This is the case in particular for I and Se.
- When comparing the risk of over-supplementation with Ca or Fe vs. Se or I, it is logical that for rare elements like Se the evolutionary need to establish an "overconsumption management strategy" was quite low (in contrast to Ca or Fe) and therefore the risk of toxicity of such elements through over-supplementation will be higher.

Minerals as essential nutrients

Mineral intake through the ingestion of plants or plant products does not guarantee adequate intake; additional supplementation is often required. The approach to macro vs. trace mineral supplementation is quite different. Macro elements are used fairly freely, provided as oxides, chlorides or sulphates. Some (e.g., $CaCl_2$) can induce mucosal damage and require either high dilution or specific coating to avoid adverse effects. A selection of commonly used mineral compounds is presented in Table 10-2.

Use of feed grade quality compounds helps to ensure safety with respect to contamination by elements that may interfere with utilization (e.g., high Fe) or the uptake of undesirable elements and substances (e.g., Pb and dioxins). The trace elements, partly due to their toxic potential, are regulated by law within the EU and, for certain trace elements (e.g., Se) also in the USA. The EU legal restrictions include the definition of permitted trace element carriers (Table 10-3) as well as the maximum concentration in the diet. Adverse effects are a substantial risk in the case of overdosage, including negative interaction with the availability of other minerals, tissue accumulation, and the impairment of cellular functions. These factors are considered in defining a safe upper limit (SUL). Current data on SULs are summarized in Table 10-4 (Anke 2004, NRC 2005, Poppenga, 2001).

Calcium (Ca)

Ca in the pure elemental form is a hard metal (density 1.55 g/cm^3); combined with organic or inorganic anions Ca is the most abundant macroelement in the mammalian body. The Ca-content of a newborn foal is close to 20 g/kg BW and decreases to ~15 g/kg BW in adults (Grace et al 1999b, Meyer & Ahlswede 1976). About 99% of total body Ca is found deposited in bone. The biochemistry of Ca in bone ensures two functions: (a) the formation of a tissue with high mechanical load capacity, and (b) buffering of changes in Ca-homeostasis. This fact ensures a high flexibility in Ca turnover via the "feeding" of the mobile Ca pool in blood or muscle by the mobilization of Ca from bone. The import and export of Ca into and out of bone is regulated by calcitonin and parathyroid hormone, respectively.

Table 10-2 Commonly used Mineral Compounds as Source for Macroelements[1]

Compound	Content of element (%)						
	Ca	P	Mg	Na	Cl	K	S
$CaCO_3$	36						
$CaCl_2$	36				64		
$Ca(H_2PO_4)_2{+}2H_2O$	15	22					
$CaHPO_4 + 2H_2O$	21	16					
$Ca_{10}(PO_4)_6(OH_2)$	35	18					
Ca-Gluconate	8.5						
Ca-Formiate	29						
Ca-Lactate	12						
Ca-Acetate	20–25						
H_3PO_4		31,6					
MgO			50				
$MgCl_2 + 6\ H_2O$			12		35		
$MgHPO_4 + 3H_2O$		16	12				
$MgSO_4 + 7\ H_2O$			9,8				13
NaCl				38	61		
$NaH_2PO_4 + 2\ H_2O$		19		13			
$Na_2HPO_4 + H_2O$		8		11			
Na_2SO_4				32			23
$Na_2SO_4 \cdot 10\ H_2O$				14			10
KCl					47	52	

[1]Beside the provision of an individual element by the compounds shown above, it is common to use a mineral supplement which combines different elements. A mineral supplement is defined in some countries by the crude ash (CA) content, e.g., Germany min. 400 g CA/kg, and requires specific labeling

Major functions

Distribution over tissues

Total body Ca is close to 15 g/kg; the bulk is found in bone. Bone ash (metacarpus, tarsus) contains 385 g Ca (Table 10-5) and 177 g P/kg with no effect of gender or age (Vervuert et al 2010). The fetus has slightly higher Ca content related to the prioritization of bone formation during gestation. Ca accretion is described by an exponential model which reflects that the most intensive bone growth occurs during the last 4 months of gestation.

Ca in bone

As Ca-hydroxyapatite ($Ca_5(PO_4)_3(OH)$), calcium is an essential contributor to the physical nature of bone and teeth. The high apatite formation and inclusion of Ca in enamel (~38% Ca (Kodaka et al 1991)) produces the highest known mechanical resistant material in the equine body, able to cope with the enormous masticatory forces of >300 N (Huthmann et al 2009). With respect to the radius and tibia, the cortical hydroxyapatite density (commonly taken as bone mineral density, BMD) is 1175 mg/cm^3 (Fürst et al 2008). This corresponds to ~470 mg Ca and 87 mg P/cm^3. Although there is a strong positive age effect on mechanical strength, at least in metacarpal and metatarsal bones (Glade

Table 10-3 Example Compounds Permitted as Carriers for Trace Elements (i.e., Registered for the Provision of Trace Elements which are in Turn Classified as Additives in EU Legislation)

Element	Compound	Content of element (%)
Fe	$FeCl_2 + 4\ H_2O$	28
	$FeSO_4 + 7\ H_2O$	20
	Fe_{II}-fumarate	32
Iodine	KJ	76
	NaJ	68
	$Ca(JO_3) + 6\ H_2O$	51
Co	$CoCl_2 + 6\ H_2O$	25
	$CoSO_4 + 7\ H_2O$	21
Cu	$CuCl_2 + 2\ H_2O$	37
	$CuSO_4 + 5\ H_2O$	25
	$CuCO_3$	58
	CuO	80
	$Cu(H_2H_3O_2)_2 + H_2O$	32
Mn	$MnCl_2 + 4\ H_2O$	28
	$MnSO_4$	36
	$MnSO_4 + 4\ H_2O$	25
	$KMnO_4$	35
Se	Na_2SeO_3	46
	Na_2SeO_4	42
Zn	$ZnCl_2$	48
	$ZnSO_4 + 7\ H_2O$	23
	ZnO	80
	$ZnCO_3$	52
	$Zn(C_2H_3O_2)_2 + 2\ H_2O$	30

et al 1986), it seems that the BMD is less sensitive to age (Fürst et al 2008). Bone is formed by collagen fibers (type I, 90% of total protein) and non-collagenous proteins. Spindle- or plate shaped crystals of hydroxyapatite ($Ca_{10}[PO_4]_6[OH]_2$) are found on the collagen fibers and in the ground substance. The mechanisms of mineralization are not fully understood. The ground substance is composed of glycoproteins plus proteoglycans. These highly anionic complexes have a high ion-binding capacity and are thought to play an important role in the calcification process and in the fixation of hydroxyapatite crystals to the collagen fibers. Osteocalcin, a non-collagenous protein which is synthesized by the osteoblasts, is thought to affect the growth or maturation of Ca^{2+}-phosphate incorporating structures. However, Mg also plays an important role in mineralization as it has been shown to bind to the surface of hydroxyapatite crystals and seems to compete with Ca for the same absorption site (Rude et al 2003, 2009). In addition, studies in laboratory animals have shown negative effects of excessive Mg intake on crystal size and structure as well. In summary, low and high Mg intake in horses has the potential to interact with Ca in the "building of proper hydroxyapatite crystals".

As a consequence of the biology of bone, Ca and P constitute a mobile component as they can be mobilized from bone on demand in case of a mismatch between intake and the need to maintain homeostasis. This means that the physical properties of bones essentially change during gestation and lactation (Glade 1993, Gruber & Stover 1994). Regardless of Ca intake, a major impact on equine bone quality and bone mineral content is caused by exercise. Stabling horses induces a reduction in BMD whereas natural exercise on pasture as well as short term training bouts induce an increase in BMD, which should result in a corresponding response in bone Ca (Bell et al 2001, Hiney et al 2004, Porr et al 1998). It is evident that the positive impact of natural exercise is underestimated in practice.

Key Points

- ~99% of Ca is deposited in bone and is key in supporting the mechanical property of bone
- Ca in bone can be rapidly mobilized to maintain blood Ca^{2+} concentrations
- There is no benefit on the mechanical properties of bone when the Ca supply in the diet exceeds requirements
- Immobility/stabling of a horse results in a loss of minerals from the bone – regardless of being provided an adequate Ca intake – and such tissue responses cannot be fully overcome by increasing the mineral supply. The stimulus of physical activity (load bearing exercise) is also required

Other functions

In addition to its contribution to ossification, Ca is involved in blood clotting, muscle contraction, enzyme activities related to energy metabolism, and digestive processes as well as the transmission of nerve signals ((Wijnberg et al 2002a, b, c).

The second highest ranked tissue for Ca content is muscle where the Ca^{2+} is essentially linked to the contractility of muscle fiber. Inside the muscle cell, Ca shows the lowest concentration, in comparison to other ions, being in the range of 4–19 mmol (160–462 mg)/kg dry matter (DM) (Gottlieb-Vedi et al 1996). Release of Ca from the sarcoplasm and reuptake drive muscle contraction and relaxation (with an impressive exchange rate of ~200 nmol/g muscle). The energy used for maintaining the Ca^{2+} gradient accounts for ~30–50% of total heat production within the muscle (Hasselbach & Oetliker 1983, Kobayashi & Sugi 1980). The Ca^{2+}-ATPase plays an important role in this aspect of muscle function (Hasselbach 1998); the Ca^{2+}-ATPase varies between 20–29 nmol/kg wet weight in gluteus medius and semitendinosus muscles. There is no influence of age but concentrations are higher in pastured animals in comparison to exercised or stabled horses (Suwannachot et al 2003). The fact that the concentration of ATPase in masseter muscle is only ~20% of the above level may indicate that there is a variable distribution of Ca^{2+}, accompanied with differences in ATPase activity, according to muscle fiber type.

Ca requirements

Using the traditional factorial approach the sum of all endogenous losses plus the amount of Ca deposited or excreted in any product divided by the rate of utilization will give the minimum requirement.

Maintenance

The maintenance requirement (see Table 10-5) is related to body weight. In contrast to ruminants there is no effect of DM intake on endogenous losses and thereby on requirements.

Table 10-4 Minimal Requirement Data and Maximum Tolerable Dietary Minerals (data from NRC 2005, Poppenga, 2001, GfE 2013)

	Maintenance	Gestation	Lactation	Growth	Exercise		
		305 days	30 days	12 months	10 l sweat		
DMI kg/day	10.6	11	15.3	7.8	13.7	Safe upper limit	Dimension
Element							
Ca	1.61	3.95	3.39	3.60	1.61	20	g/kg DM
P	1.13	1.60	2.39	2.37	1.13	10	
Mg	0.52	0.58	0.54	0.58	0.52	8	
Na	0.26	0.39	0.44	0.41	3.03	23[1]	
K	1.39	1.48	1.78	1.52	2.27	10[2]	
Cl	0.15	0.20	0.40	0.22	4.17	37[1]	
S	0.18	0.42	0.53	0.40	0.17	5	
Cu	9.6	9.6	6.8	14.4	7.4	250	mg/kg DM **Note:** consider the variation in DM intake when evaluating the potential for toxicity or when reduced DM is being provided in order to restrict energy intake
Zn	38.4	48.1	34.1	52.2	37.2	500	
Fe	38.4	48.1	34.1	104.4	29.8	500	
Mn	38.4	38.4	27.3	52.2	37.2	400	
Se	0.10	0.14	0.10	0.20	0.07	2	
I	0.10	0.19	0.14	0.26	0.15	5	
Co	0.05	0.10	0.07	0.13	0.07	25	
Cr						100	
Contaminants							
As	–					30	
Cd	–					10	
Mo	–					5	
Pb	–					10	
Hg	–					1 (organic source) 0.2 (inorganic)	

[1]ND = not determined.
[2]>500 mg/kg BW/day may increase water intake and cause diuresis.

Growth

It is evident that any type of growth results in a remarkable increase in requirement.

The Ca concentration in the conceptus increases over time because intrauterine growth shows a preference for connective tissue development in the last 4 months of gestation in order to make the newborn ready for standing and flight-fright responses. The postnatal growth curve (see Chapter 12) determines the development of Ca requirements in the growing foal. Postnatally, in relation to bone, there is a preferred growth of soft tissue and therefore the proportion of Ca in the mature body mass is lower than in a newborn. Therefore, the product "postnatal daily gain" has a lower Ca content vs. preterm gain.

Lactation

On average, Ca in mare's milk is ~1740 mg/kg but there is a continuous decrease in concentration throughout lactation. The Ca excretion via milk therefore varies according to the day of lactation and milk yield. In fact, the most demanding performance with respect to Ca requirements is milk production (see Fig. 10.2). Although milk yield in mares is

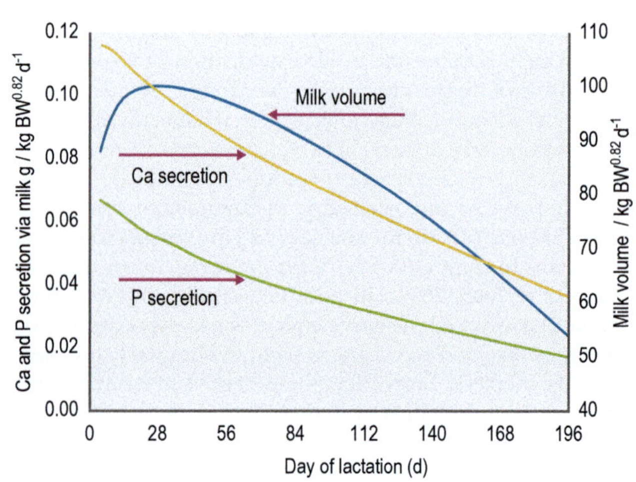

Figure 10.2 Model of milk yield in horses as well as Ca and P excretion via milk. (milk volume, g kg $BW^{0.82}$ d^{-1} = $66d^{0.1727}e^{-0.00539d}$; Ca-secretion, g kg $BW^{0.82}$ d^{-1} = $0.1161d^{0.00757}e^{-0.00599d}$; P-secretion, g kg $BW^{0.82}$ d^{-1} = $0.0700d^{-0.02276}e^{-0.00649d}$; Coenen et al 2010)

Table 10-5 Key Data on Calcium in the Equine Body and Requirements

	Item	Dimension	Value	Miscellaneous
Distribution				% of total
	total body	$g\ kg^{-1}$	14.78	100
	bone	$g\ kg^{-1}$	110.0	99.5
	muscle	$g\ kg^{-1}$	0.04	0.13
	liver	$g\ kg^{-1}$	0.05	<0.01
	kidney	$g\ kg^{-1}$	0.10	<0.01
	lung	$g\ kg^{-1}$	0.10	0.01
	heart	$g\ kg^{-1}$	0.04	<0.01
	GIT	$g\ kg^{-1}$	0.06	0.03
	skin	$g\ kg^{-1}$	0.06	0.03
	blood	$g\ kg^{-1}$	0.08	0.03
Products				
	fetus	$g\ kg^{-1}$	18.2	
		daily Ca-accretion in pregnant uterus, g/kg birth = $0.0422e^{0.0184d}$ (1)		
	daily gain	g/kg	15	
	milk	mg/l	1620–426*log(10)d(2)	
		Lactogenic daily excretion, g/kg $BW^{0.82} = 0.1161d^{0.00757}e^{-0.00599d}$ (2)		
	sweat	mg/l	120	
Balance				
	endogenous losses	mg/kg BW0.75	74	
	absorption	% of intake	60–78	prececally
			<10–43	total GIT
	utilization	% of intake	46	
	main excretion route for surplus		kidney	

[1]day of gestation.
[2]day of lactation (Coenen et al 2010; GfE 2013; Coenen & Vervuert 2003; Grace et alet al 1999a, b; McCutcheon & Geor, 1998a; McCutcheon et al 1995b; Meyer, 1990, 1987; Meyer & Ahlswede, 1976; Kienzle 2012; GfE 2011).

difficult to define, a current model based on measured milk volumes and energy requirements of the foal suggests that the maximum mineral excretion via milk occurs within the first 40 days of lactation. Taking into consideration the time dependent drop in mineral concentrations (Ca, P, Mg) in mares' milk, this results in a nonlinear description of lactogenic Ca export (Fig. 10.2).

Exercise

Weak data and conflicting recommendations exist with respect to the Ca requirements of exercising horses. Long-lasting effects of exercise on Ca are associated with an adaptation of bone; a likely temporary shift of bone formation towards resorption results in a loss of BMD which can be overridden by an elevated Ca intake. However, neither the persistence of this tissue sensitivity nor the beneficial effects of extra Ca is sufficiently defined. Short-term exercise induces changes in Ca homeostasis which are associated with PTH secretion in part to compensate for the trapping of Ca^{2+} by lactate. This temporary shrinkage in the Ca^{2+} pool indicates an extra requirement in response to exercise but it is likely that this small increase, coupled with the small increase in Ca loss via the sweat will only elevate Ca requirements for exercising animals by a small amount. Practically, it can be stated that 1.5-fold of maintenance requirements is sufficient for horses in exercise work.

Ca balance

Ca intake

The Ca-concentrations in feeds typically varies between 0.5 and 15 g/kgDM. A guide to the ranking according to content (g/kgDM) is:

legumes, whole plant	grass–legume mix	grass	grain
15	10	5	1–0.4

The contribution of roughage to total Ca intake is closely linked to the botanical composition of the ration. Alfalfa, clover or herbs like dandelion contain the highest Ca concentrations. Where such plants contribute to the plant community on a pasture, overall content will be >6 g Ca/kg DM. This provides Ca above the requirements for maintenance or exercise if the daily intake of such a pasture is ~20 g DM/kg BW. Typical grass hay provides on average around 4–5 g Ca/kg DM, but it is important to recognize that there is a wide variation in the Ca content of grass and conserved forages; a high percentage of grass forages are below this average value (Fig. 10.3) especially in the UK. This is particularly relevant to the management of Ca nutrition in lactating and growing animals. Cereals in particular are low in Ca (oats > rye & barley & wheat > corn) (Table 10-6). By-products vary between 2 (wheat bran) and >15 g Ca/kg DM (citrus pulp). Cereal straw contains ~1.8 g Ca/kg DM without major differences depending on the source. At DMIs of 80 and 130 g $kg^{0.75}$ BW for maintenance and lactation, respectively, a Ca intake concentration of 5 g/kg DM results in a Ca supply which would provide ~2 fold and ~1.1-fold of recommended requirements.

The use of mineral supplements is very common in practice, although in most circumstances the feeding of a Ca-containing supplement in addition to average pasture or hay will create a Ca intake that exceeds the requirement (Fig. 10.4).

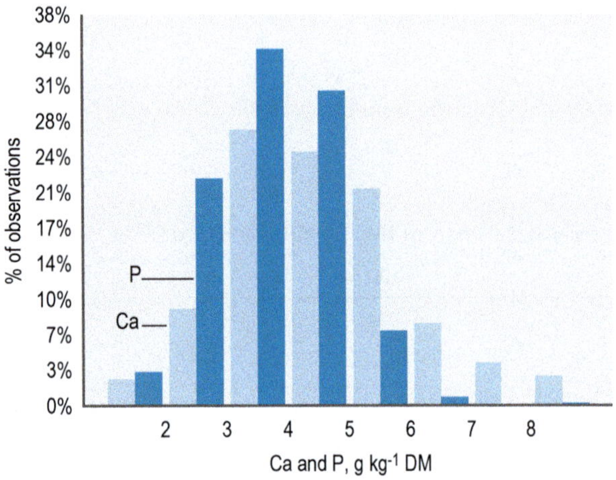

Figure 10.3 Distribution of Ca and P in grass, grass silages and hay (581 samples, northern Germany; means: Ca 4.6, P 3.7 g/kg DM).

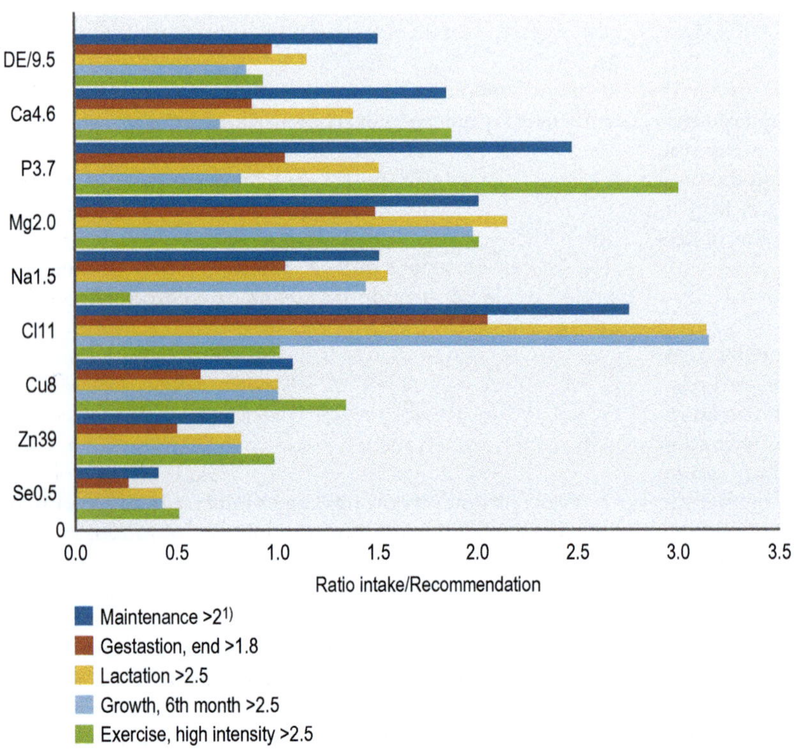

Key Points

- The presence of significant amount of legumes or certain herbal species (e.g., dandelion) in pasture or hay typically results in >6 g Ca/kg DM. This level of intake covers Ca needs in most circumstances providing that DMI is in the normal physiological range
- High grain rations are likely to provide a low intake of Ca (but high P) if not supplemented
- Typically grass or preserved grass forages may be low in overall Ca content and will require specific countermeasures, such as supplementation, especially for pregnant and lactating mares as well as growing animals

Ca secretion and absorption

Ca needs to be dissociated for transmenbrane transport; the nature of Ca in animal and plant tissue corresponds to this situation, Ca-oxalate being the exception. This Ca complex is a special form of Ca storage in some plants.

Secretion

Saliva (see Table 10-9) contains 157 g/l Ca (Coenen 1985a); assuming 6 liters of saliva production per kg DM of roughage (Meyer et al 1986); this would result in Ca

Table 10-6 Ca (g/kg DM) in Different Grains (Total Plant in Early Stage) and Several Products

Type of grain	Entire plant	Straw	Cereal	Bran
Wheat	2.6	3.1	0.7	1.8
Rye	4.1	2.9	0.9	1.7
Barley		4.8	0.7	1.8
Oats	4.4	4.1	1.2	1.8
Corn	3.8		0.4	1.7

Figure 10.4 Supply of energy and minerals to a 500 kg horse through typical preserved grass forage relative to requirements (=1). [1]For each life stage/activity level the > number represents the DM intake, kg/100 kg BW used for the calculations. The number behind each parameter on the *y*-axis is the corresponding concentration per kg hay DM in MJ, g (macroelements) and mg (trace elements) used for developing this figure.

Table 10-7 Estimated Volumes and Mineral Concentrations in Equine Gastrointestinal Secretions (Meyer & Coenen 2002)

	Volume kg/100 kg BW/day	Mineral concentrations (g/kg)					
		Na	Cl	K	Ca	Mg	P
Saliva	3–5	1.5	2–3	1.1	0.15	0.03	0.02
Gastric juice	5–10		3				
Pancreatic juice	5–10	3.3	3.2	0.2			
Bile juice	3	3.4	3.6	0.26	0.13	0.04	0.2
Mucosal secretion	2–4						

secretion of about 9.4 g/day for a horse consuming 10 kg DM of hay. There is only negligible Ca secretion in the stomach (see Table 10-7). However, the acidic environment may have an important role with respect to Ca availability. The Ca compounds that are of nutritive value (not Ca-oxalates) either from plant tissue or from added minerals are readily soluble in acids. As in other animals, the acidic gastric environment leads to dissociation of Ca, forming Ca^{2+} ions. This gastric process has two functions: (a) optimizing the solubility of Ca and thereby its absorption, and (b) modulation of gastric acid secretion via the interaction of Ca^{2+} with Ca-sensing receptors (Ca-sR) and consequent increase in gastrin secretion and gastric acid output. There is some absorption of Ca from the stomach but the majority is absorbed in the small intestine (Schryver et al 1970a, b).

The chronic administration of acid-suppressor drugs like omeprazole has been proposed to decrease Ca absorption in humans (Insogna 2009). Although there are no equine data about this interaction it should be taken as a valid hypothesis that the intensive use of antiacidic drugs will have an impact on Ca absorption. In addition, with respect to the Ca-CasR-gastrin axis, careful evaluation prior to the use of Ca containing mineral supplements is required in order to avoid requirement exceeding intake and vice versa (Shulkes et al 2006).

Ca is secreted in pancreatic juice and bile; the volumes and mineral concentrations are summarized in Table 10-7. Pancreatic Ca secretion is independent of Ca intake but is linked to DM intake (Zebrowska et al 1983). Calcium plays a role in fluid and electrolyte transfer during bile formation. The sensitivity of this function to variations in Ca intake is not known. Cholelithiasis occurs in horses but currently there are no data showing an impact of Ca intake or Ca turnover on this condition.

Absorption

Calcium absorption in the small intestine is driven by a Ca^{2+} concentration gradient in the lumen and occurs by both trans- and paracellular routes. Foals have higher capacity for Ca absorption but there is no further effect of aging on absorptive capacity. As in other species, binding of Ca^{2+} to a Ca-binding protein (Calbindin) is the first step in transport (Fullmer & Wassermann 1972). The expression of this protein has been identified in equine placenta, kidney and the intestinal tract, with highest expression in the duodenum (Rourke et al 2010, Wooding et al 2000). Calbindin expression is probably not regulated by vitamin D as Ca uptake in the horse is thought to be independent of vitamin D (Rourke et al 2010). However, recently published studies showed vitamin D receptors throughout the equine gut and an active transmucosal Ca-transport (Sprekeler et al 2011).

Prececal Ca absorption averages ~60–67% of intake (Meyer et al 1982) whereas total tract absorption varies from -5% to 50%, a lower and wider range when compared to small intestinal absorption. This is because the secretion of Ca into the hindgut is related to the amount of fiber in the diet, which obviously varies between 10–40 mg/kg BW/day (Meyer et al 1982, Schryver et al 1970b).

In contrast to ruminants, there is only a weak adaptation in Ca absorption rate in response to dietary intake. A literature survey (Kienzle & Burger 2012 in press) defined a linear relationship between Ca intake (x) and fecal excretion (y) by the following equation: $y = 32.11 + 0.54x$; $r = 0.79$, $n = 103$; intake and excretion in mg/kg $BW^{0.75}$. From these data, it can be concluded that true digestibility of Ca is ~46%. The Ca : P ratio has no impact on Ca absorption but other factors may reduce Ca absorption. For example, assisted enteral (tube) feeding decreases Ca absorption by ~50% perhaps due to increase rate of intestinal transit (Coenen 1986). Excessive Ca intake (>4-fold of requirement) also reduces the absorption rate (Kienzle & Burger 2012). Feeding fat to horses may negatively affect Ca availability via the formation of Ca salts from unsaturated fatty acids; however, no negative effect of oil feeding on preileal Ca absorption was observed in fistulated animals (Meyer et al 1997). Ca-oxalate is the only naturally occurring Ca compound in feedstuffs that has markedly reduced digestibility. Oxalic acid at >1 % of dietary DM depresses Ca absorption to <10% of intake (Walthall & McKenzie 1976, Swartzman et al 1978, Blaney et al 1981, Hintz et al 1984, Cymbaluk & Christensen 1986, Teleb 1984). Phytic acid, a member of the phosphoinositol family, also forms Ca complexes and limits absorption. Cereals like barley and oats contain up to ~8 g phytate and ~11 g total inositol phosphates per kg DM; these form complexes with P, Ca, Fe, and Zn (Brooks & Lampi 2001). The addition of phytase to the diet improves Ca absorption (van Doorn et al 2004). However, although cereals are high in phytate in typical rations they provide only a minor contribution to total Ca supply. However, the contribution of Ca from the cereal component of the diet can be assumed to be ~10% of the original Ca content. There is no routinely used analytical method for assessment of phytate content.

Ca-excretion

Fecal Ca excretion is linearly related to intake (Fig. 10.5) indicating that absorptive processes do not adapt to differences in Ca intake. Aging also does not appear to affect net absorption (Elzinga, Geor & Harris, personal communication 2011; net absorption, % of intake in mature vs. aged

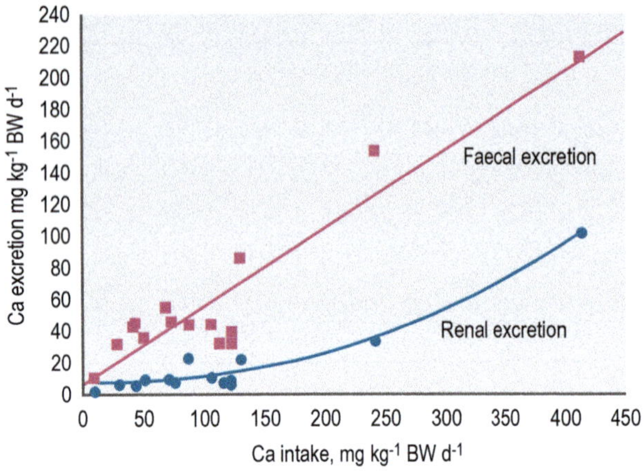

Figure 10.5 A summary of selected literature data on calcium balance in horses.

horses, 44 vs. 47). As there is no intestinal adaptation to counteract high Ca intake, the renal route becomes very important with respect to the elimination of Ca when the absorbed amount exceeds requirements and cannot be stored. As such, the kidney acts as a safety relief valve. Effectively, the Ca concentration in urine reflects intake (although sedimentation within the bladder can influence the content in voided sample) and can increase to levels which can provoke precipitation or even stone formation. Urolithiasis in the equine is mostly associated with the formation of insoluble Ca-compounds (Diaz-Espineira et al 1997, Duesterdieck-Zellmer 2007, Laverty et al 1992) as in other hindgut fermenters like manatees and rabbits (Kamphues 1991, Keller et al 2008). See Chapter 36 for more detail on urolithiasis.

A further veterinary aspect is the effect of glucocorticoid treatment in horses. In a dose dependent manner, horses develop negative Ca balance within few days of glucocorticoid treatment due to elevated fecal and renal losses (Glade et al 1982). Glucocorticoids have also been suggested to reduce the activity of the Ca-binding protein in intestinal mucosa (Glade et al 1982).

Key Points

- The small intestine is the major site for Ca absorption
- Ca absorption is not substantially modified by the level of intake
- Absorbed but not utilized Ca is excreted by the kidney

Regulation of Ca homeostasis

Blood Ca content represents the bound and ionized (Ca^{2+}) fractions. There is no distinct postprandial change in either total Ca or Ca^{2+} concentration despite the rapid flow of Ca into the extracellular fluid due to highly effective homeostatic mechanisms. In response to an increase in circulatory Ca concentrations, the hormone calcitonin (CT) is immediately secreted (Rourke et al 2009) and subsequently interacts with receptors in the gut, kidney and bone, tissues that can act as a Ca sink (Johnston et al 1989, Rourke et al 2009). The CT response is rapid but brief (Johnston et al 1989, Rourke et al 2009). A decrease in circulating Ca stimulates secretion of parathyroid hormone (PTH); the Ca^{2+} set point (the Ca^{2+} concentration at which PTH reaches 50% of its maximum concentration in response to hypocalcemia) for horses is 1.37 mmol/l (Toribio et al 2003) and is higher in comparison to other species. This indicates that feed back signals, mediated by increasing Ca^{2+} have a delayed response with respect to the reduction of PTH secretion in comparison to other species. The action of PTH on bone as well as the fractionation of Ca in blood (47.4% bound to protein, 48.5% ionized, 4.1% complexed Ca; Lopez et al 2006) restricts our ability to understand Ca homeostasis simply through analysis of blood total Ca concentrations.

Vitamin D supplementation can induce an increase in blood Ca, which suggests that there is a link between 1,25 dihydroxycalciferol and Ca homeostasis. The exclusion of vitamin D from the diet coupled with depression of sunlight-dependent activation of this vitamin resulted in bone abnormalities in horses (El Shorafa et al 1979). On the other hand, vitamin D precursors and vitamin D activity itself are very low in horses (Breidenbach et al 1998, Harmeyer & Schlumbohm 2004). Under physiological conditions, vitamin D intake has minimal effect on Ca homeostasis.

Consequences of failures in calcium intake or deranged homeostasis

There is no significant effect of Ca intake on Ca homeostasis (total vs. ionized Ca) in horses in exercise training (Vervuert et al 2002). Reference values for Ca^{2+} are lower for lactating mares and foals in comparison to adults at maintenance (Berlin & Aroch 2009). At low Ca-intakes, PTH mobilizes Ca from bone in order to maintain circulating Ca^{2+} concentration within a narrow range.

A low Ca intake may predispose to tetany, although this condition is rare in horses when compared to dairy cows (Baird 1971, Meijer 1982). Calcium absorption can be impaired by oxalic acid which complexes Ca within the GIT and reduces absorption (Laan et al 2000, Swartzman et al 1978, James & Butcher 1972). A diet providing 1% oxalic acid induced negative Ca balance (Swartzman et al 1978). Rumex species (*Rumex obtusifolius*, *R. crispius*) can contain up to ~10% DM oxalic acid (Panciera et al 1990) and this may be a relevant factor in horses on poorly managed pastures.

Under practical conditions, an imbalanced mineral intake is more likely to have an impact on Ca homeostasis than overt deficiency. A relative Ca deficiency can result from high P intake or a low Ca:P ratio. Primary and secondary hyperparathyroidism are the result of a persistent catabolic stimulus of the Ca-sensing system affecting bone. Even the very early reports of these conditions draw attention to the compensatory enlargement of bones (Brevard 1824, Hornbrook 1826). "Big head disease" or Millers disease still occurs even though we have the knowledge on Ca requirements that should prevent this condition (Luthersson et al 2005, Stewart et al 2010).

Defects in Ca-homeostasis are important for some conditions. A short-term shortage in mobile Ca^{2+} in body fluids can be the result of increased Ca export through milk. Tetanic dysfunction of the muscle in lactating mares can occur towards the peak of lactation (Montgomerie et al 1929, Richardson et al 1991). In the first weeks of lactation, milk Ca is ~1 g/l and is responsible for high losses of Ca from the mare (see Fig. 10.4). The above conditions can be treated or prevented by appropriately adjusting Ca (and P) intake to the increased requirements.

An internal shift in Ca balance via trapping of Ca^{2+} can influence Ca homeostasis. Hypocalcemia (low Ca^{2+}) occurs during exercise due to the binding of Ca^{2+} to protein and/or lactate (Vervuert et al 2002). This can result in conditions such as synchronous diaphragmatic flutter (Carlson & Mansmann 1974, Mansmann et al 1974). The exercise induced drop in Ca^{2+} occurs despite an increase in PTH during physical activity. A two- or threefold increase in Ca intake in comparison to recommendations mitigates the Ca^{2+} nadir during exercise but cannot maintain normocalcemia (Vervuert et al 2006). Decreased ionized Ca has been observed in horses with severe systemic illness (e.g., colic, endotoxemia, sepsis; Garcia-Lopez et al 2001, Delesalle et al 2005, Toribio et al 2001, 2005, 2007, Hurcombe et al 2009). Moreover, persistence of low ionized Ca was associated with poor outcome during treatment of critically ill horses (Delesalle et al 2005, Hurcombe et al 2009). In other species, some inflammatory cytokines have been shown to decrease PTH secretion, and it is possible that a similar mechanism accounts for low Ca^{2+} during inflammatory events in horses.

Key Points

- Blood Ca concentration is not useful for assessment of calcium nutrition
- Exercise results in very little change in Ca requirements
- In case of some disease PTH may not efficiently ensure Ca^{++}-homeostasis but hypocalcaemia is a critical factor for survival

Phosphorus (P)

The total body P content is around 8.6 g/kg (Table 10-8). Similar to Ca, the bulk of body P is in bone (80.8%). Bone ash is about 150–200 g P per kg (Vervuert et al 2010). The P content of bone is age insensitive. Age-related differences in bone composition mostly result from differences in the fat content. Muscle tissue is the second highest ranked tissue with respect to P partitioning in the body but has similar content per gram of tissue to the liver.

Major functions

Phosphorus is required for myriad body functions. For example, P is a component of bone hydroxyapatite and is therefore essential for bone strength. In addition, P is a key constituent of ATP and in the formation of RNA/DNA. Non-osseous body mass shows an inverse Ca:P ratio (e.g., 0.01 in liver and muscle, 0.05 in gut tissue, (Grace et al 1999b). The P concentration inside muscle cells is quite high at 282 mmol/kg DM (in comparison to Ca at 8 mmol/kg DM; Gottlieb-Vedi et al 1996), as would be expected due to the presence of several intracellular P-containing compounds such as enzymes. P is also essential for microbial digestion; low P availability depresses ruminal microbial N-synthesis and digestibility of organic matter and it has been suggested that 75–100 mg P per liter rumen fluid is required to maintain maximum degradative and synthetic microbial activities (Durand et al 1983, Komisarczuk et al 1987a, b, Breves & Schröder 1991). The P concentration in the ileal chyme of the horse is ~0.65 g/kg (Meyer et al 1982) and therefore should provide sufficient amounts for the microbial community. In horses there is substantial P absorption in the hindgut, consistent with other hindgut fermenter species. Hindgut microbes require P but under practical conditions there is no evidence that P can be a limiting resource for large intestinal fermentation.

Requirements

Endogenous losses and other factors important in determining P requirements are summarized in Table 10-8.

Maintenance

The relationship between P intake (x) and fecal losses (y) for adult horses is: $y = 7.18 + 0.85x$ ($r = 0.95$; $n = 265$; data in mg/kg $BW^{0.75}$ per day; Kienzle & Burger 2012). The reported balance data show some differences in the true digestibility related to age (adult 15% vs. young horses 39%).

Pregnancy, lactation, and growth

Lactation increases the P requirement in comparison to maintenance by ~2.8-fold, gestation by ~2.2-fold and growth by ~1.7-fold. The P expenses for lactation vary according to the stage of lactation, described by: P mg/kg milk = 948 − 283 × log day of lactation (for P excretion by milk, see Fig. 10.4) (Coenen et al 2010). The exponential intrauterine growth defines the P budget of the fetus: P g/kg birth weight $= 0.0276e^{0.0178d}$ (d = day of gestation). A constant P concentration is taken for calculating postpartum growth-related requirements. The Ca:P ratio in mare's milk is clearly below 2:1 (see Tables 10-7 and 10-8), which fits with the intensive growth in soft tissues and the delayed gain in bone mass of foals.

Exercise

The enrichment of muscles by mitochondria and other structures bearing P in response to exercise training is accompanied by retention of P in muscle cells (Guy & Snow 1977, Hoppeler 1990, Tyler 1998) and other tissues such as the liver. Regardless of the essential role of P for tissue functions associated with exercise, exercise per se does not appear to be linked to an increased requirement for P. However, young horses entering training need a higher P intake in comparison to maintenance due to tissue growth (bone and muscle). For horses up to the age of 4 years in exercise, the P requirement for yearlings is a reasonable guideline for P supply even if we cannot precisely define the fate of this additional supply.

P balance

Intake

Roughages and grain are more uniform regarding P content when compared to Ca. Forages contain ~3 g P/kg DM but levels are consistently lower in tropical grasses. Parallel to the drop in the leaf:stem ratio during plant growth, both protein and P concentrations decrease if stem mass becomes greater than leaf mass. In such circumstances, P content may fall below 1 g/kg DM. Straw is generally low in P (<1 g/kg DM). Grain typically contains around 3–3.5 g/kg DM. As P is located in the outer layer of the kernel, by-products such as bran are up to threefold higher in P in comparison to the unprocessed grain. The defatted by-products of soy or rape seed and other high fat seeds contain P at 4–10 g/kg DM.

Grouping of feeds with respect to their typical P-concentrations (g/kg DM) is:

Table 10-8 Key Data on Phosphorus in the Equine Body and Requirements

	Item	Unit	Value	Miscellaneous
Distribution				% of total
	Total body	g/kg	8.6	100
	Bone		52.3	81.4
	Muscle		3.1	16.8
	Liver		3.3	0.53
	Kidney		2.4	0.11
	Lung		2.5	0.31
	Heart		2.5	0.20
	GIT		1.2	1.13
	Skin		0.23	0.20
	Blood		0.32	0.21
Products				
	Fetus	g/kg	9.7	
		Total P in pregnant uterus, g/kg birth weight = $0.0276e^{0.0178d}$ Daily total P-accretion in pregenant uterus, g/kg birth weight = $0.00049e^{0.0178d}$ (1)		
	Daily gain	g/kg	8	
	Milk	mg/l	$948–283*\log(10)d$ (2)	
	Lactogenic daily excretion, g/kg $BW^{0.82}$		$0.07d^{-0,02276}e^{-0.00649d}$ (2)	
	Sweat	mg/l	<10	
Balance				
	Endogenous losses	$mg/kg^{0.75}$ BW/day	17	
	Absorption	% of intake	–120–25	prececally
			–120–40	total GIT
	Utilization	% of intake	15 for adults, 35 for foals	
	Main excretion route for surplus		feces + kidney	

[1]day of gestation; [2]day of lactation.
Coenen et al 2010; Coenen & Vervuert 2003; Grace et al 1999a, b; McCutcheon & Geor 1998a; McCutcheon et al 1995b; Meyer 1990, 1987; Meyer & Ahlswede 1976; Kienzle & Burger 2012; GfE 2011.

Grass, roughage	Cereals	Beans rich in protein	By products of:	
			Milling	Oil industry
3	3	5–7	9–11	6–10

The utilization of grain and their by-products in horse rations will significantly elevate P intake when compared to forage-only diets. At the recommended intakes of 80 and 130 g DMI/$kg^{0.75}$ BW for maintenance and lactation, respectively, providing 3 g P/kg dietary DM will result in 1.5-fold higher P supply with respect to maintenance requirements but even at a very high DMI the supply from a diet providing 3 g P/kg DM will be marginal or even deficient for lactating mares.

P secretion and absorption

Secretion

Phosphorus is a constituent of several secretions in the small intestine. This results in a net secretion of P prececally, the extent of which is dependent on the level of roughage intake (Teleb 1984), which increases intestinal secretions. Saliva provides ~20 mg P/l to the preileal P-flux into the gut (Table 10-9). The consumption of 1 kg hay DM is associated with ~6 liters of saliva, which in turn results in saliva-associated P secretion into the gut of 120 mg. Negligible amounts are added by the gastric secretions but the contributions by the pancreatic juice and other secretions in the upper part of small intestine are substantial. Bile secretions are a further source of P (200 mg/l; Meyer 1992). The hindgut also has the capacity for P secretion as well as absorption (Schryver et al 1972); these processes are independent of the dietary Ca:P ratio. However, P absorption in the hindgut determines external P balance (Schryver et al 1972).

Absorption

Prececal absorption is highly negative for rations high in roughage (hay and straw, 24.3 and 9.2 mg P intake per kg BW per day → prececal absorption –120 and –35% of intake) but can result in a gain of ~25% of the intake when concentrates are fed (Meyer et al 1982). Consequently, total tract absorption is highly variable depending on intake and the fiber:concentrate ratio.

In Thoroughbreds with intake of 21–22 g P/day, daily P passage through the lower small intestine and upper large

Table 10-9 Biochemical Data on Equine Saliva (Coenen 1985b, Eckersall 1984)

Constituent	Unit	Value
N	mg/l	440–585
glucose	mmol/l	34
Ca	mg/l	157–465
P	mg/l	20–54
Mg	mg/l	33–50
Na	mg/l	557–1541
K	mg/l	587–711
Cl	mg/l	780–2130
Cu	µg/l	185
Zn	µg/l	773
Fe	µg/l	3426

intestine were, respectively, ~40–60 g and ~83 g (Matsui et al 1999). A benefit of the absorption in the hindgut is that horses are able to utilize phytate phosphorus, which is made available due to microbial breakdown (Matsui et al 1999). Variation in P absorption is dependent on P intake, source and the type of ration and therefore results in an unpredictable renal excretion with regard to modelling nutrient fluxes. Low renal P excretion can be linked to low intake but also to a ration high in roughage (fiber related elevation in ileocecal P flow and fecal P-excretion). A high renal output of P may reflect different conditions: (a) high concentrate diet that provides the bulk of P intake, and (b) the liberation of P from bone in the case of Ca shortage.

Consequences of failures in P intake or deranged homeostasis

Bone is the target tissue for P deposition and mobilization that is reflected by changes in biochemical markers of bone metabolism such as bone alkaline phosphatase, hydroxyproline or osteocalcin (Lepage et al 2001, Price et al 2001). Bone responds to a dietary P shortage even though blood P concentration does not change, and P supply to the tissues will be maintained as long as bone P can be mobilized. There appears to be a strict priority to maintain P homeostasis at the expense of bone strength.

The condition of secondary hyperparathyroidism, formerly called "big head disease", arises from deranged P homeostasis due to a high or excessive P intake coupled with a marginal or even deficient Ca supply. In these circumstances, in order to maintain Ca:P balance in body fluids and cellular compartments PTH secretion induces Ca mobilisation from bone.

Key Points

- Prececally, there is net secretion of P into the gastrointestinal tract via saliva, pancreatic juice and other intestinal secretions
- Ileo-cecal P flux supports the microbial community in the hindgut
- The hindgut is the primary site of P absorption, balancing the high prececal secretion
- P intake above requirements results in increased renal P excretion

Magnesium (Mg)

Major functions

About 60% of Mg is stored in the skeleton and 32% in muscle tissue (Grace et al 1999a). In bone, magnesium is associated with the crystalline structure and its incorporation involves the same regulation as for Ca and P. Most of the Mg outside of bone is located in the intracellular space, associated with specific structures such as mitochondria or substrates such as ATP, RNA, or DNA. Most metabolic processes (e.g., oxidative phosphorylation, protein synthesis) inside the cell require Mg, which is one of the most abundant intracellular cations. Dysfunction of the Mg-dependent ATPase attached to myosin is one of the mechanisms underlying clinical signs of hypomagnesemia. Mg deficiency in horses is linked to bone weakness and abnormal mineralization in soft tissues, in particular the aorta (Harrington 1975).

There is an important interaction of Mg with the immune system that is poorly investigated in the horse and therefore the full impact of Mg nutrition on horse health is unknown. In several species, Mg depletion is associated with an increase in proinflammatory cytokines (Tam et al 2003), while increased plasma nitric oxide and lipid peroxidation in cardiac muscle have been shown in Mg-deficient rats (Bussiere et al 2002). An increase in extracellular fluid Mg concentration may be as deleterious as primary deficiency due to augmentation of apoptosis (Black et al 2001). Uterine flushings from dairy cows with abnormal embryos had higher Mg concentrations in comparison to samples from cows with normal embryos (Lamothe & Guay 1970, Wiebold 1988). Additionally, elevated amniotic fluid Mg concentration has been associated with intrauterine growth retardation (Facchinetti et al 1989). Mg is also important in brain function as it is involved in monoamine neurotransmitter synthesis and receptor binding. Mg is essential for the function of *N*-methyl-D-aspartate-type glutamate receptors that determine memory processing. Mg deficiency therefore should be linked to behavioral consequences. Indeed, studies in laboratory animals show change in fear learning and emotional disruption with Mg deficiency (Bardgett et al 2005). In addition, Mg deficiency has been proposed to play a role in Tourette's syndrome (Grimaldi 2002). There is consensus that Mg deficits induces neurological symptoms if Mg concentrations in the brain and cerebral-spinal fluid are depressed (Morris 1992). On the other hand, very high doses of Mg (e.g., administered IV) induce anesthetic effects.

Mg depletion in horses also has been associated with brain malfunction (MacKay 2004, Stewart 2011, Stewart et al 2004). However, to date there are no published data from well-designed studies to demonstrate that increased Mg intake improves brain function or ameliorates excitability in horses.

Requirements

Maintenance

Fecal and renal losses for Mg are linearly related to Mg intake (x): fecal losses$=12.17+0.54x$ ($r=0.93$, $n=258$); renal losses$=11.69+0.19x$ ($r=0.64$, $n=128$; variables expressed in mg/kg$^{0.75}$ BW/day[1]; Kienzle & Burger 2012). Average endogenous losses are 23.9 mg/kg$^{0.75}$ BW/day and the estimated utilization rate is 46%.

Table 10-10 Key Data on Magnesium in the Equine Body and Requirements

	Item	Dimension	Value	Miscellaneous
Distribution				% of total
	Total body	mg/kg	341	100
	Bone	mg/kg	1420	55.7
	Muscle	mg/kg	250	34.3
	Liver	mg/kg	188	0.77
	Kidney	mg/kg	152	0.17
	Lung	mg/kg	122	0.38
	Heart	mg/kg	244	0.48
	GIT	mg/kg	86	1.86
	Skin	mg/kg	35	0.75
	Blood	mg/kg	157	0.52
Products				
	Fetus	mg/kg	380	
		Total Mg in pregnant uterus, g/kg birth weight = $0.0012e^{0.0173d}$ (1) Daily Total Mg-accretion in pregnent uterus, g/kg birth weight = $0.00002e^{0.0173d}$ (1)		
	Daily gain	mg/kg	400	
	Milk	mg/l	$126–35.5*\log(10)d^{2}$	
		Daily lactogenic Mg-excretion, g/kg $BW^{0.82}$ = $0.0092d^{-0.0111}e^{-0.00627d}$ (2)		
	Sweat	mg/l	50	
Balance				
	Endogenous losses	$mg/kg^{0.75}$ BW/day	24	
	Absorption	% of intake	44–60	Prececally
			22–35	Total GIT
	Utilization	% of intake	46	
	Main excretion route for surplus		Kidney	

[1]Day of gestation; [2]day of lactation.
(Coenen et al 2010; GfE 2013; Coenen & Vervuert, 2003; Grace et al 1999a, b; McCutcheon & Geor, 1998a; McCutcheon et al 1995b; Meyer 1990, 1987; Meyer & Ahlswede 1976; Kapusniak et al 1988; Kienzle & Burger 2012; GfE 2011).

Gestation, lactation, and growth

Gestation and lactation result in substantial increase in Mg requirements (Table 10-10) along with needs for Ca and P. The output of Mg via milk ($mg/kg^{0.82}$ BW/day= $0.0092d^{-0.0111}e^{-0.00627d}$, d = day of lactation (Coenen et al 2010) reflects the time related decline in milk Mg concentration and the change in daily milk volume. A constant Mg concentration in daily gain is used to calculate growth related requirements. The absorption efficiency for suckling foals will be higher than the average figure for adults (see Table 10-9). Currently, the calculated requirement for growth may be overestimated in foals in the first 2 months of life.

Exercise

As for Ca and P, Mg losses via sweat are low. It has been suggested that Mg requirements are elevated by exercise (over and above the small losses in sweat) but accurate balance data to enable estimation of any additional requirement associated with exercise are lacking. Bone and muscle adaptation in early training, in particular in young horses, may induce additional Mg retention and explain the requirements being above maintenance level. As with P, for horses <4 years of age in exercise training it is recommended to provide Mg at the yearling level of intake to ensure adequate Mg supply.

Balance

Intake

Green forages contain higher Mg concentrations in comparison to cereals. The Mg content of seeds high in protein is comparable to forages. The byproducts from oil extraction and milling are good sources of Mg. The average concentrations (g/kg DM) are:

Grass, roughage	Native grain	Seed rich in protein	Byproducts	
			Milling	Oil industry
5–3	1–1.5	2.5	5	3–5.5

Feeding roughage of an average quality should result in Mg intake that will be above requirements even in lactating mares. If additional Mg is required it should be added as a phosphate or chloride because Mg-oxide is poorly absorbed. Organic Mg compounds are highly digestible. High-level supplementation, often in the form of Mg-aspartate, is widely used in the equine industry for the purpose of reducing the excitability of horses; the efficacy of this practice requires experimental confirmation.

Mg secretion and absorption

Mg secretion in the upper GIT is small (see composition of saliva and pancreatic juice) with more substantial secretion in the hindgut. The net absorption of Mg over the entire GIT tract varies between 5% and 60% of intake (Hintz & Schryver 1972, Meyer et al 1982). The small intestine is the primary site of absorption (~45–60%; Meyer et al 1982), and therefore under physiological conditions net Mg secretion occurs in the hindgut. However, Mg can be absorbed in the large intestine if the concentration in the chyme is elevated (e.g., by rectal infusion). A linear relationship between Mg intake (x) and fecal excretion over a wide range of intake (fecal Mg mg/kg BW/d=0.51+0.54+Mg intake, mg/kg BW/day (von Bieberstein 1990)) indicates the independence of absorption from intake. High Mg intake elevates Ca absorption and vice versa (Hintz & Schryver 1973). The surplus ingested Mg is excreted via the urine. The regression equation $y=2.18+0.17x$ (Meyer & Staderman 1990) describes this relationship between Mg intake (x, mg/kg BW/day) and renal output (y, mg/kg BW/day) and has been confirmed in review of literature data (Kienzle & Burger 2012).

Consequences of failures in Mg intake or deranged homeostasis

Total Mg in plasma is between 0.5 and 1.11 mmol/L; ionized Mg varies between 0.38 and 0.63 mmol/l (Berlin & Aroch 2009). In ruminants there is a negative interaction between high dietary protein intake and K plus Mg absorption in the rumen. It is not clear whether the Mg-absorption in the equine hindgut responds to the high ammonia concentration and high K influx. The link of Mg to bone and mitochondria suggests that insufficient Mg supply will affect bone strength and energy metabolism. But the dominant response in all animals to an inadequate Mg intake is poor performance (e.g., growth), increased disease risk due to immune-incompetence and muscle weakness. Animals demonstrate tetanic cramps as the most pronounced clinical sign of hypomagnesemia.

In vitro studies have shown that ^{35}S incorporation into chondrocytes is decreased when they are incubated in Mg-deficient medium (Davenport et al 2001). Mg deficiency therefore might increase risk of orthopedic diseases, particularly in growing horses, but there is no evidence linking Mg nutrition to bone abnormalities. Harrington 1975 reported hypomagnesemia and associated Mg losses from bone when horses were fed a low Mg diet (7–8 mg Mg/kg vs 390 mg Mg/kg as control). In horses with enterocolitis, both hypocalcemia and hypomagnesemia occur in association with low PTH (Toribio et al 2001) suggesting failure of regulatory mechanisms during illness. In healthy animals fed typical diets, blood Mg concentration is an insensitive indicator of Mg intake whereas reduced renal excretion may reflect marginal or deficient Mg nutrition (Stewart 2011, Stewart et al 2004).

Key Points

- The small intestine is the major site for Mg absorption
- The percentage of Mg intake that is absorbed is weakly influenced by Mg intake
- Mg absorbed in excess of requirements is excreted via urine

Electrolytes (Na, K, Cl)

Cell functions require a well controlled water-based environment, the main characteristics of which are a specific acid–base-balance and osmotic condition. The electrolytes sodium (Na), potassium (K) and chloride (Cl) are not exclusively responsible for ensuring such an environment is present, but they are indispensable. The outstanding position of Na and Cl is represented by the central regulation of salt appetite (Geerling & Loewy 2008).

Major functions

The skeleton contains ~51% of the body's Na, while K is found mainly in muscle (75%; Lindner 1983, Gürer 1985). Several tissues contain around 10–15% of total body Cl (Coenen 1991). The key data on body distribution and balance are summarized in Tables 10-11–10-13. Movement of the electrolytes Na, K and Cl across membranes are the major driving forces for the distribution of water and have a significant impact on the electrochemical properties of the body's water compartments. The osmolality of the extracellular water space (ECW) and blood plasma depends mainly on the concentration of these elements. As the most abundant cations and anions, they are major contributors to acid–base balance. Changes in the dietary profile of Na, K and Cl will induce changes in systemic pH and bicarbonate concentrations as well as urinary acidity (Baker et al 1998, 1993, Coenen 1991, Stürmer 2005, Stutz et al 1992, Wall et al 1992). The Na–K pump maintains a large difference in the intra- (K) and extracellular (Na) location of these two cations, and serves other functions regarding the substrate equilibrium in and outside the cell. Further transport functions are linked to Na-symporter systems. For example, iodine transport through the thyroid cell membrane occurs in association with Na. Muscle contraction induces a change in the intracellular/extracellular ratio through liberation of intracellular K and is reflected in an exercise intensity-dependent increase in plasma K concentration. Chloride is the most abundant inorganic anion; Cl homeostasis interacts with bicarbonate retention or excretion in order to maintain systemic acid–base balance. Cl also has a specific role in gastric hydrogen ion secretion (Shulkes et al 2006) and in respiratory CO_2 elimination. Na, K and Cl appear in most secretions in concentrations close to those in blood. Interestingly, these electrolytes have limited flexibility with respect to internal balance as there is no tissue which serves as a depot. On the other hand, there is large flexibility in external balance that is managed via renal retention and excretion depending on intake and utilization (i.e. extra output in milk or sweat). Fecal losses do not respond to these factors see Fig. 10.6A). Increased Na excretion by sweat is mirrored by a reduced renal excretion (Coenen & Vervuert 2003). By this simple strategy, Na homeostasis is maintained over a wide range

Table 10-11 Key Data on Sodium in the Equine Body and Requirements

	Item	Unit	Value	miscellaneous
Distribution				% of total
	Total body	mg/kg	1580	100
	Bone	mg/kg	3000	51.1
	Muscle	mg/kg	369	10.8
	GIT	mg/kg	806	4.3
	Skin	mg/kg	502	8.3
	Blood	mg/kg	1992	10.8
	other organs	mg/kg	1096	2.1
	Ingesta	mg/kg	1082	12.4
Products				
	Fetus	mg/kg	1900	
		Total Na in pregnant uterus, g/kg birth weight = $0.0225e^{0.0133d}$ (1) Daily total Na-accretion in uterus, g/kg Birth weight = $0.0003e^{0.0133d}$ (1)		
	daily gain	g/kg	1.7	
	Milk	mg/l	174	
		Lactogenic daily excretion, g/kg $BW^{0.82} = 0.0120d^{0.1727}e^{-0.00539d}$ (2)		
	Sweat	g/l	2.8	
Balance				
	endogenous losses	$mg/kg^{0.75}$ BW/day	19	
	Absorption	% of intake	40–90	total GIT
		% of ileocecal flow	>92	hindgut
	Utilization	% of intake	72	
	Main excretion route for surplus		kidney	

[1]day of gestation; [2]day of lactation.
Coenen et al 2010; GfE 2013; Coenen & Vervuert, 2003; Grace et al 1999a, b; McCutcheon & Geor, 1998a; McCutcheon et al 1995b; Meyer 1990, 1987; Meyer & Ahlswede 1976; Kapusniak et al 1988; Kienzle & Burger, 2012; GfE 2011.

of intakes and in the face of acute changes in utilization see Fig. 10.6B). This is extremely important in the case of sweat production; the sweat gland is unable to modify sweat Na concentration to any great extent. This is also true for Cl which can reach ~5.5 g/kg sweat and therefore cutaneous Cl losses can add up to ~20% of total body Cl. The actual changes in overall electrolyte homeostasis that occur in the face of such losses are minimal or quite small in comparison to the actual amount lost in the sweat due to the efficiency of renal conservation mechanisms. Fig. 10.6 shows the change in renal Na excretion between rest and exercise. The increase in cutaneous loss (e.g., Cl) is mirrored by a decrease in renal excretion (Fig. 10.7).

Dietary cation–anion balance (DCAB)

As mentioned, Na, K, and Cl are integral to acid-base balance. In general, the cations (in particular K) present an alkalizing potential whereas Cl (anion) acts as an acidifying force. A change in acid-base status must be followed by a response by the renal or respiratory systems (possibly underestimated e.g., breathing frequency 12 vs. 18 min^{-1} for Cl intake at 72 vs. 282 mg/kg BW/day), as most cellular functions require a narrow range in terms of environmental pH. In practical situations, respiratory and renal compensation mechanisms which act to counterbalance any alkalizing or acidifying potential of the diet will be sufficient to maintain an acceptable pH and protect cellular functions in most tissues, including muscle, but potentially not with respect to bone. As shown in laboratory animals and practically applied in dairy cows for the prevention of hypocalcemia, an acidic condition induces collagen synthesis and reduces Ca flux into the tissue but liberates Ca from bone (Bushinsky 1996, Martin-Tereso & Verstegen 2011). The non-deposited or mobilized Ca must then be excreted by the kidney. In the short term, such an acidic environment may be beneficial by helping to increase Ca mobilization from bone but chronic acidemia may lead to deterioration of bone mineral status. Therefore, although dietary N, K, and Cl balance has no influence on mineral absorption (e.g., Ca), dietary supply may impact bone Ca content via effects on acid-base balance. DCAB can influence urine pH and to a lesser extent systemic pH but the extent of any effect appears to depend on the nature of the underlying ration - in particular the amount and type of forage being fed (Coenen 1991, Stutz et al 1992, Wall et al 1992, Schwarzer 1997, Baker et al 1998, Zeyner et al 2002, Waller et al 2004, Stürmer 2005, Kienzle et al 2006, Waller & Lindinger 2007, Berchtold 2009).

Table 10-12 Key Data on Potassium in the Equine Body and Requirements

	Item	Unit	Value	Miscellaneous
Distribution				% of total
	Total body	mg/kg	2090	100
	Bone	mg/kg	652	4.7
	Muscle	mg/kg	3841	75.1
	Git	mg/kg	1843	5.6
	Skin	mg/kg	377	2.6
	Blood	mg/kg	1510	5.0
	Other organs	mg/kg	3094	5.0
	Ingesta	mg/kg	520	4.5
Products				
	Fetus	mg/kg	1900	
		Total K pregnant uterus, g/kg birth weight = $0.0246e^{0.0129d}$ (1) Daily total K-accretion in uterus, g/kg birth weight = $0.00032e^{0.0129d}$ (1)		
	Daily gain	g/kg	1.8	
	Milk	mg/l	659	
		Lactogenic daily excretion, g/kg $BW^{0.82} = 0.044d^{0.1727}e^{-0.00539d}$ (2)		
	Sweat	g/l	1.4	
Balance				
	Endogenous losses	$mg/kg^{0.75}$ BW/day	118	
	Absorption	% of intake	50–95	Total GIT
		% of ileocecal flow	28–44	Hindgut
	Utilization	% of intake	85	
	Main excretion route for surplus		Kidney+feces	

[1]day of gestation; [2]day of lactation.
Coenen et al 2010; GfE 2013; Coenen & Vervuert, 2003; Grace et al 1999a, b; McCutcheon & Geor, 1998a; McCutcheon et al 1995b; Meyer 1990, 1987; Meyer & Ahlswede 1976; Kapusniak et al 1988; Kienzle & Burger, 2012; GfE 2011.

The author believes that there is unlikely to be a long-term effect of high or low DCAB (from typical horse rations) on mineral balance which will adversely affect health or performance. The mobilization of Ca from bone during an induced metabolic acidosis may occur in horses as in other animals (Baker et al 1998); however, weanling horses consuming highly anionic diets were apparently able to compensate with no adverse effect on growth (Cooper et al 2000) although again this may depend on the rations involved. Feeding high amount of NaCl in response to sweat losses (see below) is also unlikely to create side effects on acid base balance at least with well balanced rations providing sufficient intakes of roughage (Romanowski et al 2011).

Key Points

- Regulation of body Na, K, Cl differs markedly from that for the other macro elements with control via the hypothalamus–pituitary–adrenal axis
- Na, K and Cl are major players in the maintenance of the cellular and extracellular environment and are closely involved in substrate exchange between the different compartments
- Reduced renal excretion is the primary response to Na, K and Cl loss via sweat and is essential for maintaining homeostasis

Requirements

Maintenance

Low endogenous losses (see Tables 10-11–10-13) coupled with a high absorption and utilization rates characterize the requirement figures (see Table 10-4). It should be noted that Cl provision accordingly the factorial approach may underestimated the optimal Cl provision as the Cl homeostasis in blood may become weakened associated with an acid-base-response. Most forages contain >6 g Cl/kg DM and will provide Cl highly above the calculated minimal requirement.

Growth and milk production

The concentration of Na, K, and Cl in the products of prenatal and postnatal growth, as well as lactation, have been fairly well determined (see Tables 10-10–10-12).

Exercise

Sweat production is responsible for large changes in the electrolyte requirements of exercising horses. Large amounts of total body Na, K, and Cl can be lost in a relatively short period of time (e.g., up to 25% of the total Cl within 2 hours of exercise with high sweat rate). The losses are linearly related to sweat production and thereby are linked to energy

Table 10-13 Key Data on Chloride in the Equine Body and Requirements

	Item	Unit	Value	Miscellaneous
Distribution				% of total
	Total body	mg/kg	1124	100
	Bone	mg/kg	1067	13.9
	Muscle	mg/kg	560	19.9
	GIT	mg/kg	1618	6.1
	Skin	mg/kg	2886	15.1
	Blood	mg/kg	3109	15.5
	Other organs	mg/kg	1359	15.4
	Ingesta	mg/kg	876	14.1
Products				
	Fetus	mg/kg	1200	
		Total Cl in pregnant uterus, g/kg birth weight = $0.013e^{0.0135d}$ (1) Daily total Cl-accretion in uterus, g/kg birth weight = $0.00018e^{0.0135d}$ (1)		
	Daily gain	g/kg	1.2	
	Milk	mg/l	278	
		Lactogenic daily excretion, g/kg $BW^{0.82} = 0.0183d^{0.1727}e^{-0.00539d}$ (2)		
	Sweat	g/l	5.3	
Balance[3)]				
	Endogenous losses	$mg/kg^{0.75}$ BW/day	14	
	Absorption	% of intake	90	total GIT
		% of intake	>92	hindgut
	Utilization	% of intake	99	
	Main excretion route for surplus		Kidney	

[1]Day of gestation; [2]day of lactation; [3]the Cl intake at the level calculated by the tabled data accordingly the factorial approach is rather low and may affect normochloremia and acid–base balance.
Coenen et al 2010; GfE 2013; Coenen & Vervuert, 2003; Grace et al 1999a, b; McCutcheon & Geor, 1998a; McCutcheon et al 1995b; Meyer 1990, 1987; Meyer & Ahlswede 1976; Kapusniak et al 1988; Kienzle & Burger, 2012; GfE 2011.

metabolism (although fitness and environmental conditions will influence sweating rate and sweat composition changes in a narrow change depending on sweating rate (McCutcheon et al 1995a). Roughly 80–70% of expended energy is transformed into heat and the majority (40–60% of this energy needs to be removed from the body via evaporation, with the remainder eliminated through the respiratory tract (see below, excretion) or stored in body tissues. Modeling of heat balance in the exercising horse can present a rough estimate of sweat volume; however, accuracy of these estimates are questionable due to the impact of environmental factors as well as sweat losses after exercise.

Electrolyte balance

Intake

Na is low in most feeds of plant origin; cereals and forages contain Cl at 4–8 g/kg DM while K varies between <10 (cereals) and >20 g/kg (forages). The constituents of equine diets provide the following typical amounts of electrolytes (g/kg DM):

	Grass, roughage	Native grain	Seed rich in protein	By products	
				Milling	Oil industry
Na	<1	<1			
K	>20	4–8	8–12	10–13	12–20
Cl	4–8	<1–1.5	1–1.5	1–1.5	0.4–1

Secretion and absorption

Secretion A production rate of 6 liters saliva per kg of ingested hay corresponds to 6, 3.6, and ~12 g of salivary output of Na, K, and Cl, respectively (Meyer et al 1986). For Na and Cl, there is high net prececal secretion; both are effectively absorbed in the hindgut and net absorption over the entire GIT is ~95% (Meyer et al 1982, Coenen 1991). Recent work, however, has suggested that Na has a lower overall digestibility than Cl (which means effectively that adding NaCl to the diet can have an acidifying effect under certain circumstances) (Kienzle & Burger 2012, Stürmer 2005). In contrast to Cl, K is absorbed in the small intestine (~52–74%, Meyer et al 1982) and a net secretion occurs in the hindgut so that total tract net absorption varies but is typically <50%. The fecal output of Na and Cl is independent of

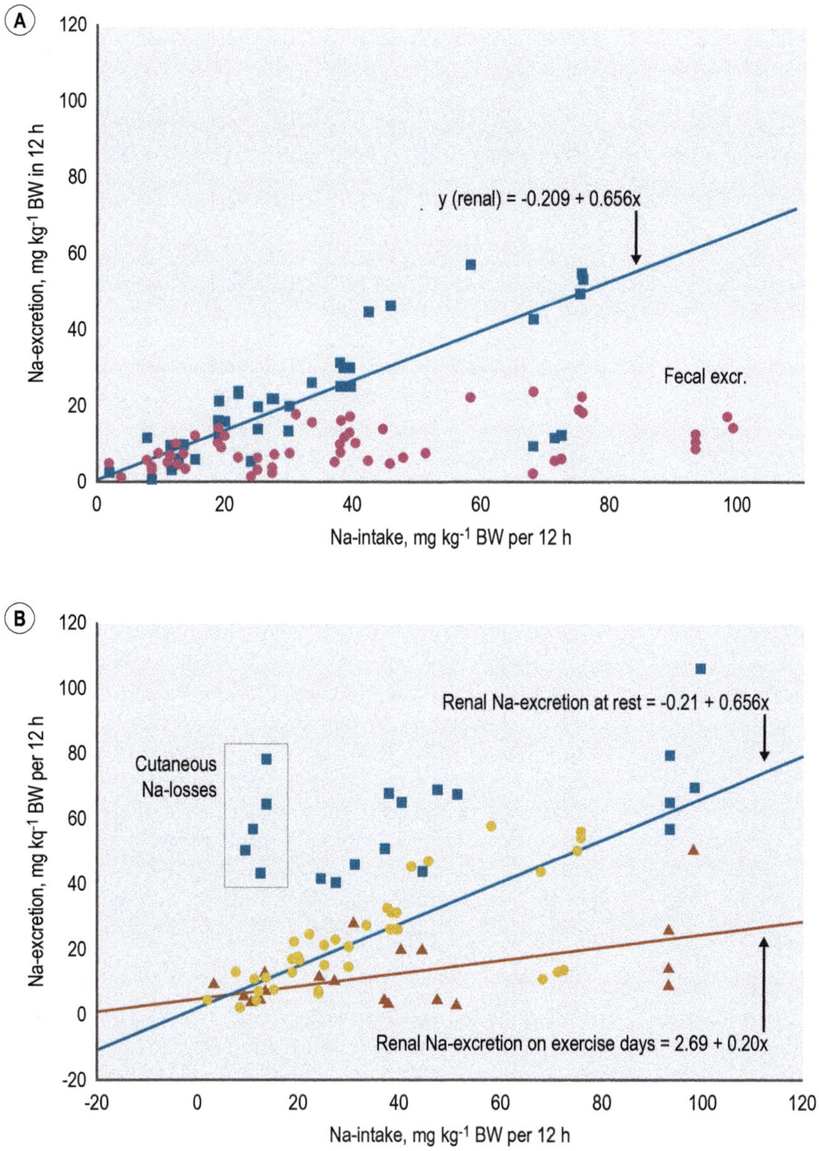

Figure 10.6 Na losses by feces, urine and sweat according to intake.
Coenen & Vervuert, 2003.

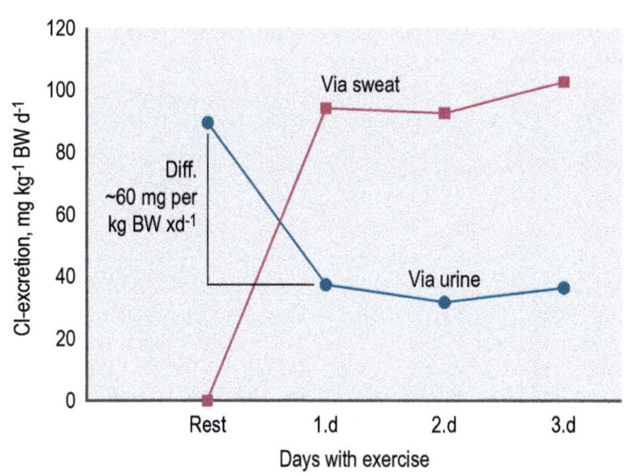

Figure 10.7 Changes in the route of Cl-excretion in response to exercise and related sweat production.
McKeever et al 2002.

intake whilst fecal K excretion increases to a limited extent with increasing intake. For all three electrolytes there exists a strong relationship between intake and renal excretion (Coenen 1991, Meyer & Stadermann 1990). Modification of renal output is the main adaptation to high or low intakes; the following models describe renal output as a function of metabolic body weight (Kienzle & Burger 2012):

Renal output, mg/kg$^{0.75}$ BW/day for

$$Na = 43.3 - 0.1345x + 0.0013x^2; r = 0.88, n = 191$$
$$K = 65.15 + 0.72x; r = 0.99, n = 200$$
$$Cl = 155.9 + 0.176x + 0.0006x^2; r = 0.80, n = 51$$

where x = intake, mg/kg$^{0.75}$ BW/day

A change in renal electrolyte excretion is an essential response to counteract sweat losses (see Figs 10.6 and 10.7). But two points need to be considered: 1. Electrolyte intake must be above maintenance level in order to enable the kidneys for electrolyte saving activity for restoration of the body electrolyte pool; and 2. Within a short period the kidney cannot compensate 100% of cutaneous losses by the mentioned electrolyte saving mechanisms but will need 2 or 3 days.

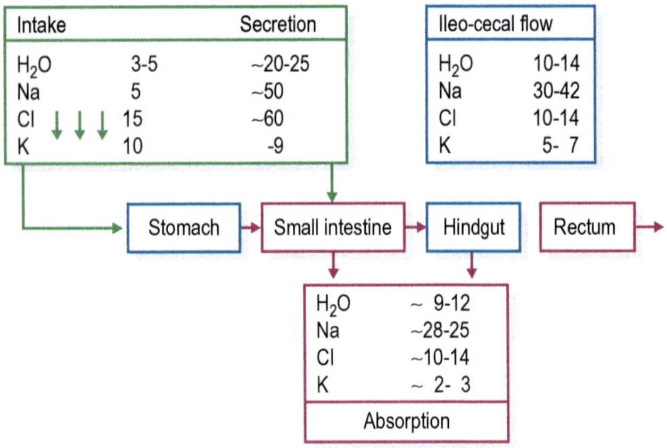

Figure 10.8 Daily intestinal flow rates for water and electrolytes in horses. Water in liters, electrolytes in g per 100 kg BW.
Data from Meyer & Coenen, 2002.

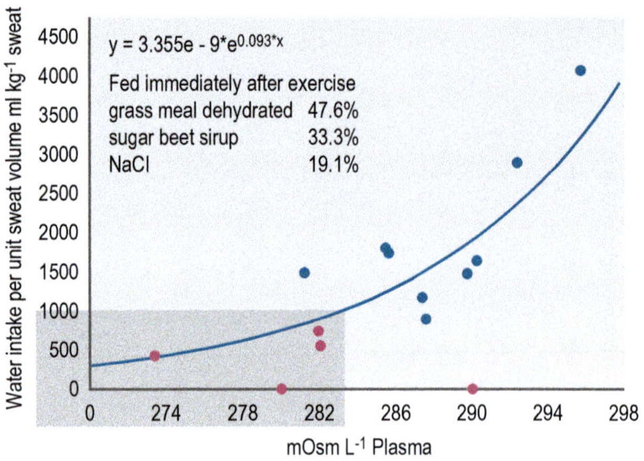

Figure 10.9 Water intake per unit of sweat volume in relation to plasma osmolality modified by provision of a salty feed immediately after exercise.

In summary, there is substantial exchange of water and electrolytes along the intestine (Fig. 10.8). Although there is capacity for electrolyte absorption in the small intestine, the high ileocecal flow of electrolytes is dealt primarily through very effective absorption in the hindgut and therefore fecal losses are quite low (except for K as the net absorption of this cation is lower in comparison to Na and Cl). Diarrhea will therefore induce large increases in fecal electrolyte losses. In contrast to the condition in ruminants, in case of diarrhea the horse is faced by high K deficits in addition to those for Na and Cl. In horses with castor oil induced diarrhea, the deficits were calculated at 108, 143, and 384 mmol Na, K, and Cl respectively per liter water deficit (Ecke et al 1998a, b, 1997), assuming that fecal Cl losses change in the same manner as Na losses do (4% via urine, 96% by feces). Horses with diarrhea should be provided rather high amounts of K (e.g., 1:1 NaCl/KCl or KCl/$NaHCO_3$ or KCl/$KHCO_3$, 30 g every 6 h; Schott 1998).

Consequences of failures in electrolyte intake or deranged homeostasis

Inadequacy of Na intake is quite common in equines. The most likely sign in the case of Na deficiency is poor performance as well as increased licking and searching for salty substances including urine. These clinical signs have been reported with experimental Na or Cl deficiency (Lindner 1983) as well as anecdotally. Such signs are not specific for NaCl deficiency as a K deficit (but not Cl deficit) also induces such behavior (Gürer 1985, Coenen 1991). As Cl concentrations are quite high in most feeds in comparison to Na, Cl deficiency is unlikely to occur in association with a Na deficit. In fact, Cl and K deficits are rare under natural conditions providing adequate amounts of forages are fed (there is an increased risk of such deficits in racehorses when low intakes of hay are replaced on a weight basis with haylage). However, diarrhea and heavy exercise may result in marked Cl and K deficits (see hypochloremia in endurance horses).

A hyponatremic state induces salt appetite. This is the product of a complex neuroendocrine response to suboptimal Na homeostasis as well as a deficit in plasma and ECW volumes (Geerling & Loewy 2008). A deranged distribution and quantity of body water and of osmolality outside and inside of cells will affect energy metabolism and neuronal communication between tissues. In contrast to a Na or K deficit, losses in Cl are associated with a stronger impact on acid-base balance. A Cl deficit induces metabolic alkalosis, as in other animals (Coenen 1991). Disrupted transmembrane electrolyte distribution and electrochemical gradients will damage cellular energy metabolism and the alkalotic condition results in loss of cellular respiration and protein turnover. This explains how an electrolyte deficit disrupts glycogen utilization and restoration in exercising horses (Lindinger & Heigenhauser 1991, Lindinger et al 1990, Mainwood & Renaud 1985, Waller & Lindinger 2007, Waller et al 2009).

Sweating can result in large electrolyte and water losses (Coenen 2005, Coenen & Vervuert 2003, Flaminio & Rush 1998, Lindinger 1999, McCutcheon & Geor 1996, 1998b, 2000, McCutcheon et al 1999, McCutcheon et al 1995a, McKeever 1998, McKeever et al 1993, Nyman et al 1996, Williamson et al 1996). Horses may not adequately replace the water and electrolyte deficit as these losses are approximately isotonic and therefore there is minimal change in ECW osmolality. However, feeding salt post-exercise will increase in ECW osmolality and effectively induce water consumption (Fig. 10.9). The threshold value is close to 283 mOsm (Coenen 1991).

Key Points

- The electrolytes (Na, K and Cl) are involved in maintaining water distribution between the fluid compartments, and a safe osmotic condition inside and outside the cell. In addition, their movement across membranes is associated with the transport of certain substrates e.g., glucose.
- Forage based diets provide sufficient intakes of K and Cl but not of Na.
- Exercise increases the requirement for electrolytes substantially. This requires specific dietary supplementation of Na and Cl .
- Renal excretion is linearly linked to electrolyte intake.
- The impact of electrolytes, in particular Na and Cl, on plasma osmolality contributes to thirst inducing mechanisms.

Sulfur (S)

Major functions

S at ~1.5 g/kg BW is found in all tissues (Table 10-14) as an organic substrate mostly associated with the S-containing amino acids methionine and cysteine. This explains the absence of a S reservoir in the body aside from body protein. As Ingenbleek and Young (2004) noted "N and S metabolism is closely interwoven throughout both the plant and animal kingdoms". In mammals, the S:N ratio is ~1:14.5 (Ingenbleek 2006). At a body S content of 1490 mg/kg BW (Table 10-14) in the horse, this corresponds to 21.6 g N or 135 g protein/kg BW. The adjustment of the urinary S:N ratio in response to the composition of feed intake reflects the tight link between S and N metabolism and the importance of the renal route for excretion (Sherman & Hawk 1900, Wilson, 1925, 1926).

S is essential for the formation of disulfide bonds in keratin that enable tertiary protein folding and thus ensure the unique strength of the hoof capsule: hardness of >70 on the Shore D scale on one hand and flexibility on the other. Minerals comprise about 5% keratin and S is present at ~15 g per kg horn DM, which means that keratin contains the most S of any tissue of the body (Table 10-15). This S-dependent organization of proteins is present in other

Table 10-14 Key Data on Body Sulfur Composition and Balance

	Item	Unit	Value	Miscellaneous
Distribution				% of total
	Total body	mg/kg	1490	100
	Bone	mg/kg	1282	11.5
	Muscle	mg/kg	2250	70.5
	GIT	mg/kg	941	4.6
	Skin	mg/kg	628	3.12
	Blood	mg/kg	1079	4.07
	Other organs	mg/kg	1918	2.5
	Ingesta	mg/kg	4000	3.73
Products				
	Fetus	mg/kg	*1750*	*Assumption*
		Total S in pregnant uterus. g/kg birth weight = $0.0657e^{0.001d}$ Daily total S-accretion in uterus, g/kg birth weight = $0.00099e^{0.001d}$ (1)		
	Daily gain	g/kg	*1.75*	*Assumption*
	Milk	mg/l	241	
		Lactogenic daily excretion, g/kg $BW^{0.82}$ = $0.0159d^{0.1727}e^{-0.00539d}$ (2)		
	Sweat	g/l	traces	
Balance				
	Endogenous losses	mg/kg BW/day	13	
	Absorption	% of intake	30–80	small intestine
		% of intake	hindgut neglectable	
		% of intake	81	total GIT
	Utilization	% of intake	*70*	*Assumption*[3]
	Main excretion route for surplus		feces+kidney	

[1]Day of gestation; [2]day of lactation; [3]as S is metabolized along with S-containing amino acids a figure for the likely utilization of protein and amino acids respectively is used here;
Original data which are expressed per kg empty body weight (EBW) are transferred to BW assuming that EBW is BW×0.85; the mineral in EBW is used for the fetus and daily gain unless it has been differently stated
Coenen et al 2010; GfE 2013; Coenen & Vervuert 2003; Grace et al 1999a, b; McCutcheon & Geor, 1998a; McCutcheon et al 1995b; Meyer 1990, 1980, 1987; Meyer & Ahlswede, 1976.

Table 10-15 Mineral in Equine Hoof Horn (Wall of the Hoof Capsule; Coenen 2012)

S	Cl	Ca	P	Mg	Na	K	Cu	Zn	Fe	Mn	Se
g/kg DM		mg/kg DM									
19.1	3.7	551	240	137	637	957	5.8 (5.4)[1]	155 (171)	567	1.7	0.23 (0.24)

[1]Data for damaged hoof horn (Coenen & Spitzlei 1996a).

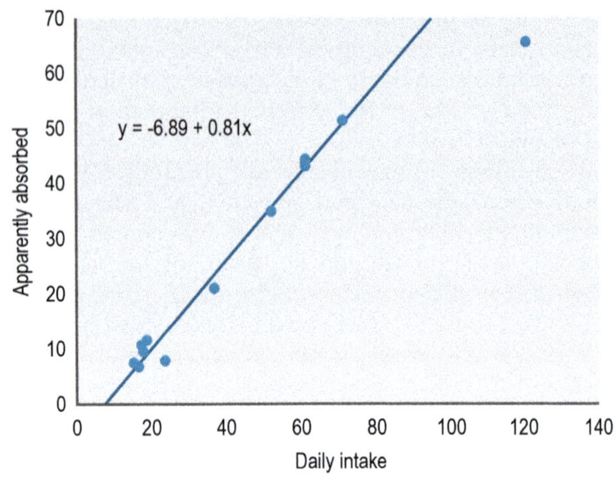

Figure 10.10 Absorbed S as a function of S intake. mg/kg BW/day; data from Grace et al 2002, 2003, Crozier et al 1997, Baker et al 1998; 121 mg intake and the corresponding absorption of 66 mg are excluded from regression analysis based on the published means of 79 balance trials.

cells, notably muscle. Feed composition and DM digestibility affect S levels in the intestinal contents; published data for the colon vary between 3.8 and 5.3 g/kg DM (Hassel et al 2004, 2009); 4 g/kg DM has been taken as the ingesta contribution to total body S in Table 10-14.

Requirements

The endogenous losses for S are not well defined. Digestion trials have yielded estimated fecal losses of 7.9–55.6 mg/kg BW/day (Fig. 10.10) while renal excretion varies between 3.9 and 8.6 mg/kg BW/day (Baker et al 1998) over a wide range of intakes (18.4–121.3 mg/kg BW/day). Assuming obligate renal losses of 6 mg/kg BW/day, total endogenous S losses can be estimated at 13 mg/kg BW/day. This combined with an assumed digestibility of 70% results in a maintenance requirement of 18.6 mg/kg BW/day. Using the S:N-ratio of 1:14.5, the calculated protein requirement is 1.7 g/kg BW/day, which is quite high; consequently the S requirement for maintenance may be overestimated.

Data on the composition of weight gain as well as growth of the conceptus and milk output enable S requirements to be estimated under different circumstances. Exercise associated protein catabolism and the breakdown of S-containing proteins such as glutathione peroxidase will result in increased S requirements for exercise even though sweat losses are negligible. Typically the increased feed intake associated with exercise will ensure an adequate S intake.

S balance

Intake

The S content of roughages varies according to the plant and its protein content (e.g., clover>grass) and the level of any artificial fertilization. Industrial activity can result in S transfer into crop production but normally S content rarely exceeds 4 g/kg DM. Any increase in crop protein content requires S fertilization and therefore high plant protein is in general linked to elevated S concentrations. The protein rich by-products from oil seeds are highest in S. The grouping of feeds according to S concentrations (g/kg DM; McDowell 2003) is:

Grass, roughage	Native grain	Beans rich in protein	By products	
			Milling	Oil industry
2–4	1–3	2–3	3–7	4–8

Absorption and excretion

As almost the total mass of S is ingested through S-containing plant protein, it can be concluded that S digestibility is a function of protein digestion and that the small intestine is the major site of S absorption (mainly as SO_4). Total tract apparent digestibility is 81% (Fig. 10.10). Overconsumption of S will be regulated by renal excretion, partly as Ca-sulfate (Diaz-Espineira et al 1995, 1996, Neumann et al 1994), which may increase the risk for the formation of uroliths, particularly when combined with overconsumption of Ca. Theoretically, the presentation of SO_4^{2-} to body water compartments should result in an acidifying effect but the type of ration (roughage vs. grain) has a dominant influence and may mask any potential impact of SO_4^{2-} on acid–base balance (Berchtold 2009).

Consequence of deficient S intake or deranged homeostasis

A deficiency in S is unlikely even in the absence of mineral supplementation by reason of the average S content in forages. The estimated maintenance requirement of 18.6 mg/kg BW/day is met by 1.86 g S/kg dietary DM even if DM intake is lowered to 1% of BW.

Marginal S-supply may occur in extensive feeding regimes based on forage with low protein (e.g., straw) or in periods of feed restriction for reduction of body weight. However no specific clinical signs are reported to be linked to S-shortage. One can conclude that hoof horn growth may be impaired and likely semen quality.

Trace elements

The quantity of knowledge on trace elements as a part of nutrition is lower in comparison to the macroelements and in contrast to the large volume of research in human and animal nutrition. Recent work in other species has revealed previously unknown or underestimated roles of trace elements in metabolic processes: e.g., iron or copper uptake during fetal development affects mental capacity of the offspring; e.g., the renewed interest in the interaction between chromium and insulin (Gambling & McArdle 2004, Mertz et al 1965, Wiernsperger & Rapin 2010).

All trace elements have the potential to be toxic. The tolerance of animals depends on the natural availability of the elements. For elements with limited natural resource (e.g., Se) there is no mechanism to counter nutritional excess. In contrast, for more available elements such as iron, animals have developed mechanisms to enable adjustment in the face of oversupply.

The factorial method for calculating requirements (using data on endogenous losses and rate of utilization) is successfully practiced for most nutrients but not established for trace elements due to a lack of data. However, for some elements preliminary estimates are presented here in order to derive recommendations for trace element provision. These data should be used cautiously as they remain incomplete (Table 10-16).

Iron (Fe)

Major functions

Blood, muscle and spleen together contain ~3/4 of the horse's body iron, similar to the reported data in humans (Munoz et al 2009). Fe is associated with: (1) the oxygen transport proteins hemoglobin and myoglobin; (2) the Fe-storing structures ferritin and hemosiderin; and (3) a small fraction is found in enzymes (Crichton & Ward 2003). A large proportion of the Fe in liver and spleen is located in macrophages and for this reason Fe is linked to immune defense mechanisms. The primary biological function of Fe is its contribution to oxygen transport. As a constituent or activator of enzymes (e.g., succinate dehydrogenase and

Table 10-16 Basic Data on Iron, Copper, Zinc, Manganese and Selenium in Horses
(a) Tissue concentrations and distribution of total body trace element (means of different publications are weighted by number of observations for presented tissue data)

	Concentration, mg kg^{-1} tissue DM									
	Fe		Cu		Zn		Mn		Se	
Muscle	204		21.55		115.0		2.421		0.2668	
Bone	81		6.62		92.3		4.612		*0.2000**	
Skin	60		6.03		16.9		3.900		*0.2000**	
Hair	55		3.47		69.7		3.840		1.1000	
Hoof	56		4.84		185.5		3.000		0.2289	
Gut	80		6.15		64.0		2.600		*0.2000**	
Blood	2381		4.31		4.5		*1.000*		*0.2000**	
Blood plasma, mg/l	2		1.33		0.9		1.119		0.1028	
Liver	558		27.46		287.3		6.013		0.8465	
Lung	415		8.20		76.6		0.997		*0.2000**	
Heart	179		17.75		108.4		1.600		0.2652	
Spleen	3091		5.72		111.9		1.769		*0.2000**	
Kidney	321		37.75		262.2		4.389		2.0905	
Pancreas	*300**		9.80		178.0		4.700		*0.5000**	
Brain	61		8.71		56.8		1.724		*0.2000**	
Spinal cord										
Thyroid gland	*300**		4.20	17	317.0	17	3.400	17	*0.2000**	

	Distribution by different tissues in mg/kg or µg/kg BW and % of total									
	Fe		Cu		Zn		Mn		Se	
	mg	%	µg	%	mg	%	µg	%	µg	%
Muscle	19.51	32.12	2065	65.97	11.02	46.71	231.90	27.91	25.56	42.46
Bone	7.79	12.82	640	20.43	8.92	37.82	445.55	53.63	19.32	32.10
Skin	1.02	1.68	103	3.30	0.29	1.23	66.86	8.05	3.43	5.70
Hair	0.05	0.08	3.1	0.10	0.06	0.27	3.46	0.42	0.99	1.64
Hoof	0.20	0.33	17.4	0.56	0.67	2.83	10.80	1.30	0.82	1.37
Gut	0.83	1.36	63.5	2.03	0.66	2.80	26.86	3.23	2.07	3.43
Blood	21.96	36.15	39.8	1.27	0.04	0.18	9.22	1.11	1.84	3.06
Liver	2.21	3.64	109	3.48	1.14	4.83	23.85	2.87	3.36	5.58
Lung	1.09	1.79	21.5	0.69	0.20	0.85	2.62	0.32	0.53	0.87
Heart	0.28	0.47	28.1	0.90	0.17	0.73	2.53	0.30	0.42	0.70
Spleen	5.55	9.13	10.3	0.33	0.20	0.85	3.18	0.38	0.36	0.60
Kidney	0.21	0.35	24.9	0.80	0.17	0.73	2.89	0.35	1.38	2.29
Pancreas	0.01	0.02	0.3	0.01	0.01	0.02	0.15	0.02	0.02	0.03

Table 10-16 *Continued*

(a) Tissue concentrations and distribution of total body trace element (means of different publications are weighted by number of observations for presented tissue data)

	Concentration, mg kg^{-1} tissue DM									
	Fe		Cu		Zn		Mn		Se	
Brain	0.03	0.05	4.5	0.14	0.03	0.12	0.88	0.11	0.10	0.17
Spinal cord										
Thyroid	0.00	0.01	0.06	0.00	0.005	0.02	0.05	0.01	0.003	0.00
Not defined										
Total quantity in mg/kg total BW										
a)[1]	60.75		3.13		23.59		0.831		0.06	
b)[2]	*94.96*		*3.25*		29.51		0.971			

*Assumptions without data from literature.
[1]Sum of quantities defined in the column above.
[2]Data from literature given directly as mg/kg BW.

(b) Concentration in products, absorption, endogenous losses and estimated utilization rate

	Fe	Cu	Zn	Mn	Se
Fetus mg/kg[2]	85–118	3.8–5.0	21–42	0.7–1.3	0.06
Milk, mg/kg [3]	0.7	0.3	2.0	0.03	0.032
Endogenous losses, mg/kg BW/day	0.09	0.035	0.16	0.11[0.27][3)]	0.63*
Absorption, side	SI[1]	SI	SI	SI	SI
Absorption, % of intake – prececally – total GIT	 12[4]	 30–50 36[4]	 4–49 32[4]	 18–44 32[4][37][3]	 59[4]
Utilization % of intake	10	30	30	30	25
Route for excretion	Bile/feces				Feces+kidney

*For Se µg/kg BW/day.
[1]small intestine; [2]for accretion in conceptus see Meyer & Ahlswede (1976); for output via milk see Coenen et al (2010); [3]data in brackets from Pagan (2001); [4]taken from the following equation ($y = a + bx$) predicts fecal losses as a function of intake, mg (for Se µg/kg BW/day:
Fe $y = 0.0880 + 0.883x$; $r = 0.995$; Cu $y = 0.0084 + 0.638x$; $r = 0.852$; Zn $y = 0.1509 + 0.643x$; $r = 0.951$; Mn $y = 0.1036 + 0.683x$; $r = 0.843$; Se $y = 0.4221 + 0.410x$; $r = 813$; 1 minus value for parameter b from these equations = absorption
Crozier et al 1997; Cymbaluk et al 1981a, 1981b; Grace et al 1999b, 2002, 2003; Meyer et al 1982; Ordakowski-Burk et al 2006; Pagan 2001; Rieker et al 2000; Schryver et al 1980, 1986; Staniar et al 2010; Wagner et al 2010.

tryptophan peroxidase-oxidase), Fe is also a driving force for multiple metabolic functions. As a component of lactoferrin, Fe is essential for the bacteriocidal activity in the mammary gland and the transfer of an effective bacteriocidal capacity to the newborn.

The recently discovered hormone hepcidin has a key role in the regulation of Fe uptake and distribution (Anderson et al 2009, Munoz et al 2009, 2010, Theurl et al 2009, Zafon et al 2011). Upregulation of hepcidin reduces Fe absorption and increases sequestration of Fe in macrophages. Hepcidin is increased by high Fe intake but also by inflammatory cytokines, in part explaining the anemia that develops with chronic inflammatory conditions (Agarwal & Prchal 2009, Borges et al 2007). The interaction between inflammation and Fe metabolism has been reported in humans with obesity or metabolic syndrome (Mojiminiyi et al 2008, Zafon et al).

Intake, absorption and requirements

A typical equine diet will provide >100 mg Fe per kg DM. Higher levels are common due to soil contamination of grass or other forages (Table 10-17). The latter is mainly associated with Fe^{3+}, which has limited bioavailability. Plants store Fe as ferritin which has higher availability (Schümann & Elsenhans 2004). Gastric acidification transforms ingested Fe into a soluble form prior to entry to the small intestine, the main site of absorption (Meyer et al 1982). Data from horse studies indicates an apparent absorption rate over the entire GIT of 20% (Fig. 10.11).

Fe uptake by enterocytes is driven by the divalent metal transporter 1 (DMT1); this protein is involved in the uptake of other elements as well (Munoz et al 2010). The Fe-laden enterocytes are sloughed and phagocytized, thereby ensuring the transfer of the incorporated Fe^{2+} to the circulation. In blood, Fe transportation requires association with a transport protein. In theory, intestinal uptake should be a function of Fe intake as hepcidin works to lower absorption if the Fe status of the animal is sufficient and vice versa. Excessive Fe intake may overwhelm the regulation of Fe-absorption; however, providing 50 mg Fe/kg BW/day to ponies resulted in an increase in tissue iron content but no adverse clinical effects were observed (Pearson & Andreasen, 2001). As renal output is negligible in healthy subjects (Schryver et al 1986), absorbed Fe must be transferred to physiological stores

Table 10-17 Ranges for Trace Elements in Groups of Feedstuffs (McDowell 2003)

	Grass, roughage	Native grain	Seeds high in protein	Byproducts from grain processing oil industry	
Fe	>100	>30–100	>150	>150	>150
Cu	4–8	6–9	10->20	>20	>20
Zn	>20	15–40	40–50	>100	>40
Mn	>30	30–40	40–60	>100	>100
Se	<0.1	0.2–0.3		0.3–0.4	0.3–0.4
J	0.05–0.1	<0.1	<0.1	0.1–0.15	0.1–0.3
Co	0.1–0.3	<0.1		0.1–0.15	0.1–0.13

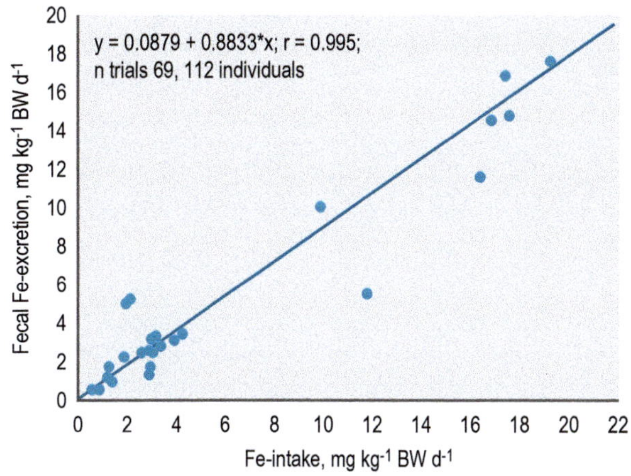

Figure 10.11 Literature data illustrating the relationship between fecal Fe excretion and Fe intake.
Crozier et al 1997; Cymbaluk et al 1981a, b; Meyer et al 1982; Ordakowski-Burk et al 2006b; Rieker et al 2000; Schryver et al 1980; Staniar et al 2010; Wagner et al 2010 plus adapted data from Rieker et al (2000).

(potentially as ferritin in the spleen). However, there is a limit with respect to tolerated Fe accumulation (Puls 1994).

Turnover of heme-carrying cells, mostly erythrocytes, liberates Fe which is in part "recycled" during erythropoiesis. Unused or liberated Fe^{2+} is excreted via bile which helps to avoid the oxidative stress that would occur with Fe^{2+} accumulation. Hepatic hemochromatosis is characterized by high tissue Fe and occurs as a consequence of primary hepatopathy; hemochromatosis is unlikely to occur as a result of Fe overconsumption (Pearson & Andreasen 2001, Pearson et al 1994). However, there is likely a risk of excessive Fe supply possibly enforced by mucosal damage and related loss in control of absorption (e.g., inflammatory bowel disease); in particular Fe provision to foals and Fe injections are reported to cause Fe toxicosis (Lavoie & Teuscher 1993, Lewis & Moyer 1977, Mullaney & Brown, 1988).

In general, 50 mg Fe/kg dietary DM (50 ppm) is appropriate for horses. The data presented in Fig. 10.13 show that balance becomes zero at 1.23 mg/kg BW/day; this results in 615 mg/d for a 500 kg horse which is close to the 50 ppm (assuming 12 kg DM intake).

The increased turnover (shorter half-life) of erythrocytes provides a basis for the recommended higher requirement in horses in athletic training. The increased requirement should be covered by the higher DM intake, particularly in view of the fact that many rations contain >100 ppm Fe. Milk yield and growth results in additional Fe requirements; however the Fe requirement for late gestation is not well defined. In the fetus, erythropoiesis may approach maximum during the last few weeks of gestation, perhaps justifying a higher Fe requirement for mares in late gestation. However, insufficient data are available to provide precise recommendations. It is known from laboratory animals that an increase in intestinally localized transport protein expression and a decrease in hepcidin occur maternally in late gestation (Millard et al 2004). However, Fe deficiency is unlikely to occur when >100 ppm Fe is fed with DM intake >1.5% BW.

Additional iron supplementation

There is little rationale for additional Fe supplementation providing horses are fed diets with at least 50 ppm Fe. There is no evidence of an increase in erythropoiesis with Fe supplementation. In humans, Fe supplementation of patients with Fe deficiency can result in small intestinal bacterial overgrowth (Fe is rate-limiting for bacterial growth).

Key Points

- Fe absorption is strictly regulated in response to intake and tissue requirements, and this is influenced by the hormone hepcidin. However, excessive Fe supply can overwhelm regulatory mechanisms.
- Forage based diets will provide sufficient amounts of Fe
- Most mineral supplements contain Fe in an available form; however, the feeding of additional Fe is generally not recommended

Copper (Cu)

Major functions

The equine body contains ~3.2 mg Cu/kg BW (±1.36, n=90 (Grace et al 1999b, Meyer & Ahlswede 1976, Schryver et al 1974); ~3/4 of total Cu is present in muscle, liver and blood. The high Cu concentration in liver (~20 mg/kg DM) reflects the importance of this organ for Cu processing. Liver is the most important site of Cu storage but, as a consequence, also the tissue most susceptible to toxicity. Cu is involved in multiple cellular functions, e.g., hemoglobin formation, myelination of neurons; keratin synthesis; bone formation. The Cu:Ca ratio in the metaphysis is constant throughout prenatal maturation but declines over this period in the epiphysis (Fig. 10.12). Obviously, the requirement for Cu to

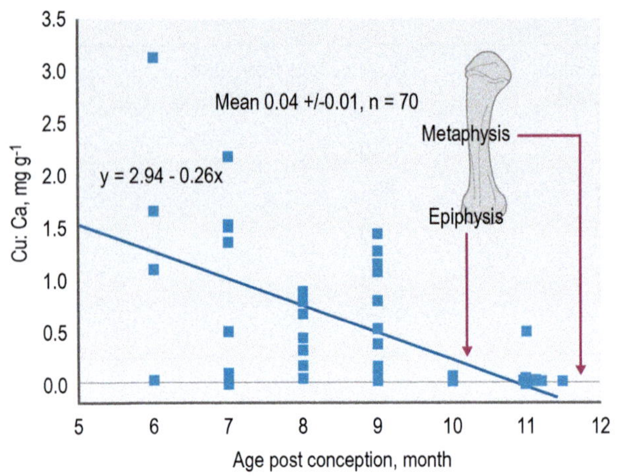

Figure 10.12 The ratio of Cu:Ca throughout gestation in fetal bone in different locations. Hebeler (1996).

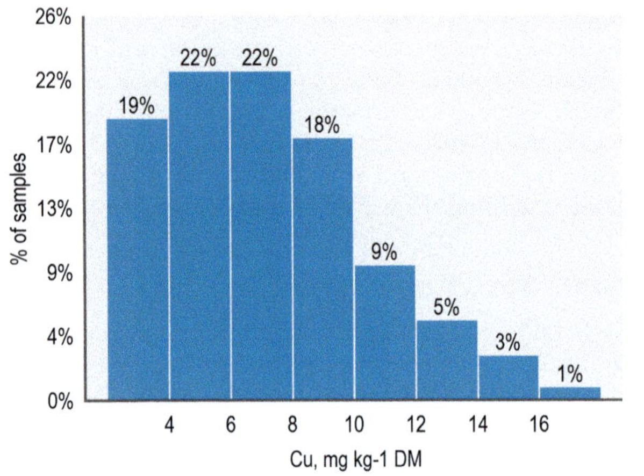

Figure 10.13 Distribution of Cu-concentrations in grass, grass silages and hay.

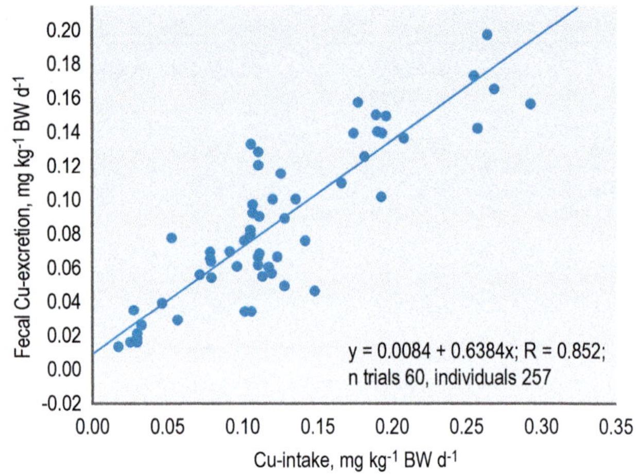

Figure 10.14 Fecal excretion of Cu in dependence on Cu intake.

(Coger et al 1987; Crozier et al 1997; Cymbaluk et al 1981a, b; Ducharme et al 1987; Günther, 1984; Meyer et al 1982; Ordakowski-Burk et al 2006b; Ralston et al 1986; Rieker et al 2000; Roose et al 2001; Schryver et al 1980, 1986, 1987; Spais et al 1978; Staniar et al 2010; Wagner et al 2010; Young et al 1987); filled dots represent horses after colon resection (Ducharme et al 1987; Ralston et al 1986).

support ossification alters with age. Particular interest in horses with respect to Cu requirements arises from its link with lysyl oxydase, a Cu-dependent enzyme that acts as a pacemaker for connective tissue formation during fetal maturation and postnatal growth (Keen et al 1998, Kothapalli & Ramamurthi 2009, Rucker et al 1999). This enzyme drives the formation of cross linkages between collagen fibers. Tyrosinase, another Cu-dependent enzyme, is responsible for the formation of pigments from tyrosine; this role explains the changes in pigmentation seen with Cu deficiency, at least in other species. Cytochrome oxydase and Cu-Zn superoxide dismutase are other key enzymes which belong to the Cu-enzyme family (Linder & Hazegh-Azam 1996, Linder et al 1999); they contribute to cell respiration and anti-oxidative capacities. Cu stores in the form of ceruloplasmin (extracellular) and Cu-thionein (intracellular) provide a buffer against a temporary shortage.

Intake, absorption and requirements

The Cu concentrations in feeds vary but tend to be below 20 mg/kg DM; ~8 mg are expected in grass and related products but it is of practical relevance that ~40% of grass-based forage has Cu at <6 mg/kg DM (Fig. 10.13). As straight grains contain 4–7 mg Cu/kg DM, nonsupplemented rations are often <8 mg/kg (8 ppm Cu) DM. It is possible that intakes between 4 and 8 ppm may be acceptable for adapted adult animals at maintenance (Cymbaluk et al 1981a, b) although the recommendation is for a minimum of 10 mg Cu/kg dietary DM and 12–15 mg/kg DM in breeding horses (Meyer 1994).

The major site for absorption and secretion is the small intestine where Cu absorption varies between 30 and 51% (Meyer et al 1982). Bile flow is responsible for Cu secretion at about 0.06 µg/kg BW (Cymbaluk et al 1981a); the net absorption therefore is above 40%. The total tract apparent digestibility of ~36% (Fig. 10.14) suggests a net secretion in the hindgut associated with microbes and mucus. Zinc and cadmium may have an effect by competing with copper binding sites and the dietary ratio between copper and zinc may also be important (Bridges & Moffitt 1990, Harris et al 2005, Spais et al 1978). Mb is argued to interfere with Cu absorption as in other species (e.g., sheep) but this is debatable in horses because the grazing of high Mb pastures (up to 15 mg/kg DM) did not have an effect on copper status, at least in weanling fillies and adult geldings (Harris et al 2005, Pearce et al 1998a, b, c, 1999).

The renal excretion of Cu is very low (4 µg/kg BW/day) even in the face of an excessive Cu load; therefore the figure of ~36% should be close to the utilization rate. The endogenous losses via feces can be set at 35 µg/kg BW/day (Cymbaluk et al 1981a, Meyer 1994). Cutaneous Cu losses will be marginal due to the low Cu concentration in hair. These data form the basis for a preliminary factorial calculation of requirements that includes information on Cu deposition in gestation and foal weight gain as well as milk output.

Absorbed Cu enters the liver. The protein transcuprein transfers Cu to the liver and bone marrow where it is used in the synthesis of ceruloplasmin and erythrocuprein. Ceruloplasmin, the primary posthepatic transport form, distributes Cu to target tissues. Plasma Cu and ceruloplasmin concentration show a close linear relationship (Pearce et al 1998b, Bell et al 1987, Okumura et al 1998). There is little published data available on ceruloplasmin metabolism in the horse; ceruloplasmin has been measured in intrauterine fluids and milk. In humans and laboratory animals, Cu in non-ceruloplasmin forms is not absorbed by the suckling neonate (Linder et al 1999). This information should be considered when discussing Cu supply in neonatal foals (e.g., via milk replacers).

Cu supply may modify the occurrence of osteochondrosis in foals given its role in connective tissue synthesis (lysyl oxydase). Several experimental studies support an interaction between Cu nutrition and osteochondrosis (OCD) (Bridges & Harris 1988, Hurtig et al 1993, Pearce et al 1998a). However, it remains unclear whether naturally-occurring OCD is due to Cu deficiency or that OCD can be prevented by Cu supply above the basic intake (Coenen et al 2003, Gee et al 2005a, b, 2007, Vervuert et al 2003). Although there is a weak link only between Cu intake by the mare, their blood and milk Cu-concentrations and the Cu-status of the foal Breedveld et al. 1988), the newborn foal reflects the Cu-supply to the dam. The mare effectively "feeds" Cu to the fetal liver; foals are born with variable liver copper stores. Liver copper concentrations of less than 400 mg/kg DM in newborn foals have been suggested to reflect inadequate uptake by the dam (Meyer 1995) allthough this has been questioned (Gee et al 2000). The transient Cu reserve is then available for the newborn foal to draw upon during the first weeks of life and helps ensure a constant source of Cu in the face of low supply from milk (colostrum 1.9, milk 0.29 mg/kg) (Coenen et al 2010). Figure 10.15 shows the physiology of Cu metabolism in foals both preterm and postpartum. Note that bile secretion does not occur in the fetus. The fetal liver likely functions as a simple Cu sink, a situation that corrects postpartum.

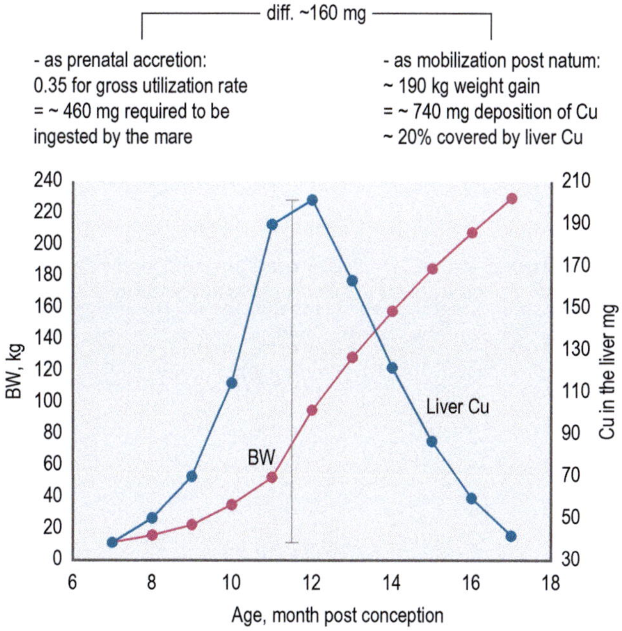

Figure 10.15 Changes in liver Cu stores in a fetus and and foal respectively of a 500 kg mare during gestation and lactation – the months for age are counting from day of fertilization. Calculations, liver weight, g/kg BW of fetus or foal $=10.1e^{4.76-0.0052x}$, x = day after fertilization; liver Cu mg/kg DM antepartum $= 1094 - 217x + 14x^2$ and postpartum $= 62.2e^{6.37-0.41x}$, where x = month after fertilization; liver dry matter is fixed at 30%, according to Gee et al (2004); 190 kg weight gain results from 240 kg BW at the age of ca. 18 month minus 50 kg birth weight.

Whether the pregnant mare requires increased dietary Cu to accommodate this fetal Cu storage remains unknown although some work supports this idea (Pearce et al 1998a, b, c). The postpartum decrease in liver Cu results in a marked change in blood Cu and ceruloplasmin; within the first month of life – with no noteworthy contribution from solid feed – Cu and ceruloplasmin increase to a plateau similar to mares values but weakly responding on additional Cu-supply (Gee et al 2004; Pearce et al 1998b).

Key Points

- The small intestine is the major site of Cu absorption
- Liver tissue acts as a Cu sink. This function is essential for Cu metabolism in foals. The Cu status of newborn foals (liver stores) likely depends on the Cu intake of the mare
- A high proportion of forages have low Cu concentrations; supplementation is often needed to ensure adequate supply

Zinc (Zn)

Zn nutrition is commonly linked with skin health although its biological function is distributed over all tissues. In some regions soil Zn is very low, explaining why Zn deficiency is one of the leading micronutrient deficiencies in humans.

Major functions

The total body Zn store in horses is ~29.5 mg/kg BW (average from 90 individuals). The highest concentrations are found in pancreatic tissue, hoof horn and liver (respectively, 242, 186, and 134 mg/kg DM) but ~56 % of total body Zn is located in muscle tissue. Zn is a constituent of many enzymes including superoxide dismutase, liver dehydrogenase, and alkaline phosphatase. Through these enzymes, Zn is involved in countless cellular processes; the most prominent role is in the replication of DNA and RNA, where Zn is critical for cell division and the conservation of genetic information. In humans, Zn nutrition is critical for normal cognitive and emotional function (Bitanihirwe & Cunningham 2009). Zn deficiency is associated with mental redardation but excessive Zn is neurotoxic.

The high concentration of Zn in pancreatic tissue is indicative of its importance to the function of this organ. Studies in humans show a significant linear association between pancreatic Zn and enzyme output (Dominguez-Munoz et al 2004). Zn is involved in cellular energy metabolism where insulin is required for GLUT-4 mediated glucose uptake (Jansen et al 2009, Wiernsperger & Rapin 2010, Kelishadi et al 2010, Marreiro et al 2006). There has been one report of a horse in which Zn deficiency was suggested to play a role in the development of a diabetes-like condition. However, any connection between Zn nutrition and insulin resistance in horses remains unproven.

Zn dependent enzymes are involved in keratinization, explaining the role of Zn in skin health. Differences in the degree of keratinization are linked to differences in Zn supply to different tissues (Lansdown & Sampson 1997). Zn deficiency causes hyperkeratosis. The Zn content of horse hoof horn varies from the capsule to the sole (hard vs. soft keratinization); low Zn concentrations have been associated with decreased horn strength and hardness (Coenen & Spitzlei 1996a).

Intake, absorption and requirements

Zn requirements are shown in Table 10-4, with the maintenance need ~40 mg/kg DM. The majority of European cultured grass species and conserved forages contain Zn of ~20–50 mg/kg DM (Fig. 10.16). Most rations based on grass-type forages have Zn <50 mg/kg and therefore may lead to marginal Zn-supply; in one survey 46% of horses were found to receive less than 75% of recommended Zn (Wichert et al 2002). Horses fed restricted amounts of roughage in order to limit energy intake will be at increased risk at marginal or deficient Zn intake unless provided appropriate supplementation. The required Zn concentration in a mineral supplement can easily be calculated; corresponding data are given in Table 10-18 based on the lower quartile for trace elements in grass.

Manufactured complementary feeds often contain >50 ppm Zn; therefore Zn intake should be adequate when roughage-concentrate rations are fed according to manufacturer's recommendations. The further addition of a mineral supplement can result in oversupply of Zn (and intake may exceed legal limits). However, the Zn requirement for horses is not well defined and possibly has been overestimated in the past. The absorption of Zn occurs predominantly in the small intestine and compensates for the high Zn losses into the gut via the secretions. A prececal absorption of around 30% was found after feeding roughage-based rations but the results for concentrates were inconsistent (Meyer et al 1982). Literature data yield a linear relationship between Zn-intake and the amount of absorbed Zn. An average total GIT absorption rate of 36% can be extracted from Fig. 10.17. As for Cu, data obtained from horses before and after colon resection are not different. As renal Zn losses are very low under physiological conditions, the slope of 0.36 in Fig. 10.17 should be close to the utilization rate. Using these data (0.16 mg/kg BW/day as endogenous losses and 35% for utilization), a preliminary estimate of the maintenance requirement is 0.46 mg/kg BW/day,

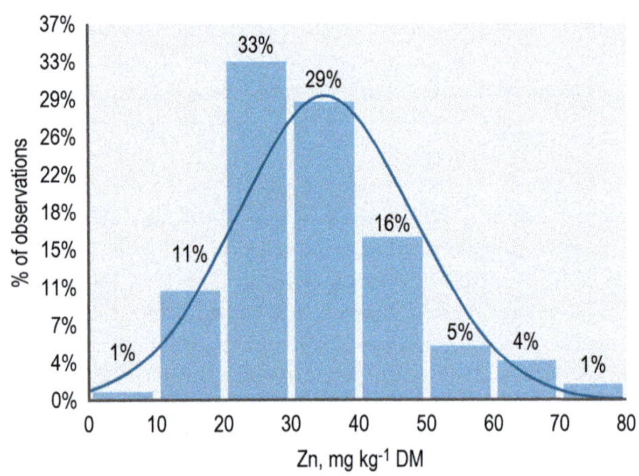

Figure 10.16 Distribution of Zn in grass, grass silages and hay.

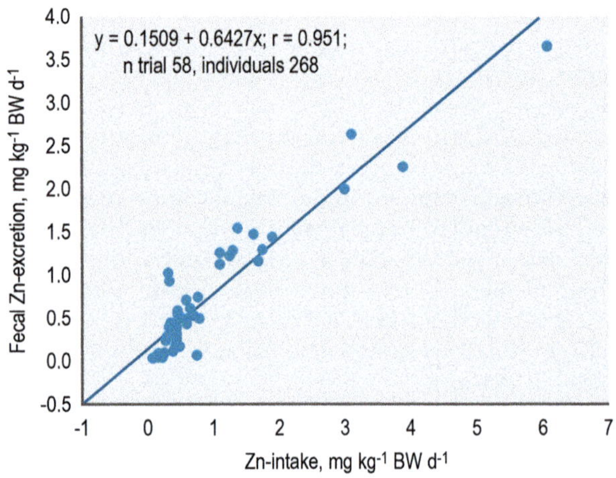

Figure 10.17 Fecal excretion of Zn in relation to Zn intake. *Data from Coger et al 1987; Crozier et al 1997; Cymbaluk et al 1981a, b; Ducharme et al 1987; Günther, 1984; Meyer et al 1982; Ordakowski-Burk et al 2006b; Ralston et al 1986; Rieker et al 2000; Roose et al 2001; Schryver et al 1980, 1986, 1987; Spais et al 1978; Staniar et al 2010; Wagner et al 2010; Young et al 1987.*

Table 10-18 Calculation of the Suitable Trace Element Concentrations in a Supplement (either Mineral Feed or Compound Feed) in Order to Ensure Sufficient Intake Based on the 25 % Quartile of Trace Element Concentration in Grass and Grass Products

		Cu	Zn	Se
			mg/kg DM	
Concentration in grass/products		5	23	0,02
Target value for total ration		12	50	0,2
Difference		7	27	0,18
Suggested amount of supplement per kg forage DM		Needed concentration per kg supplement		
Mineral supplement, g/kg forage DM	5	1400[1]	5400	36
	10	700	2700	18
	15	467	1800	12
Compound feed, kg/kg forage DM	0.2	35	135	0,9
	0.4	18	68[2]	0,5
	0.6	12	45	0,3

[1]Example: 7/5 × 1000 = 1400 mg Cu/kg Supplement dosed by 5 g/kg grass DM ⇨ ensures 12 mg Cu/kg total ration DM.
[2]27/0.4=68 mg Zn/kg compound feed dosed by 0.4 kg/kg grass DM ⇨ ensures 50 mg Zn/kg total ration.

which is ~23 mg/kg DM (using the traditional DM intake of 2% of BW).

Unlike Cu, oversupply of Zn by common supplements is unlikely to result in toxicity (despite the impact on Cu) (see Table 10-4). However, Zn oversupply may be a problem in regions where industrial activity liberates Zn into the environment. Industrially contaminated grassland with either zinc or cadmium was evaluated as being causally linked to DOD in foals (Harris et al 2005). Excessive Zn has the potential to contribute to the development of osteochondrosis (Harris et al 2005), but this needs to be confirmed.

Key Points

- Zn absorption occurs along the entire gut but the small intestine is the most important site.
- Zinc intake by rations with common forages can be marginal related to common recommendations
- Keratinized tissues may respond to increased Zn intake; however, Zn deficiency is rarely the reason for impaired keratin formation e.g. hoof quality

Manganese (Mn)

Major functions

Some enzymes contain Mn while others are activated by this cation. The manganese-superoxide-dismutase (Mn-SOD) enzyme is located in the mitochondria and, in liver tissue for example, ensures protection of DNA against superoxides (Ishida et al 1999). Mn-chloride administered by infusion increased the superoxide scavenging ability of equine blood (Singh et al 1992, 1999). However, there is not a simple relationship between Mn intake and blood SOD activity (Smith et al 1983) and alterations in dietary Mn are not constantly manifest by changes in blood SOD. The Mn^{3+} cation accumulates in the mitochondria of astrocytes where it supports antioxidant functions. For this reason, there has been interest in the evaluation of Mn status in human patients with degenerative CNS diseases. Equine motor neuron disease (EMND) is a comparable CNS disease in which oxidative tissue damage is a contributing factor. However, data on the trace mineral concentrations of spinal cord tissue from affected horses did not support involvement of a Mn deficiency. In contrast, tissue Cu concentration was higher in EMND when compared to control horses (Polack et al 2000).

There is limited evidence that Mn status affects human fertility ((Selby et al 1970, Wirth et al 2007, Zha et al 2008). Mn deficiency also has been considered as a possible reason for abnormal ovarian function in ruminants (Hidiroglou 1979), with altered steroid hormone synthesis and secretion (e.g., luteinizing hormone; Lee et al 2006, Pine et al 2005) and loss of ovarian antioxidant function (Tilly & Tilly 1995) as suggested mechanisms. The impact of Mn status on reproductive function in horses is not known.

The formation of mucopolysaccharides and chondroitin sulfate also requires Mn; this explains the effects of Mn deficiency on bone growth observed in other species (Frantz et al 2008, Gallup & Norris 1938, Tal & Guggenheim 1965). The specific effect of Mn on cartilage synthesis and integrity is not well defined (Frantz et al 2008).

There is no Mn sink or storage site in the body. Additionally, it is not clear whether Mn is stored in the fetal liver like Cu. No hepatic Mn storage is observed in the ruminant fetus but this needs to be confirmed in horses.

There is no evidence that physical conditioning status (regular exercise) alters Mn requirements.

Intake, absorption and requirements

The typical concentration of Mn in feeds is >30 mg/kg DM. Minimum Mn intake should be 0.3 mg/kg BW/day (at DM intake of at least 1% of BW). Tissue Mn concentrations are ~2–3 mg/kg tissue DM, with 90% of body total Mn (0.9 mg/kg BW) in muscle, bone, and skin (Table 10-16a). Absorption efficiency is ~30% of intake; as renal losses are low this value should be close to the utilization rate (Table 10-16b). Fecal excretion is linearly related to Mn intake. Therefore, in the range of intake shown in Fig. 10.18 there is no adaptation if the requirement exceeds Mn intake or vice versa. Most Mn is absorbed in the small intestine, evidenced by the observation that total tract absorption did not differ between control horses and horses that had undergone colon resection (Ducharme et al 1987, Ralston et al 1986).

Estimates of endogenous losses range between 0.11 mg/kg BW/day (per Fig. 10.18) and 0.27 mg/kg BW/day (from balance trials; Pagan 2001), while the true absorption rate is 32–37%. These data can be used to calculate daily requirements for maintenance as well as for lactation and postnatal growth if the Mn in milk and daily gain, respectively, is considered. The pregnancy-related requirement is likely underestimated by this approach as uterus and placenta are rich in Mn. The equine fetus contains 0.7–1.3 mg Mn/kg between days 214 and 335 of gestation (Meyer & Ahlswede 1976), which is high in comparison to body composition in adults (0.9 mg/kg BW, see Table 10-16a). The daily Mn accretion in the conceptus for a 500 kg mare at the end of gestation is ~1.6 mg/day; assuming a utilization of 30% and a gestation + maintenance requirement of 189 mg/day. The required dietary Mn concentration is 25 mg/kg DM, assuming low daily DMI of 7.5 kg (1.5 % BW).

Selenium (Se)

Se deficiency has been implicated in several diseases of humans (e.g., coronary heart disease), providing impetus for use of Se-enriched fertilizers in crop production. Data from

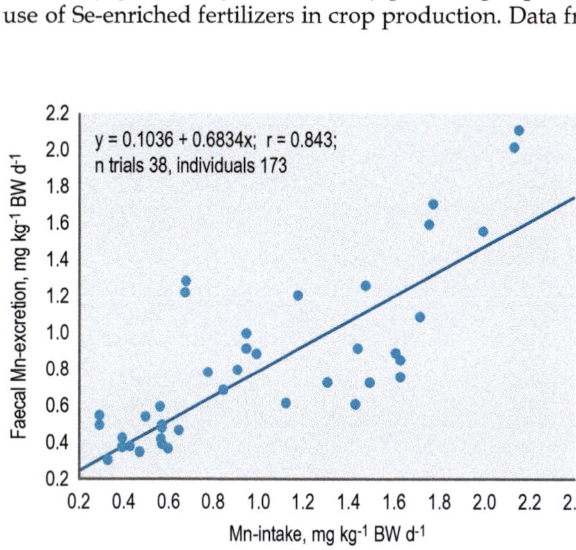

Figure 10.18 Fecal excretion of Mn as a function of intake. *Coger et al 1987; Crozier et al 1997; Cymbaluk et al 1981a, b; Ducharme et al 1987; Günther, 1984; Meyer et al 1982; Ordakowski-Burk et al 2006b; Ralston et al 1986; Rieker et al 2000; Roose et al 2001; Schryver et al 1980, 1986, 1987; Spais et al 1978; Staniar et al 2010; Wagner et al 2010; Young et al 1987.*

Finland shows the effect of Se fertilization on the Se concentration of grain (Fig. 10.19).

Major functions

The understanding that Se was an essential constituent of animal tissue came with the identification of Se as a component of glutathione peroxide, one of the most important antioxidant compounds in the body (Rotruck et al 1973). The term "radical scavenger" is often used to describe the biological function of Se as well as that of vitamin E. However, numerous other Se-containing proteins with important functions have now been identified (Table 10-19). For example, male and female fertility, mammary tissue defences, and protection from oxidant damage in cardiac and skeletal muscle and liver are all dependent on adequate Se. The activity of a deiodinase depends on Se; this function links Se to thyroid hormone availability, protein synthesis and consequently to growth. As there is no Se depot in maternal tissues, Se supply to the fetus is wholly dependent on Se intake of the dam.

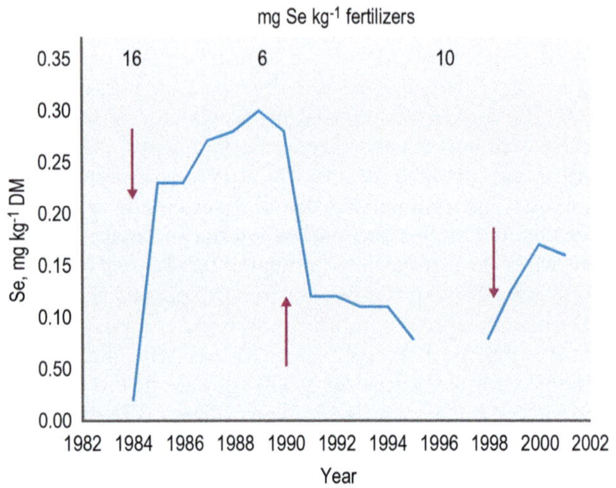

Figure 10.19 Changes in Se of spring wheat grown in Finland since the start of a Se fertilizing program.
Data from Eurola et al (2003).

Table 10-19 An Interspecies Summary of Important Selenoproteins and Identified Functions (Arthur & Beckett 1994, Brown & Arthur 2001)

Selenoprotein	Function
GSH peroxidase Cytosolic, RBC Plasma Phospholipid hydroperoxide	Hydroperoxide catabolism
Gastrointestinal	
Selenoprotein P	Se-transport, antioxidative
Iodothyronine 5′-deiodinase	T_4 activation, T_3 inactivation
Thioredoxin reductases	Protein thiol redox regulation, Vit.C recycling
Methionine sulfoxide reductase B	Reactive oxygen species removal by methionine
Sperm capsule selenoprotein	Sperm structure
Selenoprotein W	Antioxidative
58, 56 and 14 kDa Se-binding proteins	Modulation of regulatory protein for cell growth, "anticancer"

The several functions of Se require a metabolic processing of ingested and absorbed Se irrespectively from Se-source (Weiss 2003).

Compared to mature horses, the consequences of Se deficiency are more pronounced in the fetus as evidenced by white muscle disease in newborns. Se-independent peroxidases are widely distributed (Herbette et al 2007) and compensate for limitations imposed by Se deficiency in mature animals. This Se-independent peroxidase capacity becomes depressed again with aging, at least in humans (He et al 2009).

Data regarding the Se content of horse tissues are incomplete; therefore the total body Se estimate ~0.06 mg/kg BW should be taken as preliminary information (Table 10-16). Most of body Se is located in muscle, bone and skin, although liver and renal tissues become storage sites in situations of elevated Se intake, overload or toxicity (Stowe 1980, 1967).

There also is enrichment of Se in hair and hoof horn (Coenen et al 1998). The type of keratinization (soft vs. hard) is associated with differences in Se; the hoof horn from the capsule contains 0.23 mg Se/kg tissue DM whereas horn from the sole is slightly lower in Se at 0.2 mg kg^{-1} DM (Coenen & Spitzlei, 1996a). The impact of Se on keratin is based on the substitution of S during keratin synthesis, which affects normal protein folding and explains the hair and hoof damage observed with Se intoxication.

Intake, absorption and requirements

Se can reach >0.2 mg/kg DM in feeds produced on Se fertilized soil. Otherwise Se is typically <0.05 mg/kg feed DM. Balance data regarding Se in horses are scant; experimental data indicate that Se absorption is high when compared to the other trace elements (Pagan et al 1999, Spais et al 1978). The data summarized in Table 10-16 should be taken as preliminary.

The absorption rate is about 59% of intake which suggests a possible role of the kidney for elimination of Se that is not utilized. Volatile Se compounds may be exhaled, particularly in response to excessive Se intake. The Se intake in balance studies is clearly above the range of non-supplemented rations. If it is assumed that 37% Se intake is eliminated by the kidney, the maintenance requirement is 0.63 μg/kg BW/day or 1.26 mg/day for a 500 kg horse, corresponding to 0.17 mg/kg feed DM at DMI of 1.5% BW. Despite the limitations of the data used to derive this estimate, the recommended requirement seems reasonable.

Interspecies data about the availability of organic and inorganic Se-sources show no general benefit of organic Se; Se enriched yeast provide Se via amino acids. This may be linked to enforced absorption and different metabolic processing as this type of Se is trafficking through the amino acid pool.

Blood Se as well as the content of selenoproteins changes in response to altered Se intake. The activity of GSHPx in blood is linearly associated with the Se concentration in grass (GSHPx, U/g HB=19.97+2.17x, r=0.85; where x = Se μg/kg grass DM (Meyer et al 1995) although this relationship will be influenced by the duration on such rations

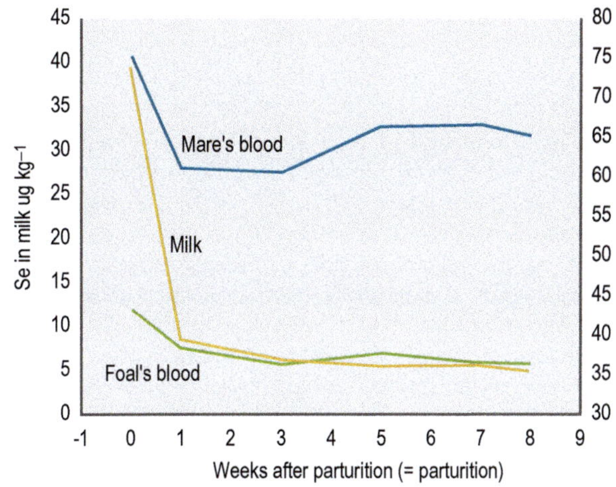

Figure 10.20 **Changes in Se in blood and milk of mares and in the blood of their associated foals.**
Data from Breedveld et al (1988).

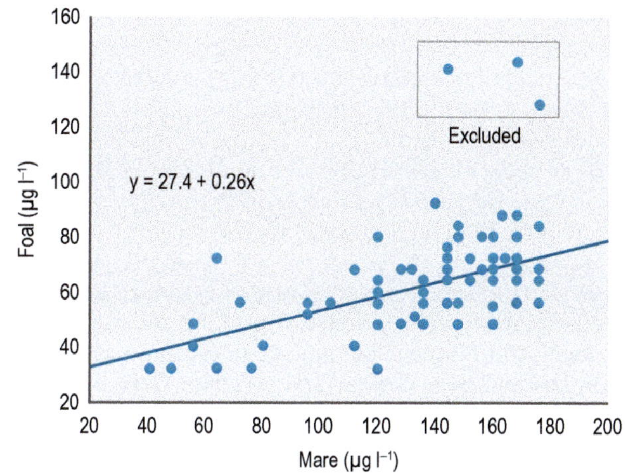

Figure 10.22 **Se in blood of lactating mares and their foals (μg/l).**
Data from Schönthaler (1998).

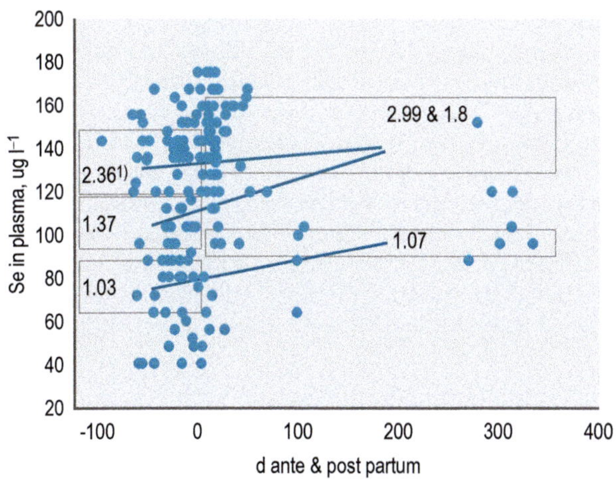

Figure 10.21 **Se in blood of Thoroughbred mares ante- and postpartum as well as the corresponding Se intake; the frames include median ±25% of blood levels on three farms and the associated daily Se-intake in mg/day.**
Data from Schönthaler (1998).

(reflecting the lifespan of red blood cells). An increase in Se intake induces a dose-dependent change in plasma Se. The GSHPx activity is poorly reflective of those changes (Shellow et al 1985).

Some horses appear able to adapt to low Se intakes. Icelandic horses that consume forages with low Se content (0.01–0.06 mg/kg DM) have average blood Se concentrations of 66 μg/l (reference range of 140–250 μg/l; Puls 1994) and no apparent signs of Se deficiency. On the other hand, low blood selenium as well as low T_4 concentrations were observed in 29 and 32% of horses in Prince Edward Island (Muirhead et al 2010). Mares and their foals are the most critical group with respect to Se nutrition. As shown in Figs 10.20–10.22, the Se concentration of mare's milk is dependent upon mare's Se-status and dictates the Se-status of the foal.

If the requirements for Se are covered by the core diet there obviously is no benefit to provide additional from a specific Se source. European legislation in fact requires that horses should not be fed more than 0.5 mg Se/kg of total diet on a DM basis – which approximates to around 1 mg/100 kg BW, i.e. 5 mg for a 500 kg horse. Organic Se sources were expected to be more efficiently utilized in comparison to Na-selenite but this has not been confirmed to date in the majority of experimental studies in horses (Calamari et al 2009, 2010, Podoll et al 1992, Richardson et al 2006, Karren et al 2010, Thorson et al 2010).

Selenium toxicity

Selenium toxicosis can occur in any age, breed or sex of animal and is most commonly seen globally in horses on pasture (Raisbeck et al 1993). In the UK at least, the selenium concentrating plants responsible for pasture based toxicosis are not present. Instead, toxicity can arise from excessive Se administration due to an error in manufacturing, high levels in the water or excessive administration by injection – *all of which are comparatively rare*. The most common cause is multiple supplementation or excessive supplementation by the owner or feeder.

Whilst acute toxicosis (blind staggers) tends to result in blindness, as well as signs relating to the gut, lungs (respiratory failure), heart and kidney (nephritis) – it is the more chronic form of toxicity (alkali disease) that causes problems for the feet (McDowell 2003). Early lesions begin as lameness and soreness of the coronary band and feet – often accompanied by reddening and swelling of the coronary band. These signs are often missed as they settle down relatively quickly. They are followed in one or more days by the development of a crack that occurs parallel to and just below the coronet (due to defective tubular horn produced by the dermal papillae of the coronary band). Interestingly, it has been reported that the hind feet often tend to be affected first. Hoof separation and lameness progress together for several months until the damaged hoof is displaced from beneath by new growth and sloughs off. Not surprisingly, affected animals are extremely lame. The hair coat initially becomes very rough and typically hair loss occurs along the nape of the neck and on the tail but in severe cases a more generalized loss of hair may be seen. The exact mechanism is unknown and there have been many theories – perhaps the earliest and commonest is that selenium replaces the sulfur in a number of sulfur-containing amino acids.

However, more recently it has been suggested that excessive selenium actually acts by causing oxidative stress and subsequent oxidative damage. Certainly it has been suggested that selenium may act by damaging developing keratinocytes (Tomlinson et al 2004).

It has been suggested that uncomplicated chronic selenium excess can be successfully treated with low selenium, high protein, high quality diets, backed by supportive care for many months. This care may include providing the horses with soft sandy footing, or equivalent, to lessen the pain associated with standing and walking, the use of heart bar shoes and frequent therapeutic hoof trimming to help minimize abnormal posture and resultant secondary joint and skeletal problems.

Such marked cases of chronic toxicity are very rare - but less severe, but still significant, effects on hoof quality due to excessive selenium supplementation have been suggested. It has also been suggested that moderately high intakes of selenium, which are not toxic enough to cause the signs described above, may affect the frog horn and be a factor in some cases of persistent thrush (Kempson 2005).

Key Points

- Se intake via typical forages does not meet requirements
- Selenium is absorbed along the entire gastrointestinal tract
- Intestinal Se uptake is not regulated and therefore excretion via the kidney and, to a lesser extent, the respiratory system (volatile forms) occurs under conditions of excess dietary supply
- Excessive Se intake depresses the utilization of S in the formation of keratin. Hair loss and hoof abnormalities are clinical signs of Se toxicosis

Iodine (I)

Goiter associated with cretinism was a common disease in humans for thousands of years. Discoveries regarding the chemistry of iodine, the links between metabolic rate and iodine metabolism (Fig. 10.23) and the role of iodine deficiency or excess in thyroid diseases began to emerge ~100 years ago. Goiter, which manifests as swelling of the neck, occurs with both over- and under-consumption of iodine.

Major functions

In humans, total body I is ~0.2 mg/kg BW with ~71% of body I located in the thyroid glands as a component of the thyroid hormones (Hays 2001). The ovary has the second highest content of I in the human body, although iodine's specific role in ovarian function is not fully understood (Slebodzinski 2005). Comparable data on body I composition and distribution for the horse are not available. The thyroid hormones are critical to basal metabolic rate as well as growth and tissue renewal and determine metabolic rate/energetic in all physiologic situations, such as hibernation, molting or exercise (Tomasi et al 1998, Ciloglu et al 2005, Vezina et al 2009). In horses, thyroid hormone concentrations differ between breeds and are related to metabolic rate, e.g., lower in ponies vs. Thoroughbreds (Malinowski et al 1996, Medica et al 2011a, b)

The thyroid glands develop early in embryo development, enabling orchestrated organogenesis in the embryo and fetus - with a crucial role in the development of the brain and spinal cord (Benton 2012, Benton & Donohoe 2011, Benton et al 2012, House 2007, Negro et al 2011, Katzen-Luchenta 2007). To ensure optimal development of the conceptus, the pregnant uterus employs two strategies related to thyroid hormone and I metabolism: (a) enrichment of T_4 and (b) I deposition in the placenta. The placenta provides a temporary I sink while the thyroid gland is still developing in the embryo. Although equine-specific data are not available, based on information from other species, it can be assumed that the iodine requirement of mares increases early in gestation even though the total mass of the conceptus and its daily gain are quite low. In addition, it is evident that iodine deficiency at this stage will adversely affect nervous system development.

Gestation is the most critical period with regard to I nutrition. Whether the disastrous congenital hypothyroidism associated with cretinism occurs in horses is uncertain. However, studies of thyroidectomized equine fetuses clearly show that defects in thyroid hormone synthesis in the equine embryo or fetus will produce clinical signs at

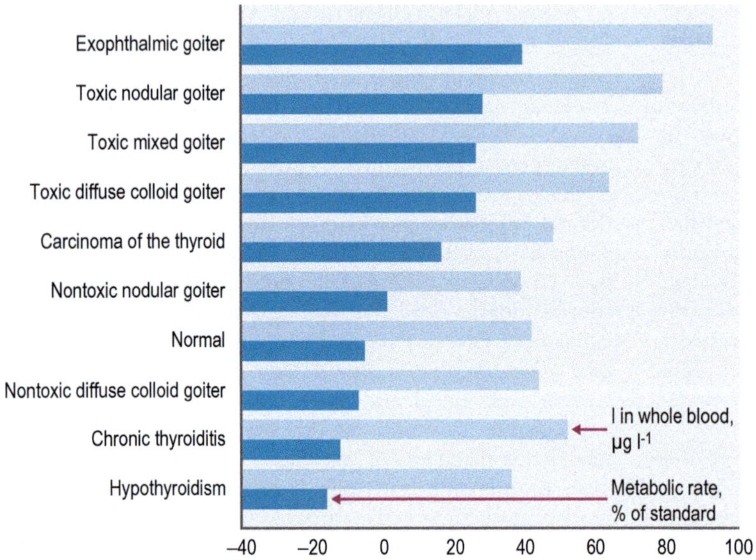

Figure 10.23 Metabolic rate (relative to a maintenance standard (*x*-axis) as defined by Boothby (1921) **In humans with deranged thyroid function and the corresponding blood iodine concentrations.**
Data according to Curtis and Fertman (1945).

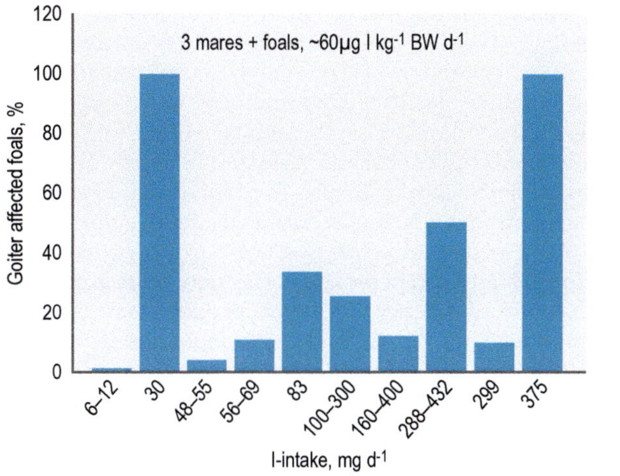

Figure 10.24 Observations on thyroid dysfunction in foals corresponding to the iodine intake of mares during gestation. *Data from Baker & Lindsey 1968; Drew et al 1975; Conway & Cosgrove 1980; Eroksuz et al 2004; Silva et al 1987a, b; Sippel 1969; Miyazawa et al 1978.*

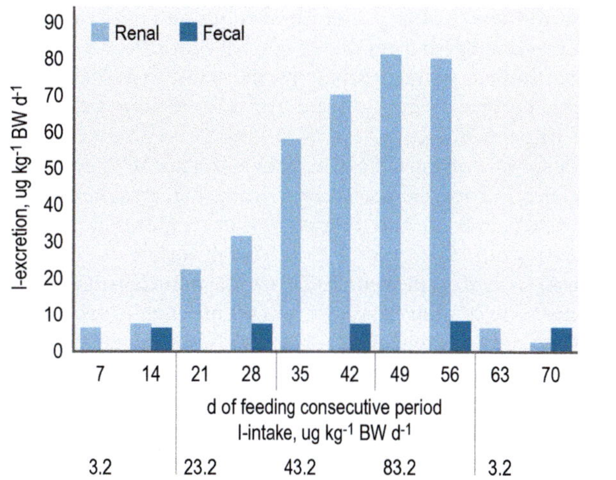

Figure 10.25 Distribution of fecal and renal iodine excretion for different levels of iodine intake in ponies. *Wehr et al (2002).*

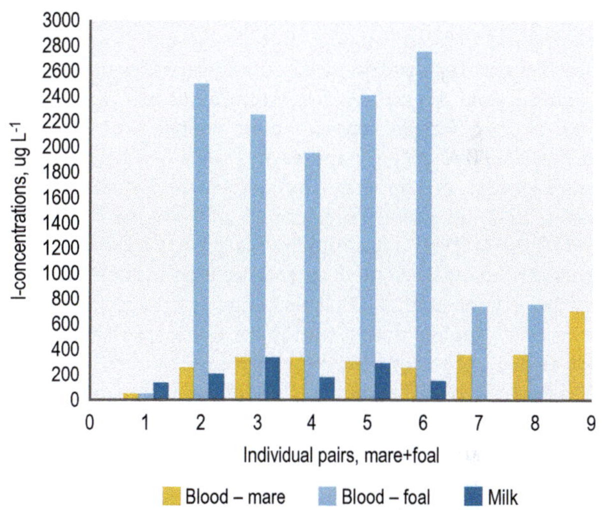

Figure 10.26 Iodine concentrations in mare's blood and milk and the blood of the corresponding foal (Silva et al 1987a, b).

birth consistent with congenital hypothyroidism, see Fig. 10.23) (Allen et al 1996, 1998).

Maternal overconsumption of I is also a concern. Iodine intake by the pregnant mare at >10 mg per day (~>40 µg/kg BW/day) increases the risk for thyroid dysfunction in the newborn foal. Weakness, muscle immaturity, tendon contraction, and skeletal abnormalities have been described in newborn foals associated with I toxicosis (Fig. 10.24).

Intake, absorption and requirements

Grass forage provides typically 0.2–0.3 mg I per kg DM (Alderman & Jones 1967). With intensive nitrogen and sulphate fertilization and an increase in plant biomass production, there will be a decrease in I content. In areas far away from the seaside, soil-based and aerogenic I transfer into feed are low (Leskova 1969). However, even in countries with a higher I availability from the ocean (e.g., Belgium), I intake of animals may not ensure adequate supply (Guyot et al 2009). Grain as well as seed rich in protein contain <0.1 mg iodine/kg DM. Naturally high sources of I are vetches, milk products, in particular, whey, algae and kelp.

The absorption of I occurs preferentially in the small intestine; in pigs ~90% of supplemented I is absorbed (Hays 2001, Herzig et al 2000) Absorption efficiency in horses is also likely to be high. In ponies, renal excretion of I is tightly linked to intake whereas fecal excretion is not associated with dietary level (Fig. 10.25; Wehr et al 2002). Indeed, renal I excretion is a sensitive method for assessment of I intake, e.g., by measurement of the creatinine: iodine ratio (Götz 2005). The mammary gland is a further route for I output and this is relevant to situation of overconsumption in mares. The data in Fig. 10.26 show parallel adjustments in the I content of mare's blood and milk as well as blood of the foal (Silva et al 1987a, b).

Iodine uptake by thyroid tissue can be impaired by endocrine disrupting substances such as nitrate, thiocyanate, glucosinolates, goitrin, thiouracil, and perchlorate. These substances impair function of the I-Na-symporter. The adverse effects of perchlorate on human health are well described (Pearce & Braverman 2009, Braverman et al 2005, Braverman & Pearce 2005, 2009, Sanchez et al 2008, Srinivasan & Viraraghavan 2009, Brent 2010). As a pollutant (primarily water contamination), perchlorate may affect animals as well. Perchlorate is normally <1 µg/l in surface water (Scheytt et al 2011) and, below this threshold, does not affect thyroid I uptake in animals. Data from India and the United States show that in industrialized areas perchlorate may occur above 1 µg/l (2.5–4% of samples; Gullick et al 2001, Kannan et al 2009).

Forage can be rich in nitrate due to uptake from soil or from the addition of nitrate-containing preservatives. Grass contains mostly <1 g nitrate/kg DM. A pregnant mare grazing intensively managed pasture may ingest 20–40 mg nitrate/kg BW (1–2 g nitrate/kg DM, intake of 20 g DM/kg BW); this level of nitrate ingestion does not appear to pose risk of nitrate toxicosis as, in general, nitrates do not promote the formation of methemoglobin in horses as occurs in ruminants. However, the possible link between nitrate in forage and the dysmaturity syndrome in foals that has clinical features consistent with hypothyroidism (Allen et al 1996) points to the possibility that nitrates are an endocrine disruptor in horses. In humans, 15 mg Na-nitrate/kg BW/day did not induce thyroid problems (Hunault et al 2007). No equine-specific tolerance limit for nitrate can be given regarding the impact on I. A "zero-nitrate" recommendation for horses is questionable as nitrate is a naturally occurring substance in forages, particularly in spring. Assessment of dietary I provision and thyroid status in mares is recommended if nitrate exceeds 2 g/kg DM of forage.

Linseed and rapeseed are possible natural sources of cyanate. The cyanate levels in linseed are legally regulated in some countries (e.g., Germany, max 150 mg/kg). Typical linseed intakes will not exceed ~2 g/kg BW/d (i.e., <10% of dietary DM intake) and are unlikely to affect I turnover. However, in other species the potential for linseed to elevate blood thiocyanate concentrations and modify thyroid status has been demonstrated (e.g., in pigs, Schöne et al 1997). The conclusion from several studies is that the inclusion of thiocyanate-generating feeds in animal diets will not impair thyroid function as long as I intake is not marginal.

Goitrin can be present in rape. In contrast to the compounds mentioned above more dietary I cannot compensate the impaired thyroid function. But the correct utilization of rape seed and rape products is unlikely to create a risk.

Equine data regarding I requirements are weak. An intake of 3 μg/kg BW/day for maintenance and exercise, and 5 μg/kg BW/day for mares and foals is a preliminary guideline that is adapted from other species (Meyer & Coenen 2002). In a study four ponies that received between 0 and 80 μg/kg BW/day supplementary I for 14-day periods, regression analysis yielded an endogenous loss of 7 μg/kg BW/day (Wehr et al 2002). This suggests an I requirement that is much higher than reported for other species; further work is needed to confirm these findings. In case of anticipated anti-thyroidal factors such as nitrate (>1 g/kg DM) or higher level inclusion of linseed, I provision should be increased but the recommended maximum amount is 10 μg/kg BW/day.

Grain contains <0.15 mg I/kg DM while forages vary between <0.2 and 0.4 mg/kg DM. As I analysis of feed is not commonly performed, it is difficult to estimate I supply from roughages. The inclusion of a mineral supplement containing e.g., 20 mg I/kg to a diet of hay plus grain at a rate of 0.2 g/kg BW/day will provide 4 μg I/kg BW/day. Consequently, the use of I-containing compound feeds or mineral supplements enables one to calculate the core I supply. If at least 50% of I requirements are provided by these feeds, there is no need to provide additional I.

Key Points

- Iodine is efficiently absorbed
- Surplus iodine is excreted via urine and milk
- Excess as well as deficient iodine provision impairs thyroid function
- Iodine uptake by thyroid tissue can be impaired by certain substances in feeds, e.g. nitrate, glucosinolates, and thiocyanate

Cobalt/vitamin B_{12}

Cobalt (Co) is a key component of vitamin B_{12}, also commonly referred to as cobalamin (although more correctly Vitamin B_{12} may be taken to refer to a group of cobalt-containing vitamer compounds known as cobalamins). The natural synthesis of vitamin B_{12} is associated with microbial activity, and therefore ruminants and hindgut fermenters are not thought to require intake of the preformed vitamin. Cobalt and cobalamin take part in energy metabolism, with methylcobalamin being a donor of methyl groups. Adenosylcobalamin is another Co-dependent complex that is involved in the formation of glucose from volatile fatty acids. The depression of β-oxidation of fatty acids in adenosylcobalamin deficiency in other species demonstrates the importance of Co and related compounds in energy metabolism. Cobalt is also involved in several other proteins and associated biological functions (Kobayashi & Shimizu 1999).

Muscles and bone contain the major portions of body Co (McDowell 2003), with 43% and 14%, respectively, while the liver is the most important site of vitamin B_{12} metabolism. Excretion of Co and vitamin B_{12} is via bile secretion. Hindgut fermenters do not appear to store cobalamin in the liver as there is equilibrium between plasma and liver concentrations (McOrist & Thomas 1984). Cobalt intake by the gravid mammal determines the cobalamin status of the newborn via effects of liver cobalamin and the supply of cobalamin in milk (Stemme et al 2002). In addition, the cobalamin supply to the embryo and the fetus depend on maternal cobalamin status (Szakmáry et al 2001).

The cobalamin concentrations in plasma and liver of ruminants increase as a function of intake (Stemme et al 2002), and a drop in intake results in rapid changes in tissue cobalamin. There is, however, minimal experimental-based information about Co in horses. Systemic absorption from the hindgut was demonstrated after administration of cyanocobalamin^{60}Co into the cecum (Stillions 1971). Cobalt is absorbed as part of the cobalamin complex formed through bacterial synthesis. A specialized plasma protein transports the cobalt-complex in blood. A constant replenishment of Co for cobalamin synthesis is therefore required; however, it is uncertain whether the utilization rate of Co for cobalamin synthesis derived from ruminant studies (~37–65% depending on cobalt intake) can be used for the equine. Nonetheless, microbial synthesis of cobalamin by the equine intestinal community occurs and obviously appears to provide sufficient cobalamin for the horse (Salminen 1975).

A sufficient Co intake is stated to be 0.1 mg/kg DM (McDowell 2003). Pasture contains 0.5–0.2 mg/kg DM; alfalfa (0.3 mg/kg DM) and yeast also are rich sources, cereals are intermediate, and straw is low in Co.

Conclusion

In summary, an adequate and balanced supply of mineral and trace elements is important to the optimal health and performance of horses, as for all animals. Whilst overt deficiencies may result in obvious clinical signs, the more subtle effects of marginal intakes are more difficult to detect but may be very important, especially in growing and exercising animals. Although some information on requirements is available, our knowledge is incomplete. Use of factorial equations provides a valuable foundation for nutrient requirements but further work in this area is needed. Some further elements are detected as essential contributors to certain cell functions in rather low quantities, e.g. Chromium (Cr) or Boron (B). Cr is becoming in the focus of the debate around the insulinresistance-obesity complex. Cr is involved in the activation of glucose transporters. However, the natural occurence of these elements will ensure the required intake.

References

Agarwal, N., Prchal, J.T., 2009. Anemia of chronic disease (anemia of inflammation). Acta Haematol 122, 103–108.

Alderman, G., Jones, D.I.H., 1967. The Iodine content of pasture. J Sci Food Agric 18, 197–199.

Allen, A.L., Townsend, H.G., Doige, C.E., et al., 1996. A case-control study of the congenital hypothyroidism and dysmaturity syndrome of foals. The Canadian veterinary journal. La revue veterinaire canadienne 37, 349–351; 354–348.

Allen, A.L., Fretz, P.B., Card, C.E., et al., 1998. The effects of partial thyroidectomy on the development of the equine fetus. Equine Veterinary Journal 30, 53–59.

Anderson, G.J., Frazer, D.M., McLaren, G.D., 2009. Iron absorption and metabolism. Curr Opin Gastroenterol 25, 129–135.

Anke, M., 2004. Essential and toxic effects of macro, trace, and ultratrace elements in the nutrition of man. In: Anke, M., Ihnat, M., Stoeppeler, M. (Eds.), Elements and their compounds in the environment No. 1. Wiley VCH Verlag GmbH, Weinheim, pp. 343–367.

Arthur, J.R., Beckett, G.J., 1994. New metabolic roles for selenium. Proc Nutr Soc 53, 615–624.

Baird, J.D., 1971. Lactation tetany (eclampsia) in a Shetland pony mare. Australian Veterinary Journal 47, 402–404.

Baker, H.J., Lindsey, J.R., 1968. Equine goiter due to excess dietary iodine. J Am Vet Med Assoc 153, 1618–1630.

Baker, L.A., Topliff, D.R., Freeman, D.W., et al., 1998. The comparison of two forms of sodium and potassium and chloride versus sulfur in the Dietary Cation-Anion Difference equation: Effects on acid-base status and mineral balance in sedentary horses. J Equine Vet Sci 18, 389–395.

Baker, L.A., Wall, D.L., Topliff, D.R., et al., 1993. Effect of dietary cation-anion balance in mineral balance in anaerobically exercised and sedentary horses. Journal of Equine Veterinary Science 13, 557–561.

Bardgett, M.E., Schultheis, P.J., McGill, D.L., et al., 2005. Magnesium deficiency impairs fear conditioning in mice. Brain Res 1038, 100–106.

Bell, J.U., Lopez, J.M., Bartos, K.D., 1987. The postnatal development of serum zinc, copper and ceruloplasmin in the horse. Comp Biochem Physiol A Comp Physiol 87, 561–564.

Bell, R.A., Nielsen, B.D., Waite, K., et al., 2001. Daily access to pasture turnout prevents loss of mineral in the third metacarpus of Arabian weanlings. J Anim Sci 79, 1142–1150.

Benton, D., 2012. Vitamins and neural and cognitive developmental outcomes in children. Proc Nutr Soc 71, 14–26.

Benton, D., Donohoe, R., 2011. The influence of creatine supplementation on the cognitive functioning of vegetarians and omnivores. Br J Nutr 105, 1100–1105.

Benton, S.J., Hu, Y., Xie, F., et al., 2012. Can placental growth factor in maternal circulation identify fetuses with placental intrauterine growth restriction? American journal of obstetrics and gynecology 206, 163 e161–e167.

Berchtold, L., 2009. Untersuchungen zum Einfluss der Anionen-Kationen-Bilanz auf den Mineralstoff- und Säure-Basen-Haushalt bei Ponys (Investigations on the influence of the cation-anion-balance on the mineral and acid-base metabolism in ponies). Ludwig-Maximillians University Munich.

Berlin, D., Aroch, I., 2009. Concentrations of ionized and total magnesium and calcium in healthy horses: Effects of age, pregnancy, lactation, pH and sample type. Vet J 181, 305–311.

Bitanihirwe, B.K., Cunningham, M.G., 2009. Zinc: the brain's dark horse. Synapse 63, 1029–1049.

Black, S., Yu, H., Lee, J., et al., 2001. Physiologic concentrations of magnesium and placental apoptosis: prevention by antioxidants. Obstet Gynecol 98, 319–324.

Blaney, B.J., Gartnera, R.J.W., McKenziea, R.A., 1981. The effects of oxalate in some tropical grasses on the availability to horses of calcium, phosphorus and magnesium. J Agric Sci 97, 507–514.

Boothby, W.M., 1921. The basal metabolic rate in hyperthyroidism. J Am Med Assoc 77, 252–255.

Borges, A.S., Divers, T.J., Stokol, T., et al., 2007. Serum iron and plasma fibrinogen concentrations as indicators of systemic inflammatory diseases in horses. J Vet Int Med 21, 489–494.

Braverman, L.E., He, X., Pino, S., et al., 2005. The effect of perchlorate, thiocyanate, and nitrate on thyroid function in workers exposed to perchlorate long-term. J Clin Endocrinol Metab 90, 700–706.

Braverman, L.E., Pearce, E.N., 2005. Comment on "Perchlorate and iodide in dairy and breast milk". Environ Sci Technol 39, 5498; author reply 5499–5500.

Breedveld, L., Jackson, S.G., Baker, J.P., 1988. The determination of a relationship between the copper, zinc and selenium levels in mares and those in their foals. J Equine Vet Sci 8, 378–382.

Breidenbach, A., Schlumbohm, C., Harmeyer, J., 1998. Peculiarities of vitamin D and of the calcium and phosphate homeostatic system in horses. Veterinary Research 29, 173–186.

Brent, G.A., 2010. The impact of perchlorate exposure in early pregnancy: is it safe to drink the water? J Clin Endocrin Metab 97, 3154–3157.

Brevard, J.F., 1824. On the disease in horses gerally called the "Big Head". New England Farmer 2, 388.

Breves, G., Schröder, B., 1991. Comparative aspects of gastrointestinal phosphorus metabolism. Nutr Res Rev 4, 125–140.

Bridges, C.H., Harris, E.D., 1988. Experimentally induced cartilaginous fractures (osteochondritis dissecans) in foals fed low-copper diets. J Am Vet Med Assoc 193, 215–221.

Bridges, C.H., Moffitt, P.G., 1990. Influence of variable content of dietary zinc on copper metabolism of weanling foals. Am J Vet Res 51, 275–280.

Brooks, S.P.J., Lampi, B.J., 2001. Problems associated with measuring phytate in infant cereals. J Agr Food Chem 49, 564–569.

Brown, K.M., Arthur, J.R., 2001. Selenium, selenoproteins and human health: a review. Public Health Nutr 4, 593–599.

Bushinsky, D.A., 1996. Metabolic alkalosis decreases bone calcium efflux by suppressing osteoclasts and stimulating osteoblasts. Am J Physiol 271, F216–F222.

Bussiere, F.I., Gueux, E., Rock, E., et al., 2002. Increased phagocytosis and production of reactive oxygen species by neutrophils during magnesium deficiency in rats and inhibition by high magnesium concentration. British Journal of Nutrition 87, 107–113.

Calamari, L., Ferrari, A., Bertin, G., 2009. Effect of selenium source and dose on selenium status of mature horses. J Anim Sci 87, 167–178.

Calamari, L., Abeni, F., Bertin, G., 2010. Metabolic and hematological profiles in mature horses supplemented with different selenium sources and doses. J Anim Sci 88, 650–659.

Carlson, G.P., Mansmann, R.A., 1974. Serum electrolyte and plasma protein alterations in horses used in endurance rides. J Am Vet Med Assoc 165, 262–264.

Ciloglu, F., Peker, I., Pehlivan, A., et al., 2005. Exercise intensity and its effects on thyroid hormones. Neuro Endocrinol Lett 26, 830–834.

Coenen, M., 1985a. Beiträge zur Verdauungsphysiologie des Pferdes; 13. Mitteilung. Verdaulichkeit und precaecale Passage einer suspendierfähigen Diät in Abhängigkeit von der Applikationsform (spontaner Futteraufnahme bzw. flüssig per Sonde (Contributions to digestive physiology in horses, 13th communication: Digestivbility and praecaecal passage of a complete diet fed as meal or via noso-gastric tube). J Anim Physiol a Anim Nutr 56, 104–117.

Coenen, M., 1985b. Beiträge zur Verdauungsphysiologie des Pferdes; 13. Mitteilung. Verdaulichkeit und precaecale Passage einer suspendierfähigen Diät in Abhängigkeit von der Applikationsform (spontaner Futteraufnahme bzw. flüssig per Sonde [Digestibility and precaecal passage of a soluble diet in dependence on its application as dry feed or tube fed in liquid form]. J Anim Physiol Anim Nutr 56, 104–117.

Coenen, M., 1986. Contributions to digestive physiology of the horse. 13. Digestibility and precaecal passage of diet in dependence on the format of provision (spontaneous intake vs. tube feeding). J Anim Physiol Nutr 56, 104–117.

Coenen, M., 1991. Chloridhaushalt und Chloridbedarf des Pferdes [Chloride turnover and chloride requirement in the horse]. Habilitationsschrift, Hannover.

Coenen, M., 2005. Exercise and stress: impact on adaptive processes involving water and electrolytes. Livestock Prod Sci 92, 131–145.

Coenen, M., 2012. Bedeutung der Fütterung für die Hufgesundheit (Impact of Nutrition on Hoof Health). Der Huf (The Hoof). L. F. Litzke und B. Rau. Enke-Verlag, Stuttgart.

Coenen, M., Spitzlei, S., 1996a. Investigation in the composition of hoof horn in dependance on age,breed and quality. Pferdeheilkunde (2nd European Conference on Horse Nutrition) 12, 279–283.

Coenen, M., Vervuert, I., 2003. Wasser- und Electrolythaushalt arbeitender Pferde [Water and Electrolyte Turnover in the Equine Athlete]. Übers. Tierernährung 31, 29–73.

Coenen, M., Kirchhof, S., Kienzle, E., et al., 2010. An update on basic data for the factorial calculation of energy and nutrient requirements in lactating mares. Übersichten Tierernährung 38, 91–121.

Coenen, M., Landes, E., Assmann, G., 1998. Selenium toxicosis in the horse – case report. Journal of Animal Physiology and Animal Nutrition-Zeitschrift Fur Tierphysiologie Tierernahrung Und Futtermittelkunde 80, 153–157.

Coenen, M., Vervuert, I., Borchers, A., et al., 2003. Feed compsition and nutrient intake in Hannoverian Warmblood marews and foals with regard to the incidence of osteochondrotic lesions in foals. Equine Nutrition & Physiology Symposium, East Lansing.

Coger, L.H., Hintz, H.F., Schryver, H.F., et al., 1987. The effect of high zinc intake on copper metabolism and bone development in growing horses. In: Equine Nutrition & Physiology Symposium. Colorado. pp 173–178.

Conway, D.A., Cosgrove, J.S., 1980. Equine goitre. Irish Vet J 34, 29–31.
Cooper, S.R., Topliff, D.R., Freeman, D.W., et al., 2000. Effect of dietary cation-anion difference on mineral balance serum osteocalcin concentration and growth in weanling horses. J Equ Vet Sci 20 (1), 39–44.
Crichton, R.R., Ward, R.J., 2003. An overview of iron metabolism: molecular and cellular criteria for the selection of iron chelators. Curr Med Chem 10, 997–1004.
Crozier, J.A., Allen, V.G., Jack, N.E., et al., 1997. Digestibility, apparent mineral absorption, and voluntary intake by horses fed alfalfa, tall fescue, and caucasian bluestem. J Anim Sci 75, 1651–1658.
Curtis, G.M., Fertman, M.B., 1945. Blood iodine studies : VII. The relation of the basal metabolic rate to the blood iodine in thyroid disease. Ann Surg 122, 963–972.
Cymbaluk, N.F., Christensen, D.A., 1986. Oxalate concentration in feeds and its metabolism by ponies. Can J Anim Sci 66, 1107–1116.
Cymbaluk, N.F., Schryver, H.F., Hintz, H.F., 1981a. Copper metabolism and requirement in mature ponies. J Nutr 111, 87–95.
Cymbaluk, N.F., Schryver, H.F., Hintz, H.F., et al., 1981b. Influence of dietary molybdenum on copper metabolism in ponies. J Nutr 111, 96–106.
Davenport, C.L., Boston, R.C., Richardson, D.W., 2001. Effects of enrofloxacin and magnesium deficiency on matrix metabolism in equine articular cartilage. Am J Vet Res 62, 160–166.
Delesalle, C., Dewulf, J., Lefebvre, R.A., et al., 2005. Use of plasma ionized calcium levels and Ca2+ substitution response patterns as prognostic parameters for ileus and survival in colic horses. Vet Q 27, 157–172.
Diaz-Espineira, M., Escolar, E., Bellanato, J., et al., 1995. Crystalline composition of equine urinary sabulous deposits. Scanning Microsc 9, 1071–1077; discussion 1077–1079.
Diaz-Espineira, M., Escolar, E., Bellanato, J., et al., 1996. Minor constituents of sabulous material in equine urine. Research in veterinary science 60, 238–242.
Diaz-Espineira, M., Escolar, E., Bellanato, J., et al., 1997. Infrared and atomic spectrometry analysis of the mineral composition of a series of equine sabulous material samples and urinary calculi. Res Vet Sci 63, 93–95.
Dominguez-Munoz, J.E., Martinez, S.M., Leodolter, A., et al., 2004. Quantification of pancreatic zinc output as pancreatic function test: making the secretin-caerulein test applicable to clinical practice. Pancreatology 4, 57–62.
Drew, B., Barber, W.P., Williams, D.G., 1975. The effect of excess iodine on pregnant mares and foals. Vet Rec 97, 93–95.
Ducharme, N.G., Burton, J.H., Van Dreumel, A.A., et al., 1987. Extensive large colon resection in the pony. II. Digestibility studies and postmortem findings. Can J Vet Res 51, 76–82.
Duesterdieck-Zellmer, K.F., 2007. Equine urolithiasis. Vet Clin North Am Equine Pract 23, 613–629, vi.
Durand, M., Beaumatin, P., Dumay, C., 1983. In vitro estimation using radioactive phosphorus of the phosphorus requirements of rumen microorganisms. Reprod Nutr Dev 23, 727–739.
Ecke, P., Hodgson, D.R., Rose, R.J., 1997. Review of oral rehydration solutions for horses with diarrhoea. Aust Vet J 75, 417–420.
Ecke, P., Hodgson, D.R., Rose, R.J., 1998a. Induced diarrhoea in horses. Part 1: Fluid and electrolyte balance. Vet J 155, 149–159.
Ecke, P., Hodgson, D.R., Rose, R.J., 1998b. Induced diarrhoea in horses. Part 2: Response to administration of an oral rehydration solution. Vet J 155, 161–170.
Eckersall, P.D.P., 1984. Equine wohle saliva: A sample collection system and biochemical analysis. Vet Rec 27, 437–438.
El Shorafa, W.M., Feaster, J.P., Ott, E.A., et al., 1979. Effect of vitamin D and sunlight on growth and bone development of young ponies. J Anim Sci 48, 882–886.
Eroksuz, H., Eroksuz, Y., Ozer, H., et al., 2004. Equine goiter associated with excess dietary iodine. Vet Hum Toxicol 46, 147–149.
Eurola, M., Alfthan, G., Aro, A., et al., 2003. Results of the Finnish selenium monitoring program 2000–2001. Agrifood Research Reports 36.
Facchinetti, F., Borella, P., Valentini, M., et al., 1989. Intra-uterine growth retardation is associated with increased levels of magnesium in amniotic fluid. European journal of obstetrics, gynecology, and reproductive biology 32, 227–232.
Flaminio, M.J., Rush, B.R., 1998. Fluid and electrolyte balance in endurance horses. Vet Clin N Am Equine practice 14, 147–158.
Frantz, N.Z., Andrews, G.A., Tokach, M.D., et al., 2008. Effect of dietary nutrients on osteochondrosis lesions and cartilage properties in pigs. American journal of veterinary research 69, 617–624.
Fullmer, C.S., Wassermann, R.H., 1972. Isolation and partial characterization of intestinal calcium-binding protein from cow, pig, horse, guinea pig and chick. Clinica Chimica Acta 159, 239–248.
Fürst, A., Meier, D., Michel, S., et al., 2008. Effect of age on bone mineral density and micro architecture in the radius and tibia of horses: an Xtreme computed tomographic study. BMC Vet Res 4, 3.
Gallup, W.D., Norris, L.C., 1938. The essentialness of manganese for the normal development of bone. Science 87, 18–19.
Gambling, L., McArdle, H.J., 2004. Iron, copper and fetal development. Proc Nutr Soc 63, 553–562.
Garcia-Lopez, J.M., Provost, P.J., Rush, J.E., et al., 2001. Prevalence and prognostic importance of hypomagnesemia and hypocalcemia in horses that have colic surgery. Am J Vet Res 62, 7–12.
Gee, E.K., Grace, N.D., Firth, E.C., et al., 2000. Changes in liver copper concentration of thoroughbred foals from birth to 160 days of age and the effect of prenatal copper supplementation of their dams. Aust Vet J 78, 347–353.
Gee, E., Davies, M., Firth, E., et al., 2007. Osteochondrosis and copper: histology of articular cartilage from foals out of copper supplemented and non-supplemented dams. Vet J 173, 109–117.
Gee, E.K., Morel, P.C.H., Mogg, T.D., et al., 2004. Liver copper kinetics in Thoroughbred foals at pasture from birth to 160 days of age. New Zea J Agric Res 47, 109–118.
Gee, E.K., Firth, E.C., Morel, P.C., et al., 2005a. Articular/epiphyseal osteochondrosis in Thoroughbred foals at 5 months of age: influences of growth of the foal and prenatal copper supplementation of the dam. N Z Vet J 53, 448–456.
Gee, E.K., Firth, E.C., Morel, P.C., et al., 2005b. Enlargements of the distal third metacarpus and metatarsus in Thoroughbred foals at pasture from birth to 160 days of age. N Z Vet J 53, 438–447.
Geerling, J.C., Loewy, A.D., 2008. Central regulation of sodium appetite. Exp Physiol 93, 177–209.
GfE, 2013. Gesellschaft für Ernährungsphysiologie der Haustiere, Ausschuss für Bedarfsnormen – Society of Physiology in Animals, Committee for feeding standards; Energie- und Nährstoffbedarf landwirtschaftlicher Nutztiere – Energy and nutrient Requirements in Animals; Empfehlungen zur Energie- und Nährstoffversorgung der Pferde – Recommendation for Energy and Nutritent Provision to Horses – in press. Frankfurt/Main, DLG-Verlag.
Glade, M.J., 1993. Effects of gestation, lactation, and maternal calcium intake on mechanical strength of equine bone. J Am Coll Nutr 12, 372–377.
Glade, M.J., Krook, L., Schryver, H.F., et al., 1982. Calcium metabolism in glucocorticoid-treated pony foals. J Nutr 112, 77–86.
Glade, M.J., Luba, N.K., Schryver, H.F., 1986. Effects of age and diet on the development of mechanical strength by the third metacarpal and metatarsal bones of young horses. J Anim Sci 63, 1432–1444.
Gottlieb-Vedi, M., Dahlborn, K., Jansson, A., et al., 1996. Elemental composition of muscle at rest and potassium levels in muscle, plasma and sweat of horses exercising at 20 degrees C and 35 degrees C. Equine Vet J Suppl, 35–41.
Götz, C., 2005. Iodine supply in horses – a field study. Ludwig-Maximillians University, Munich.
Grace, N.D., Pearce, S.G., Firth, E.C., et al., 1999a. Concentrations of macro- and micro-elements in the milk of pasture-fed thoroughbred mares. Aust Vet J 77, 177–180.
Grace, N.D., Pearce, S.G., Firth, E.C., et al., 1999b. Content and distribution of macro- and micro-elements in the body of pasture-fed young horses. Aust Vet J 77, 172–176.
Grace, N.D., Gee, E.K., Firth, E.C., et al., 2002. Digestible energy intake, dry matter digestibility and mineral status of grazing New Zealand Thoroughbred yearlings. N Z Vet J 50, 63–69.
Grace, N.D., Rogers, C.W., Firth, E.C., et al., 2003. Digestible energy intake, dry matter digestibility and effect of increased calcium intake on bone parameters of grazing Thoroughbred weanlings in New Zealand. N Z Vet J 51, 165–173.
Grimaldi, B.L., 2002. The central role of magnesium deficiency in Tourette's syndrome: causal relationships between magnesium deficiency, altered biochemical pathways and symptoms relating to Tourette's syndrome and several reported comorbid conditions. Med Hypotheses 58, 47–60.
Gruber, H.E., Stover, S.J., 1994. Maternal and weanling bone: the influence of lowered calcium intake and maternal dietary history. Bone 15, 167–176.
Gullick, R.W., Lechevallier, M.W., Barhorst, T.S., 2001. Occurrence of perchlorate in drinking water sources. Am Water Works Assoc 93, 66–77.
Günther, C., 1984. Untersuchungen über die Verdaulichkeit und Verträglichkeit von Hafer, Quetschhafer, Gerste und Mais beim Pferd [Investigation on digestibility and combatability of oats, rolled oats, barley and corn in horses]. University of Veterinary Medicine, Hannover.
Gürer, G., 1985. Untersuchungen zum Kaliumstoffwechsel des Pferdes bei marginaler Versorgung und zusätzlicher Belastung (Investigation on potassium metabolism in horses during marginal potassium supply and exercise). University of Veterinary Medicine, Hannover.
Guy, P.S., Snow, D.H., 1977. The effect of training and detraining on muscle composition in the horse. The Journal of physiology 269, 33–51.
Guyot, H., Saegerman, C., Lebreton, P., et al., 2009. Epidemiology of trace elements deficiencies in Belgian beef and dairy cattle herds. J Trace Elements Med Biol 23, 116–123.
Harmeyer, J., Schlumbohm, C., 2004. Effects of pharmacological doses of Vitamin D3 on mineral balance and profiles of plasma Vitamin D3 metabolites in horses. J Steroid Biochem Mol Biol 89–90, 595–600.
Harrington, D.D., 1975. Influence of magnesium deficiency on horse foal tissue concentraion of Mg, calcium and phosphorus. Br J Nutr 34, 45–57.
Harris, P.A., Staniar, W.B., Ellis, A.D., 2005. Effect of exercise and diet on the incidence of DOD. In: Juliand, V., Martin-Rosset, W. (Eds.), The growing horse: nutrition and prevention of growth disorders No. EAAP publication No. 114. Wageningen Academic Publishers pp. 273–290.
Hassel, D.M., Rakestraw, P.C., Gardner, I.A., et al., 2004. Dietary risk factors and colonic pH and mineral concentrations in horses with enterolithiasis. J Vet Intern Med 18, 346–349.

Hassel, D.M., Spier, S.J., Aldridge, B.M., et al., 2009. Influence of diet and water supply on mineral content and pH within the large intestine of horses with enterolithiasis. Vet J 182, 44–49.
Hasselbach, W., 1998. The Ca(2+)-ATPase of the sarcoplasmic reticulum in skeletal and cardiac muscle. An overview from the very beginning to more recent prospects. Ann N Y Acad Sci 853, 1–8.
Hasselbach, W., Oetliker, H., 1983. Energetics and electrogenicity of the sarcoplasmic reticulum calcium pump. Annu Rev Physiol 45, 325–339.
Hays, M.T., 2001. Estimation of total body iodine content in normal young men. Thyroid: official journal of the American Thyroid Association 11, 671–675.
He, T., Joyner, M.J., Katusic, Z.S., 2009. Aging decreases expression and activity of glutathione peroxidase-1 in human endothelial progenitor cells. Microvasc Res 78, 447–452.
Hebeler, D., 1996. Zum Zn-, Cu- und Se-Gehalt in Organen und Geweben abortierter Pferdefeten bzw. post natum verendeter Fohlen aus Norddeutschland [Zn, Cu and se concentration in tissues of aborted equine fetusses and non surviving foals in Northern Germany University of Veterinary Medicine, Hannover.
Herbette, S., Roeckel-Drevet, P., Drevet, J.R., 2007. Seleno-independent glutathione peroxidases. More than simple antioxidant scavengers. Febs J 274, 2163–2180.
Herzig, I., Pisarikova, B., Kursa, J., et al., 2000. Utilisation of iodine from different sources in pigs. Archiv fur Tierernahrung 53, 179–189.
Hidiroglou, M., 1979. Manganese in ruminant nutritiion. Can J Anim Sci 59, 217–236.
Hiney, K.M., Nielsen, B.D., Rosenstein, D., 2004. Short-duration exercise and confinement alters bone mineral content and shape in weanling horses. J Anim Sci 82, 2313–2320.
Hintz, H.F., Schryver, H.F., 1972. Magnesium metabolism in the horse. J Anim Sci 35, 755–759.
Hintz, H.F., Schryver, H.F., 1973. Magnesium, calcium and phosphorus metabolism in ponies fed varying levels of magnesium. J Anim Sci 37, 927–930.
Hintz, H.F., Schryver, H.F., Doty, J., et al., 1984. Oxalic acid content of alfalfa hays and its influence on the availability of calcium, phosphorus and magnesium to ponies. J Anim Sci 58, 939–942.
Hohenheim, D.d.U., 1976. Spurenelemente mit toxischer Wirkung: Tabellen über Gehalte in Futtermitteln = Trace elements with toxic effect in feeds. Stuttgart.
Hoppeler, H., 1990. The different relationship of VO2max to muscle mitochondria in humans and quadrupedal animals. Respiration physiology 80, 137–145.
Hornbrook, S., 1826. Big head. New England Farmer 5, 150–151.
House, S.H., 2007. Nurturing the brain nutritionally and emotionally from before conception to late adolescence. Nutr Health 19, 143–161.
Hunault, C.C., Lambers, A.C., Mensinga, T.T., et al., 2007. Effects of subchronic nitrate exposure on the thyroidal function in humans. Toxicol Lett 175, 64–70.
Hurcombe, S.D., Toribio, R.E., Slovis, N.M., et al., 2009. Calcium regulating hormones and serum calcium and magnesium concentrations in septic and critically ill foals and their association with survival. J Vet Intern Med 23, 335–343.
Hurtig, M., Green, S.L., Dobson, H., et al., 1993. Correlative study of defective cartilage and bone growth in foals fed a low-copper diet. Equine Vet J S16, 66–73.
Huthmann, S., Staszyk, C., Jacob, H.G., et al., 2009. Biomechanical evaluation of the equine masticatory action: calculation of the masticatory forces occurring on the cheek tooth battery. J Biomech 42, 67–70.
Ingenbleek, Y., 2006. The nutritional relationship linking sulfur to nitrogen in living organisms. J Nutr 136, 1641S–1651S.
Ingenbleek, Y., Young, V.R., 2004. The essentiality of sulfur is closely related to nitrogen metabolism: a clue to hyperhomocysteinaemia. Nutr Res Rev 17, 135–151.
Insogna, K., 2009. The effect of proton pump-inhibiting drugs on mineral metabolismproton pump-inhibiting drugs and mineral metabolism. Am J Gastroenterol 104, S2–S4.
Ishida, N., Katayama, Y., Sato, F., et al., 1999. The cDNA sequences of equine antioxidative enzyme genes Cu/Zn-SOD and Mn-SOD, and these expressions in equine tissues. The Journal of veterinary medical science/the Japanese Society of Veterinary Science 61, 291–294.
James, L.F., Butcher, J.E., 1972. Halogeton poisoning of sheep: effect of high level oxalate intake. J Anim Sci 35, 1233–1238.
Jansen, J., Karges, W., Rink, L., 2009. Zinc and diabetes–clinical links and molecular mechanisms. J Nutr Biochem 20, 399–417.
Johnston, J.K., Divers, T.J., Reef, V.B., et al., 1989. Cholelithiasis in horses: ten cases (1982–1986). J Am Vet Med Assoc 194, 405–409.
Kamphues, J., 1991. Calcium metabolism of rabbits as an etiological factor for urolithiasis. J Nutr 121, S95–S96.
Kannan, K., Praamsma, M.L., Oldi, J.F., et al., 2009. Occurrence of perchlorate in drinking water, groundwater, surface water and human saliva from India. Chemosphere 76, 22–26.
Kapusniak, L.J., Greene, L.W., Potter, G.D., 1988. Calcium, magnesium and phosphorus absorption from the small and large intestine of ponies fed elevated amounts of aluminum. J Equine Vet Sci 305–309.
Karren, B.J., Thorson, J.F., Cavinder, C.A., et al., 2010. Effect of selenium supplementation and plane of nutrition on mares and their foals: selenium concentrations and glutathione peroxidase. J Anim Sci 88, 991–997.
Katzen-Luchenta, J., 2007. The declaration of nutrition, health, and intelligence for the child-to-be. Nutr Health 19, 85–102.
Keen, C.L., Uriu-Hare, J.Y., Hawk, S.N., et al., 1998. Effect of copper deficiency on prenatal development and pregnancy outcome. Am J Clin Nutr 67, 1003S–1011S.
Kelishadi, R., Hashemipour, M., Adeli, K., et al., 2010. Effect of zinc supplementation on markers of insulin resistance, oxidative stress, and inflammation among prepubescent children with metabolic syndrome. Metabolic syndrome and related disorders 8, 505–510.
Keller, M., Moliner, J.L., Vasquez, G., et al., 2008. Nephrolithiasis and pyelonephritis in two West Indian manatees (Trichechus manatus spp.). J Wildl Dis 44, 707–711.
Kempson, S.A., 2005. Nutritional management of horses with hoof diseases. Applied Equine Nutrition: Equine nutrition Confenrence (ENUCO) 2005. A. Lindner: 105–112.
Kienzle, E., Burger, A., 2012. Maintenance requirements of major minerals in horses. Übersichten Tierernährung in press.
Kienzle, E., Sturmer, K., Ranz, D., et al., 2006. A high roughage/concentrate ratio decreases the effect of ammonium chloride on acid-base balance in horses. J Nutr 136, 2048S–2049S.
Kobayashi, T., Sugi, H., 1980. Measurement of heat production during the summation of isometric contraction in frog skeletal muscle with an infrared radiometer. Jpn J Physiol 30, 617–629.
Kobayashi, M., Shimizu, S., 1999. Cobalt proteins. Eur J Biochem 261 (1), 1–9.
Kodaka, T., Debari, K., Yamada, M., 1991. Physico-chemical and morphological studies of horse dentin. J Electron Microsc (Tokyo) 40, 385–391.
Komisarczuk, S., Durand, M., Beaumatin, P., et al., 1987a. Effects of phosphorus deficiency on rumen microbial activity associated with the solid and liquid phases of a fermentor (Rusitec). Reprod Nutr Dev 27, 907–919.
Komisarczuk, S., Merry, R.J., McAllan, A.B., 1987b. Effect of different levels of phosphorus on rumen microbial fermentation and synthesis determined using a continuous culture technique. The British Journal of Nutrition 57, 279–290.
Kothapalli, C.R., Ramamurthi, A., 2009. Lysyl oxidase enhances elastin synthesis and matrix formation by vascular smooth muscle cells. J Tissue Eng Regen Med 3, 655–661.
Laan, T.T., Spoorenberg, J.F., van der Kolk, J.H., 2000. Hypocalcemia in a four-week-old foal. Tijdschr Diergeneeskd 125, 185–187.
Lamothe, P., Guay, P., 1970. Electrolytes in bovine intrauterine secretions in infertility sine material. Can J Comp Med 34, 167–176.
Lansdown, A.B., Sampson, B., 1997. Trace metals in keratinising epithelia in beagle dogs. Vet Rec 141, 571–572.
Laverty, S., Pascoe, J.R., Ling, G.V., et al., 1992. Urolithiasis in 68 horses. Vet Surg 21, 56–62.
Lavoie, J.P., Teuscher, E., 1993. Massive iron overload and liver fibro sis resembling haemochromatosis in a racing pony. Equine Vet J 25, 552–554.
Lee, B., Pine, M., Johnson, L., et al., 2006. Manganese acts centrally to activate reproductive hormone secretion and pubertal development in male rats. Reprod Toxicol 22, 580–585.
Lepage, O.M., Carstanjen, B., Uebelhart, D., 2001. Non-invasive assessment of equine bone: an update. Veterinary journal 161, 10–22.
Leskova, R., 1969. Iodine supply of dairy cattle in Austria. Wien Tierarztl Monatsschr 56, 369–374.
Lewis, H.B., Moyer, W.A., 1977. Iatrogenic iron overload in the horse. Proceedings. 1st Intern Symp Equine Hematol 1, 258–261.
Linder, M.C., Hazegh-Azam, M., 1996. Copper biochemistry and molecular biology. Am J Clin Nutr 63, 797S–811S.
Linder, M.C., Lomeli, N.A., Donley, S., et al., 1999. Copper transport in mammals. Adv Exp Med Biol 448, 1–16.
Lindinger, M.I., 1999. Exercise in the heat: thermoregulatory limitations to performance in humans and horses. Can J Appl Physiol 24, 152–163.
Lindinger, M.I., Heigenhauser, G.J., 1991. The roles of ion fluxes in skeletal muscle fatigue. Can J Physiol Pharmacol 69, 246–253.
Lindinger, M.I., Heigenhauser, G.J., Spriet, L.L., 1990. Effects of alkalosis on muscle ions at rest and with intense exercise. Can J Physiol Pharmacol 68, 820–829.
Lindner, A., 1983. Untersuchungen zum Natriumstoffwechsel des Pferdes bei marginaler Versorgung und zusätzlicher Bewegungsbelastung (Investigation on sodium metabolism in horses with marginal sodium supply and exercise). University of Veterinary Medicine, Hannover.
Lopez, I., Felsenfeld, A.J., Estepa, J.C., et al., 2006. Effect of changes in ionized calcium concentration in arterial blood and metabolic acidosis on the arterial partial pressure of oxygen in dogs. Am J Vet Res 67, 801–808.
Luthersson, N., Chumekamrai, S., Estepa, J.C., et al., 2005. Secondary hyperparathyroidism in ponies in Northern Thailand. Pferdeheilkunde 21, 97–98.
MacKay, R.J., 2004. Brain injury after head trauma: pathophysiology, diagnosis, and treatment. Vet Clin North Am Equine Pract 20, 199–216.

Mainwood, G.W., Renaud, J.M., 1985. The effect of acid-base balance on fatigue of skeletal muscle. Can J Physiol Pharmacol 63, 403–416.

Malinowski, K., Christensen, R.A., Hafs, H.D., et al., 1996. Age and breed differences in thyroid hormones, insulin-like growth factor (IGF)-I and IGF binding proteins in female horses. J anim Sci 74, 1936–1942.

Mansmann, R.A., Carlson, G.P., White, N.A., 2nd, et al., 1974. Synchronous diaphragmatic flutter in horses. J Am Vet Med Assoc 165, 265–270.

Marreiro, D.N., Geloneze, B., Tambascia, M.A., et al., 2006. Effect of zinc supplementation on serum leptin levels and insulin resistance of obese women. Biol Trace Elem Res 112, 109–118.

Martin-Tereso, J., Verstegen, M.W., 2011. A novel model to explain dietary factors affecting hypocalcaemia in dairy cattle. Nutr Res Rev 24, 228–243.

Matsui, T., Murakami, Y., Yano, H., et al., 1999. Phytate and phosphorus movements in the digestive tract of horses. Equine veterinary journal 31, 505–507.

McCutcheon, L.J., Geor, R.J., 1996. Sweat fluid and ion losses in horses during training and competition in cool vs. hot ambient conditions: implications for ion supplementation. Equ Vet J Suppl 54–62.

McCutcheon, L.J., Geor, R.J., 1998a. Sweating. Fluid and ion losses and replacement. Vet Clin North Am Equine Pract 14, 75–95.

McCutcheon, L.J., Geor, R.J., 1998b. Sweating. Fluid and ion losses and replacement. The Veterinary Clinics of North America. Equ Pract 14, 75–95.

McCutcheon, L.J., Geor, R.J., 2000. Influence of training on sweating responses during submaximal exercise in horses. J Appl Physiol 89, 2463–2471.

McCutcheon, L.J., Geor, R.J., Ecker, G.L., et al., 1999. Equine sweating responses to submaximal exercise during 21 days of heat acclimation. Journal of applied physiology 87, 1843–1851.

McCutcheon, L.J., Geor, R.J., Hare, M.J., et al., 1995a. Sweating rate and sweat composition during exercise and recovery in ambient heat and humidity. Equine Veterinary Journal Supplement, 153–157.

McCutcheon, L.J., Geor, R.J., Hare, M.J., et al., 1995b. Sweat composition: Comparison of collection methods and effects of exercise intensity. Equine Veterinary Journal 18, 279–284.

McDowell, L.R., 2003. Minerals in Animal and Human Nutrition, second ed. Elsevier Science B.V., Amsterdam.

McKeever, K.H., 1998. Effect of exercise on fluid balance and renal function in horses. Equine Practice 14, 23–44.

McKeever, K.H., Hinchcliff, K.W., Reed, S.M., et al., 1993. Plasma constituents during incremental treadmill exercise in intact and splenectomised horses. Equine Veterinary Journal 25, 233–236.

McKeever, K.H., Scali, R., Geiser, S., et al., 2002. Plasma aldosterone concentration and renal sodium excretion are altered during the first days of training. Equine Vet J Suppl 524–531.

McOrist, S., Thomas, K.W., 1984. Levels of trace elements in the liver and diet of free-living koalas, Phascolarctos cinereus (Goldfuss). J Wildl Dis 20 (3), 220–225.

Medica, P., Cravana, C., Fazio, E., et al., 2011a. 24-Hour endocrine profiles of Quarter Horses under Resting Conditions. Journal of Equine Veterinary Science 31, 35–40.

Medica, P., Fazio, E., Cravana, C., et al., 2011b. Influence of endemic goitre areas on thyroid hormones in horses. Animal 5, 82–87.

Meijer, P., 1982. Two cases of tetany in the horse. Tijdschrift Voor Diergeneeskunde 107 (9), 329–332.

Merian, E., Anke, M., Ihnat, M., et al., 2004. Wiley-VCH Verlag GmbH&Co KGaA, second ed, Weinheim.

Mertz, W., Roginski, E., Schroeder, H.A., 1965. Some Aspects of Glucose Metabolism of Chromium-Deficient Rats Raised in a Strictly Controlled Environment. The Journal of Nutrition 86, 107–112.

Meyer, H., 1980. Na-Stoffwechsel und Na-Bedarf des Pferdes. Übers. Tierernährung 8, 37–64.

Meyer, H., 1987. Nutrition of the equine athlete. Equine Exercise Physiology 2, 644–673.

Meyer, H., 1990. Contributions to water and mineral metabolism of the horse. Parey, Hamburg.

Meyer, H., 1992. Intestinaler Wasser- und Elektrolytstoffwechsel beim Pferd (Intestinal Water and Electrolyte metabolism in horses). Übersichten Tierernährung 20, 135–156.

Meyer, H., 1994. Kupferstoffwechsel und Kupferbedarf beim Pferd [Copper - Metabolism and Requirements in Horses]. Übersichten Tierern 22, 363–394.

Meyer, H., Ahlswede, L., 1976. Über das intrauterine Wachstum und die Körperzusammensetzung von Fohlen sowie den Nährstoffbedarf tragender Stuten. Übersichten Tierernährung 4, 263–292.

Meyer, H., Coenen, M., 2002. Pferdefütterung [Horse nutrition]. Parey Verlag, Berlin.

Meyer, H., Stadermann, B., 1990. Möglichkeiten zur Bestimmung der Mineralstoffversorgung des Pferdes durch Harnanalysen (On the evaluation of mineral intake in horses by analyses of urine). In: Meyer, H. (Ed.), Advances in animal physiology and animal nutrition - Contributions to water and mineral metabolism of the horse No. 21. Parey, Hamburg, pp 102.

Meyer, H., Schmidt, M., Lindemann, G., et al., 1982. Praecaecale und postileale Verdaulichkeit von Mengen- (Ca, P, Mg) und Spurenelementen (Cu, Zn, Mn) beim Pferd (Prececal and postileal absorption of macro- (Ca, P, Mg) and trace elements (Cu, Zn, Mn) in horses). In: Meyer, H. (Ed.), Contribution to Digestive Physiology of the Horse. Verlag Paul Parey, Hanburg, Berlin, pp. 61–69.

Meyer, H., Coenen, M., Probst, D., 1986. Beiträge zur Verdauungsphysiologie des Pferdes, 14. Mitteilung: Futtereinspeichelung und -passage im Kopfdarm des Pferdes (Contributions to digestive physiology in horses, 14. communication: Saliva production during feed ingestion and oro-esophageal feed passage). J Anim Pysiol a Anim Nutr 56, 266–275.

Meyer, H., Zentek, J., Heikens, A., et al., 1995. Untersuchungen zur Selenversorgung von Pferden in Norddeutschland (Investigation on the selenium intake in horses in Northern Germany). Pferdeheilkunde 11, 313–321.

Meyer, H., Flothow, C., Radicke, S., 1997. Preileal digestibility of coconut fat and soybean oil in horses and their influence on metabolites of microbial origin of the proximal digestive tract. Archiv fur Tierernahrung 50, 63–74.

Millard, K.N., Frazer, D.M., Wilkins, S.J., et al., 2004. Changes in the expression of intestinal iron transport and hepatic regulatory molecules explain the enhanced iron absorption associated with pregnancy in the rat. Gut 53, 655–660.

Miyazawa, K., Motoyoshi, S., Usui, K., 1978. Nodular goiters of three mares and their foals, induced by feeding excessive amount of seaweed. Nippon Juigaku Zasshi 40, 749–753.

Mojiminiyi, O.A., Marouf, R., Abdella, N.A., 2008. Body iron stores in relation to the metabolic syndrome, glycemic control and complications in female patients with type 2 diabetes. Nutr Metab Cardiovasc Dis 18, 559–566.

Montgomerie, R.F., Savage, W.H., Dodds, E.C., 1929. Tetany in Welsh mountain ponies. Vet Rec 9, 319–334.

Morris, M.E., 1992. Brain and CSF magnesium concentrations during magnesium deficit in animals and humans: neurological symptoms. Magnes Res 5, 303–313.

Muirhead, T.L., Wichtel, J.J., Stryhn, H., et al., 2010. The selenium and vitamin E status of horses in Prince Edward Island. Can Vet J 51, 979–985.

Mullaney, T.P., Brown, C.M., 1988. Iron toxicity in neonatal foals. Equine Vet J 20, 119–124.

Munoz, M., Villar, I., Garcia-Erce, J.A., 2009. An update on iron physiology. World J Gastroenterol 15, 4617–4626.

Munoz, M., Garcia-Erce, J.A., Remacha, A.F., 2010. Disorders of iron metabolism. Part 1: molecular basis of iron homoeostasis. J Clin Pathol.

Negro, R., Soldin, O.P., Obregon, M.J., et al., 2011. Hypothyroxinemia and pregnancy. Endocrine practice: official journal of the American College of Endocrinology and the American Association of Clinical Endocrinologists 17, 422–429.

Neumann, R.D., Ruby, A.L., Ling, G.V., et al., 1994. Ultrastructure and mineral composition of urinary calculi from horses. American Journal of Veterinary Research 55, 1357–1367.

NRC., 2005. National Research Council, Mineral Tolerance of Animals, second revised ed. National Academies Press, Washington DC.

Nyman, S., Jansson, A., Dahlborn, K., et al., 1996. Strategies for voluntary rehydration in horses during endurance exercise. Equine Veterinary journal Supplement, 99–106.

Okumura, M., Asano, M., Tagami, M., et al., 1998. Serum copper and ceruloplasmin activity at the early growing stage in foals. Can J Vet Res 62, 122–126.

Ordakowski-Burk, A.L., Quinn, R.W., Shellem, T.A., et al., 2006a. Voluntary intake and digestibility of reed canarygrass and timothy hay fed to horses. Journal of Animal Science 84, 3104–3109.

Ordakowski-Burk, A.L., Quinn, R.W., Shellem, T.A., et al., 2006b. Voluntary intake and digestibility of reed canarygrass and timothy hay fed to horses. J Anim Sci 84, 3104–3109.

Pagan, J., 2001. Micomineral Requirements in Horses. In: Pagan, J., Geor, R.J. (Eds.), Advances in Equne Nutrition II. Nottingham University Press, Nottingham, pp. 317–327.

Pagan, J.D., Karnezos, P., Kennedy, M.A.P., et al., 1999. Effect of selenium source on selenium digestibility and retention in exercised Thoroughbreds. Proc Equine Nutrition and Physiology Society 16, 135–140.

Panciera, R.J., Martin, T., Burrows, G.E., et al., 1990. Acute oxalate poisoning attributable to ingestion of curly dock (Rumex crispus) in sheep. Journal of the American Veterinary Medical Association 196, 1981–1984.

Pearce, E.N., Braverman, L.E., 2009. Environmental pollutants and the thyroid. Best Pract Res Clin Endocrinol Metab 23, 801–813.

Pearce, S.G., Firth, E.C., Grace, N.D., et al., 1998a. Effect of copper supplementation on the evidence of developmental orthopaedic disease in pasture-fed New Zealand Thoroughbreds. Equine Vet J 30, 211–218.

Pearce, S.G., Grace, N.D., Wichtel, J.J., et al., 1998b. Effect of copper supplementation on the copper status of pasture-fed young Thoroughbreds. Equine Veterinary journal 30, 204–210.

Pearce, S.G., Grace, N.D., Wichtel, J.J., et al., 1998c. Effect of copper supplementation on copper status of pregnant mares and foals. Equine Veterinary Journal 30, 200–203.

Pearce, S.G., Firth, E.C., Grace, N.D., et al., 1999. The effect of high pasture molybdenum concentrations on the copper status of grazing horses in New Zealand. New Zealand Journal of Agricultural Research 42, 93–99.

Pearson, E.G., Andreasen, C.B., 2001. Effect of oral administration of excessive iron in adult ponies. Journal of the American Veterinary Medical Association 218, 400–404.

Pearson, E.G., Hedstrom, O.R., Poppenga, R.H., 1994. Hepatic cirrhosis and hemochromatosis in three horses. Journal of the American Veterinary Medical Association 204, 1053–1056.

Pine, M., Lee, B., Dearth, R., et al., 2005. Manganese acts centrally to stimulate luteinizing hormone secretion: a potential influence on female pubertal development. Toxicol Sci 85, 880–885.

Podoll, K.L., Bernard, J.B., Ullrey, D.E., et al., 1992. Dietary selenate versus selenite for cattle, sheep, and horses. J Anim Sci 70, 1965–1970.

Polack, E.W., King, J.M., Cummings, J.F., et al., 2000. Concentrations of trace minerals in the spinal cord of horses with equine motor neuron disease. Am J Vet Res 61, 609–611.

Poppenga, R.H., 2001. Risks associated with the use of herbs and other dietary supplements. The Veterinary Clinics of North America. The Veterinary Clinics of North America Equine Practice 17, 455–477, vi-vii.

Porr, C.A., Kronfeld, D.S., Lawrence, L.A., et al., 1998. Deconditioning reduces mineral content of the third metacarpal bone in horses. J Anim Sci 76, 1875–1879.

Price, J.S., Jackson, B.F., Gray, J.A., et al., 2001. Biochemical markers of bone metabolism in growing thoroughbreds: a longitudinal study. Research in veterinary science 71, 37–44.

Puls, R., 1994. Mineral Levels in Animal Health Diagnostic Data. Sherpa International, Clearbrook, Canada.

Raisbeck, M.F., Dahl, E.R., Sanchez, D.A., et al., 1993. Naturally occurring selenosis in Wyoming. J Vet Diagn Invest 5, 84–87.

Ralston, S.L., Sullins, K.E., Stashak, T.S., 1986. Digestion in horses after resection or ischemic insult of the large colon. Am J Vet Res 47, 2290–2293.

Richardson, J.D., Harrison, L.J., Edwards, G.B., 1991. Two horses with hypocalcaemia. Vet Rec 129, 98.

Richardson, S.M., Siciliano, P.D., Engle, T.E., et al., 2006. Effect of selenium supplementation and source on the selenium status of horses. J Anim Sci 84, 1742–1748.

Rieker, J.M., Cooper, S.R., Topliff, D.R., et al., 2000. Copper balance in mature geldings fed supplemental molybdenum. Journal of Equine Veterinary Science 20, 522–525.

Romanowski K, HAcke S, Vernunft A, et al. 2011. Effects of different doses of oral sodium chloride on acid-base and mineral balance of exercised horses fed a haybased diet. Proceedings of the 15th ESVCN Congress p 83.

Roose, K.A., Hoekstra, K.E., Pagan, J.D., et al., 2001. Effect of an aluminium supplement on nutrient digestibility and mineral metabolism in thoroughbred horses. In: Pagan, J., Geor, R.J. (Eds.), Advances in Equine Nutrition II. Nottinghasm University Press, Nottingham. pp. 119–126.

Rotruck, J.T., Pope, A.L., Ganther, H.E., et al., 1973. Selenium: biochemical role as a component of glutathione peroxidase. Science 179, 588–590.

Rourke, K.M., Coe, S., Kohn, C.W., et al., 2010. Cloning, comparative sequence analysis and mRNA expression of calcium-transporting genes in horses. Gen Comp Endocrinol 167, 6–10.

Rourke, K.M., Kohn, C.W., Levine, A.L., et al., 2009. Rapid calcitonin response to experimental hypercalcemia in healthy horses. Domest Anim Endocrinol 36, 197–201.

Rucker, R.B., Rucker, B.R., Mitchell, A.E., et al., 1999. Activation of chick tendon lysyl oxidase in response to dietary copper. J Nutr 129, 2143–2146.

Rude, R.K., Gruber, H.E., Wei, L.Y., et al., 2003. Magnesium deficiency: effect on bone and mineral metabolism in the mouse. Calcif Tissue Int 72, 32–41.

Rude, R.K., Singer, F.R., Gruber, H.E., 2009. Skeletal and Hormonal Effects of Magnesium Deficiency. J Am Coll Nutr 28, 131–141.

Salminen, K., 1975. Cobalt metabolism in horse. Serum level and biosynthesis of vitamin B12. Acta Vet Scand 16 (1), 84–94.

Sanchez, C.A., Blount, B.C., Valentin-Blasini, L., et al., 2008. Perchlorate in the feed-dairy continuum of the southwestern United States. J Agric Food Chem 56, 5443–5450.

Scheytt, T., Freywald, J., Ptacek, C., 2011. Untersuchung ausgewählter Oberflächen-, Grund- und Bodenwasserproben auf Perchlorat in Deutschland: Erste Ergebnisse. Grundwasser 16, 37–43.

Schöne, F., Kirchheim, U., Tischendorf, F., et al., 1997. Prüfung von Leinfuttermitteln (Saat, Extraktionsschrot) an wachsenden Schweinen – Futterwert, Thiocyanat- und Schilddrüsenhormonstatus. Lipid / Fett 99, 15–18.

Schönthaler, S., 1998. Untersuchungen zur Selenversorgung von Vollblutstuten und deren Fohlen während Trächtigkeit, Laktation und Aufzucht (Investigation on Selenium intake in Thoroughbred mares and foals during gestation and lactation). Freie Universität, Berlin.

Schott, H.C., 2nd., 1998. Oral fluids for equine diarrhoea: an underutilized treatment for a costly disease? Vet J 155, 119–121.

Schryver, H.F., Craig, P.H., Hintz, H.F., 1970a. Calcium metabolism in ponies fed varying levels of calcium. J Nutr 100, 955–964.

Schryver, H.F., Craig, P.H., Hintz, H.F., et al., 1970b. The site of calcium absorption in the horse. J Nutr 100, 1127–1131.

Schryver, H.F., Hintz, H.F., Craig, P.H., et al., 1972. Site of phosphorus absorption from the intestine of the horse. The Journal of Nutrition 102, 143–147.

Schryver, H.F., Hintz, H.F., Lowe, J.E., 1980. Absorption, excretion and tissue distribution of stable zinc and 65zinc in ponies. J Anim Sci 51, 896–902.

Schryver, H.F., Hintz, H.F., Lowe, J.E., et al., 1974. Mineral composition of the whole body, liver and bone of young horses. J Nutr 104, 126–132.

Schryver, H.F., Millis, D.L., Soderholm, L.V., et al., 1986. Metabolism of some essential minerals in ponies fed high levels of aluminum. Cornell Vet 76, 354–360.

Schryver, H.F., Parker, M.T., Daniluk, P.D., et al., 1987. Salt consumption and the effect of salt on mineral metabolism in horses. Cornell Vet 77, 122–131.

Shulkes, A., Baldwin, G.S., Giraud, A.S., 2006. Regulation of gastric acid secretion; in Johnson, L.R. (editor in chief). Physiology of the gastrointestinal tract, fourth ed. Academic Press, New York, pp. 1223–1258.

Schümann, K., Elsenhans, B., 2004. The iron group. In: Merian, E., Anke, M., Ihnat, M., et al. (Eds.), Elements and their compounds in the environment. Wiley-VCH Verlag GmbH & Co.KGaA, Weinheim.

Schwarzer, U., 1997. Untersuchungen zum Säure-Basen-und Elektrolythaushalt bei Stuten unter besonderer Berücksichtigung der Säuren-und Basenausscheidung im Harn (Investigation on Electrolytes balance in mares with special regard to the elimination of acids and bases by urine). Thesis Veterinary Medicine, University Leipzig.

Selby, L.A., Marienfeld, C.J., Pierce, J.O., 1970. The effects of trace elements on human and animal health. J Am Vet Med Assoc 157, 1800–1808.

Shellow, J.S., Jackson, S.G., Baker, J.P., et al., 1985. The influence of dietary selenium levels on blood levels of selenium and glutathione peroxidase activity in the horse. J Anim Sci 61, 590–594.

Sherman, H.C., Hawk, P.B., 1900. On the elimination of nitrogen, sulphates, and phosphates after the ingestion of proteid food. Am J Physiol 4, 25–49.

Silva, C.A., Merkt, H., Bergamo, P.N., et al., 1987a. Consequence of excess iodine supply in a Thoroughbred stud in southern Brazil. J Reprod Fertil Suppl 35, 529–533.

Silva, C.A.M., Merkt, H., Bergamo, P.N.L., et al., 1987b. Jodvergiftung beim Vollblutfohlen [Intoxication of iodine in Thoroughbred foals]. Pferdeheilkunde 3, 271–276.

Singh, R.K., Kooreman, K.M., Babbs, C.F., et al., 1992. Potential use of simple manganese salts as antioxidant drugs in horses. Am J Vet Res 53, 1822–1829.

Singh, A.K., Dobashi, K., Gupta, M.P., et al., 1999. Manganese superoxide dismutase in rat liver peroxisomes: biochemical and immunochemical evidence. Molecular and cellular biochemistry 197, 7–12.

Sippel, W.L., 1969. A Veterinarian's Approach to Stud Farm Nutrition. Equine Veterinary Journal 1, 203–211.

Slebodzinski, A.B., 2005. Ovarian iodide uptake and triiodothyronine generation in follicular fluid. The enigma of the thyroid ovary interaction. Domest Anim Endocrinol 29, 97–103.

Smith, P., Stubley, D., Blackmore, D.J., 1983. Measurement of superoxide dismutase, diamine oxidase and caeruloplasmin oxidase in the blood of thoroughbreds. Res Vet Sci 35, 160–164.

Spais, A., et al., 1978. Studies on iron, manganese, zinc, copper and selenium retention and interaction in horses. In: 3. Int. Kongreß Spurenelemente bei Mensch und Tier.

Sprekeler, N., Muller, T., Kowalewski, M.P., et al., 2011. Expression patterns of intestinal calcium transport factors and ex-vivo absorption of calcium in horses. BMC veterinary research 7, 65.

Srinivasan, A., Viraraghavan, T., 2009. Perchlorate: health effects and technologies for its removal from water resources. Int J Environ Res Public Health 6, 1418–1442.

Staniar, W.B., Bussard, J.R., Repard, N.M., et al., 2010. Voluntary intake and digestibility of teff hay fed to horses. J Anim Sci 88, 3296–3303.

Stemme, K., Meyer, U., Flachowsky, G., et al., 2002. Die Kobalt-Versorgung von Wiederkäuern – Bedeutung, Bedarf und Bewertung (The Cobalt Uptake in Ruminants – Physiology, Requirement, Evaluation). Übersichten Tierernährung 30, 1–36.

Stewart, A.J., 2011. Magnesium disorders in horses. Vet Clin North Am Equine Pract 27, 149–163.

Stewart, A.J., Hardy, J., Kohn, C.W., et al., 2004. Validation of diagnostic tests for determination of magnesium status in horses with reduced magnesium intake. American journal of veterinary research 65, 422–430.

Stewart, J., Liyou, O., Wilson, G., 2010. Bighead in Horses - Not an Ancient Disease. Australian Equine Vet 29, 55–62.

Stillions, 1971. Stowe, H. D. 1967. Serum selenium and related parameters of naturally and experimentally fed horses. J Nutr 93, 60–64.

Stowe, H.D., 1980. Effects of copper pretreatment upon toxicity of selenium in ponies. Am J Vet Res 41, 1925–1928.

Stürmer, K., 2005. Investigations on the effects of feeding on acid-base balance in ponies. Ludwig-Maximillians-University, Munich.

Stutz, W.A., Topliff, D.R., Freeman, D.W., et al., 1992. Effects of dietary cation-anion balance on blood parameters in exercising horses. Journal of Equine Veterinary Science 12, 164–167.

Suwannachot, P., Verkleij, C.B., Van Weeren, P.R., et al., 2003. Ca2+ ATPase in Dutch warmblood foals compared with Na+, K+ ATPase: intermuscular differences and the effect of exercise. J Vet Med A Physiol Pathol Clin Med 50, 385–390.

Swartzman, J.A., Hintz, H.F., Schryver, H.F., 1978. Inhibition of calcium absorption in ponies fed diets containing oxalic acid. Am J Vet Res 39, 1621–1623.

Szakmáry, E., Ungváry, G., Hudák, A., et al., 2001. Effects of cobalt sulfate on prenatal development of mice, rats, and rabbits, and on early postnatal development of rats. J. Toxicol. Environ. Health, Part A367–A386.

Tal, E., Guggenheim, K., 1965. Effect of Manganese on Calcification of Bone. Biochem J 95, 94–97.

Tam, M., Gomez, S., Gonzalez-Gross, M., et al., 2003. Possible roles of magnesium on the immune system. Eur J Clin Nutr 57, 1193–1197.

Teleb, H., 1984. Investigation on the intestinal Calcium metabolism in horses after different Calcium intake and additional oxalate. University of Veterinary Medicine-Foundation, Hannover.

Theurl, I., Aigner, E., Theurl, M., et al., 2009. Regulation of iron homeostasis in anemia of chronic disease and iron deficiency anemia: diagnostic and therapeutic implications. Blood 113, 5277–5286.

Thorson, J.F., Karren, B.J., Bauer, M.L., et al., 2010. Effect of selenium supplementation and plane of nutrition on mares and their foals: foaling data. J Anim Sci 88, 982–990.

Tilly, J.L., Tilly, K.I., 1995. Inhibitors of oxidative stress mimic the ability of follicle-stimulating hormone to suppress apoptosis in cultured rat ovarian follicles. Endocrinology 136, 242–252.

Tomasi, T.E., Hellgren, E.C., Tucker, T.J., 1998. Thyroid hormone concentrations in black bears (Ursus americanus): hibernation and pregnancy effects. Gen Comp Endocrinol 109, 192–199.

Tomlinson, D.J., Mülling, C.H., Fakler, T.M., 2004. Invited review: formation of keratins in the bovine claw: roles of hormones, minerals, and vitamins in functional claw integrity. J Dairy Sci 87, 797–809.

Toribio, R.E., Kohn, C.W., Chew, D.J., et al., 2001. Comparison of serum parathyroid hormone and ionized calcium and magnesium concentrations and fractional urinary clearance of calcium and phosphorus in healthy horses and horses with enterocolitis. Am J Vet Res 62, 938–947.

Toribio, R.E., Kohn, C.W., Sams, R.A., et al., 2003. Hysteresis and calcium set-point for the calcium parathyroid hormone relationship in healthy horses. Gen Comp Endocrinol 130, 279–288.

Toribio, R.E., Kohn, C.W., Hardy, J., et al., 2005. Alterations in serum parathyroid hormone and electrolyte concentrations and urinary excretion of electrolytes in horses with induced endotoxemia. Journal of Veterinary Internal Medicine / American College of Veterinary Internal Medicine 19, 223–231.

Toribio, R.E., Kohn, C.W., Rourke, K.M., et al., 2007. Effects of hypercalcemia on serum concentrations of magnesium, potassium, and phosphate and urinary excretion of electrolytes in horses. Am J Vet Res 68, 543–554.

Tyler, C.M., Golland, L.C., Evans, D.L., et al., 1998. Skeletal muscle adaptations to prolonged training, overtraining and detraining in horses. Pflugers Archiv : European journal of physiology 436, 391–397.

van Doorn, D.A., Everts, H., Wouterse, H., et al., 2004. The apparent digestibility of phytate phosphorus and the influence of supplemental phytase in horses. J Anim Sci 82, 1756–1763.

Vervuert, I., Coenen, M., Wedemeyer, U., et al., 2002. Calcium homeostasis and intact plasma parathyroid hormone during exercise and training in young Standardbred horses. Equine Vet J 34, 713–718.

Vervuert, I., Coenen, M., Borchers, A., et al., 2003. Growth rate and incidence of osteochondrotic lesions in Hannoverian Warmblood foals. Equine Nutrition & Physiology Symposium, East Lansing.

Vervuert, I., Stanik, K., Coenen, M., 2006. Effects of different levels of calcium and phosphorus intake on calcium homeostasis in exercising horses. Equine Vet J Suppl, 659–663.

Vervuert, I., Junge, J., Martin-Rosset, W., et al., 2010. Assessment of bone mineral density by dual X-ray absortiometry in the horse: A methodological approach. In: European Workshop on Equine Mutrition.

Vezina, F., Gustowska, A., Jalvingh, K.M., et al., 2009. Hormonal correlates and thermoregulatory consequences of molting on metabolic rate in a northerly wintering shorebird. Physiol Biochem Zool 82, 129–142.

von Bieberstein, S.R., 1990. Prüfung von verschiedenen Magnesium-Verbindungen beim ruhenden und arbeitenden Pferd (Investigation on different Magnesium-soureces in sedentary and exercising horses). University of Veterinary Medicine-Foundation, Hannover.

Wagner, E.L., Potter, G.D., Gibbs, P.G., et al., 2010. Copper and zinc balance in exercising horses fed two forms of mineral supplements. J Anim Sci 89, 722–727.

Wall, D.L., Topliff, D.R., Freeman, D.W., et al., 1992. Effect of dietary cation-anion balance on urinary mineral excretion in exercised horses. Journal of Equine Veterinary Science 12, 168–171.

Waller, A., Lindinger, M.I., 2007. The effect of oral sodium acetate administration on plasma acetate concentration and acid-base state in horses. Acta Vet Scand 49, 38.

Waller, A., Armstrong, S., Smithurst, K.-J., et al., 2004. Effects of diet, feeding and daily variation on acid-base balance in horses. Equine and Comp. Exercise Physiol. 1, 153–165.

Waller, A.P., Heigenhauser, G.J., Geor, R.J., et al., 2009. Fluid and electrolyte supplementation after prolonged moderate-intensity exercise enhances muscle glycogen resynthesis in Standardbred horses. Journal of Applied Physiology 106, 91–100.

Walthall, J.C., McKenzie, R.A., 1976. Osteodystrophia fibrosa in horses at pasture in Queensland: field and laboratory observations. Australian Veterinary Journal 52, 11–16.

Wehr, U., Englschalk, B., Kienzle, E., et al., 2002. Iodine Balance in Relation to Iodine Intake in Ponies. The Journal of Nutrition 132, 1767S–1768S.

Weiss, W.P., 2003. Selenium nutrition of dairy cows: comparing responses to organic and inorganic selenium forms. In: Lyons, T.P., Jacques, K.A. (Eds.), Proc. Alltech's Nineteenth Annual Symposium, Nutritional Biotechnology in the Feed and Food Industries No. 19. Nottingham University Press, UK. pp. 333–343.

Wichert, B., Frank, T., Kienzle, E., 2002. Zinc, copper and selenium intake and status of horses in Bavaria. J Nutr 132, 1776S–1777S.

Wiebold, J.L., 1988. Embryonic mortality and the uterine environment in first-service lactating dairy cows. J Reprod Fertil 84, 393–399.

Wiernsperger, N., Rapin, J., 2010. Trace elements in glucometabolic disorders: an update. Diabetology & metabolic syndrome 2, 70.

Wijnberg, I.D., Franssen, H., van der Kolk, J.H., et al., 2002a. Quantitative analysis of motor unit action potentials in the subclavian muscle of healthy horses. American Journal of Veterinary Research 63, 198–203.

Wijnberg, I.D., Franssent, H., van der Kolk, J.H., et al., 2002b. Quantitative motor unit action potential analysis of skeletal muscles in the Warmblood horse. Equine Veterinary Journal 34, 556–561.

Wijnberg, I.D., van der Kolk, J.H., Franssen, H., et al., 2002c. Electromyographic changes of motor unit activity in horses with induced hypocalcemia and hypomagnesemia. American Journal of Veterinary Research 63, 849–856.

Williamson, L.H., Andrews, F.M., Maykuth, P.L., et al., 1996. Biochemical changes in three-day-event horses at the beginning, middle and end of Phase C and after Phase D. Equine veterinary journal Supplement, 92–98.

Wilson, H.E.C., 1925. The Relation between Sulphur and Nitrogen Metabolism. Biochem J 19, 322–337.

Wilson, H.E.C., 1926. Studies in Nitrogen and Sulphur Metabolism. Biochem J 20, 76–83.

Wirth, J.J., Rossano, M.G., Daly, D.C., et al., 2007. Ambient manganese exposure is negatively associated with human sperm motility and concentration. Epidemiology 18, 270–273.

Wooding, F.B., Morgan, G., Fowden, A.L., et al., 2000. Separate sites and mechanisms for placental transport of calcium, iron and glucose in the equine placenta. Placenta 21, 635–645.

Young, J.K., Potter, G.D., Greene, L.W., et al., 1987. Copper balance in minature horses fed varying amounts of zinc. Equine Nutrition & Physiology Symposium.

Zafon, C., Lecube, A., Simo, R., 2011. Iron in obesity. An ancient micronutrient for a modern disease. Obes Rev 11, 322–328.

Zebrowska, T., Low, A.G., Zebrowska, H., 1983. Studies on gastric digestion of protein and carbohydrate, gastric secretion and exocrine pancreatic secretion in the growing pig. Br J Nutr 49, 401–410.

Zeyner, A., Kirbach, H., Fürll, M., 2002. Effects of substituting starch with fat on the acid-base and mineral status of female horses. Equine Veterinary Journal 34, 85–91.

Zha, S.W., Yu, J.Q., Liu, J.Y., et al., 2008. Contents of lead, cadmium, zinc and manganese in the follicular fluid and semen of non-professionally exposed infertile couples. Zhonghua nan ke xue = National journal of andrology 14, 494–497.

Section B

Nutrition for Lifestage, Type or Function

11 Feeding stallions and broodmares

Laurie M. Lawrence

Introduction

Horses are most commonly kept for performance activities and less commonly for breeding. Not surprisingly there is a relative lack of research on factors influencing optimal reproductive efficiency in horses. Similarly, there is a lack of information on feeding the pregnant mare to allow optimal fetal development. The following chapter reviews the current knowledge on the nutrient requirements of stallions and broodmares. In addition to providing information on recommended feeding programs, this chapter attempts to draw attention to areas in which information is lacking or where new information is needed. The recommendations that follow should be considered as starting points and should be modified when necessary to accommodate different management systems as well as differences among breeds and individual horses.

Stallions

Requirements

The nutrient requirements of breeding stallions are assumed to be similar to those of other adult horses, with allowances for level of activity. Level of activity should be considered the sum of breeding frequency and voluntary (and/or imposed) physical activity. Popular thoroughbred stallions may breed more than 150 mares in a season; often mounting 2 or 3 mares a day during the peak periods (Umphenour et al 2011). Conversely, some stallions may only breed a few mares in an entire year. Popular stallions used in artificial insemination programs may mount a phantom once a day, or more commonly, three or four times per week. An assessment of physical activity should include any imposed exercise (riding, driving, etc.) as well as voluntary exercise. Individual temperament can greatly influence level of voluntary physical activity. For example, some stallions may run or walk along a paddock fence during turnout periods while others may graze or rest quietly. Housing can also impact voluntary activity as stallions maintained primarily in stalls will often have a lower level of activity than stallions kept in pastures, particularly if they are used in a pasture-breeding system.

The effect of body condition on stallion libido or semen quality has not received much attention, but in humans, both very low and very high body mass index is associated with increased risk for infertility (Nguyen et al 2007). Obese men have been reported to have increased incidence of oligozoospermia, increased incidence of low progressively motile sperm and increased risk of sperm DNA fragmentation (Hammoud et al 2008a, b). The effects of obesity on fertility in men may be mediated by changes in several reproductive hormones including testosterone, estrogen and inhibin (Hammoud et al 2008a). It is also possible that changes to antioxidant status are related to the changes in semen quality observed in obesity-related infertility.

Based on the observations in humans, it would seem prudent to utilize a feeding program that prevents stallions from becoming too thin or too fat. Henneke and coworkers (1983) developed a 9-point body condition scoring system in which "moderate" body condition was associated with a score of 5. Many performance horses are maintained at condition scores between 4 and 6, while optimal reproductive efficiency in mares occurs at condition scores above 5. Therefore, a target condition score range for breeding stallions could be between 5 and 6.

Energy intake is the primary nutritional variable affecting body condition. Mature, inactive stallions with docile temperaments may have digestible energy requirements that are similar to any other mature horse at maintenance. However, very active breeding stallions probably have higher energy requirements. Siciliano and coworkers (1993) reported that commercial thoroughbred stallions (~ 600 kg) received about 26 Mcal of digestible energy per day during early spring (March). This estimate of digestible energy intake was subject to several sources of error (intake was calculated from farm-reported amounts of hay and concentrate offered to the stallions and did not include any pasture consumed during 3 hours of turn-out each day). Nonetheless these observations suggest that the energy requirements of active breeding stallions are substantially above maintenance and may be similar to the requirements of horses in light or moderate work (20 to 40% above average maintenance). Table 11-1 provides daily recommended nutrient intakes for inactive and active breeding stallions.

Feeding programs

Table 11-2 provides several examples of diets that could be fed to stallions at different levels of activity. These examples should be considered as starting points and should be

Table 11-1 Recommended Daily Nutrient Intakes for Breeding and Nonbreeding Stallions (600 kg) with Various Levels of Voluntary Activity

	Nonbreeding Sedentary[a]	Nonbreeding[b]	Breeding[b]	Breeding Very active[c]
Digestible energy (Mcal/day)	18.2	21.8	26.1	28
Crude protein (g/day)	648	864	947	921
Lysine (g/day)	28	37	41	40
Calcium (g/day)	24	24	36	42
Phosphorus (g/day)	17	17	22	25
Copper (mg/day)	120	120	120	135
Iron (mg/day)	480	480	480	540
Zinc (mg/day)	480	480	480	540
Iodine (mg/day)	4.2	4.2	4.2	4.7
Selenium (mg/day)	1.2	1.2	1.2	1.35
Vitamin A (IU/day)	18000	18000	27000	27000
Vitamin E (IU/day)	600	600	960	1080

[a]Source: NRC (2007): Adult horse, minimal voluntary activity, no work (600 kg).
[b]Source: NRC (2007): Average nonbreeding and breeding stallions (600 kg).
[c]Source: NRC (2007): Adult horse in moderate work (600 kg). This category would apply to breeding stallions with very high activity levels, either from breeding or from self-imposed exercise.

Table 11-2 Example Daily Rations for Nonbreeding and Breeding Stallions (600 kg) with Various Levels of Voluntary Activity

	Nonbreeding Sedentary	Nonbreeding	Breeding	Breeding Very active
Forages[a,b]				
Grass (mid–late maturity)	9–11 kg			
Grass/legume mix (midmaturity)		10–12 kg	10–12 kg	
Grass/legume mix (early maturity)				10–12 kg
Concentrate[c]	0	0	2–3 kg	2–4 kg
Supplement[d]	0.5–1.0 kg	0.5–1.0 kg	0	0
Comments	The amount and quality of forage should be adequate to maintain a body condition score of 5–6	The amount and quality of forage should be adequate to maintain a body condition score of 5–6	The amount of concentrate should be adjusted to maintain a body condition score of 5–6	The amount of concentrate should be adjusted to maintain a body condition score of 5–6

[a]Based on a late maturity grass hay containing (90% dry matter basis) 1.6–1.7 Mcal DE/kg, 7–11% CP, 0.3–0.4% Ca, 0.25–0.3% P, 6–9 ppm Cu; a mid-maturity grass/legume mix containing 1.8–2.0 Mcal DE/kg, 11–14% CP, 0.6–0.9% Ca, 0.25–0.35% P, 6–9 ppm Cu; and an early maturity legume/grass mix containing 2.0–2.1 Mcal DE/kg, 14–16% CP, 0.6–0.9% Ca, 0.25–0.35% P, 6–9 ppm Cu.
[b]Hay can be replaced with equivalent pasture.
[c]Based on concentrates containing (as fed basis) 3.2 Mcal DE/kg; 12–14% CP; 0.5% Ca; 0.3% P; 30 ppm Cu; 0.3 ppm Se.; 0.5 ppm I. Daily concentrate intakes should be divided into meals of less than 1.5 kg. When total daily concentrate intake is less than 2 kg/day, 1 kg of supplement may be used instead to provide adequate mineral intakes.
[d]Based on supplements containing (as fed basis) 14–30% CP; 2–4% Ca; 1–2% P; 100–150 ppm Cu; 0.6–1.0 ppm Se; 1–2 ppm I. A higher protein supplement should be selected if the hay contains less than 10% crude protein.

implemented in concert with a regular body condition scoring or weighing program. Dietary adjustments should be made whenever a stallion begins to become too thin or too fat. Adjustments to feeding programs should be made gradually. In the case of a stallion that is too fat, the goal should be to reduce calorie intake while maintaining adequate intake of protein, vitamins and minerals. Inactive stallions may be able to maintain body weight on a diet consisting of good quality hay or pasture and a small amount of a fortified supplement. Pasture availability and quality should always be considered when the diet is evaluated. For example, as pasture becomes available in the spring, or as weather conditions permit longer periods of turnout in good quality pastures, the amount of other feeds in the diet should be adjusted appropriately to prevent the stallion from becoming too fat.

It is the author's observation that it is possible for some stallions to lose weight and become somewhat thin (condition score <5) during the breeding season. If a stallion is too thin, forage quality and quantity should be increased first. If a stallion is very active in its paddock, reducing turnout time may be indicated. The amount of concentrate should be increased when changes to the forage component of the diet do not produce the desired effect. Large amounts of grain-based concentrates should be fed cautiously because of the potential for digestive upset. It has been suggested that substantial starch bypass to the large intestine may occur when a concentrate meal contains more than 2 g starch/kg BW (1200 g for a 600 kg horse). Grain-based concentrates (*complementary feeds*) may contain 40–60% starch; therefore a conservative guideline is to divide daily concentrate intakes of 0.4–0.6% of BW into two meals per day. Concentrate intakes between 0.6–1.0% of BW should be divided into three meals per day. Thin stallions may benefit from concentrates with added fat that have an increased energy density. If stallions are not able to maintain a body condition score of at least 4 during the breeding season despite changes in diet, then it may be desirable for the stallion to start each breeding season at a body condition slightly above 6.

Semen quality

Despite the importance of semen quality to reproductive performance, very few studies have examined the effects of diet on sperm concentration, morphology or motility in fresh, cooled or frozen stallion semen. Sperm are relatively high in lipid content and changes in the lipid composition of the diet may have implications for sperm physiology (Wathes et al 2007). The addition of n-3 fatty acids to the diet has been shown to alter the fatty acid content of sperm in several species, but effects on sperm characteristics are variable (Cerolini et al 2006, Gliozzi et al 2009). The effects of fatty acid supplements on stallions have also been inconsistent. Supplementing the diet of stallions with 8 to 11 g of n-3 fatty acids from either fish oil or from a combination of flax seed and algae did not affect semen quality (Grady et al 2009). However, other researchers found that a supplement containing n-3 fatty acids altered semen fatty acid composition and resulted in improved 48 h motility in cooled semen and in frozen semen (Brinsko et al 2005). The authors noted that the supplement appeared to be of most benefit to stallions that started the study with relatively low progressive motility in cooled semen. Stallions that received a supplement containing 30 g of docosahexanoic acid (DHA) for 80 days had increased sperm number, increased motility and reduced percentage of abnormal sperm (Elhordoy et al 2008). These authors also reported that the stallions that exhibited the greatest improvements had the poorest semen quality at the beginning of the experiment.

Interaction between sperm and reactive oxygen species (ROS) appears to facilitate capacitation but exposure to excessive ROS may damage sperm DNA and reduce sperm viability (Ball 2008). To combat ROS, semen contains a variety of endogenous antioxidants, several of which may be susceptible to dietary manipulation. Short term supplementation of fertile pony stallions with an antioxidant supplement containing 300 mg vitamin E, 300 mg vitamin C, 4000 mg L-carnitine and 12 mg of folic acid had no effect on total sperm, percentage total motility or percentage progressive motility. Motility following 24 h storage was not affected, but there was a small decrease in the percentage of sperm with morphological defects (Deichsel et al 2008). Daily supplementation of stallions with 5000 IU of D,L α-tocopheryl acetate did not affect total sperm or percentage progressive motility in fresh semen but effects on sperm viability after storage were not investigated (Rich et al 1983). Although these studies demonstrated limited benefit from antioxidant supplements, it has been suggested that antioxidant therapy in men may be beneficial only in selected cases of infertility (Zini et al 2009). Vitamin E supplementation (3000 IU D-α-tocopherol/day) of stallions with poor post-thaw progressive sperm motility did not affect total or progressive motility in raw, 24 h cooled or frozen semen (Gee et al 2008). However, vitamin E supplementation improved motility in cooled semen after 48 h in that study. As noted above, the response to n-3 fatty acid supplementation also appeared to be most pronounced in stallions with low sperm motility in cooled semen. These results suggest that the relationship of dietary lipids and dietary antioxidants to semen quality in subfertile stallions should be explored further. The efficacy of n-3 fatty acid and antioxidant supplementation in the stallion should be considered in the context of the basal diet. In the studies mentioned above that observed benefits to supplementation, the basal diets consisted predominantly of stored feeds that would have been low in natural sources of vitamin E, vitamin A, β-carotene and n-3 fatty acids. The effect of n-3 supplementation or antioxidant supplementation could be expected to be less pronounced in stallions that have access to good quality pasture which is an excellent source of these compounds.

The relationship of semen quality to a variety of other nutrients (vitamin C, β-carotene, zinc, selenium, B-vitamins) has been studied in humans and other animals (Audet et al 2004, Eskenazi et al 2005, Ebisch et al 2007, Colagar et al 2009). Severe deficiencies are likely to detrimentally affect sperm production and/or semen quality but the response to supplementation above requirements is often variable. Inconsistent results may arise from differences in experimental conditions such as the levels of nutrients in the basal diets or length of the supplementation period.

In general the relationship of nutrition and feeding management to stallion fertility has received little attention. Several factors could explain this lack of research, one of which is that most stallions have acceptable fertility. Live foal rates reported by the Jockey Club for thoroughbred stallions average above 60% for the population, and may be above 80% for some individuals. With normal stallions, it seems likely that only very large studies would be able to detect differences in fertility in response to nutritional modifications. However, as indicated by some of the previously mentioned studies, subfertile stallions may be more responsive to dietary modifications than normal stallions. Particularly where subfertility is linked to a specific semen characteristic, a targeted nutritional intervention could be useful.

Key Points – Stallions

- The nutrient requirements of stallions are similar to other horses with adjustments for level of activity.
- Feeding programs should focus on balanced diets fed in amounts to maintain a body condition between 5 and 6.
- A variety of nutritional supplements have been fed to stallions in an attempt to affect semen quality but results are inconsistent.
- Stallions with normal fertility appear to be less likely to respond to nutritional supplements than subfertile stallions.

Pregnant mares

Requirements

The daily nutrient intakes of pregnant mares should meet the maintenance requirement of the mare and the nutrient needs for the synthesis and maintenance of the products of conception. Gestational weight gain is expected to be 12–16% of a mare's initial body weight, most of which is attributed to the fetus and placental tissues. Since 1978, most feeding standards for pregnant mares have relied on the estimates of nutrient deposition in the fetus that were published by Meyer and Ahlswede in 1978. Their data (Table 11-3) were obtained from compositional analyses of stillborn and aborted fetuses presented to a veterinary college. A few other studies have also reported fetal weights from aborted fetuses but weights and compositional analyses from normal fetuses in various stages of development are not available.

Table 11-3 Chemical Composition of the Equine Fetus at 7, 8, 9, 10, and 11 Months of Gestation[a]

Month of gestation		7	8	9	10	11
Dry matter	g	175	199	238	262	273
Crude ash	g	36	42	49	60	56
Crude protein	g	104	120	147	154	171
Crude fat	g	19	19	20	21	26
Energy	MJ	3.36	3.74	4.48	4.74	5.20
Calcium	g	10.5	12.9	15.4	19.8	18.2
Phosphorus	g	6.0	6.4	8.5	10.3	9.7
Magnesium	g	0.2	0.3	0.4	0.4	0.4
Sodium	g	1.9	2.1	2.0	2.0	1.9
Potassium	g	1.8	1.7	1.8	1.8	1.9
Chloride	g	1.2	1.2	1.2	1.2	1.2
Copper	mg	3.8	4.3	3.9	5.8	5.0
Zinc	mg	21	30	27	46	42
Iron	mg	86	65	82	85	118
Manganese	mg	0.7	0.9	0. 8	1.2	1.3

[a]Per kg on as is basis
Source: Meyer and Ahlswede (1978).

Most fetal weight gain occurs during the third trimester of gestation but the nutrient needs of pregnant mares begin to increase before then (Table 11-4). The vitamin E and vitamin A intakes of pregnant mares are elevated above maintenance throughout pregnancy (NRC 2007). It is suggested that calcium and phosphorus requirements do not increase until the 7th month of gestation (NRC 2007) even though the available data on fetal composition suggest that calcium and phosphorus have been deposited into the fetus before then. The normal maintenance intakes may be sufficient to meet calcium and phosphorus needs before the 7th month of gestation or the current recommendations for calcium and phosphorus may be somewhat low. In the 6th revised edition of the Nutrient Requirements of Horses, the recommended intakes of copper and iodine were increased for mares in late gestation. However the recommended intakes for several other nutrients (iron, manganese, zinc, selenium) were not changed. An increase in the recommended copper intake was based on the studies that suggested copper supplementation of pregnant mares might influence the copper status of foals and their subsequent susceptibility to developmental cartilage lesions (NRC 2007). The change in the iodine requirement was based on a review of a published study that had been misquoted in an earlier publication (NRC 1989) and the recommendations of Donoghue et al (1990).

Several studies have examined the effect of vitamin and mineral supplementation of the pregnant mare on the passive transfer of immunoglobulins to neonatal foals. There does not appear to be a relationship between maternal vitamin E status and colostral immunoglobulin G (IgG) concentration or foal serum IgG when mares have adequate vitamin E status at foaling (Siciliano et al 2009). However, in mares that were kept in dry lots prior to parturition vitamin E supplementation at twice the recommended concentration resulted in increased colostral IgG concentrations and increased serum IgG concentrations in foals (Hoffman

Table 11-4 Nutrient Requirements of Pregnant Mares (500–600 kg Mature Weight)

	0–4 months	5th month	6th month	7th month	8th month	9th month	10th month	11th month
Digestible Energy (Mcal/day)	16.7–20.0	17.1–20.5	17.4–20.9	17.9–21.5	18.5–22.2	19.2–23.1	20.2–24.2	21.4–25.7
Crude Protein (kg/day)	0.63–0.76	0.69–0.82	0.70–0.85	0.73–0.87	0.76–0.91	0.80–0.96	0.84–1.01	0.89–1.07
Lysine (g/day)	27.1–32.5	29.5–35.3	30.3–36.3	31.3- 37.6	32.7–39.2	34.3–41.1	36.2–43.4	38.4–46.1
Calcium (g/day)	20.0–24.0	20.0–24.0	20.0–24.0	28.0–33.6	28.0–33.6	36.0–43.2	36.0–43.2	36.0–43..2
Phosphorus (g/day)	14.0–16.8	14.0–16.8	14.0–16.8	20.0–24.0	20.0–24.0	26.3–31.5	26.3–31.5	26.3–31.5
Copper (mg/day)	100–120	100–120	100–120	100–120	100–120	125–150	125–150	125–150
Zinc (mg/day)	400–480	400–480	400–480	400–480	400–480	400–480	400–480	400–480
Iodine (mg/day)	3.5–4.2	3.5–4.2	3.5–4.2	3.5–4.2	3.5–4.2	4.0–4.8	4.0–4.8	4.0–4.8
Selenium (mg/day)	1.0–1.2	1.0–1.2	1.0–1.2	1.0–1.2	1.0–1.2	1.0–1.2	1.0–1.2	1.0–1.2
Vitamin A (IU/day)	30 000–39 600	30 000–39 600	30 000–39 600	30 000–39 600	30 000–39 600	30 000–39 600	30 000–39 600	30 000–39 600
Vitamin E (IU/day)	800–960	800–960	800–960	800–960	800–960	800–960	800–960	800–960

Source: NRC (2007).

et al 1999). Colostral IgG concentration was increased when mares were given a marine source supplement containing DHA compared to a corn oil supplement. However, foal IgG concentrations were not affected (Kruglik et al 2006). In another study colostral IgG concentrations were lower in mares receiving a marine based *n*-3 fatty acid supplement (Stelzleni et al 2006), whereas a linseed-based *n*-3 fatty acid supplement did not alter colostral immunoglobulin concentrations in comparison to a rapeseed-based oleic acid supplement (Duvaux-Ponter et al 2004).

Selenium supplementation above the requirement has been reported to increase serum IgG concentrations (Janicki et al 2000), but in another study selenium supplementation did not affect colostral or foal IgG concentrations (Thorson et al 2010). In addition, time to expulsion of the placenta was not affected by selenium supplementation in either study. Replacing sulfated sources of copper, zinc, manganese, and cobalt with amino acid complexes resulted in increased colostral IgA concentrations but did not affect colostral or foal IgG concentrations (Vickers et al 2009). Clearly the effects of diet on passive transfer are variable. Some of the variation may relate to characteristics of the basal diet that are not always considered during the design of the study such as availability of natural sources of vitamins or minerals from the forage and even the level of nutrient intake by the mare. Pagan and Hintz (1986) observed that energy intake was inversely correlated with the concentration of several milk components. Thorson et al (2010) found that Brix percentage and colostral IgG concentrations were higher in mares that received pasture only compared to mares that received pasture and concentrate. Therefore it is possible that well-fed mares produce more dilute milk or colostrums and comparisons among various treatments should be adjusted to a dry matter basis or another component.

The amount of protein and energy needed to fuel the products of conception increase above maintenance in the 5th month of gestation and continue to increase throughout the gestation period. Feeding excess energy in late gestation will increase body weight and condition but does not result in larger birth weights (Kubiak et al 1988). Similarly, moderate energy restriction in late gestation does not affect birth weight (Banach & Evans 1985, Thorson et al 2010) but it may result in prolonged gestation (Hines et al 1987).

Less than 40% of fetal weight gain occurs before the 9th month of gestation but appreciable increases in body weight have been reported during early or mid-gestation in mares maintained in both research and commercial settings (Lawrence et al 1992, Cassill et al 2009). Increases in condition score occur simultaneously with weight gain in early and mid-lactation (Lawrence et al 1992). The optimal body condition score for a pregnant mare at any stage of gestation has not been established. One group attempted to study the effect of moderate and high rates of weight gain in early and mid-gestation on pregnant mares (Wilsher & Allen 2006, Ousey et al 2008). The study was confounded by an outbreak of *Streptococcus equi* in the mares at about 100–140 days of gestation, so the authors inadvertently studied the effect of illness and marked weight loss (approximately 8–11%) on pregnant mares. When the authors compared the data obtained from all mares that had been sick to historical data on normal mares they concluded that the placental efficiency of the infected mares had been reduced (Wilsher & Allen 2006). Interestingly, mares that had gained more weight prior to getting sick appeared to sustain fewer long-term effects of illness and weight loss on measures of placental efficiency. In addition the foals from the fatter mares appeared to have more normal responses to an insulin sensitivity test administered at 2–4 days of age. The mares that had been fed for high weight gain had a body condition score of 7 at the onset of illness, compared to a body condition score of 5 for the mares that had been fed for moderate weight gain. The authors suggested that feeding mares to a higher condition score could have mitigated the effects of the acute nutritional deprivation that occurred during the infection with *Streptococcus equi* (Ousey et al 2008). It is not suggested that mares be fed to obesity, but these observations suggest that allowing mares to gain weight in early and mid-gestation creates a nutritional buffer in the event that nutritional resources become scarce in later gestation. A mare that is rebred at 30 days after foaling may reach mid-gestation and weaning at the same time. Changes in feed intake are expected at weaning and it is possible that mares with higher condition scores might be able to buffer the effect of these changes on the fetus more effectively than mares with low condition scores. Feed withdrawal can affect prostaglandin production by the uterus, therefore mares should be managed carefully at weaning to prevent an extended period of feed deprivation (Silver & Fowden 1982).

Feeding programs

Table 11-5 gives example diets for mares in early, mid and late gestation, using either mature grass hay or early maturity legume grass hay. It is not always necessary to feed concentrate to mares in early gestation. The energy and protein requirements of mares in early gestation will be met if a mare consumes adequate good quality forage. However, forage alone may not meet the mineral needs of gestating mares. Some horses may obtain adequate mineral support from free-choice use of a trace mineralized salt block or a mineral block. However, mineral intake from a block is likely to be erratic and some horses will not meet their requirements. A better practice is to feed each mare a small amount of a fortified ration balancer pellet each day (Table 11-5) to complement the forage. If abundant good quality forage is not available to mares in early and mid-gestation then a fortified concentrate may be necessary. When the horses receive more than 2 to 3 kg of a fortified concentrate, the ration balancer pellet is not usually needed.

The nutrient requirements of mares in late gestation can be met with good quality forage and a fortified concentrate. There has been some research on the effects of dietary energy source of the maternal diet on the energy metabolism of the foal. At this time there do not appear to be great differences in the glucose or insulin responses of foals raised by mares that were fed diets high in starch and sugar or high in fat and fiber during gestation (George et al 2009). Mares that are bred in February, March, and April (Northern Hemisphere) will reach late gestation when winter weather is most severe and it may be necessary to increase energy intake above the recommendations in Table 11-5 by 20 to 50%.

The nutrient recommendations for pregnant mares in Table 11-4 and the example feeding programs in Table 11-5 do not account for any effects of a previous or concurrent

Table 11-5 Example Feeding Programs for 500–600 kg Mares During Gestation

	0–4 months	5–7 months	8–9 months	10–11 months
Forages[a,b]				
Grass (mid-late maturity)	10–12 kg			
Grass/legume mix (midmaturity)		9–11 kg	8–10 kg	
Legume/grass mix (early maturity)				8–10 kg
Concentrate[c]	0	0	1–2 kg	2–3 kg
Supplement[d]	0.5–1.0 kg	0.5–1.0 kg	0	0
Comments	The amount and quality of forage should be adequate to maintain a body condition score of 5–6	The amount and quality of forage should be adequate to maintain a body condition score of 5–6	The amount of concentrate should be adjusted to maintain a body condition score of 5–6[e]	The amount of concentrate should be adjusted to maintain a body condition score of 5–6[e]

[a]Based on a late maturity grass hay containing (90% dry matter basis) 1.6–1.7 Mcal DE/kg, 7–11% CP, 0.3–0.4% Ca, 0.25–0.3% P, 6–9 ppm Cu ; a mid-maturity grass/legume mix containing 1.8–2.0 Mcal DE/kg, 11–14% CP, 0.6–0.9% Ca, 0.25–0.35% P, 6–9 ppm Cu; and an early maturity legume/grass mix containing 2.0–2.1 Mcal DE/kg, 14–16% CP, 0.6–0.9% Ca, 0.25–0.35% P, 6–9 ppm Cu.
[b]Hay can be replaced with equivalent pasture.
[c]Based on concentrates containing (as fed basis) 3.2 Mcal DE/kg; 12–14% CP; 0.5% Ca; 0.3% P; 30 ppm Cu; 0.3 ppm Se.; 0.5 ppm I. Daily concentrate intakes should be divided into meals of less than 1.5 kg. When total daily concentrate intake is less than 2 kg/day, 1 kg of supplement may be used instead to provide adequate mineral intakes.
[d]Based on supplements containing (as fed basis) 14–30% CP; 2–4% Ca; 1–2% P; 100–150 ppm Cu; 0.6–1.0 ppm Se; 1–2 ppm I. A higher protein supplement should be selected if the hay contains less than 10% crude protein.
[e]Higher concentrate amounts may be necessary during winter.

Table 11-6 Approximate Amount of Nutrients Secreted into Milk Each Day by a 550 kg Mare[a,b]

Days of lactation	Energy (Mcal/day)	Protein (kg/day)	Lysine (g/day)	Calcium (g/day)	Phosphorus (g/day)
30	9.2	0.366	31	22.0	13.7
60	8.6	0.344	29	20.6	12.9
120	7.1	0.284	24	17.0	10.7

[a]Sources: NRC 2007; Wickens et al (2002).
[b]Daily nutrient intakes to meet the needs for milk production can be calculated if the efficiency of use of the absorbed nutrient and digestibility of the nutrient is known.

lactation, so they do not include increments for the replenishment of energy stores, lean body mass or bone mineral that were depleted during lactation. In addition, the nutrient recommendations for Table 11-4 do not account for the potential effects of winter weather on the maintenance energy requirements of pregnant mares. All of these factors should be considered when feeding programs for pregnant mares are designed.

Key Points – Pregnant mares

- Nutrient requirements increase as early as 5 months of gestation
- In early and midgestation, good quality forage may meet energy and protein requirements but some mineral supplementation may be needed
- In late gestation, many mares will require concentrate, particularly if they are housed out of doors during the winter months
- Pregnant mares entering late gestation in a body condition of 6 will have body stores available to buffer periods of scarce resources during late gestation
- Mares should have adequate condition (condition score >5) at foaling to promote subsequent reproductive efficiency.

Lactating mares

Requirements

Lactation is the most nutritionally demanding period for a broodmare. Fluid milk contains approximately 500 kcal/kg, 2% CP, 0.12% Ca and 0.075% P (NRC 2007). Milk yield varies over the course of lactation and may be estimated from the following equation (NRC 2007):

$$\text{Milk yield (kg/day)} = (0.0274287 \times \text{BW}) \times d^{0.0953} \times e^{-0.0043d};$$
where, d = day of lactation and BW is reported in kg.

The nutrients secreted into milk each day can be estimated from milk composition and milk yield. Although the average amounts of energy, protein, calcium and phosphorus that are deposited in milk can be estimated relatively easily (Table 11-6), additional adjustments must be made to extrapolate these values into dietary recommendations. Nutrient digestibility varies by nutrient and by feedstuff. In addition, the efficiency of use of absorbed nutrients for milk production is not always 100%. The efficiency of converting digestible energy into milk energy by horses has been estimated to be about 60% (NRC 2007). However, various absorbed substrates (glucose, volatile fatty acids, etc.) are probably used with different efficiencies. The efficiency of converting crude protein to milk protein has been estimated to approximately 35–40% (NRC 1989, 2007) but protein quality could affect this value. If dietary protein is poorly digested or if it contains an unbalanced amino acid profile, the efficiency of conversion to milk protein will be reduced.

The effect of lactation on the amino acid requirements of the broodmare has received limited study. Wickens and colleagues (2002) calculated the digestible lysine requirement for milk production to be 2.62 g/kg fluid milk. A mare producing 15 kg of fluid milk would require 39 g of digestible lysine in addition to the amount needed for maintenance. The average digestibility of crude protein in equine diets has been estimated to be 79% (NRC 2007), therefore the dietary lysine needed to produce 15 kg of milk would be estimated at 49 g/day (above maintenance), or about 3.3 g dietary lysine/kg fluid milk. Wickens et al (2002) also estimated the required amounts of digestible arginine, histidine, isoleucine, leucine, methionine, phenylalanine, threonine, and valine to be 1.81, 0.86, 2.04, 3.85, 0.84, 1.39, 1.88, and 2.54 g/kg fluid milk, respectively. Wickens et al (2002) measured amino acid concentrations in milk collected at 30 days of lactation. A subsequent study has reported somewhat lower amino acid concentrations in milk obtained at 7 weeks of lactation (Matsui et al 2005). The lysine concentration in fluid milk at 7 weeks of lactation was 1.2 g/kg which would yield an estimate of 2.33 g of dietary lysine per kg of fluid milk. The current lysine recommendations assume that mares require 3.3 g lysine/kg fluid milk throughout lactation. Based on the available information it seems likely that this recommendation may overestimate the lysine needs of mares after the first month of lactation. Additional studies will be necessary to define the amino acid requirements of lactating mares more accurately.

A lactating mare must consume enough nutrients to meet the needs of lactation and to maintain her own body stores. Thus, suggested daily requirements of lactating mares (Table 11-7) take into account not only milk production, but also the maintenance requirements of the mare. Some feeding standards have assumed that lactation does not change the nutrient requirements for maintenance (NRC 1973, 1978, 1989). However it has also been suggested that lactation may increase the maintenance requirement for some nutrients such as protein and/or energy (NRC 1949, 2007, Blaxter 1989). The amount of energy required for maintenance is determined by basal metabolism, voluntary activity, thermal regulation, product synthesis, waste excretion and digestive processes. Several of these components of maintenance are probably increased in the lactating mare, such as the energy needed for digestive and waste processes associated with increased feed intake and possibly increased voluntary activity associated with maternal behavior (NRC 1949, 2007, Blaxter 1989). Increased feed intake might also be expected to increase the protein and amino acid requirements associated with maintenance by increasing endogenous fecal nitrogen losses. The maintenance requirements of lactating mares for energy and protein are estimated to be about 10% higher than the same requirements for sedentary adult horses of the same body weight (NRC 2007). The increased maintenance requirement is based on the assumption that lactating mares will have higher voluntary feed intakes and higher voluntary activity than the average horse.

Failure to meet the dietary requirements of lactating females can result in the use of body stores to maintain milk production and composition. Foals from pony mares fed an energy restricted diet grew at the same rate as foals from non-restricted mares (Pagan et al 1984) even though their dams lost weight (Pagan et al 1984). However, energy restriction of lactating mares and/or the accompanying weight loss can reduce subsequent reproductive performance (Henneke et al 1984). There is some indication that mares mobilize body protein at the onset of lactation to meet the needs for milk production even when dietary protein requirements are met (Manso Filho et al 2008). However, severe or prolonged restriction of dietary protein should be avoided during lactation. In other species lactating females mobilize body protein stores to meet the needs for milk production, but only to a point. Sows fed protein and amino acid deficient diets used protein to maintain normal milk production until body protein losses reached 12%. When body protein losses exceeded 12%, detrimental effects on pig

Table 11-7 Nutrient Requirements of Lactating Mares with a Mature Body Weight of 500–600 kg[a]

	1st month	3rd month	5th month
Digestible energy (Mcal/day)	31.7–38.1	30.6–36.7	28.3–34.0
Crude Protein (kg/day)	1.54–1.84	1.47–1.76	1.33–1.6
Lysine (g/day)	84.8–101.7	80.3–96.4	71.2–85.5
Ca (g/day)	59.1–70.9	55.9–67.1	39.5–47.4
P (g/day)	38.3–45.9	38.1–43.2	24.7–29.6
Copper (mg/day)	125–150	125–150	125–150
Zinc (mg/day)	500–600	500–600	500–600
Iodine (mg/day)	4.4–5.3	4.4–5.3	4.4–5.3
Selenium (mg/day)	1.25–1.5	1.25–1.5	1.25–1.5
Vitamin A (IU/day)	30 000–36 000	30 000–36 000	30 000–36 000
Vitamin E (IU/day)	1000–1200	1000–1200	1000–1200

[a]Source: NRC 2007.

growth and sow ovarian activity were observed (Clowes et al 2003). Similarly, mares that received low protein diets during gestation and lactation had foals that weighed the same at 30 and 60 days of age as foals from mares receiving adequate protein. However, by 90 days of age the foals from mares receiving a low protein diet during lactation were smaller than foals from mares receiving adequate protein, even though both groups had received protein restricted diets during gestation (Gill et al 1983). In addition, mares fed a diet with poor quality protein were not able to produce as much milk as mares fed a protein adequate diet over an 150-d lactation (Gibbs et al 1982).

The effect of lactation on bone mineral turnover has been studied using measures of bone mineral density and serum markers of bone turnover. Nursing women experience a reduction in bone mineral density and an increase in markers of bone demineralization during lactation (More et al 2001, Akesson et al 2004) but these changes occur even when calcium intake is relatively high (Prentice 2000). Cassill et al (2005) reported that a marker of bone demineralization increased in mares during early lactation and then declined. A low calcium diet will exacerbate bone demineralization in lactating mares (Glade 1993) but supplementing calcium and phosphorus above the recommended level does not mitigate the apparent demineralization (Ott & Asquith 1983, Cassill et al 2004). The long-term ramifications of bone mobilization during lactation in mares are not known. It is possible that mares regain bone mineral after lactation ends.

The mare has the ability to buffer the effects of mild dietary insufficiency on the output of many milk nutrients. Similarly, she has the ability to buffer the effect of excess nutrients on milk nutrient output. The foals of pony mares fed excess energy grew at the same rate as foals from mares fed a normal energy intake, but the mares gained weight (Pagan et al 1986). Interestingly, the concentrations of several milk components were inversely correlated with energy intake. Because foal growth was not depressed by the lower concentration of nutrients, the authors suggested that overfeeding energy might have resulted in higher yields of less concentrated milk (Pagan et al 1986). Dietary energy source may affect the composition of the milk as well. The addition of fat to the diet of lactating mares altered the fat concentration in the milk but did not alter average daily gain in foals (Davison et al 1991). Diet composition can also alter the fatty acid profile of the milk (Hoffman et al 1998; Spearman et al 2005), but the impact of these changes on the health or growth of the foal has not been determined.

The mineral composition of milk appears to be resistant to dietary modification, with a few exceptions. Increasing the amount of copper and zinc in the diet of the mare above recommended levels did not alter the concentration of copper or zinc in milk (Kavazis et al 2002). Similarly increasing calcium and phosphorus intakes of lactating mares did not affect milk calcium and phosphorus concentrations (Cassill et al 2004). Supplementation of lactating mares with silicon in the form of sodium zeolite A increased milk silicon concentrations but bone metabolism and bone density of the foals were not affected (Lang et al 2001). At this time there is little evidence that supplementation of the lactating mare above current nutrient recommendations has beneficial effects on the bone development in the foal. The addition of organic selenium (selenium yeast) to the diets of lactating mares increased milk selenium concentration and foals from supplemented mares had higher selenium status than foals from mares receiving inorganic selenium (Janicki et al 2001). However, the average daily gain of supplemented foals was not affected by selenium supplementation of the mare and other indicators of foal performance (health status, bone density, etc.) were not measured. Selenium supplementation of pregnant mares resulted in higher serum and muscle selenium concentrations in foals but muscle glutathione peroxidase activity was not affected (Karren et al 2010).

Feeding programs

The recommendations for daily nutrient intakes in Table 11-7 should be applied with an understanding of the factors that can result in elevated or decreased requirements. Optimal feeding programs should account for individual differences in horses as well as management differences among farms or stables. There may be large differences in the milk production of individual mares, and there will also be differences in environmental conditions or individual temperament that alter maintenance requirements. The suggested energy intakes may be somewhat high for breeds of horses prone to obesity including some draft breeds or pony breeds. Regular measurement of body weight and/or regular monitoring of body condition are helpful tools to assess the appropriateness of feeding programs for lactating mares and their foals.

Example feeding programs for lactating mares are shown in Table 11-8. Although the examples specify hay as the forage source, pasture should be utilized whenever possible. Pasture is a better source of many vitamins than conserved forage. Seasonal changes in vitamin A and vitamin E status have been reported to coincide with access to actively growing pasture in mares and foals (Maenpaa et al 1988). When broodmares have no access to pasture for an extended period of time it is important to provide adequate vitamin fortification through the concentrate portion of the diet.

Table 11-8 Example Rations for 600 kg Mares in Early Lactation

	Forage type[a]	
	Early maturity legume-grass hay	Middle maturity grass hay
Daily forage intake[b]	11–13 kg	9–11 kg
Daily Concentrate Intake[c]	4–5 kg	6–7 kg
Comments	Estimated from a DM intake of at least 2.5% BW. If DM intake is higher forage can be increased and concentrate decreased	Estimated from a DM intake of at least 2.5% BW. If DM intake is higher forage can be increased and concentrate decreased

[a]Based on a mid-maturity grass/legume mix containing (90% dry matter basis)1.8–2.0 Mcal DE/kg, 11–14% CP, 0.5–0.7% Lys; 0.6–0.9% Ca, 0.25–0.35% P, 6–9 ppm Cu; and an early maturity legume/grass mix containing 2.0–2.1 Mcal DE/kg, 14–16% CP, 0.8–1.0% Lys; 0.6–0.9% Ca, 0.25–0.35% P, 6–9 ppm Cu.
[b]Hay can be replaced by equivalent pasture.
[c]Based on concentrates containing (as fed basis) 3.2 Mcal DE/kg; 14–16% CP; 1.0% Lys;0.9% Ca; 0.6% P; 40 ppm Cu; 0.5 ppm Se.; 0.5 ppm I. Daily concentrate intakes should be divided into meals of less than 2.0 kg each.

An increase in daily dry matter intake is expected once lactation begins. Dry matter intakes for most lactating mares will exceed 2% of BW, and some will consume more than 3 kg DM/100 kg BW. As the mare transitions from the diet fed in late gestation to the higher feed intakes of lactation, all dietary changes should be made gradually to reduce the risk of digestive upset. The higher the quality of forage that is available, the lower the amount of concentrate that will be needed to meet nutrient needs. Voluntary dry matter intake is related to forage quality so horses will consume more of high quality forage (St. Lawrence et al 2001). Pasture dry matter consumption by lactating mares has been reported to be about 2.4% BW (Grace et al 2002). The pasture in that study contained 19% CP and 2.58 Mcal DE/kg DM, therefore many lactating mares grazing very high quality pasture can meet their energy and protein requirements with minimal amounts of concentrate. It should be noted that forage-only diets may not meet all of the mineral needs of a lactating mare and a small amount of supplement may still be necessary.

Forage alone will not be sufficient to meet the energy and protein needs of lactating mares in many situations. When forage quality is moderate, concentrate intakes will range from 0.5 to 1.0 kg/100 kg BW/day (Table 11-8). If low quality forages are used or if voluntary intake is below 2.25% of BW, it may be difficult to meet energy needs without feeding large amounts of concentrate (>1 kg/100 kg BW). High intakes of grain-based concentrates may increase the risk of digestive disturbances, therefore to minimize the need for concentrate, higher quality forages should be selected for lactating mares. When high concentrate intakes are necessary, the concentrate should be divided into two or three meals per day. As noted previously, all dietary changes, including an increase in concentrate offered should be made gradually to reduce the risk of colic and other digestive disturbances.

Feeds for lactating mares must contain good quality protein or it may be difficult to meet amino acid needs. A 500 kg mare requires about 1.5 kg of crude protein and 84 grams of lysine in early lactation. To meet this requirement the crude protein must contain more than 5% lysine. Many common feed ingredients contain protein that has less than 5% lysine (Table 11-9). Therefore commercial feeds for lactating mares often rely on soybean meal as a protein supplement. Some commercial feeds also contain a lysine supplement to ensure that lysine requirements are met. Many byproduct ingredients may be relatively high in protein but relatively low in essential amino acids. In addition, factors that limit the small intestinal availability of amino acids in feeds and forages should be considered when a diet is formulated. A discussion of the factors affecting dietary protein quality and protein digestibility can be found in Chapter 6. It is more important to meet amino acid needs than to meet crude protein requirements. Therefore, if a diet contains protein with a low level of lysine the amount of protein in the diet should be increased to meet the lysine need. Even when soybean meal is included in the concentrate it may be difficult to meet the lysine needs for early lactation unless the recommended crude protein allowance is exceeded.

The nutrient needs of the lactating mare will decrease in late lactation when milk yield declines. Therefore as mares enter late lactation it would be expected that the amount of concentrate needed by the mare will decrease. However, if mid or late lactation coincides with a period of reduced forage availability (slow pasture growth) then it may be necessary to maintain concentrate intakes. Also, a 4–6-month-old foal could easily consume 1–2 kg of concentrate per day. Therefore if the foal has access to the dam's feed, the total amount of feed offered to the mare–foal pair may not decrease (and could possibly increase) in late lactation.

Some managers may withdraw all concentrate from mares at the time of weaning in an attempt to decrease milk production. There is no documentation that the cessation of milk production by mares is hastened by dietary restriction. If a mare has been rebred, it is possible that weaning will coincide with the middle of gestation when the demands of the subsequent pregnancy will start to increase. Feed withdrawal can alter uterine prostaglandin production in pregnant mares (Silver & Fowden 1982). It is the author's opinion that it is prudent to avoid sudden changes in a broodmares's diet at any point in gestation to ensure that nutrient availability to the fetus remains relatively constant. Changes to the diet should be made gradually before and after weaning to provide a smooth transition during the weaning period.

The nutrient requirements of mares in the post-weaning period have received little attention from researchers. However, this period may be a critical time of replenishment for mares that will experience subsequent gestation-lactation cycles. Mares that end lactation with a condition score below 5 should be fed to achieve a condition score above 5 before

Table 11-9 Lysine Content of Some Common Forages and Other Ingredients Used in Horse Diets[a]

	% CP (DM Basis)	% Lysine (DM Basis)	% Lysine in CP
Hay – mostly legume, immature	20.5	0.97	4.73
Hay – mostly legume, mature	17.2	0.8	4.65
Hay – grass, cool season, mid-maturity	10.8	0.38	3.51
Hay, Bermudagrass – Coastal	10.4	0.36	3.46
Oat grain – rolled	13.2	0.55	4.17
Corn grain – cracked	9.4	0.27	2.87
Barley grain – rolled	12.4	0.45	3.63
Soybean meal – solvent extracted, 44% CP	49.9	3.13	6.27
Canola meal – mechanical extraction	37.8	2.12	5.6
Sunflower meal – solvent extraction	28.4	1.01	3.56
Sugar beet pulp-molassed	10.0	0.42	4.20
Wheat middlings	18.5	0.67	3.62
Distillers dried grains w/solubles (DDGS)[b]	28.4	0.85	2.99

[a]Source: NRC 2007.
[b]Urriola et al 2009.

the onset of winter. As noted above, mares may mobilize amino acids and minerals during lactation as well as energy. Feeding programs for mares that lost weight and body condition during lactation should probably be more nutrient dense than diets for horses at maintenance.

Key Points – Lactating mares

- Nutrient requirements increase after foaling in order to meet the needs of milk production
- Mares fed inadequate rations will mobilize body stores to meet the needs of lactation and may lose body condition
- Mares that are in suboptimal body condition may have reduced rebreeding efficiency
- Feed intake will usually increase after foaling. Mares should be transitioned to higher levels of feed intake gradually to reduce the risk of digestive disturbance
- Changes in feed intake should also be made gradually at weaning. Mares that are weaned at 5 months post-foaling may be entering mid-gestation when nutrient requirements begin to increase again

Reproductive efficiency in the mare

It seems likely that vitamin and mineral deficiencies have the potential to affect reproduction in the mare, but documented cases appear to be infrequent (NRC 2007). In addition there are no convincing studies to suggest that supplementing any vitamin or mineral above the recommended level will enhance mare fertility. Robl and Forfa (1987) reported that a supplement containing chelated minerals resulted in earlier dates of conception in mares, but the nutritional treatment was confounded with application of artificial lights. Variable responses to the amount and/or form of trace mineral supplements have been reported in other studies (Ley et al 1990, Vickers et al 2009). The administration of vitamin A and E to barren mares improved reproductive performance but it was not clear whether the basal diet was adequate or deficient in these nutrients (Stowe 1967). Mares grazing pasture have been reported to have high vitamin E and vitamin A status therefore any potential benefits of supplementation are more likely to be observed in animals fed stored feeds that do not provide the required amounts of these vitamins. Similarly reproductive responses to supplements containing various fatty acids have been variable and could be related to the fatty acid composition of other feeds in the diet (Poland et al 2006, Canibal et al 2008).

There is some evidence that protein quality may be important to equine reproduction (van Niekerk & van Niekerk 1997) but energy intake and body condition are much more critical. The relationship between energy status and reproductive efficiency in the mare was recently reviewed in depth (NRC 2007). Nonpregnant mares in good body condition (condition score at or above 5) at the onset of the breeding season will generally have higher conception rates and will require fewer cycles to conceive. Mares in thin body condition have a longer anovulatory or transitional period, resulting in a later date of first ovulation in the spring. Pregnant mares that foal in a thin body condition and mares that lose body condition at the onset of lactation may also have reduced reproductive efficiency. Fat mares (body condition above 7) do not appear to have reduced reproductive efficiency in comparison to mares in moderate or thin body condition (Henneke et al 1984, Cavinder et al 2005).

Body condition

Frequent body condition scoring is an important management tool for broodmare managers. Condition scoring of pregnant mares may be more useful than weighing because it assesses changes in the mare as opposed to the total maternal-fetal unit. Visual appraisal of body condition is effective in many cases but better assessments of changes in the body stores will be obtained by physical appreciation of the various areas of fat deposition. Palpation of the fat cover on the ribs, tail head and spine of the broodmare is especially important in the winter when a thick hair coat and extended abdomen may create the impression of adequate body condition.

Initial assessment of body condition should be made at least 3 months prior to the onset of the breeding season. A 3-month period allows dietary adjustments to be made in a gradual and conservative manner, thus reducing the risk of digestive disturbances. In order for a mare to lose weight, she must be in negative energy balance (energy intake is less than energy expenditure) and for weight gain a mare must be in positive energy balance (energy intake is greater than energy expenditure). If a mare is perceived to be too fat, late fall and winter weather will increase the amount of energy expended for thermoregulation so weight loss can be accomplished without drastic reductions in feed intake. Conversely, late fall and winter are the most difficult times to increase body weight and condition. The easiest time to accomplish weight gain in mares is in the late summer and early fall when the climate is mild and energy expenditure is relatively low. The amount of weight gain needed to raise body condition score from a 4 to a 5 has been estimated to be 16 to 20 kg for a 500 kg horse (NRC 2007). Each kilogram of gain requires about 20 Mcal of DE above maintenance. Therefore, increasing a mare's concentrate intake by 1–2 kg per day for 60–90 days should result in enough weight gain to raise condition score by about 1 unit. Less concentrate can be fed if high quality forage is available.

Key Points – Reproductive efficiency in mares

- The variable most likely to affect reproductive efficiency in the mare is body condition
- Mares in thin body condition take longer to cycle in the spring, require more cycles to conceive and may have reduced conception rates
- Mares intended for breeding in the spring should be evaluated for body condition in the early fall so that dietary interventions can be imposed gradually
- The addition of vitamin and mineral supplements above required levels of these nutrients has not been shown to enhance reproductive efficiency in the mare

Conclusion

Feeding programs for stallions and mares should focus on feeding balanced diets in amounts that maintain body weight and condition. Stallions that are inactive may have requirements that are similar to any mature horse at maintenance; however, stallions that are very active may have requirements similar to adult horses performing light or moderate work. An assessment of activity should include breeding frequency as well as the amount of exercise a stallion receives (either forced or voluntary). An appropriate body condition for a breeding stallion may be between 5 and 6 (1 to 9 scale; 5 = moderate), although the optimal condition for a stallion has not been studied. Several studies have demonstrated that broodmares should generally be maintained at a body condition of at least 5 (moderate). Mares should be evaluated in early fall and dietary changes made well in advance of winter. It may be desirable for mares that winter outside to begin winter at a higher body condition score in order to ensure adequate stores to buffer any periods when feed intake may not meet requirements. The nutrient needs of gestating mares begin to increase in mid-gestation and peak in late gestation. At foaling, feed intake will generally increase and this increase should be transitioned gradually to minimize the risk of digestive upset. Lactation is the most nutritionally demanding period for the mare. Mares will utilize their own body tissues to maintain the amount and composition of milk so adequate feeding programs are necessary to maintain body condition during lactation. Feed intake should be changed gradually prior to and after weaning to ensure that nutrient intake for the next gestation cycle is adequate. Few research studies have been able to demonstrate positive effects of nutrient supplements on fertility when horses are already receiving a nutrient adequate diet. However, further research on nutrient supplements that target specific causes of infertility (such as oxidative damage to sperm) may be warranted.

References

Akesson, A., Vahter, M., Berglund, M., et al., 2004. Bone turnover from early pregnancy to postweaning. Acta Obstet Gynecol Scand 83, 1049–1055.

Audet, I., Laforest, J.P., Martineau, G.P., et al., 2004. Effect of vitamin supplements on some aspects of performance, vitamin status and semen quality in boars. J Anim Sci 82, 626–633.

Ball, B.A., 2008. Oxidative stress, osmotic stress and apoptosis: Impacts on sperm function and preservation in the horse. Anim Reprod Sci 107, 257–267.

Banach, M.A., Evans, J.W., 1985. Effects of inadequate energy during gestation and lactation on the estrous cycle and conception rates of mares and on their foal weights. Proc 9th Equine Nutr Physiol Symp., East Lansing MI. Equine Nutrition and Physiology Society, Savoy, IL, pp. 97–100.

Blaxter, K., 1989. Energy Metabolism in Animals and Man. Cambridge University Press, Cambridge UK.

Brinsko, S.P., Varner, D.D., Love, C.C., et al., 2005. Effect of feeding a DHA enriched nutriceutical on the quality of fresh, cooled and frozen stallion semen. Theriogenology 63, 1519–1527.

Canibal, M.C.H.B., Neves, A.P., Castro, F.S., et al., 2008. Effect of a fatty acid supplement on the estrus cycle and pregnancy rates of Brazilian pony mares. Pferdeheilkunde 24, 23 (English abstract).

Cassill, B., Hayes, S., Ringler, R., et al., 2004. The effect of dietary calcium on indicators of bone turnover in mares. J Anim Sci 82 (Suppl 1), 330.

Cassill, B., Hayes, S., Ringler, J., et al., 2005. Changes in serum markers of bone turnover during pregnancy and lactation. Proc. 19th Equine Sci Soc. Equine Science Society, Tucson AZ. Equine Science Society, Champaign, IL, pp. 63–64.

Cassill, B., Jackson, S., Lawrence, L., 2009. Body weight changes in pregnant mares. J Equine Vet Sci 29, 400–401.

Cavinder, C.A., Vogelsang, M.M., Forrest, D.W., et al., 2005. Reproductive parameters of fat vs moderately conditioned mares following parturition. Proc. 19th Equine Sci Soc., Tucson AZ. Equine Science Society, Champaign, IL, pp. 65–69.

Cerolini, S., Zaniboni, L., Maldjian, A., et al., 2006. Effect of docosohexaenoic acid and alpha tocopherol enrichment in chicken sperm on semen quality, sperm lipid composition and susceptibility to peroxidation. Theriogenology 66, 877–886.

Colagar, A.H., Marzony, E.T., Chaichi, M.J., 2009. Zinc levels in seminal plasma are associated with sperm quality in fertile and infertile men. Nutr Res 29, 82–88.

Clowes, E.J., Aherne, F.X., Foxcroft, G.R., et al., 2003. Selective protein loss in lactating sows is associated with reduced litter growth and ovarian function. J Anim Sci 81, 753–764.

Davison, K.E., Potter, G.D., Greene, L.W., et al., 1991. Lactation and reproductive performance of mares fed added dietary fat during late gestation and early lactation. J Equine Vet Sci 11, 111–115.

Deichsel, K., Palm, F., Koblischke, P., et al., 2008. Effect of a dietary antioxidant supplementation on semen quality in pony stallions. Theriogenology 69, 940–945.

Donoghue, S., Meacham, T.N., Kronfeld, D.S., 1990. A conceptual approach to optimal nutrition of broodmares. Vet Clin N Am: Equine Pract 6 (2), 373–391.

Duvaux-Ponter, C., Tournie, M., Detrimont, L., et al., 2004. Effect of a supplement rich in linolenic acid added to the diet of mares on the fatty acid composition of mammary secretions and the acquisition of passive immunity in the foal. Anim Sci 78, 399–407.

Ebisch, I.M.W., Thomas, C.M.G., Peters, W.H.M., et al., 2007. The importance of folate, zinc and antioxidants in the pathogenesis and prevention of subfertility. Hum Reprod Update 13, 163–174.

Elhordoy, D.M., Cazales, N., Costa, G., et al., 2008. Effect of dietary supplementation with DHA on the quality of fresh, cooled and frozen stallion semen. Anim Reprod Sci (abstract #17).

Eskenazi, B., Kidd, S.A., Marks, A.R., et al., 2005. Antioxidant intake is associated with semen quality in healthy men. Hum Reprod 20, 1006–1012.

Gee, E.K., Bruemmer, J.E., Siciliano, P.D., et al., 2008. Effects of dietary vitamin E supplementation on spermatozoa quality in stallions with suboptimal post-thaw motility. Anim Reprod Sci 23–24 (abstract).

George, L.A., Staniar, W.B., Treiber, K.H., et al., 2009. Insulin sensitivity and glucose dynamics during pre-weaning foal development and in response to maternal diet composition. Domestic Anim Endocrinol 37, 23–29.

Gibbs, P.G., Potter, G.D., Blke, R.W., et al., 1982. Milk production of Quarter Horse mares during 150 days of lactation. J Anim Sci 54, 496–499.

Gill, R.J., Potter, G.D., Kreider, J.L., et al., 1983. Postpartum reproductive performance of mares fed various levels of protein. Proc 8th Equine Nutr Physiol Symp, Lexington KY. Equine Nutrition and Physiology Society, Lexington, KY, pp. 311–316.

Glade, M.J., 1993. Effects of gestation, lactation and maternal calcium intake on mechanical strength of equine bone. J Amer Coll Nutr 372–377.

Gliozzi, T.M., Zaniboni, L., Maldjian, A., et al., 2009. Quality and lipid composition of spermatozoa in rabbits fed DHA and vitamin E rich diets. Theriogenology 71, 910–919.

Grace, N.D., Shaw, H.L., Gee, E.K., et al., 2002. Determination of the digestible energy intake and apparent absorption of macroelements in pasture fed lactating Thoroughbred mares. N Z Vet J 50, 182–185.

Grady, S.T., Cavinder, C.A., Brinsko, S.P., et al., 2009. Dietary supplementation of 2 sources of n-3 fatty acids and subsequent effects on fresh, cooled and frozen seminal characteristics of stallions. The Prof Animal Scientist 27, 768–773.

Hammoud, A.O., Gibson, M., Peterson, M., et al., 2008a. Impact of male obesity on infertility: a critical review of the current literature. Fertil Steril 90, 897–904.

Hammoud, A.O., Wilde, N., Gibson, M., et al., 2008b. Male obesity and alteration in sperm parameters. Fertil Steril 90, 2222–2493.

Henneke, D.R., Potter, G.D., Kreider, J.L., et al., 1983. Relationship between condition score, physical measurements and body fat percentage in mares. Equine Vet J 15, 371–372.

Henneke, D.R., Potter, G.D., Kreider, J.L., 1984. Body condition during pregnancy and lactation and reproductive efficiency of mares. Theriogenology 21, 897–909.

Hines, K.K., Hodge, S.L., Kreider, J.L., et al., 1987. Relationship between body condition and levels of serum luteinizing hormone in postpartum mares. Theriogenology 28, 815–825.

Hoffman, R.M., Kronfeld, D.S., Herbein, J.H., et al., 1998. Dietary carbohydrates and fat influence milk composition and fatty acid profile of mare's milk. J Nutr 128, 2708S–2711S.

Hoffman, R.M., Morgan, K.L., Lynch, M.P., et al., 1999. Dietary vitamin E supplemented in the periparturient period influences immunoglobulins in equine colostrums and passive transfer in foals. Proc 16th Equine Nutr. Physiol Symp., Raleigh NC. Equine Nutrition and Physiology Society, Savoy, IL, pp. 96–97.

Janicki, K.M., Lawrence, L.M., Barnes, T., et al., 2000. The effect of dietary selenium source and level on broodmares and their foals. J Anim Sci 83 (Suppl. 1), 172.

Janicki, K.M., Lawrence, L.M., Barnes, T., et al., 2001. The effect of dietary selenium source and level on selenium concentration, glutathione peroxidase activity and influenza titers in broodmares and their foals. Proc 17th Equine Nutr Physiol Symp. Lexington KY, Equine Nutrition and Physiology Society, Savoy, IL, pp. 43–44.

Karren, B.J., Thorson, J.F., Cavinder, C.A., et al., 2010. Effect of selenium supplementation and plane of nutrition on mares and their foals: Selenium concentrations and glutathione perioxidase. J Anim Sci 88, 991–997.

Kavazis, A.N., Kivipelto, J., Ott, E.A., 2002. Supplementation of broodmares with copper, zinc, iron, manganese, cobalt, iodine and selenium. J Equine Vet Sci 22, 460–464.

Kruglik, V.L., Kouba, J.M., Hill, C.M., et al., 2006. Effect of feeding protected N-3 polyunsaturated fatty acids on plasma and milk fatty acid levels and

IgG concentrations in mares and foals. Proc. 19th Equine Sci Soc. Equine Sci, Tucson AZ. Equine Science Society, Champaign, IL, pp. 635–136.

Kubiak, J.R., Evans, J.W., Potter, G.D., et al., 1988. Parturition in the multiparous mare fed to obesity. J Equine Vet Sci 8, 135–140.

Lang, K.J., Nielsen, B.D., Waite, K.L., et al., 2001. Supplemental silicon increases milk silicon concentrations in horses. J Anim Sci 79, 2627–2633.

Lawrence, L.M., DiPietro, J., Ewert, K., et al., 1992. Changes in body weight and condition in gestating mares. J Equine Vet Sci 12 (6), 355–358.

Ley, W.B., Thatcher, C.D., Swecker, W.S., et al., 1990. Chelated mineral supplementation in the barren mare: A preliminary trial. J Equine Vet Sci 10, 176–181.

Manso Filho, H.C., McKeever, K.H., Gordon, M.E., et al., 2008. Changes in glutamine metabolism indicate a mild catabolic state in the transition mare. J Anim Sci 86, 3424–1054.

Maenpaa, P.H., Pirhonen, A., Koskinen, E., 1988. Serum profiles of vitamins A, E and D in mares and foals during different seasons. J Anim Sci 66, 1418–1423.

Matsui, A., Inoue, Y., Asai, Y., 2005. Effects of acute changes in the energy and protein intake levels over the short-term on the maternal milk amino acid concentrations in lactation mares. Asian-Aust J Anim Sci 18, 855–860.

Meyer, H., Ahlswede, L., 1978. The intra-uterine growth and body composition of foals and the nutrient requirements of pregnant mares. Anim Res Devel 8, 86–111.

More, C., Bettembuk, P., Bhattoa, H.P., et al., 2001. The effects of pregnancy and lactation on bone mineral density. Osteoporosis Int 12, 732–737.

Nguyen, R.H.N., Wilcox, A.J., Skjaerven, R., et al., 2007. Men's body mass index and infertility. Hum Reprod 22, 2488–2493.

NRC, 1949. Recommended Nutrient Allowances for Horses. National Research Council, Washington DC.

NRC, 1973. Nutrient Requirements of Horses, third revised ed. National Academy Press, Washington DC.

NRC, 1978. Nutrient Requirements of Horses, fourth revised ed. National Academy Press, Washington DC.

NRC, 1989. Nutrient Requirements of Horses, fifth revised ed. National Academy Press, Washington DC.

NRC, 2007. Nutrient Requirements of Horses, sixth revised ed. National Academy Press, Washington DC.

Ousey, J.C., Fowden, A.L., Wilsher, S., et al., 2008. The effects of maternal health and body condition on the endocrine responses of neonatal foals. Equine Vet J 40, 673–679.

Ott, E.A., Asquith, R.L., 1983. Calcium and phosphorus supplementation of foaling mares. Proc 8th Equine Nutr Physiol Symp., Lexington KY. Equine Nutrition and Physiology Society, Savoy, IL, pp. 317–322.

Pagan, J.D., Hintz, H.F., Rounsaville, T.R., 1984. The digestible energy requirements of lactating pony mares. J Anim Sci 58, 1382–1387.

Pagan, J.D., Hintz, H.F., 1986. Composition of milk from pony mares fed various levels of digestible energy. Cornell Vet 76, 139–148.

Poland, T.A., Kouba, J.M., Hill, C.M., et al., 2006. Effects of fatty acid supplementation on plasma fatty acid concentrations and characteristics of the first postpartum estrous. J Anim Sci 84 (Suppl 1), 393.

Prentice, A., 2000. Calcium in pregnancy and lactation. Annu Rev Nutr 20, 249–272.

Rich, G.A., McGlothlin, D.E., Lewis, L.D., et al., 1983. Effect of vitamin E on stallion sexual characteristics and sexual behavior. Proc 8th Equine Nutr Physiol Symp., Lexington KY. Equine Nutrition and Physiology Society, Savoy, IL, pp. 85–89.

Robl, M.G., Forfa, R.J., 1987. Effects of metallosates on conception rates of thoroughbred mares. Proc 10th Equine Nutr Physiol Symp., Ft Collins CO. Equine Nutrition and Physiology Society, Savoy, IL, pp. 637–641.

Siciliano, P.D., Wood, C.H., Lawrence, L.M., Duren, S.E., 1993. Utilization of a field study to evaluation digestible energy requirements of breeding stallions. Proc 13th Equine Nutr. Physiol. Symp. Equine Nutrition and Physiology Society, Savoy, IL, pp. 293–298.

Siciliano, P.D., Dowler, L.E., Hayes, S.H., et al., 2009. Relationship between colostral IgG, foal serum IgG and mare vitamin E status. J Equine Vet Sci 29, 392–394.

Silver, M., Fowden, A.L., 1982. Uterine prostaglandin F metabolite production in relation to glucose availability in late pregnancy and a possible influence of diet on time of delivery in the mare. J Reprod Fert Suppl. 32, 511–519.

Spearman, K.R., Ott, E.S., Kivapelto, J., et al., 2005. Effect of fatty acid supplementation of the mare on milk and foal plasma composition and foal growth. Proc. 19th Equine Sci Soc., Tucson AZ. Equine Nutrition and Physiology Society, Savoy, IL, pp. 3–4.

Stelzleni, E.L., Warren, L.K., Kivipelto, J., 2006. Effect of dietary n-3 fatty acid supplementation on plasma and milk composition and immune status of mares and foals. J Anim Sci 84 (Suppl 1), 392–393.

St. Lawrence, A.C., Lawrence, L.M., Coleman, R.J., 2001. Using an empirical equation to predict voluntary intake of grass hays by mature equids. Proc 17th Equine Nutr Physiol Symp., Lexington KY. Equine Nutrition and Physiology Society, Savoy, IL, pp. 99–100.

Stowe, H.D., 1967. Reproductive performance of barren mares following vitamin A and E supplementation. Proc 13th Amer. Assoc. Equine Pract., New Orleans LA. American Association of Equine Practitioners, Lexington, KY, p. 81.

Thorson, J.F., Karren, B.J., Bauer, M.L., et al., 2010. Effect of selenium supplementation and plane of nutrition on mares and their foals: Foaling data. J Anim Sci 88, 982–990.

Umphenour, N.W., McCarthy, P., Blanchard, T.L., 2011. Management of stallions in natural service programs. In: McKinnon, A.O., Squires, E.L., Vaala, W.E., et al (Eds.), Equine Reproduction, Blackwell Publishing, Oxford, pp 1208–1227.

Urriola, P.E., Hoehler, D., Pedersen, C., et al., 2009. Amino acid digestibility of distillers dried grains with soluble produced from sorghum, a sorghum-corn blend and corn fed to growing pigs. J Anim Sci 87, 2574–2580.

van Niekerk, F.E., van Niekerk, C.H., 1997. The effect of dietary protein on reproduction in the mare. III. Ovarian and uterine changes during the anovulatory, transitional and ovulatory periods in the non-pregnant mare. J South African Vet J 68, 86–92.

Vickers, J.G., Warren, L.K., Kivipelto, J., et al, 2009. Replacement of sulfate trace minerals with amino acids complexes in mare diets and its effects on innate and acquired immunity in nursing foals. J Equine Vet Sci 29, 394–396.

Vickers, J.G., Warren, L.K., Silva, L.A., et al., 2009. Replacement of sulfate trace minerals with amino acid complexes in mare diets and effects on early postpartum reproductive performance. J Equine Vet Sci 29, 392–394.

Wathes, D.C., Abayasekara, D.R.E., Aitken, R.J., 2007. Polyunsaturated fatty acids in male and female reproduction. Biol Reprod 77, 190–201.

Wickens, C.L., Ku, P.K., Trottier, M.L., 2002. An ideal protein for the lactating mare. J Anim Sci 80 (Suppl. 1), 155.

Wilsher, S., Allen, W.R., 2006. Effects of a *Streptococcus equi* infection-mediated nutritional insult during mid-gestaton in primiparous Thoroughbred fillies. Part 1: Placental and fetal development. Equine Vet J 38, 549–547.

Zini, A., San Gabiel, M., Baazeem, A., 2009. Antioxidants and sperm DNA damage: a clinical perspective. J Assist Reprod Genet 26, 427–432.

12

Feeding the growing horse

William B. Staniar

Introduction

The diet of the growing horse can be broken down into its simple components of colostrum, milk, water, forage, and concentrates (complementary or supplementary feed). The percentage, within the diet, that each of these account for will change in relation to age and circumstances. The final ration should ideally provide all the energy substrates, building materials, and solvents (including, for example, carbohydrates, protein, and water, respectively) that facilitate life and growth. Those in charge of the care of the growing horse have varying degrees of control over the intake and format of these different components. For example, the amount and type of concentrate fed to a horse can be precisely determined, while the intake of fresh forage from pasture is much more difficult to evaluate. A related example would be that the nutrient make-up of a manufactured feed should be much more consistent than that of forages or even individual grains. This does not mean that manufactured feeds are better than grains or forages, but those responsible for feeding need to be aware of where they do or do not have control over their growing horse's diet. Through knowledgeable management of the different dietary components, the horse owner/feeder can have a significant impact on the current and future health and athletic potential of the growing horse.

It is assumed within this chapter that the ultimate objective of those feeding the growing horse is optimal growth. Optimal growth being the increase in size of the horse from birth that allows for maximum health and performance at designated stages of life. As a corollary to this, a cessation of growth during a horse's early years (generally the first three years) is an obvious indication that there is some sort of health problem or nutritional deficit present. The definition of performance depends on the horse owner, and may vary considerably from breed to breed and even owner to owner within a breed. An interesting example of this would be the 14.1 hand Shetland, Arabian, and Thoroughbred cross, Theodore O'Connor. "Teddy" was a pony that by all measures competed quite well in the sport of top level three day eventing.

This chapter first addresses several basic questions about equine growth; what defines and characterizes equine growth, how does it change over time, what is the composition of that growth, and are there breed differences that can be identified? All of this will be examined in the context of understanding what the optimal nutrition is for the growing horse. A section discussing the energy and nutrient requirements of growth then logically follows, in which there is some theoretical discussion of these requirements, particularly in regard to the great genetic and phenotypic variability that represents the horse today. Finally, there is a section on the practical application of nutrition to growing horses during different stages of their development.

Growth

Growth is critical to the eventual development of a horse's athletic potential. A very general definition of growth is an increase in size. Genetics and environment both play important roles in the expression of growth related traits. Each horse has a certain genetic potential for growth that is inherited from its sire and dam. This genetic potential relates mostly to the overall shape of the lifetime growth pattern and the mature size of the animal. As an example, the heritability of withers height has been estimated to be between 0.25 to 0.28 (Stock et al 2005). This can be interpreted to mean that roughly 26% of the phenotypic variation in withers height can be attributed to genetic variation. Environment, and nutrition as a component of environment, has a very important role to play. Nutrition's impact on the lifetime growth pattern is likely to be seen more in short-term deviations from the longer-term genetically determined growth pattern. The short-term fluctuations seen in Figs 12.1 and 12.2 are examples of these short-term deviations.

At a cellular level, growth occurs both through an increase in the number as well as the size of cells. The mechanisms that control cell number and size are complex and still not well understood, but generally differences in size between animals can be accounted for by differences in the total number of cells. The cells themselves are not notably different in size between animals. The decrease in the rate of growth as an animal approaches mature size is mainly accounted for by a decrease in cell proliferation (Lui & Baron 2011). Some measures of growth that are commonly recorded for horses are body weight, wither height, body length, and cannon circumference (Hintz et al 1979, Staniar et al 2004a). Each of these measures will have a different pattern of

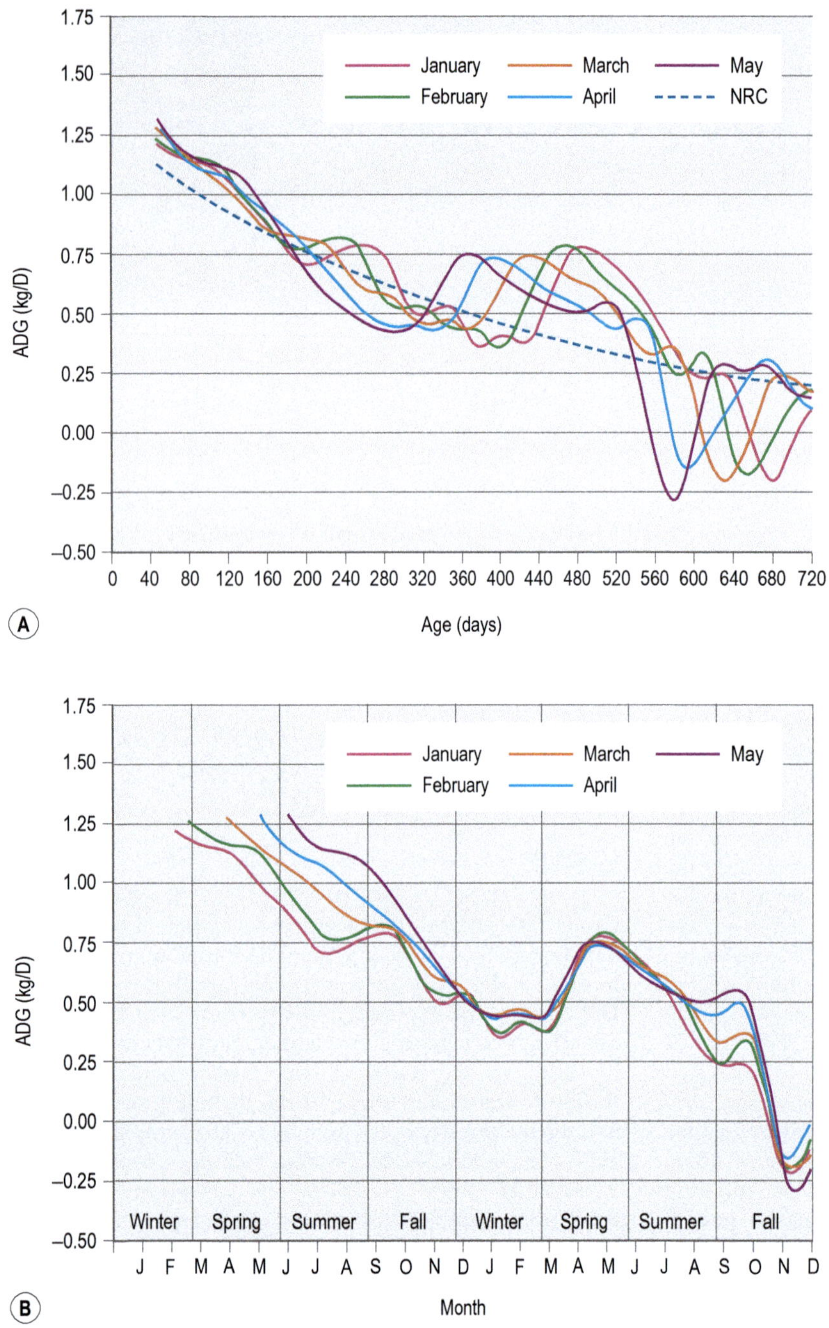

Figure 12.1 Average daily weight gain (kg/day) of Thoroughbred foals (n = 2096) over a period of approximately 2.5 years. The x-axis is labeled with either the age of the foals in days A) or the month of the year B). The different lines represent foals born in January, February, March, April, or May, and are the same for (A) or (B). The line labeled NRC represents the predicted rate of gain of a growing horse with an expected mature weight of 550 kg. These foals were raised in the northern hemisphere, and the seasons are listed as such.

growth, based on the tissues involved and the nutrients and energy being supplied (Hammond 1950).

Growth curves

Taking what we know of equine growth, it is difficult to develop a single all inclusive model to accurately describe the growth of all horses. The range of breeds, management scenarios, and owner objectives are part of what make this such a challenge. The pattern of equine growth from conception to maturity (5–7 years) can generally be described as a sigmoid curve. There are several examples of sigmoid curves fitting well to equine data (Walton & Hammond 1938, Staniar et al 2004b, NRC 2007). The point of inflection for most of these curves indicates that the horse is different from cattle, in that the most rapid rate of gain occurs just prior to parturition. This emphasizes the point that sufficient attention should be paid to the nutrition of the broodmare throughout gestation. Another characteristic of equine growth is a sine wave like pattern superimposed on the sigmoid curve (Staniar 2001). This sine wave pattern is likely associated with seasonal fluctuations in nutrient availability and ambient temperature and is commonly seen in horses raised away from the equator and kept outside (Dawson et al 1945, Pagan et al 1996). The presence of this pattern suggests that energy requirements should be adjusted based on local environmental conditions. Dr. Nadia Cymbaluk has conducted extensive research studying horses under changing climatic conditions and has suggested that digestible energy in the diet of growing horses should be increased by 1.3% for each degree Celsius below the lower critical temperature specific to the particular life stage of that horse

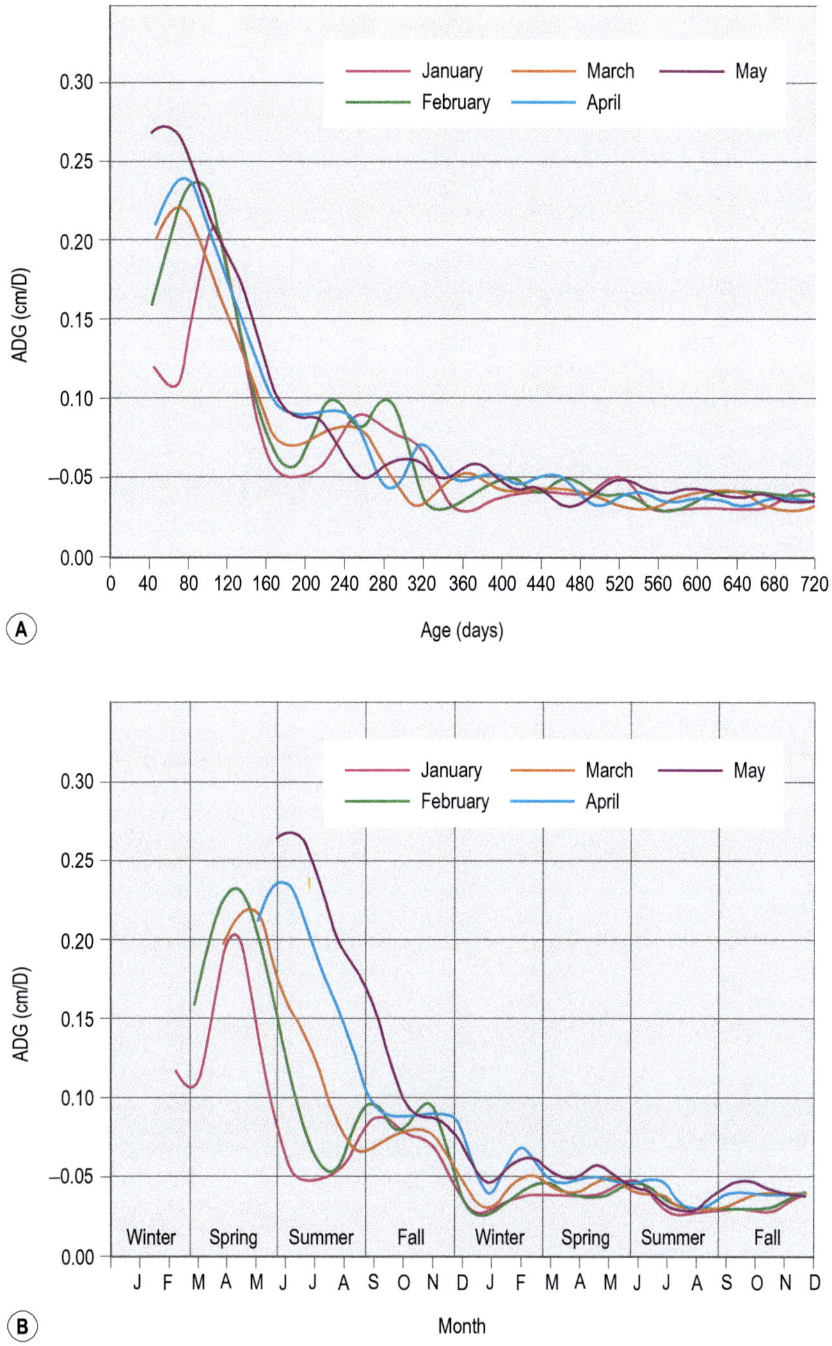

Figure 12.2 **Average daily wither height gain (cm/day) of Thoroughbred foals (n = 2096) over a period of approximately 2.5 years.** The x-axis is labeled with either the age of the foals in days **A)** or the month of the year **B)**. The different lines represent foals born in January, February, March, April, or May, and are the same for **A)** or **B)**. These foals were raised in the northern hemisphere, and the seasons are listed as such.

(Cymbaluk 1994). Examples of these lower critical temperatures for a newborn foal are 16 to 26°C, for a week-old foal, 13 to 23°C, and as an adult –20 to 5°C (NRC 2007). In conclusion, equine growth can be described as following a sigmoid pattern, with an exponential increase in size occurring in utero, followed by a post parturition period during which the rate of growth slows as the mature size is approached.

Growth rate

Any evaluation of growth has to include a measure of the time over which that growth has occurred. Age in months or days is commonly used as a measure of time, and is often measured more precisely than body weight, a measure that is often estimated as most farms do not have access to a calibrated weighing machine/scale. As an example, in one of the few studies to use a body mass index, Donaldson et al (2004) used an estimate of body weight based on heart girth and body length. The fact that body weight was estimated makes it possible that the accuracy of these published data is not as good as it could be if actual weights had been used. No published studies have used this body mass index in growing horses, although it may be useful in further characterizing growth. Time is often implied when growth is defined as rapid, moderate, or slow. After all, it is the rate of growth that is being described with each of these modifiers, and that rate also changes with age. So a rapid growth rate for a 2- or 6-month-old Thoroughbred foal might be 1.2 or 0.9 kg/day, respectively, while moderate growth for the same foal at these time points might be 1 or 0.8 kg/day. There are a multitude of factors that can influence the rate of growth, making the definition of rapid, moderate, or slow a tricky business. Three factors that are probably necessary in defining these terms are breed, age, and date of birth. Figure 12.1(A) is an illustration of the rate of body weight gain in Thoroughbred foals, and is broken into average daily gain patterns based on the foals' month of birth. Figure 12.1(B) provides a different perspective, by looking at the same data on a month of year basis. This figure makes it clear that it is not only age that influences the rate of gain but also time of year and that it is therefore important to examine growth using both these different time scales. Finally whilst the potential for growth decreases with age, during the first 2 years changes in the environment, particularly nutrition, continue to have the potential to have a large impact. This means that, in general, modifications to nutrition during the first two years of life may have a greater impact on the growth and development of tissues such as bone than in older horses. Finally, there has been relatively little comparison of the growth curves of horse breeds that might be expected to have significantly different patterns of growth (see Box 12.1).

It is worth noting that the majority of growth analysis of horses has focused on changes in body weight, but the growth pattern of individual organs may be quite different from that of the whole body. Some examples of the percentage increase in size of different components of growth from birth to maturity in Thoroughbreds have been estimated based on sigmoid models of growth (Staniar et al 2005). Maturity in this case is defined as the asymptote of the sigmoid curve for each growth variable:

- An 18% increase in the length of the front cannon bones.
- A 130% increase in body length measured from the point of the shoulder to the point of the buttocks.
- A 50% increase in wither height.

These differences highlight the different patterns of growth for each of these anatomical characteristics. It is likely that more attention needs to be give to the pattern of growth for some of these other characteristics, as they may be as, if not more important than weight in realizing the full athletic potential of the horse.

Box 12.1 Do Different Breeds of Horse Have Different Patterns of Growth?

The horse of today is the product of breeding choices associated with its domestication and use. The horse is quite different from other livestock species in regard to the diversity of objectives its owners have, and in this way is similar to the dog. In both the dog and the horse, there is a wide phenotypic range in measurable size characteristics. This variability in mature size, leads to questions about associated differences in the pattern of growth between breeds (NRC 1987). The measurement of thousands of horses is required to develop growth curves that can be used to precisely compare different breed's patterns of growth. While there are a large number of studies characterizing the growth of breeds like the Thoroughbred, or Warmblood-type horses, data for other breeds is scarce if not completely lacking. As was pointed out, information on the weight and rate of gain at different ages is critical to determining the energy and nutrient requirements. Most assume that all growing horses follow a common pattern of growth that is characterized by a sigmoid curve of the percent of mature size attained at different ages.

Because the nutrient and energy requirements for growth are based on weight and rate of gain, it is probably less important to focus on different breeds of horse, and instead understand something about the variation in growth patterns expressed over all horses. If the variation in these patterns is wide enough, one could argue that the energy and nutrient requirements for growth would be different for horses in one percentile versus another. For example, horses such as Thoroughbreds, Standardbreds, and Quarter Horses might be characterized as light-build horses, whereas Hanoverians, Trakehners, and Oldenburgs would be medium-build horses (these are arbitrary designations, and only relate to the known relative growth data and mature size of these particular animals). Perhaps the medium-build horses take longer to mature and have a higher rate of gain at an earlier age than the light-build. Do these differences in growth mean that there are substantial differences in the way requirements should be calculated? This difference may be more substantial if a heavy-build horse, such as a Percheron, is compared with a light-build, such as an Arabian. Isn't it likely that the accretion patterns for protein and lipids are different in these animals? These questions remains to be answered, but in application can be bypassed by careful attention to the condition, health and growth rates of individual animals. It is unlikely that an equation or table will ever be a substitute for the keen eye of those raising the horse. However more precise designation of energy and nutrient requirements for growth will benefit owners with less experience and those managing a large number of animals.

Growth composition

Growth composition can be described in tissue or chemical specific terms. When discussing energy and nutrient requirements for the growing horse, it is useful to describe tissue development in terms of adipose, muscle, and skeletal tissues. The building materials and energy required for each of these are generally different, and therefore the nutrition required for the optimal growth and development of these tissues changes, based on the growth rates of each tissue at the time the horse is being fed. Generally, the horse follows a tissue development pattern similar to other livestock species in that tissue specific maximum growth rates occur in the following sequence; bone followed by muscle, and then adipose. There is a relatively small body of literature on the actual body composition of growing horses (Martin-Rosset et al 1983, Doreau et al 1986, Martin-Rosset, 2005) An overview of the data indicates that both muscle and adipose tissue undergo significant growth in the 2 years following birth. This highlights the importance of both dietary protein and energy to supply the requirements of these large developing tissues. In relative terms the chemical composition of 1 kg of gain in a weanling will consist of more protein and less lipid than the same 1 kg in a 2-year-old, or said another way the older the horse is the greater the percentage of fat in every kg of gain.

Tangential data on weight and linear measures of growth support the concepts discussed above. As an example, body weight and wither height growth patterns for approximately 2000 Thoroughbred foals from birth to 2 years of age are shown in Fig. 12.3 (Staniar, unpublished). The difference in these two patterns is likely due to the fact that changes in body weight reflect changes in all tissues, while wither height is more reflective of the skeletal structure and form

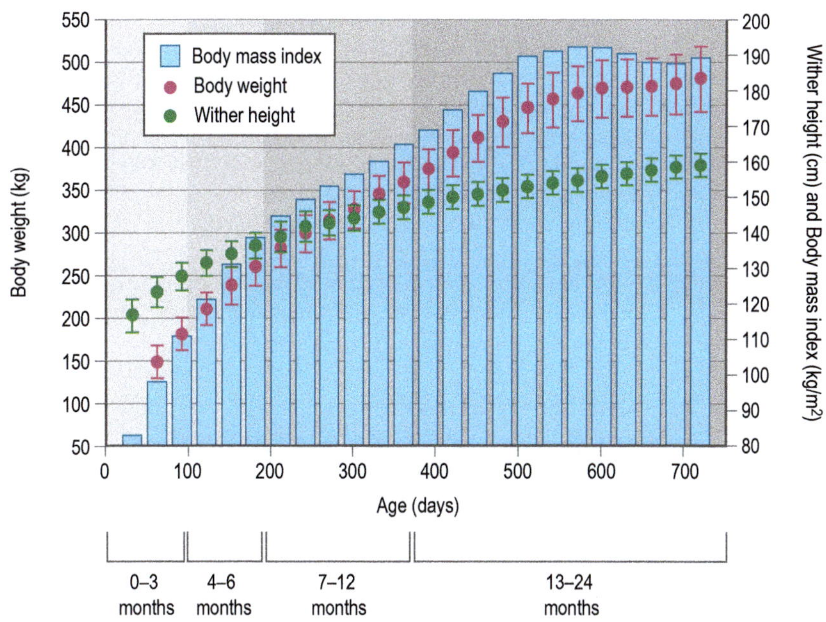

Figure 12.3 Weight, height, and body mass index changes in Thoroughbred foals (*n* = 2096) in 30-day intervals from one month of age through 2 years. Shaded regions represent important periods in the growth of the horse.

of the horse's forelimb. The body mass index (BMI) is a mathematical relationship of body weight divided by height^2, and is commonly and effectively used as a measure of relative weight in humans (Keys et al 1972). An analogous equine body mass index has been developed for use in the horse, in which body weight is divided by the wither height^2. It is of interest to note that the equine BMI between 1.5 and 2 years of age (Fig. 12.3) has reached 190 kg/m^2 which is close to the median value of 196 kg/m^2 calculated for a group of 82 horses representing at least 10 different breeds and ranging in age from 1 to 23 years of age (average, 10 years) (Donaldson et al 2004). While it is unlikely that overall growth has ceased in the 2-year-old, the relationship between body weight and wither height has stabilized. Based on this, body weight may not be the best indicator of nutrition's impact on development during the first two years of life. Assuming that skeletal development is a priority for those raising equine athletes, measures such as withers height or other skeletal variables should be used in addition to body weight when evaluating the impact of nutrition on early equine growth. Body condition scoring is a technique used in adult horses that uses a subjective scaling of subcutaneous adipose stores to evaluate energy balance (Henneke et al 1983). A similar system for young growing horses has not yet been developed. Initially, a problem with using any of these measures of equine growth is that optimal patterns of development for each have not been defined. Future studies need to examine the relationships between observed patterns of growth and measures of success or failure, such as racing ability or occurrence of skeletal abnormalities.

Key Points – Growth

- Genetics and environment both play critical roles in the pattern of equine growth.
- Growth can be measured in many different ways including most commonly changes in body weight and withers height. Other measures, such as girth or cannon circumference may also be useful
- Equine growth is most rapid near parturition, highlighting the importance of properly feeding the broodmare
- There are short term fluctuations in growth that are likely associated with changes in the growing horse's environment, and these are overlaid on a long term genetically determined sigmoid pattern. The combination of these results in the observed pattern of growth

The above discussion of growth leads to the seemingly simple concept that the period during which growth occurs is a period of constant change. Therefore, the amount of energy and nutrients needed at one particular time point during this process may be different from those needed at another time point. One approach to determining the energy and nutrient requirements during growth therefore is to use information about the quantity (body weight), rate of gain, body composition (generally described in terms of protein, fat, and major minerals), and the utilization rate of energy or nutrients for building the individual components of the growing horse. While there is a large amount of data characterizing bodyweight and rate of gain, body composition and utilization rates are not well characterized. Martin-Rosset (Martin-Rosset 2005) summarizes the relative growth rates of different components of the equine body, breaking these down by anatomical designations and chemical composition. Using these data plus that collected by the German Society of Nutritional Physiology (M. Coenen, personal communication), it is possible to develop gross estimates of the protein and lipid gain during different phases of growth (Table 12-1). Protein and lipid gain are going to be the main sinks for dietary energy required for growth. It should be noted that the specific energy requirements for this gain needs to be added to the core primary maintenance requirement (see next section). Based on limited data, estimates of protein as a percentage of daily gain range from 18 to 30% and lipids from 4 to 22%. However, care should be taken not to over interpret these numbers, as there are many factors that are estimated, and the data supporting them is limited.

Table 12-1 Approximate Percentages of Muscle, Bone, and Adipose in Carcasses of Horses at 0, 12, and 30 Months of Age (Martin-Rosset 2005).

	Tissue component as a percentage of carcass weight		
Age, months	% Muscle	% Bone	% Adipose
0	59	32	6
12	70	16	11
30	70	15	11

As an example, it is not always clear whether compositions are described as a percentage of total body weight, empty body weight, or carcass weight. These designations need to be clear as the percent composition will change based on what is being examined. Having said this, the general changes over time are likely to hold for important substances such as protein and lipid. Understanding the chemical composition of gain is important because the dietary energy required will change based on the relative amounts of protein and lipid being deposited.

Generally, it appears that the horse follows a growth pattern similar to what is seen in other livestock species, with muscle reaching a peak in rate of gain prior to adipose tissue (Hammond 1950). Based on the fact that water content decreases from birth to maturity, it is likely that the contribution of protein initially and then mainly lipid, as a proportion of daily gain, will increase and so the energy requirement for gain will increase with age (Martin-Rosset 2005). The lack of data decreases our ability to make precise estimates of the requirements for key dietary constituents such as the individual amino acids. Research in this area would likely lead to improved precision feeding of horses to not only reduce the risk of diet related developmental problems, but also potentially improve the ability to realize the full athletic potential of a greater number of horses at maturity.

Energy requirements

Energy requirements for the growing horse are split between those for maintenance and those for growth. The split is relatively even early on, but as the foal gains weight, and growth slows, the maintenance component becomes proportionally larger than that for growth. The equation that defines the digestible energy (DE) requirement for growing horses published in the National Research Council's nutrient requirements for horses contains components for maintenance (in bold) and growth (NRC 2007).

$$\text{DE (Mcal/d)} = \{[(56.5x^{-0.145}) \times \text{BW})/1000] + [(1.99 + 1.21x - 0.021x^2) \times \text{ADG}]\}$$

Those interested in calculating the DE requirements of their growing horse can enter the horse's age in months (x), body weight (kg), and average daily gain (ADG; kg/day) in the above equation. There are numerous computer spreadsheet programs that once this equation has been entered into, will calculate an estimated DE requirement based on the data entered. This equation is a best estimate of energy requirements for growth based on an extensive review of research conducted prior to 2007 (NRC 2007). There are certainly still questions as to more precise estimates of the energy requirement for growth, but it is unlikely that any improved precision is going to come from a single equation. It is more likely that calibrations based on factors such as breed, date of birth, and climatic conditions will allow for improved precision at the cost of increased complexity. The complexity of growth is highlighted by the patterns of growth illustrated in Figs 12.1 and 12.2. Questions remain as to the exact reason each of these deviations occurs and whether additional energy alone could smooth the growth curves.

Dietary energy source

Nutrition supports growth through the supply of energy and nutrients. While the nutrients can be thought of as building materials and supplies, energy is found stored in the chemical bonds in the nonstructural and structural carbohydrates, fats or oils, and protein, within the feedstuffs of the foal and growing animal.

It may be more practical to consider how the energy supplied via the diet changes with age by looking at typical dietary ingredients. For the young foal, milk composed of lactose, fat, and protein is going to provide most if not all of its energy needs. However, as the foal ages forage will comprise an increasing proportion of its diet, and most of the energy derived from forages comes from the volatile fatty acids produced via fermentation in the growing horse's cecum and colon.

There are limited data on exactly how the foal's diet changes while still with their dam and numerous factors affect how this change in diet progresses including frequency of suckling, length of each suckling bout, milk production, milk nutrient composition, dam temperament, and alternative feed availability. Regardless, it is generally accepted that foals will begin to ingest ingredients other than milk as early as 1 week of age and will slowly decrease the percent of their ration that the dam's milk composes up until weaning (Crowell-Davis et al 1985). Another factor that influences the source of energy available to the foal is the decrease in lactase and increase in sucrase and maltase activity in the small intestine as the foal ages (Roberts, 1975). This integrates well with the transition from a milk-based to a plant-based diet and enables the growing horse to efficiently utilize the nonstructural carbohydrates in grains and other plant materials (see Box 12.2).

Excessive energy intake

High concentrations of dietary energy will increase the rate of growth up to the genetic potential. Dietary energy provided above this requirement will either be stored in adipose tissue or potentially contribute to a more subjective characteristic of heightened excitability. Periods of rapid growth have been associated with skeletal abnormalities in the horse as well as other livestock species (Hill 1990, Van Weeren 2006). While most horse owners would generally choose to avoid anything described as skeletal abnormalities, the group of conditions that fall under this set of terms range from mild angular limb deformities that may be generally considered a normal part of equine development to osteochondritis dessicans that may require surgery for a

Box 12.2 An Evolutionary Perspective on Feeding the Growing Horse

Nutrition plays an obvious role in the evolutionary success of any species. The horse has evolved as a nonruminant herbivore, taking advantage of forages as its primary source of nutrients and energy. In so doing, it has adapted to a diet consisting of feeds with a relatively low nutrient and energy content. For example, most grasses that would have been a part of a feral horse's diet would probably have less than 10% crude protein on a dry matter basis. Taken further, it could be said that the horse is adapted to a relatively low quality diet which it then eats in sufficient quantity to meet its nutrient and energy needs. How would a rapidly growing young horse possibly survive or prosper in such an environment?

If we assume that the recent ancestors of most modern horses evolved on the grasslands of North America, they were adapted to a temperate dry savannah environment. They were seasonally polyestrous, fitting their reproductive cycle with the climatic and nutritional environments in which they lived. The very end of gestation would correspond with the growth of forages in the spring, supplying the dams with the energy and nutrients to support the rapid late development of the fetus and prepare for early lactation. If energy and nutrients were lacking, the mare would sacrifice her body condition first with the likely implication that she would not be bred back for the following year, an appropriate safeguard for her own survival for when nutrients would be available to support another pregnancy. The early growth of the newborn foal is supported by its diet of nearly 100% milk, but it quickly begins to sample forages and hence begin the development of the bacterial microflora that will enable it to derive energy from structural carbohydrates in the grasses that surround it. Over the next 6 months, the growing foal makes a gradual change from milk to forage, while maintaining a relatively rapid and constant rate of growth. While it is unlikely that horses weaned themselves by 6 months of age, it is likely that by 6 months the majority of the young horse's diet consists of grass. The fall flush of energy and nutrients in the grass further help to maintain growth, supply for adipose stores and a winter coat for the coming harsh winter. The rapid maturation of size in the horse during the first spring and summer is an advantage when the cold and nutrient poor winter environment sets in. The larger body size means less surface area for the dissipation of heat and generally a lower energy requirement on a weight basis. During these winter months most young horses would not have grown much, utilizing energy and nutrients for thermoregulation and maintenance. However, with the coming spring and the energy and nutrient flush in the grasses, horses would undergo a period of compensatory growth, again pushing to reach mature body size and the survival advantages that large size provides. This cycle of harvesting forages in the spring, summer, and fall to allow for body growth and winter energy stores would then continue for the next 5 to 7 years, until mature size was reached. It is beyond the scope of this chapter to consider all the implications of taking the horse that has adapted to the environment and life described here, and placing it in the variety of very different environments that horse owners do today.

horse to remain sound. Research has demonstrated dyschondroplasia, one form of skeletal abnormality, in horses fed dietary energy as low as 129% of NRC (1989) recommendations (Savage et al 1993). In this same study, there was also a group fed 126% of NRC (1989) recommendations for crude protein, and a control group that was fed 100% of both dietary energy and protein. The rate of growth and presence of dyschondroplasia was only significantly higher in those horses fed 129% of the dietary energy requirement. Yet there are certainly horses that are fed this much energy or more that do not develop lesions. It is therefore very important to have a basic understanding of causation in order to appropriately evaluate the role nutrition potentially plays in increasing or reducing the risk of skeletal abnormalities as well as in supporting optimal growth (see Box 12.3).

Compensatory growth

Compensatory or catch-up growth is a period of rapid growth that a young horse goes through after a period where its rate of growth has decreased significantly below genetic potential. The decrease and subsequent increase can be caused by a number of different factors, but generally these factors result in a change in the partitioning of energy and nutrients for growth. Examples might include ambient temperature, weaning or other psychological stress, and decreased availability of dietary energy. Energy is likely to be the first limiting component of the diet with respect to growth rate. It is important to re-emphasize here that growth is not just affected by the diet. There is instead the classic interaction between genetics and the environment over the lifetime of the horse. If energy is the first limiting component of the diet, it only plays this role until it is provided in an amount that results in another component of the diet becoming limiting. Another way of expressing this in terms of the requirements of the growing horse would be to examine ratios of nutrients like protein or calcium with dietary energy. However, dietary energy below that required will result in the growth rate dropping below the genetic potential. It has been hypothesized that it is these changes in energy availability that cause most of the short term deviations in equine growth patterns (Staniar et al 2004b).

Most mammals, including the horse, will undergo a period of compensatory growth when energy becomes available after a period of energy depravation (Gafni & Baron 2000, Staniar et al 2004b). This ability to undergo compensatory growth will decrease with age. As an example, a weanling that has dietary energy restriction during the winter will exhibit a decreased growth rate, but will then exhibit a significant compensatory growth rate in the following spring if energy and nutrients are no longer limiting. However, dietary restriction over a longer period (e.g. a year or more) may limit attainment of genetic potential for mature size because the ability to undergo compensatory growth is no longer sufficient. Understanding what components of a growing horse's environment can cause short term changes in the rate of growth provides a tool to those raising the horse to more precisely control growth at different ages and under different conditions.

Figures 12.1 and 12.2 offer a useful example of the fluctuations in growth of body weight and withers height in Thoroughbred horses born at different times of year. There are numerous important facts that are illustrated by these figures, but in essence, those raising young horses can look at these as indicators of opportunities to adjust nutrition to cause beneficial changes in the pattern of growth. This will

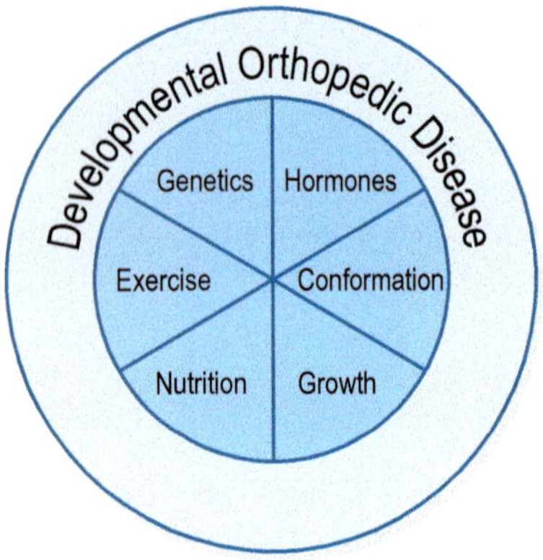

Figure 12.4 DOD is often discussed as a multifactorial disease, with factors such as nutrition, genetics, and exercise interacting with one another to cause the disease. The pie chart seen here might be taken as a rudimentary illustration of this.

> **Box 12.3 A Layman's Description of Sufficient Causation**
>
> While the following discussion could be applied to understanding the causes of any outcome, here we will focus on developmental orthopedic disease (DOD) due to its importance to the growing horse. DOD is often discussed as a multifactorial disease, with factors such as nutrition, genetics, and exercise interacting with one another to cause the disease. The pie chart shown in Fig. 12.4 might be taken as a rudimentary illustration of this.
>
> In his book on epidemiology (Rothman 2002), Dr. Rothman discusses causal components and mechanisms. Examples of causal components in this example would be each of the pie pieces in Fig. 12.5. A causal mechanism is the combination of components that are sufficient to result in the outcome, in this case DOD. The causal mechanism is the complete pie or in this case some combination of genetics, exercise, nutrition, growth, conformation, and hormones that will result in DOD occurring. Basic take home messages? (1) There are likely a number of different causal mechanisms made up of various combinations of causal components that will result in a particular outcome. (2) No known causal component by itself defines a causal mechanism. Therefore it is unlikely that nutrition, genetics, or exercise by themselves are sufficient to cause DOD. (3) By modifying individual causal components, such as nutrition, the risk of the causal mechanism being complete or sufficient can be raised or lowered. Therefore, changes in nutrition can increase or decrease the risk of DOD, but never prevent it completely. The reason it can never prevent DOD completely is because there are likely causal mechanisms that do not include nutrition.

be commented on further in a moment, but first a few comments about the figures. Depending on the metric of growth that is used, the pattern of growth can be very different. For example it is clear that there is a more rapid decline in the rate of growth for withers height than body weight. Having said this, there are also characteristics of these growth curves that are similar. The influence of nutrient and energy supply during the first year of life has a similar impact on the rate of gain for both measures. The foals born in January have a more erratic pattern of growth than those born in April and May. But the question remains as to what is the most beneficial or optimal pattern of growth. Most would suggest that

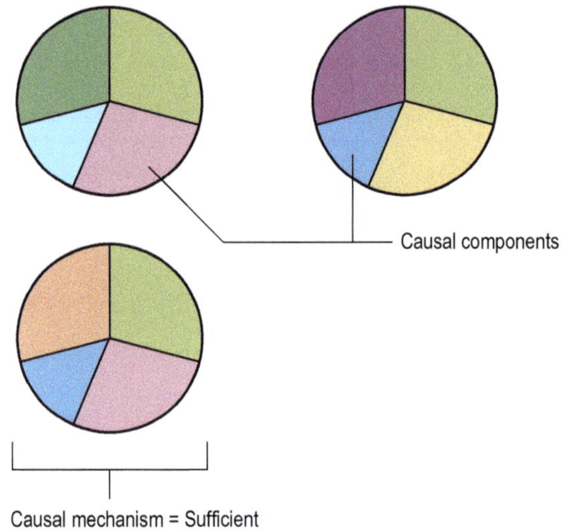

Figure 12.5 Examples of causal components in this example would be each of the pie pieces.

the less erratic pattern of the April or May born foal may be better to reduce the risk of developmental orthopedic disease, but the scientific evidence supporting this theory is still lacking. If a more moderate pattern of growth is beneficial, Figs 12.1 and 12.2 could be used to develop a proactive feeding program that may be able to diminish; to a certain degree, the fluctuations seen in the January-born foals. It remains to be shown that this is truly beneficial to the ultimate health and performance of the mature horse.

A common recommendation for feeding the growing horse is to provide energy and nutrients in manner that allows for a moderate and consistent rate of growth. Moderate and consistent growth may be viewed as something approaching the pattern of average daily gain predicted by the NRC (2007) (Fig. 12.1A). It is unlikely that an absolutely smooth growth pattern will be achieved, nor should it be interpreted that an absolutely smooth growth curve is the best. Instead, the naturally occurring increases and decreases in the rate of growth can be influenced by alterations in dietary energy and nutrient supply.

A final thought on dietary energy and its relationship with growth is that it can be seen as analogous to fuel supply and speed in a car. When more fuel (energy from the diet) is available speed (growth) will increase up to a maximum, when less is available speed (growth) will decrease. But there is no brake on growth, and maximum growth like maximum speed may not be optimal. For those that might be thinking that this suggests that a pony could be fed to become a horse, there are two additional points to remember: (1) by definition a maximum means there is a limit to the rate at which growth can occur, and (2) growth rate does not influence the genetically pre-determined mature size.

> **Key Points – Energy**
>
> - Energy requirements of the growing horse are primarily dependent on age, body weight, and rate of growth
> - An oversupply of other nutrients cannot overcome a limited energy supply
> - If energy is not limiting, the supply of other nutrients need to be sufficient to meet the requirements of the rate of growth

supported by the energy supply or growth abnormalities are likely to occur
- The maximum growth rate may not be the optimal growth rate, as the optimum integrates the objectives of athletic performance, longevity, and soundness, while the maximum is simply the most rapid rate of gain

Protein requirements

Dietary proteins, and more specifically the amino acids that are the building blocks of proteins, are critical nutrients for the growing horse. Proteins are central to structural molecules such as collagen, but they are also key components of the enzymes required for the development of various tissues and in addition they facilitate metabolism. Dietary crude protein (CP) concentrations of 9 to 20% on a dry matter basis have been investigated for their appropriateness to support growth in the horse (Jordon et al 1972, Ott et al 1979, Schryver et al 1987). A rudimentary analysis of the results from these past studies suggests that a CP intake within the range of 13 to 17% will maintain the highest growth rates in foals between 4 and 6 months of age, from a number of different breeds.

Protein quality/amino acid composition

In the 20 to 30 years since these studies were conducted there have been a number of studies investigating what is the most appropriate dietary amino acid composition for growth. A useful starting point could be the amino acid composition of equine muscle or mare's milk (Bryden 1991). A logical approach to decreasing the total amount of CP needed in the diet would be through enhancement in protein quality, achieved by simply improving protein digestibility and amino acid composition to more closely match that of muscle or milk. Protein quality is defined by the similarity between the composition of amino acids required for maintenance and growth and the composition of dietary amino acids. Protein quality may be improved by supplementation with amino acids that are limiting to protein synthesis. By more closely matching the amino acid composition needed for growth, it is possible to make more efficient use of all amino acids and therefore protein in the diet. Therefore if quality is improved the total quantity of protein can often be decreased. This could be a benefit both from an economic standpoint, as protein tends to be one of the more expensive ingredients in the diet, and an environmental standpoint, as efficient use of protein will lead to less nitrogen in feces and urine.

Lysine was identified as the first limiting amino acid when growing horses were fed a diet of Bermuda grass and alfalfa hay (Breuer et al 1971) as well as several other common diets (Potter et al 1975, Ott et al 1981). Threonine was found to be the second limiting amino acid in horses consuming a corn plus oats concentrate and Bermuda grass hay (Graham et al 1994). Dietary fortification with the free forms of lysine and threonine will influence the rate of growth in horses, supporting more rapid growth when energy is not limiting (Staniar et al 2001). In the study by Staniar et al (2001), a group of Thoroughbreds fed a concentrate containing 9% CP fortified with 0.6% lysine and 0.4% threonine grew more rapidly during the spring than a group fed a 14% CP concentrate. Care should be taken that all other nutrients are available in sufficient quantity when energy and protein are no longer limiting. The rapid skeletal growth of a foal on a high energy and high quality protein diet may still be compromised if minerals and vitamins are not at the concentrations required to support the increased rate of growth.

There is a growing body of evidence that particular amino acids play a role in metabolic regulation (Poso & Hyyppä 1999, Urschel et al 2010). This highlights the importance of considering what impact amino acid supplementation may have on the regulation of glucose, insulin, and other hormones and metabolites involved in growth.

Common ingredients used to improve the protein quality of diets for the growing horse include milk proteins, soybean meal, and alfalfa meal (Pugh & Williams 1992). Again this is because the amino acid composition of these ingredients is similar to that required for growth. There are high lysine corn varieties available that due to their improved amino acid composition may be useful in decreasing the total dietary crude protein in growing horse diets, although no research has examined this potential option in equine diets (Azevedo & Arruda 2010). Lowering the crude protein content of the diet while still meeting the amino acid requirements of the growing animal has potential benefits that include decreased metabolic processing of excess nitrogen, decreased nitrogen excretion into the environment, and potential cost savings as protein is often one of the more expensive components of the diet. Examples of ingredients that generally have a lower quality dietary protein include most cereal grains and forages. Another simple and straightforward technique to improve the bioavailability of dietary protein is to provide more frequent and smaller meals (NRC 2007). This approach more closely mimics the natural feeding behavior of the horse, allowing for a more constant low flow/supply of proteins and amino acids to be digested and absorbed predominantly in the small intestine.

Amino acids and bone quality

There is some evidence that alteration in the dietary supply of specific amino acids may enable moderation of growth rate (Ott et al 1979, Graham et al 1994). Whether such modifications can also have an impact on the quality of growth, particularly on muscle, bone and cartilage is unknown. Approximately 30% of bone is made up of organic compounds; of which 90 to 95% are collagen and the majority of the rest are other protein-based molecules, with the protein makeup of cartilage being similar. Both bone and cartilage have optimized levels of stiffness and flexibility to maximize strength and usability. Collagen in bone and cartilage and proteoglycans in cartilage are key compounds that contribute to the flexibility component, while the inorganic mineral matrix provides much of the stiffness in bone. Major amino acids in collagen molecules include glycine, proline, and hydroxyproline. Studies in rabbits have shown that intra-articular injection of these amino acids along with other nutrients may enhance cartilage healing (Park et al 2007). This leads to the concept that a particular dietary amino acid composition may be more beneficial to the quality of cartilage and bone than another. If skeletal quality is defined as the ability of cartilage and bone to function under the stresses of athletic performance, we may be able to improve that quality through the focused dietary supply of amino acids that influence bone and cartilage function. For example, during periods of rapid growth it may be appropriate to fortify a diet with glycine, proline, and hydroxyproline to better support collagen formation in the rapidly developing skeleton. However, there is currently no research to support this hypothesis.

Key Points – Protein

- In general, common feed sources for horses that contain 13 to 17% CP on a dry matter basis fit within a broad optimal range for growth
- Providing a dietary amino acid composition that is closer to that required for optimal growth, thereby improving protein quality, has the potential to decrease the total amount for protein needed by the growing horse

Mineral and vitamin requirements

Energy and protein are generally the first two limiting dietary components with respect to supporting growth, but this does not diminish the importance of other nutrients. It is worth noting that the requirements for most of these other nutrients are usually estimated according to some calculation of average daily gain (NRC 2007). Simply put, the nutrient requirements for the more rapidly growing foal are likely to be higher than those for a similarly aged slowly growing counterpart (Schryver et al 1974). The appropriate intake of minerals and vitamins is therefore critical for optimal growth and development. The use of the word appropriate may be somewhat misleading, as it hides the complexity of excesses, deficiencies, and interactions. Classic examples that are often highlighted in the growing horse include the Ca:P and Cu:Zn dietary ratios, which we believe should be balanced to allow for optimal skeletal development. The complexity lies in the fact that these mineral interact with one another in the gastrointestinal tract, and through this interaction can impact each other's absorption. Hence, a diet that provides the requirement of Ca, but has more P than Ca may result in a Ca deficiency due to the excess phosphorus negatively impacting Ca absorption. The concentrations of these should be tailored to the rate and stage of growth. The nutrients highlighted as being key for the growing horse include minerals important to skeletal development, such as Ca, P, Mg, Cu, Zn, Mn, and Si, as well as the fat-soluble vitamins, A, D, and E.

In brief, minerals can act as structural components of bone or cartilage extracellular matrix or as functional components of the enzymes that help to build or breakdown skeletal tissues. Most of the minerals listed are important structural components of bone or cartilage. Bones store over 99% of Ca, 80% of P, 62% of Mg that is present in the horse's body (Grace et al 1999). Calcium, P, and Mg make up between 45 to 60% of bone matrix while Cu and Zn play important roles in collagen and proteoglycan synthesis in both cartilage and bone. In the fetus during gestation, over 80% of the Mg and 90% of the Ca and P that make up the total present at birth are deposited between the 8th and 11th month of gestation (Coenen 2001). These facts highlight the importance of a dietary supply of these minerals from conception through two years of life due to the sheer volume of skeletal development occurring.

Due to their important roles in the development of skeletal tissues, mineral requirements have been the focus of a significant amount of equine related research (Knight et al 1985, Hurtig et al 1993, O'Connor et al 2008). A problem has been that defining mineral requirements for the growing horse is fraught with pitfalls due to the complex nature of growth and the challenge of designing studies capable of examining individual minerals. Having said this, there are some broad concepts that can be identified. The balance of Ca and P should be a priority (Hintz 1996). Diets with more P than Ca can induce a Ca deficiency (Schryver et al 1971). Such a diet is possible with a high ratio of grain to forage. On the other hand, foals fed primarily forages may have an insufficient P intake. Monitoring the dietary concentrations of these minerals is a straightforward and useful recommendation for those feeding growing horses.

Minerals like Cu, Zn, Mn, and Si make up smaller portions of bone and cartilage, but also play important functional roles in facilitating the dynamic nature of skeletal tissue. Copper requirements have an interesting recent history of debate within the equine nutrition field (see NRC 2007). Copper is a critical cofactor for the lysyl oxidase enzyme that aids in the crosslinking of collagen with elastin in connective tissues such as bone and cartilage (Rucker et al 1998). Through this relationship, one can understand why dietary Cu requirements for the growing horse have received considerable attention. This author concludes from these studies that the dam should receive 0.25 mg Cu/kg body weight in months 9, 10 and 11 of gestation to support the development of liver copper stores in the fetus. It is thought that these Cu stores will help to reduce the risk of skeletal abnormalities (van Weeren et al 2003). This same dietary concentration is recommended for the lactating mare and growing horse (NRC 2007). Zinc's role in skeletal development is both as a component of enzymes involved in skeletal metabolism and also as an antagonist of copper absorption or action. Manganese is required for the formation of chondroitin sulfate, and hence critical for cartilage formation, but there is little evidence to suggest that the current requirements need to be increased, although it is worth noting that there has been limited work conducted examining Mn requirements in growing horses. Silicon is another mineral important to both cartilage and bone development. To date, the data from research into different dietary sources of silicon and its impact on dependent varaiables such as radiographic aluminum equivalents associated with bone mineral density remains equivocal (Frey et al 1992, Nielsen et al 1993). Additional studies on Si have focused on the availability of different sources for absorption (O'Connor et al 2008, Turner et al 2008). While most horses are likely to meet their requirements for Si, there is some thought that skeletal development may be improved at higher intakes but currently there are no data to support this contention. Future research should focus on various sources of Si and the impact of supplemental Si on measures of skeletal health.

Minerals are not the only nutrients important to skeletal development. Vitamins also play an important role in the active metabolism of the growing foal. Probably the most effective way of assuring that both mare and foal are receiving adequate vitamins is to provide them with access to appropriate amounts of good quality fresh forages. However, once cut and preserved, forages begin to lose much of their vitamin content (Kellems & Church, 2010). Care needs to be taken to avoid over as well as under supplementation as described in the paragraphs below.

Vitamin A is an example of where over-supplementation has been suggested to have negative consequences to the growing horse (Kienzle 2005). This evaluation was based on the onset of general unthriftiness, ataxia, and hyperextension of various joints in growing foals provided an intoxication dose of 35 000 IU vitamin A/kg body weight (Donoghue et al 1981). The upper safe limit for dietary vitamin A is listed as 16 000 IU/kg dry matter but is based on a very limited amount of research (NRC 2007). Data collected from pigs and cattle indicates that most livestock show no signs of toxicity when fed dietary concentrations of vitamin A as high as 220 000 IU/kg dry matter (Anderson et al 1966). So while very high concentrations of vitamin A may be detrimental, deficiency is unlikely as long as growing horses and their dams have sufficient access to fresh forages (Griewe-Crandell et al 1995). However, when fresh forages are not available, dietary vitamin A may fall below the concentrations required to maintain proper immune and reproductive function and supplementation is necessary (Griewe-Crandell et al 1995). An example would be the young racehorse in training, being kept at the track and fed a diet consisting mainly of preserved forages and oats. In this case there may be the potential for an increased risk of problems such as respiratory infection, associated with vitamin A's role in the immune system. A simple solution in this case would be to either provide a vitamin supplement with the oats or feed a formulated concentrate that contains added vitamin A in place of the oats. There are a number of forms of vitamin A available, but research has demonstrated differences in the ability of some of these forms (retinyl palmitate and water soluble β-carotene), to replenish vitamin A status in depleted mares (Greiwe-Crandell et al 1997) (see Chapter 9).

Vitamin D is a nutrient that may be worth further investigation as its role in skeletal metabolism in the horse remains unclear. It is of particular interest that the available data indicates that the horse is significantly different from other mammalian species in regard to vitamin D metabolism (Breidenbach et al 1998). The current requirements for vitamin D are based mainly on a study with a limited number of ponies (El Shorafa et al 1979). This study did indicate that growing ponies kept out of the sunlight and fed a vitamin D deficient diet had a decrease in the quality of skeletal development when compared to those kept outside or supplemented. Recent research in human skeletal development highlights the integrated role of vitamin D with some of the metabolic signals for growth such as growth hormone and insulin-like growth factor-I (Fernandez-Cancio et al 2009). While vitamin D may be worth another look from a research perspective, it is unlikely that most growing horses maintained outside with access to fresh forages will be deficient. The recommended intakes for vitamin D for growing horses range from 500 to 800 IU/kg of air dry material (Kienzle 2005, NRC 2007). The presumed safe upper limit has been given as 44 IU/kg BW/day (NRC 1987).

For specific requirements, those formulating diets should refer to the relevant chapters in this book as well as to publications such as the *Nutrient Requirements of the Horse* (NRC 2007) and other similar references. Such publications can provide an excellent starting point for formulating diets, but it is the responsibility of the person who sees the growing horse daily to adjust the components of the diet to achieve the chosen end objective for an individual animal. No table or equation can be written to account for every scenario.

While the dietary mineral and vitamin requirements of the growing horse are an obvious place to start in formulating an optimal diet, the concentrations in various feedstuffs is variable. Here we have focused on minerals and vitamins that are centered on skeletal development, but other nutrients like iodine should also be considered due to their fundamental role in the basic health and physiology. It is imperative that all components of the diet are analyzed to determine if a deficiency or excess is a concern. For the farm manager or veterinarian that is managing the day to day nutrition of growing horses, it may make more sense to monitor the seasonal ranges in the nutrient make up of diet ingredients. By using the lower end of the range, deficiency can be avoided, and the upper limits will also provide some guidance as to when supplementation can be reduced. As an example, the crude protein content of grass forages in a pasture may range from a low of 10% to a high of 25% on a dry matter basis, depending on the ambient growing environment. At the low end of this range, a 9-month-old growing horse (expected mature weight of 550 kg) consuming approximately 2.5% of their bodyweight may not be ingesting the required crude protein for their expected rate of gain. In this case, supplementation with a higher protein preserved forage, or with a concentrate may be appropriate. For the horse owner with a background in economics, a technique akin to sensitivity analysis may be a way to optimize rations to best handle the normal fluctuations in nutrients (Kronfeld 2001).

Key Points – Minerals and vitamins

- Mineral and vitamin requirements will change according to the rate of growth. If dietary energy and protein are increased to support a more rapid rate of gain, minerals and vitamins should also be increased
- During the first two years of growth, high priority should be given to nutritional support of skeletal development
- Interactions between nutrients and physiologic regulation mean that supplying the appropriate amounts of minerals and vitamins should not be approached with a "more is better" strategy. Careful attention should be paid to well-known ratios, such as Ca:P and Cu:Zn
- When possible, the incorporation of fresh forages into the growing horse's diet will help to meet many of the mineral and particularly vitamin requirements. Having said this, there are numerous scenarios where this is not possible and supplementation is required

Practical application

A practical approach to feeding the growing horse should take into account the fact that there are numerous changes occurring over a relatively short period of time. Many references can be found that point to the concept that aging occurs most rapidly when an animal is youngest (Minot 1908). To be practical, some middle ground needs to be found between changing the diet on a daily basis, and feeding the same diet throughout the whole growth period. This chapter divides growth into a number of discrete time periods. These were chosen based on factors such as changing growth patterns, diet and seasonal changes, as well as the influence of weaning, and training. The period from birth to 3 months represents when milk is likely to make up a large portion of the foal's diet. The season is likely to be spring, with fresh forage beginning to become available. The period from 4 to 6 months represents a period of time when milk intake has decreased significantly with a concurrent increase in forage and grain intake. In many cases, non-natural, weaning occurs between 4 to 8 months of age, so the period from 6 to 12 months of age represents the weanling phase when milk is no longer part of the diet. The stress of weaning also needs to be considered as intake may decrease in the early post-weaning period. This can compound with a change in the seasons, resulting in a significant decrease in growth rate. Finally, the yearling and 2-year-old are discussed. Growth has slowed considerably after 1 year of age, but is still progressing at a rate that means nutrition can significantly impact the quality of that growth. During these later stages, attention begins to shift from the skeletal system to overall athletic development. Consider these phases as critical periods within which the diet of the growing horse can be re-evaluated to take into account significant changes in the horse and its environment. Table 12-2 provides guidelines for nutrient intake by growing horses, while Table 12-3 describes example feeding strategies for achievement of these nutritional goals.

Birth to 3 months

At birth, the normal growing horse is about 10% of its eventual mature body weight, and grows to approximately 30% of its mature weight by 3 months of age. During this period the young foal is therefore growing fairly rapidly (Figs 12.1 and 12.2) and relies mainly on the mare's milk as a dietary source of energy and nutrients. As noted above, studies of equine growth indicate that the most rapid period of growth in body size occurs either in the days immediately before or after parturition, highlighting the importance of nutrition during this period (Staniar et al 2004b). The manager's ability to impact the nutrition provided to the foal is directed through feeding the broodmare to support milk production. The energy and nutrient requirements of the mare during this early stage of lactation are high. While the foal relies mainly on milk during this early period of growth, foals start to sample all the other feedstuffs available to them almost immediately after being born (Crowell-Davis 2008).

One of the earliest nutritional transitions for the foal occurs at birth. The newborn foal moves from an environment where the placenta effectively transports energy and nutrients from the mare to the "passive" fetus, to an environment in which the foal needs to actively search out the mare's udder and suckle. Foals may consume as much as 15 and 25% of their bodyweight in milk per day within the first week following parturition (Ousey et al 1996). The first milk that a foal will receive from their dam is colostrum. Immediately following birth, the foal should have an intake of colostrum sufficient to ensure adequate passive transfer of immunity and to supply energy and nutrients for maintenance, activity, and continued growth. This initial intake of colostrum is dependent on the foal standing, finding the mare's udder and successfully suckling, or the colostrum being provided to the foal via a bottle or nasogastric tube. Generally the quality of colostrum is defined by the concentration of immunoglobulins present. An effective test, based on its accuracy and ease of use, is the estimation of dissolved solids, in the available colostrum, using a refractometer (Cash 1999). Intake of immunoglobulins from colostrum

Table 12-2 Recommended Daily Nutrient Intakes[a] for Growing Horses (Expected Mature Weight of 550 kg) at 3, 6, 9 and 12 Months of Age

	3 months	6 months	9 months	12 months	24 months[b]
Estimated weight (kg)	156	237	302	353	472
Estimated average daily gain (kg/day)	1.0	0.79	0.63	0.50	0.20
Digestible energy (Mcal/day)	13	17.1	19.5	20.7	27.3
Crude protein (g/day)	731	744	833	930	977
Lysine (g/day)	31	32	36	40	42
Calcium (g/day)	43	42	42	41	40
Phosphorus (g/day)	24	24	23	23	22
Copper (mg/day)	39	59	76	88	118
Iron (mg/day)	156	238	302	353	472
Zinc (mg/day)	125	190	242	283	378
Iodine (mg/day)	1.1	1.7	2.1	2.5	3.3
Selenium (mg/day)	0.31	0.47	0.60	0.71	0.94
Vitamin A (IU/day)	7021	10686	13594	15900	21246
Vitamin E (IU/day)	312	475	604	707	944

[a]Source: NRC (2007): Growing horse at designated ages.
[b]Source: NRC (2007): Growing horse at 24 months of age with a moderate work load.

Table 12-3 Example Daily Rations for Growing Horses (Expected Mature Weight of 550 kg) at 3, 6, 9 and 12 Months of Age. Ration Components are Expressed in the Table on an as Fed Basis

	3 months	6 months	9 months	12 months	24 months[a]
Bodyweight (kg)	156	237	302	353	472
Average daily gain (kg/day)	1.0	0.79	0.63	0.50	0.20
Forages[b, c, d]					
Grass pasture (cool season, vegetative)	6 kg		6 kg		
Grass pasture (mixed mostly grass, mid-maturity)		4.5 kg			
Grass hay (cool season, mid-maturity)	1 kg	1.5 kg	3.5 kg	5 kg	8 kg
Concentrates					
Growth formula[e]	1.75 kg	3.5 kg	4 kg	4.5 kg	
Training formula[f]					5 kg
Milk[g]	13 kg	0	0	0	0

[a]Nutrient and energy requirements for 24 month old horse based on moderate exercise training.
[b, c, d]Forage choice will depend on availability (values are on a 100% dry matter basis). Grass pasture (vegetative); 20% DM, 2.4 Mcal/kg, 26% CP, 0.92% lysine, 0.56% Ca, 0.44% P, 10 mg/kg Cu, 36 mg/kg Zn. Grass pasture (mid-maturity); 47% DM, 2.6 Mcal/kg, 18% CP, 0.50% lysine 0.50% lysine, 0.60 Ca, 0.33 P, 8.8 mg/kg Cu, 34 mg/kg Zn. Grass hay (mid maturity); 84% DM, 2.2 Mcal/kg, 13% CP, 0.46% lysine, 0.66% Ca, 0.29% P, 9.0 mg/kg Cu, 25 mg/kg Zn.
[e]Growth formula concentrate (values are on a 100% dry matter basis): 90% DM, 3.0 Mcal/kg, 15% CP, 0.85% lysine, 0.70% Ca, 0.70% P, 75 mg/kg Cu, 200 mg/kg Zn, 12 000 IU/kg vitamin A, 300 IU/kg vitamin E.
[f]Training formula concentrate (values are on a 100% dry matter basis): 90% DM, 3.0 Mcal/kg, 12% CP, 0.70% lysine, 0.60% Ca, 0.50% P, 50 mg/kg Cu, 150 mg/kg Zn, 12 000 IU/kg vitamin A, 300 IU/kg vitamin E.
[g]Milk (values are on an as fed basis): 11% DM, 0.42 Mcal/kg, 17 g/kg CP, 3.3 g/kg lysine, 0.88 g/kg Ca. 0.55 g/kg P.

should occur between 1 to 6 hours following parturition with an emphasis on the earlier end of this range. It is difficult to measure the exact volume that a foal has consumed, but a newborn foal from a 500 to 600 kg dam should probably consume between 1 and 2 liters of colostrum in these 6 hours following birth.

Monitoring suckling behavior early can be helpful in evaluating the general health and nutrition of a newborn foal. Generally, once a foal has found the mare's udder and successfully suckled the first time, they will suckle in regular short bouts. The frequency of suckling will generally decrease as the foal gets older. At one day old the foal may suckle up to 10 times per hour with this rate decreasing to between 1.5 to 2 times per hour at 2 to 3 months of age (Smith-Funk & Crowell-Davis 1992). Suckling bouts should last for approximately 1 minute (NRC 2007). Usually foals will rest or play between these suckling bouts. If the foal is not receiving sufficient milk they may continue to try to suckle without taking a rest or suckle more frequently. Examination of the mare's udder and teats can provide another indication if the foal is drinking the available milk. If the mare continues to drip milk between suckling bouts, it is possible that the foal is not drinking sufficiently – however it is hard to know exactly how much milk a foal is getting during each suckling bout simply based on bout frequency and length (Cameron et al 1999). Attention to general suckling behavior as well as the attitude and condition of the foal for the first few weeks may be the best indicators of whether the foal is receiving adequate nutrients and energy (see also Chapter 40).

Just before the foal is born, its gastrointestinal tract is effectively free of microbes, but evidence indicates that there is relatively rapid population of the gut following birth (Doreau et al 1986). This is an expanding area of investigation, as the role of the gastrointestinal microbial population in the young foal is still not well understood. Yet, it is well documented that the symbiotic relationship between the horse and the microbes throughout its gastrointestinal tract is important to health and performance (Julliand 1992). It is common that young foals will be seen eating their dam's or less frequently, other horses' fecal material (coprophagy), and the process may serve to aid in populating the foal's gastrointestinal tract with microbes from their dam. Generally, foals less than 2 months of age will eat fecal material once every 4 to 9 hours (Crowell-Davis & Houpt 1985, Crowell-Davis & Caudle 1989). While it is clear that developing a microbial population in the gastrointestinal tract is important, and these microbes can come from a number of sources in the foal's environment, there are still not any clear recommendations on how this process could be improved or modified to improve the health of the foal. In fact recent research emphasizes caution towards the use of probiotics in foals (Weese & Rousseau 2005). However, overall it would seem that attention to microbial development in the gastrointestinal tract of the growing foal warrants further research. As in the adult, the microbiota ecosystem in the foal's hindgut will play an important role in the foal's ability to digest certain feedstuffs, absorb energy in the form of volatile fatty acids, and maintain their metabolic health.

A final component to consider in the newborn foal is its thermoregulatory capabilities depending on the ambient environment into which it is born. There is relatively limited work studying the impact of ambient temperature on the early nutrient and energy requirements of the newborn foal. Some of that which has been done indicates an average lower critical temperature of the thermoneutral zone of approximately 20°C (Ousey et al 1992). This indicates that foals entering an environment below this temperature are likely to expend additional energy above the maintenance requirements to thermoregulate. While the young foal is certainly capable of this thermoregulatory activity, energy used in this manner will not be available for growth. This is probably part of the reason that foals born in cold environments exhibit slower rates of early growth when compared to those born in warmer temperatures. A more consistent pattern of growth may therefore be obtained during this early period of growth if foals that are born during the late winter are maintained at ambient temperatures closer to their thermoneutral zone and their dams are provided sufficient dietary energy and nutrients to support early lactation.

Months 4 to 6

By 4 months of age, the foal may be approximately 35% of its mature size and will mature to ~45% by 6 months of age. During this period both the growth rate of the foal and the milk production of the mare have declined. Concurrently, the foal's intake of other feedstuffs such as forage and concentrates has increased. Because of this transition, the capability of those feeding to directly influence the nutrition of the growing horse is increased. It is during this period that every effort should be made to begin to introduce the foal to feedstuffs that will be a part of its diet after weaning. It is also during this period when creep feeding can help to increase growth rate and potentially lessen the decrease in growth rate often associated with weaning (Pugh and Williams, 1992) (see Box 12.4).

Prior to weaning it is beneficial to give foals some access to either a creep feed or the concentrate that they will be receiving after weaning. This access will firstly provide their gastrointestinal tract and the microbes therein an opportunity to adapt to the new diet. Secondly it offers a secondary source of dietary energy at a time when energy availability from the mare's milk is decreasing. An investigation using Thoroughbred foals demonstrated greater average daily gains in foals offered access to creep feeds prior to weaning (Coleman et al 1999). The nutritional composition of the creep feed that is offered is dependent on the other components of the foal's diet and the age of the foal. There is evidence that the composition of the diet of foals prior to and during weaning may have an influence on behavior and level of stress (Nicol et al 2005). The data from this study provides subtle indications that horses that were fed a concentrate with fat and fiber as opposed to sugar and starch as the main sources of dietary energy were less distressed during periods such as weaning.

Weanlings

Weaning is both a nutritional and psychological transition for the growing horse. Weaning can occur at a range of different ages and for a host of different reasons, but for the

Box 12.4 Creep Feeding

Creep feed is usually a concentrate that is offered to young animals while they are not yet weaned. The term creep refers to the enclosure where the feed is placed so that only the young animal and not the mother has access to the feed. Practices for creep feeding growing horses range from offering none to beginning at 2 to 4 weeks of age (Pugh & Schumacher 1993). One objective of offering a creep feed is to make up for any nutrient or energy deficiencies due to decreasing milk quantity or quality, insufficient access to the dam's daily grain ration, or poor forage quantity or quality. A second objective is to allow for consistent optimal growth in the face of a changing nutrient environment. Creep feeds can range from milk replacer pellets to a grain mix and combinations of both depending on the age of the foal. Generally, the milk replacer pellets will be approximately 18 to 20% crude protein, and the grain mix fed to foals during months 1–3 will be 16 to 18% crude protein. The protein in these early feeds should be from ingredients known to have high quality protein, such as whey or soybeans. These are generally highly digestible and provide an amino acid composition that is most appropriate for growth. For the foals that are 4–6 months of age, dietary protein in the creep feed may decrease to 14%. A very common recommendation for horses likely to have a mature weight between 500 and 600 kg is to feed 1 pound of creep feed per day to a growing horse for each month of age.

Development of the microbial ecosystem in the cecum and colon of the growing horse is an area of active research (Doreau et al 1986, Philippeau et al 2011). This is an area of equine nutritional science that has not received significant attention, and yet holds numerous potential benefits for the growing horse. Creep feeding offers a unique opportunity for those managing horses to control the substrate supply to the growing horse's hindgut, and therefore have some control over the microbial development therein. Many experienced breeding farm managers will tell stories about feeding yogurt to young foals to help with gastrointestinal issues, but the research to support these practices and explain the mechanisms are lacking. There are a myriad of potential opportunities, of which just a few are listed here.

- Foal scours (diarrhea often see in the first month of life) are likely associated with early changes in the gastrointestinal tract as it adapts to milk, forage, and grain. Perhaps there is a way to more precisely guide this developmental process to reduce the risk of scours.
- Foals born in winter or very early spring conditions may have a very different exposure to microbes that populate the gut than those born in mid to late spring.
- Nutritional strategies incorporated into the creep feeding process that are aimed at optimizing the microbial development of the gut to handle the diet of the young horse after weaning may decrease nutritional problems associated with the weaning process.

Creep feeding aimed at development of a robust (robust refers to the ability of this population of microbes to handle changes in the day to day diet) microbial population in the young horse's gastrointestinal tract should certainly incorporate important nutritional substrates. These include a range of different carbohydrate and protein sources. In the carbohydrate fraction, the emphasis should be on medium and slowly fermentable sources, but a small fraction of rapidly fermentable is not to be completely avoided (everything in moderation). Protein is an important source of amino acids and nitrogen for microbes, and a good source should be included. Minerals and vitamins can be balanced as appropriate for the animals being raised. As a simple example one might mix 35% mid-maturity grass hay, 20% alfalfa hay, 10% beet pulp, 5% soybean hulls, 10% crimped oats, 5% soybean meal, 5% mineral and vitamin mix. This combination would be mixed with an attempt to maintain a fiber length of between ¾ to 1½ inches of the major fiber components.

purposes of this chapter we will assume this represents the time from 6 to 12 months of age. At the beginning of this period the foal may have reached nearly 50% of its mature weight. Generally, foals will reach ~65% of their mature weight at 12 months of age. Weaning represents both a nutritional and a psychological stress: nutritional because milk will no longer be a part of the diet and psychological because the foal is separated from its mother. Both of these factors need to be taken into consideration in feeding the growing horse during this period. One of the basic recommendations in feeding the growing horse is to avoid large fluctuations in growth rate. Weaning can be one period when the growth rate can decrease primarily due to the stresses mentioned above. Every effort should be made to maintain growth and decrease "stress" during this period, because a decrease in growth at this early stage in growth will inevitably be followed by a period of compensatory growth when the stressor(s) has gone and nutrients plus energy are available.

A common recommendation to reduce the risk of developmental orthopedic disease in growing horses is to avoid substantial changes in the rate of growth, yet separating growth rate and nutrition remains a difficult hurdle (Donabedian et al 2006). There are however some basic strategies that can be put in place around weaning to help minimize the impact on the rate of growth. Stress in many different forms will cause animals to reduce their dry matter intake. This reduction in intake is likely one of the main reasons that a foal's growth rate will drop around the time of weaning. Strategies to avoid this should address both the stress and the reduction in intake in order to be most effective.

First, prior to weaning, foals should be introduced to the concentrate and forages they will be offered as a weanling. By providing foals access to these diets at least one month prior to weaning, their gastrointestinal tracts and the microbial populations within them should have sufficient time to adapt to the new diet. Offering a concentrate will also help to support growth. Second, every effort should be made to wean foals on to the best quality forages available. This means avoiding weaning in midsummer or winter. However, it is not uncommon to wean in mid-summer, and if this is necessary, good highly digestible forage should be offered as well as a suitable concentrate to support the growth rate during this period.

Finally, it is likely that during this 6-month period the weanling will go through a winter and the spring that follows. The changes in the rates of growth around both of these events can be larger than that around weaning (Staniar et al 2004b). Every effort should be made to maintain as consistent a growth rate during this time, through appropriate supplementation during the winter and cutting back the dietary energy in the spring. It is also important to point out that it is unlikely that all fluctuations in growth can be removed, nor is it suggested that such a pattern of growth is optimal. It is likely that some seasonal fluctuation will always occur.

Key Points – Weanlings

- Weaning is a period of psychological and nutritional stress for the foal. This stress can impact feed intake and growth
- Weaning often occurs when the foal is being maintained in what is often a poor nutritional environment (mid summer or winter). This should be taken into account when formulating the weanling's diet
- To optimize nutrition for the weanling:
  - Introduce them prior to weaning to the concentrate they will be maintained on post weaning
  - Wean them onto or into the best nutritional environment possible. For a foal born in the spring, this is often the flush of pasture that occurs in the fall.
  - Use a weaning strategy that reduces psychological stress

Yearlings

Depending on the breed of horse, the term yearling can mean different things. For most, a yearling is a horse that is between 12 and 24 months old. However, Thoroughbreds are considered a yearling on 1 January following their birth date. For the purposes of this chapter a yearling will be a horse that is 365 days or 12 months old. Based on this, yearlings will start this period weighing ~65% of their mature body weight. As an 18-month-old long yearling they will have reached ~78% of their mature body weight. It is likely that yearlings will have been weaned 6 to 8 months prior to this time point, so they should be well adapted to their diet. The growth rate of a yearling has generally slowed to approximately one-third of what it was at birth, although there is still potential for that growth rate to increase significantly when energy and protein are readily available (Staniar et al 2001, 2004b) (Figs 12.1 and 12.2). Nutritional objectives for those raising yearlings should be to provide a diet that is formulated to support continued musculoskeletal development while also avoiding an exaggerated compensatory growth period. The pattern of average daily gain in Thoroughbreds over a period of two years is illustrated in Fig. 12.1. During the yearling year the horses go through more changes in the rate of growth than during the first 12 months. There is no clear scientific evidence that the changes in growth during this period have any negative impact on skeletal development. However, there is also no clear benefit to these fluctuations. Nutrition can be used as a tool to allow for more consistent growth during this period and potentially decrease the risk of abnormalities in skeletal development.

Yearlings should be fully adapted to a diet similar to that for an adult horse. Most of the dietary energy and nutrients they eat are being used for maintenance and any exercise due to the slow rate of growth at this point. The appropriate diet for the yearling should consist of a foundation of digestible forage supplemented with a concentrate. By supplying the yearling with good quality fresh forage or early or mid-maturity grass hay, they will be able to take full advantage of the energy from structural and nonstructural carbohydrates. The concentrate should include a quality source of protein, such as soybean meal, to support continued development of both bone and muscle. Especially when preserved forage is fed, additional vitamins and minerals are also likely needed to meet requirements.

Two-year-olds

The normally growing 2-year-old will have reached between 85 and 89% of their mature body weight, and at 36 months will have reached nearly 95% of their mature body weight. When does a horse stop growing? This is a common question, and at some point, you are no longer feeding a growing horse. However, maturity occurs at different times depending on the measure that is being used to define it (Staniar et al 2005). In the study by Staniar and colleagues (2005), sigmoid curves were used to estimate the ages at which various different measures of equine growth reached 75, 90, 95, and 100% maturity in Thoroughbreds. Maturity was defined as the asymptote of the sigmoid growth curve. For wither height, the mature size of which was estimated at 157 cm and was reached at 1519 days of age, but reached 90% maturity at 225 days of age. Body weight, the mature size of which was 542 kg and was reached at 2571 days of age, reached 90% maturity at 731 days of age. In fact weight was the only measure of growth that had not reached 90% of maturity by 2 years of age, and it was only 11 days over. So horses are still growing at the age of two, but they are doing so very slowly. For this reason the nutrition of the two year old should be focused more on maintaining healthy musculoskeletal structure and meeting the requirements of any exercise and training that the horse is more likely to be involved in at this point.

Conclusions

Growth

- Equine growth can be described as following a sigmoid pattern, with an exponential increase in size occurring in utero, followed by a post parturition period during which the rate of growth follows an exponential decline. A sine wave like pattern of increases and decreases in growth is overlaid on the sigmoid curve, representing the short term changes in growth caused by the growing horse's environment.
- There are many aspects of equine growth that are similar to growth in other livestock, although the end objective of that growth, i.e. athletic performance and longevity for the horse, are likely to be quite different. Therefore, feeding protocols for the growing horse need to fit those objectives.
- To this end, a focus on bodyweight alone is not warranted. Instead, to evaluate the impact of nutrition or other management strategies on growth, linear measures such as withers height, body length, girth circumference, and cannon circumference should be measured along with body weight. In addition, indexes and scoring systems such as an improved equine specific BMI or a young horse body condition scoring system could be useful in evaluating the impact of nutrition on the growing horse.
- Finally, equine growth follows a sigmoidal pattern such that the majority of growth occurs between the 8th month of gestation and the 2nd year post parturition. It is during this period that nutrition can have a large impact due to the rapid rate of tissue turnover associated with growth.
- If a pattern of growth that is relatively free of short term deviations is desired, a proactive feeding plan that takes into account predictable changes in the environment may be able to significantly moderate growth fluctuations.

Requirements

- Dietary energy is critical during equine growth to support the development of energy dense tissues such as muscle and adipose. The main sources of this energy are lactose and lipid in milk, starch and fat in concentrates, and fiber in forages. Understanding where, when, and how much energy is available is an important step in controlling the growth of the horse.
- Dietary protein and more appropriately amino acids supply the molecular building blocks for most tissues and enzymes in the growing horse. High quality protein sources may be of benefit in young growing horses because of their capability to reduce the total amount of dietary crude protein required due to amino acid composition closer to that of developing tissues. Having said this, a growing horse with access to a quality forage source and sufficient milk from their dam, or a concentrate with an ingredient such as soybean meal is unlikely to be protein deficient.
- Minerals and vitamin balance is best addressed by a qualified nutritionist. In many cases, the traditional diets fed to growing horses will be meeting these requirements, but deficiencies or excesses can go unnoticed until clinically apparent signs of deficiency or excess appear. The most common nutrients examined include Ca, P, Cu, Zn, and the vitamins A, D, and E.

References

Anderson, M.D., Speer, V.C., McCall, J.T., et al., 1966. Hypervitaminosis A in young pigs. J Anim Sci 25, 1123–1127.

Azevedo, R.A., Arruda, P., 2010. High-lysine maize: the key discoveries that have made it possible. Amino Acids 39, 979–989.

Breidenbach, A., Schlumbohm, C., Harmeyer, J., 1998. Peculiarities of vitamin D and of the calcium and phosphate homeostatic system in horses. Vet Res 29, 173–186.

Breuer, L.H., Golden, D.L., 1971. Lysine requirement of the immature equine. J Anim Sci 33, 227.

Bryden, W.L., 1991. Amino acid requirements of horses estimated from tissue composition. In: Costa, N.D., Perth, W.A. (Eds.), Proceedings of the Nutrition Society of Australia Sixteenth Annual Scientific Meeting. The Society, Australia, 1991. p. 53.

Cameron, E.Z., Stafford, K.J., Linklater, W.L., et al., 1999. Suckling behaviour does not measure milk intake in horses, Equus caballus. Anim Behav 57, 673–678.

Cash, R.S.G., 1999. Colostral quality determined by refractometry. Equine Vet Educ 11, 36–38.

Coenen, M., 2001. German Feeding Standards. Pages 365–378. In: Pagan, J.D., Geor, R.J. (Eds.), in Advances in equine nutrition II. Nottingham University Press, Nottingham.

Coleman, R.J., Mathison, G.W., Burwash, L., 1999. Growth and condition at weaning of extensively managed creep-fed foals. J Equine Vet Sci 19, 45–50.

Crowell-Davis, S.L., 2008. Understanding foal development and its relevance to raising orphaned foals. Vet Tech 29, 116.

Crowell-Davis, S.L., Caudle, A.B., 1989. Coprophagy by foals: recognition of maternal feces. Applied Anim Behav Sci 24, 267–272.

Crowell-Davis, S.L., Houpt, K.A., 1985. Coprophagy by foals: effect of age and possible functions. Equine Vet J 17, 17–19.

Crowell-Davis, S.L., Houpt, K.A., Carnevale, J., 1985. Feeding and drinking behavior of mares and foals with free access to pasture and water. J Anim Sci 60, 883–889.

Cymbaluk, N.F., 1994. Thermoregulation of horses in cold, winter weather: A review. Livestock Prod Sci 40, 65–71.

Dawson, W.M., Phillips, R.W., Speelman, S.R., 1945. Growth of horses under western range conditions. J Anim Sci 4, 47–54.

Donabedian, M., Fleurance, G., Perona, G., et al., 2006. Effect of fast vs. moderate growth rate related to nutrient intake on developmental orthopaedic disease in the horse. Anim Res 55, 471–486.

Donaldson, M.T., McFarlane, D., Jorgensen, A.J., et al., 2004. Correlation between plasma alpha-melanocyte-stimulating hormone concentration and body mass index in healthy horses. Am J Vet Res 65, 1469–1473.

Donoghue, S., Kronfeld, D.S., Berkowitz, S.J., et al., 1981. Vitamin A nutrition of the equine growth serum biochemistry and hematology. J Nutr 111, 365–374.

Doreau, M., Boulot, S., Martin-Rosset, W., et al., 1986. Relationship between nutrient intake, growth and body-composition of the nursing foal. Reprod Nutr Devel 26, 683–690.

El Shorafa, W.M., Feaster, J.P., Ott, E.A., et al., 1979. Effect of vitamin D and sunlight on growth and bone development of young ponies. J Anim Sci 48, 882–886.

Fernandez-Cancio, M., Audi, L., Carrascosa, A., et al., 2009. Vitamin D and growth hormone regulate growth hormone/insulin-like growth factor (GH-IGF) axis gene expression in human fetal epiphyseal chondrocytes. Growth Horm IGF Res 19, 232–237.

Frey, K.S., Potter, G.D., Odom, T.W., et al., 1992. Plasma silicon and radiographic bone-density in weanling Quarter Horses fed sodium zeolite A1. J Equine Vet Sci 12, 292–296.

Gafni, R.I., Baron, J., 2000. Catch-up growth: possible mechanisms. Pediatr Nephrol 14, 616–619.

Grace, N.D., Pearce, S.G., Firth, E.C., et al., 1999. Concentrations of macro- and micro-elements in the milk of pasture-fed Thoroughbred mares. Aust Vet J 77, 177–180.

Graham, P.M., Ott, E.A., Brendemuhl, J.H., et al., 1994. The effect of supplemental lysine and threonine on growth and development of yearling horses. J Anim Sci 72, 380–386.

Griewe-Crandell, K.M., Kronfeld, D.S., Gay, L.A., et al., 1995. Seasonal variation in Vitamin A status of grazing horses is assessed better by the relative dose response test than by serum retinol concentration. J Nutr 125, 2711–2716.

Greiwe-Crandell, K.M., Kronfeld, D.S., Gay, L.S., et al., 1997. Vitamin A repletion in Thoroughbred mares with retinyl palmitate or beta-carotene. J Anim Sci 75, 2684–2690.

Hammond, J., 1950. Measuring growth in farm animals. Proc R Soc Lond B Biol Sci 137, 452–461.

Henneke, D.R., Potter, G.D., Kreider, J.L., et al., 1983. Relationship between condition score, physical measurement, and body fat percentage in mares. Equine Vet J 15, 371–372.

Hill, M.A., 1990. Causes of degenerative joint disease (osteoarthrosis) and dyschondroplasia (osteochondrosis) in pigs. J Am Vet Med Assoc 197, 107–113.

Hintz, H.F., 1996. Mineral requirements of growing horses. Pferdeheilkunde 12, 303–306.

Hintz, H.F., Hintz, R.L., Vleck, L.D., 1979. Growth rate of thoroughbreds: Effect of age of dam, year and month of birth, and sex of foal. J Anim Sci 48, 480–487.

Hurtig, M., Green, S.L., Dobson, H., et al., 1993. Correalative study of defective cartilage and bone growth in foals fed a low copper diet. Equine Vet J 16, 66–73.

Jordon, R.M., Myers, V., 1972. Effects of protein levels on the growth of weanling and yearling ponies. J Anim Sci 34, 578–581.

Julliand, V., 1992. Microbiology of the equine hindgut. Pferdeheilkunde 12, 42–47.

Kellems, R.O., Church, D.C., 2010. Mineral and vitamin supplements. Pages 160–172. In: Kellems, R.O., Church, D.C. (Eds.), in Livestock feeds and feeding. Prentice Hall, New York.

Keys, A., Fidanza, F., Karvonen, M.J., et al., 1972. Indices of relative weight and obesity. J Chronic Dis 25, 329–343.

Kienzle, E., 2005. Evaluation of mineral and vitamin requirements for growing horses. Pages 199–206. In: Julliand, V., Martin-Rosset, W. (Eds.), in The growing horse: nutrition and prevention of growth disorders No. 114. Wageningen Academic Publishers, Wageningen, Netherlands.

Knight, D.A., Gabel, A.A., Reed, S.M., et al., 1985. Correlation of dietary mineral to incidence and severity of metabolic bone disease in Ohio and Kentucky. In: Proceedings of the American Association of Equine Practitioners. American Association of Equine Practitioners, Lexington, KY, pp. 445–461.

Kronfeld, D.S., 2001. A practical method for ration evaluation and diet formulation: an introduction to sensitivity analysis. Pages 1–12. In: Pagan, J.D., Geor, R.J. (Eds.), in Advances in Equine Nutrition II. Nottingham University Press, Nottingham, UK.

Lui, J.C., Baron, J., 2011. Mechanisms limiting body growth in mammals. Endocr Rev 32, 422–440.

Martin-Rosset, W., 2005. Growth and development in the equine. Pages 15–50. In: Julliand, V., Martin-Rosset, W. (Eds.), in The growing horse: nutrition and prevention of growth disorders No. 114. Wageningen Academic Publishers, Wageningen.

Martin-Rosset, W., Boccard, R., Jussiaux, M., et al., 1983. Relative growth of carcass tissues, organs and carcass joints in different heavy horse breeds between 12 and 30 months. Ann Zootech 32, 153–174.

Minot, C., 1908. The problem of age, growth, and death. G. P. Putnam's Sons, New York.

Nicol, C.J., Badnell-Waters, A.J., Bice, R., et al., 2005. The effects of diet and weaning method on the behaviour of young horses. Applied Animal Behaviour Science 95, 205–221.

Nielsen, B.D., Potter, G.D., Morris, E.L., et al., 1993. Training distance to failure in young racing quarter horses fed sodium zeolite-a. J Equine Vet Sci 13, 562–567.

NRC, 1987. Vitamin tolerance of animals. National Academy Press, Washington, DC.

NRC, 1989. Nutrient requirements of horses, fifth rev. ed. National Academy Press, Washington, D.C.

NRC, 2007. Nutrient Requirements of Horses, sixth rev. ed. National Academy Press, Washington, DC.

O'Connor, C.I., Nielsen, B.D., Woodward, A.D., et al., 2008. Mineral balance in horses fed two supplemental silicon sources. J Anim Physiol Anim Nutr (Berl) 92, 173–181.

Ott, E.A., Asquith, R.L., Feaster, J.P., et al., 1979. Influence of protein level and quality on the growth and development of yearling foals. J Anim Sci 49, 620–628.

Ott, E.A., Asquith, R.L., Feaster, J.P., 1981. Lysine supplementation of diets for yearling horses. J Anim Sci 53, 1496–1503.

Ousey, J.C., Mcarthur, A.J., Murgatroyd, P.R., et al., 1992. Thermoregulation and total-body insulation in the neonatal foal. J Therm Biol 17, 1–10.

Ousey, J.C., Holdstock, N., Rossdale, P.D., et al., 1996. How much energy do sick neonatal foals require compared with healthy foals? Pferdeheilkunde 12, 231–237.

Pagan, J.D., Jackson, S.G., Caddel, S., 1996. A summary of growth rates of thoroughbreds in Kentucky. Pferdeheilkunde 12, 285–289.

Park, Y.S., Lim, S.W., Lee, I.H., et al., 2007. Intra-articular injection of a nutritive mixture solution protects articular cartilage from osteoarthritic progression induced by anterior cruciate ligament transection in mature rabbits: a randomized controlled trial. Arthritis Res Ther 9, R8.

Philippeau, C., Faubladier, C., Sadet-Bourgeteau, S., et al.,2011. Changes in *in vitro* fermentative capacity in foals from birth to 2 months old. Journal of Equine Veterinary Science 31, 278–279.

Poso, A.R., Hyyppä, S., 1999. Metabolic and hormonal changes after exercise in relation to muscle glycogen concentrations. Equine Vet J 31, 332–336.

Potter, G.D., Huchton, J.D., 1975. Growth of yearling horses fed different sources of protein with supplemental lysine. Proceedings of the 4th Equine Nutrition and Physiology Society, Pomona, CA, pp. 19–20.

Pugh, D.G., Schumacher, J., 1993. Feeding and nutrition of brood mares. Compendium on Continuing Education for the Practicing Veterinarian 15, 106–115.

Pugh, D.G., Williams, M.A., 1992. Feeding foals from birth to weaning. Compendium on Continuing Education for the Practicing Veterinarian 14, 526

Roberts, M.C., 1975. Carbohydrate digestion and absorption studies in the horse. Res Vet Sci 18, 64–69.

Rothman, K.J., 2002. Epidemiology: an introduction. Oxford University Press, New York, N.Y.

Rucker, R.B., Kosonen, T., Clegg, M.S., et al., 1998. Copper, lysyl oxidase, and extracellular matrix protein cross-linking. Am J Clin Nutr 67, 996S-1002S.

Savage, C.J., McCarthy, R.N., Jeffcott, L.B., 1993. Effects of dietary energy and protein on induction of dyschondroplasia in foals. Equine Vet J 16, 74–79.

Schryver, H.F., Hintz, H.F., Craig, P.H., 1971. Calcium metabolism in ponies fed a high phosphorus diet. J Nutr 101, 259–264.

Schryver, H.F., Hintz, H.F., Lowe, J.E., et al., 1974. Mineral-composition of whole-body, liver and bone of young horses. J Nutr 104, 126–132.

Schryver, H.F., Meakim, D.W., Lowe, J.E., et al., 1987. Growth and calcium metabolism in horses fed varying levels of protein. Equine Vet J 19, 280–287.

Smith-Funk, E.D., Crowell-Davis, S.L., 1992. Maternal behavior of draft mares (*Equus caballus*) with mule foals (*Equus asinus* X *Equus caballus*). Applied Animal Behaviour Science 33, 93–119.

Staniar, W.B., 2001. Growth and the somatotropic axis in young Thoroughbreds. Dissertation, Virginia Polytechnic Institute and State University, Blacksburg, VA.

Staniar, W.B., Kronfeld, D.S., Cubitt, T.A., et al., 2005. Growth in linear measures of Thoroughbreds: Maturation rates and points of maturity. In: Proceedings of the 19th Equine Science Society Symposium, Tucson, AZ. Equine Science Society, Champaign, IL, pp. 226–227.

Staniar, W.B., Kronfeld, D.S., Wilson, J.A., et al., 2001. Growth of thoroughbreds fed a low-protein supplement fortified with lysine and threonine. J Anim Sci 79, 2143–2151.

Staniar, W.B., Kronfeld, D.S., Hoffman, R.M., et al., 2004a. Weight prediction from linear measures of growing Thoroughbreds. Equine Vet J 36, 149–154.

Staniar, W.B., Kronfeld, D.S., Treiber, K.H., et al., 2004b. Growth rate consists of baseline and systematic deviation components in Thoroughbreds. J Anim Sci 82, 1007–1015.

Stock, K.F., Hamann, H., Distl, O., 2005. Estimation of genetic parameters for the prevalence of osseous fragments in limb joints of Hanoverian Warmblood horses. J Anim Breed Genet 122, 271–280.

Turner, K.K., Nielsen, B.D., O'Connor-Robison, C.I., et al., 2008. Tissue response to a supplement high in aluminum and silicon. Biol Trace Elem Res 121, 134–148.

Urschel, K.L., Geor, R.J., Waterfall, H.L., et al., 2010. Effects of leucine or whey protein addition to an oral glucose solution on serum insulin, plasma glucose and plasma amino acid responses in horses at rest and following exercise. Equine Vet J 38, 347–354.

Van Weeren, P.R., 2006. Etiology, diagnosis, and treatment of OCD. Clinical Techniques in Equine Practice 5, 248–258.

van Weeren, P.R., Knaap, J., Firth, E.C., 2003. Influence of liver copper status of mare and newborn foal on the development of osteochondrotic lesions. Equine Vet J 35, 67–71.

Walton, A., Hammond, J., 1938. The maternal effects on growth and conformation in shire horse-shetland pony crosses. Proceedings of the Royal Society of London, Series B. Biological Sciences 125, 311–335.

Weese, J.S., Rousseau, J., 2005. Evaluation of Lactobacillus pentosus WE7 for prevention of diarrhea in neonatal foals. J Am Vet Med Assoc 226, 2031–2034.

13

Practical considerations for feeding racehorses

Brian D. Nielsen

To be successful in short duration, high-speed or strength-oriented activities such as racing, a horse needs to be able to perform at a high intensity and maintain that intensity longer than its competitors. There are many factors that can contribute to the ability to perform in this manner. Physical conditioning and soundness are perhaps the two primary factors that enable a horse to be in the position to perform successfully, but the nutritional program can also play a critical role in assisting a horse to achieve its athletic potential. A basic understanding of the typical racing and training programs associated with some of the more popular racing breeds, as well as some of the advantages and limitations of the various dietary constituents commonly fed, can aid in designing a feeding program which can support optimal performance.

Performance metrics

Even for the high intensity racehorse, there can be tremendous differences in the distances raced and speeds reached. Standardbred racing in the US, for example, is typically over a distance of 1609 m at speeds of ~48 km/h, whereas Thoroughbreds generally race over 1006 m to 2414 m at faster speeds around 64 km/h, although this does depend on the race distance (Harkins & Kamerling 1993, Nunamaker et al 1989). Slower speeds typically are associated with the longer races and quicker speeds often are achieved in shorter races. The true equine sprinters, the racing Quarter Horse, routinely compete at distances of 402 m or less (Nielsen et al 2006). Interestingly over 402 m, the record times for both Quarter Horses and Thoroughbreds are similar, in the range of 20.7 s (Nielsen et al 2006). Granted, this similarity is due to Quarter Horse races being timed from a standing start when the starting gates open while Thoroughbred races are officially begun and timed from a point in front of the starting gates, when the horses are already running. Although Thoroughbreds typically try to maintain a consistent speed throughout a race, Quarter Horses are accelerating through the first half of the race and have been reported to reach speeds near 90 km/h (Nielsen et al 2006, Pratt 1991).

With such differences in racing distances and speeds, training programs also vary widely. Typically, Thoroughbreds train over relatively short distances at race pace while Standardbreds are trained over longer distances (Nunamaker et al 1989). Standardbreds may spend 60 minutes of their 140 minutes weekly exercise (~40%) being worked at a high intensity (Hamlin & Hopkins 2003). A small survey of racing Thoroughbreds in England reported that they were exercised over a mean distance of 10 km per week with fast work only being performed for 1.4 km suggesting that the horses on average performed at racing speed for less than 2 minutes per week (Verheyen et al 2009). Gallagher et al (1992a) reported that although Thoroughbreds and Standardbreds were exercised over similar daily distances (6.9 km/day vs 7.7 km/day, respectively), overall intensity of exercise was higher for the Standardbreds. Thoroughbreds walked 72% of the distance traveled as compared to only 58% for Standardbreds (Gallagher et al 1992a). The distance walked is not always considered as part of the exercise protocol for Thoroughbreds and Standardbreds and is used as a means of cooling a horse out after exercising or simply a means to get the horse to and from a racetrack for training. Nonetheless, walking can make a substantial contribution to the total exercise load as well as daily energy requirements. Pagan and Hintz (1986) estimated that walking requires 2.5 kcal digestible energy (DE)/kg/h above maintenance in riding horses and thus should be considered when evaluating energy requirements even of the racehorse.

The racing Quarter Horse is generally trained over the shortest distance – 5 km or less per week – and also does not undertake significant amounts of exercise at racing speeds. Though the distance can vary, it is common to work a horse at race speeds over a distance of 229 m only once every two or three weeks if a horse is not actively racing. If racing on a regular schedule, they may not be worked at speed at all in-between races. The duration of "all-out" galloping is often no more than 30 s during racing or training sessions. Compared to Thoroughbreds and Standardbreds, walking often constitutes a significant portion of the training program for racing Quarter Horses and, for many, walking is their only exercise for several days per week. In comparison, both Standardbreds and Thoroughbreds are often exercised at the jog, canter, or at a fast walk five to six days per week and would accumulate substantially greater distances trained monthly (Table 13-1).

Nutrition and performance

Body condition

Regardless of breed, for horses performing high intensity exercise the goal is to minimize excess weight whilst not

Table 13-1 Average Monthly Distances (km) Trained by English Thoroughbreds and New Zealand Standardbreds

Thoroughbreds		Standardbreds	
Canter	37.5	Jog	177
Fast Work	4.4	Fast Work	25.7
Race	1.7	Race*	5.1
Total	43.6	Total	207.8

*Standard race distance of 2.4 km
Data adapted from Verheyen et al 2009 and Shearman & Hopkins 1996.

sacrificing energy stores or their availability. Energy requirements for a mature horse in intense training are reported to be over twice that of a similar horse at maintenance (NRC 2007). Inadequate energy intakes, even of a short duration, potentially will result in a more rapid onset of fatigue and reduced performance. This highlights the importance of dietary energy, as a short-term inadequate intake of most nutrients usually does not have such a dramatic impact on performance.

Unlike in man, the relationship between body fatness, fat-free mass, and running performance has not been studied extensively in the horse. The optimal bodyweight of racehorses, however, appears to be highly correlated with performance and the optimal bodyweight of a racehorse only has a range of ±1.5% with performance appearing to be less affected by being overweight as compared to underweight (Lim 1981). Rider and equipment weight, in addition to the weight of the horse, also needs to be factored into the energy requirements needed to run so anything increasing the overall weight increases the energy cost of locomotion (Harris & Harris 2005). Thornton et al (1987) demonstrated that a 10% increase in weight load, increased oxygen consumption by 15% in horses exercising on a horizontal treadmill. By contrast, the acute reduction in bodyweight after administration of furosemide resulted in decreased anaerobic energy expenditure during brief high-intensity work and may be responsible for any improvement in performance (Hinchcliff et al 1996). Frape (1994) suggested Thoroughbreds of moderate fatness use depot fat as a source of energy more effectively than thin or fat horses. Webb et al (1990) reported horses in fleshy condition require more DE for maintenance (an additional 11.1 kcal/kg BW/day) than do horses in moderate condition and that the optimal body condition for the performance horse might vary according to ambient temperature and humidity at the time of performance.

Gaining or losing weight may alter lean mass as well as percentage body fat. As speed is linked, to a certain extent, to fat-free mass, this may alter performance as well (Kearns et al 2002). Therefore, during conditioning, a balance is needed to maximize lean body mass while minimizing excessive body fat, rather than just restricting calorie intake in an attempt to produce a very lean animal without the appropriate exercise and nutritional regimens.

To practically assess the adequacy of energy intake, a body condition score (BCS; Henneke et al 1983) should be determined on a regular basis (see Chapter 22). Even if the BCS remains unchanged, it does not guarantee that the animal is at the optimal BCS. Having a BCS that is either too high or too low can impair performance. For most athletic horses, the goal should be to have a BCS between 4 and 6 on a scale of 1 to 9 (Becvarova et al 2009) though it would be rare, and probably disadvantageous, to have a racehorse with a BCS as high as 6. When a horse is in a thin condition, glycogen stores may be lower than when they are in a moderate or fat condition (Jones et al 1992, Scott et al 1992) contributing to an earlier onset of fatigue. Given that glycogen is a preferred substrate for energy transduction during short-term, high-intensity predominantly anaerobic exercise such as racing, maximizing glycogen stores would seem advisable (see Chapter 26).

A small over-consumption of most nutrients may be wasteful but it is unlikely to impair performance. However, a horse in continual or frequent positive energy balance will store this excess energy as fat which can be detrimental to athletic performance. Glycogen storage does not appear to increase with BCS once over a certain level (Jones et al 1992) and there appears to be no performance benefit for an athletic horse having a BCS much higher than 5 (on a scale of 1 to 9). Indeed, a higher BCS may be detrimental to athletic performance. A Thoroughbred racehorse at BCS 6 and weighing 500 kg, for example, would be expected to weigh 16 to 20 kg more than a similarly built horse that has a BCS of 5 (NRC 2007) – "natural handicapping". By being overweight, animals also put additional load on their limbs and, potentially, fat deposition in the thoracic cavity could reduce or limit lung expansion. Additionally, extra subcutaneous fat serves as insulation increasing the challenge for the horse to dissipate heat (Morgan 1997). All of these factors may prevent the horse from performing optimally. Trainers will often attempt to determine the optimal racing weight for an individual and then try to maintain this weight. A weighbridge, calibrated appropriately, is the ideal way to determine the weight of racehorses as weight tapes (heart girth measurement) tend to have reduced accuracy in very fit lean animals (personal observation). Even if weighbridges are used, it is still recommended that racehorses are scored for body condition as that will aid in determining whether the weight is appropriate or if weight needs to be gained or lost. Use of weight tapes in combination with body condition scoring is another approach to monitoring.

Protein

Due to the anabolic changes in muscle associated with the start of physical conditioning and the need to repair any resultant muscle damage as well as enable muscle hypertrophy, protein requirements of athletic horses are increased compared to sedentary horses (Custalow 1991; see Chapter 6). Quantifying this additional demand has been challenging, in part because variation in conditioning programs likely results in different protein needs. Furthermore, while requirements are established as a minimum to replace losses and prevent health problems, the amount needed for optimal performance is likely to be greater. As a result, many trainers feed protein greatly in excess of published requirements (Gallagher et al 1992a, b). This, however, may not be desirable, as discussed below.

Although horses in exercise have a higher protein requirement, as evidenced by an increase in nitrogen retention in association with greater exercise load (Freeman et al 1988), the increase is not as dramatic as many would believe. Even without raising the actual concentration of protein in the feed, any increase in the protein requirements is often met simply by the enhanced dry matter (DM) intake (NRC 2007). Recently, however, with the increased practice of switching to energy-dense, oil-supplemented diets at the start of training, this increase in DM intake may not occur. Consequently, it is important to estimate how much protein an animal is receiving in order to determine whether its protein requirements are being met. High quality hay (particularly legume hay) can provide substantial amounts of protein, often equaling or exceeding the amount provided by the grain portion of the diet (Connysson et al 2006). Under these circumstances it is often unnecessary to provide a high protein complementary/concentrate feed. A complete ration evaluation is therefore recommended. It is, however, important to take into account that published requirements for protein, as well as other nutrients, as established by the NRC (2007) are minimum requirements, as opposed to optimal amounts, and were established for a population of horses. Individual requirements may vary greatly and extra allowances to account for individual variation may be warranted (Becvarova et al 2009).

Providing excess dietary protein may be undesirable because of the potential adverse effects on heat production, acid-base balance (especially at maximal exercise), and possibly respiratory health due to ammonia accumulation under confinement housing conditions (Graham-Thiers et al 2000). Excess protein intake has been shown to result in increased urine production and possible evaporative fluid losses that could result in an unnecessary challenge for horses during prolonged exercise (Connysson et al 2006). However, potential benefits have been shown by Essen-Gustavsson et al (2010) who reported that trotters in training fed a high CP (16.6%) forage-only diet had greater glycogen and free leucine concentrations in the muscle than when fed a forage-only diet containing CP close to the 1989 NRC-recommended concentrations (12.5%). It was suggested that the higher muscle glycogen concentrations were due to either greater synthesis or lower degradation and that possibly the additional amino acids provided via the diet were used for oxidation in the muscle, thus sparing the glycogen.

Additionally, there is some evidence that substantial amounts of nitrogen may be lost through sweat (Freeman et al 1986), possibly in the range of 1 to 1.5 g of N/kg of sweat and estimates of sweat losses have been as high as 5 kg/100 kg of BW (Meyer 1987). Nitrogen losses of that magnitude would equate to losses of over 200 g of crude protein. This demonstrates the potential for protein requirements to be influenced by the ambient environmental conditions and not just the duration and intensity of the exercise.

Finally, as discussed in Chapter 6 (Protein and Amino Acids), the quality of the dietary protein (the amino acid profile) is important. Unfortunately, there is minimal published research on this subject (Antilley et al 2007) especially in exercising horses. Hence, knowledge regarding the true amino acid requirements for exercise is limited but research has suggested that exercising horses can successfully be fed lower concentrations of crude protein if their diets are fortified with limiting amino acids (Graham-Thiers et al 2001). Some commercial concentrates are now including lysine and threonine in their formulations.

In both humans and horses, protein is needed in the repair and recovery process so an adequate intake of quality protein is necessary. Both arginine and ornithine have been reported to stimulate growth hormone release and promote increased lean tissue (Clarkson 1998). The effect is small and, despite several amino acids being sold as "anabolic agents" for humans, it is doubtful that amino-acid supplements will promote gains in muscle mass (Clarkson 1998) unless the core diet is deficient or marginal in amino acid composition (O'Connor et al 2002). Still, it is not known whether supplementation of certain amino acids could cause subtle long-term benefits on muscle structure, including repair and recovery from exercise. For instance, L-arginine supplementation in rats appears to reduce oxidative damage and inflammatory response to the myocardium after exhaustive exercise (Lin et al 2006).

Branched-chain amino acid (BCAA) supplementation had no influence on the metabolic response to exercise in Standardbreds (Casini et al 2000, Stefanon et al 2000), though any potential role in recovery nor other types of exercise was not explored. Additionally, timing of ingestion may play a role in the response of exercise to nutritional supplements. In humans, net muscle protein synthesis was greater when an essential amino acid-carbohydrate supplement was given before, rather than after, resistance exercise (Tipton et al 2001). Recent pilot work in the horse, however, suggests that post- rather than pre-exercise amino acid supplementation results in higher plasma amino acid concentrations (Graham-Thiers & Bowen, 2011) which, in turn, may results in increased protein synthesis and decreased protein degradation (Matsui et al., 2006). More work is needed in this area.

Minerals

Mineral requirements of athletic horses vary considerably according to a number of factors including the management of the animals during training, as well as the stage and intensity of the training (Nielsen et al 1997).

Calcium is usually considered first when discussing mineral nutrition in racing animals due to its importance in bone health. There is an added dimension in high-intensity exercising animals due to the dynamic nature of bone, which tends to respond fairly rapidly to the forces that are applied to it. In essence the skeleton tries to achieve a balance between bone that is strong enough to withstand frequently encountered strain loads and maintaining an energetically efficient skeleton without storing excess mineral. In response to sprint exercise (whether forced or free-choice), bone becomes stronger or, if already strong, maintains its strength. By comparison, when no high-speed exercise is performed, there is no signal to increase, or even maintain, bone mineral content and skeletal strength is lost. For racehorses competing at high speeds, maintaining skeletal strength is critical.

During periods of training when high-speed exercise is being introduced, the demand for calcium is increased. In contrast, when the forces placed upon the skeleton are decreased (i.e. when horses are stall-rested without a requirement for high-speed exercise or when the training intensity is decreased), the demand for calcium is decreased (Nielsen et al 1998). Even when fed dietary Ca at twice the recommended levels, bone loss decreased when conditioned horses were stall-rested for 12 weeks (Porr et al 1998). These variations in mineral requirements associated with stage of training or management of horses makes it difficult to provide firm guidelines as to the specific calcium requirement of an individual horse. This probably also applies with respect to the requirements for phosphorus (Elmore-Smith et al 1999) and magnesium (Stephens et al 2001). Again, it is important to note that the guidelines established by the NRC (2007) attempt to ensure that minimum requirements for minerals are met, regardless of the stage of exercise and the type of management used.

As with the protein content of the diet, full ration analysis is required when evaluating mineral intake vs. requirements. Generally, if a commercial fortified complementary feed/concentrate is being fed at the recommended levels, the risk of deficiency is low.

Electrolytes

In comparison to the other macrominerals, hard working horses have a substantially increased requirement for the electrolytes sodium, chloride, and potassium due to the need to replace the electrolytes lost in sweat (Coenen 2005). The NRC (2007) provides estimates based on perceived intensity of exercise performed by the horse (see also Chapter 10 and Chapter 14). This estimate is, however, quite subjective and contains an inherent flaw because ambient environmental conditions can greatly influence sweat rates. Additionally, though many would consider all racehorses to be in heavy work, if work load is based on distance trained weekly, Standardbreds are in fact likely to be subjected to a greater work load than most Thoroughbreds or Quarter Horses and thus in theory would have greater electrolyte requirements. It also is important to recognize the potential importance of sweat loss during any transportation to a race.

Fortunately, if allowed free access to salt (sodium chloride), fed a commercial fortified concentrate grain mix that contains about 1% salt, and provided with sufficient access to good-quality forage, most horses will consume enough electrolytes to meet their needs. This is particularly true for the horse exercising at a high-intensity as the length of their exercise bout tends to be shorter than, for instance, an endurance horse. However, even with free access to salt, there is no guarantee that adequate quantities will be consumed and, particularly with some extremely hard-working horses in hot climates, additional electrolyte supplementation may be justified. Some horses can consume substantially more salt than they need if allowed free access. Thus, it is critical that adequate water is available. Electrolyte deficiency or imbalance can arise when forage intake is restricted, especially when haylage replaces hay on a weight to weight basis as potassium intake may become inadequate.

Key Points

- Electrolyte demands can increase dramatically due to exercise-related sweat losses
- Ambient conditions influence the rate of sweat fluid losses. Electrolyte requirements are higher for horses working in hot vs. cool or moderate ambient conditions.
- For most racehorses, electrolyte requirements will be met by a ration that includes free-choice salt (NaCl), good quality roughage, and a commercial fortified concentrate

Vitamins

Development of a vitamin deficiency is unlikely provided horses are fed green, high quality hay that has been relatively recently harvested or allowed access to good pasture, and are exposed to sunlight (Saastamoinen & Harris 2008; see also Chapter 9). Additionally, commercial feeds used in racehorse diets are usually highly fortified with vitamins, further decreasing risk of a vitamin deficiency. However, inadequate intakes of some vitamins, especially the fat-soluble vitamins, may occur if horses are fed a diet consisting of unfortified grains and conserved forage for an extended period of time (Saastamoinen & Harris 2008). Additionally, inappetence may occur in some hard working horses and it has been speculated that in these circumstances supplementation with B-vitamins, thiamin in particular, may help restore appetite and improve cellular energy (Carroll et al 1949, Wolter 1987). Although B-vitamins are normally synthesized in sufficient amounts by the microflora in the hindgut, given their role as co-factors involved in energy metabolism, such supplementation may be justified especially when DM intake is depressed. While some vitamins can be stored by the body for extended periods, storage is much shorter for others, e.g. thiamin reserves may last only 1–2 weeks (Saastamoinen & Harris 2008). This provides perhaps additional justification for supplementation if it is believed that endogenous synthesis is not keeping up with the demand in the intensely exercising horse.

The important antioxidant role that certain vitamins play, especially vitamin E, is obviously important to the exercising horse. There is, however, little published work showing specific benefits to the intensely exercising horses of enhanced supplementation and it is unclear if additional supplementation to a horse fed a balanced diet is warranted (see also Chapter 9).

Water

Water is an essential nutrient for exercising horses and the requirement for water increases as the extent of sweat fluid losses increase, which in turn will be influenced by the intensity and duration of exercise, as well as ambient conditions. Water intake by a 500-kg horse in work has been estimated to be in the range of 36 to 92 liters per day depending upon the environmental conditions and the exercise performed (NRC 2007; see also Chapter 4).

Traditionally, allowing horses to drink water (especially large volumes of very cold water) soon after exercise has been discouraged due to a perceived increased risk of colic. However, there is little hard evidence of an association between postexercise water consumption and colic. Furthermore, the withholding of water during the early postexercise period can delay rehydration (Butudom et al 2003). The author recommends that a horse should be allowed to drink water within 30 minutes of completing a high-intensity exercise bout. However, given the uncertainty regarding health risks associated with large volume water intake after a maximal or near maximal exercise bout, it may be advisable to allow frequent intakes of smaller volumes rather than unlimited access until the horse is fully "cooled down".

There is little published work on strategies for electrolyte replenishment after high intensity exercise (see Chapter 14 with respect to electrolyte provision after endurance type exercise). However, if electrolytes are to be provided in the drinking water, it is recommended that a source of fresh, non-supplemented water also be available. Interestingly, oral water and electrolyte supplementation provided after exercise has been shown to modestly enhance the rate of muscle glycogen resynthesis, thus leading to the speculation that dehydration after exercise may be a contributing factor to the slow rate of postexercise muscle glycogen replenishment observed in horses (Waller et al 2009). This is potentially another reason why the practice of withholding water after an intense exercise bout should be abolished.

Typical feeding programs

Depending upon the energy density of the dietary constituents, as well as the intensity and duration of exercise, athletic horses would be expected to consume between 2 and 2.5% of their BW as DM per day (NRC 2007) though this can vary greatly depending upon the individual. Most racehorses typically receive a diet consisting of hay (or equivalent long fiber source) and some form of grain or grain-based complementary/concentrate feed. As they are usually housed in stalls, access to pasture is often limited thus highlighting the need for the trainer to provide an appropriately balanced ration that meets all nutrient requirements. Assessment of workload is one of the key issues when evaluating feeding programs and requirements for racehorses. Due to their heavy training schedule, Standardbreds would be expected to have a higher energy requirement when compared to Thoroughbred or Quarter Horse racehorses. Another key issue is expected daily DM intake, specifically how best to provide sufficient digestible energy without compromising health and behavior. While racehorses are commonly provided a rather substantial portion of their diet in the form of a concentrate feed, a concurrent decrease in the roughage portion may result in "boredom", colic, and possibly gastrointestinal ulcers.

A field survey reported that racing Standardbreds (mean BW = 449 kg) consumed an average of 14.4 kg DM/day – about 4 kg DM more than was estimated by the 1989 NRC (Gallagher et al 1992a). In comparison, Thoroughbreds (mean BW = 506 kg) consumed 12.3 kg DM – approximately 1 kg DM more than was predicted (Gallagher et al 1992b). The core basis of the feeding program for racing Quarter Horses does not tend to be substantially different from that of racing Thoroughbreds, although intake is likely to be less due to a lower workload. The concentrate:forage ratio of the ration is obviously important; Standardbreds have been reported to receive ~ 35% of the ration as concentrate vs. ~45% for flat-racing Thoroughbreds (Gallagher et al 1992b). This may in part explain the observed higher DM intake by Standardbreds as they were receiving less nutrient-dense concentrate and more roughage (Gallagher et al 1992a). However, even when adjusted for body weight, Standardbreds still consumed 27% more digestible energy than did Thoroughbreds (Gallagher et al 1992a). An example feeding program for adult racehorses is provided in Table 13-2.

Conserved forages

Globally, a variety of forages are fed to racehorses, including straight grass, mixed hay, and alfalfa (lucerne). Use of locally grown or commercial haylages has increased in some countries in recent years. Typically, as the percent neutral detergent fiber (NDF) in hay increases, the energy and digestibility decrease along with palatability (see Chapter 17). Additionally, as roughages mature, NDF digestibility decreases. Given the importance of meeting the energy requirement of a racehorse, choosing hay that was harvested while immature and has low NDF would be advisable. While it has been recommended that horse diets contain at least 20% NDF (Wolter 1993), hays with an NDF under 40% would be considered to be prime, between 41 and 46% would be premium, and between 47 and 53% would be considered to be good (Kapper 2004). Feeding hays that would be of this quality will help to insure adequate DM and DE intake. When an increase in DE intake is desired, the first step should be provision of higher quality roughage (typically lower NDF) rather than the common practice of increasing the concentrate portion of the diet. The first consideration in meeting the energy needs of a racehorse should be optimization of roughage nutritional quality, which will provide a substantial portion of daily DE intake (Fig. 13.1). If provided with unlimited roughage, some horses will eat too much and may develop a "hay belly" (Huff et al 1985), especially if not in hard work. While not detrimental to the health of the horse, it may prove to be disadvantageous to racing performance and should be avoided.

Table 13-2 Example Ration for an Adult Racehorse being Fed Timothy Hay and a 12% CP Grain

	Timothy hay	Grain mix	Timothy hay	Grain mix
	Composition		Daily intake	
DM	93.8%	88.0%	6.0 kg	6.5 kg
DE	2.1 Mcal/kg	3.1 Mcal/kg	12.5 Mcal	20.3 Mcal
CP	8.0%	12.0%	480 g	785 g
Lysine	0.24%	0.65%	14.4 g	42.2 g
Calcium	0.34%	0.60%	20.4 g	39.0 g
Phosphorus	0.21%	0.52%	12.6 g	33.8 g

Adapted from Pagan and Nash (2009).

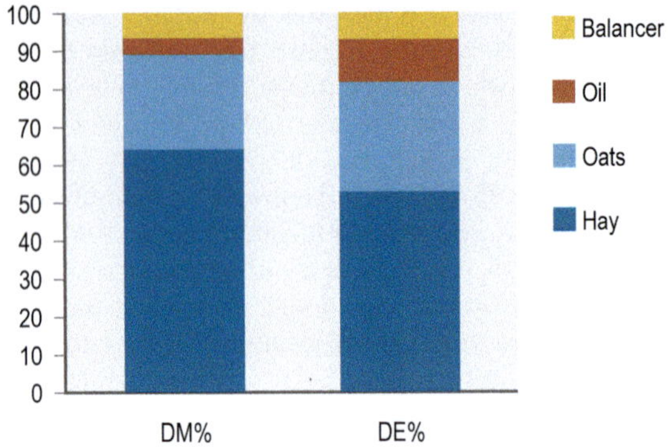

Figure 13.1 A "typical" ration for a high performance horse (without NaCl) consisting of 10 kg hay, 4 kg oats, 1 kg concentrate balancer, and 0.5 kg oil (13.7 kg DM, 159 MJ DE). Although concentrate feed constitutes about 35% of the diet, the roughage portion contributes about half of the total DE – demonstrating the substantial contribution roughage plays in meeting the energy needs of a racehorse and the value of providing roughage of high nutritional quality in situations where DM intake is limited. Such a ration can be adjusted in terms of optimizing the "chemical" origin of energy (% from cellulose, starch, or fat) and the amount of energy provided can be adjusted to obtain a desired BCS.

Complementary feed/concentrate

The type and quality of hay or other forage fed, obviously influences the amount as well as the nutrients required from the concentrate portion of the diet. In most circumstances, a horse should be able to consume sufficient DM to meet its energy demands although the forage to concentrate ratio may need to be adjusted. Often the available high forage diet cannot meet the energy needs of high performing athletic horses (Harris 2009), necessitating the feeding of relatively large amounts of concentrate to avoid excessive weight loss and decreased performance. Dividing the concentrate portion of the ration into as many feedings as practical may reduce the risk of certain health and behavior-related problems which are associated with high grain/concentrate, low forage diets

While most trainers feed a commercially prepared concentrate, some also choose to add oats to the diet (Gallagher et al 1992a, b). This is not a recommended practice unless further analysis of the ration is done to verify the overall nutrient balance of the diet. This is particularly true for young horses in training as oats may not be nutrient-dense enough to meet the requirements for both growth and exercise.

High starch versus high oil or fat diets

Despite recent work suggesting that Standardbred trotters can be trained and raced on diets consisting of only high nutritional quality forage (Essen-Gustavsson et al 2010), most racehorse trainers feed some form of energy-dense complementary/concentrate feed. This practice allows energy requirements to be met in animals with a limited appetite and also may improve performance. Typical feeding programs for most racehorses, therefore, provide a variety of feedstuffs in addition to forage, including high starch providing straight grains (e.g., oats, cracked corn) and/or blended concentrates that often contain added oil.

The ability to delay the onset of fatigue often determines how well a horse performs in a race (Worth 1985). Many biochemical and physiological factors contribute to the onset of fatigue in a race but one reason can be the depletion of muscle glycogen stores. High intensity exercise, particularly when repeated, can reduce muscle glycogen by up to 50% (Lacombe et al 2001). However, Thoroughbred racehorse muscle glycogen concentrations only decreased 23 to 32% following a 1600 m exercise bout (Harkins et al 1992). These findings would seem to support the conclusions reached by Snow et al (1987) that fatigue during short, intense exercise bouts is not related to glycogen depletion. However, despite the absence of marked glycogen depletion within such muscle samples, it is possible that glycogen depletion in given muscle fibers may contribute to an overall decrease in performance. Hence, the continued interest in manipulating muscle glycogen stores.

Jose-Cunilleras et al (2006) unsuccessfully attempted to alter muscle glycogen through the feeding of starch-rich meals. In another study feeding horses a diet high in nonstructural carbohydrates (50.9% starch) resulted in higher muscle glycogen concentrations 48 and 72 hours after intense exercise compared to the feeding of diets with low (4.3% starch) or moderate (26.4%) amounts of nonstructural carbohydrate (Lacombe et al 2004). However, to accomplish this, the "high" diet consisted of only 21% hay, with the rest of the diet consisting primarily of 37% corn, 20% oats, and 20% cracked barley. Such a diet would not be typically recommended. In conclusion, attempts to enhance glycogen stores through the feeding of a starch-rich diet have either been unsuccessful or require the feeding of starch at concentrations so great as to raise health concerns. Similarly, attempts to hasten glycogen replenishment after exercise by feeding high levels of carbohydrates have been met with mixed results. Snow and Harris (1991) reported a return to resting muscle glycogen concentrations 2–3 days after 1600 m gallops when horses consumed a mixed diet of pelleted feed and hay. This rate of glycogen replenishment was similar to that observed in an earlier study in which horses were fed a low carbohydrate diet consisting mainly of hay (Snow et al 1987) providing 20.8 Mcal DE per day, but not as fast as when the horses of this earlier study were fed a normal or high carbohydrate diet providing about 32.5 Mcal DE per day.

Generally it is the concentrate portion of the diet that is considered to be high in nonstructural (or "soluble") carbohydrates though, under certain circumstances, it may be possible for performance horses to obtain sufficient amounts from the roughage they consume, particularly if they are consuming young, fresh vegetation. Although not common practice, there have been racehorses that have successfully competed while receiving minimal or no grain. They were able to meet their energy requirements on forage alone.

It has been suggested that since horses evolved as a hindgut fermenter, that use low to moderate quality fermentable roughage carbohydrates as their main energy source, they have a relatively limited ability to utilize large amounts of nonstructural carbohydrates in a manner that would allow glycogen synthesis to occur as rapidly as is seen in humans and rodents (Waller & Lindinger 2010). Another potential explanation for the limited benefits seen with trying to enhance glycogen storage in horses may be due to the short duration of the studies reported, as horses have been shown to only gradually increase glucose transport rates over a 2-month period while on a high nonstructural carbohydrate diet as compared to a forage-only diet (Dyer et al 2009). Therefore, a rapid change in diet from one low in nonstructural carbohydrates to one high in nonstructural carbohydrates may not have the same effect as if the horses had been maintained on that diet for an extended period.

Horses also did not evolve eating diets containing substantial amounts of fat or oil. However, it is now common to add fat or oil to the diet as one way to increase the energy density of the ration and ensure adequate DE intake. Some intensely exercising horses seem not to be able to consume sufficient quantities of a traditional diet consisting of hay and grain to meet requirements. Adding oil or fat to the diet also is typically accompanied by a decrease in the amount of nonstructural carbohydrates in the ration, which might be advantageous (Julliand et al 2006 see also Chapter 7). Even feeding high fat containing oats, as compared to regular oats, has been proposed as a way to decrease the amount of grain, and accompanying starch, that needs to be fed to meet dietary energy requirements (Lindberg et al 2006; Chapter 17).

Feeding diets containing elevated amounts of oil or fat has been shown in some (but not all studies) to result in an increase in muscle glycogen stores (Potter et al 1992, Geelen et al 2001). Likewise, it has also been suggested to have a glycogen-sparing effect in which fat is used preferentially to glycogen when a horse is working aerobically allowing glycogen to be spared for when a horse is working anaerobically (Pagan et al 2002, Treiber et al 2008). Plasma lactate has also been shown to be decreased post-exercise in horses fed a high fat diet (11.8% fat on a total DM basis) as compared to a low-fat diet (1.5% fat) suggesting the potential to enhance performance by delaying lactate accumulation and the onset of fatigue (Sloet van Oldruitenborgh-Oosterbaan et al 2002).

Fermentation of carbohydrates is accompanied by the release of heat. This can be useful in cold climates in helping to keep the horse warm. However, in warmer climates, or for the exercising horse that already has a challenge in dissipating extra heat generated through muscle contractions, this can be a disadvantage. Reducing the fiber fraction of the diet by replacing with calories from fat or oil, results in less heat being generated in the hindgut, potentially assisting with overall management of heat load (Potter et al 1990, Kronfeld 1996).

Fat can be included at the upper limits of cost effectiveness and practicality, having been shown to have no negative effects on digestibility at the inclusion rate of up to 20% (Swinney et al 1995). Issues associated with feed handling, palatability, and diminished benefits relative to the cost are reasons why high-end inclusion rates are typically limited to 10% of the total diet. One could expect greater benefits for higher inclusion rates for racehorses in heavy training that would be training and racing greater distances, such as Thoroughbreds and Standardbreds, than one would expect for horses with lower energy requirements that race short distances such as racing Quarter Horses. However, direct comparisons between breeds for ideal inclusion rate have not been made. Additionally, most studies have examined only one form of fat or oil at a time (the common ones tested include corn oil, vegetable oil, and rendered animal fat). Without specific research documenting advantages to performance of one form of fat or oil over another, decisions are often made on cost, availability, and palatability with corn oil often being considered (anecdotally) the most palatable.

Despite health concerns for humans consuming a high-fat diet, no adverse effects have been reported when feeding a high-fat diet (up to 10% of total diet) for over a year compared to horses fed a moderate starch (19%) diet (Zeyner et al 2002). One of the reasons may simply be that a high-fat diet for a horse is usually considered to be around 10% of the total intake, which would be considered a relatively low-fat diet in human nutrition.

Key Points

- Racehorses are often fed diets containing large amounts of concentrate or grain mixes to aid in meeting energy needs
- High nutritional quality roughages should be provided as they contribute greatly to the energy content of the diet
- Nonstructural (soluble) carbohydrates are often incorporated into the diet through the inclusion of grain and may enhance glycogen storage
- Diets high in fats or oils can aid in meeting energy requirements while lowering dietary starch and risk of conditions associated with high starch feeding

Recommendations for pre-exercise feeding

Besides the importance of providing a balanced diet, time of feeding with respect to an exercise bout may influence performance (Harris & Graham-Thiers 1999). Restricting hay intake to about 1% of body weight for three days prior to exercise, compared to allowing horses ad libitum access to hay, resulted in a 2% decrease in body weight (Rice et al 2001). Hay restriction also resulted in an increase in the mass specific rate of oxygen consumption during sprint exercise and a corresponding decrease in anaerobic energy expenditure. However, as very few horses in intense performance work are currently fed ad libitum forage, further work is needed to determine optimal forage feeding practices in the days leading up to a race.

Likewise, there is not sufficient published information to give precise advice on when to feed concentrates in the immediate pre-race period. Nonetheless, current recommendations include keeping pre-exercise meals small (typically less than 1 kg) and typically not within 2–3 hours of a race. If fed a grain meal within 3 hours of exercise, elevated insulin and decreased glucose concentrations have been reported to occur in research studies and these alterations may affect performance. There is reason to believe that the psychological response to actual competition might override any negative effect of the hypoglycemia that may accompany the feeding a grain meal shortly before exercise. Even if that is true, other physiological changes that accompany meal feeding may still have an influence on performance including a large decrease in plasma volume (Clarke et al 1990). To avoid potential performance-limiting physiological changes, grain should be withheld from horses for a few hours prior to exercise though small quantities of hay (again, perhaps a kilogram or less) can be fed (Pagan & Harris 1999). The roughage can promote chewing and salivation without excessive gut fill and can also help prevent "boredom" and aid in keeping a horse calm. There has been recent work suggesting feeding alfalfa hay can aid in gastric buffering (Nadeau et al 2000, Vervuert & Coenen 2004) so using a roughage that includes alfalfa may be helpful.

Water is also often withheld for a period of time before races, often up to 4 hours (Pinchbeck et al 2004). Withholding water during this period will not cause performance-limiting dehydration (although potentially more subtle adverse effects have not been evaluated) but should prevent unnecessary weight carriage. After a race and before a horse has cooled down, it is advisable to provide water to the horse. Allowing the horse to take short drinks while hot will aid in rehydrating the horse and likely will shorten recovery time.

Supplements

There are few dietary supplements provided to racehorses that have been scientifically shown to have an effect on performance. Part of the reason is that it is difficult to design a study that can detect differences in performance that may be small, but still economically important. A 2% improvement in performance may be difficult to demonstrate in a research setting without a large number of horses, but it can result in a difference of a couple of seconds in a race lasting 2 minutes – which could mean the difference between winning a race and losing by a large margin. This may explain why trainers still use supplements even if no actual evidence exists as to their efficacy (or safety!) in the horse. Certainly given the cost of most supplements, the author recommends trying to determine if there is any basis to the marketing claims of new supplements prior to using.

Below are a few personal comments on supplements more commonly used within the racing industry. Commercial iron supplements or iron-containing tonics are commonly used to improve an apparent anemia (even though iron deficiency anemia in the adult horse is rare) or with the intent of improving oxygen utilization by increasing the percent hemoglobin or packed cell volume even though research has not shown any such effect (Loch et al 1984). In humans, oral administration of creatine has been shown to increase muscle total creatine pool (Harris et al 1992) and enhanced sprinting performance (Harris et al 1993). However, no studies appear to support the use of creatine in horses. Dimethylglycine (DMG) is an ergogenic agent marketed to horse owners and trainers as a method of reducing lactate accumulation (Warren et al 1999). At this time, controlled and well-designed studies do not support use of DMG. Bee pollen is frequently fed to racehorses with the belief that it improves athletic performance and increases appetite. A study by Turner et al (2006) did not detect an effect on performance but did find that the horses supplemented with bee pollen had greater dry matter intake while on a digestibility trial than did control horses. As that study was done with a limited number of horses, it is necessary to repeat the work before conclusions can be drawn.

Other supplements that have been studied and that are commonly provided to racehorses include agents to calm horses. Anecdotally, L-tryptophan has been reported to have a calming effect on horses and is included in many "calming" products sold (Harris 2005, see Chapter 25). Ironically, the low doses found in many commercial products may actually induce mild excitement while high doses seem to reduce endurance capacity (Grimmett & Sillence 2005). Thus, at this time, its use could not be justified, though research will undoubtedly continue to determine tryptophan's ability to alter behavior. Supplemental magnesium and thiamin have also been suggested to have a calming effect. While magnesium sulfate was used as an intravenous anesthetic agent many years ago and, hence, there is some basis to the belief (but no current evidence), there is no work to show that thiamin supplementation has any effect on behavior.

One supplement that has reported benefits is sodium zeolite A, which has been shown to be a bio-available source of silicon (Nielsen et al 1993). Silicon deficiency has been linked with abnormal connective and bone tissue metabolism and may result in skeletal abnormalities (Pérez-Granados & Vaquero 2002). Silicon is the second most common element of the Earth's crust and is found throughout the environment, so it is unlikely a horse would become deficient. However, providing a source that can be readily absorbed may be useful as absorption varies widely amongst sources (Sripanyakorn et al 2009). Additionally, in man, several factors including exercise appear to reduce the ability to absorb silicon suggesting athletes may require increased silicon in the diet (Pérez-Granados & Vaquero 2002). Utilizing 53 horses in race training in a controlled, blinded study, reductions in injury rates, increased training distance until injured and reduced race times were observed in treated horses (particularly in the medium dosage group consuming diets containing 1.32% sodium zeolite A) as compared to controls (Nielsen et al 1993). However, there are a number of concerns with the supplementation of sodium zeolite A. It seems to require a fairly large dosage to achieve the optimal response. In addition, supplementation currently is associated with high intakes of aluminum. Whilst no detrimental effects have been shown in horses, if the positive effects are truly due to silicon and not some other part of the sodium zeolite A molecule, a silicon source that limits aluminum intake may be preferable (O'Connor et al 2008). Orthosilic acid is one such source that appears to have beneficial effects in a laboratory setting (Sripanyakorn et al 2005) and may prove useful in the horse.

Poor appetite

Racehorses in heavy training anecdotally often seem to lose their appetite and "go off feed". Given their high-energy requirements, this can lead to weight loss and reduced performance. Poor appetite is a commonly accepted clinical sign of gastric ulceration (van den Wollenberg & Sloet van Oldruitenborgh-Oosterbaan 2000) and therefore it is important to eliminate this as a cause. However, beyond that, little research has been done to examine the issue of exercise-induced inappetance (Gordon et al 2006) although there has been work undertaken on the "overtraining syndrome" (Rivero et al 2008), which can be associated with depressed appetite (Tyler et al 1996). As mentioned above anecdotal evidence suggests supplementation with B-vitamins may help to restore appetite in heavily exercising horses. Thiamin requirements have been suggested to be elevated in exercising horses (Topliff et al 1981) and dietary supplementation with a thiamin-containing product has been linked to increased feed intake (Turner et al 2006). Additionally, when a high starch diet is consumed, as is the case with many racehorses, greater amounts of propionate is produced. Vitamin B_{12} is necessary to metabolize the propionate and, if deficient in the diet, potentially could result in an accumulation of propionate and a resultant decrease in appetite (Frape 1989). While strong scientific proof does not yet exist to substantiate it, providing supplemental B-vitamins to a horse that has lost its appetite is one approach that may be helpful.

Conclusion

Despite the importance of optimal nutrition to athletic performance, many questions remain unanswered in terms of optimal feeding of the racehorse. As with the research into supplements, determining if dietary manipulations alter performance can be challenging due to the many other factors that influence performance. These can vary from trial to trial and include the rider/driver, track surface, weather conditions, and even the other horses that a research subject may be competing against! While treadmill studies are able to remove some of these variables, conditions would not be considered "real world" and it can still be difficult to pick up small treatment differences that could have a meaningful impact on actual race results.

That being said, it is recognized that an inadequate intake of energy will compromise racing performance, as will continued excessive energy intake. While it is unclear if providing large amounts of nonstructural carbohydrates can aid in enhancing glycogen stores, attempting to do so through such means carries certain health risks. In contrast, meeting energy needs through providing diets containing up to 10% fat or oil may provide benefits with limited risks. Quality, highly digestible forage plays an important role in meeting energy demands and should not be overlooked. Such forage can also provide a substantial amount of the protein required by the exercising horse and aid in meeting the amino acid requirements.

Mineral requirements can vary greatly with the stage and intensity of training but usually are increased in the exercising horse. In particular, the requirements for electrolytes can increase dramatically due to their loss through sweat. With training programs that involve substantial amounts of exercise or with horses trained in hot environments, electrolyte requirements can be substantially greater than those for maintenance. Specific additional requirements for vitamins associated with an increased exercise load are less well defined. Fortunately, if horses are provided access to fresh pasture or recently harvested green hay, and/or if provided a balanced fortified commercial concentrate, the vitamin requirements of most athletic horses should be met.

References

Antilley, T.J., Potter, G.D., Gibbs, P.G., et al., 2007. Evaluating the technique of using nitrogen retention as a response criterion for amino acid studies in the horse. Journal of Equine Veterinary Science 27 (12), 525–530.

Becvarova, I., Pleasant, R.S., Thatcher, C.D., 2009. Clinical assessment of nutritional status and feeding program in horses. Veterinary Clinics of North America 25 (1), 1–21.

Butudom, P., Axiak, S.M., Nielsen, B.D., et al., 2003. Effect of varying initial drink volume on rehydration of horses. Physiology & Behavior 79 (2), 135–142.

Carroll, F.D., Goss, H., Howell, C.E., 1949. The synthesis of B vitamins in the horse. Journal of Animal Science 8, 290–296.

Casini, L., Gatta, D., Magni, L., et al., 2000. Effect of prolonged branched-chain amino acid supplementation on metabolic response to anaerobic exercise in standardbreds. Journal of Equine Veterinary Science 20, 120–123.

Clarke, L.C., Roberts, M.S., Argenzio, R.A., 1990. Feeding and digestive problems in horses. Veterinary Clinics of North American: Equine Practice 6, 433–449.

Clarkson, P.M., 1998. Nutritional supplements for weight gain. Sports Science Exchange 11 (1), 1–2.

Coenen, M., 2005. Exercise and stress: impact on adaptive processes involving water and electrolytes. Livestock Production Science 92 (2), 131–245.

Connysson, M., Muhonen, S., Lindberg, J.E., et al., 2006. Effects on exercise response, fluid and acid-base balance of protein intake from forage-only diets in Standardbred horses. Equine Veterinary Journal 36 (Suppl.), 648–653.

Custalow, B., 1991. Protein requirements during exercise in the horse. Journal of Equine Veterinary Science 11 (1), 65–266.

Dyer, J., Al-Ramahi, M., Waterfall, L., et al., 2009. Adaptive response of equine intestinal Na+/glucose co-transporter (SGLT1) to an increase in dietary soluble carbohydrates. Pflugers Archiv European Journal of Physiology 458, 419–430.

Elmore-Smith, K.A., Pipkin, J.L., Baker, L.A., et al., 1999. The effect of aerobic exercise after a sedentary period on serum, fecal, and urine calcium and phosphorus concentrations in mature horses. In: Proceedings 16th Equine Nutrition and Physiology Society Symposium. Raleigh, NC, USA, 2–2 June 1999, pp. 106–107.

Essen-Gustavsson, B., Connysson, M., Jansson, A., 2010. Effects of crude protein intake from forage-only diets on muscle amino acids and glycogen levels in horses in training. Equine Veterinary Journal 42 (Suppl. 38), 341–346.

Frape, D.L., 1989. Nutrition and the growth and racing performance of thoroughbred horses. Proceedings of the Nutrition Society 48, 141–252.

Frape, D.L., 1994. Diet and exercise performance in the horse. Proceedings of the Nutrition Society 53, 189–206.

Freeman, D.W., Potter, G.D., Schelling, G.T., et al., 1986. Nitrogen metabolism in the mature physically conditioned horse I. Response to conditioning. Equine Practice 8 (5), 6–29.

Freeman, D.W., Potter, G.D., Schelling, G.T., et al., 1988. Nitrogen metabolism in mature horses at varying levels of work. Journal of Animal Science 66, 407–412.

Gallagher, K., Leech, J., Stowe, H., 1992a. Protein, energy and dry matter consumption by racing Standardbreds: a field survey. Journal of Equine Veterinary Science 12 (6), 382–388.

Gallagher, K., Leech, J., Stowe, H., 1992b. Protein, energy and dry matter consumption by racing Thoroughbreds: a field survey. Journal of Equine Veterinary Science 12 (1), 43–48.

Geelen, S.N., Sloet van Oldruitenborgh-Oosterbaan, M.M., Beyen, A.C., 2001. Supplemental fat in the diet of horses…is it advantageous? Tijdschr Diergeneeskd 126 (9), 310–315.

Gordon, M.E., McKeever, K.H., Bokman, S., et al., 2006. Training-induced energy balance mismatch in Standardbred mares. Equine and Comparative Exercise Physiology 3 (2), 73–82.

Graham-Thiers, P.M., Bowen, L.K., 2011. The effect of time of feeding on plasma amino acids during exercise and recovery. Journal of Equine Veterinary Science 31, 281–282.

Graham-Thiers, P.M., Kronfeld, D.S., Kline, K.A., et al., 2000. Protein status of exercising Arabian horses fed diets containing 14% or 7.5% crude protein fortified with lysine and threonine. Journal of Equine Veterinary Science 20, 516–521.

Graham-Thiers, P.M., Kronfeld, D.S., Kline, K.A., et al., 2001. Dietary protein restriction and fat supplementation diminish the acidogenic effect of exercise during repeated sprints in horses. Journal of Nutrition 131, 1959–1964.

Grimmett, A., Sillence, M.N., 2005. Calmatives for the excitable horse: a review of L-tryptophan. Veterinary Journal 170, 24–32.

Hamlin, M.J., Hopkins, W.G., 2003. Retrospective trainer-reported incidence and predictors of health and training-related problems in Standardbred horses. Journal of Equine Veterinary Science 23 (10), 443–452.

Harkins, J.D., Morris, G.S., Tulley, R.T., et al., 1992. Effect of added dietary fat on racing performance in Thoroughbred horses. Journal of Equine Veterinary Science 12, 123–129.

Harkins, J.D., Kamerling, S.G., 1993. Effect of race distance and competition on performance of Thoroughbred racehorses. Journal of Equine Veterinary Science 13 (1), 41–45.

Harris, P.A., 2005. Nutrition, behaviour and the role of supplements for calming horses: The veterinarian's dilemma. The Veterinary Journal 170, 10–21.

Harris, P.A., 2009. Feeding management of elite endurance horses. Veterinary Clinics of North America: Equine Practice 25, 137–153.

Harris, P.A., Graham-Thiers, P.M., 1999. To evaluate the influence that "feeding" state may exert on metabolic and physiological responses to exercise. Equine Veterinary Journal 30 (Suppl.), 633–636.

Harris, P.A., Harris, R.C., 2005. Ergogenice potential of nutritional strategies and substances in the horse. Livestock Production Sciences 92, 147–165.

Harris, R.C., Sodehund, K., Hultman, E., 1992. Evaluation of creatine in resting and exercised muscle of normal subjects by creatine supplementation. Clinical Science 83, 367–374.

Harris, R.C., Viru, M., Greenhaff, P.L., et al., 1993. The effect of oral creatine supplementation on running performance during short-term exercise in man. Journal of Physiology 467, 74P.

Henneke, D.R., Potter, G.D., Kreider, J.L., et al., 1983. Relationship between condition score, physical measurements and body fat percentages in mares. Equine Veterinary Journal 15 (4), 371–372.

Hinchcliff, K.W., McKeever, K.H., Muir, W.W., et al., 1996. Furosemide reduces accumulated oxygen deficit in horses during brief intense exertion. Journal of Applied Physiology 81, 1550–1554.

Huff, A.N., White, H.E., Meacham, T.N., 1985. Hays for horses. Journal of Equine Veterinary Science 5, 173–175.

Jones, D.L., Potter, G.D., Greene, L.W., et al., 1992. Muscle glycogen in exercised miniature horses at various body conditions and fed a control or fat-supplemented diet. Journal of Equine Veterinary Science 12 (5), 287–291.

Jose-Cunilleras, E., Hinchcliff, K.W., Lacombe, V.A., et al., 2006. Ingestion of starch-rich meals after exercise increases glucose kinetics but fails to enhance muscle glycogen replenishment in horses. Veterinary Journal 171, 468–477.

Julliand, V., De Fombelle, A., Varloud, M., 2006. Starch digestion in horses: the impact of feed processing. Livestock Science 100, 44–52.

Kapper, D.R., 2004. Applied nutrition. In: Reed, S., Bayly, W.M., Sellon, C. (Eds.), Equine Internal Medicine, second ed. Saunders, St. Louis, Missouri, pp. 1543–1605.

Kearns, C.F., McKeever, K.H., Kumagai, K., et al., 2002. Fat-free mass is related to one-mile race performance in elite Standardbred horses. Veterinary Journal 163, 260–266.

Kronfeld, D.S., 1996. Dietary fat affects heat production and other variables of equine performance, under hot and humid conditions. Equine Veterinary Journal 22 (Suppl.), 24–34.

Lacombe, V.A., Hinchcliff, K.W., Geor, R.J., et al., 2001. Muscle glycogen depletion and subsequent replenishment affect anaerobic capacity of horses. Journal of Applied Physiology 91, 1782–1790.

Lacombe, V.A., Hinchcliff, K.W., Kohn, C.W., et al., 2004. Effects of feeding meals with various soluble-carbohydrate content on muscle glycogen synthesis after exercise in horses. American Journal of Veterinary Research 65, 916–923.

Lim, A.S., 1981. Body weight and performance in racehorses. In: Bourke, J.M., Ashelford, P.J. (Eds.), Proceedings 4th International Conference on Control of the Use of Drugs in Racehorses. Victorian Racing Club, Melbourne, Australia, pp. 93–94.

Lindberg, J.E., Essen-Gustavsson, B., Dahlborn, K., et al., 2006. Exercise response, metabolism at rest and digestibility in athletic horses fed high-fat oats. Equine Veterinary Journal 36 (Suppl.), 626–630.

Lin, W.-T., Yang, S.-C., Tsai, S.-C., et al., 2006. L-arginine attenuates xanthine oxidase and myeloperoxidase activities in hearts of rats during exhaustive exercise. British Journal of Nutrition 95, 67–75.

Loch, W.E., Brockschmidt, L., Harmon, H., 1984. Effect of supplemental iron, live saccharomyces cerevisiae yeast and exercise on hemoglobin and packed cell volume of the blood of horses. Journal of Equine Veterinary Science 4 (3), 125–127.

Matsui, A., Ohmura, H., Asai, Y., et al., 2006. Effect of amino acid and glucose administration following exercise on the turnover of muscle protein in the hindlimb femoral region of Thoroughbreds. Equine Veterinary Journal 36 (Suppl.), 611–616.

Meyer, H., 1987. Nutrition of the equine athlete. In: Gillespie, J.R., Robinson, N.E. (Eds.), Equine Exercise Physiology 2. ICEEP Publications, Davis, CA, pp. 644–673.

Morgan, K., 1997. Thermal insulance of peripheral tissue and coat in sport horses. Journal of Thermal Biology 22 (3), 169–175.

Nadeau, J.A., Andrews, F.M., Mathew, A.G., et al., 2000. Evaluation of diet as a cause of gastric ulcers in horses. American Journal of Veterinary Research 61 (7), 784–790.

Nielsen, B.D., Potter, G.D., Morris, E.L., et al., 1993. Training distance to failure in young racing Quarter Horses fed sodium zeolite A. Journal of Equine Veterinary Science 13 (10), 562–567.

Nielsen, B.D., Potter, G.D., Morris, E.L., et al., 1997. Changes in the third metacarpal bone and frequency of bone injuries in young Quarter Horses during race training – observations and theoretical considerations. Journal of Equine Veterinary Science 17 (10), 541–549.

Nielsen, B.D., Potter, G.D., Greene, L.W., et al., 1998. Response of young horses in training to varying concentrations of dietary calcium and phosphorus. Journal of Equine Veterinary Science 18 (6), 397–404.

Nielsen, B.D., Turner, K.T., Ventura, B.A., et al., 2006. Racing speeds of Quarter Horses, Thoroughbreds and Arabians. Equine Veterinary Journal 36 (Suppl.), 128–132.

NRC., 1989. Nutrient requirements of horses, fifth rev. ed. National Academy Press, Washington, DC.

NRC., 2007. Nutrient requirements of horses, sixth rev. ed. National Academy Press, Washington, DC.

Nunamaker, D.M., Butterweck, D.M., Provost, M.T., 1989. Some geometric properties of the third metacarpal bone: a comparison between the Thoroughbred and Standardbred racehorse. Journal Biomechanics 22 (2), 129–134.

O'Connor, C.I., Nielsen, B.D., Schott, H.C., et al., 2002. Effects of weight carrying exercise and a myo-anabolic supplement on growth and muscle. Equine Veterinary Journal 34 (Suppl.), 178–181.

O'Connor, C.I., Nielsen, B.D., Woodward, A.D., et al., 2008. Mineral balance in horses fed two supplemental silicon sources. Journal of Animal Physiology and Animal Nutrition 92, 173–181.

Pagan, J.D., Harris, P.A., 1999. The effects of timing and amount of forage and grain on exercise response in Thoroughbred horses. Equine Veterinary Journal 30 (Suppl.), 451–457.

Pagan, J.D., Hintz, H.F., 1986. Equine energetics. II. Energy expenditure in horses during submaximal exercise. Journal of Animal Science 63, 822–830.

Pagan, J.D., Nash, D., 2009. Nutrition of the young equine athlete. In: Pagan, J.D. (Eds.), Advances in Equine Nutrition IV. Nottingham University Press, United Kingdom, pp. 161–171.

Pagan, J., Geor, R., Harris, P., et al., 2002. Effects of fat adaptation on glucose kinetics and substrate oxidation during low intensity exercise. Equine Veterinary Journal 34 (Suppl.), 33–38.

Pérez-Granados, A.M., Vaquero, M.P., 2002. Silicon, aluminium, arsenic and lithium; essentiality and human health implications. Journal of Nutrition, Health, and Aging 6, 154–162.

Pinchbeck, G.L., Clegg, P.D., Proudman, C., et al., 2004. Horse injuries and racing practices in National Hunt racehorses in the UK: the results of a prospective cohort study. Veterinary Journal 167, 45–52.

Porr, C.A., Kronfeld, D.S., Lawrence, L.A., et al., 1998. Deconditioning reduces mineral content of the third metacarpal bone in horses. Journal of Animal Science 76, 1875–1879.

Potter, G.D., Hughes, S.L., Julen, T.R., et al., 1992. A review of research on digestion and utilization of fat by the equine. Pferdeheilkunde Sonderheft 1, 119–123.

Potter, G.D., Webb, S.P., Evans, J.W., et al., 1990. Digestible energy requirements for work and maintenance of horses fed conventional and fat-supplemented diets. Journal of Equine Veterinary Science 10 (3), 214–218.

Pratt, G.W., 1991. Clocking the fastest horses on earth. Quarter Racing Journal 4, 36–40.

Rice, O., Geor, R., Harris, P., et al., 2001. Effects of restricted hay intake on body weight and metabolic responses to high-intensity exercise in Thoroughbred horses. In: Proceedings 17th Equine Nutrition and Physiology Society Symposium. Lexington, KY, USA, 31 May-2 June 2001, pp. 273–279.

Rivero, J.L.L., van Breda, E., Rogers, C.W., et al., 2008. Unexplained underperformance syndrome in sport horses: classification, potential causes and recognition. Equine Veterinary Journal 40, 611–618.

Saastamoinen, M.T., Harris, P.A., 2008. Vitamin requirements and supplementation in athletic horses. In: Saastamoinen, M.T., Martin-Rosset, W. (Eds.), Nutrition of the Exercising Horse. EAAP Publication No. 125. Wageningen Academic Publishers, Netherlands, pp. 233–255.

Scott, B.D., Potter, G.D., Greene, L.W., et al., 1992. Efficacy of a fat-supplemented diet on muscle glycogen concentrations in exercising Thoroughbred horses maintained in varying body conditions. Journal of Equine Veterinary Science 12 (2), 109–213.

Shearman, J.P., Hopkins, W.G., 1996. Training of Standardbred maiden pacers. Journal of Equine Veterinary Science 16, 116–219.

Sloet van Oldruitenborgh-Oosterbaan, M.M., Annee, M.P., Verdegaal, E.J., et al., 2002. Exercise- and metabolism-associated blood variables in Standardbreds fed either a low- or a high-fat diet. Equine Veterinary Journal 34 (Suppl.), 29–32.

Snow, D.H., Harris, R.C., 1991. Effects of daily exercise on muscle glycogen in the Thoroughbred racehorse. In: Persson, S.G.B., Lindholm, A., Jeffcott, L.B. (Eds.), Equine Exercise Physiology 3. ICEEP Publications, Uppsala, Sweden, pp. 299–304.

Snow, D.H., Harris, R.C., Harman, R.C., et al., 1987. Glycogen repletion following different diets. In: Gillespie, J.R., Robinson, N.E. (Eds.), Equine Exercise Physiology 2. ICEEP Publications, CA, pp. 701–710.

Sripanyakorn, S., Jugdaohsingh, R.,Thompson, R.P.H., et al., 2005. Dietary silicon and bone health. Nutrition Bulletin 30, 222–230.

Sripanyakorn, S., Jugdaohsingh, R., Dissayabutr, W., et al., 2009. The comparative absorption of silicon from different foods and food supplements. British Journal of Nutrition 102, 825–834.

Stefanon, B., Bettini, C., Guggia, P., 2000. Administration of branched-chain amino acids to Standardbred horses in training. Journal of Equine Veterinary Science 20, 115–119.

Stephens, T.L., Potter, G.D., Mathiason, K.J., et al., 2001. Mineral balance in juvenile horses in race training. In: Proceedings 17th Equine Nutrition and Physiology Society Symposium. Lexington, KY, USA, 30 May-2 June 2001, pp. 26–31.

Swinney, D.L., Potter, G.D., Greene, L.W., et al., 1995. Digestion of fat in the equine small and large intestine. In: Proceedings 14th Equine Nutrition and Physiology Society Symposium. Ontario, CA, USA, January 19–21, pp. 30–35.

Thornton, J., Pagan, J., Persson, S., 1987. The oxygen cost of weight-loading and inclined treadmill exercise in the horse. In: Equine Exercise Physiology 2. ICEEP Publications, CA, pp. 206–215.

Tipton, K.D., Rasmussen, B.B., Miller, S.L., et al., 2001. Timing of amino acid-carbohydrate ingestion alters anabolic response of muscle to resistance exercise. American Journal of Physiology – Endocrinology and Metabolism 281, E197–E206.

Topliff, D.R., Potter, G.D., Kreider, J.L., et al., 1981. Thiamin supplementation for exercising horses. In: Proceedings 7th Equine Nutrition and Physiology

Society Symposium. Warrenton, VA, USA, April-2 May 1981, pp. 167–172.
Treiber, K.H., Geor, R.J., Boston, R.C., et al., 2008. Dietary energy source affects glucose kinetics in trained Arabian geldings at rest and during endurance exercise. Journal of Nutrition 138, 964–970.
Turner, K.K., Nielsen, B.D., O'Connor, C.I., et al., 2006. Bee pollen product supplementation to horses in training seems to improve feed intake: a pilot study. Journal of Animal Physiology and Animal Nutrition 90, 414–420.
Tyler, C.M., Golland, L.C., Evans, D.L., et al., 1996. Changes in maximum oxygen uptake during prolonged training, overtraining, and detraining in horses. Journal of Applied Physiology 81, 2244–2249.
van den Wollenberg, L., Sloet van Oldruitenborgh-Oosterbaan, M.M., 2000. Gastric ulceration in horses: etiology, diagnosis, and therapy: a review. Tijdschrift voor Diergeneeskunde 125 (21), 642–647.
Verheyen, K.L.P., Price, J.S., Wood, J.L.N., 2009. Exercise during training is associated with racing performance in Thoroughbreds. Veterinary Journal 181, 43–47.
Vervuert, I., Coenen, M., 2004. Nutritional risk factors of equine gastric ulcer syndrome. Pferdeheilkunde 20, 349–352.
Waller, A.P., Heigenhauser, G.J., Geor, R.J., et al., 2009. Fluid and electrolyte supplementation after prolonged moderate-intensity exercise enhances muscle glycogen resynthesis in Standardbred horses. Journal of Applied Physiology 106, 91–100.
Waller, A.P., Lindinger, M.I., 2010. Nutritional aspects of post exercise skeletal muscle glycogen synthesis in horses: a comparative review. Equine Veterinary Journal 42, 274–281.
Warren, L.K., Lawrence, L.M., Thompson, K.N., 1999. The influence of betaine on untrained and trained horses exercising to fatigue. Journal of Animal Science 77, 677–684.
Webb, S.P., Potter, G.D., Evans, J.W., et al., 1990. Influence of body fat content on digestible energy requirements of exercising horses in temperate and hot environments. Journal of Equine Veterinary Science 10, 116–120.
Wolter, R., 1987. La nutrition de l'animal de sport. Science Sports 2 (2), 63–73.
Wolter, R., 1993. Fibre in the feeding of horses. Practique Veterinaire Equine 25, 45–49.
Worth, M., 1985. Muscle fatigue in the horse: a review. Journal of Equine Veterinary Science 5, 276–278.
Zeyner, A., Bessert, J., Gropp, J.M., 2002. Effect of feeding exercised horses on high-starch or high-fat diets for 390 days. Equine Veterinary Journal 34 (Suppl.), 50–57.

14 Nutritional management of elite endurance horses

Patricia A. Harris, Harold C. Schott II

The sport of endurance racing is probably the most demanding of the equine athletic disciplines, with horses required to complete distances of up to 160 km in a single day (and over longer distances during multi-day races). In the past, races tended to be over longer distances and at relatively slow speeds e.g. the winner in an event in Berlin in 1892 travelled 597 km at an average speed of 8.4 km/h, but recently, particularly at the international level, the trend has been for very high racing speeds. The winner of the 2005 World Equine Endurance Championship race in Dubai, for example, covered the 160 km distance at an average speed of 22.5 km/h (~14 miles/h) and the winner of the 2010 World Equestrian Games (WEG) race in Lexington competed at an average speed of 21 km/h (~13 miles/h). In addition, the top three finishers of the 2010 WEG competition completed the final loop at speeds of 30 km/h (~18 miles/h)! These high work rates pose several challenges for the endurance horse. First, high energy demands may result in depletion of substrate stores, particularly muscle and liver glycogen, resulting in a decline in performance. Second, as the evaporation of sweat is the major mechanism for heat dissipation during exercise, there is a substantial loss of body water and electrolytes (especially sodium and chloride). Failure to mitigate the resultant dehydration and electrolyte losses via replacement strategies is another potential reason for poor performance and elimination from the race. Additionally, dehydration and electrolyte imbalances may increase risk for the development of metabolic problems including heat stress, synchronous diaphragmatic flutter, ileus and rhabdomyolysis. In a survey of horses that participated in 16 CEI or CEN events in France, depending on the ride 27.8–69% (mean 50%) were disqualified and between 4.6–17.6% (mean 10.5%) had to be treated (Robert 2004). The frequency of elimination for lameness (~41%) and for metabolic reasons (~40%) was very similar in this survey. The most common clinical diagnoses were dehydration (~26%), colic (~17%), exhaustion syndrome (~13%) and tying up (~13%). It can be argued that appropriate nutritional management may help reduce the incidence of metabolic problems that result in race disqualification and/or the need for veterinary intervention.

It is important to consider that whilst only mature horses (at least 5 years old) can compete in FEI affiliated endurance races (even as novices) these horses will have been trained for many years in order to be fit both "mentally" and physically for such competitions and there are age restrictions for each level of competition (e.g., for the top 4-Star competitions and Championships horses must be at least 8 years of age). If we take the perfect endurance horse as being one that "stays healthy and sound" and wins then many factors are involved, the most obvious being: genetics (intrinsic ability), conformation, training, and veterinary and paraprofessional support. However, nutrition and management have both enabling and supporting roles to play. Appropriate nutrition during the training period and the race itself can help to reduce the incidence of metabolic problems. One major nutritional challenge is to adjust the feeding in harmony with the individual and its level of training exercise; the other is the race itself. It is therefore very important for all those involved in this complex sport to have a good understanding of nutritional practices. However, it must be realized that sound nutrition will only help a horse to be able to compete optimally – it will not improve the intrinsic ability of the horse. Poor or inappropriate nutrition, on the other hand, may impose limits on an animal's ability to perform.

A number of factors will influence the choice of feeding program for an individual endurance horse (e.g., temperament, housing [pasture vs. confinement], level of training and competition, and owner/rider preference) such that there is no single correct way to feed "an endurance horse." Nonetheless, there are a few general principles that should guide development of a diet and feeding plan. The purpose of this chapter is to review guidelines for feeding management of endurance horses.

Energy metabolism

For athletic horses, the supply of energy from the diet is crucial to maintenance of body weight plus condition as well as the storage and availability of substrates needed to fuel muscular work. Thus, an increase in energy (i.e. caloric) intake is required for avoidance of weight loss, and probably loss of performance, in the face of the increased energy demands of training and competition. In addition, there is some evidence that the source of dietary energy can affect storage and utilization of the primary substrates used to fuel muscular work, namely glycogen (liver, skeletal muscle) and fat.

Body condition score (BCS) reflecting body fat content, (see Chapter 22) may influence performance during endurance rides. In one study of horses that competed in a 240 km (150 mile) ride, over 2 days, the average BCS (scale 1–9) was 4.7 and the percentage of body fat, estimated from ultrasound assessment (see Chapter 22) of rump fat thickness, was 7.8% (Lawrence et al 1992). Among the top finishers the estimated total fat was ~6.5% of body mass, whereas the fat content of non-finishers averaged ~11%. In another study, mean BCS of horses that completed the 160 km (100 mile) Tevis cup ride was 4.5 (measurement taken pre-ride), while all horses with a BCS less than three failed to finish (Garlinghouse & Burrill 1999). Horses eliminated for metabolic reasons had a mean pre-ride BCS of 2.9 as compared to a BCS of 4.5 in those disqualified for nonmetabolic problems such as lameness. The authors of this study suggested that, at least in more difficult rides such as the Tevis Cup, thin horses (i.e., BCS <3) might be at a disadvantage because of lower energy reserves (and potentially lower muscle mass) when compared to horses with higher body condition. Over-conditioned horses (BCS >6) also could have problems due to the extra weight carried plus the insulating effect (impairment to heat dissipation) of the additional subcutaneous adipose tissue (Garlinghouse & Burrill 1999, Langlois & Robert 2008). Similarly, in a recent study (Barnes et al 2010) of an Australian 160 km ride, horses that were eliminated for metabolic reasons weighed less pre-ride than those that completed (and interestingly appeared more dehydrated with greater electrolyte depletion at the mid-ride checkpoint). In general, feeding programs for endurance horses should target a BCS of around 4–4.5 on the 9-point scale. There are many potential pitfalls in trying to determine accurately, using theoretical equations, an individual's energy requirements (see Chapter 5). It is therefore important to appreciate the value in the functional "energy" check that the assessment of an individual animal's body condition provides.

The capacity for endurance exercise is dependent on the availability of substrate for the synthesis of adenosine triphosphate (ATP), the cell's energy "currency." Stored energy, in the form of muscle and liver glycogen, intramuscular and adipose triglycerides, along with glucose and fatty acids derived from the feed ingested during longer rides are used for ATP synthesis in working tissues. It has been estimated that a 450-kg horse has around 1400–2800 g muscle triglyceride, 40,000 g adipose triglyceride, 3000–4000 g muscle glycogen (1–2% skeletal muscle weight) and 100–200 g liver glycogen (Harris 1997). Fat stores are therefore comparatively larger, and it is currently thought depletion of muscle and liver glycogen stores (Farris et al 1998, Lacombe et al 2001) combined with fluid and electrolyte disturbances (Pösö et al 2004) are factors that contribute to fatigue in endurance racing.

Traditional aerobic conditioning endurance training is associated with an increase in skeletal muscle oxidative capacity and a decrease in anaerobic metabolism as well as alterations in fiber type and mitochondrial respiratory function (Serrano et al 2000, Votion et al 2010). Further work is needed to understand the type of training best suited to achieve the higher speeds of recent elite competitions. At low to moderate work intensities, oxidative phosphorylation (*aerobic metabolism*) of glucose and fatty acids is an efficient mechanism for regeneration of ATP. At higher workloads (e.g., canter and gallop), however, ATP demand cannot be met by oxidative metabolism alone and non-oxidative breakdown (*anaerobic metabolism*) of glycogen and glucose (fatty acids cannot be metabolized by anaerobic mechanisms) also contributes to ATP resynthesis. However, anaerobic glycolysis is far less efficient in terms of ATP yield per gram of glucose metabolized and also results in lactic acid accumulation within skeletal muscle, that may also contribute to the development of fatigue (Pösö et al 2004). Historically, aerobic metabolism of fatty acids was thought to predominate during endurance rides undertaken at an average speed of 12–14 km/h (8–9 miles/h) – with increasing contributions from anaerobic metabolism for only brief periods of time, e.g., during controlled "sprints" that some riders use at the beginning or at the end of the ride or when hill climbing. However, this assumption may not apply to modern, elite level endurance racing wherein the more sustained periods of high speed running will invoke a larger contribution from anaerobic metabolism and, therefore, greater demands for use of the more limited body glycogen stores. Even with the low rate of glycogen utilization during submaximal exercise (<15 km/h), if such exercise is continued for several hours, muscle glycogen stores may be depleted by more than 50–75% (Snow et al 1982). Therefore, there is increasing interest in the application of strategies (e.g. diet, training, racing strategy) that might reduce the rate or extent of glycogen utilization.

Key Points

- In general, feeding programs for endurance horses should target a BCS of around 4 – 4.5 on the 9 point scale
- Fatigue during endurance racing is likely to be due to depletion of muscle and liver glycogen stores combined with fluid and electrolyte disturbances
- The increasing speeds now expected at certain international rides challenge traditional concepts of the training and feeding of endurance horses

Energy requirements

Energy requirements for horses are most commonly expressed as megacalories (Mcal) or megajoules (MJ) of digestible energy (DE), where 1 Mcal = 4.184 MJ. For an endurance horse, energy needs depend not only on work duration and intensity but also on environmental conditions, terrain, weight of the rider and tack, ability of the rider, and fitness of the horse, etc. (Harris 1997, NRC 2007). In general terms, the requirement is the sum of *maintenance requirements plus an allowance for the work being undertaken*. Maintenance DE requirements for a 450 kg endurance horse (NRC 2007) are around 13.6–16.3 Mcal/day (~57–68 MJ/day). Training or competition requirements depend on the weight of the horse plus rider and tack as well as the speed of work (Harris 1997, NRC 2007). As illustrated in Table 14-1 (adapted from Pagan & Hintz 1986) a 450 kg horse (plus 75 kg for the rider and tack) performing a 3 h training ride at a medium trot (~250 m/min) would have an estimated additional DE requirement of 15 Mcal (63 MJ) giving a total requirement of ~29–31 Mcal (~120–130 MJ) for that day. The National Research Council (NRC)

Table 14-1 A Guide to Potential Digestible Energy (DE) Requirements above Maintenance at Various Speeds (Adapted from Pagan & Hintz 1986: DE (kJ per kilogram of Horse, Rider and Tack) $= 4.184 \times \{[e^{(3.02+0.0065y)} - 13.92] \times 0.06\}/0.57$ Where *y* is the Speed (Meters per Minute) and 0.57 Accounts for the Efficiency of Utilization of DE)

Gait	Speed (meters/min)	DE MCal/kg BW (of horse plus rider plus tack)/h	DE MJ/kg BW (of horse plus rider plus tack)/h
Slow walk	59	0.0017	0.0071
Fast walk	95	0.0025	0.0105
Slow trot	200	0.0065	0.0272
Medium trot	250	0.0095	0.03975
Fast Trot/slow canter	300	0.0137	0.0573
Medium canter	350	0.0195	0.0816

publication on nutrient requirements for horses (NRC 2007), uses a multiplier (1.9) over maintenance in order to estimated the requirements for elite endurance horses, which are included in the very heavy work load category. In this category maintenance requirements are taken at the elevated level, which might reflect the increased voluntary activity of such animals or perhaps help compensate for any extra energy costs associated with restoring and maintaining body energy stores. This also gives an estimated requirement value of ~31 Mcal/day (129 MJ/day) for a 450 kg horse. In a US survey of aspiring international level competitors (Crandell 2002) average estimated daily DE intake (from forage and supplementary feeds) during training was 24 Mcal (~100 MJ) for horses with an average body weight (BW) of 460 kg. However, many of the horses surveyed were kept at pasture and the estimate did not account for DE intake from pasture forage.

Horses are individuals and therefore actual DE requirements may deviate from calculated estimates, and vary widely among horses of similar bodyweight undertaking the same amount and type of work. From a practical aspect, weekly or biweekly monitoring and assessment of bodyweight and/or BCS (see Chapter 22) will enable the feeding program to be individually tailored.

Meeting energy requirements

The four main sources of energy (Harris 1997) in horse feeds are:

1. Fermentable fiber (includes cellulose, hemicellulose and pectins): these components are not digestible by mammalian enzymes but can be fermented by microorganisms predominantly located in the hindgut. Speed of fermentation as well as site likely influence the energy value to the horse.
2. Hydrolyzable carbohydrates (e.g., simple sugars and starches): these can be digested by mammalian enzymes to hexoses which are absorbed from the small intestine (SI) or, if they "escape" digestion in the SI, they are rapidly fermented in the hindgut, i.e., cecum and colon.
3. Oils/fats: although horses evolved on diets with low concentrations of oils and fats, they are able to digest and utilize up to 20% of the diet (dry matter basis) as oil, if suitably introduced (see further comments below).
4. Protein: protein is not primarily fed as an energy source because metabolism of amino acids to useable energy is inefficient relative to metabolism of carbohydrates and fats (see below for specific comments re protein requirements to support exercise activity and recovery).

Different feeds and feedstuffs contain differing amounts of gross energy. The efficiency of conversion from gross to useable or net energy also differs widely (Martin-Rosset et al 1994), both between the feedstuffs and between individual animals. Vegetable oils provide proportionally more net energy than the cereal grains (~2.5 times as much DE as maize/corn and three times as much as oats). Cereal grains, in turn, provide more net energy than hay, while the net energy from hay is twofold higher than that available from straw (Martin-Rosset et al 1994).

Forage should be the foundation

Forage should be the foundation of the diet for all horses. In the aforementioned US survey of feeding practices (Crandell 2002), about 80% of the horses had 24 h pasture turnout (with additional preserved forage provided some of the year). On average, 78% of the ration was forage which is higher in comparison to other sports horses (e.g. the ration of racehorses may be no more than 30% forage). Although there is currently no agreed upon requirement for dietary fiber, the inclusion of some long stem roughage in the diet is thought to be important for maintenance of hindgut function and health as well as for reduction in risk of gastric ulceration and abnormal behaviours (Goodwin et al 2002, Shirazi-Beechey 2008) and the authors currently recommend a minimum of 1.5% BW on a dry matter (DM) basis of long stem roughage or chopped long fiber (see also Chapter 26). Fiber may provide energy during an endurance ride via absorption of volatile fatty acids (acetate, propionate) produced by fermentation that continues long after the fiber has been ingested. Propionic acid from hindgut fermentation of fiber is also an important substrate for gluconeogenesis (Ford & Simmons 1985).

Some fiber sources (e.g., beet pulp, soya hulls) may augment the size of the large intestinal fluid reservoir, which may represent as much as 8–10% of bodyweight and 10–20% of total body Na, K and Cl (Meyer & Coenen 1989, Warren et al 2001, Parsons et al 2011). This may assist in the maintenance of hydration during exercise by acting as a reservoir for both water and electrolytes (Meyer & Coenen 1989). Extrapolating from studies in ponies (Meyer & Coenen 1989) during low intensity exercise, approximately 10 liters of water, 19 g of Na and 10 g of Cl may be absorbed from the gastrointestinal tract of horses during 2–3 h of exercise, potentially offsetting some of the sweat water and electrolyte losses that occur during endurance rides (Geor & Harris 2005). Recent work has suggested that differences in dietary fiber type, which affect total body water, may also influence core temperature during endurance type exercise (Spooner et al 2007). However, the potential benefits of a high-fiber diet with respect to improved water and electrolyte balance must be weighed against possible energetic disadvantages associated with an increase in hindgut weight (bowel ballast: Kronfeld 2001a, Chapter 26). The optimal mix of dietary fiber types is not known but it is common for endurance horses to consume a variety of fiber sources, including long stem hay, beet pulp and soya hulls (Kronfeld 2001b). Recent work has suggested that organic matter, DM and neutral detergent fiber digestibility may be higher after endurance conditioning but these adaptations were not systematically associated with a longer total tract mean retention time nor an increase in microbial fibrolytic activity (Goachet et al 2010).

Key Points – Forage feeding

Practical recommendations include:

- Feeding preferably 1.5–2.0 kg (DM basis) per 100 kg bodyweight of long stem roughage or chopped long fiber
- Avoiding overly mature forages, due to reduced digestibility and possibly reduced water reservoir capacity.
- Selecting hay with a low to moderate protein content (i.e., grass hay with crude protein [CP] of 8–14%) rather than a legume hay (often with CP >20%) because of concerns regarding a high protein intake (*see below*). A good quality grass hay or a grass/alfalfa mix in which alfalfa is no more than 30% of the mix is recommended
- Avoiding high intakes of calcium-rich forages (i.e., alfalfa) due to the perceived increased risk of synchronous diaphragmatic flutter ("thumps") during endurance rides when horses are fed a high calcium ration
- Appropriate vitamin/mineral and possibly protein fortification will be required especially in highly forage based rations

Supplemental energy sources

Cereal grains

Many endurance horses are Arabian, at least in part, and tend to be "easy keepers". However, even good quality pasture/preserved forage may not be sufficient to maintain bodyweight and condition during endurance training and competition. Therefore, some cereals are commonly required – the average amount in the aforementioned survey (Crandell 2002) was 2.27 kg/day. However, even higher quantities are likely to be required by horses engaged in heavier training and higher level racing.

Starch, a hydrolyzable carbohydrate, is the principal component of cereal grains (~50% of oats and 70% of corn). Recommendations with respect to starch intake per meal have been reduced for various reasons (link with increased risk of equine gastric ulcer syndrome, insulin response, etc.), in recent years from 4 to 1 g/kg BW or even less under specific clinical circumstances (Potter et al 1992, Kienzle 1994, McLean 2000, De Fombelle et al 2001, Luthersson et al 2009, Vervuert et al 2009, see Chapters 8 and 26), although this may depend to some extent on the source and processing of the starch. It is also advisable to limit the size of individual grain-based meals to no more than 1.5 kg (for a 450 kg horse). Some nutritionists also advocate providing grain-based meals separately from a large meal of *long* fibrous hay due to potential concerns of lower prececal starch digestibility when these feeds are ingested together (Pagan & Harris 1999), although no effect on the glycemic response has been reported with the addition of short chopped fiber (Harris et al 2005).

Highly digestible fiber sources

As mentioned, the feeding of sugar beet pulp and soya hulls to horses has gained popularity recently (Crandell et al 1999, Palmgren Karlsson et al 2002). When compared to more traditional fiber sources like hay, these highly digestible or "super fibers" contain less indigestible material (e.g., lignin) and higher amounts of non-starch polysaccharides, pectins and gums which can be digested to a large extent within the time period that they remain within the gastrointestinal tract (see Chapter 17). This translates to a higher energy yield. In addition, there may be beneficial effects on hydration due to improved water holding and releasing capacities (Warren et al 2001). In addition, work with resting horses showed that replacing hay with sugarbeet pulp resulted in a decreased water intake and retention but an increase in the proportion of water lost via the urine. During exercise it is possible that these increased urinary losses may be more easily and "safely" reduced providing more water to support sweat losses.

Vegetable oils

Energy-rich vegetable oils contain no starch or sugar and potentially may provide other advantages, including reduced heat production (important in conditions of high heat and humidity) (see Box 14.1), reduced amount of feed needed to achieve desired energy intake, and possible behavioural advantages (Harris 1997, Harris & Harris 1998, Holland et al 1996, Harris & Kronfeld 2003, NRC 2007). Reduced bowel ballast, due to the substitution of some cereals by oil, helps to balance to a certain extent the recommendation for a high fiber intake (which creates more bowel ballast) in endurance horses. Of perhaps more interest is the potential for oil supplemented diets to provide a direct performance advantage. More than 30 years ago, it was reported that horses fed a diet containing 12% fat (9% added corn oil) and ridden 67 km over mountainous terrain for 8–10 h performed better and had higher blood glucose concentrations at the end of the ride than horses fed the control diet (3% fat) (Slade et al 1975). Subsequent studies have demonstrated that oil supplementation is characterized by a dose-dependent increase in the activity of lipoprotein lipase and, in some reports, an increase in the activity of skeletal muscle citrate synthase and beta-hydroxy acyl-CoA dehydrogenase (Orme et al 1997, Dunnett et al 2002). These alterations in enzyme activities may result in increased uptake and oxidation of free fatty acids in skeletal muscle (Pagan et al 2002). Horses fed a diet supplemented with oil to provide 25–30%

Box 14.1

If you need to supply 10 MJ of maintenance net or useable energy then (based on Harris 1997) as a guide to the amounts of feed needed and the amount of waste heat the horse needs to remove:

- 10 MJ would require feeding 1.8 kg of timothy hay and would produce 3.8 MJ waste heat from metabolism plus 1.1 MJ of fermentation heat = 4.9 MJ
- 10 MJ would require feeding 1.14 kg of oats and would produce 2.6 MJ waste heat from metabolism plus around 0.4 MJ of heat of fermentation = 3 MJ
- 10 MJ would require feeding 0.36 kg of oil and would produce 1.44 MJ waste heat from metabolism and nothing from fermentation = 1.44 MJ

of DE had a lower respiratory exchange ratio (Dunnett et al 2002, Pagan et al 2002) and decreased glucose utilization (Pagan et al 2002) during low intensity exercise (~ 25–35% VO_{2max}) than horses fed a control (nonsupplemented) ration. Investigators that used compartmental modeling techniques to evaluate glucose kinetics also observed that horses adapted to and fed an oil- and fiber-rich complementary feed utilized less glucose during exercise (4 m/s on a treadmill) when compared to horses fed a starch-rich complementary feed (Treiber et al 2008). Theoretically, enhancement of lipid oxidation and sparing of plasma glucose utilization should result in muscle glycogen sparing and could perhaps improve (or prolong) endurance performance. Preliminary work also suggests that adaptation to fat- and fiber-rich feeds lowers serum insulin concentration during endurance rides in association with improved performance (Hess et al 2007). Overall, however, the effect of diet composition on performance during endurance races currently remains uncertain (Harris 1997, NRC 2007).

The ideal type (including fatty acid profile) and amount of vegetable oil for supplementation of horse diets has not been determined. Corn oil tends to be one of the more palatable oils (Holland et al 1998) but several vegetable oils show acceptable palatability providing they are fresh, not rancid and of a good quality - preferably human grade. Individual horse preferences also occur. Any supplemental oil should be introduced slowly (over 14–21 days) to avoid intestinal disturbances as the capacity to hydrolyse lipids requires time to adapt (Kronfeld et al 2004). However, the equine pancreas has high lipase activity (Lorenzo-Figueras et al 2007) which might explain why horses are able to digest and utilize up to 20% or more of the diet as oil (Kronfeld et al 2004) if introduced appropriately. Supplementation with soya oil (15% DM intake; ~ 35% of daily energy intake) was reported to decrease fiber digestibility in one study (Jansen et al 2007); however the evidence is conflicting as several other studies (analyzed in Kronfeld et al 2004) suggested no effect of fat supplementation on fiber digestibility (see Chapter 7).

Practical recommendations for endurance horses in hard training/competition are that vegetable oil should be 5–8% of the total diet (with 10% as an upper limit) on an as fed basis. An alternative recommendation is to feed up to 1 ml/1 kg BWt/day. For reference, 450 ml of oil (~420 g) provides about 3.4 Mcal (14 MJ) of DE. This daily amount should be divided into two to three portions and mixed in with the other complementary feed. Supplemental oil should be introduced gradually (e.g., starting at 50 ml/day) and to obtain optimal metabolic benefits of dietary oil, it has been recommended that the oil be fed for several weeks if not months before competition (Pagan et al 2002). High fat diets are commonly linked with reduced exercise performance in humans, but it is important to note that "normal" baseline human diets tend to contain >10% fat whereas the additional of 500 ml of oil to a 9 kg DM ration in a 450 kg endurance horse is only just >5%.

With the exception of vitamin E (variable amounts), vegetable oils do not provide other nutrients. Indeed, adding oil to an existing ration has the potential to create multiple imbalances, because it adds energy but no accompanying micronutrients, vitamins or amino acids. Therefore, it is recommended to feed a diet in which the inclusion of oil has been balanced with respect to other essential nutrients. Alternatively a vitamin/mineral supplement may be needed to achieve the desired balance and ensure that nutrient requirements are met. Although oil supplementation may enhance vitamin E absorption in horses (Siciliano & Wood, 1993) studies in humans suggest that the requirement for vitamin E increases with increasing dietary polyunsaturated fatty acid content (Wardlaw 1999). The increased fat oxidation that occurs during submaximal exercise following fat supplementation (Dunnett et al 2002) is likely to increase the production of peroxyl free radicals and hence the need for additional dietary antioxidants. Based on studies in other species, it has been estimated that the vitamin E requirement is 0.6 mg α-tocopherol per g linoleic acid and around 3 mg α-tocopherol per g of omega-3 polyunsaturated fatty acid (NRC 1987). Currently, the author (P.H.) recommends an additional 1–1.5 IU per 1 ml of added vegetable oil.

Key Points

- Supplementary energy if required can be provided by a mixture of highly digestible fibers, cereal grains and vegetable oil
- Although not proven to improve performance, it is currently recommended that up to 1 ml/kg BW vegetable oil may provide a number of metabolic advantages. Additional Vitamin E should be provided at consistency of 1–1.5 IU/1 ml supplemental oil
- If required any additional starch should be provided at <1 g/kg BW starch/meal

Muscle glycogen storage

During exercise, horses appear to rely more heavily on carbohydrate for energy transduction (from muscle glycogen and blood glucose) than humans (Jose-Cunilleras et al 2006). Suboptimal liver and muscle glycogen content at the onset of exercise may therefore reduce performance (Snow et al 1982, Lacombe et al 1999), However, the carbohydrate based nutritional strategies employed by human marathon runners to raise muscle glycogen levels (exercise-linked depletion followed by a high carbohydrate meal) do not appear to be of any value in the horse. Several studies have shown that diet has minimal impact on the slow rate of muscle glycogen restoration in the horse following glycogen depleting exercise (Essen-Gustavsson et al 1991, Pösö et al 2004, Lacombe et al 2004, Jose-Cunilleras et al 2006). See Chapter 2 for more details.

A recent study reported that oral administration of a hypotonic electrolyte solution after prolonged moderate intensity exercise enhanced the rate of muscle glycogen storage when compared to no fluid treatment (Waller et al 2009). The authors suggested that post-exercise dehydration may be one factor that contributes to the slow muscle glycogen replenishment in horses. This may be a very important consideration in the endurance horse.

Timing of feeding relative to exercise

There is evidence from several studies that the timing and composition of a meal consumed before exercise can influence metabolic responses and possibly distribution of body fluids in horses (Harris & Graham-Thiers 1999). In particular, hyperglycemia and insulinemia associated with digestion and absorption of grain meals affects the mix of substrates utilized during a bout of exercise. Insulin is a potent inhibitor of lipolysis and fatty acid oxidation in skeletal muscle, and also promotes glucose uptake into muscle via recruitment of the glucose transporter protein GLUT4 to the sarcolemma. Thus, an elevated circulating insulin concentration at exercise onset will suppress free fatty acid availability as well as lipid oxidation and increase reliance on carbohydrate stores (including plasma glucose) for energy transduction. The resultant decrease in plasma glucose concentrations that occurs when horses are exercised 2–3 hr following a grain meal tends to be relatively transient (Pagan & Harris 1999). However, plasma free fatty acids concentrations and lipid oxidation rate may remain lower in fed animals when compared to the fasted state throughout certain types of exercise (Jose-Cunilleras et al 2002). The impact of feeding may be more complex in endurance horses because they are also offered carbohydrate-rich feeds at rest stops during rides. In this circumstance exercise-associated alterations in hormones (e.g., increased catecholamines, decreased insulin) may counterbalance the effect of any hormonal changes induced by feeding.

Large meals (hay or grain/concentrate or mixtures) may result in a decrease in plasma volume, reflected by an increase in plasma protein concentration, as a result of a fluid shift into the lumen of the gastrointestinal tract (Pagan & Harris 1999) and should therefore be avoided shortly prior to exercise. Although the effects of pre-exercise grain feeding on endurance exercise performance in the field have not been reported, the potential acceleration in carbohydrate oxidation and suppression of fat oxidation lead to a current recommendation that grain or concentrate based meals should not be fed within 3 h of a race.

Protein nutrition

Additional protein over maintenance requirements may be needed with exercise and training because of the accompanying muscular development, the need for muscle repair and to replenish nitrogen lost in sweat (~20–25 g/kg sweat loss). The precise protein requirements for exercise, however, are unknown and the current NRC recommendations (NRC 2007) are 1.26 g CP/kg BW/day for maintenance plus between 0.089 and 0.354 g CP/kg BW/day depending on the exercise level and sweat nitrogen loss (see also Chapter 6). The author's (P.H.) current recommendations are to feed 2.0–2.5 g CP/kg bodyweight/day (providing stable hygiene is good and water intake is not restricted). There is some evidence that dietary protein level may alter urea metabolism in horses. It has been estimated that a change in dietary CP from 10% to 15% of DM intake would increase water requirement by approximately 5% because of an obligate increase in urine production for clearance of endogenous urea (Kronfeld 1996). Higher protein diets may also be undesirable because of the effects of excess dietary protein on heat production, acid-base balance (especially as speeds increase), and possibly respiratory health (due to ammonia accumulation in confinement housing) (Graham-Thiers et al 2000). However, in Standardbred trotters it has recently been reported that feeding a forage only diet with a high CP intake (16.6%) increased glycogen and leucine concentrations in the muscle of trained animals compared with a lower CP forage (12.5%) and had no effect on plasma lactate and blood pH during exercise tests performed to mimic a race. The authors concluded that the higher protein intake might be beneficial for muscle recovery following intensive exercise (Essen-Gustavsson et al 2010). It is important to note that the responses were not compared with those from animals fed a forage cereal/sweet feed based diet and these were trotters rather than endurance horses.

It has in fact been recommended (Meyer 1987) that athletic horses should not be fed more than 2 g of digestible protein/kg BW/day (around 3–4 g CP/kg BW/day depending on the feedstuffs). Some potential advantages during more short term exercise (Graham-Thiers et al 2000) have been demonstrated with a restricted protein diet (7.5% CP with added lysine and threonine) but this has not been proven in the field to date. Further work is needed with respect to the optimal protein requirements for endurance horses racing under different environmental conditions and speeds.

The quality and nature of the protein fed is important, especially in growing horses and those in hard or repetitive work (NRC 2007, see also Chapter 6). Recent work in humans suggests that the timing and type of protein/amino acid supplementation may influence protein synthesis and degradation in muscle (Phillips 2011). However, detailed information for the endurance horse is not currently available. At the present time it is therefore recommended that as a start, the lysine and possibly threonine content of the diet of actively exercising horses at least should be considered. A recommended allowance (PH) for lysine in hard working endurance horses is 0.08–1.0 g/kg BW/day. Soya bean meal or flakes are a good source of lysine. The amount of additional lysine needed will depend on the hay and pasture being fed – for example, alfalfa and other legumes have higher lysine content than many meadow hays and grasses.

Branch chain amino acids (BCAA)

Supplementation with BCAA (valine, leucine, and isoleucine) has been advocated as a strategy to improve performance. One theory suggests that BCAA supplementation increases the concentration of trichloroacetate intermediates (anaplerosis) available for condensation with acetyl-CoA, enabling an increase in the turnover rate of the cycle. A second theory is that BCAA may attenuate fatigue during exercise by limiting the rise of free, unbound plasma tryptophan which results in elevated brain serotonin and development of central fatigue. However, this theory has been disputed (Grimmett & Sillence, 2005) and research in the horse has failed to show any beneficial effect of BCAA supplementation on exercise performance (Casini et al 2000, Steffanon et al 2000). Certainly, changes in plasma BCAA concentrations have been observed in horses during treadmill (Trottier et al 2002) and field (Nery et al 2005) endurance exercise, which may suggest some value during recovery. However, further studies are needed before recommendations can be given regarding BCAA supplementation.

Antioxidants

Metabolic reactions that produce free radicals are responsible for many key biochemical events and under controlled circumstances they are essential for life. However, free radicals can cause irreversible denaturation of essential cellular components and result in a number of degenerative disease processes (Halliwell 1994). During exercise there is a marked increase in free radical production in the horse due to increased activity of xanthine oxidase during anaerobic exercise, degradation of purine nucleotides and the partial reduction of oxygen during oxidative phosphorylation within the mitochondria. It has been suggested that free radical production may play a role in muscle damage and fatigue if the production exceeds the capacity of natural defense mechanisms (Marlin et al 2005). A system of natural antioxidant defenses is present in the body to help counteract such free radical-induced damage, including vitamins E and C as well as the selenium containing enzyme, glutathione peroxidase (GSHPx). Glutathione peroxidase reduces the production of hydroxyl radicals, vitamin E scavenges free radicals, and vitamin C assists by reducing the tocopheroxyl radicals formed by during this scavenging process. In addition, vitamin E helps to block lipid peroxidation and may also form an important part of membrane structure. Recent work has suggested that basal oxidative stress markers, circulating cytokines and anti-inflammatory neuroendocrine hormones appear to correlate with endurance performance in horses, but further work is needed (Holbrook et al 2010).

All horses, but especially those in hard work such as the endurance horse, need vitamin E and selenium. The levels of plasma antioxidants throughout an endurance race may depend to some extent on the difficulty of the race and the environmental conditions. Additional antioxidant supplementation above the levels recommended by the NRC (NRC 2007) may be of value before and during the race (Hargreaves et al 2002, Marlin et al 2002, Williams et al 2004). The author (P.H.) recommends providing vitamin E at ~2000 IU/day and selenium at ~2 mg/day (for a 450 kg endurance horse). In the total ration, selenium should not exceed 1 mg/100 kg BW/day. Note that additional vitamin E is required if the horse is fed a vegetable oil supplemented diet.

Key Points

- Protein quality (i.e. amino acid profile) and timing of ingestion may be important in optimally supporting muscle development and recovery post exercise
- An adequate antioxidant intake is recommended and although not proven to improve performance enhanced intakes of vitamin E and possibly vitamin C may be advantageous

Fluid and electrolyte losses accompanying endurance exercise

Evaporation of sweat and respiratory water is the major mechanism for removal of excess heat produced as a consequence of substrate utilization during exercise (Hodgson et al 1993, Jose-Cunilleras 2004). Development of hyperthermia and disturbances to fluid, electrolyte and acid-base homeostasis consequent to these body fluid losses may contribute (Fielding et al 2009) to elimination of the horse from competition (so called "metabolic failure"). The amount of sweat produced depends on environmental conditions, nature of the work performed (which also depends on the rider's ability and terrain) and the animal's fitness (Jose-Cunilleras 2004, Ecker & Lindinger 1995). Total body fluid loss during endurance exercise can be closely estimated by measuring BW loss, as long as food and water are not provided during the exercise bout and urine as well as faecal losses are taken into consideration (Kingston et al 1999). However, BW loss during actual and urine as well as fecal losses are taken into consideration endurance competitions reflects the balance between sweat, urine and respiratory fluid losses, changes in gastrointestinal tract content plus food and water intake. In both human and equine endurance athletes, loss of body fluid during prolonged exercise typically exceeds voluntary fluid replacement despite the fact that water, other rehydration solutions and food are frequently made available during competition. In contrast to pure dehydration (a pure water deficit), athletes lose both water and electrolytes in sweat; consequently, increases in plasma osmolality are less than with a pure water deficit and the osmotic thirst stimulus is blunted. This condition, in which body fluid losses are only partially replaced by drinking during and shortly after the exercise bout, has been termed "involuntary dehydration" (Greenleaf 1992).

In most human marathon and ultraendurance competitions, mean BW loss of successful competitors is typically in the range of 2–4% (Noakes 1995, Sharwood et al 2004). However, a common finding is a wide range of BW loss in successful competitors; for example, losses ranging from more than 10% to actual weight gain were observed in a group of 767 successful Ironman triathletes (Sharwood et al 2004). Studies that have measured BW loss in horses competing in endurance races have found mean values ranging from 2–7% by the end of competition (Table 14-2: Lawrence et al 1992, Andrews et al 1994, Ecker & Lindinger 1995, Schott et al 1996, 1997, 2006, Barton et al 2003, Sampieri et al 2006, Barnes et al 2010). Overall, a value of ~5% BW loss is approached by the end of endurance competition, somewhat regardless of the competition distance and duration. Again, this BW loss develops despite the fact that horses have been offered water and various feeds at rest stops to promote fluid, electrolyte, and fuel replacement. As with human athletes, a wide range of BW loss has also been documented in equine endurance athletes with some successful competitors losing in excess of 10% during the event (Lawrence et al 1992, Ecker & Lindinger 1995, Barton et al 2003, Schott et al 2006). The large variation in BW loss is more likely related to variation in replacement, by voluntary eating and drinking, rather than differences in fluid losses during the race. Further, the BW loss is only partially replaced during overnight recovery from endurance competition, likely due to a persistent decrease in the amount of ingesta in the large intestine and depletion of body fluid and electrolyte stores (Schott et al 1997, Barnes et al 2010). Incomplete restoration of fluid and electrolyte losses is further reflected by an even greater increase in serum aldosterone concentration after overnight recovery from the race, as compared to values at the finish (Schott et al 1997). As with human endurance athletes, ingestion of several meals over 3–5 days is likely required for full recovery from challenging endurance competitions (Fellman et al 1989).

Two factors appear to contribute to a greater magnitude of involuntary dehydration, and mean BW loss, in equine as compared to human endurance athletes. First, equine sweat remains isotonic during prolonged exercise while human

Table 14-2 Bodyweight Loss in Horses Competing in Endurance Competitions during Which They Had Access to Water and Feed

Type of ride	Distance	Mean BW loss	Reference
Endurance	240 km over 2 days	6.3%	Lawrence et al 1992
Endurance (13 rides)	Variable	2–7%	Ecker & Lindinger 1995
Endurance	80–90 km/day, 424 km over 5 days	6.2%	Schott et al 1996
Endurance	80 km	3.6%	Schott et al 1997
Endurance	160 km	4.9%	Schott et al 1997
Endurance	48 km	4.9%	Barton et al 2003
Endurance	83 km	1.7%	Barton et al 2003
Endurance	159 km	3.7%	Barton et al 2003
Endurance, elite*	160 km	6.1%	Schott et al 2006
Endurance	80 km	4.0%	Sampieri et al 2006
Endurance	80 km	4.2%	Wilson et al (unpublished data)
Endurance	160 km	6.5%	Wilson et al (unpublished data)
Endurance, elite*	120 km	5.7%	Schott et al (unpublished data)
Endurance	160 km	4.1%	Barnes et al 2010
	Overall mean	4.8%	

*Endurance, elite – refers to international competitions at speeds >15 km/h.

sweat becomes hypotonic, in comparison to plasma osmolality (Hodgson et al 1994). Thus, horses lose a comparatively greater amount of electrolytes in each liter of sweat produced. As a consequence, plasma osmolality rises more slowly in horses than human endurance athletes and produces a lesser osmotic thirst stimulus. Second, fluid reserves in the lumen of the equine gastrointestinal tract are substantially greater (8–10% of bodyweight) in comparison to those in human athletes (1–2% of bodyweight) (Jose-Cunilleras 2004). Thus, the equine athlete has a larger "fluid reserve" that can be called upon to replace sweat fluid losses during endurance exercise. As mentioned above this intestinal fluid reserve as discussed above may provide 10 liters of water containing 19 g of Na and 10 g of Cl (800–900 mmol Na^+ and 350 mmol Cl^-) in a 450 kg horse that could be absorbed to replace sweat losses during endurance exercise (Schott et al 1997).

In studies in which bodyweight loss has been measured at multiple times during the competition, a consistent finding in endurance horses has been that the majority of BW loss occurs during the first half of the event and BW remains fairly steady or can even increase from that point onward (Schott et al 1997, 2006, Barton et al 2003). Because sweating continues throughout exercise, maintenance of BW during the later stages of the race is best explained by water and feed intake at a rate nearly matching ongoing fluid losses. This statement is supported by the finding of greater voluntary water intake during the later stages of treadmill endurance exercise tests (Kingston et al 1997, Düsterdieck et al 1999). Further, it suggests that horses that lose the greatest amount of BW during the competition are not actually losing more body fluid; rather, they are more likely failing to replace lost fluids by eating and drinking.

In humans, variation in the magnitude of involuntary dehydration observed during exercise has led to a threshold value of ~2% BW loss being used to separate individuals that are considered "better drinkers" from those that are considered "poorer drinkers" (Sandick et al 1984, Szlyk et al 1989). Although data in horses is limited, cluster analysis of bodyweight loss in several cohorts of 2-year-old Arabian horses that performed several 60 km treadmill exercise tests also allowed separation into groups of good drinkers, average drinkers, and poor drinkers (Schott et al 2003). These data support inherent (or genetic) differences in voluntary fluid replacement by endurance athletes.

Sweat electrolyte losses

Under mild ambient conditions horses (~500 kg BW) may lose 5–7 liters of sweat per hour of steady totting and cantering (McCutcheon et al 1995a, Kingston et al 1997). However, under conditions of high heat and humidity, sweat rates may approach 10–12 l/hr (Carlson, 1983, McCutcheon et al 1995a). In addition, to the large amounts of water that can be lost in sweat by horses performing several hours of endurance exercise, equine sweat contains 110–130 mmol Na^+ (2.5–3.0 g), 120–140 mmol Cl^- (4.3–5.0 g), and 30–40 mmol K^+ (1.2–1.6 g) per liter (McCutcheon et al 1995b, Kingston et al 1997). Thus, during exercise horses can lose 500 to >1000 mmol of Na^+ per hour in sweat and equine endurance athletes thereby have substantially greater dietary requirements to replace such losses (McCutcheon & Geor, 1996). As an example of the magnitude of sweat losses that can occur during endurance exercise, approximately 25 liters of sweat containing ~3000 mmol Na^+, ~3250 mmol Cl^-, and ~750 mmol K^+ was produced by horses completing 45 km of treadmill exercise during a ~3.5 hour treadmill exercise test (Kingston et al 1997). These values are equivalent to loss of ~175 g of NaCl and ~55 g of KCl in sweat and represent losses of ~20%, ~27.5%, and ~2.5% of exchangeable Na^+, Cl^-, and K^+, respectively, from body fluid compartments. Similarly, sweat losses of ~1500 mmol Na^+, ~1700 mmol Cl^-, and ~400 mmol K^+ were estimated during an ~2 hour treadmill exercise test simulating the speed and endurance phase of a 3-day event under cool, dry ambient conditions (McCutcheon & Geor 1996). These estimated losses were nearly doubled when the same exercise test was performed under conditions of high heat and humidity. Clearly, horses performing endurance exercise on a regular basis, especially in hot and humid climates, require salt supplementation in the diet to replace sweat losses. Further, many riders actively attempt to replace sweat electrolyte losses during competition by offering horses water containing electrolytes for voluntary drinking or by oral administration of hypertonic oral electrolyte slurries.

Attenuation of involuntary dehydration

Active cooling during exercise

To limit sweat fluid losses, enhancement of metabolic heat dissipation by conductive and convective heat transfer has been pursued through active cooling strategies during equine competitions. These include use of misting fans, shaded areas to limit solar radiation heat gain, and intense sponging and washing with cold water at rest breaks (Jeffcott & Kohn 1999, Jeffcott et al 2009). These strategies have been demonstrated to produce a more rapid decline in core temperature and are an effective tool for limiting sweat loss under conditions of high heat and humidity (Jeffcott & Kohn 1999).

Fluid and electrolyte supplementation

Over the past two decades the variety of sports drinks and electrolyte supplements marketed to correct dehydration in both human and equine athletes has expanded dramatically. However, it is generally acknowledged that little, if any, fluid replacement is needed for human endurance exercise lasting 2 h or less. For exercise lasting several hours human endurance athletes have been encouraged to drink about 500 ml a couple of hours prior to exercise and small amounts (150–300 ml) of a sports drink containing both electrolytes and carbohydrate every 15–20 min during exercise in an attempt to limit dehydration from exceeding a 2% BW loss (Convertino et al 1996, Latzka & Montain 1999). This frequent fluid replacement is not driven by thirst but by a conscious effort to drink in the absence of thirst. Of interest, this trend toward "excessive" fluid replacement (drinking that is not driven by thirst) is not without controversy in human sports medicine as it has become clear that excessive drinking of water or hypotonic sports drinks is the cause of exercise-associated hyponatremia (EAH) (Hew et al 2003, Noakes 2007, Beltrami et al 2008). EAH and and EAH-associated encephalopathy, now recognized as the leading cause of death in human endurance athletes, is particularly a problem for slower athletes that exercise for a longer period and have a greater opportunity (more time) for excess fluid replacement (Hew et al 2003, Ayus et al 2005). Thus, perhaps it is fortunate that "you can lead a horse to water, but you can't make it drink" because horses cannot be trained to drink in the absence of thirst.

Exercise scientists opposed to the recommendation for excessive drinking by human endurance athletes cite the fact that no data exist to demonstrate that dehydration >2% BW loss negatively affects performance in endurance competitions or significantly increases the risk of development of medical problems during or after competition (Noakes 1995, 2007). In fact, the study of 767 successful Ironman triathletes mentioned previously found that athletes that lost the most BW actually finished faster (Sharwood et al 2004). Further, some exercise physiologists have gone so far as to state that promulgation the "excessive drinking doctrine" has been driven by bias induced by research funding support provided by the sports drink industry to researchers that have been involved in preparing consensus statements about recommendations for hydration during endurance exercise (Convertino et al 1996) as well as misleading marketing information used by the sports drink industry (Noakes 2011).

Although electrolyte supplementation of horses competing in endurance events or under adverse environmental conditions of high heat and humidity has become a common practice, it warrants emphasis that, similar to their human counterparts, convincing data to document that fluid and electrolyte depletion adversely affects performance is currently lacking in endurance horses. Further, despite the favorable clinical responses observed with use of intravenous fluids for treatment of horses that either are eliminated for metabolic disorders or develop medical problems after competition (Fielding et al 2009), no data currently exist to document that affected horses are any more dehydrated than successful horses. In all likelihood, metabolic elimination and development of medical problems after competition are multifactorial in origin and, at present, our understanding of the development of these disorders is limited.

Despite the lack of data, supplementation of endurance horses with oral electrolyte slurries before, during, and after competition is widely practiced and there is evidence to support that this practice could enhance recovery. Investigations to date have largely addressed the question of whether or not supplemental electrolyte administration would increase voluntary water intake (drinking) by exercising horses. Horses completing a 60 km simulated endurance ride on a treadmill, with water offered at multiple points during the test were studied with and without electrolyte supplementation (Düsterdieck et al 1999). When horses ran without electrolyte supplementation, they lost about 25 kg of fluid as sweat and replaced a little more than half of this loss by drinking ~13 liters of water. However, when they ran with electrolyte supplementation (salts were given as a slurry dosed into the mouth before and during the run) the horses drank ~23 liters of water, replacing nearly all of the fluid lost in sweat. In addition, to "tricking" horses into drinking a greater total amount of water by giving electrolytes, supplementation also resulted in horses starting to drink earlier during the course of the endurance test and abolished the increase in aldosterone concentration following the test. In this study, horses were given an amount of electrolytes that would be expected to be lost in 25 liters of sweat (~175 g NaCl and 55 g KCl). This was a much larger dose than typically used by competitors; nevertheless, no adverse effects of supplementing with this large amount of electrolytes were observed, although urine Na^+ concentration increased after the exercise test in electrolyte supplemented horses.

Next, to determine if horses would drink salt water, horses were exercised for 30 or 45 km on a treadmill at a walk, trot and canter, again simulating endurance racing. However, unlike the prior investigation, further dehydration was induced by administration of furosemide (1 mg/kg, IV) 90 min before the exercise test and horses were not offered anything to drink until the end of exercise. At the end of the test, horses were randomly offered either water or two concentrations of salt water (0.45% and 0.9% NaCl solutions) for the initial 5 min of recovery (while still standing on the treadmill) and then further water intake was measured from 20–60 min of recovery with the horse washed off and placed free in a stall (Butudom et al 2002). The initial drink volume (10–12 liters, containing 90–110 g of NaCl for the 0.9% solution) was similar for all the fluids offered and was consistent with the capacity of the equine stomach. More importantly, the initial drink of salt water was followed by further drinking of ~4 liters of water from 20–60 min of recovery. In contrast, when horses were initially offered plain water, they did not drink further during the initial hour of recovery despite the fact that they remained partially dehydrated. Because drinking is stimulated by an increase in plasma osmolality, an initial drink of water dilutes ECF Na^+ concentration and abolishes the drinking stimulus. In contrast, with an initial drink of salt water, ECF Na^+ concentration remains elevated and horses wanted to drink again when provided water only a few minutes later. Thus, an initial drink of salt water "tricked" the horses into drinking a greater total amount of fluid during the initial hour of recovery. In a subsequent study by the same group, temperature preference was investigated by offering horses an initial drink of 0.9% NaCl at 10, 20, or 30°C, followed by water at the same temperatures in a stall from 20–60 min of recovery (Butudom et al 2004). When different temperatures of salt water were compared, horses drank the greatest amount, and took longer drinks, when it was 20°C, near the temperature water comes out of a hose on a warm summer day.

To determine whether or not dehydrated horses would voluntarily drink solutions at tonicities exceeding that of plasma, horses were dehydrated by furosemide administration and overnight water deprivation (but not exercise) to induce a BW loss of 5% or more. Initial drinks of plain water, isotonic solutions including 0.9% NaCl or 5% dextrose solution, or hypertonic solutions including 1.8% NaCl, 2.5% dextrose in 0.9% NaCl, or 5% dextrose in 0.9% NaCl were offered, in a randomized fashion. Horses drank similar amounts of water or the isotonic solutions with an initial drink of 8–12 liters, again approaching stomach capacity, while initial drink volume was reduced by 50% or more with all hypertonic solutions offered (Fig. 14.1, Schott, unpublished data). Thus, when salt water is initially offered to horses, tonicity should not exceed that of plasma. In further support of limiting tonicity of replacement fluids to that of plasma, nasogastric administration of a hypertonic (628 mOsm/kg) rehydration solution to furosemide-dehydrated horses appeared to delay intestinal absorption, indirectly assessed as a further rise in plasma protein concentration during the initial 2 h after fluid administration, as compared to administration of water or an isotonic rehydration solution (Sosa-León et al 1995). A long-standing concern has been whether or not administration of hypertonic oral electrolyte slurries could have similar adverse effects on gastric emptying and intestinal absorption of electrolytes and water – this controversy remains unresolved. However, a critical point is that when these hypertonic slurries are used during endurance races, riders must pay attention to ensure that their horses continue to drink after the electrolytes are administered. If drinking ceases, no further electrolytes should be administered and a horse that stops drinking is likely at risk for metabolic elimination.

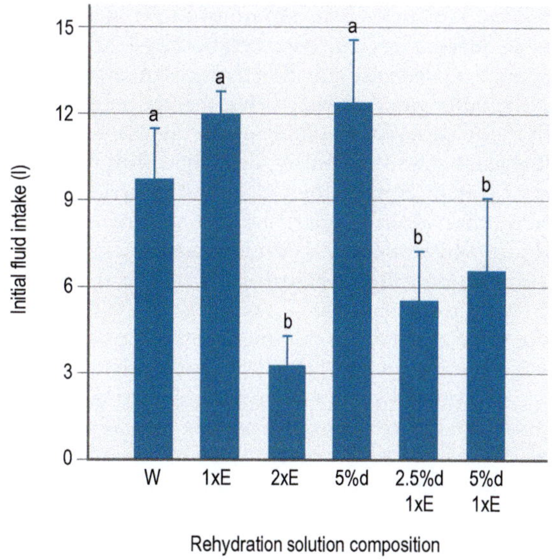

Figure 14.1 Effect of fluid composition and tonicity on the volume of the initial drink (over a 5 min period) imbibed by horses that had been dehydrated to a ≥5% body weight loss by overnight water deprivation and furosemide administration. W = water, 1xE = 0.9% NaCl solution, 2xE = 1.8% NaCl solution, 5%d = 5% dextrose solution, 2.5%d 1xE = 2.5% dextrose solution in 0.9% NaCl solution, and 5%d 1xE = 5% dextrose solution in 0.9% NaCl solution (Schott, unpublished data).

In theory, greater intake of water and electrolytes, either by oral administration of hypertonic electrolyte slurries followed by voluntary drinking or by initially offering salt water, followed by plain water, should limit dehydration and enhance recovery. However, it again warrants mention that limited data exist to support that limiting dehydration either lessens the risk of metabolic elimination or development of medical problems following ride completion. An early study in Australia found higher plasma protein concentrations at both the ride finish and after 30 min of recovery in horses with heart rates >60/min, as compared to horses with heart rates <60/min (Rose et al 1977). The investigators concluded that horses with higher heart rates were more dehydrated, yet BW loss was not measured. A recent report of 30 horses receiving veterinary treatment after metabolic elimination also described higher plasma protein and lower serum electrolyte concentrations in "pulled" horses, as compared to successful competitors but again BW loss was not measured (Fielding et al 2009). Recently, Barnes et al (2010) also reported higher plasma protein and lower serum electrolyte concentrations at the mid-ride checkpoint in horses that were subsequently eliminated for metabolic problems in a 160 km race, as compared to successful horses or horses subsequently eliminated for lameness. Although the findings of these two studies could also support greater dehydration and electrolyte losses as risk factors for subsequent metabolic elimination, BW loss at the mid-ride in the latter study was not different (actually tended to be less) in horses eliminated for metabolic problems, again when compared to successful horses or horses subsequently eliminated for lameness. It is important to recognize that increases in plasma protein concentration and heart rate only support a decrease in effective circulating blood volume. The latter can decrease with either dehydration or a fluid shift; for example, fluid movement into the intestinal tract in the early stages of ileus or, arguably, with repeated oral administration of hypertonic electrolyte slurries. All in all, these studies again support the fact that our current knowledge of why some horses develop metabolic problems during endurance racing is limited.

What also remains unclear in horses is whether or not electrolyte supplementation can improve performance. To investigate the effects of electrolyte supplementation on performance, ride times were compared in a group of endurance horses that received oral slurries containing the amounts of NaCl and KCl expected to be lost in 30 liters of sweat (high dose) or expected to be lost in 10 liters of sweat (low dose) during an 80 km ride. There was no difference in ride completion times or other subjective performance factors assessed in horses that were given the higher dose of electrolytes; however, the study was limited because it was performed in nonelite horses competing in 80 km rides under moderate ambient conditions (Sampieri et al 2006). Further, some of the horses administered the high dose of electrolytes developed serum Na^+ and Cl^- concentrations exceeding 150 and 115 mmol/l, respectively. Although no adverse consequences were observed, these high values suggest that the high dose may have provided more electrolytes than were needed by these horses. As mentioned earlier, recent work also demonstrated that nasogastric administration of a rehydration solution following treadmill endurance exercise enhanced the rate of glycogen resynthesis (Waller et al 2009). This novel finding provides support that electrolyte administration may enhance recovery and warrants further study under actual race conditions.

Factorial approach to estimating requirements

Using a typically applied factorial approach to replenishment based on BW loss, however, seems to practically overestimate the daily requirements of horses, especially those that lose large quantities of sweat fluid. Several factors may contribute to this overestimation. First, and perhaps most importantly, sweat electrolyte losses may be offset by absorption of ions in the large intestinal fluid reservoir (as discussed below). Second, respiratory water loss (devoid of electrolytes) is included in estimates derived from BW loss (Butudom et al). Third, some movement from other body stores such as bone and muscle may occur and renal losses of certain electrolytes such as sodium can be significantly reduced. Finally, the electrolyte content of sweat fluid may be lower in some animals vs. values derived from research studies. In addition, not all losses may need to be replenished immediately.

As an example, the sodium requirements for a horse at rest have been estimated at 20 mg/kg BW/day (NRC 2007). Sodium requirements for exercise would then take into consideration the sodium content of sweat (allow for replacement ~3.1 g/l). If we take a horse in training losing 8 kg of weight as having lost 8 kg of sweat on a factorial basis, then, a 500 kg horse should receive ~10 g + 25 g = 35 g of Na or ~100 g of salt/day. This calculation assumes that the sodium sources are 90% available which may be an overestimate (Zeyner et al 2008). Such a level of supplementation has been demonstrated to affect acid–base balance (Zeyner et al 2008) at least in the short term. If we assume, however, that 20% of the weight loss is due to respiratory non-electrolyte containing fluid then actual sweat losses could be ~ 6.5 kg, requiring 30 g of Na/day. Of course some of this will come from the diet itself – and if we assume this provides an intake of 20 g of sodium per day, therefore as the losses do not need to be replenished all at once as they are not large, 18 g of this can be absorbed from the gastrointestinal tract (90% availability) then the requirement for replacement is around 12 g of Na or around 36 g of salt (at 90% availability) – approximately a third of the amount calculated initially. If correct, therefore the goal in such circumstances may be to replace only about a third to a half of the electrolytes estimated as being lost in sweat based on body weight changes as the horses can also draw on the electrolyte reserves in the large intestine during and after exercise. If the horse only exercises at this level on an infrequent basis it is possible that provision of a fortified feed daily with free access to a salt lick alone may be adequate and additional supplementation is not required.

Difficulties, however, with this method arise when the horse is allowed to eat and drink between weighings – as the change in weight can no longer be taken to represent sweat losses and when the losses are more continuous and potentially more extreme. In these circumstances typical sweating rates of around 0.5–1 liter, 1–2 liters, 2–5 liters and 7–8 liters per 100 kg BW for light, moderate, hard and very heavy exercise may need to be used (Harris et al 2006) or for a 500 kg horse undertaking light/moderate work ~5 liters per hour (15.5 g of Na/h) may be used as estimates. Again, an allowance for horses that are being fed fortified meals (every 3 to 4 hours) is to base on 1 g/100 kg BW of Na to be absorbed per hour from the core diet and to estimate that a further 1 g/kg BW/h can be derived from other stores. So for our 500 kg horse 15.5 g of sodium is being lost in the sweat per hour (endogenous losses may very well be reduced as urinary losses will decrease and the losses in sweat are already accounted for – therefore for these purposes they can be considered to be negligible) and 10 g/h is being taken up from the feed reservoir in the gut and from bone and muscle, leaving 5.5 g/h to be replenished. We have to assume that additionally provided free electrolytes will be taken up, in addition to the Na obtained from the feed reservoirs. Availability of 5.5 g Na at 90% means 6 g Na or ~14 g NaCl/h. Again, this works out at around a third to a half of the estimated losses based on sweat loss. This methodology makes a number of assumptions including that any changes in blood flow to the gut as a result of the combination of exercise and regular feeding do not significantly influence uptake of Na.

Further work is required to confirm the estimations made.

Practical recommendations for electrolyte supplementation

The forage-based diet should provide an adequate reserve for potassium and therefore the main concern should be for salt replenishment during training. Recently it has been suggested that as moderate to fast exercise can result in hyperkalemia, the provision of potassium containing electrolyte formulations during fast loops of an endurance ride may increase the risk of cardiac arrhythmia and muscle cramping

(Hess et al 2006, 2008). However, more research in the field is required before firm recommendations can be made.

Most commercial feeds, and home mixed rations, do not provide adequate Na and Cl for horses that lose substantial sweat during training. For those horses in little or no work the provision of a salt block or free choice salt may be adequate (placed so that its use by that individual horse can be monitored). When a commercial feed or a vitamin-mineral supplement is being fed, the block should be pure salt rather than a salt-mineral type. Owners should be advised to *not* use blocks formulated for other species. However, adequate salt intake from licking a block cannot be guaranteed (Jose-Cunilleras 2004, Jansson & Dahlborn 1999, Jansson et al 1996, Kennedy et al 1998). For this reason, it is generally recommended to provide loose salt to horses in hard training - either added to feed or provided in a separate vessel. Salt should be introduced or removed from a feed gradually.

A simple approach for endurance horses in regular training would be to add 28 g of salt (note that using kitchen volumetric measures 1 volumetric ounce of NaCl powder ≈ 30 ml of NaCl powder ≈35 g of NaCl because the bulk density of NaCl powder is ~1.15 g/cm^3, as compared to the absolute NaCl density of 2.165 g/cm^3) to the concentrate feed being fed with plenty of forage once or twice daily (depending on the amount of training and sweating). During times of the year when it is hot and more humid, more may be required. Any excess that is not needed to replace losses would be excreted in urine and a simple test to assess adequacy of supplementation would be to measure urine Na^+ concentration in a morning urine sample collected before the concentrate meal is fed. Adequate supplementation should result in a urine Na^+ concentration >30 mmol/l while a value <20 mmol/l would indicate that more salt could be provided. A value >100 mmol/l would indicate excessive supplementation and the amount being fed could be decreased in half. At present, there is no recommendation for supplementation with additional potassium, calcium, or magnesium as adequate amounts of these minerals should be available through the forage/feed (providing adequate forage etc. is fed).

During competition

What remains unclear in horses is whether or not electrolyte supplementation can improve performance and whether or not equine athletes could also benefit from electrolyte supplementation during endurance competition. In an attempt to answer the former question, performance in a group of horses that received either a high or a low dose of electrolytes during a 80-km ride was compared (owners would not enroll for a nonsupplemented control group). In this study, there was no improvement in performance in horses that were provided the higher dose of electrolytes; however, the study was limited because it was performed in non-elite horses competing in 80-km rides under favorable ambient conditions (Sampieri et al 2006).

Regardless if additional electrolytes are going to be administered during competition as oral electrolyte slurries or by offering salt water as an initial drink, these practices should be started during training to familiarize the horse with this type of supplementation and to ensure that it does not cause possible problems. Usually, oral electrolyte slurries are a mixture of NaCl and KCl powders (at a 3:1 ratio) and about 35 g (~1 volumetric oz) is administered with each dose (mixed in corn oil, apple sauce, or yoghurt). For a 2 h training ride, one dose could be administered 1–2 h before the ride and an additional dose could be administered after 60–90 min of work. Horses should then be provided opportunities to drink while on the trail. Horses appear to have variable responses to oral electrolyte supplementation and if administering slurries before and during the training exercise bout does not result in an appreciable increase in voluntary water intake, this form of electrolyte supplementation during competition may not be advisable. An alternative approach in this situation could be to offer an initial drink of 0.9% NaCl at the end of the workout, always followed by plain water. Further, if electrolytes are administered in this fashion, there may be no need for further supplementation in concentrate meals.

During competition in 160-km endurance races with four veterinary checkpoints, administration of ~35 g (i.e., ~ one volumetric oz) of a 3:1 NaCl/KCl mixture at each checkpoint, in addition to ~70 g in a meal before the ride start provides about 160 g of NaCl and 50 g of KCl (an amount that would be lost in ~20 liters of sweat). Assuming that horses may lose 50 liters of sweat during the ride, this would replace about 40% of estimated losses and would seem a reasonable goal as 10 or more liters can also be replaced by absorption of water and electrolytes from the intestinal reservoir (Fig. 14.2), leading to a net deficit of ~20 liters at the end of the ride. The goal is not to replace all sweat electrolyte losses during the competition and attempts to do so may result in undesirable hypernatremia and hyperchloremia.

Practically, oral electrolyte slurries are commonly administered at the end of the rest period at veterinary checkpoints because they can have a bad taste and stop the horse from eating at the checkpoint and they can also be irritating to oral membranes. When administered in this fashion, it is important that riders stop along the trail to allow horses to drink as well as allow them to drink as soon as they enter

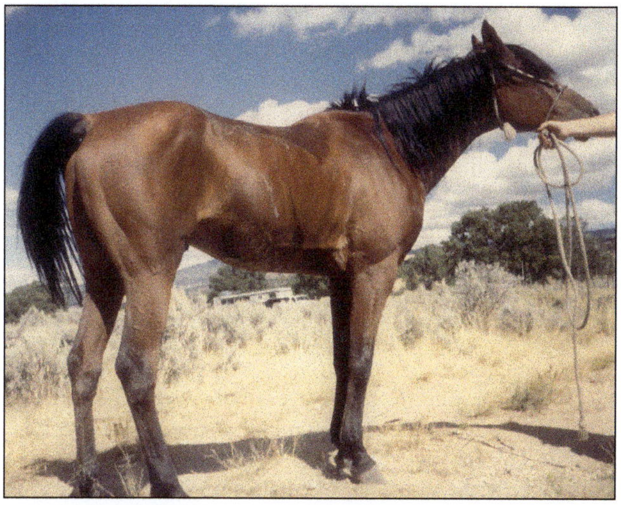

Figure 14.2 "Tucked-up" appearance to the abdomen of an endurance horse that successfully completed 80 km of endurance exercise over three consecutive days, supporting that absorption of water and electrolytes from the large intestinal reservoir is an important mechanism by which endurance horses maintain adequate hydration during prolonged exercise.

the next checkpoint. Other alternatives that can be used to avoid this problem are to train horses to initially drink an isotonic NaCl/KCl solution (4 liters would approximate one dose of an oral slurry) or to provide the additional electrolytes in a mix of concentrate feed at the checkpoints.

What remains unclear is whether or not horses can be administered "too much electrolytes" and whether or not there truly can be adverse effects of electrolyte supplementation. In theory, excess electrolyte administration should not be a problem as long as competing horses are provided frequent access to water and continue to drink because excessive electrolytes should be excreted in urine. However, as mentioned above, when electrolytes were administered in a high dose to fully replace anticipated sweat losses in an 80 km ride, mild hypernatremia and hyperchloremia developed in some horses (Sampieri et al 2006). Although no clinical problems were observed with these electrolyte changes, this finding provides support to recommend limiting electrolyte replacement to 30–40% of the anticipated losses. Again, another 20% of anticipated losses may be replaced by intestinal reserves resulting in an overall deficit of 40–50%, approximating a 4–5% BW loss. Finally, whether or not supplementation with hypertonic oral electrolyte slurries may exacerbate gastric ulcer disease is another concern. A recent gastroscopic survey of high-level endurance horses found ulcers in 93% of horses during the competitive season as compared to only 48% during the short rest period between seasons (Tamzali et al 2011). To assess whether or not electrolyte supplementation could possibly exacerbate gastric ulcer disease, groups of non-exercised horses were administered either eight doses of hypertonic oral salt slurries or a placebo (water) at hourly intervals. In comparison to gastroscopic findings 24 h before treatments were started, blinded scores for both number and severity of gastric ulcers were increased on gastroscopic examination 12 h after the last dose of electrolytes or placebo in both groups. However, scores for the horses treated with oral electrolyte slurries increased to a greater extent than for the horses administered the placebo (Holbrook et al 2005). It would certainly be of interest to repeat this type of study in a group of endurance horses completing a 160 km race.

Our discussion of electrolyte supplementation so far has been limited to additional NaCl during training or a mix of NaCl and KCl during competition. Although concerns about KCl supplementation during competition have been raised (potassium supplementation could exacerbate the mild increase in plasma K^+ concentration that occurs during endurance exercise and increase the risk of neuromuscular irritability [synchronous diaphragmatic flutter and cardiac arrhythmias]), more evidence to support this concern in practice is required (Hess et al 2005, 2006, 2008). The large amount of K^+ lost in sweat would support that supplementation during prolonged endurance exercise is warranted. Many commercially available electrolyte supplements also contain calcium and magnesium salts as well as varying amounts of carbohydrate (glucose and others). Although 8–10 g of calcium and 4–5 g of magnesium may be lost in 50 liters of sweat, no research to date has specifically investigated whether supplementation with these minerals is of benefit. Of interest, when a mixture of NaCl and KCl was administered to horses completing a 60 km treadmill endurance exercise test, the mild decrease in ionized calcium concentration and mild increase in venous blood pH observed during control (non-supplemented) runs were abolished with NaCl and KCl supplementation alone (Düsterdieck et al 1999).

Last, carbohydrate supplementation, in addition to offering various concentrate feeds during the rest breaks, has also become more common over the past decade, especially in elite endurance athletes. Marathon runners appear to benefit from ingestion of carbohydrate gels during the latter half of the race, likely due to limiting glycogen depletion. In horses, there has been little research in this area although a continuous rate intravenous glucose supplementation was demonstrated to prolonged endurance exercise performance on a treadmill in a few studies (Farris et al 1995, 1998). With the increasing speeds of elite competitions, as well as the even greater speed during the final loop of the recent WEG 160 km race, investigation of potential benefits of carbohydrate supplementation may be warranted. Unfortunately, such studies would ideally be performed on elite endurance athletes, rather than in non-elite horses or horses running on a treadmill, to adequately answer this research question. Similarly, it would be of great benefit to study these high-level equine athletes competing over 160 km with and without electrolyte supplementation to assess potential performance enhancing effects of this common practice.

Finally, the optimal amount of salt supplementation likely varies between horses and some may be able to successfully complete 80 and 160 km rides without any supplementation, other than that provided in feed at the checkpoints.

Key Points

- This area remains controversial and the authors do not feel that precise generic recommendations can be made
- The optimal level of salt supplementation likely varies between horses, and will depend on many factors during a race including the environmental conditions and the fitness of the horse, etc.
- In practice, although it is not ideal, currently riders tend to establish the most appropriate replacement strategy for their horse by a process of trial and error, ideally through the evaluation of different approaches during training rides

Suggested feeding and management strategies for race days

Pre-ride

An endurance horse should start the competition fully hydrated with optimal amounts of liver and muscle glycogen and, after appropriate physical conditioning, with metabolic processes primed for efficient energy utilization. Exercise training increases the amount of glycogen in muscle and to some extent influences the metabolic characteristics of muscle, both of which help to increase the workload/running speed before onset of substantial anaerobic metabolism (i.e. delays the onset of the lactate threshold).

- Training should be light for the 4–5 days before a race – which combined with regular feeding will help to ensure that the glycogen stores are "topped" up.
- Forage intake should be high before a ride and good quality forage should be used during the ride.

- Ensure adequate antioxidant and micronutrient provision.
- A high glycemic meal (in a grain adapted horse) the night before may be helpful to top up liver glycogen stores – however, it is important not to overload the digestive capacity of the small intestine.
- Avoid changes in the ration in the period leading up to the race.
- The practice of "electrolyte loading" during the 2–3 day period leading up to a race is not recommended (most of the administered electrolyte will be relatively quickly excreted: Coenen et al 1995) but an additional 70 g (2 volumetric oz) of a 3:1 NaCl/KCl in the concentrate meal around 2 h before the ride (providing adequate water is also provided and the horse is adequately hydrated) may be of benefit.
- The horse should be allowed to ingest small amounts (1–2 kg as fed) of hay or other forage in the 1–3 h period prior to the race. Given the recent work suggesting some advantage, with respect to gastric buffering, of feeding alfalfa hay (Lybbert et al 2007) the inclusion of alfalfa in the forage may be helpful. However, more work is needed in this area before firm recommendations can be made.
- Grain-based concentrates should not be fed within 3 h of the ride but short chopped fiber (e.g., hay chop) or grazing pasture grass may be advantageous.

During the ride

- Water should be provided at frequent intervals during a ride (e.g., every 30–40 min), especially in hot weather. Ideally horses should be trained to take any opportunity to drink either plain water or appropriate salt/electrolyte solutions.
- Electrolytes can be added to the feed if this does not discourage eating. Alternatively, electrolyte slurries can be given after the horse has consumed feed and water. The administration of hypertonic electrolyte pastes is contraindicated in horses with a poor drinking response or potentially those with or prone to gastric ulceration.
- Small amounts of calcium and magnesium can be provided during the ride but predominantly sodium, potassium and chloride are required
- Anecdotally, unlike in humans, there have been reports of detrimental effect (e.g., poor heart rate recovery at vet checks) in horses receiving certain carbohydrate supplements during rides (e.g., as glucose polymers). Fructose is absorbed in the horse and at low levels at least may be used as an alternative or partial substitute for glucose if required during exercise, although, unlike in other species, the horse does respond to ingestion of fructose with an insulin response (Bullimore et al 2000, Vervuert et al 2004).
- There are in fact no hard and fast rules on what to feed during a race – it does depend to a large extent on what the horse will eat. Certainly, the horse should be offered high quality feedstuffs and plenty of water. Typically a *smorgasbord* of feeds is provided as the primary goal is to encourage feed consumption. Appetite is an indicator of overall health and feed intake may assist in the maintenance of normal gastrointestinal motility. Consumed feed also helps to support work performance by providing a source of energy and perhaps water and electrolytes. Mash or slurry mixtures are popular; ingredients often used include alfalfa meal, cereals, wheat bran, stabilized rice bran, and some molasses. Most riders will also provide plain forage (often soaked). It has been suggested, but not proven, that forage based pellets or cubes may be advantageous as they may be consumed faster and reach the cecum more quickly – where they can be fermented to produce volatile fatty acids resulting in enhanced energy availability. Ideally all feeds offered should be ones the horse has recently been fed.
- If available and the horse shows interest, grazing grass would also be recommended.

Post-ride

- Water immediately. It may be beneficial, in horses adapted to consumption of saline solutions, to offer salt water (0.9% NaCl, 9 g in 1 liter of water) immediately after exercise and then plain water free choice The temperature of the water may also be of importance for some horses.
- If the horse exhibits an appropriate drinking response a further dose of an electrolyte supplement may be given, preferably in feed.
- Provide free choice hay followed by some cereal or mash (as per the ride) then maintain on normal diet for the next few days – do not attempt to replenish all the lost energy in the immediate (12–24 h) post ride period. Most endurance horses are only given light exercise (e.g., walking, pasture turnout) for a few days post race combined with a return to a normal feeding pattern.
- Provide supplementary electrolytes over at least the 24 h post race period – it is essential to include potassium in this supplement. Rations with an appropriate level of electrolytes should be provided in the 2–3 days following a race.

Conclusion

The optimal feeding and management of the endurance horse remains a challenge especially with the changing nature of the sport. However, individually targeted nutrition offers a practical way to help support the horse during training and competition as well as a means to reduce the incidence and severity of certain metabolic causes of disqualification. Finally, the magnitude of dehydration can be attenuated by administration of electrolytes as concentrated oral slurries or dissolved in water provided before and during the competition. However, whether or not electrolyte supplementation improves (or at least helps maintain) performance remains unclear and potential adverse effects of excess electrolyte supplementation may exist.

Acknowledgment

Some parts of the chapter were included in the chapter published by Elsevier Saunders in the Vet Clinics series: Harris PA (2009) Feeding management of elite endurance horses. In Veterinary Clinics of North America (Equine Practice) Geor RJ (ed) Elsevier Saunders Philadelphia, pp 137–154.

References

Andrews, F.M., Ralston, S.L., Williamson, L.H., Maykuth, P.L., White, S.L., Provenza, M., 1994. Weight loss, water loss and cation balance during the endurance test of a 3-day event. Equine Vet J 27 (S18), 294–297.

Ayus, J.C., Arieff, A., Moritz, M.F., 2005. Hyponatremia in marathon runners. N Engl J Med 353, 427–428.

Barnes, A., Kingston, J., Beetson, S., et al., 2010. Endurance veterinarians detect physiologically compromised horses in a 160km ride. Equine Vet J 42 (suppl. 38), 6–11.

Barton, M.H., Williamson, L., Jacks, S., et al., 2003. Body weight, hematologic findings, and serum and plasma biochemical findings of horses competing in a 48-, 83-, or 159-km endurance ride under similar terrain and weather conditions. Am J Vet Res 64, 746–753.

Beltrami, F.G., Hew-Butler, T., Noakes, T.D., 2008. Drinking policies and exercise-associated hyponatremia: is anyone still promoting overdrinking? Br J Sports Med 42, 796–801.

Bullimore, S.R., Pagan, J.D., Harris, P., et al., 2000. Carbohydrate supplementation of horses during endurance exercise: Comparison of fructose and glucose. J Nutr 120, 1760–1765

Butudom, P., Schott II, H.C., Davis, M.W., et al., 2002. Drinking salt water enhances rehydration in horses dehydrated by frusemide administration and endurance exercise. Equine Vet J Suppl 34, 513–518.

Butudom, P., Axiak, S.M., Nielsen, B.D., et al., 2003. Effect of varying initial drink volume on rehydration of horses Physiology & Behavior 79, 135–142.

Butudom, P., Barnes, D.J., Davis, M.W., Nielsen, B.D., Eberhart, S.W., Schott II, H.C., 2004. Rehydration fluid temperature affects voluntary drinking in horses dehydrated by furosemide administration and endurance exercise. The Veterinary Journal 167 (1), 2–80.

Carlson, G.P., 1983. Thermoregulation and fluid balance in the exercising horse. In: Snow, D.H., Persson, S.G.B., Rose, R.J. (Eds.), Equine Exercise Physiology. Granta Editions, Cambridge, pp. 291–309.

Casini, L., Gatta, L., Magni, B., et al., 2000. Effect of prolonged branch chain amino acid supplementation on metabolic responses to anaerobic exercise in standardbreds. J Equine Vet Sci 20, 120–123.

Coenen, M., Meyer, H., Steinbrenner, B., 1995. Effects of NaCl supplementation before exercise on metabolism of water and electrolytes Equine Vet J 18, 270–273.

Convertino, V.A., Armstrong, L.E., Coyle, E.F., et al., 1996. American College of Sports Medicine position stand, Exercise and fluid replacement. Med Sci Sports Exerc 28, i–vii.

Crandell, K., 2002. Trends in feeding the American Endurance horse. In Proceedings of the 2002 Kentucky Equine Research Equine Nutrition Conference, Kentucky, pp. 135–139. Online. http://www.ker.com/library/advances/315.pdf (accessed 6 July 2012).

Crandell, K., Pagan, P., Harris, P., et al., 1999. A comparison of grain oil and beet pulp as energy sources for the exercised horse. Equine Vet J Suppl 30, 485–490.

Düsterdieck, K.F., Schott II, H.C., Eberhart, S.W., et al., 1999. Electrolyte and glycerol supplementation improve water intake by horses performing a simulated 60 km endurance ride. Equine Vet J Suppl 18, 418–424.

De Fombelle, A., Frumholtz, P., Poillion, D., et al., 2001. Effect of botanical origin of starch on its prececal digestibility measured with the mobile bag technique. Proceedings of the 17th Equine Nutrition & Physiology Society Conference, Lexington, KY. Equine Nutrition & Physiology Society, Savoy, IL, pp. 153–155.

Dunnett, C., Marlin, D.J., Harris, R.C., 2002. Effect of dietary lipid on response to exercise: relationship to metabolic adaptation. Equine Vet J Suppl 34, 75–80.

Ecker, G.L., Lindinger, M.I., 1995. Effects of terrain, speed, temperature and distance on water and ion losses. Equine Vet J Suppl 18, 298–305.

Essen-Gustavsson, B., Blomstrand, E., Karlstroom, K., et al., 1991. Influence of diet on substrate metabolism during exercise. In: Persson, S.G.B., Lindholm, A., Jeffcott, L.B. (Eds.), Equine Exercise Physiology 3. ICEEP Publications, Davis, California, pp. 288–298.

Essen-Gustavsson, B., Connysson, M., Jansson, A., 2010. Effects of crude protein intake from forage only diets on muscle amino acids and glycogen levels in horses in training. Equine Vet J 42 (suppl. 38), 34–346.

Farris, J.W., Hinchcliff, K.W., McKeever, K.H., et al., 1995. Glucose infusion increases duration of prolonged treadmill exercise in Standardbred horses. Equine Vet J Suppl 18, 357–361.

Farris, J., Hinchcliff, K.W., McKeever, K.H., et al., 1998. Effect of tryptophan and of glucose on exercise capacity of horses. J Appl Physiol 85, 807–816.

Fellmann, N., Bedu, M., Giry, J., et al., 1989. Hormonal, fluid, and electrolyte changes during a 72-h recovery from a 24-h endurance run. Int J Sports Med 10, 406–412.

Fielding, C.L., Magdesian, K.G., Rhodes, D.M., et al., 2009. Clinical and biochemical abnormalities in endurance horses eliminated from competition for medical complications and requiring emergency medical treatment: 30 cases (2005–2006). J Vet Emerg Crit Care 19, 473–478.

Ford, E.J.H., Simmons, H.A., 1985. Gluconeogenesis from caecal propionate in the horse. Br J Nutr 53, 55–60.

Garlinghouse, S.E., Burrill, M.J., 1999. Relationship of body condition score to completion rate during 160km endurance races. Equine Vet J Suppl 30, 591–595.

Geor, R., Harris, P.A., 2005. Nutritional management of endurance horses. In: Harris, P.A., Mair, T.S., Slater, J.D. (Eds.), Equine Nutrition for All. Proceedings of the 1st BEVA & WALTHAM Nutrition symposi, a Harrogate, UK, pp. 15–24.

Goachet, A-G., Varloud, M., Philippeau, C., et al., 2010. Long-term effects of endurance training on total tract apparent digestibility, total mean retention time and faecal microbial ecosystem in competing Arabian horses. Equine Vet J 42 (suppl. 38), 387–392.

Goodwin, D., Davidson, H.P.B., Harris, P., 2002. Foraging enrichment for stabled horses: effects on behaviour and selection. Equine Vet J 34, 686–691.

Graham-Thiers, P.M., Kronfeld, D.S., Kline, K.A., et al., 2000. Dietary protein level and protein status in Arabian horses during interval training and repeated sprints. J Equine Vet Sci 20 (8), 516–521.

Greenleaf, J.E., 1992. Problem: thirst, drinking behavior, and involuntary dehydration. Med Sci Sports Exerc 24, 645–656.

Grimmett, A., Sillence, M.N., 2005. Calmatives for the excitable horse: A review of L-tryptophan. Vet J 170 (1), 24–32.

Halliwell, B., 1994. Free radicals and antioxidants: a personal view. Nutr Rev 52, 253–265.

Hargreaves, B.H., Kronfeld, D.S., Waldron, J.E., et al., 2002. Antioxidant status and muscle cell leakage during endurance exercise. Equine Vet J Suppl 34, 116–121.

Harris, P.A., 1997. Energy sources and requirements of the exercising horse. Annu Rev Nutr 17, 185–210.

Harris, P.A., Harris, R., 1998. Nutritional ergogenic aids in the horse – uses and abuses. In: Lindner, A. (Ed.), Proceedings of the Conference on Equine Sports Medicine and Science. Wageningen Press, The Netherlands, pp. 203–218.

Harris, P.A., Graham-Thiers, P., 1999. To evaluate the influence that "feeding" state may exert on metabolic and physiological responses to exercise. Equine Vet J Suppl 30, 633–636.

Harris, P.A., Kronfeld, D.K., 2003. Influence of dietary energy sources on health and performance. In: Robinson, N.E. (Ed.), Current Therapy in Equine Medicine 5. WB Saunders Co., Philadelphia, pp. 698–704.

Harris, P.A., Sillence, M., Inglis, R., et al., 2005. Effect of short (<2cm) lucerne chaff addition on the intake rate and glycaemic response to an oat meal. In: Tuscon, A.Z. (Ed.), Proceedings of the 19th Equine Science Society symposium. Equine Science Society, Champaign, IL, pp. 151–152.

Harris, P.A., Coenen, M., Frape, D.L., et al., 2006. Equine nutrition and metabolic disease. In: Higgins, A., Snyder, J. (Eds.), Equine Manual. Elsevier Saunders, London, pp. 151–222.

Hess, T.M., Kronfeld, D.S., Williams, C.A., et al., 2005. Effects of oral potassium supplementation of acid-base status and plasma ion concentrations of horses during endurance exercise. Am J Vet Res 66, 466–473.

Hess, T.M., Kronfeld, D.S., Carter, R.A., et al., 2006. Does usefulness of potassium supplementation depend on speed. Proceedings of the 7th International Conference of Equine Exercise Physiology (B Essen Gustavvson, E Barrey, PM Lekeux, DJ Marlin, eds). Equine Veterinary Journal Suppl 36, 74–82.

Hess, T.M., Kronfeld, D.S., Treiber, K.H., et al., 2007. Fat adaptation affects insulin sensitivity and elimination of horses during an 80km endurance ride. Pferdeheilkunde 23 (3), 241–246.

Hess, T.M., Greiwe-Crandell, K.M., Waldron, J.E., et al., 2008. Potassium-free electrolytes and calcium supplementation in an endurance race. Comp Exerc Physiol 5 (1), 33–41.

Hew, T.D., Chorley, J.N., Cianca, J.C., et al., 2003. The incidence, risk factors, and clinical manifestations of hyponatremia in marathon runners. Clin J Sports Med 13,41–47.

Hodgson, D.R., McCutcheon, L.J., Byrd, S.K., et al., 1993. Dissipation of metabolic heat in the horse during exercise. J Appl Physiol 74, 1161–1170.

Hodgson, D.R., Davis, R.E., McConaghy, F.F., 1994. Thermoregulation in the horse in response to exercise. Br Vet J 150, 219–235.

Holbrook, T.C., Simmons, R.D., Payton, M.E., et al., 2005. Effect of repeated oral administration of hypertonic electrolyte solution on equine gastric mucosa. Equine Vet J 37 (6), 501–504.

Holbrook, T.C., McFarlane, D., Schott II, H.C., 2010. Neuroendocrine and non-neuroendocrine markers of inflammation associated with performance in endurance horses. Equine Vet J 42 (suppl. 38), 123–128.

Holland, J., Kronfeld, D.S., Rich, G.A., et al., 1998. Acceptance of fat and lecithin containing diets by horses. Appl Anim Behav Sci 56, 91–96.

Holland, J.L., Kronfeld, D.S., Meacham, T.N., 1996. Behavior of horses is affected by soy lecithin and corn oil in the diet. J Anim Sci 74, 1252–1255.

Jansen, W.L., Sloet van Oldruitenborgh-Oosterbaan, M.M., Cone, J.W., et al., 2007. Studies on the mechanism by which a high intake of soybean oil depresees the apparent digestibility of fibre in horses. Anim Feed Sci Technol 138, 298–308.

Jansson, A., Dahlborn, K., 1999. Effects of feeding frequency and voluntary salt intake on fluid and electrolyte regulation in athletic horses. J Appl Physiol 86, 1610–1616.

Jansson, A., Rytthammar, Å., Lindberg, J.E., et al., 1996. Voluntary salt (NaCl) intake in Standardbred horses. Pferdeheilkunde 12, 443–445.

Jeffcott, L.B., Kohn, C.W., 1999. Contributions of equine exercise physiology research to the success of the 1996 Equestrian Olympic Games: a review. Equine Vet J 31, 347–355.

Jeffcott, L., Leung, W.M., Riggs, C., 2009. Managing the effects of the weather on the equestrian events of the 2008 Beijing Olympic Games. Vet J 182, 412–429.

Jose-Cunilleras, E., 2004. Abnormalities of body fluids and electrolytes in athletic horses. In: Hinchcliff, K.W., Kaneps, A.J., Geor R.J. (Eds.), Equine Sports Medicine and Surgery. Elsevier, London. pp. 898–917.

Jose-Cunilleras, E., Hinchcliff, K.W., Sams, R.A., et al., 2002. Glycemic index of a meal fed before exercise alters substrate use and glucose flux in exercising horses. J Appl Physiol 92, 117–128.

Jose-Cunilleras, E., Hinchcliffe, K.W., Lacombe, V.A., et al., 2006. Ingestion of starch – rich meals after exercise increases glucose kinetics but fails to enhance muscle glycogen replenishment in horses. Vet J 171, 468–477.

Kennedy, M.A.P., Entrekin, P., Harris, P.A., et al., 1998. Voluntary intake of loose versus block salt and its effect on water intake in mature idle thoroughbreds. In: Pagan, J.D., Geor, R.J. (Eds.), Advances in Equine Nutrition II. Nottingham University Press, Nottingham, pp. 147–149.

Kienzle, E., 1994. Small intestinal digestion of starch in the horse. Revue Med Vet 145 (2), 199–204.

Kingston, J.K., Geor, R.J., McCutcheon, L.J., 1997. Rate and composition of sweat fluid losses are unaltered by hypohydration during prolonged exercise in horses. J Appl Physiol 83, 1133–1143.

Kingston, J.K., McCutcheon, L.J., Geor, R.J., 1999. Comparison of three methods for estimation of exercise-related ion losses in sweat of horses. Am J Vet Res 60 (10), 1248–1254.

Kronfeld, D.S., 1996. Dietary fat affects heat production and other variables of equine performance under hot and humid conditions. Equine Veterinary Journal Suppl 22 (11), 24–35.

Kronfeld, D., 2001a. Body fluids and exercise: Influences of nutrition and feeding management. J Equine Vet Sci 21, 417–428.

Kronfeld, D., 2001b. Body fluids and exercise: replacement strategies. J Equine Vet Sci 21, 368–375.

Kronfeld, D.S., Holland, J.L., Rich, V., et al., 2004. Fat digestibility in *Equus caballus* follows increasing first order kinetics. J Anim Sci 82, 1773–1780.

Lacombe, V.A., Hinchcliff, K.E., Geor, R.J., et al., 1999. Exercise that induces substantial muscle glycogen depletion impairs subsequent anaerobic capacity. Equine Vet J suppl 30, 29–297.

Lacombe, V., Hinchcliff, K.W., Geor, R.J., et al., 2001. Muscle glycogen depletion and subsequent replenishment affect anaerobic capacity of horses. J Appl Physiol 91, 1782–1790.

Lacombe, K.W., Hinchcliffe, K.W., Kohn, C.W., et al., 2004. Effects of feeding meals with various soluble carbohydrate content on muscle glycogen synthesis after exercise in horses. Am J Vet Res 65, 916–923.

Langlois, C., Robert, C., 2008. Epidemiology of metabolic disorders in endurance racing horses. Pratique Veterinaire Equine Editions du Point Veterinarire 157, 51–60.

Latzka, W.A., Montain, S.J., 1999. Water and electrolyte requirements for exercise. Clin Sports Med 18, 513–524.

Lawrence, L.M., Jackson, S., Kline, K., et al., 1992. Observations on body weight and condition of horses in a 150 mile endurance ride. J Equine Vet Sci 12, 320–324.

Lorenzo-Figueras, M., Morisset, S.M., Morisset, J., et al., 2007. Digestive enzyme concentrations and activities in healthy pancreatic tissue of horses. Am J Vet Res 68 (10), 1070–1072.

Luthersson, N., Nielsen, K.H., Harris, P., et al., 2009. Risk factors associated with equine gastric ulceration syndrome in 201 horses in Denmark. Equine Vet J 41 (7), 625–630.

Lybbert, T., Gibbs, P., Cohen, N., et al., 2007. Gastric ulcer syndorme in exercising horses fed different types of hay. Proceedings Equine Science Symposium, Equine Science Society, Champaign, IL, pp. 128–129.

Marlin, D.J., Fenn, K., Smith, N., et al., 2002. Changes in circulatory antioxidant status in horses during prolonged exercise. J Nutr 132, 1622S-1627S.

Marlin, D.J., Dunnett, C.E., Deaton, C.M., 2005. The role of antioxidants. In: Harris, P.A., Mair, T.S., Slater, J.D. (Eds.), Proceedings of the 1st BEVA & Waltham Nutrition Symposia. Equine Veterinary Journal Ltd, Newmarket, pp. 39–48.

Martin-Rosset, W., Vermorel, M., Doreau, M., et al., 1994. The French horse feed evaluation systems and recommended allowances for energy and protein. Livestock Production Sci 40, 37–56.

McCutcheon, L.J., Geor, R.J., Hare, M.J., et al., 1995a. Sweating rate and sweat composition during exercise and recovery in ambient heat and humidity. Equine Vet J Suppl 20, 153–157.

McCutcheon, L.J., Geor, R.J., Hare, M.J., et al., 1995b. Sweat composition; comparison of collection methods and effects of exercise intensity. Equine Vet J Suppl 18, 279–284.

McCutcheon, L.J., Geor, R.J., 1996. Sweat fluid and ion losses in horses during training and competition in cool vs hot ambient conditions: implications for ions supplementation. Equine Vet J Suppl 22, 54–62.

McLean, B.M.L., Hyslop, J.J., Longland, A.C., et al., 2000. Physical processing of barley and its effects on intra-caecal fermentation parameters in ponies. Animal Feed Sci Technol 85, 79–87.

Meyer, H., 1987. Nutrition of the equine athlete. In: Robinson, N.E. (Ed.), Equine Exercise Physiology 2. ICEEP Publications, Davis, California, pp. 644–673.

Meyer, H., Coenen, M., 1989. Influence of exercise on the water and electrolyte content of the alimentary tract. In: 11th Conference of the Equine Nutrition and Physiology Symposium, Stillwater, OK. Equine Nutrition and Physiology Society, Savoy, IL, pp. 3–7.

Nery, J., Assenza, A., Pinna, W., et al., 2005. A study of horse's blood constitutents and weight variations during endurance competitions. Pferdeheilkunde 21, 103–104.

Noakes, T.D., 1995. Dehydration during exercise: What are the real dangers? Clin J Sports Med 5, 123–128.

Noakes, T.D., 2007. Hydration in the marathon – using thirst to gauge safe fluid replacement. Sports Med 37, 463–466.

Noakes, T.D., 2011. Changes in body mass alone explain almost all of the variance in the serum sodium concentrations during prolonged exercise. Has commercial influence impeded scientific endeavor? Br J Sports Med (published online December 22, 2010, 10.1136/bjsm 2010.075697).

NRC, 1987. Omega 3 fatty acids. Roche Report. National Academy Press, Washington DC, pp. A5, 1–5.

NRC, 2007. National Research Council Nutrient Requirements of Horses, 6th edn. National Academy Press, Washington DC.

Orme, C.E., Harris, R.C., Marlin, D.J., et al., 1997. Metabolic adaptation to a fat supplemented diet in the thoroughbred horse. Br J Nutr 78, 443–458.

Pagan, J.D., Hintz, H.F., 1986. Equine energetics. II. Energy expenditure in horses during submaximal exercise. J Anim Sci 63, 822–830.

Pagan, J.D., Harris, P.A., 1999. The effects of timing and amount of forage and grain on exercise response in Thoroughbred Horses. Equine Vet J Suppl 30, 451–458.

Pagan, J.D., Geor, R.J., Harris, P.A., et al., 2002. Effects of fat adaptation on glucose kinetics and substrate oxidation during low intensity exercise. Equine Vet J Suppl 34, 33–38.

Palmgren Karlsson, C., Jansson, A., Essen-Gustavsson, B., et al., 2002. Effect of molassed sugar beet pulp on nutrient utilisation and metabolic parameters during exercise. Equine Vet J Suppl 34, 44–49.

Parsons, A.M., Nielsen, B.D., Shcott, H.C., et al., 2011. Effects of fiber type, particle size and soak time on water hydration and estimated potential water releasing capacities of roughages fed to horses. J Equine Vet Sci 31, 261.

Phillips, S.M., 2011. Exercise and protein nutrition The science of muscel hypertrophy: making dietary protein count. Proceedings of the Nutrition Society 70, 100–103.

Pösö, A.R., Hyyppa, S., Geor, R., 2004. Metabolic responses to exercise and training. In: Hinchcliff, K.W., Kaneps, A.J., Geor, R.J. (Eds.), Equine Sports Medicine and Surgery. Saunders, London, pp. 771–792.

Potter, G., Arnold, F., Householder, D., et al., 1992. Digestion of starch in the small or large intestine of the equine. Pferdeheilkunde (1. European Conference on Horse Nutrition), 109-111.

Robert, C., 2004. Risk factors for horses developing metabolic troubles in long distance endurance rides: update of epidemiological data collected at French endurance rides. In: Proceedings of International Endurance Veterinary Seminar, Newmarket, pp. 5–8.

Rose, R.J., Purdue, R.A., Hensley, W., 1977. Plasma biochemistry alterations in horses during an endurance ride. Equine Vet J 9, 122–126.

Sampieri, F., Schott, H.C., Hinchcliff, K.W., et al., 2006. Effects of sodium chloride and potassium chloride supplementation on endurance horses competing in 80 km rides. Equine Vet J Suppl 36, 19–26.

Sandick, B.L., Engell, D.B., Maller, O., 1984. Perception of drinking water temperature and effects for humans after exercise. Physiol Behav 32, 851–855.

Schott, H.C., McGlade, K.S., Molander, H.A., et al., 1997. Body weight, fluid, electrolyte, and hormonal changes in horses during and after recovery from 50- and 100-mile endurance rides. Am J Vet Res 58, 303–309.

Schott II, H.C., McGlade, K.S., Hines, M.T., et al., 1996. Bodyweight, fluid and electrolyte, and hormonal changes in horses that successfully completed a 5 day, 424 kilometer endurance competition. Pferdeheilkunde 12, 438–442.

Schott, H.C., Butudom, P., Cardoso, F.F., et al., 2003. Innate variability in voluntary drinking in Arabian horses. J Vet Int Med, Abstract 314: 17–456.

Schott, H.C., Marlin, D.J., Geor, R.J., et al., 2006. Changes in selected physiological and laboratory parameters in elite horses competing in a 160 km endurance race. Equine Vet J Suppl 36, 37–42.

Serrano, A.L., Quiroz-Rothe, E., Rivero, J.-L.L., 2000. Early and long-term changes of equine skeletal muscle in response to endurance training and detraining. Pflügers Archiv European Journal of Physiology 441 (2–3), 263–274.

Sharwood, K.A., Collins, M., Goedecke, J.H., et al., 2004. Weight changes, medical complications, and performance during an Ironman triathlon. Br J Sports Med 38, 718–724.

Shirazi-Beechey, 2008. Molecular insights into dietary induced colic in the horse. Equine Vet J 40 (4), 414–421.

Siciliano, P.D., Wood, C.H., 1993. The effect of added dietary soybean oil on vitamin E status of the horse. J Anim Sci 71, 3399–3402.

Slade, L.M., Lewis, L.D., Quinn, C.R., et al., 1975. Nutritional adaptations of horses for endurance performance. Proceedings of the Equine Nutrition and Physiology Symposium, Pomona, CA. Equine Nutrition and Physiology Society, Savoy, IL, p. 114.

Snow, D.H., Kerr, M.G., Nimmo, M.A., et al., 1982. Alterations in blood, sweat, urine and muscle composition during prolonged exercise in the horse. Vet Rec 110, 377–384.

Sosa León, L.A., Davie, A.J., Hodgson, D.R., et al., 1995. The effects of tonicity, glucose concentration and temperature of an oral rehydration solution on its absorption and elimination. Equine Vet J Suppl 20, 140–146.

Spooner, H.S., Nielsen, B.D., Harris, P.A., et al., 2007. Hydration status of horses during endurance exercise as affected by dietary fiber type. In: Proceedings of the 20th Equine Science Symposium, Maryland. Equine Science Society, Champaign, IL, pp. 24–25.

Steffanon, B., Bettini, C., Guggia, P., 2000. Administration of branched chain amino acids to standardbred horses in training. J Equine Vet. Sci 20, 115–119.

Szlyk, P., Sils, I.V., Francesconi, R.P., et al., 1989. Effects of water temperature and flavoring on voluntary dehydration in men. Physiol Behav 45, 639–647.

Tamzali, Y., Marguet, C., Priymenko, N., et al., 2011. Prevalence of gastric ulcer syndrome in high-level endurance horses. Equine Vet J 43, 141–144.

Treiber, K.H., Geor, R.J., Boston, R.C., et al., 2008. Dietary energy source affects glucose kinetics in trained Arabian geldings at rest and during endurance exercise. J Nutr 138, 964–970.

Trottier, N.L., Nielsen, B.D., Lang, K.L., et al., 2002. Equine endurance exercise alters serum branched chain amino acid and alanine concentrations. Equine Vet J 34, 168–172.

Vervuert, I., Coenen, M., Bichmann, M., 2004. Comparison of the effects of fructose and glucose supplementation on metabolic responses in resting and exercising horses. J Vet Med series A 51 (4), 171–177.

Vervuert, I., Voigt, K., Hollands, T., et al., 2009. Effect of feeding increasing quantities of starch on glycaemic and insulinaemic responses of healthy horses. Vet J 182, 67–72.

Votion, D.M., Fraipont, A., Goachet, A., et al., 2010. Alterations in mitochondrial respiratory function in response to endurance training and endurance racing. Equine Vet J 42 (suppl. 38), 268–274.

Waller, A., Heigenhauser, G.J.F., Geor, R.J., et al., 2009. Fluid and electrolyte supplementation after moderate intensity exercise enhances muscle glycogen resynthesis in Standardbred horses. J Appl Physiol 106, 91–100.

Wardlaw, G.M., 1999. Perspectives in nutrition, 4th ed. WBC Mc Graw-Hill, New York.

Warren, L., Lawrence, L.M., Roberts, A., 2001. The effect of dietary fiber on gastrointestinal fluid volume and the response to dehydration and exercise. In: 17th Conference of the Equine Nutrition and Physiology Symposium. Equine Nutrition and Physiology Society, Savoy, IL, pp. 148–149.

Williams, C.A., Kronfeld, D.S., Hess, T.M., et al., 2004. Antioxidant supplementation and subsequent oxidative stress of horses during an 80-km endurance race. J Anim Sci 82, 588–594.

Zeyner, A., Romanowski, K., Müller, A.-M., et al., 2008. Effects of different doses of sodium chloride on the acid–base balance of horses. Institute of Nutrition, Department for Farm Animals and Veterinary Public Health, University of Veterinary Medicine Vienna, Vienna, Austria, September 25–27, 2008 (Iben C, Wagner E, Handl S, eds). Printed by Reumiller & Reumiller, Vienna, Austria, p. 29.

15

Nutritional considerations for aged horses

Sarah L. Ralston, Patricia A. Harris

Introduction

Aging has been defined as "an irreversible, progressive and time-dependent decline of overall body functions, resulting from the interaction of genetic and stochastic factors" (Figuieredo et al 2008). One theory regarding the cause of aging and eventual death of multicellular organisms is related to macromolecular damage caused by reactive oxygen species produced by mitochondria, the so-called "mitochondrial theory of aging" (Terman et al 2010). The decay of metabolically relevant structures that occurs with age appears to be linked with total energy intake, in that dietary energy restriction is accepted as an interspecies factor for longevity (as discussed below). Regardless of the cause, aging in mammals is usually associated with changes in body composition, physical strength and physiological function. These are a result of a combination of intrinsic factors associated with the aging process itself, as well as factors indirectly associated with age, in particular degenerative diseases secondary to environmental or physical insults that progress with time and physical inactivity. However, it has been noted in the human literature that "a healthy lifestyle, incorporating a well-balanced diet and physical activity, cannot stop the years advancing, but may play a useful part in a healthful, active and independent old age" (Phillips 2003). We should have a similar goal of optimal nutrition and physical activity for the horses in our care, based on what we know about the aging process and the individual's circumstances. More importantly perhaps, different dietary approaches may be required, depending on whether the horse is just old in years or is afflicted with one or more age related problems. This chapter will, start by outlining some key aspects of aging in humans and other species, followed by conditions associated with aging in the horse. It will then go on to discuss nutritional and management recommendations for the horse.

Key aspects of aging in humans and other species

Body composition changes as age increases in most species studied to date. A principal change is a decrease in skeletal muscle mass, often referred to as "sarcopenia", which is often associated with loss of physical strength (Evans 1995, Thompson 2009) and reportedly occurs in all humans, even if they remain active (Phillips 2003). Sarcopenia of aging, in healthy individuals, may be the result of an inability to maintain muscle protein synthesis after feeding (*anabolic resistance*), which is exacerbated by physical inactivity (Rennie et al 2010). A recent review of age-related changes in body mass concluded that the reduction in resting metabolic rate which favors weight gain due to fat accumulation with concomitant loss of fat free mass may be due in part to reduction in specific organ mass and metabolic rate (i.e., liver) (St-Onge & Gallagher 2010), although in the very elderly (over 75 years) body fat also tends to decrease, probably due to altered dietary habits (Phillips 2003). In humans, aerobic capacity is estimated to decline by about 1% per year and anaerobic capacity, as well as muscle strength, by about 0.5% per year between 30 and 70 years of age (Sutton & Brook 1986). Appropriate exercise training (Sutton & Brook 1986, Raj et al 2010) can reduce the rate of decline and have positive anabolic effects, even in frail (Aagaard et al 2010) and malnourished elderly patients (Hebuterne et al 2001). Resistance, as well as aerobic training, is generally considered to be safe for elderly people to improve strength and increase muscle mass (Graves et al 1994, Phillips 2003), but it is also usually recognized that a sensible exercise regimen throughout life is most advantageous in the reduction or inhibition of age related sarcopenia. Recent work has shown that 80 yr old humans who have partaken in lifelong aerobic or strength training regimens have maximal aerobic capacities and muscle strength that are comparable to that of sedentary individuals around 50 yrs of age (Booth & Zwetsloot 2010).

In elderly people, loss of weight is common and a low body mass index linked with unintentional weight loss is associated with an increased mortality risk (Phillips 2003, Dorner et al 2010), as is obesity (Dorner et al 2010) though for different reasons. The decline in food intake and loss of the motivation to eat, which is seen in many elderly people, may be related to a reduction in the central feeding drive, possibly secondary to increased effectiveness of cholecystokinin (Donini et al 2003), as well as physical problems such as poor dentition or social factors such as isolation. In addition, alterations in taste and olfactory perception have been suggested to reduce feed intake in older people and perhaps lead to inappropriate diet selection leading to inadequate protein and/or calorie intake (Schiffman 1997, Pelchat 2000). Protein-energy malnutrition in turn leads to impaired muscle function, poor wound healing, delayed recovery from surgery and ultimately increased morbidity and mortality (Donini et al 2003).

Chronic dietary restriction, however, appears to be the only nutritional intervention that consistently extends the life span of the animals evaluated (e.g., dogs, Kealy et al 2002; rats, Wohlgemuth et al 2010). Labrador Retrievers fed 25% less, than that consumed by those given *ad libitum* access, from weaning to 3.25 years of age, after which both were fed for maintenance, had increased median life span and delayed onset of signs of chronic disease (Kealy et al 2002, Lawler et al 2008). Dogs with a body condition score (BCS) of 5 or less (on a 9-point scale) at middle age (6–8 years of age) were more likely to live beyond 12 years of age compared to middle aged dogs with a higher BCS. Looking at the group as a whole, high fat mass and declining lean body mass were strongly correlated with death within 1 year (Lawler et al 2008).

The immune system becomes less competent with increasing age, which is often referred to as "immunosenescence". This change in immune function is thought to increase susceptibility to opportunistic infections, cancer and autoimmune conditions (Campbell et al 2004, Henson & Akbar 2009) and may reflect in particular a decline in T cell immune function (Henson & Akbar 2009). Aging is also associated with increased markers of chronic inflammation (Bruunsgaard & Pedersen 2003, Grimble 2003, Salminen et al 2007).

It has been recognized that stress is associated with proteolysis and a negative nitrogen balance that erodes cell mass (Hebuterne et al 2001), and older people may have a reduced capacity to respond in situations that require the mobilization of amino acids for protein synthesis in vital organs and the immune system. Studies also suggest a lack of adaptation to severe malnutrition in the elderly, with a preferential use of their fat-free mass and body cell mass as a fuel (Hebuterne et al 2001). A reduction in maximal mitochondrial ATP production rate (MAPR) and mitochondrial DNA abundance occurs with age in association with muscle weakness and reduced endurance in elderly people (Tatpati et al 2010). In a recent study an 8 hr infusion of branched chain amino acids resulted in an increased MAPR in young adults compared with the elderly suggesting that the response to amino acid supplementation may not be the same across all ages (Tatpati et al 2010). Dardevet et al (2002) showed a defect in the postprandial stimulation of protein synthesis in geriatric rats. Supplementation of leucine overcame this defect, possibly by enhancing the efficiency of translation during the protein synthesis process.

Osteoarthritis (OA) is the most commonly occurring musculoskeletal disease in people, and there is a strong relationship between age and the development of OA (Verzijl et al 2003). From about the age of 30 years, the matrix of minerals and collagen are removed from bone more rapidly than new bone tissue is put down, resulting in weakened structural support and increased risk of fractures, although the rate of age-related bone loss is influenced by many factors including level of physical activity (Phillips 2003).

Age-related differences were found in the microflora composition within the cecum, colon and rectum of beagles, but not in the stomach or small intestine (Hayek et al 1997). Whether such differences occur in the horse and what clinical relevance this might have is currently unknown, but probably warrants further evaluation. Similarly age-related changes in vagal afferents innervating the gastrointestinal tract have been reported in other species (Phillips et al 2010).

Definition and prevalence of the "geriatric" or "aged" horse

The term "geriatrics" was derived from the Greek words meaning "old men" and "medical treatment" and implies that there are health or physical problems, whether age-related or not, that need special attention as one ages. There is, however, considerable variation in the aging process (e.g., humans: Phillips 2003) and there is no set age at which an individual is automatically considered to be "geriatric" as opposed to "aged but healthy". Some horses remain physically active and healthy well into their twenties and yet others become "geriatric" by mid teens. These individual differences need to be taken into consideration when determining optimal management and feeding practices. For the purposes of this chapter therefore we will refer in general to the aged horse rather than use the perhaps more specific term "geriatric".

In a paper by Brosnahan and Paradis (2003b), in which the management and activity of 218 older horses was surveyed, the owners perceived their horses as being "old" at approximately 22 years of age. They also found that, in horses aged 16.5 years or more, age became a negative factor in a proposed purchase. The proportion of horses over 20 years of age has increased in recent years. One retrospective study reported that in 1989 only around 2% of the equine referral cases at a university veterinary hospital were over 20 years of age, but this had increased to 12.5% by 1999 (Brosnahan & Paradis 2003a) and approximately 20% by 2003 (Brosnahan & Paradis 2003b). Pony breeds were significantly over represented in the ≥30 years of age group. This progressive increase in old horses presented for veterinary care is probably due to both improved health care and nutrition as well as an increased willingness of owners to maintain older horses (NRC 2007).

In a survey of the horse population in the United States done in 2005, 7.6% of the total population was reported to be over 20 years old (National Animal Health Monitoring System 2006). Previous studies suggested that a quarter of those horses might have been 30 years or older (Paradis 2002). It has been estimated that around 30% of the UK equine population is aged 15 years or older (Hotchkiss et al 2007, Ireland et al 2011a), with 11% between 20–30 years and 2% over 30 years (Ireland et al 2011a). Horses over the age of 40 years are no longer uncommon in the United States (Ralston, personal observation). An Arabian-cross gelding, Elmer Bandit, competed successfully in competitive trail rides until his demise at 38 years (Hayes 2010).

Note

The oldest horse we could find record of was apparently 62 years old when he died in 1822: "Old Billy" a Cleveland/Eastern blood cross who was apparently still pulling boats up to 1819.

Key Points

- Aged horses comprise an increasing proportion of horses in developed countries
- Not all aged horses are compromised
- Public perception and expectations regarding aged horses is changing

Common causes of mortality in aged horses

A 2002 study on causes of mortality in older horses in the UK reported that cardiovascular deficiencies were the major cause of death (41%), followed by injuries of the locomotor system (18%, 61% of which were degenerative disorders) and colics (11%) (Leblond et al 2002). In Australia, a survey of horses and ponies over 15 years old (McGowan et al 2010), reported that mortality rate was 9.4 per 100 horse years with the majority being euthanized (89%) due to musculoskeletal disorders (21%), weight loss (13%) and colic (12%). In the general aged horse population, 43% had cardiac murmurs, 50% were lame, 69% had hoof abnormalities and 96% were found to have some form of dental abnormality. A recent study in the UK reported similar findings (Ireland et al 2009, Stevens et al 2009). Ireland et al 2009 found a slightly higher overall mortality rate (11.1 per 100 horse years at risk) and the most frequent reasons for death were musculoskeletal disorders (28.8%), colic (19.5%) and chronic diseases (19.5%). At a UK equine charity in 2009 the average age of the horse requiring euthanasia was 20 years with 66.3% due to osteoarthritis (average age 21.9 years), 11% colic and the remaining 22.7% due to respiratory or hepatic problems, laminitis, ocular lesions and neoplasia (Jarvis 2010).

Clinical conditions most commonly associated with aging (not necessarily mortality) in horses

In the Brosnahan and Paradis (2003a, b) papers, gastrointestinal, musculoskeletal and respiratory problems were the most frequently reported problems in horses ≥20 years of age. A survey in Australia found that owners considered ~43% of horses >20 years to be suffering from a health disorder compared with ~33% in the 6–10 year age group (Cole et al 2005). In a more recent survey (McGowan 2009), owners of elderly horses were most concerned about weight loss (maintaining the horse's body condition), arthritis/lameness and dental care.

Clinical conditions that are most commonly seen in the older horse include:

- Neoplasia: Pituitary pars intermedia dysfunction (PPID) and thyroid tumors are common in horses over 20 years of age (Beech 1987, Ralston et al 1988, Dybdal 1997, Brosnahan & Paradis 2003a, Mcfarlane et al 1998, McFarlane & Cribb 2005) see Box 15.1. Although prevalence in the general population has not been documented, in one study of 24 horses over the age of 20 years, only one mare did not have neoplastic

Box 15.1 Pituitary Pars Intermedia Dysfunction (PPID)

PPID is a common endocrine disorder of old horses. Key features of this condition are summarized below (see also reviews by McFarlane et al 1998, Schott 2002, McFarlane 2011):

- A neurodegenerative disease characterized by hyperplasia, hypertrophy, and cellular atypia of the pars intermedia with a single large adenoma or multiple small adenomas.
- A slowly progressive condition associated with loss of dopaminergic inhibitory input to the melanotropes of the pars intermedia.
- Of unknown etiology although oxidative stress and/or abnormal accumulations of misfolded proteins such as α-synuclein may contribute to the neuronal damage and cell death. Research does not suggest that systemic oxidative stress or antioxidant failure contributes to the development of PPID but mitochondrial antioxidant dysfunction and increased mitochondrial reactive oxygen species production may play a role.
- Although minimal descriptive epidemiological data are available, the disease is thought to affect between 15 and 30% of aged equids of both sexes.
- Typically recognized on the basis of associated clinical signs in animals from 15 years upwards – and rarely in animals <10 years of age.
- Possibly more prevalent in ponies, Arabians and Morgans but more work is needed to clarify the influence of breed and type.
- Difficult to definitively diagnose in the early stages and especially in those animals without the classic signs of hypertrichosis (previously referred to as hirsutism – recent work has confirmed that there is persistence of hair follicles in anagen). There are profound effects of season on many of the diagnostic tests currently used.
- Hypertrichosis is a common clinical sign (with a 90% positive predictive value for identification of PPID using post-mortem examination as the gold standard). Owner surveys suggest 14–30% of aged horses have hair coat abnormalities.
- Other clinical features include: muscle atrophy, increased risk of laminitis, polyuria, polydipsia, hyperhidrosis, abnormal fat distribution, and insulin resistance (although whether this is specific to PPID horses or aged animals or the horse population as a whole is currently unknown), increased risk for opportunistic infections, behavioral abnormalities (including lethargy), other neurological conditions as well as raised basal ACTH concentrations. Not all are present in every case.

changes in the pituitary and/or thyroid (Ralston et al 1988). Other tumors such as intestinal lipomas, melanomas, and squamous cell carcinomas also are more commonly found in the older horse (Howarth et al 1991, Brosnahan & Paradis 2003b, Springer et al 2010).

- Increased incidence of colics, especially impactions: In one survey, impactions comprised 88% of colic episodes in the older horse versus 29% of episodes in horses of all ages (Carson-Dunkerley & Hanson 1996), and an increased incidence of strangulating lipomas has also been recorded in aged horses (Edwards & Proudman 1994). In contrast, increasing age was not associated with an increased incidence of colic in a recent study in the UK (Ireland et al 2011b).
- Dental abnormalities: Loss of teeth and abnormal wear patterns are extremely common with advancing age because the teeth of the horse continue to erupt throughout life until approximately 20 years of age, after which time they begin to loosen and are shed (Graham 2002). With age, the enamel ridges of the cheek teeth, considered by many to be essential to efficient mastication of forage, become worn, and the resultant marble-like occlusal surface is known as a "smooth mouth". This can lead to "quidding" (inadequate mastication with wads of partially chewed feed dropped from the mouth) of long fiber forages, weight loss (Knottenbelt 2003) and potentially an increased risk of choke (Ralston & Breuer 1996).
- Increased incidence of glaucoma (Chandler et al 2003, Ollivier et al 2009).
- Reduced maximal contractile function of the aortic valve: This abnormality is associated with an increase in collagen content of the valve (Bowen et al 2006) and a high incidence of valvular regurgitation (Stevens et al 2009).
- Alterations in respiratory function: Changes include lower partial pressures of arterial oxygen and carbon dioxide plus, potentially, impaired transfer of oxygen across the alveoli (Aguilera-Tejero et al 1998). The incidence of recurrent small airway obstruction is higher in the older horse (Deaton et al 2004, Hotchkiss et al 2007) .
- Increased risk for and severity of bacterial and viral infections, potentially due to decreased immunocompetence. For example, more severe clinical signs of equine viral arteritis infection were seen in aged (over 20 years old) vs. young animals kept in similar conditions (Traub-Dargatz et al 1985). The ability of horses to produce antibodies in response to viral antigens in a vaccine gradually decreases with age (Goto et al 1993, Horohov et al 1999). It has been suggested that low plasma ascorbic acid concentrations associated with pituitary dysfunction may adversely impact immunocompetence (Ralston et al 1988).
- Increased risk of tendon and ligament damage: There is reportedly a reduction in the crimp pattern of collagen fibrils and a decrease in overall fibril diameter associated with advanced age (Patterson-Kane et al 1997, 1998). In the horse, unlike man, the biochemical characteristics of the collagen component of equine cartilage are apparently not influenced by age alone (Brama et al 1999); however osteoarthritis is a very common cause of lameness and poor performance in horses of all ages (Kidd et al 2001) and is commonly observed in the joints of older horses (Brama et al 1999). Degenerative joint disease was reported to be a frequent reason for euthanasia in old horses (Leblond et al 2002). In a report of horses housed at a welfare facility, 55.4% of horses ≥ 15 years of age were treated with a nonsteroidal anti-inflammatory drug (NSAID) because of osteoarthritis, while 62.2% of animals ≥ 20 years and 65.3% older than 25 years were treated with an NSAID (Jarvis 2010).
- Increased risk of death when undergoing general anesthesia for surgery: It was reported that horses over 12 years of age had a higher risk of death during general anesthesia than younger horses (Johnston et al 1995). The reasons were thought to be multifactorial and may reflect the types of surgery older horses are presented for (predominantly emergency colics as opposed to elective orthopedic or cosmetic procedures) as well as overall effects of aging.
- Decline in mare fertility: The reproductive cycles of mares change as they age, probably associated with pituitary dysfunction leading to altered ovarian function and loss of primordial follicles (Carnevale et al 1993). Eventually many old mares will enter a period of reproductive senescence with reduced oocyte viability (Madill 2002).
- Parenchymal and vascular lesions in the brain: A variety of lesions have been reported by Capucchio et al (2010) and another study suggested that there are a number of age related changes in the brain of horses, including lipofuscin deposition (Jahns et al 2006).

Age, exercise, muscle tone and skeletal strength

Maximal heart rate during exercise reportedly decreases with age (McKeever & Kearns 2001). It also has been suggested that unfit older horses may not be able to thermoregulate during exercise as well as can younger unfit horses due to changes in resting plasma volume and cardiac deficits (McKeever & Kearns 2001). More recent work has confirmed that aging may compromise the ability to handle the combined demands of exercise and thermoregulation perhaps due in part to a decreased absolute pre-exercise plasma volume (McKeever et al 2010). Aged horses may also have altered endocrine responses to exercise (McKeever & Malinowski 1999).

Mares over 20 years old had significantly lower maximal aerobic capacity and exercise capacity than young mares maintained under the same conditions and levels of training (McKeever & Malinowski 1997, see also Walker et al 2010). In a retrospective study of unfit Standardbred mares (McKeever et al 2010), a statistically significant reduction in maximal aerobic capacity was estimated to have occurred between 18 and 20 years of age, regardless of diet or exercise history. However, the old horses tested at 20 to 30 years old were still able to complete strenuous standardized treadmill tests and no special feeds or training regimens were provided to them. In the recent UK review ~61% of owners reported a decrease in intensity of exercise with increasing age but around 21% of horses were still competing with a median age of 18 years (Ireland et al 2011a) and the majority of horses were still in some ridden exercise. Similarly, Brosnahan and Paradis (2003b) reported that around 60% of the old horse population in the New England region of the USA were used regularly in some form of athletic activity, with 10% of old horses in active competition. This underscores the fact that many old horses can be maintained in good body condition and continue to be used for athletic endeavors well into their 20s and even 30s, despite reduced exercise tolerance.

Age, body condition and body composition

Prior to the 1980s, it was commonly accepted that horses over 16 years of age (the American Quarter Horse Association definition for "aged") were in some way geriatric, and the general public perception was that there was little value in applying interventions to reverse or prevent age related deterioration in health (Ralston, personal observations). It was rare to see a horse over 30 years of age and most of these animals were thin and frail. However, recently these perceptions have changed. This is likely to be the result of a number of factors including increased use of more effective, easily administered anthelmintics as well as improved overall health care since the late 1970s and the introduction of "senior" feed formulations in the 1990s. In addition, the increased prevalence of people owning horses purely for pleasure/leisure activities as opposed to commercial purposes such as draught or high level competition may have resulted in more owners being willing to maintain their "faithful companion" as a "pasture ornament" and continue to care for them into old age. Though there is some evidence that reduced frequency of some routine management practices such as farrier care and anthelmintic administration may occur in older horses (Mellor et al 2001), the highly popular use of high priced "senior" feeds is evidence that a significant proportion of owners are willing to spend extra to maintain an old horse's health (Brosnahan & Paradis, 2003b).

In a survey of 165 non-hospitalized horses over 20 years of age (mean age of 26.5 years, the oldest being 44 years old) initiated in 1998, only 4% were reported by their owners to be in poor body condition (scored on a scale of 0 to 5 with 0 = very poor, 5 = very fat; Brosnahan & Paradis 2003b). In this population of old horses in the Northeastern United States, 68% were considered to be in moderate to good body condition and 28% were reported as fat or very fat. In Australia, owners of horses and ponies aged ≥15 years (mean 20.5 years) reported that 30% were overweight (BCS 3/5) and only 2% were underweight (BCS<2/5; McGowan et al 2010). In a UK survey, ~8% of old horses were reported to be underweight and 10.5% overweight (Ireland et al 2011b). Weight loss or difficulty in maintaining adequate body condition is, however, not uncommon in elderly horses and in the survey study of Ireland et al (2011b) 17% of owners reported weight loss in their horse within the last 12 months. Weight loss may arise for many reasons such as dental abnormalities, renal and hepatic disease, and PPID. Risk of weight loss may be higher in the cold winter months. Horses over 20 years of age were reported to require higher feed intake during winter months, when maintained outdoors in 3 sided shelters in Colorado, than did middle aged mares housed under the same conditions (Ralston et al 1988). As noted above, aged mares also had difficulty with thermoregulation during exercise (McKeever & Kearns 2001) Therefore, ration and general management may be contributory factors in the failure of old horses to maintain acceptable body condition, especially in the winter months. Similarly, with the apparent increase in the prevalence of obesity in the general horse population (see Chapter 28) it may be expected that an increasing proportion of horses over 20 years of age may be overweight with the associated complications of lameness, laminitis and insulin resistance.

Age and digestive function

Chronic parasitism may impair digestive ability due to scarification of the intestinal mucosa in both the large and small intestines. It has been hypothesized (Ralston et al 2001b) that chronic parasitic scarring of the large intestine contributed to the apparent malabsorption and/or maldigestion reported in some earlier studies of digestion in aged horses (Ralston 1989, Ralston & Breuer 1996). This type of lesion could cause a reduction in the absorption of nutrients if a sufficient percentage of the absorptive surface area is affected, although this has not been documented in horses. Reduced apparent digestion of fiber, protein and phosphorus was reported in horses over 20 years of age, based on studies done in the 1980s and early 1990s (Ralston 1989, Ralston & Breuer 1996). The horses used in the original studies, however, had not had the lifelong benefit of modern intestinal parasite control, having been born in the 1960s and 1970s, before paste anthelminthics were commonly available. The digestive deficits reported were essentially the same as those reported for horses that had had their entire left and right colons surgically removed, leaving only the cecum and small colon for absorption (Ralston et al 1986, Bertone et al 1989). Similar deficits were not found in aged horses studied in the 1990s that had had good gastrointestinal parasite control all of their lives (Ralston et al 2001b). This was recently confirmed by Elzinga et al (2011) in a study that showed no age by diet differences in 8 adult (5–12 years) and 9 aged (19–28 years) mares of similar stock-type breeding, all of which had received regular anthelmintic treatment and had normal dentition. They were evaluated after 5 weeks on three different commonly fed formulated diets (high roughage, high fat and fiber, and high cereal).

The observed reduction in fiber digestion also might have been due in part to abnormal dentition, since dentition was not assessed in the first two studies (Ralston 1989, Ralston & Breuer 1996) and major abnormalities were not present in the third (Ralston et al, 2001b). However, common dental abnormalities such as points or hooks <3 mm in size did not adversely affect digestion of nutrients in middle aged (10 to 15 years old) horses (Ralston et al 2001a) and may not affect fecal particle size or apparent digestibility of nutrients (Ralston et al 2001b, Carmalt & Allen 2008). However, both groups of researchers did note that extremely poor dentition might adversely impact feed intake and may contribute to weight loss through reduced feed intake. Carmalt and Allen (2008) also speculated that there may be a minimum amount of tooth necessary for effective mastication, but that the morphological limit is currently unknown. In addition, there is evidence that age is associated with increasing severity of degenerative changes in the equine temporohyoid joint

(Naylor et al 2010), which may predispose horses to temporohyoid osteoarthropathy, which in turn causes difficulty in chewing. More work is needed into the link between dentition, digestion and weight maintenance.

Pelleted and extruded "complete" feeds that require little or no mastication, especially when soaked in water, are commonly fed to older horses. Clinical observations have indicated that use of these feeds has facilitated maintenance of good body condition in old horses, even in the face of severe dental abnormalities. Ralston and Breuer (1996) looked at the effect of a feed formulated specifically for old horses on weight gain, body condition score (BCS) and various blood parameters in horses >20 years of age at a large equine retirement facility. Half of the horses were fed a maintenance ration (mixed grains with molasses, 8.5% protein) and the other half were given a product formulated for geriatric horses (pelleted, processed to enhance digestibility, grain-based mix with added protein (14%) and fat (7%)) for 3 winter months. Horses and ponies with initial BCS ≤3 in both groups were fed ~10% more than NRC (NRC 1989) recommended energy requirements. Horses with BCS ≤3 and fed the geriatric formula had greater weight gain and higher final BCS (as well as higher plasma protein concentrations) than those fed the standard grain mix. However, the old horses with initial condition scores >3 did not differ in their final blood parameters, condition scores or weight gains. The authors concluded that "geriatric horses, especially those unable to maintain adequate weight on standard rations in the absence of hepatic or renal disease, appear to benefit from the special formulation", but those that were able to maintain good condition on a conventional ration did not benefit in any way from dietary intervention. This study confirms the individuality of the older horse and the requirement to assess the needs of each horse based on current condition and activity.

The feeding of alfalfa to older horses is controversial. It has been suggested that the feeding of alfalfa hay, with higher leucine and crude protein when compared to grass forage, may help to prevent loss of muscle mass in older horses, although no studies have tested this hypothesis (Siciliano 2002). However, if used as the sole or major source of roughage/forage, alfalfa may promote the formation of calculi/enteroliths due to the high calcium plus protein content and perhaps exacerbate renal and/or hepatic dysfunction (Ralston & Breuer 1996). There may be some advantages of including a small amount of alfalfa in an older horse's diet where there is no renal or hepatic compromise.

Although more work is needed in this area, current evidence suggests that advanced age (>20 years) alone does not significantly affect digestive efficiency in horses (Ralston 2007, Elzinga et al 2011). As long as healthy old horses are fed rations that provide calories and nutrients in quantities that meet or exceed the recommended amounts for their body size and physiologic status (NRC 2007), adjusted for environmental conditions and with adequate anthelminthic administration and dental care, old horses can easily maintain good body condition well into their 20s and even 30s.

Age, inflammation and immunity

A few studies have looked at age-associated changes in lymphocyte populations in otherwise healthy light-breed aged horses (20 years and older) (McFarlane et al 2001, Horohov et al 2002, Campbell et al 2004). These studies have reported an age-related decline in total lymphocyte count, as well as lymphocyte subset cell counts ($CD5^+$, $CD4^+$, $CD8^+$ and B cells), as seen in other species (McFarlane et al 2001, Horohov et al 2002, Campbell et al 2004). There was no significant difference in the immunoglobulin (Ig) isotypes in aged horses compared to the younger controls, although there was a trend towards a higher concentration of IgA and IgG. In other species, changes in immunoglobulins have also been reported, although in the cat higher levels of IgA and IgM were noted (Campbell et al 2004). In the study by Horohov et al (2002), the peripheral blood mononuclear cells also showed a reduced proliferative response to challenge with mitogens. These changes have been suggested to reflect a down-regulation of the cellular component of the acquired immune response with age. An earlier study had shown that, although older horses overall had reduced immune function, they appeared to be more resistant to the exercise-induced immune suppression seen in young horses (Horohov et al 1999).

More recently, work has suggested that aged horses, like humans, show evidence of a pro-inflammatory state (i.e., "inflamm-aging") that may contribute to the development of age-associated diseases (McFarlane & Holbrook 2008). Older horses have been reported to have significantly higher levels of the inflammatory interleukins, IL-1, IL-15, IL-18, and tumor necrosis factor (TNF-α) gene expression in peripheral blood, increased levels of TNFα protein and increased frequency of interferon gamma (IFN-γ) and TNF-α producing cells in circulation (Adams et al 2008). While peripheral blood mononuclear cells from old horses have increased inflammatory cytokine production compared with those from young animals, obese old horses have even greater frequencies of lymphocytes and monocytes producing inflammatory cytokines than do thin old horses (Adams et al 2009). This suggests that obesity may play an important role in the apparent age-related dysregulation of inflammatory cytokine production (Adams et al 2009). Reduction of body weight and body condition in fat old horses significantly reduced the percent of IFN-γ- and TNF-α-positive lymphocytes and monocytes as well as circulating concentrations of TNF-α. (Adams et al 2009).

Insulin resistance and age

In humans, there is a progressive decrease in insulin sensitivity with age, while in rats there is evidence that the insulin resistance (IR) in adipose tissue precedes the development of IR in liver and muscle (Serrano et al 2009). A survey of geriatric horses in the Northeastern part of the USA suggested that older horses were more likely to have higher resting blood glucose and insulin concentrations but also a lower BCS and to be undertaking less exercise than their younger counterparts (Costa et al 2010). Mares >20 years of age with documented pituitary pars intermedia adenomas had higher resting insulin concentrations than younger mares fed the same feeds, possibly associated with the higher resting cortisol (Ralston et al 1988). In a recent study (Rapson et al 2011) no difference in the glycemic response to a sweet feed meal was seen in association with age (19–28 yrs vs 5–12 yrs). However, healthy aged horses had a greater peak insulin concentration and area under the curve for insulin, than adult horses, regardless of the background diet they had been fed for 5 weeks prior to the meal challenge.

Key Points

- Aged horses have an increased risk of certain conditions, e.g., PPID and dental abnormalities. However, they can remain healthy and physically active well into their 20s
- Aged horses may be in a pro-inflammatory state (i.e., "inflamm-aging"), which may contribute to the development of certain age-associated diseases
- There appears to be an increase in insulin resistance and a reduction in immunocompetence with age
- Aged horses may be under or overweight, although very old horses more typically have difficulties in maintaining weight
- Advanced age per se (>20 years), however, does not significantly affect digestive efficiency in horses

Changes in nutritional requirements with age

Resting metabolic rate, total energy expenditure and energy requirements are thought to decrease with age in people. In dogs, there may be a decline in energy requirements with age (with no change in overall efficiency of nutrient digestion), but cats may require the same or higher intakes, perhaps due to reduced protein and fat digestibility with increasing age (Burkholder 1999). The authors are not aware of any specific work on this in the horse although a variety of external factors may influence energy requirements of clinically healthy aged horses, including activity level and environmental conditions. As noted above, aged horses may require higher energy intakes in cold weather due to their reduced thermoregulatory ability, but requirements will also be influenced by current body condition and level of activity, for example old horses that are fat or obese should not necessarily be supplemented with extra energy sources just because it is cold.

It has also been suggested that the skeletal systems of horses at different ages respond differently to calcium and phosphorus supplementation, as well as to exercise and periods of inactivity (Mansell et al 2001), however horses over 21 years of age have not been investigated in this respect. Reduced phosphorus retention was documented in old horses in the 1980s (Ralston et al 1988) and skeletal fragility not associated with calcium deficits has been reported in old horses with PPID (Dybdal 1997). Reduced phosphorus retention has been observed in horses following extensive resection of the large colon (Bertone et al 1989) which would be expected since the large colon is a major site of phosphorus absorption in the horse (NRC 2007). In an old horse which is failing to maintain weight/is losing weight and/or has an unknown history with respect to parasite control there may well be justification for a higher intake of protein and phosphorus (Ralston & Breuer 1996, Ralston 2006).

Even in humans it is still not known whether the elderly have different nutritional requirements than their younger counterparts (Lesourd 2006). However, it is important to note that even if energy expenditure and energy requirements decrease with age, requirements for the daily intake of many essential vitamins and minerals do not decline in proportion, and therefore intake of these nutrients should at least meet normal maintenance amounts. Similarly, a specially formulated diet may be indicated for horses with suboptimal caloric intake (e.g. providing a palatable "balancer" product as a concentrated source of vitamins and minerals).

General considerations regarding feeding and management of the old horse

This chapter will only address old horses with common age-associated problems that can be supported through alterations in feeding management. These include reduced mobility due to chronic lameness, inadequate dentition, increased sensitivity to extremes of temperature, apparent malabsorption/maldigestion, recurrent impaction colic, and PPID (also commonly known as equine Cushing's disease). Clinical evaluation of weight loss in an old horse should rule-out common causes such as pain associated with arthritis (especially of the neck), acute or chronic diarrhea, or inflammation associated with infections (Ralston 2007). Before "old age" dietary changes are instituted, renal or hepatic function should be evaluated by assessment of standard indices because dietary recommendations for renal or hepatic conditions are often contrary to those given below (Ralston et al 1988, McFarlane et al 1998). Similarly otherwise healthy old horses that are obese and/or insulin resistant that do not have evidence of pituitary dysfunction should be managed as described elsewhere in this book.

Management considerations

When asked for nutritional recommendations for a horse over 20 years old, an important first step is a thorough assessment of the horse's environment. As noted above, old horses apparently are sensitive to extremes of weather and are poorer at thermoregulation than they were when they were younger (Ralston et al 1988, McKeever et al 2010). Therefore old horses, especially those that are still being exercised regularly, should have protection from extremes of temperature if at all possible. Shelter from direct sun, wind and precipitation should be easily accessible during extremes of temperature. However, prolonged confinement to a stall may exacerbate orthopedic problems and stiffness due to arthritic changes (Ralston, personal observation) and should be used only if necessary. Continuous turnout with free access to a deep run-in shelter is usually the ideal situation. Some old horses may have limited mobility due to chronic arthritis or old injuries which should be taken into account when deciding where to place feeders/water sources.

Heat stress may reduce feed intake (Cymbaluk & Christison 1990) and feed intakes should be carefully monitored. If feeds are being fed soaked in water, any feed left after one or two hours in hot weather should be discarded to prevent spoilage. Since hypertrichosis secondary to PPID is extremely common in old horses and, in view of their reduced thermoregulatory capacity, "hirsute" horses should have their hair coats clipped during hot and humid weather conditions, especially if still being used for athletic endeavors. In extremely hot weather, taking measures to keep both sedentary and exercising old horses as cool as possible (e.g., application of cool water, providing shade and fans) will improve comfort and perhaps reduce any heat-related inappetance. Temperatures below the lower critical temperature

(LCT) of any horse will increase caloric needs (NRC 2007, Cymbaluk et al 1990). The LCT has been reported to vary between -20 to 9.4°C in adult horses and can change within an individual through adaptation (NRC 2007, Cymbaluk et al 1990). Specific feeding guidelines for cold weather, therefore, are not possible since the increase in requirements will depend on the climate to which the horse is adapted, shelter availability, hair coat and body fat, and perhaps even individual differences in metabolic rate and tolerance. However, it has been recommended for adult horses at maintenance that the caloric intake be increased by 2.5% for each degree celsius below the LCT (McBride et al 1985, as quoted in Cymbaluk & Christison 1990) which is usually estimated to be -1 to -5°C for horses in northern, temperate climates that are adapted to being outdoors. For old horses the increase in digestible energy (DE) needed may be even higher if they are thin and not hirsute. Therefore, body condition should be monitored carefully during prolonged bouts of cold weather and the amount of feed adjusted according to condition loss or gain.

Key Points

General management considerations in the elderly horse include:

- Provision of adequate shelter but avoidance of prolonged confinement to stalls if possible
- Thorough, regular dental care and strict attention to control of internal parasites
- Clipping long hair coats in hot weather if necessary
- Water and feed containers at an appropriate location and height to optimize access
- Monitoring bodyweight/condition
- Choosing field companions carefully to avoid bullying
- Regular foot trimming and choosing a flat paddock, free from poaching and ruts, to decrease strain on joints
- Regular blood work/veterinary evaluations to detect onset of common disease/aging infirmities.

The last two points may be especially important as recent work has suggested that as horses age there is a reduction in the provision of preventive health care measures including vaccinations, farrier care and routine veterinary checks (Ireland et al 2011b).

Box 15.2 Classification of old horses with respect to their nutritional needs.

Old horses can be divided into four groups with respect to their nutritional needs:

1. **Apparently "Normal"** Those that are maintaining good body condition, clinically normal and "in use", i.e., the horse that is old in years but has no apparent age-related or clinically important disorders and is still being used for performance and/or reproduction. Such horses can maintain optimal bodyweight and condition on a standard "adult" ration formulated for their level of activity and reproductive status.

   Nutritional advice: Continue on current management regimen, assuming it is balanced for their needs, but continue to monitor weight and to maintain routine vaccination, dental and parasite control programmes.
2. **Apparently "Normal" but overweight** Those that are overweight/obese but clinically normal, i.e., the horse that is old in years and still functioning normally, but has a reduced level of physical activity and a tendency to gain weight.

   Nutritional advice: Consider following the recommendations for weight loss given in Chapter 28. Continue to monitor weight and to maintain routine vaccination, dental and parasite control programmes
3. **Apparently "Normal" but underweight** Those with difficultly to maintain weight but clinically normal, i.e.. the horse that is old in years, *clinically normal* but no longer able to maintain weight on a normal diet.

   Nutritional advice: Confirm that teeth and parasite control programs are adequate and that hepatic and renal functions are within normal limits. Gradually change to a more calorie- and nutrient-rich diet. Commercial feeds designed to prevent weight loss and restore optimal condition in older horses are now commonly available. Ideally these should provide good quality protein (10–14% typically with soybean meal or legumes as the main sources), added oil (7–10%), phosphorus (0.3–0.45%) and restricted calcium (0.45–1.0%).
4. **The Geriatric Horse** The truly geriatric horse, which has one or more physical or metabolic abnormalities as well as old age.

   Nutritional advice: Provide treatment and support for the specific underlying conditions as discussed below and in other chapters in this book. It may not be possible to address all of the issues in such horses adequately. It is better to feed something that reasonably meets the horse's nutritional needs and that it will consume voluntarily than to feed a ration it will not consume or nothing at all.

Nutritional considerations

Many old horses do not need special feeds or rations as a consequence of age alone (see Box 15.2). Under maintenance conditions, many old horses will maintain body weight and condition when provided 1.5 to 2.5% of body weight (BW) of good quality hay/forage with free access to water and salt together with any forage balancer (vitamins, minerals and trace-elements) as required. Forage- or grain-based concentrates are only needed when the horse is unable to maintain weight on forage alone or if the horse can no longer chew long stem hay or grass effectively. Depending upon their physiologic status (sedentary, exercising, pregnant, or lactating), most old horses, especially those in their early 20s, can be fed adult (not geriatric or senior) formulations for their specific physiologic states (see Fig. 15.1).

Water

Due to the increased risk of impaction colic in all horses with insufficient water intake (NRC 2007) adequate water intake is of major concern. In freezing weather it is especially important that the horse be encouraged to ingest as much water as possible. Strategies to promote water consumption include the soaking of feeds in water and providing the horses with free access to unlimited amounts of unfrozen water, especially in winter (Cymbaluk et al 1990, Ralston 2006). Addition of 30 to 60 g of salt (NaCl) to feed or water may encourage water intake but avoid excessive forced supplementation of feed or water since it may actually reduce voluntary intake (NRC 2007, Ralston 2006). If the old horse is housed in a group situation it is important that the water source is adequate for the number of horses present and is located such that a horse cannot be excluded by more dominant, aggressive individuals.

Forage

For all old horses, even those with severely compromised dentition, the ration should be based on forage/high fiber feeds (as for all horses). Unless choke is a problem, hay, preferably high quality grass or grass/legume mix, can be

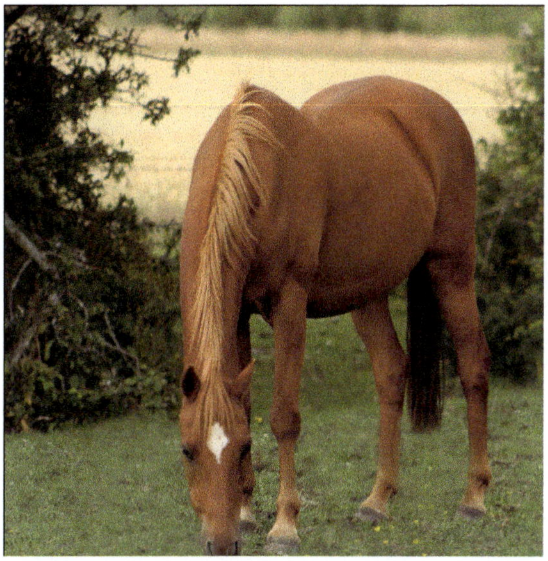

Figure 15.1 Picture of a healthy active 23yr old horse – out at grass during the summer, with additional hay if required and a vitamin/mineral balancer. In winter out all day, in all night, with hay and fed a standard low energy coarse mix, chaff (short chopped forage) and a small amount of soaked sugarbeet pulp.
© *Hannah Briars: MARS Horsecare.*

offered free choice. If, however, the horse cannot adequately masticate long stem hay as evidenced by persistent quidding and even choke, the use of chopped or cubed hays should be considered. If choke is a problem, these alternate forms of roughage can be soaked in water to form easily swallowed slurries.

Feed

In the UK survey of Ireland et al (2011a), 40% of owners of animals ≥15 years of age reported making major changes to the horse's diet as they had aged. The median age for this group was significantly higher (21.8 years) when compared to the group of horses with no reported dietary changes (19 years). The median age of the horses fed "senior" feeds was 22.7 years, significantly higher than those animals not receiving such feeds (19 years). Horses were also more likely to receive complete mash feeds as they aged. Senior feeds were provided to 51% of horses aged ≥20 years in a survey conducted in the USA (Brosnahan & Paradis 2003b).

Most major feed companies offer feeds designed specifically for old horses ("Senior" type feeds). These feeds typically contain 12–16% crude protein, restricted calcium (0.6–0.8%) and increased phosphorus (0.45–0.6%) based on the reduction in protein and phosphorus retention reported in the 1980s (Ralston 1989) and concern about renal excretion of excess calcium in horses that might have reduced renal function. Old horses fed only alfalfa containing >1.5% calcium on a dry matter basis had high incidence of renal medullary calculi and bladder stones (Ralston, unpublished data, 1985–1988). "Senior" formulas in the US are usually either "predigested" (as described by the manufacturer often without full details) or extruded to increase digestibility, but the majority are of moderate caloric density as most are designed as "complete" feeds to be fed as the primary or sole source of nutrition at the rate of 1.0 to 2.0% BW per day. Some "senior" feeds also contain between 3 and 5% added molasses for palatability and/or are grain-based with a nonstructural carbohydrate (NSC – which includes starch, sugars and fructans) content well over 30% (Ralston, unpublished data,1989–2010). Such products should be used with caution if pituitary function of the horse has not been evaluated or if PPID with associated chronic laminitis has been diagnosed.

All dietary changes should be implemented gradually, depending on how different the new ration will be in NSC and fiber content. If the horse cannot maintain good body condition on 2.0% to 2.5% BW of the ration currently fed divided into three or four feedings, it may be necessary to provide a feed with higher caloric density. High-fat stabilized rice bran products are commonly used in equine rations but should be used with caution in old horses if they are on a calcium- restricted ration, as bran products contain high (>1%) concentrations of phosphorus that may or may not be balanced with an equally high concentration of calcium.

Specific considerations

Horses with PPID

Chronic laminitis, skin infections, hyperinsulinemia with or without hyperglycemia following a glucose challenge, polyuria/polydypsia and hypertrichosis (hirsutism) and failure to control cortisol secretion are commonly associated with PPID (Beech 1987, Dybdal 1997, Ralston 2006). Hyperinsulinemia in response to glucose challenges and low plasma vitamin C concentrations were observed in horses with documented (on post mortem) adenomas of the pars intermedia (Ralston et al 1988). Decreased immune function (Dimock et al 1999, Horohov et al 2002) is also associated with aging, perhaps secondary to the elevated cortisol and reduced plasma vitamin C concentrations associated with PPID.

If a horse has clinical evidence of PPID but has not had laminitic episodes, it can be maintained on good quality forage (pasture and/or hays) with the addition of a low starch adult or "senior" product, that has <3% added molasses and restricted starch from grains, if necessary to maintain body weight/condition. The acceptable threshold for % NSC under such circumstances has yet to be established, but is generally assumed to be <20% NSC, with some recommending as low as 10%, although this degree of restriction is probably only necessary for the overweight, laminitis-prone or chronically laminitic horses.

If the PPID horse has had laminitic episodes and/or clinical signs are not being successfully managed with drug therapy, more dramatic restrictions in carbohydrate intake and supplementation will be necessary. Chronic laminitis also can be exacerbated by high fructan/NSC content of grasses and some hays (NRC 2007). If pasture is available, horses predisposed to laminitis should have restricted pasture access during periods when NSC accumulation is greatest: e.g early spring and late fall (especially after midday if not cloudy), after periods of drought or freezing weather, especially if the pasture is overgrazed (Watts 2000, NRC 2007). More details on the nutritional management of horses at high-risk for laminitis can be found elsewhere in this book (Chapter 27 and Chapter 18). If the horse is hirsute, it will have increased sweat losses in warm weather and these animals should have free access to both water and salt.

Old horses with PPID were documented to have higher fecal gastrointestinal parasite egg counts than healthy age-matched controls or younger animals (McFarlane et al 2010). Heavy intestinal parasite burdens may contribute to weight loss in these animals and the implementation of a more rigorous anthelmintic treatment regimen is indicated in these circumstances. Adequate control of intestinal parasitism may or may not enable resolution of weight loss without the need for major dietary changes.

Horses with inadequate dentition

Dental abnormalities are common in older equids and can lead to difficulties with mastication (Lowder & Mueller 1998). Donkeys start to develop serious dental disorders from age 16–20 years (du Toit et al 2009). In a population of 349 donkeys where the average age was 30 years, 93% were found to have significant dental abnormalities (DuToit et al 2008). Thorough examination of the oral cavity is an important part of the clinical evaluation of old horses. McGowan (2009) reported that while owners of aged horses reported only 0.5% dental disease, veterinary evaluation confirmed that moderate to severe dental disease occurred in 46% of the horses examined (a subpopulation of the original population). Observations of ingestive and masticatory behavior can provide useful information (e.g., evidence of quidding that suggests a dental/oral cavity abnormality; see Figs 15.2A + B). The teeth and oral cavity of old horses should be evaluated using a mouth speculum to adequately assess the condition of even the most caudal molars. Correctable dental abnormalities (sharp points, hooks, broken or infected molars) should be addressed but over-correction or aggressive rasping should be avoided if possible (Ralston 2006). Based on one study, it appears that the angle of the occlusal surface of the molars and premolars should be between 72–80° relative to the lateral surface of the tooth for optimal mastication (Ralston et al 2001a). If dental abnormalities are not correctable, dietary changes may be necessary, even though the actual nutrient requirements are not altered. Even if significant dental abnormalities are not present (Carmalt & Allen 2008), periodontal disease (inflamed gums and buccal/lingual lesions) can be painful and affected horses may demonstrate a reduced rate of feed intake (an issue with group feeding in particular) with partial or even complete anorexia (Knottenbelt 2003).

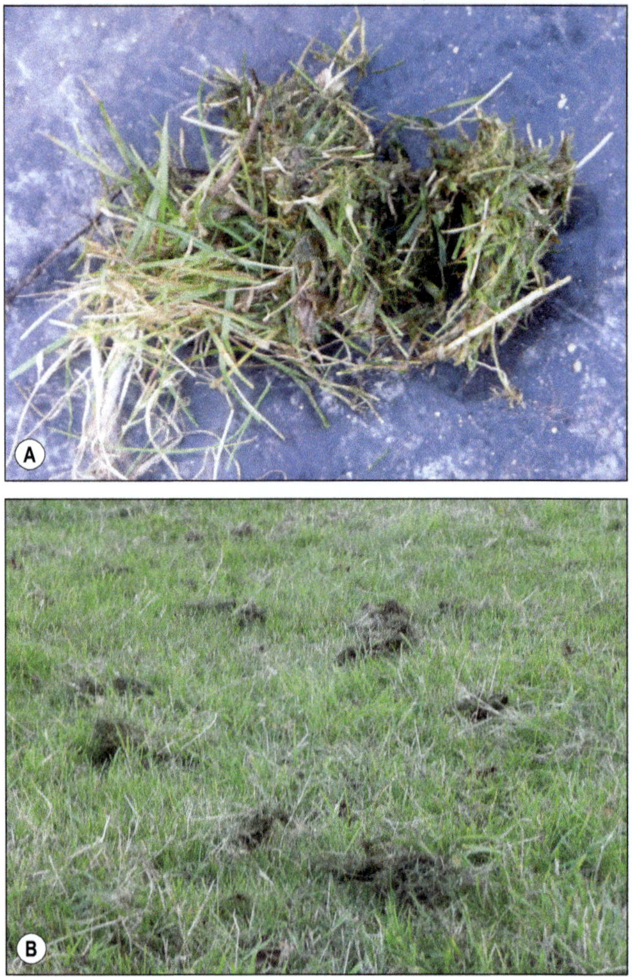

Figure 15.2 (A) Fresh grass 'quid' (food dropped from mouth in semi-chewed state sometimes referred to as 'Corn Dollies') plus evidence of quidding (dysmastication) in a paddock **(B).** Such dysmastication could be neurologic, muscular, pain related or physical in origin and therefore the cause needs to be determined via a thorough oral examination. In older animals it is commonly due to physical reduction in masticatory efficiency . If no resolution is possible, allowing the aged animal to grass and quid can be positive (re behaviour/welfare) and may not be an issue unless it causes choke or other adverse effects as long as adequate amounts of feed that can be assimilated (e.g. soaked fibre based feed) is provided. © *MARS Horsecare.*

Horses with uncorrectable dental abnormalities, such as multiple missing molars and premolars, should still receive at least 1.5% body weight of forage/roughage-based feed per day. However, these animals may not be able to adequately masticate long stem hays. When available, and if laminitis is not an issue, pasture turnout may be the most appropriate forage source, as grass appears to require less mastication than dried long stem forages and is usually an excellent source of most of the nutrients required by healthy adult horses. Alternatively, chopped hays or haylages, beet pulp, or hay cubes divided into at least two or, preferably, three feedings per day can be used. These processed fiber and nutrient sources, especially the latter two, can be soaked in water to reduce the risk of choke and increase water intake (see Fig 15.3). Pelleted or extruded "complete" feeds that are designed to be fed without hay may also be used, especially for horses that have little or no ability to masticate even chopped hays adequately. These should also be soaked in water to reduce the risk of choke. The soaked feeds should be offered in limited amounts (sometimes as little as 0.05–0.1% BW on a DM basis) per feeding to prevent spoilage and maximize intake. If grain-based pellet or extruded feeds are offered, the amount should not exceed 0.5% body weight per feeding in order to maximize the efficiency of digestion, as larger meals of high starch feeds have been documented to increase small intestinal bypass, with a resultant decrease in digestive efficiency and alterations in large intestinal fermentation (NRC 2007). Whole grains and even textured grain mixes are not suitable for horses with severe dental abnormalities.

Table 15-1 Sample Rations Recommended (SR) for Aged Horses That Are Otherwise Healthy[a] and Have Protection from Extremes of Temperature. These Recommendations Apply to Horses with No or Limited Access to Pasture and Will Need to be Adapted to the Individual Circumstances

	Forage	Grain-based concentrate	Supplements	Alternate feed types
Maintenance Aged, healthy, BCS 5 to 7	2.0 to 2.5% BW DM per day of good quality grass or legume mix hay/haylage that provides 7.5–8.5 MJ (~1.8 to 2 Mcal) DE/kg DM, with 10 to 12% crude protein.	None usually required but if desired or in work, choose one with restricted starch/ sugar, perhaps added fat (4–7%)	Free access to NaCl and water plus perhaps an additional mineral mix to balance the ration taking into account the forage and the amount of any fortified concentrate	Forage based pellets or cubes could be used to replace 10 to 50% of the long stem/chopped forages
Aged, healthy, Thin BCS <4[b]	2.0 to 2.5% BW DM good to excellent quality grass or grass/legume mix hay/haylage providing 8–10 MJ/kg (~2–2.4 Mcal) DE/kg and 12 to 14% crude protein	0.5 to 1% BW of a commercial product formulated for the aged horse with 12 to 14% crude protein, 4 to 7% fat. Divide into two or more feedings. Minimize starch and sugar intake if prone to laminitis or have PPID.	As above	Forage based pellets or cubes could be used to replace 10% to 50% of the long stem/chopped forages–these tend to be higher calorie/ digestibility
Poor dentition	Free access if choke not a problem	0.5 to 1% BW divided into two or more feedings of a commercial product formulated for the aged horse with 12 to 14% crude protein, 4 to 7% fat. See above re starch and sugar	As above	1.5 to 2.5% BW forage based pellets or cubes divided into three or more feedings. Can be soaked in water

[a]For horses with reduced immune competence/chronic inflammation, e.g., recurrent skin infections, hoof abscesses, respiratory problems may benefit from including 0.3 g/kg BW of an omega-3 rich oil as well as vitamin C (0.01 g/kg BW), vitamin E (to provide in total 2–3 mg/kg BW), and B-complex vitamins in the form of brewers yeast (30 to 60 g/day) or commercial supplement in recommended amounts.
[b]Once the desired weight/condition is achieved the horse should be switched to the maintenance ration.

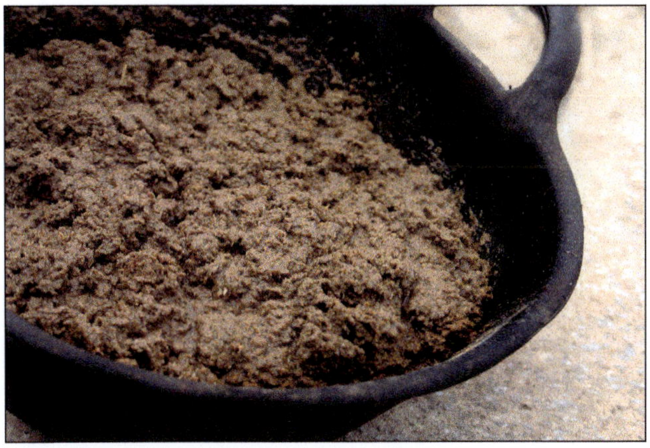

Figure 15.3 Picture of a typical soaked meal (of a high fibre fortified cube/pellet) for an aged horse with poor dentition.
© Hannah Briars: MARS Horsecare.

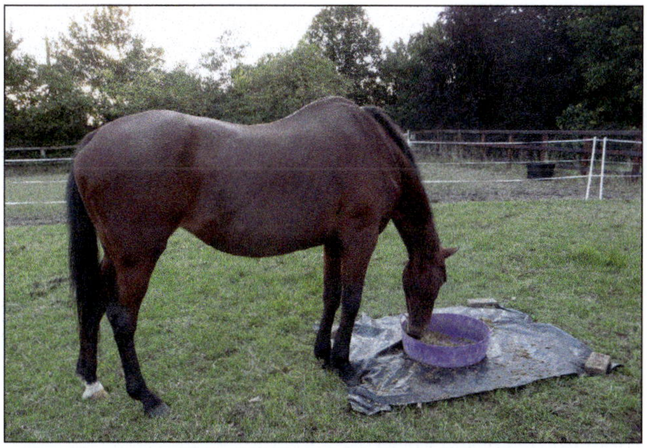

Figure 15.4 Practical example of a washable "plastic tablecloth" being used for an aged (~30 yrs) horse with marked quidding enabling her to lick up any spillage without problems (rubber mats are more durable alternatives but can be more difficult to keep clean).
© MARS Horsecare.

Access to long stem hay or pasture, however, should not be restricted unless choke or chronic impaction is a problem or in cases of horses with few teeth or with major periodontal disease, where long fiber feeds are not tolerated. In such cases a soaked mixture of commercial senior feeds, hay cubes and sugar beet pulp can be used, again offering at least 1.5 to 2.0% BW in dry feed weight divided into two or more feedings per day (see Fig 15.4). Additional vegetable oil can be added if required to help maintain weight (see below). Examples of recommended diets are shown in Table 15-1.

Possible additional nutritional support

Vitamins and other antioxidants

It has been suggested that free radical accumulation is closely involved in aging and many of the age-related conditions including sarcopenia; however, there is limited evidence as to the benefits of synthetic anti-oxidant supplementation in aged humans (Van der Horst-Graat et al 2004, Phillips 2003). One study in mice suggested that conjugated linoleic acid may help to prevent sarcopenia during aging but further work to confirm this in other species and over longer periods is needed (Rahman et al 2009). However, healthy Standardbred mares that were >20 years old had similar measures of oxidative stress (plasma lipid hydroperoxide concentrations) and concentrations of the major plasma antioxidant, glutathione, as younger animals provided the same diet and undergoing the same fairly intense exercise regimen (Williams et al 2008). In another study, there was no apparent effect of age (groups were <3, 4–6, 7–10 and >10 years old) on a number of antioxidant parameters including superoxide dismutase, glutathione peroxidase and apparent total antioxidant status, as determined by the trolox equivalent antioxidant capacity method (Gorecka et al 2002). However, the aged horse was not specifically studied, as their oldest animal was 17 years of age. These findings suggest that age alone, even in exercising horses, does not increase the need for anti-oxidant supplementation. More work is needed before specific advice on the need for antioxidant supplementation in healthy old horses can be given.

The incidence of recurrent airway obstruction (RAO, chronic obstructive pulmonary disease, heaves) does increase with age in horses and the concentration of ascorbic acid in plasma and pulmonary epithelial lining is significantly reduced in RAO-affected horses, in both crisis and remission compared to healthy control animals (Deaton et al 2004). It has been postulated that specific targeted dietary antioxidant supplementation may be of benefit in horses prone to RAO, as well as potentially to stabled horses in general (Deaton et al 2002, 2005; Kirshvink et al. 2002). One study has reported lower plasma vitamin C in old horses when compared to younger animals fed the same feed and housed under the same conditions (Ralston et al 1988). None of the old horses in that study had chronic respiratory disorders but all but one had pituitary or thyroid tumors. The one mare that did not have tumors on post mortem examination was also the only old horse that had plasma vitamin C concentrations in the same range as the younger horses in the study (Ralston et al 1988, and unpublished data, 1986). It was hypothesized (Ralston 2006) that low plasma vitamin C may be the result of PPID and/or thyroid dysfunction in old horses and may contribute to the reduction in immune function discussed above.

Vitamin C supplementation (0.02 g ascorbic acid/kg BW twice a day) has been observed to increase antibody response to vaccine administration in aged horses, (Ralston & Dimock, unpublished data) and administration may help if chronic infections are a problem (S Ralston personal observations). However, supplementation of vitamin C for 5 or 10 days in weanling horses subjected to prolonged (36 hours+) transportation stress suppressed plasma ascorbic acid concentrations after the supplementation was stopped acutely, to below normal for up to 3 weeks, in the horses supplemented for 10 days (Ralston & Stives 2012). In the horses supplemented for only 5 days there was an apparent reduction in the incidence and severity of "shipping fever" compared to non-supplemented control animals and no suppression of plasma ascorbic acid after the supplementation was stopped (Ralston & Stives 2012). More work is needed in this area but it is important to note that at the present time it is recommended that vitamin C supplementation should not be stopped abruptly, but instead tapered off slowly over the course of a week or so.

Recent studies in aged rats have suggested that a high intake of folic acid improves the normal liver morphology in older animals (Roncales et al 2004). Whether or not this information is relevant to the horse is unknown, but it is possible that any changes in microbiota as found in other species (Hayek et al 1997) may influence supplemental folic acid as well as other B-vitamin requirements with age.

Some authors have suggested that increased levels of vitamin E and beta-carotene may be beneficial in the preservation of immune status in other species (Hayek et al 1997, Chandra 2002). A recent study suggested that vitamin E status may be associated with immune function and quality of life in elderly people (Capuron et al 2009). In the horse a recent study suggested that there was a significant decrease in IFN and TNF-α production in resveratrol (2000 mg/day) supplemented aged horses post 4 weeks supplementation compared to non-supplemented control horses. Interestingly there was an increase in neutrophil ROS activity in the resveratrol group which might be advantageous (Adams et al 2010).

It has recently been suggested that, in older people, micronutrient deficiencies are common and supplementation appears to be of benefit (Lesourd & Mazari 1999, Chandra 2002). It has been suggested that the nutrient recommendations should be increased (in particular for vitamins B_6, B_{12}, C, D and E, folic acid, β-carotene and zinc) in the elderly, for a number of reasons (Blumberg 1994, Flood & Carr 2004). It is unlikely that this would be the case in old horses provided with an appropriately fortified and balanced diet with the exceptions noted above. Over supplementation with trace minerals, such as chromium (Dimock et al 1999) and zinc (NRC 2007) may actually be detrimental to immune function.

Oral chondroprotective agents

Recently, there has been a relative explosion in the number and variety of nutraceutical products on the market, targeted at the management of lameness related to OA. Although there have been many anecdotal reports about the efficacy of these products, there has been a lack of published clinical trials, especially in the older horse. See Chapter 33.

Conclusion

Considering horses as individuals as they age and providing them with targeted nutrition, and appropriate management as well as veterinary attention will help to support them to have as healthy and active a life as possible as they age.

References

Aagaard, P., Suetta, C., Caserotti, P., et al., 2010. Role of the nervous system in sarcopenia and muscle atrophy with aging: Strength training as a countermeasure. Scandinavian Journal of Medicine and Science in Sports 20 (1), 49–64.

Adams, A.A., Breathnach, C.C., Katepalli, M.P., et al., 2008. Advanced age in horses affects divisional history of T cells and inflammatory cytokine production. Mechanisms of Ageing and Development 129, 656–664.

Adams, A.A., Katepall, M.P., Kohler, K., et al., 2009. Effect of body condition, bodyweight and adiposity on inflammatory cytokine responses in old horses. Vet Immunology and Immunopathology 127, 286–294.

Adams, A.A., Betancourt, A., Brummer, M., et al., 2010. In vitro and in vivo immunomodulatory effects of resveratrol on immune function in aged horses. In: Proceedings of the Havemeyer Equine Geriatric Workshop. Cambridge, MA, pp. 63.

Aguilera-Tejero, E., Estepa, J.C., Lopez, I., et al., 1998. Arterial blood gases and acid base balance in healthy young and aged horses. Equine Veterinary Journal 30, 352–354.

Beech, J., 1987. Pituitary tumors. In: Robinson, N.E. (Ed.), Current Therapy in Equine Medicine 2. Saunders, Philadelphia, pp. 182–185.

Bertone, A.L., van Soest, P.J., Stashak, T.S., 1989. Digestion, fecal and blood variables associated with extensive large colon resection in the horse. American Journal of Veterinary Research 50, 253–258.

Blumberg, J., 1994. Nutrient requirements of the healthy elderly - should there be specific RDAs? Nutrition Reviews 52, IIS15–S18.

Booth, F.W., Zwetsloot, K.A., 2010. Basic concepts about genes, inactivity and aging. Scandinavian Journal of Medicine and Science in Sports 20 (1), 1–4.

Bowen, I.M., Marr, C.M., Wheeler-Jones, C.P.D., et al., 2006. The effects of aging on the structure and function of the equine aortic valve. Proceedings of the American College of Veterinary Internal Medicine 20, 742.

Brama, P.A.J., TeKopple, J.M., Bank, R.A., 1999. Influence of site and age on biochemical characteristics of the collagen network of equine articular cartilage. American Journal of Veterinary Research 60, 341–345.

Brosnahan, M.M., Paradis, M.R., 2003a. Demographic and clinical characteristics of geriatric horses: 467 cases (1989–1999). JAVMA 223, 93–98.

Brosnahan, M.M., Paradis, M.R., 2003b. Assessment of clinical characteristics, management practices and activities of geriatric horses. JAVMA 223, 99–103.

Bruunsgaard, H., Pedersen, B.K., 2003. Age related inflammatory cytokines and disease. Immunology and Allergy Clinics of North America 23, 15–39.

Burkholder, W.J., 1999. Age related changes to nutritional requirements and digestive function in adult dogs and cats. JAVMA 215, 625–629.

Campbell, D.J., Rawlings, J.M., Koelsch, S., et al., 2004. Age-related differences in parameters of feline immune status. Veterinary Immunology and Immunopathology 100, 73–80.

Capuron, L., Moranis, A., Combe, N., et al., 2009. Vitamin E and quality of life in the elderly: influence of inflammatory processes. British Journal of Nutrition 102, 1390–1394.

Capucchio, M.T., Marquez, M., Pregel, P., et al., 2010. Parenchymal and vascular lesions in aging equine brains: Histological and immunohistochemical studies. Journal of Comparative Pathology 142 (1), 61–73.

Carmalt, J.L., Allen, A., 2008. The relationship between cheek tooth occlusal morphology, apparent digestibility, and ingesta particle size reduction in horses. Journal of the American Veteterinary Medicine Association 233 (3), 452–455.

Carnevale, E.M., Bergfelt, D.R., Ginther, O.J., 1993. Aging effects on follicular activity and concentrations of FSH, LH and progesterone in mares. Animal Reproductive Science 31, 287–299.

Carson-Dunkerley, S.A., Hanson, R.R., 1996. Survival from colic in aged horses. Proceedings of the American Association of Equine Practitioners 42, 262–263.

Chandler, K.J., Billson, F.M., Mellor, D.J., 2003. Ophthalmic lesions in 83 geriatric horses and ponies. Veterinary Record 153, 319–322.

Chandra, R.K., 2002. Nutrition and the immune system from birth to old age. European Journal of Clinical Nutrition 56, S73–S76.

Cole, F.L., Hodgson, D.R., Reid, S.W.J., et al., 2005. Owner reported equine health disorders: results of an Australia-wide postal survey. Australian Veterinary Journal 83 (8), 490–405.

Costa Lais, R.R., Hermida, P., Sanchez, A.L., et al., 2010. Age related differences in resting glucose and insulin, body characteristics and exercise management of horses in New England. Proceedings of the Havemeyer Equine Geriatric Workshop, Cambridge, MA, pp. 55.

Cymbaluk, N.F., Christison, G.I., 1990. Environmental effects on thermoregulation and nutrition of horses. Veterinary Clinics of North America 6 (2), 355–372.

du Toit, N., Gallagher, J., Burden, F.A., et al., 2008. *Post mortem* survey of dental disorders in 349 donkeys from an aged population (2005–2006). Part 1: Prevalence of specific dental disorders. Equine Veterinary Journal 40 (3), 204–208.

du Toit, N., Burden, F.A., Dixon, P.M., 2009. Clinical dental examinations of 357 donkeys in the UK: Part 2 - Epidemiological studies on possible relationship between different dental disorders, and between dental disease and systemic disorders. Equine Veterinary Journal 41, 395–400.

Dardevet, D., Sornet, C., Bayle, G., et al., 2002. Postprandial stimulation of muscle protein synthesis in old rats can be restored by a leucine supplemented meal. Journal of Nutrition 132, 95–100.

Deaton, C., Marlin, D., Roberts, C., et al., 2002. Antioxidant supplementation and pulmonary function at rest and exercise. Equine Veterinary Journal, Supplement 34, 58–65.

Deaton, C.M., Marlin, D.J., Smith, N.C., et al., 2004. Pulmonary epithelial lining fluid and plasma ascorbic acid concentrations in horses affected by recurrent airway obstruction. American Journal of Veterinary Research 65, 80–87.

Deaton, C.M., Marlin, D.J., Smith, N.C., et al., 2005. Effect of acute airway inflammation on the pulmonary antioxidant status. Experimental Lung Research 31, 653–670.

Donini, L.M., Savina, C., Cannella, C., 2003. Eating habits and appetite control in the elderly: the anorexia of aging. International Psychogeriatrics 15, 73–87.

Dimock, A.N., Ralston, S.L., Malinowski, K., et al., 1999. The effect of supplemental chromium on the immune status of geriatric mares. In: Proceedings of the 16th Equine Nutrition and Physiology Symposium, North Carolina, USA, pp. 10–11.

Dorner, T.E., Schwarz, F., Kranz, A., et al., 2010. Body mass index and the risk of infections in instutionalised geriatric patients. British Journal of Nutrition 103, 1830–1835.

Dybdal, N., 1997. Pituitary pars intermedia dysfunction (equine Cushings-like disease). In: Robinson, N.E. (Ed.), Current Therapy in Equine Medicine, 4th ed. W.B. Saunders Co., Philadelphia, pp. 499–501.

Edwards, G.B., Proudman, C.J., 1994. An analysis of 75 cases of intestinal obstruction caused by pedunculated lipomas. Equine Veterinary Journal 26, 18–21.

Elzinga, S., Nielsen, B.D., Schott, H.C., et al., 2011. Effect of age on digestibility of various feedstuffs in horses. Journal of Equine Veterniary Science 31, 268–269.

Evans, W.J., 1995. What is sarcopenia? Journal of Gerontology A Biological Science and Medical Science 50, 5–8.

Figueriedo, P.A., Mota, M.P., Appell, H.J., et al., 2008. The role of mitochondria in aging of skeletal muscle. Biogerontology 9, 67–84.

Flood, K.L., Carr, D.B., 2004. Nutrition in the elderly. Current Opinion in Gastroenterology 20, 125–129.

Gorecka, R., Sitarska, E., Klucinski, W., 2002. Antioxidant parameters of horses according to age, sex, breed and environment. Polish Journal of Veterinary Science 5, 209–216.

Goto, H., Yamamoto, Y., Ohta, C., 1993. Antibody responses of Japanese horses to influenza viruses in the past few years. Journal of Veterinary Medical Science 55, 33–37.

Graham, B.P., 2002. Dental care in the older horse. Veterinary Clinics of North America: Equine Practice 18, 509–522.

Graves, J.E., Pollock, M.L., Carroll, J.F., 1994. Exercise, age and skeletal muscle function. Southern Medical Journal 87, S17–S22.

Grimble, R.F., 2003. Inflammatory response in the elderly. Current Opinion in Clinical Nutrition and Metabolic Care 6, 21–29.

Hayek, M.G., Sunvold, G.D., Reinhart, G.A., 1997. Aging, physiology and nutritional considerations in geriatric dogs and cats. Proceedings ACVIM 15, 21–24.

Hayes, M., 2010. Competitive Trail Horse Elmer Bandit, 38, Euthanized. TheHorse, http://www.thehorse.com/ViewArticle.aspx?ID=15827

Hebuterne, X., Bermon, S., Schneider, S.M., 2001. Aging and muscle: the effects of malnutrition, re-nutrition and physical exercise. Current Opinion in Clinical Nutrition and Metabolic Care 4, 295–300.

Henson, S.M., Akbar, A.N., 2009. KLRG1 - more than a marker for T cell senescence. Age 31, 285–291.

Horohov, D.W., Dimock, A., Guirnalda, P., et al., 1999. Effect of exercise on the immune response of young and old horses. American Journal of Veterinary Research 60, 643–647.

Horohov, D.W., Kydd, J.H., Hannant, D., 2002. The effect of aging on T cells responses in the horse. Developmental and Comparative Immunology 26, 121–128.

Howarth, S., Lucke, V.M., Pearson, H., 1991. Squamous cell carcinoma of the equine external genitalia. Equine Veterinary Journal 23, 53–55.

Hotchkiss, J.W., Reid, S.W.J., Christley, R.M., 2007. A survey of horse owners in Great Britain regarding horses in their care, Part 1: Horse demographic characteristics and management. Equine Veterinary Journal 39 (4), 294–300.

Ireland, J.L., Clegg, P.D., McGowan, C.M., et al., 2009. Demographic charcteristics, health and management in geriatric horses in the UK - a cross sectional study. Proceedings of the 12th International Symposium on Veterinary Epidemiology and Economics, Durban South Africa.

Ireland, J.L., Clegg, P.D., McGowan, C.M., et al., 2011a. A cross sectional study of geriatric horses in the United Kingdom. Part 1: Demographics and management practices. Equine Veterinary Journal 43 (1), 30–36.

Ireland, J.L., Clegg, P.D., McGowan, C.M., et al., 2011b. A cross sectional study of geriatric horses in the United Kingdom. Part 2: Health care and disease. Equine Veterinary Journal 43 (1), 37–44.

Jahns, H., Callanan, J.J., McElroy, M.C., et al., 2006. Age-related and non-age-related changes in 100 surveyed horse brains. Veterinary Pathology 43 (5), 740–750.

Jarvis, N., 2010. Demographics of equine residents at the UK's largest Equine Charity. In: Proceedings of the Havemeyer Equine Geriatric Workshop. Cambridge MA, pp. 27–28.

Johnston, G.M., Taylor, P.M., Holmes, M.A., et al., 1995. Confidential enquiry of perioperative equine fatalities (CEPEF-1): preliminary results. Equine Veterinary Journal 27, 193–200.

Kealy, R.D., Lawler, D.F., Ballam, J.M., et al., 2002. Effects of diet restriction on life span and age related changes in dogs. JAVMA 220, 1315–1320.

Kidd, J.A., Fuller, C., Barr, A.R.S., 2001. Osteoarthritis in the horse. Equine Veterinary Education 13, 160–168.

Kirschvink, N., Fievez, L., Bougnet, V., et al., 2002. Effect of nutritional antioxidant supplementation on systemic and pulmonary antioxidant status, airway inflammation and lung function in heaves affected horses. Equine Veterinary Journal 34 (7), 705–712.

Knottenbelt, D.C., 2003. The systemic effects of dental disease. In: Baker, G.J., Easley, J. (Eds.), Equine Dentistry. WB Saunders, Philadelphia, pp. 127–138.

Lawler, D.F., Larson, B.T., Ballam, J.M., et al., 2008. Diet Restriction and aging in the dog: major observations over two decades. British Journal of Nutrition 99, 793–805.

Leblond, A., Corbin-Gardey, C., Cadore, J.L., 2002. Studies of the pathology and causes of mortality of the old horse. In: Proceedings of the 41st British Equine Veterinary Association Congress. Equine Veterinary Journal Ltd., Newmarket, pp. 202–203.

Lesourd, B., 2006. Nutritional factors and immunological aging. Proceedings of the Nutrition Society 65, 319–325.

Lesourd, B., Mazari, L., 1999. Nutrition and immunity in the elderly. Proceedings of the Nutrition Society 58, 685–695.

Lowder, M.Q., Mueller, E., 1998. Dental disease in geriatric horses. Veterinary Clinics of North America Equine 14 (2), 365–380.

Madill, S., 2002. Reproductive considerations: mare and stallion. Veterinary Clinics Equine 18, 591–619.

Mansell, B.J., Baker, L.A., et al., 2001. The effect of calcium and phosphorus supplementation on bone metabolism in young, mature and aged horses during inactivity and subsequent aerobic training. Journal of Equine Veterinary Science 21, 445–450.

McBride, G.E., Christopherson, R.J., Sauer, W., 1985. Metabolic rate and plasma thyroid hormone concentrations of mature horses in response to changes in ambient temperature. Canadian Journal of Animal Science 65, 375–382.

McFarlane, D., 2011. Equine Pituitary Pars Intermedia Dysfunction. Vet Clin Equine 27, 93–113.

McFarlane, D., Cribb, A.E., 2005. Systemic and pituitary pars intermedia antioxidant capacity associated with pars intermedia oxidative stress and dysfunction in horses. American Journal of Veterinary Research 66 (12), 2065–2072.

McFarlane, D., Holbrook, T.C., 2008. Cytokine dysregulation in aged horses and horses with pituitary pars intermedia dysfunction. Journal of Veterinary Internal Medicine 22 (2), 436–442.

McFarlane, D., Sellon, D.C., Gaffney, D., et al., 1998. Hematologic and serum biochemical variables and plasma corticotrophin concentrations in aged horses. American Journal of Veterinary Research 59, 1247–1251.

McFarlane, D., Sellon, D.C., Gibbs, S.A., 2001. Age-related quantitative alterations in lymphocyte subsets and immunoglobulin isotypes in healthy horses. American Journal of Veterinary Research 62, 1337–1512.

McFarlane, D., Hale, G.M., Johnson, E.M., et al., 2010. Fecal egg counts after anthelminthic administration to aged horses and horses with pituitary pars intermedia dysfunction. JAVMA 236, 330–334.

McGowan, T.W., 2009. Aged Horse Health, Management and Welfare. PhD thesis University of Queensland, Brisbane, Australia.

McGowan, T.W., Pinchbeck, G.L., Hodgson, D.R., et al., 2010. Clinical disease and mortality in geriatric horses: an Australian Perspective. In: Proceedings of the Havemeyer Foundation Equine Geriatric Workshop, Cambridge, MA, Oc. 24–27, pp. 23.

McKeever, K.H., Malinowski, K., 1997. Exercise capacity in young and old horses. American Journal of Veterinary Research 58, 1468–1472.

McKeever, K.H., Kearns, C.F., 2001. Aging induced alteration in plasma volume in horses. Medical Science Sports and Exercise 33, S257.

McKeever, K.H., Malinowski, K., 1999. Endocrine response to exercise in young and old horses. Equine Veterinary Journal (suppl. 30), 561–566.

McKeever, K.H., Eaton, T.L., Geiser, S., et al., 2010. Age related decreases in thermoregulation and cardiovascular function in horses. Equine Veterinary Journal 42 (suppl. 38), 220–227.

Mellor, D.J., Love, S., Walker, R., et al., 2001. Sentinel practice-based survey of the management and health of horses in northern Britain. Veterinary Record 149, 417–423.

National Animal Health Monitoring System, 2006. Equine 2005, Part II: Changes in the US Equine Industry, 1998–2005. USDA-APHIS-VS, Fort Collins, Colorado.

National Research Council (NRC), 1989. National Research Council Nutrient Requirements of Horses, 5th ed. National Academy Press, Washington DC.

National Research Council (NRC), 2007. National Research Council Nutrient Requirements of Horses, 6th ed. National Academy Press, Washington DC.

Naylor, R.J., Perkins, J.D., Allen, S., et al., 2010. Histopathology and computed tomography of age-associated degeneration of the equine temporohyoid joint. Equine Veterinary Journal 42 (5), 425–430.

Ollivier, F.J., Sanchez, R.F., Monclin, S.J., 2009. Equine glaucomas: a review. Equine Veterinary Education 21 (5), 232–235.

Paradis, M.R., 2002. Demographics of health and disease in the geriatric horse. Veterinary Clinics of North America: Equine Practice 18, 391–401.

Patterson-Kane, J.C., Wilson, A.M., Firth, E.C., et al., 1997. Comparison of collagen fibril populations in the superficial digital flexor tendons of exercised and non-exercised Thoroughbreds. Equine Veterinary Journal 29, 121–125.

Patterson-Kane, J.C., Wilson, A.M., Firth, E.C., et al., 1998. Exercise related alterations in crimp morphology in the central regions of superficial digital flexor tendons from young thoroughbreds: a controlled study. Equine Veterinary Journal 30, 61–64.

Pelchat, M.L., 2000. You can teach an old dog new tricks: olfaction responses to novel food by the elderly. Appetite 35, 153–160.

Phillips, F., 2003. Nutrition for healthy ageing. Nutrition Foundation 28, 253–263.

Phillips, R.J., Walther, G.C., Powley, T.L., 2010. Age-related changes in vagal afferents innervating the gastrointestinal tract. Autonomic Neuroscience: Basic and Clinical 153 (1–2), 90–98.

Rahman, M.M., Halade, G.V., El Jamali, A., et al., 2009. Conjugated linoleic acid (CLA) precents age- associated skeletal muscle loss. Biochemical and Biophysical Research Communications 383, 513–518.

Raj, I.S., Bird, S.R., Shield, A.J., 2010. Ageing and the force–velocity relationship of muscles. Experimental Gerontology 45 (2), 81–90.

Ralston, S.L., 1989. Digestive alterations in aged horses. Journal of Equine Veterinary Science 9, 203–205.

Ralston, S.L., 2001. Effect of vitamin supplementation post-transportation in weanlings. Proceedings of the 17th Equine Nutrition and Physiology Symposium May, 2001, University of Kentucky, Lexington, KY, pp. 131.

Ralston, S.L., 2006. Nutrition of the geriatric horse. In: Bertone, J. (Ed.), Equine Geriatric Medicine and Surgery. Elsevier Publishing, St. Louis, MO, pp. 169–171.

Ralston, S.L., 2007. Evidence-based equine nutrition. Veterinary Clinics of North America Equine 23 (2), 365–384.

Ralston, S.L., Breuer, L.H., 1996. Field evaluation of a feed formulated for geriatric horses. Journal of Equine Veterinary Science 16, 334–338.

Ralston, S.L., Stives, M., 2012. Supplementation of ascorbic acid in weanling horses following prolonged transportation. Animals 2, 184–194 (Special issue: Monogastric Animal Nutrition and Metabolism) http://www.mdpi.com/2076-2615/2/2/184/.

Ralston, S.L., Nockels, C.F., Squires, E.L., 1988. Differences in diagnostic test results and hematologic data between aged and young horses. Am J Vet Res. 49, 1387–1392.

Ralston, S.L., Sullins, K.E., Stashak, T.S., 1986. Digestion in horses after resection or ischemic insult of the large colon. American Journal of Veterinary Research 47 (10), 2290–2293.

Ralston, S.L., Foster, D.L., Divers, T., et al., 2001a. Effect of dental correction on feed digestibility in horses. Equine Veterinary Journal 33 (4), 390–393.

Ralston, S.L., Malinowski, K.M., Christensen, R., et al., 2001b. Digestion in the aged horse-re-visited. Journal of Equine Veterinary Science 21 (7), 310–311.

Rapson, J., Schott II, H.C., Nielsen, B.D., et al., 2011. Effects of age and diet on glycemic and insulinemic responses of horses to a concentrate meal. Proceedings of the American College of Veterinary Internal Medicine Forum, Denver, CO.

Rennie, M.J., Selby, A., Atherton, P., et al., 2010. Facts, noise and wishful thinking: muscle protein turnover in aging and human disuse atrophy. Scandinavian Journal of Medicine and Science in Sports 20 (1), 5–9.

Roncales, M., Achon, M., Manzarbeitia, F., et al., 2004. Folic acid supplementation for 4 weeks affects liver morphology in aged rats. Journal of Nutrition 134, 1130–1133.

Schott, H.C., 2002. Pituitary pars intermedia dysfunction: equine Cushing's Disease. Veterinary Clinics of North America Equine Practice 18, 237–270.

Salminen, A., Huuskonen, J., Ojala, J., et al., 2007. Activation of innate immunity system during aging: NK-κB signaling is the molecular culprit of inflamm-aging. Ageing Research Reviews 7 (2), 83–105.

Schiffman, S.S., 1997. Taste and smell losses in normal aging and disease. JAVMA 278, 1357–1362.

Serrano, R., Villar, M., Gallardo, N., et al., 2009. The effect of aging on insulin signaling pathway is tissue dependent central role of adipose tissue in the insulin resistance of aging. Mechanisms of Ageing and Development 130 (3), 189–197.

Siciliano, P., 2002. Nutrition and feeding of the geriatric horse. Veterinary Clinics of North America: Equine Practice 18, 491–508.

Springer, T., Elce, Y.A., Green, E., 2010. Treatment of an osteoblastic osteosarcoma in an aged gelding. Equine Veterinary Education 22, 159–162.

Stevens, K.B., Marr, C.M., Horn, J.N.R., et al., 2009. Effect of left-sided valvular regurgitation on mortality and causes of death among a population of middle-aged and older horses. Veterinary Record 164, 6–10.

St-Onge, M.P., Gallagher, D., 2010. Body composition changes with aging: The cause or the result of alterations in metabolic rate and macronutrient oxidation? Nutrition 26 (2), 152–155.

Sutton, J.R., Brook, R.M., 1986. Sports Medicine for the Mature Athlete. Brown and Benchmark, Dubuque, Iowa.

Tatpati, L.L., Irving, B.A., Tom, A., et al., 2010. The effect of branched chain amino acids on skeletal muscle mitochondrial function in young and elderly adults. Journal of Clinical Endocrinology and Metabolism 95 (2), 894–902.

Terman, A., Kurz, T., Navratil, M., et al., 2010. Mitochondrial turnover and aging of long-lived postmitotic cells: the mitochondrial-lysosomal axis theory of aging. Antioxidants and Redox Signaling 12 (4), 503–535.

Thompson, L.V., 2009. Age related muscle dysfunction. Experimental Gerontology 44 (1–2), 106–111.

Traub-Dargatz, J.L., Ralston, S.L., Collins, J.K., 1985. Equine viral arteritis. Compendium on Continuing Education for the Practicing Veterinarian 7, S490–S496.

Van der Horst-Graat, J.M., Kok, F.J., Schouten, E.G., 2004. Plasma carotenoid concentrations in relation to acute respiratory infections in elderly people. British Journal of Nutrition 92, 113–118.

Verzijl, N., Bank, R.A., TeKoppele, J.M., et al., 2003. Ageing and ostoarthritis: a different perspective. Current Opinion in Rheumatology 15, 4616–4622.

Walker, A., Arent, S.M., McKeever, K.H., 2010. Maximal aerobic capacity (VO_{2max}) in horses: a retrospective study to identify the age-related decline. Comparative Exercise Physiology 6, 177–181.

Watts, K., 2000. Factors affecting NSC in grasses. http://www.safergrass.org/articles/nfcfactors.html

Williams, C.A., Gordon, M.E., Betros, C.L., et al., 2008. Apoptosis and antioxidant status are influenced by age and exercise training in horses. Journal of Animal Science 86, 576–583.

Wohlgemuth, S.E., Seo, A.y., Marzettis, E., et al., 2010. Skeletal muscle autophagy and apoptosis during ageing: Effects of calorie restriction and life-long exercise. Experimental Gerontology 45 (2), 138–148.

16

Practical donkey and mule nutrition

David G. Smith, Faith A. Burden

The donkey

The domestic donkey is a descendant of the African wild ass and was first domesticated in approximately 3000 BCE (Rossel et al 2008). Current estimates of the worldwide donkey population are approximately 44 million (Starkey & Starkey 2000) with the majority of donkeys providing transport and draught power in developing countries. Donkeys are tractable animals that come in a variety of sizes, with breeds ranging from miniatures of less than 91 cm to mammoth jacks and Andalusian donkeys reaching over 1.6 m (Svendsen 2009). The donkey evolved in desert areas and has adapted to eating poor quality fibrous plant material (Izraely et al 1989). The donkey and its hybrid offspring the mule and hinny are renowned for their stoic natures and ability to survive in tough environments on poor quality food making them the work animals of choice in inhospitable areas of the world (Svendsen 2009, Starkey & Starkey 2000).

Donkeys and mules are also used for leisure and competition in developed countries and are popular as children's ride and drive animals or as mounts for trail riding. Keeping donkeys and mules in temperate environments as leisure animals can, however, put them at risk of diseases associated with obesity or inappropriate management. They therefore require careful feeding to help to prevent conditions such as laminitis, hyperlipemia, and gastric ulceration.

Donkeys, for many reasons, should not be considered as if they were small horses; studies have shown physiological (Hill et al 2001, Liberatore et al 2001) as well as pharmacological and pharmacokinetic differences between donkeys and horses (Lizarraga et al 2004). Unfortunately, however, little specific detailed information about the nutritional needs of donkeys and mules is available and although some fundamental research has been carried out it is still far behind the field of horse nutrition. Much of the information in this chapter draws on scientific research but also the extensive experience of the authors in managing herds of both working and non-working donkeys as well as mules.

The structure of the donkey's gut

The structure and function of the donkey's gut is similar to that of the horse. In post-mortems carried out on working donkeys in Ethiopia, the intestine of the average sized donkey (100 kg) was ~24 m long and has a total maximal capacity of ~160 liters (S. Yoeseph, personal communication, Ethiopian Agricultural Research Organisation). Donkeys may have enhanced digestive efficiency compared with the horse due to improved digestibility of dry matter (DM), energy and fiber; longer gastrointestinal mean retention times of feed residues on high-fiber diets (Pearson et al 2006), higher volatile fatty acid (VFA) production per kg DM intake in the large intestine and enhanced recycling of urea (Suhartanto et al 1992, Faurie & Tisserand 1994).

One additional way in which donkeys may adapt to high-fiber diets, as mentioned above, is to use the full capacity of their large intestine (cecum and colon) so forage can be retained for longer and be digested more thoroughly. This increased capacity of the large intestine may give donkeys a "pot belly", which conspires with their angular body frame to give the appearance of ill thrift. Consequently, donkey keepers should always use a body condition scoring system developed specifically for donkeys.

Key Points

- Donkeys have increased digestive efficiency when compared to horses
- Donkeys use the full capacity of the cecum and colon so forage can be retained for longer and digested more thoroughly
- Donkey's teeth should be checked by a qualified professional and rasped if appropriate once per year or more frequently if problems dictate

Physical breakdown

Before digestion can start, donkeys must first physically break down their food by the action of chewing. It has been recommended that every kilogram of hay that the donkey consumes should be chewed more than 2000 times in order to reduce the forage to fragments of approximately 1.6 mm in length (Frape 2004). Smith (1999) compared the number of chews per kg of feed ingested in donkeys, ponies and cattle across three different diets (straw, haylage and chopped alfalfa). All species of herbivore chewed the more fibrous forages for longer, but on a given diet, donkeys tended to chew food less than ponies and obtained a faster rate of intake relative to body size (Smith 1999).

Concentrate feeds require less chews per kilogram (1000–1500) whilst poorer quality feeds like straw require more chews per kilogram (2500+). The condition of the teeth has a large effect on chewing efficiency; donkeys with dental disease will spend longer chewing and chew less efficiently than a donkey with healthy teeth. It is therefore very important that owners keep a careful eye on the condition of their donkey's teeth, especially in mature donkeys that have all their permanent teeth. Donkeys should have their teeth rasped at least once a year by a qualified equine dental technician; the frequency of rasping will need to increase as the donkey gets older. Checking the donkey's mouth should be an essential part of any routine veterinary examination of working donkeys; surveys have shown up to 62% of working donkeys have dental disease (Du Toit et al 2008a, b). A few minutes spent rasping the teeth of a working donkey can make an immeasurable long-term improvement to its tough life.

Water requirements

On average approximately 60% of the donkey's body is made up of water, about 82% of the blood volume is water and even 25% of the weight of bone is water. Donkeys have evolved in semiarid environments and are well adapted to cope with thirst and rapid rehydration (Maloiy 1973). They are able to tolerate body water losses of up to 30% of their normal body weight, then rehydrate rapidly by drinking 24–30 liters of water in 2–5 minutes without apparent ill effect (Maloiy 1973). Donkeys are more thirst tolerant than ponies, and will maintain food intake even when deprived of water for long periods (Mueller et al 1997). Work has suggested that donkeys may be able to reduce water and energy turnover rates, as well as sweating rates and reduce water excretion whilst maintaining feed intake (Yousef 1991, Sneddon et al 2006). It has been reported that when given access to water after withdrawal of food and water donkeys will eat first and then drink (Houpt 1993). However, this short-term tolerance of thirst should not be confused with the long-term requirement for water.

The overall water requirement of donkeys is believed to be similar to that of horses. The general rule is that animals should always be provided with free access to clean water throughout the day. The best way to provide this is by self-filling water troughs that should be regularly cleaned. Donkeys can be particularly finicky about water temperature so care must be taken to provide water that is not too cold (>15°C) especially to geriatric animals (generally those older than 20 years). Donkeys may refuse to drink rather than take water from a trough with icy water, leading to problems such as impaction colic. Provision of water for working donkeys and mules is an essential part of preventive healthcare, donkeys and mules should be taken to water as frequently as possible during the day and at least every 4 hours.

Key Points

- Water requirements for donkeys are the same as those for a similar sized horse
- Donkeys are more thirst tolerant than horses and are capable of maintaining food intake even when deprived of water for relatively long periods
- Water provided must be clean, palatable and of a reasonable temperature, in particular, very cold water will often be refused leading to potential health issues such as impaction colic

Table 16-1 Digestible Energy Requirements and Dry Matter Intake of Donkeys of Different Body Weights Fed on a Low Energy Density Diet Such as Straw (5.5–6.5 MJ/kg DM of Food)

Donkey live weight (kg)	Daily requirement for digestible energy (MJ/day)	Daily dry matter intake (kg/day)
150	12–14	2.3
175	14–17	2.6
200	16–19	3
225	18–22	3.4
250	20–24	3.8

Energy requirements

It is important to appreciate the energy requirements of donkeys in order to avoid under- or over-feeding. Research carried out by the Donkey Sanctuary has established scientifically validated guidelines for donkeys kept in temperate and in tropical climates (Wood et al 2005, Carretero-Roque et al 2005).

Mature donkeys that are kept at maintenance levels require between 80 and 95 kJ of digestible energy (DE) per kilogram of live weight per day (see Table 16-1). The upper value will apply during winter months when the energy requirement of donkeys tends to increase. The lower value will apply during the height of summer.

In order to formulate an appropriate ration for donkeys it is necessary to estimate how much dry matter a donkey will eat per day. In a study at the Donkey Sanctuary, total daily dry matter intakes of between 1.3–1.7% of live weight were measured in donkeys fed on straw and hay (straw was available ad libitum). Other published studies have reported dry matter intake values in donkeys of between 0.9 and 2.5% that were given a variety of feeds (Smith & Pearson 2005) the higher values in this range were recorded in donkeys fed chopped lucerne. Much higher values of daily dry matter intakes have been recorded in horses fed chaff based diets (Dugdale et al 2008) and in donkeys fed chopped lucerne (Smith 1999). However, for donkeys fed unchopped forage a reasonable estimate of the appetite limits of a typical donkey is approximately 1.5% of its live weight in dry forage per day (Smith & Pearson 2005).

It is important to satisfy the energy requirement of donkeys, their appetite and their psychological need to spend much of the day foraging. For most of the year a ration that contains 70–75% barley straw or other fibrous forage such as maize stover and 25–30% of moderate quality grass hay, grazing or green fodder will supply all the energy requirements of donkeys. During the winter when energy requirements increase the proportion of hay or green fodder may need to be increased to 50–75% and the proportion of straw fed decreased to 25–50%. In practice, donkeys select hay in preference to straw, therefore by limiting the amount of hay fed and offering straw ad libitum animals are unlikely to exceed their energy requirements. It is important to select straw with few cereal heads or retained loose grain in order to prevent excess energy and starch intake, this is particularly important when owners are trying to manage the weight of obese animals and in order to prevent laminitis. A mineral supplement will also be required and some source of vitamins either in the form of a small quantity of fresh green fodder (200 g of chopped fresh alfalfa) or a commercial vitamin mix.

Little work has been done to compare the metabolism of donkeys with horses. As both species are hind-gut fermenters they have been said to exhibit better glucose tolerances than fore-gut fermenters such as ruminants (Frape 2004). Preliminary work by McLean et al (2009) suggests that donkeys have similar insulin sensitivity to adult horses of similar body condition score; this is particularly interesting when contrasted to adult ponies who generally have lower levels of insulin sensitivity when compared to both groups.

In terms of energetics donkeys have higher energy requirements for maintenance per kilogram of body weight than ponies but expend less energy per metre travelled than ponies relative to their body weight (Smith et al 1994). This greater locomotive efficiency may reflect the relatively larger proportion of "endurance" muscle fibers in donkey muscles (Marlin & Nankervis 2002). Endurance muscle fibers use metabolic energy more efficiently and fatigue more slowly than sprint muscle fibers.

There is little published research on the microbial activity of the donkey gut. One paper suggested that in the caecum the microbial cellulolytic activity is higher in donkeys than in ponies (Faurie & Tisserand 1994), whilst the same group has shown that greater quantities of VFAs are produced in the cecal fluid of hay-fed ponies 12 hours feeding than in donkeys fed the same diet (Tisserand et al 1991). In terms of the diversity of microbial species and their total number there is little difference across a wide variety of mammal herbivore species including fore and hind gut fermenters although they did not include the donkey (Stevens & Hume 2004). Gut flora is affected by diet, and horses that are adapted to a hay diet are reported to digest fiber more efficiently than horses that are adapted to a grain diet (Frape 2004). As donkeys tend to be fed on higher-fiber diets than horses, better microbial adaptation would be expected. When fed straw alone or with corn, in one study the VFA production was significantly higher in donkeys than in ponies (Suhartanto et al 1992) and the relative concentrations of butyric, isobutyric, valeric and isovaleric acids were higher. The pH of the cecal fluid was lower (6.7–6.9) than in ponies (7–7.3) when on the same diet. Explanations for the improved digestibility of high fiber forages in donkeys compared with ponies have previously included higher dry matter intakes per day coupled with faster mean retention time (Pearson et al 2006) and more efficient microbial digestion in the cecum (Suhartanto et al 1992, Faurie & Tisserand 1994). However, more recently the improved digestibility was associated with reduced dry matter intakes but longer gut retention times (Smith & Pearson (2005). Whether these differences in the explanations for the improved digestibilities recorded are due to differences in diet, intake, experimental study design, feeding regimen or breed is unknown. One study, in which the ponies and donkeys were fed almost identical dry matter intakes of either pelleted hay or straw, suggested a higher digestibility of the organic matter and the cell walls in the donkey (Faurie & Tisserand 1994) (%organic matter digestibility of 41.7±1.2 and 48.3±2.3 for straw in the pony and donkey respectively). More work is needed in this area.

The adaptation of the donkey to consume highly fibrous diets, especially those high in lignin, would suggest that the microbial community is specific to these substrates; an important consequence of this adaptation may be that this community is even more sensitive to dietary change to feedstuffs high in starch. This may make the feeding of high starch diets difficult to achieve safely in donkeys due to the sensitive nature of their microbiota; such diets are therefore actively discouraged.

Feeding for pregnancy, lactation and growth

When donkeys are growing, pregnant or lactating extra energy is needed. Research in this area is still to be conducted but general guidelines are provided below.

Key Points

- Mature donkeys that are kept at maintenance levels require between 80–95 kJ of digestible energy (DE) per kilogram of body weight per day
- For donkeys fed unchopped forages a reasonable estimate of the appetite limits of a typical donkey is approximately 1.5% of its body weight in dry forage per day

Ideally immature growing donkeys should be provided with sufficient energy to allow them to grow at a steady rate, avoiding periods of rapid growth or retardation. Providing too much energy to a growing donkey, especially when not balanced with adequate protein, calcium and phosphorus may result in the development of orthopedic problems. The available time for young donkeys to attain their mature stature is 2–3 years. Growing donkeys may face problems at weaning and during their first winter and some supplementation with concentrate feed may be required in order to avoid prolonged growth checks or permanent stunting. Pasture-fed immature donkeys are unlikely to require energy supplements, but should be given access to mineral licks formulated for equines, use of molassed mineral licks is discouraged as donkeys are likely to gorge on these products and may risk developing laminitis.

In pregnant donkeys the demands of the growing fetus only exceed the normal requirements in the final three months of pregnancy. Current advice, based on horse/pony information but shown to be effective in practical situations, is that digestible energy allowances should be increased by 11% above maintenance in the 9th month, 13% in the penultimate month and 20% in the final month of pregnancy. Pregnant and lactating jennies should have new feeds introduced very gradually over a period of 4–6 weeks, consideration should always be given to supplying additional requirements by increasing the hay or haylage proportion of the ration before introducing less suitable grain or concentrate rations.

Lactating jennies are likely to lose weight (½–1 body condition score point/5; based on Fig. 16.1) during the first 2 months that their foals are suckling, even when they are receiving moderate feed supplementation. Preparation for this loss should be made in the final months of pregnancy by allowing pregnant jennies of body condition score 3 to

C/S		Neck and shoulders	Withers	Ribs and belly	Back and loins	Hindquarters
1. Poor	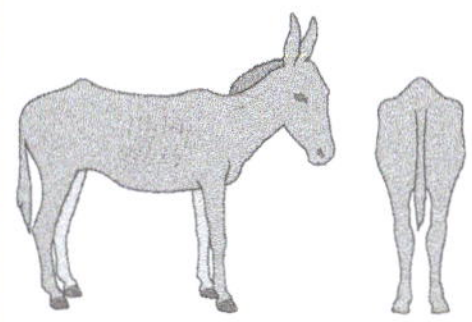	Neck thin, all bones easily felt. Neck meets shoulder abruptly, shoulder bones felt easily, angular.	Dorsal spine of withers prominent and easily felt.	Ribs can be seen from a distance and felt with ease. Belly tucked up.	Backbone prominent, can feel dorsal and transverse processes easily.	Hip bones visible and felt easily (hock and pin bones). Little muscle cover. May be cavity under tail.
2. Moderate	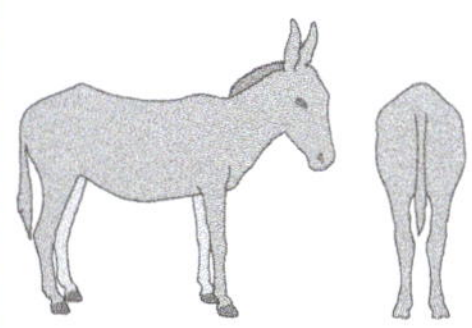	Some muscle development overlying bones. Slight step where neck meets shoulders.	Some cover over dorsal withers, spinous processes felt but not prominent.	Ribs not visible but can be felt with ease.	Dorsal and transverse processes felt with light pressure. Poor muscle development either side midline.	Poor muscle cover on hindquarters, hip bones felt with ease.
3. Ideal	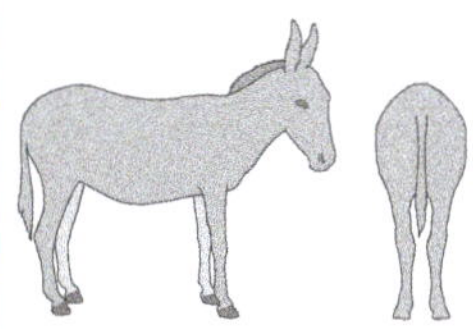	Good muscle development, bones felt under light cover of muscle/fat. Neck flows smoothly into shoulder, which is rounded.	Good cover of muscle/fat over dorsal spinous processes, withers flow smoothly into back.	Ribs just covered by light layer of fat/muscle, ribs can be felt with light pressure. Belly firm with good muscle tone and flattish outline.	Cannot feel individual spinous or transverse processes. Muscle development either side of midline is good.	Good muscle cover in hindquarters, hip bones rounded in appearance, can be felt with light pressure.
4. Fat (show condition ?)	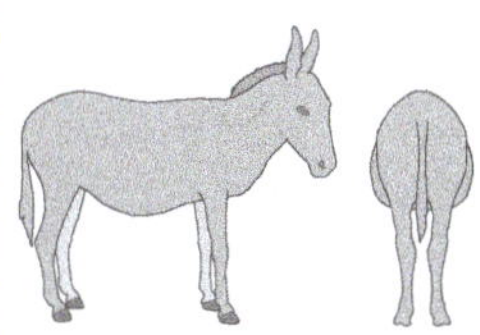	Neck thick, crest hard, shoulder covered in even fat layer.	Withers broad, bones felt with firm pressure.	Ribs dorsally only felt with firm pressure, ventral ribs may be felt more easily. Belly overdeveloped.	Can only feel dorsal and transverse processes with firm pressure. Slight crease along midline.	Hindquarters rounded, bones felt only with firm pressure. Fat deposits evenly placed.
5. Obese	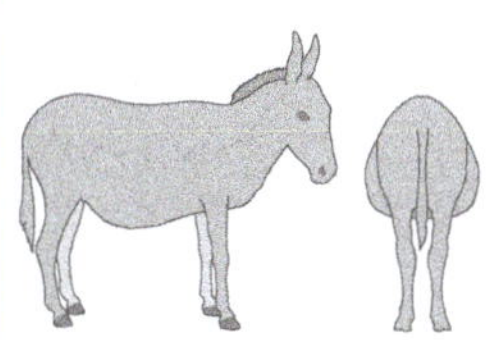	Neck thick, crest bulging with fat and may fall to one side. Shoulder rounded and bulging with fat.	Withers broad, unable to feel bones.	Large, often uneven fat deposits covering dorsal and possibly ventral aspect of ribs. Ribs not palpable. Belly pendulous in depth and width.	Back broad, unable to feel spinous or transverse processes. Deep crease along midline bulging fat either side.	Cannot feel hip bones, fat may overhang either side of tail head, fat often uneven and bulging.

Figure 16.1 Body condition chart for donkeys.
Copyright The Donkey Sanctuary.

gain ½ to 1 point of body condition by additional feeding (i.e., at foaling they should have a body condition of 3½–4). If the pregnant jenny is already in such condition then attention must be paid to maintaining this whilst not allowing the jenny to become more overweight as this may increase the risk of her becoming hyperlipemic. The jenny should receive sufficient additional feeding during the first 2–3 months of lactation to minimize body weight losses aiming at a stable body condition score of 3 for the remainder of the preweaning period.

Key Points

- Immature growing donkeys should be provided with sufficient energy to allow them to grow at a steady rate, avoiding periods of rapid growth or retardation
- In pregnant donkeys the demands of the growing fetus only exceed the normal requirements in the final three months of pregnancy. Digestible energy allowances should be increased by 11% above maintenance in the 9th month, 13% in the penultimate month and 20% in the final month of pregnancy
- Lactating jennies should receive sufficient additional feeding during the first 2–3 months of lactation to minimize body weight losses aiming at a stable body condition score of 3. The jenny may be allowed to put on a little extra weight (BCS 3.5) before foaling to allow for the expected drop in condition

Protein requirements

Proteins are required by all living creatures for growth and repair of body tissues. The ability of donkeys to thrive and grow on the very low protein forages found in many tropical

Table 16-2 Vitamin Dietary Allowances for Donkeys*

Required vitamin level per 100 kg/BW	Maintenance	Pregnant and lactating jennies	Growing donkeys	Working donkeys
Vitamin A (IU/100 kg BW)	3000	6000	2310	4500
Vitamin D (IU/100 kg BW)	660	660	1025	660
Vitamin E (IU/100 kg BW)	100	100	105	160
Thiamine (mg/100 kg BW)	6	6	4	6
Riboflavin (mg/100 kg BW)	4	4	2.5	4

*These are based on recommendations for horses.
Data from NRC (2007).

countries does provide some anecdotal evidence that processes of protein digestion and metabolism in donkeys are more complex than is currently perceived.

As a general rule, once the energy requirements of a donkey or mule are satisfied by the diet then the protein requirements tend also to be satisfied. This has been confirmed by studies at the Donkey Sanctuary which have estimated the digestible crude protein (DCP) requirements for adult donkeys at 26±1.3 g DCP per 100 kg bodyweight (BW) per day (approximately 40 g CP/100 kg BW). In practice this amount of DCP would be comfortably supplied from a diet of hay and ad libitum straw. More detailed measurements of DCP requirement for pregnant, lactating and growing donkeys have not been carried out. Standard methods for measuring apparent DCP of the typically low quality diets fed to donkeys are likely to be prone to error because fecal protein content often exceeds that of the feed. In order to improve the accuracy of DCP requirements more detailed nitrogen balance trials are required in which the contribution of microbial and endogenous protein to the faecal protein is determined.

Key Points

- Anecdotal evidence suggests donkeys have the ability to survive on lower protein diets than horses
- As a general rule, once the energy requirements of a donkey or mule are satisfied by the diet then the protein requirements tend also to be satisfied

Vitamin requirements

Many vitamins are abundant in green forage; pasture-fed donkeys or those fed fresh forage are highly unlikely to suffer from vitamin deficiency. Young or geriatric animals may be vulnerable to vitamin deficiency particularly when intake of green forage is restricted or they are housed for prolonged periods of time.

The levels of vitamins in conserved forages are generally low and diminish as storage time increases. Animals that are fed conserved forages and concentrates are most at risk from vitamin deficiency, particularly toward the end of the winter when the vitamin levels in food are lowest. Allowing donkeys some time to graze during the winter may be beneficial for their vitamin intake and/or the provision of an appropriate vitamin/mineral supplement. Specific vitamin allowances for donkeys are unknown, accordingly recommendations are given based on published horse recommendations (NRC 2007) as shown in Table 16-2. In the authors' experience these levels of vitamins are optimal for donkeys but in reality donkeys are likely to do very well on slightly reduced levels.

Key Points

- Pasture fed donkeys or those with access to fresh forage are unlikely to develop vitamin deficiencies
- Specific vitamin allowances for donkeys are unknown; recommendations are based on those for horses

Minerals

Calcium and phosphorus are major constituents of bone, and both have a major metabolic role. Bones act as a reservoir of calcium and phosphorus, when dietary levels of the elements are low. If these deficiencies are prolonged the bones can become weakened. In young donkeys lack of calcium and phosphorus can result in developmental orthopedic disease resulting in permanent bone deformity and weakness. Excessive dietary phosphorus has been suggested to interfere with the absorption of calcium which can lead to secondary nutritional hyperparathyroidism (also known as Miller's disease, big head disease, or bran disease) in equids (McDowell 2003). Luthersson et al (2005) reported that 60% of working ponies in Northern Thailand showed clinical signs of big head disease. There have also been anecdotal reports of big head disease in donkeys in West Africa where animals are maintained almost entirely on wheat bran, nutritional status must always be assessed during clinical examination of such animals. Levels of phosphorus relative to calcium are particularly high in some crop by-products such as rice bran and cotton seed that are commonly fed to working donkeys in developing countries. Moreover, common tropical grasses (such as *Panicum maximum*, *Setaria anceps*, Digitaria spp., *Pennisetum clandestinum*, *Cenchrus ciliaris*) have high oxalate contents which can interfere with calcium absorption (Stewart 2005). Feeding crop by-products and the above grass species often form part of improved donkey husbandry programs promoted by animal welfare charities. It is therefore important that these programs encourage donkey keepers to provide appropriate mineral licks to prevent imbalance and deficiencies in calcium and phosphorus. Although the provision of mineral licks is less than ideal as it is often difficult to monitor daily intake it is often the only feasible way for donkey owners, particularly those in developing countries, to provide

Table 16-3 Mineral Dietary Allowances for Donkeys*

Mineral	Maintenance	Pregnant jennies (last trimester)	Lactating Jennies (1st month)	Growing donkeys (based on mature weight)	Working donkeys
Major minerals (g/100 kg BW)					
Calcium	4	7	12	8	6
Phosphorus	3	5	8	4	4
Magnesium	1.5	1.5	2.3	1	1.9
Potassium	5	5.2	9.6	2.9	5.7
Sodium	2	2.2	2.6	1.1	2.8
Trace elements (mg/100 kg BW)					
Iron	60	75		39	60
Manganese	60	60		31	60
Copper	20	25		13	20
Zinc	60	60		31	60
Selenium	0.15	0.15		0.1	0.15
Iodine	0.5	0.6		0.3	0.5
Cobalt	0.1	0.1		0.1	0.1

*These are based on recommendations for horses.
Data from NRC (2007).

mineral supplementation in a cost-effective and practical way. To avoid problems the mineral lick provided should be one specifically designed for equids and one which has a full statement of ingredients (Table 16-3).

Sodium and chloride ions are lost in sweat to a greater extent than other minerals. Consequently, demands for sodium chloride are higher in working donkeys in hot environments. Care should be taken to offer working animals salt to allow them to make up for these losses. Donkeys do not appear to sweat as much as horses, although objective data are not available. Losses are still likely to be significantly greater when animals are worked hard or deprived of shade (McDowell 2003). McDowell (2003) cites sodium and chlorine losses in working horses of 2.9 and 5.2 g/l respectively, and estimates of sweat production ranged from 5 ml/kg BW under light work to 50 ml/kg BW under heavy work. Unfortunately, specific information is not available for the donkey. Based on this information salt levels of 0.25–1.0% of the total diet should be adequate to meet demand for sodium and chlorine working donkeys even under hot conditions. Maximum tolerable salt should not exceed 3% of the total diet of donkeys (McDowell 2003).

Donkeys in tropical countries may be forced to drink highly saline ground water, which can become more concentrated if left to stand in troughs for long periods of time (McDowell 2003). Ideally, total soluble salt content of drinking water should not exceed 3000 ppm, levels above this are likely to cause digestive upsets and may initially be refused by animals. Levels of total soluble salt in drinking water above 7000 ppm are not fit for donkeys, especially animals that are heavily worked or heat stressed.

Mineral requirements for donkeys are based upon those published by NRC (2007) for horses and it is the authors' opinion that although these are likely to be optimal levels, donkeys are able to do very well on slightly lower levels of both vitamins and minerals than those determined for horses. Example diets (as shown in Table 16-3) used for donkeys at maintenance that provide lower levels of vitamins and minerals are, in the authors' opinions, adequate.

Key Points

- Diets either lacking in or having an imbalanced ratio of calcium : phosphorus can lead to orthopedic disease, bone deformity and secondary nutritional hyperparathyroidism
- Careful consideration must be given to the high levels of phosphorus in commonly fed crop by-products such as rice bran, wheat bran and cotton seed and the oxalate levels (which interferes with calcium absorption) of some tropical grasses
- Working animals should be provided with free-choice, equine designated, non-molassed, mineral licks, particularly when working hard to replenish minerals lost through sweating

Body condition scoring

When feeding donkeys it is important not to forget that animals are individuals and their responses to scientifically formulated rations are not entirely predictable. To fine-tune diets to the individual requirements body condition scoring is a useful tool.

The Donkey Sanctuary has developed a practically useful system, which uses a five-point scale to body condition score (see Fig. 16.1). Body condition score systems rely on the operator developing a practiced eye and hand to detect small changes in the subcutaneous fat covering. It is important for the operator to maintain objectivity when carrying out scoring to avoid the temptation to over or under score in order to give a more "acceptable" result. Regular monitoring of body condition is important and should be carried out monthly, particularly in spring when there is abundant pasture and in winter when extra fat may assist in helping to maintain body temperature.

Initially when condition scoring, place the donkey in one of the three fat classes (thin, moderate, or fat) then look for specific indicators given in Fig. 16.1 for a more precise condition score. It is important to manually and visually determine the fat covering over the neck, shoulders, back, ribs, rump, and barrel. Donkeys frequently develop a fatty crest which may even fall over to one side. The development of such a crest is a sure indication that the donkey is becoming overweight. However, care must be taken when scoring animals with such a crest, donkeys that have been dieted and lost significant body fat may still retain a large cresty neck, once gained such crests rarely disappear. Donkeys deposit fat in different areas compared to horses (see Fig. 16.2) with large fat pads (which may become calcified and extremely hard) on the buttocks, barrel ("saddle pannier" region) and neck, abdominal fat covering can also be significant with reports of up to 8 cm of fat. With this in mind it is important to assess these deposition sites detailed above rather than use a scoring system designed for horses. Mules lie somewhere between their parents, and in the experience of the authors their rump should be scored as would a horse and the middle and neck sections as one would a donkey; however, a little flexibility and discretion is required! Finally, care must be taken when condition scoring donkeys of a finer build, these tend to be larger donkeys with a more angular body frame (e.g., Poitou, Andalusian, Mammoth Jackass), rather than concentrating on the angularity of hips, spine and shoulders attention should be directed at fat and muscle coverage on the points outlined above.

A nomogram (see Fig. 16.3) has also been developed to allow estimation of bodyweight by using a heart girth measurement and height measurement, this is particularly useful when bodyweight is needed for drug dosage purposes or when monitoring bodyweight changes when dieting or conditioning animals.

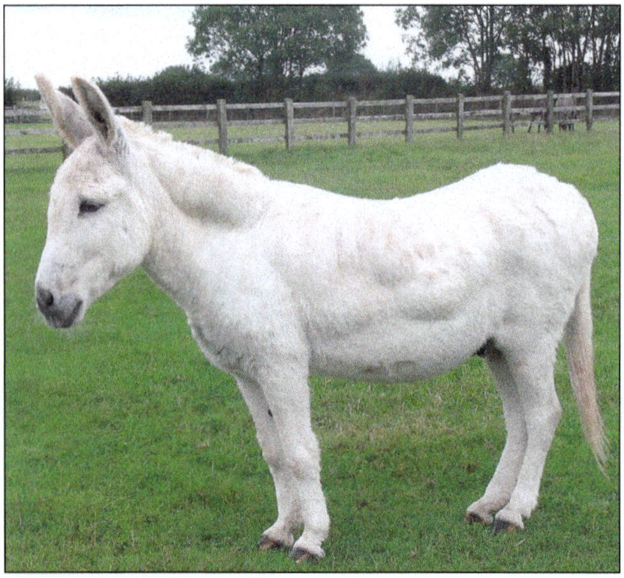

Figure 16.2 A donkey of body condition score 5 showing defined fat deposition sites commonly seen in obese donkeys and mules.

Key Points

- A condition scoring system developing for donkeys and mules must always be used; weight may be estimated using a donkey nomogram
- Donkeys deposit fat in different areas to those seen in horses. Deposit sites include the barrel, crest, rump and abdomen. Long-standing deposits may become hard and calcified and once in this state will not be lost
- Mules have features of both parents, generally the rump should be scored as one would a horse with the middle and neck sections scored as one would a donkey

Practical feeding

The donkey's natural feeding behavior

Under feral conditions donkeys will spend virtually all the hours of daylight and some of the night (14–16 hours per day) foraging for food (Smith & Pearson 2005). They are highly selective feeders and, when allowed to roam in their natural environment, dedicate a significant amount of time to finding preferred morsels particularly graminoids before eventually resigning themselves to eating less nutrient-rich fodders such as forbs and woody plants (Lamoot et al 2005). When donkeys are domesticated these natural conditions are difficult to replicate, especially under temperate conditions where fodder is abundant and often of high quality. Moreover, donkeys are more efficient at digesting fibrous food than horses (Pearson 2005), this difference is particularly marked with poor quality feeds and, as a consequence they can thrive on less forage than a similar-sized pony (Wood et al 2005). The challenge for keepers is to provide donkeys with enough food to keep them busy in their favorite activity (eating) but not to allow them to become obese, which puts them at risk of developing serious and often fatal diseases such as hyperlipemia and laminitis.

Key Points

- Donkeys have evolved to eat for 14–16 hours per day; domestic feeding practices should mimic this as much as possible
- Donkeys form strong bonds and may need to be fed with, or in sight of, their companion; refusal to follow this rule may lead to a nervous and inappetant animal
- Sham eating is a trait seen commonly in sick donkeys where food appears to be mouthed and swallowed and yet intake is negligible; careful observation is key
- Equine feedstuffs based on cereals or containing high levels of molasses are unsuitable for donkeys
- For most of the year a ration that contains 70–75% barley or wheat straw or other fibrous forage such as maize stover and 25–30% of moderate quality grass hay, grazing or green fodder will supply all the energy requirements of donkeys
- During the winter when energy requirements increase the proportion of hay or green fodder may need to be increased to 50–75%
- A mineral supplement will also be required and some source of vitamins either in the form of a small quantity of fresh green fodder (200 g of chopped fresh alfalfa) or a commercial vitamin mix
- Feedstuffs suitable for donkeys must be low in non-structural carbohydrates (<15%) and high in fiber (>20%)

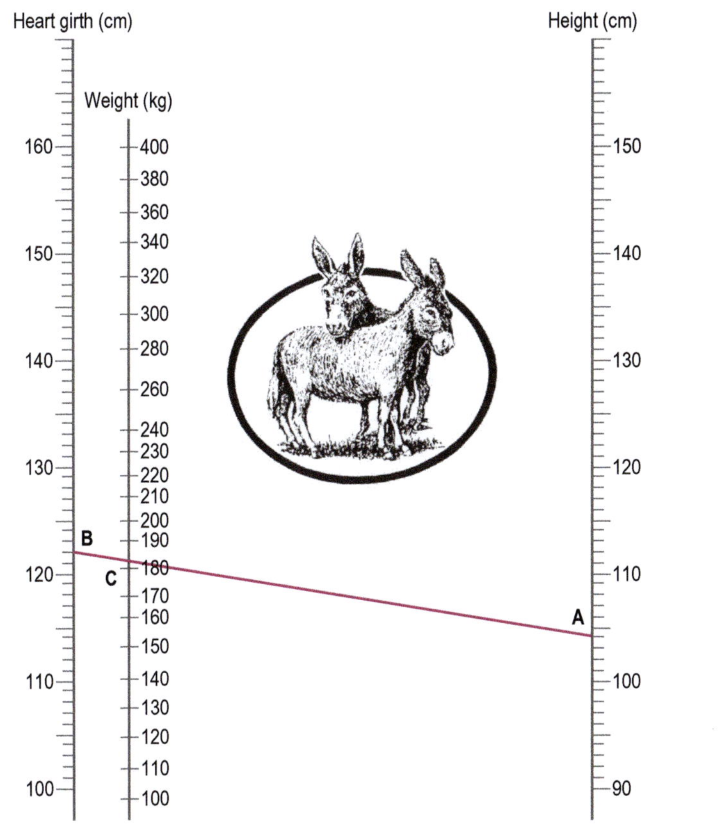

A donkey 104 cm tall (A) and with a heart girth 122 cm (B) should weigh 181 kg (C). The nomogram is accurate to within 10 kilograms.

Weight table for donkeys under 2 years:

Heart Girth cm	75	76	77	78	79	80	81	82	83	84	85	86	87	88	89	90	91	92	93	94	95	96	97	98	99	100
Weight kg	46	47	49	51	53	55	57	59	61	63	65	67	69	71	74	76	78	81	83	86	88	91	94	96	99	102

For adult donkey; weight = 0.000252 x height$^{0.240}$ x heart girth$^{2.575}$
For donkey under 2 years; weight = 0.000283 x heart girth$^{2.778}$

Figure 16.3 Donkey nomogram. *Copyright The Donkey Sanctuary.*

When feeding donkeys it is important to consider the donkey's surroundings. Donkeys are gregarious animals that form strong bonds. When feeding a bonded donkey it is essential to have the friend at least within sight (some donkeys will not even tolerate being separated by a fence) otherwise one or both animals may refuse to eat in spite of their hunger. Another unique donkey trait of note is that of "sham eating," which is frequently seen in sick donkeys and mules. Donkeys will often sham eat for considerable periods of time; the animal appears to mouth and swallow food or may simply nudge it but invariably intakes virtually none. Such behavior is often a sign of a serious illness and should be investigated fully by a veterinarian who must be particularly mindful of hyperlipemia.

Donkeys may be fed successfully in a group and generally tolerate the presence of other equids well. Dominant donkeys may bully other animals lower in the hierarchy and care should be taken to provide ample feeder space to prevent reduced intake by submissive animals. Further consideration must be given to other animals who may be present whilst donkeys are feeding. Invariably donkeys are bullied at feed time by horses, ponies plus mules and may end up injured or unable to access enough feed to satisfy their requirements. In such situations the donkey's natural preference for highly fibrous forages such as straw can be used to their advantage as many other equids will be less inclined to bully for access to such low-quality fiber.

Practical rationing

Donkeys on a maintenance diet require little more than a limited amount of moderate quality grass hay (as discussed previously) or moderate quality grazing, free access to good clean wheat, barley or oat straw to fill them up, a mineral/vitamin balancer and plenty of clean water (Table 16-4). Keepers should avoid over-complicating a donkey's diet by the addition of various mixes to rectify apparent dietary problems or because the donkey likes them! Most complementary feedstuffs and legume hays are energy rich and even small quantities will exceed the energy requirements of the donkey. Studies on pasture fed donkeys in temperate climates (Wood 2010), indicate that overfeeding is a bigger

Table 16-4 An Example Ration for Maintenance in a Healthy Donkey of 200 kg BW Fed at 1.3% BW DM Basis Providing 19 MJ of DE per Day Based on 75% Barley Straw and 25% Low Energy Forage

Ration/day	As fed	DM intake	Crude protein	Fat	CF	Nitrogen free extract	Digestible crude protein	DE	Ca	P	Mg	Na	K	Cl
	kg	kg/day	g/day					MJ/day	g/day					
Roughage	3	2.6	167	45	1023	1179	76	19.1	11	4	3	3	35	22
NRC for horses 200 kg/day			*216*						8	5.6	4	4	10	16
Total ration per day	3	2.6	167	45	1023	1179	76	19.1	11	4	3	3	35	22
Total ration per kg DM			65	17	395	455	29	7.4	4	2	1	1	13	9

Note that although NRC recommendations for protein, phosphorus and sodium are not met by this ration in the authors' experience these diets are sufficient for maintenance in donkeys and mules.

risk than underfeeding. Under most conditions it is recommended that pasture fed donkeys are provided with free-access to clean straw but are not provided with hay. Body condition score should be regularly monitored.

Donkeys are prone to developing conditions such as laminitis (Crane 2008), gastric ulceration (Burden et al 2009), fatty liver disease and hyperlipemia (Morrow et al 2010). Inappropriate feeding may lead to the development of these problems or further exacerbate pre-existing problems. Equine feedstuffs based upon cereals or containing high levels of molasses should be strictly avoided, they have been shown to be risk factors for the development of gastric ulceration (Burden et al 2009), colic (Cox et al 2009) as well as laminitis in donkeys and are unsuitable for donkeys unless worked very hard.

Key Points

- Do not resort to proprietary equine senior feeds or conditioning feeds for underweight or sick animals, they will over supply energy and do not provide enough fiber
- Low energy hay replacement products made from chopped straw, grass and alfalfa are useful for individuals with poor dentition
- High-fiber nuts, unmolassed sugar beet and alfalfa chops may be useful as supplementary feeds. Supplementing with oil may also increase the energy content of the donkey's diet, rice bran products, soya and corn oil may all be fed in small quantities (up to 150 ml) but must be fed with care to animals with liver disease
- If sick donkeys become inappetant it is essential to stimulate feeding to prevent hyperlipemia developing, useful products include peppermint cordial, dried mint, ginger, carrots, bananas and yeast extract. The donkey's wish to browse is also very useful and donkeys may eat hedgerows over any other offering

Practical feeding for problem donkeys

Although the vast majority of donkeys can be fed adequately on a diet of straw and limited grass hay or grazing, some animals do require supplementary feeding due to advancing age or health problems. When devising a diet for these animals it is important to satisfy the "trickle feeding" requirements of the donkey whilst taking into account underlying health problems such as poor dentition, liver disease and kidney disease. It is important not to resort to proprietary equine senior feeds and other high energy feeds as these will tend to over supply energy and typically do not provide the level of fiber intake that is essential for the digestive health of the donkey. Feedstuffs suitable for donkeys must be low in nonstructural carbohydrates (<15%) and high in fiber (>20%).

Elderly and sick donkeys

Research has shown that elderly donkeys frequently suffer from dental disease, with a prevalence of 98% being reported (Du Toit et al 2008b). They may not be able to chew long fiber forages effectively potentially leading to weight loss, colic and depression. It is essential to replace these long fibers with alternative fiber sources that can be easily chewed and digested. Low-energy hay replacement products made from chopped straw, grass and alfalfa are ideal and many of these products can be used to completely replace all other fiber sources. For donkeys that do not require such drastic feed changes high fiber products such as high-fiber nuts, alfalfa chops, and unmolassed sugar beet all designed to be suitable for laminitic equines are ideal supplementary feeds. Supplementing with oil is a useful way of increasing the energy content of the donkey's diet, rice bran products, soya and corn oil may all be fed in small quantities (up to 150 ml) but must be fed with care to animals with liver disease. If high levels (>100 ml) are to be fed consideration must be given to supplying additional vitamin E (100–150 IU per 100 ml oil), particularly if the animal has limited access to fresh grazing. It is often possible to source products already fortified with appropriate levels of vitamin E where simplicity is needed. Introduction of oil to the diet must be gradual and carried out over a number of weeks as it can lead to feed refusal in large quantities when donkeys and mules are unused to it. Mixing oil well in to feeds will help, rather than allowing clumps to form.

Sick donkeys and mules frequently present with anorexia, which may lead to life-threatening hyperlipemia, it is essential to stimulate the appetite in such cases. Most donkeys can be tempted with additives such as peppermint cordial, bananas, dried or fresh mint leaf, ginger, grated or chopped carrots and apples, and yeast extracts. It is important not to underestimate the donkey's natural instinct as a browser. Donkeys that have shown no interest in tasty proprietary mixes and treats will often be tempted to eat if led to a nearby hedgerow to browse on the brambles and herbs available, this natural instinct can often be used successfully in the worst of cases.

Feeding obese donkeys

Perhaps the biggest donkey welfare issue in developed countries is their propensity to obesity when fed high-energy diets by well-meaning owners, coupled with the fact that very few are worked. Dieting an overweight donkey is extremely difficult and needs to be tackled carefully; changes to the diet must be made very gradually (4–6 weeks). The diet of the animal is often only part of the problem with lack of exercise, companion issues and mental stimulation all needing to be addressed as well. Grazing must be very tightly restricted by strip grazing and owners must be encouraged to be guided more by reducing the area of land the donkey has available rather than the amount of time the donkey spends grazing, studies have shown that donkeys are able to eat the same amount in 8 hours as they would if given access to pasture 24 hours a day (Smith & Pearson 2005). If there are concerns about vitamin and mineral deficiency then supplements may be fed to balance the diet. In order to help donkeys lose weight they must be exercised and encouraged to work for their food. Ridden or in hand exercise is ideal but, where this is inappropriate, other methods can be employed. Donkeys can be encouraged to "work" for their food by using sloping pastures, placing feedstuffs in different locations (i.e., spread in four to five different locations in the field), providing stable toys and employing long, narrow, strip grazing areas.

Key Points

- Dieting donkeys must be undertaken with care and be done very gradually
- Grazing must be tightly restricted, restriction of the area of pasture rather than amount of time at grazing is essential
- Donkeys must be exercised alongside a reduced energy intake, for example a diet of ad lib wheat straw with very restricted grazing or limited grass hay, vitamin and mineral supplements can be offered if appropriate
- Donkeys should be condition scored and have heart girth measurements taken once per month

Animals should be scored for body condition weekly and records kept of their heart girth measurements, estimation of weight may be possible using a nomogram (Fig. 16.3). In the author's experience a typical 180 kg donkey with good dentition should be provided with ad lib wheat or barley straw with very little access to pasture (no more than 0.2 acres per donkey of short cropped pasture) or grass hay, the diet may then be supplemented with a proprietary vitamin and mineral supplement to avoid malnutrition. Consideration may also be given to providing additional protein to the diet to ensure that muscle loss is not an unfortunate side-effect of weight loss; many proprietary balancers are available containing excellent sources of quality protein, vitamins and minerals but little energy. In other situations supplementation with small amounts of alfalfa and soya hulls may be required. In such cases it is particularly important to ensure that exercise is increased to account for the increased dietary energy supplied by these feeds. Whilst providing straw ad libitum is important to fulfill the appetite of the donkey or mule, it is important not to allow the donkey to be too fussy and pick out the most palatable morsels. To avoid this occurring, providing new straw every 2–3 days is generally sufficient (some will always be left over as donkeys never eat all offered, so do not be guided by this) and if the straw has much retained grain then shaking over a plastic sheet before feeding to discard as much as possible is useful. The natural changes in seasons can be used to the donkey owner's advantage, energy requirements for the donkey increase in the winter and this period can be used to naturally assist the donkey to lose weight. Progress when dieting donkeys is slow and perseverance is important, changes in body condition scores may take months to achieve and visible changes may not be obvious despite actual weight loss. It often takes time for the first weight to be lost and it is neither realistic nor healthy to expect more than 2% of bodyweight to be lost per month, once weight loss begins it should be gradual and not excessive and care must be taken to stop when the donkey has reached the target body condition score (Table 16-5).

Feeding mules

Mules are the hybrid resulting from the mating between a horse mare and a donkey jack. Less frequently encountered are hinnies, the result of a mating between a donkey jenny and a horse stallion. Mules are said to possess "hybrid vigour" and enthusiasts believe they possess the best traits

Table 16-5 The Daily Digestible Energy (DE) and Digestible Crude Protein Requirement of Different Types of Donkeys with Various Body Condition Score (BCS) and Under Different Environmental Conditions

Donkey type	Environmental conditions	DE requirements per day (MJ/day)	DCP requirements per day (g/day)
Typical donkey (BCS 3, 175 kg BW)	Temperate summer climate Temperate winter climate	14 17	46 46
Overweight donkey (BCS 4, 220 kg) – Allowing for safe weight loss	Temperate summer climate Temperate winter climate	12 16	46 46
Typical working donkey in developing country (BCS 2, 150 kg BW) – Allowing for some weight gain	Tropical dry season Tropical wet season	16 + 8 (work) 12 + 6 (work)	39 39
Larger breeds of donkey (e.g. Poitou = 350 kg)	Temperate summer climate Temperate winter climate	28 34	92 92

of both species. Nutritionally, mules should be treated like their donkey parent. Little research has been carried out to determine the nutritional needs of mules, but in the authors' experience mules thrive on rations similar to those described for the donkey. Owners of mules will often state that mules will not overeat even if given the opportunity and hence will not suffer from laminitis and obesity. This does appear to be true to a certain extent with lower incidences of laminitis and obesity in the mule populations known to the authors. However, obese, laminitic mules can and do occur so care must be taken to restrict feed. It has been reported that feeding a mule as one would a horse leads to significant behavioral changes. Experienced mule owners often keep animals on "dry lots" with supplementary straw and hay.

Mules make excellent working animals and are valued for their physical and mental strength and ability to survive harsh conditions. Mules possess the physical stature and strength of their horse mother along with the ability to cope with cold, wet conditions that the donkey would not thrive in. The mule has also gained the digestive efficiency of the donkey and has many times been the last survivor on long journeys when horses and oxen have starved. Working mules should have supplementary feed supplied as required, as with donkeys, feeds low in nonstructural carbohydrates and high in fiber are most suitable.

Key Points

Nutritionally mules should be treated like their donkey parent.

Special considerations for working donkeys

Appropriate feeding of working donkeys is essential to sustain working activities, disease resistance and longevity. It also contributes towards reducing work-related saddle and harness sores as donkeys in poor body condition suffer from sores more frequently than those in good condition (Burden et al 2009).

Key Points

- Under certain working conditions working donkeys may require five times more water than a sedentary individual (up to 35 liters per day)
- An average donkey with a pack or pulling a cart travelling 20 km will require 100% more energy than a sedentary animal, and one travelling 30 km will require 160% more energy
- Where distance is less easily discerned work hours can be used to estimate requirements; 4 hours work will require 50% more energy and 6 hours work will require 100% more energy
- Nutrition is an important component of preventive healthcare and must be addressed alongside matters such as parasite control, harnessing and infectious diseases

Working donkeys must receive adequate water to enable them to work and digest their food effectively; water will be lost through sweating and under certain conditions working donkeys may require five times more water than a sedentary individual (up to 35 liters per day). However, one potential benefit of the working donkey over the horse is their ability to continue to work and maintain appetite with reduced water intakes. The gut fluid pool apparently depletes by up to 50% during severe dehydration (25% dehydration: see Sneddon et al 2006) and plasma volume is apparently maintained in dehydrated donkeys even when they lose 20% of normal body water (Matthews et al 1998). Work, however, has suggested that when experiencing mild chronic dehydration (6% drop in BW) whilst working, fermentation activity in the caecum increases and there is enhanced fluid retention in the ventral colon (Sneddon et al 2006). The enhanced fermentation activity associated with the enhanced mucosal absorptive or secretory capacity within the hindgut may help to maintain appetite.

When donkeys are working their energy requirements can be considerably higher than those quoted for maintenance. Requirements will vary according to the work done, access to feed, quality of feed and length of period worked. Previous work has shown that an average donkey with a pack, or pulling a cart travelling 20 km, will require 100% more energy than a sedentary animal, and one travelling 30 km will require 160% more energy. Where distances are difficult to estimate, length of time that the donkey is worked for can be used as a guideline: 4 hours work will require 50% more energy and 6 hours work will require 100% more energy (Pearson 2005).

Donkeys with such increased energy requirements may struggle to obtain all their requirements from highly fibrous roughages as they may be unable to eat enough quantity either due to lack of digestive tract capacity or lack of time to physically eat. Such donkeys may require higher energy feedstuffs or access to good quality grazing. Grazing is often limited in tropical areas for much of the year so locally available crop by-products or standing hay crops are frequently fed. Cereals such as barley, oats, maize and sorghum are often fed (Fig. 16.4).

However, care must be taken not to feed in excess and to ensure that the cereal is crushed, cracked or rolled to promote small intestinal digestion. The use of molasses or oils to increase the energy level of the diet may be helpful; highly digestible oils such as sunflower, soya, corn and palm oils can add energy to the diet but must be added gradually to a base feed of cereal or vegetable matter to avoid feed refusal. Addition of up to 150 ml of oil, split in to two feeds,

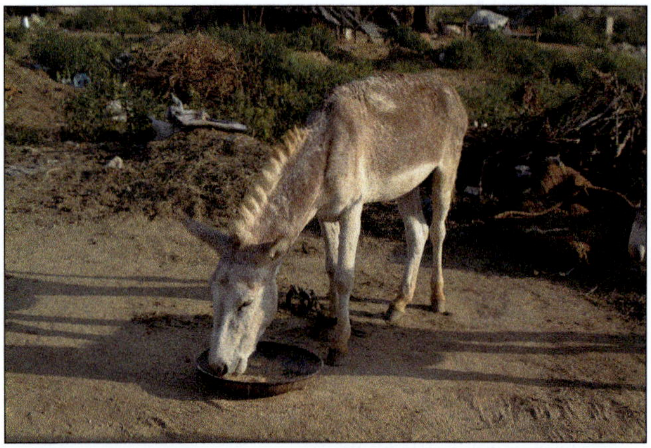

Figure 16.4 A working donkey receiving supplementary bran feeding, care must be taken to provide a balanced diet and to allow the animal adequate time to feed.

for a 180 kg donkey or 250 ml for a large donkey or mule is sufficient to make a significant contribution to the energy content of the diet. Finally, protein-rich legumes such as alfalfa (lucerne), berseem and faba beans can be fed alongside roughages to enhance the energy and protein content of the diet, all are highly palatable to donkeys and mules. Inclusion rates of up to 25% of the dry matter intake for the donkey or mule working 4–6 hours per day are recommended, higher inclusion rates are likely to oversupply energy and protein and are therefore wasteful.

Essential to the nutritional management of the working donkey or mule is educating owners on suitable, locally available feedstuffs and the importance of frequent body condition scoring. Nutrition is an important component of preventive healthcare and must be addressed alongside matters such as parasite control, harnessing and infectious diseases.

Summary

- The energy and protein requirements of donkeys are generally lower than those of a similar sized pony. Donkeys fed to maintenance (neither gaining nor losing weight) require limited amounts of grass hay or restricted grazing and free access to straw.
- For stabled donkeys a diet of 25% medium quality grass hay and 75% barley, oat or wheat straw should be adequate in the spring and autumn. The level of hay should be slightly decreased in the summer and increased to 75% in midwinter.
- Body condition scoring should be used to fine-tune a donkey's diet.
- Pasture fed donkeys normally require no supplementary hay except in harsh winter conditions, especially if they are given free access to straw.
- Unmolassed equine specific mineral licks and a plentiful supply of clean water should always be provided.
- Provide an energy-free vitamin and mineral supplement during the winter, especially if the donkey has no access to fresh grazing at this time.

References

Burden, F.A., Gallagher, J., Thiemann, A., et al., 2009. Necropsy survey of gastric ulcers in a population of aged donkeys: prevalence, lesion description and risk factors. Animal 3 (2), 287–293.

Carretero-Roque, L., Colunga, B., Smith, D.G., et al., 2005. Digestible energy requirements of Mexican donkeys fed oat straw and maize stover. (Special issue: Nutrition and health of donkeys in the tropics). Tropical Animal Health and Production 37, (Supplement 1), 123–142.

Crane, M., 2008. The donkey's foot. In: Svendsen, E.D., Duncan, J., Hadrill, D. (Eds.), The Professional Handbook of the Donkey, fourth ed. Whittet Books, Yatesbury, Chapter 10.

Cox, R., Burden, F., Gosden, L., et al., 2009. Case control study to investigate risk factors for impaction colic in donkeys in the UK. Preventive Veterinary Medicine 92 (3), 179–187.

Du Toit, N., Burden, F.A., Dixon, P.M., 2008a. Clinical dental findings in 203 working donkeys in Mexico. Veterinary Journal 178, 380–386.

Du Toit, N., Burden, F.A., Dixon, P.M., 2008b. Clinical dental examinations of 357 donkeys in the UK: Part 1: Prevalence of dental disorders. Equine Veterinary Journal 41 (4), 390–394.

Dugdale, A.H.A., Curtis, G.C., Knottenbelt, D.C., et al., Argo CMcG, 2008. Changes in body condition and fat deposition in ponies offered an ad libitum chaff based diet. Proceedings of 12th Congress of the European Society of Veterinary and Comparative Nutrition, September 25–27, 2008. University of Veterinary Medicine Vienna, Austria.

Faurie, F., Tisserand, J-L., 1994. Comparative study of the cellulytic activity of caecum microbes in ponies and donkeys. Annals of Zootechnology 43, 281.

Frape, D., 2004. Equine Nutrition and Feeding, third ed. Blackwell Publishing, Oxford.

Hill, E.M., Greene, H.M., Wickler, S.J., et al., 2001. Hematological responses to high altitude exposure (3800 m) in donkeys. In: Proceedings of Equine Nutrition and Physiology Society, pp. 440–441.

Houpt, T.R., 1993. Water and electrolytes. In: Dukes, H.H., Swenson, M.J., Reece, W.O. (Eds.), Physiology of Domestic Animals. Cornell University Press, Ithaca NY, p. 9.

Izraely, H., Choshniak, I., Stevens, C.E., et al., 1989. Factors determining the digestive efficiency of the domesticated donkey (*Equus asinus asinus*). Quarterly Journal of Experimental Physiology 74, 1–6.

Lamoot, I., Callebaut, J., Demeulenaere, E., et al., 2005. Foraging behaviour of donkeys grazing in a coastal dune area in temperate climate conditions. Applied Animal Behaviour Science 92 (1), 93–112.

Liberatore, G.A., Wickler, S.J., Greene, H.M., 2001. Effect of acute altitude exposure (3800 Meters) on the metabolic capacity of the middle gluteal muscle of the donkey (*Equus asinus*). In Proceedings of the Equine Nutrition and Physiology Society, pp. 377–381.

Lizarraga, I., Sumano, H., Brumbaugh, G.W., 2004. Pharmacological and pharmacokinetic differences between donkeys and horses. Equine Veterinary Education 16 (2), 102–112.

Luthersson, N., Chunekamrai, S., Estepa, J.C., et al., 2005. Secondary nutritional hyperparathyroidism in ponies in Northern Thailand. Pferdeheilkunde 21, 97–98.

Marlin, D., Nankervis, K., 2002. Equine Exercise Physiology. Blackwell Publishing, Oxford.

Maloiy, G.M.O., 1973. The effect of dehydration and heat stress on intake and digestion of food in the Somali Donkey. Environment, Physiology and Biochemistry 3, 36–39.

Matthews, N.S., Taylor, T.S., Potter, G.D., 1998. Physiologic responses during exhaustive driving test in donkeys: effects of conditioning. Applied Animal Behaviour Science 59, 31–38.

McDowell, L.R., 2003. Minerals in Animal and Human Nutrition, second ed. Elsevier, Amsterdam.

McLean, A.K., Nielsen, B.D., Yokoyama, M., et al., 2009. Insulin resistance in standard donkeys (*Equus asinus*) of three body conditions – thin, moderate and obese. Journal of Equine Veterinary Science 29, 406–407.

Morrow, L.D., Smith, K.C., Piercy, R.J., et al., 2010. Retrospective analysis of post-mortem findings in. 1444. aged donkeys. Journal of Comparative Pathology Doi: 10.1016/j.jcpa.2010.08.005.

Mueller, P.J., Brockmann, K.A., Houpt, K.A., et al., 1997. Water intake by donkeys: is it affected by accessibility? Proceedings of the Fifteenth Equine Nutrition and Physiology Symposium, Fort Worth, Texas, USA, 28–31 May, 1997, pp. 193–194.

National Research Council, 2007. Nutrient Requirements of Horses, sixth ed. National Academy Press, Washington DC.

Pearson, R.A., 2005. Nutrition and feeding of donkeys. In: Mathews, N.S., Taylor, T.S. (Eds.), Veterinary Care of Donkeys. International Veterinary Information Service, Ithaca, NY, pp. 1–5 (http://www.ivis.org).

Pearson, R.A., Archibald, R.F., Muirhead, R.H., 2006. A comparison of the effect of forage type and level of feeding on the digestibility and gastrointestinal mean retention time of dry forages given to cattle, sheep, ponies and donkeys. British Journal of Nutrition 95, 88–98.

Rossel, S., Marshall, F., Peters, J., et al., 2008. Domestication of the donkey: timing, processes, and indicators. Proceedings of the National Academy of Sciences USA 105 (10), 3715–3720.

Smith, D.G., 1999. The impact of grazing time allowance on the dry matter intake and foraging behaviour of cattle and donkeys managed under Traditional African grazing systems. PhD Thesis, University of Edinburgh.

Smith, D.G., Nahius, A., Archibald, R.F., 1994. A comparison of the energy requirements for work in donkeys, ponies and cattle. In: Bakkoury, M., Prentis, R.A. (Eds.), Working Equines. Second International Colloquium, Rabat, Morocco, 20–22 April 1994, (Actes Éditions, Rabat, Morocco), pp. 17–22.

Smith, D.G., Pearson, R.A., 2005. A review of the factors affecting the survival of donkeys in semi-arid regions of sub-Saharan Africa. (Special issue: Nutrition and health of donkeys in the tropics). Tropical Animal Health and Production 37 (Supplement 1), 1–19.

Sneddon, J.C., Boomker, E., Howeard, C.V., 2006. Mucosal surface area and fermentation activity in the hind gut of hydrated and chronically dehydrated working donkeys. Journal of Animal Science 84, 119–124.

Starkey, P., Starkey, M., 2000. Regional and world trends in donkey populations. In: Starkey, P., Fielding, D. (Eds.), Donkeys, People and Development. A resource book of the Animal Traction Network for Eastern and Southern Africa (ATNESA). ACP-EU Technical Centre for Agricultural and Rural Cooperation (CTA), Wageningen, The Netherlands, pp. 10–21.

Stevens, C.E., Hume, I.D., 2004. Comparative Physiology of the Vertebrate Digestive System, second ed. Cambridge University Press, Cambridge.

Stewart, J.H., 2005. Big head or bran disease. http://www.mitavite.com.au/mitavite06/PDF/Nutritional%20Information%20PDF/Vet%20notes/Big%20Head%20or%20Bran%20Disease.pdf (accessed 24 June 2010).

Suhartanto, B., Julliand, V., Faurie, F., et al., 1992. Comparison of digestion in donkeys and ponies. In: Proceedings of the 1st European Conference on Horses. Pferdeheikund Sondersgabe, Hannover, pp. 158–161.

Svendsen, E.D., 2009. The Complete Book of the Donkey. Kenilworth Press Ltd, Shrewsbury.

Tisserand, J-L., Faurie, F., Toure, M., 1991. A comparative study of donkey and pony digestive physiology. In: Fielding, D., Pearson, R.A. (Eds.), Donkeys, Mules and Horses in Tropical Agricultural Development. Alexander Ritchie & Son, Edinburgh, pp. 67–72.

Wood, S.J., 2010. Some factors affecting the digestible energy requirements and dry matter intake of mature donkeys, PhD Thesis, Edinburgh University.

Wood, S.J., Smith, D.G., Morris, C.J., 2005. Seasonal variation of digestible energy requirements of mature donkeys in the UK. Pferdeheilkunde 21, Conference, 39–40.

Yousef, M.K., 1991. Physiological responses of the donkey to heat stress. In: Fielding, D., Pearson, R.A. (Eds.), Donkeys, Horse and Mules in Tropical Agricultural Development. Alexander Ritchie & Son, Edinburgh, p. 96.

Applied Nutrition – Feeds

C

SECTION

17

Feedstuffs for horses

Jan Erik Lindberg

Introduction

Practical horse feeding differs between countries, mainly due to the availability of feedstuffs and the existence of long held beliefs over what can/should or cannot/should not be fed, i.e. traditions. Whilst a large number of feedstuffs are available and can be used in the formulation of diets for horses (Axelsson 1943, Nehra et al 2005, Olsson & Ruudvere 1955, Sauvant et al 2004) because of "tradition", most horse owners only use a limited number of feedstuffs and are reluctant to try alternatives. However, in compounded concentrate feeds (complementary feeds) the range of feedstuffs used is larger and there is a great interest in the feed industry to find alternatives to the traditional feed ingredients.

There are different ways to classify feedstuffs depending on the criteria used to formulate diets (Axelsson 1943). The international feed identification system classifies feedstuffs into the following eight categories (Kellems & Church 2010):

1. Dry roughage
2. Pasture and range grasses
3. Ensiled roughages
4. High-energy concentrates
5. Protein sources
6. Minerals
7. Vitamins
8. Additives.

This classification is useful in many cases but there is a need for additional information about energy and nutrient content for optimal diet formulation. From a nutritional point of view the classification should be based on properties (coarse, fiber-rich, bulky) and/or on nutrient content (protein-rich, fat-rich, rapidly fermentable, carbohydrate-rich). In horse feeding practice, classification of feedstuffs is often based on the type of feeds commonly used (i.e. roughage, concentrate, sweet feed, etc.), and it is understood that roughage has different properties and nutrient content than concentrate/sweet feed.

Roughage

Roughage should always be the foundation of a horse's diet. Any additional grains or protein/vitamin/mineral supplements should be used only to supply additional energy and/or essential nutrients not supplied by the roughage. Through the well-developed symbiosis with the hindgut microbiota, and its production of energy yielding substrates in the form of volatile or short-chain fatty acids (SCFA), it should be possible to provide the energy needs of most horses with a forage-only diet (NRC 2007). However, the most common feeding practise for performance horses world-wide today is to supplement the roughage part of the diet (hay, haylage, silage, straw) with a cereal-based concentrate (*complementary*) feed (Gallagher et al 1992, Lindner & Gansen 1995, Richards et al 2006). Concentrate is included in diets for athletic horses in order to increase the energy density and thereby make it possible to meet increased energy requirements. Roughage can be grazed or fed post harvesting in the fresh or more commonly a preserved/conserved form. Many roughage sources may potentially be used in horse feeding (Kellems & Church 2010), but the most commonly used roughages for stall-fed horses are various forages (hay, silage, haylage) of different botanical composition (grasses, legumes, herbs) and straw (NRC 2007, Nehra et al 2005).

Grazed forage forms the basis of diets for wild equids and can constitute the entire diet for domesticated horses (NRC 2007). In northern Europe, pasture generally cannot be provided all year round due to the cold climate and snow cover. In southern Europe, as well as in many other parts of the world, low precipitation and/or periods of drought may be reasons for limited forage supply from pasture. Therefore, forage has to be harvested and preserved either by drying or by ensiling to provide a year-round source of roughage.

Nutritional properties

Forages are composed of cell contents (protein, fat, soluble carbohydrates) and cell walls (cellulose, hemicellulose, lignin); the relative proportions of which vary according to the forage source and maturity at the time of harvest. The cell content is highly digestible (80–100%; Fonnesbeck 1968, 1969), while the true digestibility of the cell wall is more limited (40–50%; Fonnesbeck 1968, 1969). Thus, the energy and nutritive value of forages can vary considerably (Ragnarsson & Lindberg 2008, 2010) and will to a large extent be determined by fiber content and fiber quality (Van Soest 1994). This implies that the forage used in horse feeding should be carefully selected in order to provide appropriate levels of energy and nutrients, and not just the fiber necessary to support hindgut function.

Table 17-1 Chemical Composition (g/kg Dry Matter), Proportion of Lysine (% of Crude Protein), and Content of Linoleic and Linolenic Acid (g/kg Dry Matter) and Energy (MJ/kg Dry Matter) in Cereals and Cereal by-Products[a,b]

	Oats		Barley	Wheat			Maize			Rice		
	Regular	Dehulled	Grain	Grain	Bran	Middlings	Grain	Bran	Feed flour	Grain	Bran	Bran, extr.
Crude protein	111	124	116	121	170	176	94	123	103	88	153	160
Crude fat	55	29	21	17	39	41	43	41	62	14	182	34
Starch	411	614	602	697	227	314	742	340	522	882	304	335
Sugars	12	14	24	28	77	70	18	25	29	5	32	25
NDF	372	135	216	143	455	355	120	594	293	59	227	267
Crude fiber	138	47	53	25	106	79	25	146	66	13	87	103
Lysine	4.2	4.2	3.8	3.1	3.9	4.0	3.0	3.7	4.1	3.7	4.4	4.5
Linoleic acid	19	10	9	7	18	18	21	20	30	4	52	8
Linolenic acid[c]	0.7	0.4	0.9	0.7	1.8	1.9	0.4	0.3	0.5	0.2	2.2	0.4
GE	19.5	18.8	18.3	18.2	18.8	18.9	18.7	18.9	19.4	18.1	21.5	17.6
DE	13.1	14.7	14.7	15.4	11.7	13.1	15.9	11.0	13.7	15.7	14.2	12.2
ME	11.9	13.7	13.7	14.5	10.1	11.4	15.2	9.9	12.6	15.4	12.3	10.7
NE	9.3	10.8	10.8	11.6	8.1	9.1	12.2	8.1	10.1	12.5	10.0	8.8

[a]Data from Sauvant et al (2004).
[b]GE = gross energy, DE = digestible energy, ME = metabolizable energy, NE = net energy.
[c]α-linolenic acid.

The stage of maturity will have a profound effect on the energy and nutrient content of the forage and on the ability of the horse to consume offered quantities (NRC 2007). By selecting high-quality forage (high energy content) the required proportions of forage and concentrate can be markedly affected, and made more favorable with regards to voluntary feed intake and digestive function (Willard et al 1977, Julliand et al 2001). The daily intake of starch and dietary fiber will be markedly affected by the cereal source used in the diet (Table 17-1), as will the digestion of the cereal carbohydrate within the small intestine (Kienzle 1994) and the quantities of rapidly fermentable carbohydrates reaching the hindgut (Julliand et al 2006). This in turn will affect the ratio of fermentable starch to dietary fiber in the digesta reaching the hindgut, and thus the composition and activity of hindgut microbiota.

Country of origin may also influence the nutritive value of a particular forage type. It was recently shown for example that forage grown in Iceland (timothy and mixed grass forage) and fed to Icelandic horses had high digestibility values for all dietary components, including the fiber fraction (Ragnarsson & Lindberg 2008, 2010). Moreover, although the energy content in the forages declined with advancing maturity, late cuttings maintained high energy values (Fig. 17.1) compared to other reported values (NRC 2007). This could be due to the combination of high latitude, long photoperiod and cool climate, resulting in a slower rate of phonological development (Bertrand et al 2008, Deinum et al 1981, Heide et al 1985, Van Soest 1994) with subsequent changes in chemical composition and in fiber digestibility (Bertrand et al 2008, Thorvaldsson et al 2007).

Forage protein quality is comparable with that of cereal grains (lysine representing 3.5–4.5% of crude protein (CP); NRC 2007, Reverter et al 1999) and can be sufficient to cover the lysine needs of most adult horses not being used for reproductive purposes (NRC 2007) provided that the CP requirements can be met. Although crude fat content is low (approximately 30 g/kg dry matter (DM), NRC 2007), the fat "quality" is high with linoleic acid and α-linolenic acid making up 15–20 and 35–50 g/100 g total fatty acids (FA) (Woods & Fearon 2009). Thus, a forage-only diet will provide the minimum recommended intake of linoleic acid (5 g/kg DM) suggested by NRC (2007).

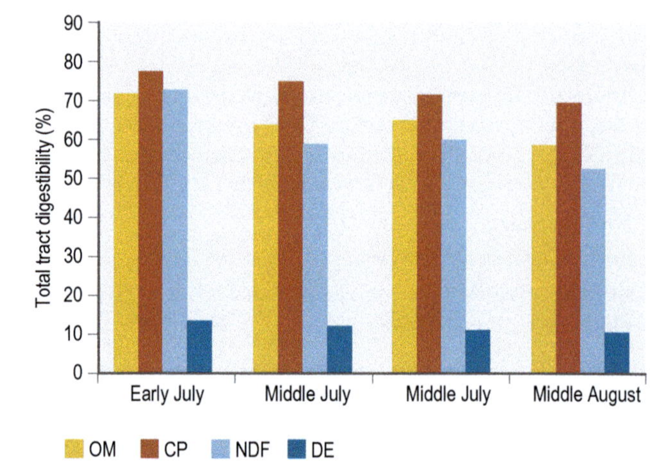

Figure 17.1 **Impact of stage of maturity of mixed grass haylage produced on Iceland on the total tract digestibility (%) of organic matter (OM), crude protein (CP) and neutral detergent fiber (NDF), and the content of digestible energy (DE; MJ per kg dry matter).**
Data from Ragnarsson and Lindberg (2010).

In general, leguminous species are richer than grasses in macrominerals (Ca in particular) and trace elements under

Table 17-2 Mineral Content (in Dry Matter) in Selected Feedstuffs and Mineral Requirements in Horses (Per Dry Matter)[a,b]

	Forage[a]		Cereal grains[b]								
	Grass	Legume	Oats	Barley	Maize	Wheat bran	Beet pulp	SBM[c]	Pea	CDDG[d]	Requirements[a,e]
Ca, g	4.7–7.2	12.2–15.6	1.2	0.8	0.5	1.6	14.8	3.9	1.3	2.4	2.0–4.7
P, g	2.6–3.4	2.8–3.1	3.6	3.9	3.0	11.4	1.0	7.1	4.6	9.5	1.4–3.0
Mg, g	1.8–2.3	2.7–3.3	1.1	1.3	1.1	4.8	2.0	3.3	1.6	3.3	0.7–1.2
K, g	20–26	24–28	5.2	5.5	3.7	14.1	4.8	24	11.3	14.1	2.5–4.2
Na, g	0.2–0.8	0.2–0.3	0.1	0.1	0.05	0.1	3.2	0.3	0.1	6.1	1.0–3.3
S, mg	1.7–2.4	2.3–3.1	2.0	1.5	1.3	2.2	2.7	4.5	2.3	3.6	1.5
Fe, mg	180–200	200–250	120	182	37	164	674	322	106	119	40–50
Mn, mg	70–90	45–50	45	18	9	128	78	43	10	21	40
Cu, mg	8–9	9–10	3	10	2	19	6	20	8	11	10
Zn, mg	25–27	24–26	26	35	22	85	21	53	37	74	40
Se, mg	0.06	0.2	0.2	0.1	0.1	0.5	0.1	0.2	0.2	0.4	0.1

[a]NRC 2007; [b]Sauvant et al 2004; [c]SBM = soybean meal; [d]CDDG = corn distillers dried grains.
[e]Based on NRC 2007.

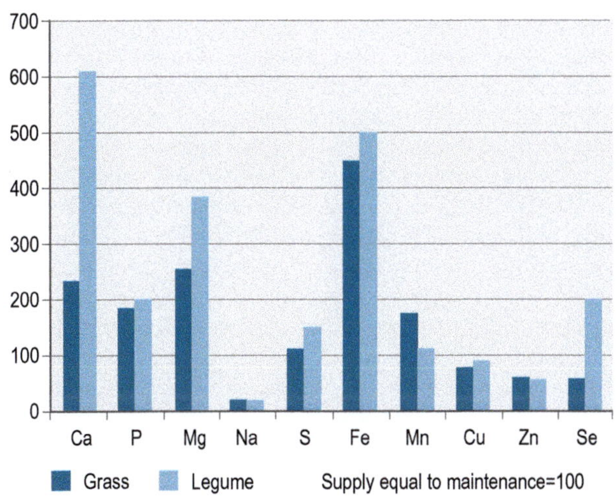

Figure 17.2 Supply of minerals from forage-only diets based on grass or legumes relative to the maintenance requirements (supply equal to maintenance = 100) of adult horses according to NRC (2007).

both temperate and tropical conditions (Suttle 2010). In forage-only and forage-cereal diets based on temperate forages (Table 17-2), the dietary content of most macrominerals will in general be sufficient to cover the needs of most horses if an adequate amount of forage is fed. However, the dietary content of Na will be below requirements and must be supplied. In forage-only and forage-cereal diets, the dietary content of K will be in excess of requirements, while the dietary content of Cu and Zn may be limiting. In Scandinavian countries, and also certain low selenium areas in other parts of the world, this will also apply to Se when feeding grass-dominated forage diets (Fig.17.2).

Fresh forage has a high content of β-carotene (vitamin A) and α-tocopherol (vitamin E), which should be sufficient to meet the requirements of all horses fed forage-only and high forage diets. However, during conserving and especially ensiling the content of both β-carotene and α-tocopherol may be reduced (Müller et al 2007), which can lead to marginal supply of vitamin E for horses fed non-vitamin supplemented diets.

Forage protein utilization

Gibbs et al (1988) reported high true digestibility values of forage protein in cannulated ponies over the total GI tract, but very low true ileal digestibility values (37%). However, nitrogen retention was high (42–59% of nitrogen digested) on all forage sources in the referred study. The ponies were fed at 2% of body weight with Coastal bermuda grass hay (11.7% CP in DM), low-protein alfalfa hay (15.0% CP in DM) and high-protein alfalfa hay (18.1% CP in DM). The low ileal digestibility values for forage protein in horses are in contrast to data on forage utilization in pigs showing high ileal digestibility values for both protein and amino acids (Phuc & Lindberg 2001, Reverter et al 1999) and high portal net appearance of amino acids (Reverter et al 2000). Therefore, since horses grow and develop satisfactorily on diets based entirely of forage (Duncan 1991), provided that energy and nutrient requirements are met (Forsmark 2006), it is difficult to accept that the true small intestinal digestibility should be as poor as indicated from the work by Gibbs et al (1988).

Impact of preservation

Historically, sun-drying in the field to produce hay was the predominant method for preservation of forage (Wilkins 1988). However, in many European countries with unstable weather conditions at harvest, barn-drying was introduced as a way of minimizing the risk for poor nutritional and hygienic quality of hay. Over the years, this has gradually been replaced by preservation by ensiling which is built on the principle of anaerobic fermentation (McDonald et al 1991). In the horse industry, use of silage with a high DM content (≥500 g DM), and called haylage, has become the common practice (Müller 2005). The extent of fermentation in the silage/haylage is influenced by the moisture content, resulting in less fermentation with increasing DM content. Thus, haylage will have a lower content of fermentation products (including lactic acid) and a higher pH compared to silage with a lower DM content (Müller 2005). The lower content of fermentation products in haylage may reduce the aerobic stability after opening of the bales. Moreover, the aerobic stability may be affected by the harvest date of the forage (Müller 2009). The common theory is that aerobic stability is shorter for stemmy material because of retention of air pockets in poorly compacted material. Moreover, a porous material may result in low haylage density and a greater gas exchange with the surrounding air. This will allow yeast growth, and if these are lactate-degrading yeast species the aerobic stability may be affected. In the referred study (Müller 2009), the aerobic stability was longer for haylage from herbage harvested in August than in haylage from herbage harvested in May and June. This was in contrast to the common theory that a late cut material, which is stemmy, is more difficult to compact and would contain more air pockets.

With an increased use of ensiled forage in horse feeding the impact of the ensiling process on the nutritional quality will become an issue. There are several indicators regularly used to evaluate silage quality in ruminant feeding (i.e., pH, organic acids, ammonia), which may also be useful in evaluating the nutritional properties of silage for horses (McDonald et al 1991, Müller 2005). Ammonia level in ensiled forage can be used as an indicator of silage quality and will also indicate if the protein fraction in the ensiled forage has been subjected to degradation during the ensiling process (McDonald et al 1991). High levels of ammonia may indicate a reduced protein quality (Table 17-3).

It has been shown that the palatability of forage may be affected by the method of preservation (Müller & Udén 2007). Horses fed the same grass crop preserved as hay (88% DM), silage (31% DM) or haylage (58% DM), had the highest rate of consumption and the longest eating time on silage followed in descending order by haylage and hay. The reason for these differences remains to be explained.

Horses, at maintenance, fed grass forage-only diets from the same crop, harvested at the same time and preserved as hay, silage (34% DM) or haylage (55% DM), did not show any differences in fermentation kinetics in the large colon (Müller et al 2008, Muhonen et al 2009). However, colonic lactobacilli counts increased on the silage diet and were greater than on the haylage diet, while colonic streptococci counts decreased on the haylage diet and were less than on the silage diet (Muhonen et al 2009). Perhaps most importantly, an abrupt change of the forage type (same crop) had only marginal effects on microbial composition of colonic contents (Muhonen et al 2009).

Impact of forage on performance

The nutritional quality of the forage will have a major impact on bodyweight gain and body development in young growing horses fed limited amounts of forage together with concentrate (Ott & Kivipelto 2002). Feeding forage high in both energy and protein will increase the chances of meeting the daily nutrient and energy needs of growing yearling horses. If, on the other hand, the forage is low in energy and protein and is given in limited amounts together with concentrate to growing yearling horses, there is a risk for poor bodyweight gain and body development (Ott & Asquith 1986).

It was recently shown that Standardbred trotters in race condition fed a high-quality forage-only diet could perform at a comparable level to those fed a typical forage:concentrate diet (Jansson & Lindberg 2008). This indicates that it should be possible to minimize the need for supplementing the performing horse with concentrate, provided that the nutritional quality of the forage is high. However, muscle glycogen content was approximately 13% lower before and after a standardized exercise test (treadmill) in horses fed the forage-only diet, while the extent of glycogen depletion was similar between diets. Moreover, while plasma glucose concentrations remained unaffected by diet composition, pre- and post-exercise plasma acetate concentrations were higher and insulin concentrations lower when Standard bred trotters in race condition were fed forage-only diets (Jansson & Lindberg 2012). These findings indicate a diet-induced shift in metabolism and substrate availability at a whole-body level that may affect performance. Interestingly, oral acetate supplementation of a hay:grain diet enhanced the rate of glycogen resynthesis during the early phase (0–4 h) of recovery after muscle glycogen depletion (Waller et al 2009). These data suggests that acetate, which is the major SCFA produced during hindgut fermentation of dietary fiber, may be an important substrate for energy metabolism in skeletal muscle.

Key Points

- The stage of maturity of forage has a major impact on forage utilization and on the need for supplemental feeds
- A major part of the energy and nutrient requirements for performance horses can be met with high-quality forage

Concentrate ingredients

Cereals

The content of carbohydrates, protein and fat varies considerably between cereal sources (Table 17-1). It is sometimes

Table 17-3 Selected Criteria to Assess Silage Quality

Criteria	Silage type	Good	Acceptable	Poor
Ammonia nitrogen (NH_3-N), % of total N	All	<8	8–12	>12
Butyrate, % of fresh matter	All	<0.1	0.1–0.3	>0.3
pH	Direct cut Prewilted, DM <35 % Prewilted, DM >35 %	<4.2 <4.5 Not applicable		

claimed that the country of origin has an impact on the nutritional properties of cereal grains (i.e., oats). However, differences in nutritional properties are related to variation in chemical composition which could be the result of variations in climate, agronomic factors and the variety used (Åman et al 1985, Pettersson & Åman 1987, Åman 1987, 1988). Thus, it appears likely that factors other than country of origin will be of importance for nutritional properties of cereal grains (Åman & Newman 1986).

The protein content is highest in wheat, followed in descending order by oats and barley, and with the lowest content in rice and maize. However, the protein quality is higher in oats, barley and rice (3.7–4.2% lysine of CP) than in wheat and maize (3.0–3.1% lysine of CP). In addition, the lysine content of oats is only affected to a minor extent with an increase in grain protein content, while the lysine content in barley and wheat decrease with an increase in grain protein content (Thomke 1970, Degussa 1996). For most horses (sedentary, pregnant, growing, or exercising) fed a mixed forage and straight cereal grains with barley, oats or rice as the cereal source, the supply of lysine should be sufficient to meet requirements (4.3% lysine of CP intake, NRC 2007). However, when wheat and maize are used as cereal sources in this type of diet there is a risk for marginal lysine supply. For lactating mares, a forage/cereal-based diet will not meet the lysine requirements (5.0–5.5% lysine of CP intake) and the diet must be supplemented with a protein source. In addition, there may be a risk for marginal supply of histidine for growing and exercising horses receiving unfortified forage/cereal diets (Table 17-4).

Oats and maize are relatively high in fat content (4–5.5%) and contain more than twice the amount present in wheat and rice (Table 17-1). This is also reflected in the content of individual postulated essential FA (linoleic and α-linolenic acid). All grain sources listed in Table 17-1, except rice, would meet the minimum linoleic acid requirement for horses (5 g/kg DM) suggested by the NRC (2007).

Based on existing data it can be estimated that in regular oats, fat provides approximately 14% of digestible energy (DE) content, a value which will be further increased up to approximately 18% in de-hulled and high fat oats (Lindberg et al 2006). In contrast, in other cereals commonly used in monogastric diets, fat provides around 3–5% of DE content.

Rice is high in starch content, and is followed in descending order by maize, wheat, barley, and oats. Starch consists of polymers of glucose, which occur in two forms: amylose and amylopectin. The former is a linear α-(1–4) linked molecule, whereas the latter is a larger molecule, being highly branched containing both α-(1–4) and α-(1–6) linkages. Starch contains varying proportions of amylose and amylopectin, the ratio depending upon the botanical origin of the starch. For example, in wheat flour amylose is around 30% of the total starch, whereas maize can contain up to 70% amylose. In addition, to the variation in the ratio of amylose and amylopectin, the molecular weight of starch can vary greatly which may influence digestibility. Glucose availability tends to be higher with the amylopectin type of starch.

Oats have the highest fiber content, followed in descending order by barley, wheat, maize and rice (Table 17-1). However, when oats are de-hulled there is a marked increase in the starch content and a marked decrease in the fiber content, resulting in a carbohydrate composition comparable to barley and wheat (Bach Knudsen 1997). De-hulling of oats will improve the digestibility of nutrients (Särkijärvi & Saastamoinen 2006) and will result in a higher energy value. Not only the fibre content, but also the fiber quality differs between cereals. For example, the fiber fraction in oats and barley is rich in β-glucans, while the fiber fraction in wheat, rye and triticale is rich in arabinoxylans (Bach Knudsen 1997). It is known that both soluble β-glucans and arabinoxylans have viscous properties, which may affect the gut environment and may therefore interfere with the digestive processes. In diets with high inclusion of oats and barley (high in soluble β-glucans), and in diets with high inclusion of wheat, rye and triticale (high in soluble arabinoxylans), this may be one of the factors that can contribute to disturbed gut function. This may be less of a problem in diets where the cereal sources are maize (corn) or rice, as they contain low levels of both soluble β-glucans and arabinoxylans.

Table 17-4 Essential Amino Acid Profile (Relative to Lysine; Lysine = 100) in Selected Feedstuffs and in Horse Milk and Horse Muscle

	Forage[a]		Cereal grains[a]									
	Grass	Legume	Oats	Barley	Maize	Wheat bran	Beet pulp	SBM[b]	Pea	CDDG[c]	Milk[d]	Muscle[d]
Lysine	100	100	100	100	100	100	100	100	100	100	100	100
Arginine	100	96	161	126	158	157	62	121	119	162	70–82	76
Histidine	55	47	51	58	100	65	47	43	35	108	29–37	58
Isoleucine	97	84	90	95	125	81	56	75	57	131	53–79	55
Leucine	164	151	176	182	425	157	89	120	98	395	127–147	107
Methionine	34	32	44	45	71	40	23	23	13	69	29–35	27
Phenylalanine	108	97	119	129	167	100	58	82	65	166	53–59	60
Threonine	93	88	83	92	125	81	62	64	52	139	53–68	61
Valine	122	119	127	137	171	115	86	78	65	187	64–97	62

[a]Sauvant et al 2004; [b]SBM = soybean meal; [c]CDDG = corn distillers dried grains; [d]based on NRC 2007.

As discussed in other chapters, high starch intake may result in a number of important equine diseases such as colic, gastric ulcers, tying-up and laminitis (Beyer 1998, Clarke et al 1990, Valberg 1998). It is generally accepted that certain forms of colic and laminitis are the result of changes in the microbial population and fermentation profile in the hindgut (Bailey et al 2004, Julliand et al 2008) which may be influenced by the amount of dietary starch.

Standardbred horses in training, fed a conventional forage:concentrate diet with a starch intake of 0.54 g/kg bodyweight (BW) per day, showed a reduced microbial stability and an increase in the fecal flora of lactic acid bacteria and members of the *Streptococcus bovis/equis* complex when compared to the feeding of a forage-only diet (Willing et al 2009). Therefore, there may be justification for a decrease in the previously suggested upper limit for starch intake (2 g starch/kg BW; Kienzle 1994, Potter et al 1992a) to avoid digestive problems in horses and support equine health and welfare, as discussed elsewhere.

The replacement of starch-rich cereal grains with non-starch based carbohydrate feeds (Lindberg 2005) and/or fat or oil (Potter et al 1992b) may be an alternative way of avoiding problems related to high starch intakes.

In forage-cereal diets, the dietary content of Fe, Mn and Cu may be too low when maize (corn) is used as the cereal source (Table 17-2). Moreover, cereal grains are low in Ca and high in P which will result in imbalanced Ca:P ratios in forage-cereal-based diets. This has to be corrected with Ca supplementation. If barley is used as the cereal source, the dietary content of Mn may not meet requirements, and the dietary content of Cu may be limiting with oat feeding.

Key Points

- The energy value of cereals is closely related to the fiber and starch content, with the highest energy values for rice followed in descending order by maize, wheat, barley and oats
- Cereals are generally low in lysine and have an imbalanced Ca:P ratio

Impact of processing of cereals

There are several factors related to the macro- and microstructure of the cereal grain that will affect starch utilization in the horse. The grain macrostructure (i.e., shape, size, husks) will largely determine the utilization of unprocessed cereal grains, while in mechanically processed grains the macrostructure will be more or less destroyed. The grain microstructure (i.e., structure of starch granules, length and branching of the starch molecule, hydrogen bonds between molecular chains) will to a lesser extent be affected by mechanical processing, while hydrothermal processing (i.e., steam flaking, micronizing, popping, extrusion) may destroy the grain microstructure (Kellems & Church 2010).

The ileal digestibility of cereal starch varies with grain source and with the processing of the grain (Kienzle 1994, Julliand et al 2006). In contrast, the total tract digestibility of cereal starches is high and often marginally affected by the grain source or processing (Meyer 1992). The highest ileal starch digestibilities are found for oats, while maize starch appears to be less digestible (Kienzle, 1994). The lowest ileal starch digestibilities have been recorded for barley. A rough mechanical processing of the grain (such as rolling or crushing) does not change the ileal starch digestibility, while fine grinding (<2 mm particle size) will generally improve the ileal starch digestibility. In general, thermal and hydrothermal processing (i.e. micronizing, popping) of cereal grains will improve the ileal starch digestibility (Julliand et al 2006). However, heat-treatment did not improve the total tract digestibility of other dietary components (protein, fat, and fiber) in oats (Särkijärvi & Saastamoinen 2006).

Feeding horses with cereal starch (1.2–1.5 g starch/kg BW), resulted in a significant increase in plasma glucose and insulin concentrations but the responses were not clearly altered by different types of processing (untreated, fine grinding, steaming, steam-flaking or popping) of either oats (Vervuert et al 2003), barley (Vervuert et al 2007) or maize (Vervuert et al 2004). Differences in the extent of small intestinal starch digestibility were expected based on the degree of gelatinization of the starch in the processed cereal grain products. Possibly, the extent of starch modification by the processing methods applied in the above cited studies, in combination with a moderate starch intake, were not sufficient to affect the extent of small intestinal starch digestibility. In addition, pre-cecal (stomach and small intestine) microbial digestion of starch will be another factor to consider, and the extent of these processes may vary with starch availability and level of starch intake (Coenen et al 2006, Vervuert et al 2008), However, feeding horses differently processed barley (rolled, micronized or extruded) at a higher level of starch intake (2.0 g/kg BW) resulted in a higher glycemic and insulinemic response in the extruded and micronized barley as compared with the rolled barley (Vervuert et al 2008). Interestingly, there appears to be only a moderate glycemic and insulinemic response to starch intakes <1.1 g/kg BW in horses (Vervuert et al 2009), even if highly processed cereals are used.

Key Points

- Starch digestibility varies with grain source and type of processing
- Plasma glucose and insulin responses do not appear to be affected by processing method at starch intake <1.5 g/kg BW. However, cereal processing method may modify glycemic and insulinemic responses at starch intake >2 g/kg BW

Cereal by-products

In general, cereal by-products such as wheat bran, rice bran and maize feed flour are higher in crude protein, crude fat and fiber, and lower in starch, as compared with their parent cereal grain (Table 17-1). However, protein quality (lysine as a % of crude protein) and fat quality (linoleic and linolenic acid as a % of total FA) will be maintained at a similar level as the parent cereal grain. Due to the increased content of fiber in cereal by-products the energy value will decrease compared with the parent cereal grain.

Replacing cereals with wheat bran will improve the dietary content of most minerals, in particular with respect to P, Mg, Fe, Mn, Cu, and Zn (Table 17-2) but has the potential to result in a reversed Ca:P ratio.

Key Point

- Cereal by-products are higher in fiber compared to their parent cereal grain and lower in energy. However, protein and fat quality and the Ca : P ratio are comparable to the parent cereal grain

Protein feedstuffs

Apart from being high in protein, the content of crude fat, starch, sugars and fiber varies considerably between protein feedstuffs (Tables 17-5 & 17-6). The protein quality (lysine, as a % of CP) is high in rapeseed, soybean, peas, faba bean, and potato protein, while for other protein feedstuffs the protein quality is only slightly better than in cereals and cereal by-products.

Pulse seeds (pea, bean, lentil, chickpea) may contain protein inhibitors of hydrolases which are active against proteases, amylases, lipases, glycosidases and phosphatases (Boye et al 2010, Campos-Vega et al 2010). In addition, lectins are found in most plant foods, with beans being the most important source; lectins also can interfere with digestive processes in the gut. The content of protein inhibitors and lectins varies between plants and between cultivars (Campos-Vega et al 2010). Thus, depending on the content of these anti-nutritional factors in the seed, there may be a negative impact on the utilization of nutrients in the diet due to reduced digestibility if they are fed raw and unprocessed (Boye et al 2010, Campos-Vega et al 2010). Cooking and fermentation are simple methods that appear efficient in inactivating protein inhibitors and lectins in pulses (Campos-Vega et al 2010).

The crude fat content is high in the oil seeds (211–480 g/kg DM), but low in peas, faba beans, lupins and potato protein, and in oil seed meal. There is considerable variation in the content of individual essential FA (linoleic and α-linolenic acid) amongst protein feedstuffs. All protein feedstuffs listed in Tables 17-5 and 17-6, except linseed meal, rapeseed meal, peas and potato protein, would meet the minimum linoleic acid requirement for horses (5 g/kg DM) suggested by NRC (2007). It should be noted that linseed has a very high content of α-linolenic acid (Table 17-5).

All protein feedstuffs contain water soluble sugars (10–100 g/kg DM), while starch is only found in peas and faba beans. The fiber content varies considerably among protein feedstuffs depending on source and processing. This also applies to the energy content, which range from high to moderate values (13–23 MJ DE per kg DM).

The need to supplement the diet with protein-rich feedstuffs will depend primarily on the requirements of the horse and the quality of the roughage source as well as the proportion of roughage in the diet. A diet based on grass-dominated forage with 6–10% CP and a cereal-based concentrate (12–13% CP; 0.56% lysine), for example could not provide enough protein and lysine for a high body weight gain and body development in yearling (11-month-old) horses (Ott & Kivipelto 2002). However, if the forage is higher in CP content (>16% CP), sufficient quantities of protein and essential amino acids will be provided to support high body weight gain (Ott & Kivipelto 2002).

Several protein-rich feedstuffs that can be used to supplement horse diets (Tables 17-5 & 17-6). Earlier studies have shown that soybean meal can be replaced with brewer's grains (Ott et al 1979a, 1981), linseed meal (Hintz et al 1971) and rape seed meal (Cymbaluk 1990) in the diet of yearling horses without any negative impact on growth and development. However, for feedstuffs with a low content of lysine compared with soybean meal, such as brewer's grains and linseed meal, the diet has to be supplemented with lysine to the same levels as in soybean meal in order to reach comparable performance in yearlings (Hintz et al 1971, Ott et al

Table 17-5 Chemical Composition (g/kg Dry Matter), Proportion of Lysine (% of Crude Protein), and Content of Linoleic and Linolenic Acid (g/kg Dry Matter) and Energy (MJ/kg Dry Matter) in Oil Seeds[a]

	Cottonseed		Linseed			Rapeseed		Soybean		Sunflower seed	
	Full fat	Meal	Full fat	Expeller	Meal	Full fat	Meal	Full fat	Meal	Full fat	Meal
Crude protein	233	467	250	342	359	207	380	397	516	172	372
Crude fat	211	32	362	90	34	455	26	217	22	480	19
Starch	0	0	0	0	0	0	0	0	0	0	0
Sugars	16	69	38	39	51	55	87	99	94	26	63
NDF	423	272	245	259	257	191	319	132	139	310	400
Crude fiber	258	130	102	113	111	89	140	63	68	167	236
Lysine	4.5	3.9	3.9	3.8	3.7	6.2	5.3	6.2	6.1	3.9	3.5
Linoleic acid	105	12	50	12	4	89	4	109	9	296	9
α-Linolenic acid	0.4	0.05	186	44	14	42	2	15	1	1	0.04
GE	24.1	20.5	26.8	20.5	19.3	28.6	19.3	23.5	19.7	28.7	19.4
DE	14.9	13.6	20.6	15.4	14.5	22.8	14.3	19.9	17.4	19.9	11.6
ME	12.2	12.8	14.4	12.9	11.9	19.6	10.0	16.7	14.1	16.4	10.1
NE	8.3	9.0	11.3	8.9	8.3	13.5	7.0	11.7	8.6	12.2	6.0

[a]Data from Sauvant et al (2004).
GE = gross energy, DE = digestible energy, ME = metabolizable energy, NDF = neutral detergent fiber, NE = net energy.

Table 17-6 Chemical Composition (g/kg Dry Matter), Proportion of Lysine (% of Crude Protein), and Content of Linoleic and Linolenic Acid (g/kg Dry Matter) and Energy (MJ/kg Dry Matter) in Legume Seeds and Various by-Products[a]

	Pea	Faba bean	Lupin	Potato protein	CDGS[b]	WDGS[c]	BDG[d]	Soybean hulls	Pulp		Molasses	
									Beet	Citrus	Beet	Cane
Crude protein	238	311	385	841	279	375	262	134	91	70	145	54
Crude fat	11	13	95	10	44	72	73	25	10	25	3	15
Starch	514	433	0	7	130	42	75	0	0	32	0	0
Sugars	45	43	72	10	6	9	10	17	74	227	616	639
NDF	138	159	213	65	356	421	574	631	454	216	0	0
Crude fiber	60	87	129	9	83	102	166	382	194	135	0	0
Lysine	7.3	6.4	4.9	7.6	2.5	3.1	3.2	5.9	7.9	4.1	1.5	0.4
Linoleic acid	4	5	16	2	19	26	18	13	2	5	-	6
α-Linolenic acid	0.9	0.4	8	1.6	0.3	3	1.8	1.7	0.4	1.0	-	-
GE	18.2	18.7	21.2	22.2	19.4	21.4	20.5	18.2	17.1	17.6	15.4	14.9
DE	16.1	16.3	18.3	19.4	15.3	15.2	12.3	12.6	13.8	14.4	13.2	12.4
ME	14.3	14.0	15.6	13.8	12.3	11.6	10.0	8.7	12.3	12.8	12.1	11.7
NE	10.4	10.4	9.9	9.8	9.3	8.9	8.0	6.5	8.0	9.9	11.1	11.2

[a]Data from Sauvant et al (2004).
[b]Corn distiller's grains with solubles; [c]wheat distiller's grains with solubles; [d]brewer's dried grains.
GE = gross energy, DE = digestible energy, ME = metabolizable energy, NDF = neutral detergent fiber, NE = net energy.

1979b, 1981). This may not be needed for other classes of horses (apart from lactating mares) as the lysine requirements will be met by most forage-only diets and by forage-concentrate diets with almost all combinations of ordinary feedstuffs (Tables 17-1, 17-5 and 17-6). NRC (2007) have estimated that the lysine requirements for maintenance, growth, exercise and pregnancy is 4.3% of the dietary crude protein content, and for milk production 3.3 g lysine per kg of milk in addition to the maintenance lysine requirements.

Replacing the cereal part of the diet with protein feedstuffs to increase the dietary protein content will in general have a limited impact on the dietary mineral content (Table 17-2). This may change if large amounts of cereals are replaced and if protein feedstuffs with more extreme contents of specific minerals are used.

Key Point

- Many different protein-rich feedstuffs can be used in horse diets but they vary in their energy value, protein content and protein quality

Non-starch carbohydrate feedstuffs

In contrast to cereals, non-starch carbohydrate feeds are characterized by having a carbohydrate fraction that is composed of water soluble sugars and/or dietary fiber (Table 17-6). They are low in crude fat and often also in crude protein. The feeds classified into this category are mainly industrial by-products.

Sugar-rich feedstuffs

Molasses (beet and cane) and syrup (hydrolyzed starch) mainly contain sugars and are low in fat. The crude protein content varies, and is markedly lower in cane molasses than in beet molasses (Table 17-6). The ash content is high in molasses products (12–14% DM), and potassium in particular is high compared with other common feedstuffs (apart from roughage). In general, the energy content in this group of feedstuffs is high.

Simple sugars (glucose and fructose) are well utilized by the horse and are absorbed in the small intestine (Meyer 1992). This is reflected in a rapid increase in plasma glucose values, with a similar response for both glucose and fructose (Bullimore et al 2000). As shown by Jansson et al (2002) adult horses have no problems to digest and utilize hydrolyzed starch (glucose:maltose:maltotriose proportion of 83:15:2) at levels of 2.5 g/kg BW per day. In contrast, there are limitations in the digestive capacity of certain disaccharides depending on age and the change in secretion of digestive enzymes (Meyer 1992). Thus, in the foal lactose is well utilized due to a high activity of lactase, while sucrose is less efficiently utilized due to a limited activity of sucrase. The situation is the reverse in the adult horse. According to Meyer (1992), the upper limit to dietary inclusion of lactose in the adult horse is 1 g/kg BW per day if digestive disturbances are to be avoided.

Pectin-rich feedstuffs

In feedstuffs such as beet pulp, citrus pulp and soybean hulls a large part of the dietary fiber fraction is made up of pectin (uronic acid). In general, the energy content in this group of feedstuffs is high. The energy value for beet pulp (13.8 MJ DE and 12.3 MJ metabolizable energy (ME)) and citrus pulp (14.4 MJ DE and 12.8 MJ ME) are comparable to the energy value for regular oats (13.1 MJ DE and 11.9 MJ ME) (Tables 17-1 and 17-6).

Soaking in water prior to feeding is often recommended when larger meals (>0.5 kg) of beet pulp is fed in order to minimize the risk of esophageal obstruction due to impaction with dry feed. However, esophageal impaction is a problem that has been reported to occur when ingesting other feedstuffs and may also be related to other factors (Feige at al 2000).

Pectin-rich feedstuffs, as well as fructo-oligosaccharides, sugar-alcohols and gums, are extensively fermented in the hindgut (Sunvold et al 1995, Coenen et al 2006). However, the rate and extent of fermentation will vary considerably between fiber sources and has to be considered when formulating rations for performance horses. Inclusion levels of up to 3.0 g sugar beet pulp/kg BW per day (in dry form) has been used to adult horses without any negative effects on overall nutrient utilization and performance (Lindberg & Jacobsson 1992, Lindberg & Palmgren Karlsson 2001, Palmgren Karlsson et al 2002). Moore-Colyer et al (2000) concluded that sugar beet pulp could be used as an alternative to hay as the forage component of the diet without compromising hindgut function. However, sugar beet pulp is more completely and rapidly fermented by the cecal microflora than is hay (Hyslop et al 1999). In addition, it has been shown that a significant proportion of the sugar beet pulp (18% of the organic matter and 13% of the total NSP) is disappearing in the small intestine during transit to the hindgut (Moore-Colyer et al 2002). In contrast to sugar beet pulp, citrus pulp appears to have low palatability when given separately as a replacement to oats. However, citrus pulp was used to replace up to 15% of the oat content without any impact on concentrate intake when included in a complete pelleted diet (Ott et al 1979a).

Soybean hulls are potentially useful as feedstuff for horses and have successfully been used to feed ruminants for a long time. The carbohydrate component in soybean hulls is characterised by a high content (~80% in DM) of dietary fiber, and with a high content (~30% in DM) of pectin (Karr-Lilienthal et al 2005, Monsoor 2005) in this fiber fraction. In contrast, the content of water soluble carbohydrates and starch is low (Karr-Lilienthal et al 2005, Rodiek & Stull 2007). Horses fed soybean hulls have a lower glycemic index compared to feeding with cereal grains and sweet feed (Rodiek & Stull 2007). Soybean hulls are more completely and rapidly fermented by the cecal microflora than is hay but are less fermentable than sugar beet pulp (Hyslop et al 1999). Moreover, a significant proportion of the soybean hulls (24% of the organic matter and 8% of the total NSP) are degraded in the small intestine during transit to the hindgut (Moore-Colyer et al 2002). Increasing substitution of alfalfa/bromegrass hay with soybean hulls (0, 25, 50, or 75% on as-fed basis) in the diet of cecally cannulated Quarter horses linearly increased cecal volatile FA production and the molar proportion of propionate, while the molar proportion of butyrate and cecal pH (7.00 to 6.45) decreased (Coverdale et al 2004). The drop in cecal pH suggests that the inclusion level of soybean hulls should be limited, probably to less than 50% of the diet.

When part of the cereal portion of the diet is replaced with beet pulp, there is an increased risk for a low dietary content of P, Cu and Zn (Table 17-2).

Cellulose-rich feedstuffs

Barley hulls, oat hulls and rye bran are examples of non-starch carbohydrate feedstuffs, which are characterized by a high content of dietary fiber and high cellulose content (Bach Knudsen 1997). The dietary fiber fraction in these feedstuffs is largely insoluble and has high lignin content. Feedstuffs rich in cellulose, such as cereal fiber sources, are fermented to a limited extent by the equine hindgut microflora (Sunvold et al 1995, Coenen et al 2006). In general, the energy content in this group of feedstuffs is low.

Key Points

- Sugar-rich feedstuffs containing glucose, fructose and sucrose are well utilized by horses and can be used to replace starch-rich feedstuffs. However, these feedstuffs may not be suitable for equids prone to laminitis
- Pectin-rich feed feedstuffs are well utilized by horses and are well suited as replacement for starch-rich feedstuffs

Distillery by-products

This group of feedstuffs is characterized by high contents of crude protein, crude fat and fiber, and low contents of starch and sugars (Table 17-6). The protein quality (lysine, % of CP) and fat quality are comparable with the grain source used in the process. However, if the product is over-heated during the drying process the availability of lysine will be impaired (Shurson et al 2000, Stein et al 2006). The energy content in distillery products is moderate and comparable to cereal bran products (Table 17-1).

Young horses (7–12 months old) fed timothy hay and a concentrate based on oats and barley protein (by-product from ethanol/starch production) had a lower BW gain and poorer body development than young horses fed a concentrate based on oats and milk powder (Saastamoinen & Koskinen 1993). The daily intake of CP was similar in both groups of horses, but the intake of lysine was markedly lower in horses fed barley protein (7.0 g/day) compared with those fed milk powder (17.8 g/day).

Wheat dried distillers grains can replace soybean meal in diets for young horses (18–22 months old) fed forage (> 12% CP) ad libitum without a negative impact on BW gain and body development (Lindberg 2008). The concentrate was composed of crushed barley and oats (30:70), and dried wheat distillers grains or soybean meal. Hill (2002) found that high inclusion levels of distillery products in the concentrate decreased the palatability.

Corn dried distillers grains could replace soybean meal in diets for adult horses fed at maintenance without any negative impact on the digestibility of dry matter, cellulose and energy (Leonard et al 1975). However, the digestibility of CP was reduced when corn dried distillers grains replaced soybean meal in the diet, while the utilization of digested CP was improved. Bonoma et al (2008) found no effect on BW gain in weanling Standardbred horses (8 months of age) fed diets (50:50 ratio of alfalfa and concentrate) where 30% of the concentrate (corn and soybean meal) was replaced with corn dried distillers grains.

Key Point

- Distillery by-products are high in fiber, protein and fat, and with energy values slightly lower than or comparable with the parent cereal grain source

Fats and oils

The fat content in pasture and in a diet based on roughage only or roughage plus concentrate (based on ordinary feedstuffs) is low (3–4% crude fat in DM) and the total amount of digestible energy (DE) coming from fat is less than 10%. By feeding supplemental fat it is possible to increase the energy density of the diet, to reduce the amount of concentrate needed to meet the energy needs and to decrease the heat load coming from the diet as more of the DE is coming from fat. This feeding strategy may be of particular interest for exercising horses with a high energy requirement and where the ordinary diet cannot meet energy needs.

The fat content in the diet can be increased by selecting feedstuffs in the concentrate part of the diet with a high fat content or by adding fats or oils. Examples of regular feedstuffs rich in fat are maize and oats (4–7% in DM), high-fat oats (10–14% in DM), rice bran (15–18% in DM), full fat oil seeds (20–50% in DM), oil seed expeller, distillers grains (4–7% in DM) and brewers grains (7% in DM) (Tables 17-1, 17-5, 17-6). Fat sources used for supplementing the diet have varied among studies, but has mainly been in the form of oil obtained from different plant sources (mostly corn oil and soybean oil). The fat quality (i.e., FA composition) varies between fat and oil sources (Table 17-7), with a wide range in the proportions of saturated (SFA), mono-unsaturated (MUFA) and poly-unsaturated (PUFA) fatty acids.

The main focus has been on the amount of fat added to the diet (on weight basis or on energy basis) without consideration of the fat quality in terms of the FA composition of the used fat source. Horses fed a diet supplemented with fish oil, a PUFA oil rich in eicosapentaenoic acid (EPA) and docosahexaenoic acid (DHA), had a lower heart rate, and tended to have lower packed cell volume, lower serum insulin and higher glucose:insulin ratios during exercise (O'Connor et al 2004). Thus, the FA composition of supplemental fat sources may be one additional factor to consider with respect to potential performance capacity in exercising horses, although more work is needed to confirm this.

In addition to the energy provided from fat and oils, there may be "extra-caloric" effects of feeding some fat or oils in exercising horse (NRC 2007, Potter et al 1992b). The NRC (2007) are currently recommending a minimum dietary content of 5 g linoleic acid for all horses, while there is no recommendation for α-linolenic acid. However, data from other animal species suggest that an increased intake of n-3 PUFA will be beneficial for the maintenance of optimal pre- and post-natal growth and development (Innis 1991), as well as in the prevention of certain diseases in horses (Bauer 1994). This could be due to a high content of PUFA in spleen, thymus and macrophages, and a selective and preferential uptake of long chain PUFA by the placenta and by intestinal enterocytes (Leskanich & Noble 1999). Again further work is needed before precise recommendations can be made; see also Chapter 7.

Key Point

- In addition to energy, there are potential "extra-caloric" effects of fat or oils that may affect performance, reproduction and health

Mineral and vitamin supply

Minerals

The mineral requirements of horses can be supplied by regular feedstuffs and by mineral supplements. The need for mineral supplements will be determined by ingredient composition of the diet. However, it should be noted that there may be large variations in mineral content between batches of the same feedstuffs due to plant genotype, soil environment, climate and the stage of maturity at feeding and/or harvest (NRC 2007, Suttle 2010). Therefore, if possible, the forage as well as other feedstuffs used should be analyzed for their specific mineral content in order to facilitate ration formulation.

Mineral supplements are available in inorganic and organic forms (Suttle 2010). Historically, in animal nutrition minerals have been supplemented as inorganic salts, mainly in the form of oxides and sulfates. However, mineral salts tend to dissociate at the low pH in the upper digestive tract, which may result in antagonism with other dietary components that may reduce bioavailability. Therefore, chelated mineral supplements in which the mineral is bound to an organic ligand have been developed. The idea is that the chelated mineral complex will be stable in the upper digestive tract, thereby minimizing antagonism and improve bioavailability.

Foal growth, development and bone mineral content were not affected by trace mineral supplementation (Fe, Zn,

Table 17-7 Fatty Acid Composition (% of Total Fatty Acids) in Selected Feedstuffs and Oils[a]

	Oats	Maize and CDDG[b]	Barley and BDG[c]	Wheat and WDDG[d]	Rice bran	Plant oils: Soybean	Coconut	Rapeseed	Sun flower
SFA	23.7	15.2	27.0	20.8	22.1	17.1	91.2	10.9	14.4
MUFA	37.3	27.3	12.0	16.9	40.5	22.4	6.9	58.8	20.7
PUFA	39.0	57.5	61.0	62.3	37.4	60.5	1.9	30.3	65.2
C18:2 ω-3	37.5	56.5	55.4	56.2	35.9	53.1	1.8	20.5	64.9
C18:3 ω-6	1.5	1.0	5.6	5.9	1.5	7.4	0.1	9.8	0.3

[a]Sauvant et al 2004.
[b]CDDG = corn distillers dried grains; [c]BDG = brewers dried grains; [d]WDDG = wheat distillers dried grains.
SFA = saturated fatty acids; MUFA = mono-unsaturated fatty acids; PUFA=poly-unsaturated fatty acids.

Mn, Cu, Co, and I) either as organic (proteinates) or in the inorganic form to the mares. While serum concentrations of Zn and Cu were increased in the foals when the mares received the chelated trace minerals, inorganic trace mineral supply of the mares had no effect on foal serum minerals (Ott & Asquith 1994).

Yearlings fed a 12% CP concentrate containing a trace mineral premix (Cu, Mn, and Zn) providing either inorganic or organic (proteinate) minerals, showed no difference in BW gain and body measurements (Ott & Johnson 2001). No difference in bone mineral content and bone mineral deposition were detected, while hip height gain and hoof growth was greater for yearlings fed organic (proteinate) trace minerals.

It was recently shown that Se yeast (organic) is more effective than Na selenite (inorganic) in increasing the total blood Se concentration of mature horses (Calamari et al 2009), mares and foals (Karren et al 2010). However, whole blood glutathione peroxidase activity (GPX) in mature horses and plasma GPX in mares and foals were not affected by the form of Se supplementation. In mature horses, plasma metabolites related to energy, protein and mineral metabolism, acute phase proteins, and enzyme activities related to hepatocellular, hepatobiliary and muscle damage were unaffected by Se source (Se yeast or Na selenite) and dose (Calamari et al 2010). Moreover, there were no effects of Se supplementation (Se yeast or Na selenite) on reactive oxygen metabolites or thiol group concentrations in plasma (Calamari et al 2010). There was no effect of Se supplementation (0.3 mg/kg of DMI) on foaling variables in Quarter horse mares allocated to pasture or pasture plus grain diets (Thorson et al 2010).

Vitamins

Information regarding vitamin nutrition of horses is limited and requirements have only been estimated for vitamins A, D, E, thiamin (B_1) and riboflavin (B_2) (NRC 2007). However, no deficiency symptoms have been reported in the horse for vitamin K, riboflavin, niacin, folate, pyridoxine (B_6) and cyanocobalamin (B_{12}) (NRC 2007), suggesting that these vitamins will be provided in sufficient amounts from the diet and by intestinal bacteria.

In forage-only diets and high forage diets based on well preserved forage, the dietary supply of β-carotene (Müller et al 2007) should be sufficient to meet the vitamin A requirements for all horses. Furthermore, in the same type of diets the dietary supply of α-tocopherol (Müller et al 2007) should be sufficient to meet the vitamin E requirements for horses at maintenance level. However, for growing, exercising, pregnant and lactating horses the α-tocopherol in forage may not be sufficient to meet the requirements. For long-term stored forage and in poorly preserved forage, there may be insufficient content of both β-carotene and α-tocopherol, which can result in deficiencies.

With increasing proportion of cereals in the diet the dietary content of β-carotene and α-tocopherol will decrease, which will increase the risk for marginal supply. The β-carotene content in barley and oats (NRC 1998) is in the range 10–15% of the content in forage (Müller et al 2007), and the corresponding content in maize and wheat is in the range 3–5%. The α-tocopherol content in cereal grains (barley, oats, maize, wheat) (NRC 1998) is in the range 20–30% of the content in forage (Müller et al 2007). Replacing the cereal part of the diet with protein feedstuffs to increase the dietary protein content will not improve the dietary content of β-carotene and α-tocopherol (NRC 1998).

Vitamin D is found in plants (ergocalciferol, D_2) and in animals (cholecalciferol, D_3), but the content in feedstuffs commonly used for horses is low. However, there is no known minimum vitamin D requirement for horses exposed to sunshine (NRC 2007).

The dietary supply of thiamin and riboflavin (NRC 1998, Sauvant et al 2004) in forage-only diets, and in forage-cereal diets, should be sufficient to meet the requirements for all horses. In addition to dietary supply, there is microbial synthesis in the intestine of horses of both thiamin and riboflavin (NRC 2007). Replacing the cereal part of the diet with protein feedstuffs to increase the dietary protein content will not markedly change the supply of thiamin and riboflavin. Brewers dried yeast is an excellent source of thiamin and riboflavin, as well as other vitamins in the B-complex (NRC 1998, Sauvant et al 2004).

Key Point

- In horses exposed to sunshine and fed good quality forage-based diets, the need for supplemental vitamins is minimal, with the possible exception of vitamin E, especially for exercising animals

References

Åman, P., 1987. The variation in chemical composition of Swedish oats. Acta Agriculturae Scandinavica 37, 347–352.

Åman, P., 1988. The variation in chemical composition of Swedish wheats. Swedish Journal of Agricultural Research 18, 27–30.

Åman, P., Newman, C.W., 1986. Chemical composition of some different types of barley grown in Montana, U.S.A. Journal of Cereal Chemistry 4, 133–141.

Åman, P., Hesselman, K., Tilly, A.-C., 1985. The variation in chemical composition of Swedish barleys. Journal of Cereal Science 3, 73–77.

Axelsson, J., 1943. Hästarnas utfodring och skötsel. Nordisk Rotogravyr, Stockholm.

Bach Knudsen, K.E., 1997. Carbohydrate and lignin contents of plant materials used in animal feeding. Animal Feed Science and Technology 67, 319–338.

Bailey, S.R., Marr, C.M., Elliott, J., 2004. Current research and theories on the pathogenesis of acute laminitis in the horse. Veterinary Journal 167, 129–142.

Bauer, J.E., 1994. The potential for dietary polyunsaturated fatty acids in domestic animals. Australian Veterinary Journal 71, 342–345.

Bertrand, A., Tremblay, G.F., Pelletier, S., et al., 2008. Yield and nutritive value of timothy as affected by temperature, photoperiod and time of harvest. Grass and Forage Science 63, 421–432.

Beyer, M., 1998. Colic. In: Pagan, J.D. (Ed.), Advances in Equine Nutrition. Nottingham University Press, Nottingham, UK, pp. 483–488.

Bonoma, T.A., Brogren, A.C., Kline, K.H., et al., 2008. Effects of feeding distillers dried grains with soluble on growth and feed efficiency of weanling horses. Journal of Equine Veterinary Science 28, 725–727.

Boye, J., Zare, F., Pletch, A., 2010. Pulse proteins: processing, characterization, functional properties and application in food and feed. Food Research International 43, 414–431.

Bullimore, S.R., Pagan, J.D., Harris, P.A., et al., 2000. Carbohydrate supplementation of horses during endurance exercise: comparison of fructose and glucose. Journal of Nutrition 130, 1760–1765.

Calamari, L., Ferrari, A., Bertin, G., 2009. Effect of selenium source and dose on selenium status of mature horses. Journal of Animal Science 87, 167–178.

Calamari, L., Abeni, F., Bertin, G., 2010. Metabolic and hematological profiles in mature horses supplemented with different selenium sources and doses. Journal of Animal Science 88, 650–659.

Campos-Vega, R., Loarca-Pina, G., Oomah, B.D., 2010. Minor components of pulses and their potential impact on human health. Food Research International 43, 461–482.

Clarke, L.L., Roberts, M.C., Argenzio, R.A., 1990. Feeding and digestive problems in horses - physiological-responses to a concentrated meal. Veterinary Clinics of North America-Equine Practice 6, 433–450.

Coenen, M., Mössler, A., Vervuert, I., 2006. Fermentative gases in breath indicate that inulin and starch start to be degraded by microbial fermentation in the stomach and small intestine of the horse in contrast to pectin and cellulose. Journal of Nutrition 136, 2108S–2110S.

Coverdale, J.A., Moore, J.A., Tyler, H.D., et al., 2004. Soybean hulls as an alternative feed for horses. Journal of Animal Science 82, 1663–1668.

Cymbaluk, N.F., 1990. Using canola meal in growing horse diets. Equine Practice 12, 13–19.

Degussa, 1996. The amino acid composition of feedstuffs. Degussa AG, Frankfurt am Main, Germany.

Deinum, B., Debeyer, J., Nordfeldt, P.H., et al., 1981. Quality of herbage at different latitudes. Netherlands Journal of Agricultural Science 29, 141–150.

Duncan, P., 1991. Horses and grasses–The Nutritional Ecology of Equids and their Impact on the Camargue. Springer-Verlag, New York.

Feige, K., Schwarzwald, C., Fürst, A., et al., 2000. Esophageal obstruction in horses: a retrospective study of 34 cases. Canadian Veterinary Journal 41, 207–210.

Fonnesbeck, P.V., 1968. Digestion of soluble and fibrous carbohydrates of forages by horses. Journal of Animal Science 27, 1336–1344.

Fonnesbeck, P.V., 1969. Partitioning the nutrients of forage for horses. Journal of Animal Science 28, 624–638.

Forsmark, P., 2006. Effects of diet composition on growth in foals. Swedish University of Agricultural Sciences, Department of Animal Nutrition and Management, Examensarbete 223 (in Swedish).

Gallagher, K., Leech, J., Stowe, H., 1992. Protein, energy and dry matter consumption by racing Standardbreds–a field survey. Journal of Equine Veterinary Science 12, 382–388.

Gibbs, P.G., Potter, G.D., Schelling, G.T., et al., 1988. Digestion of hay protein in different segments of the equine digestive tract. Journal of Animal Science 66, 400–406.

Heide, O.M., Hay, R.K.M., Baugerod, H., 1985. Specific daylength effects on leaf growth and dry-matter production in high-latitude grasses. Annals of Botany 55, 579–586.

Hill, J., 2002. Effect of level of inclusion and method of presentation of a single distillery by-product on the process of ingestion of concentrate feeds by horses. Livestock Production Science 75, 209–218.

Hintz, H.F., Schryver, H.F., Lowe, J.E., 1971. Comparison of a blend of milk products and linseed meal as protein supplements for young growing horses. Journal of Animal Science 33, 1274–1276.

Hyslop, J.J., Stefansdottir, G.J., McLean, B.M.L., et al., 1999. In situ incubation sequence and its effect on degradation of food components when measured in the caecum of ponies. Animal Science 69, 147–156.

Innis, S.M., 1991. Essential fatty acids in growth and development. Progress in Lipid Research 30, 39–103.

Jansson, A., Lindberg, J.E., 2008. Effects of a forage-only diet on body weight and response to interval training on a track. In: Saastamoinen, M.T., Martin-Rosset, W. (Eds.), Nutrition of the Exercising Horse, EAAP Publication No 125. Wageningen Academic Publishers, The Netherlands, pp. 345–349.

Jansson, A., Lindberg, J.E., 2012. A forage-only diet alters the metabolic response of horses in training. Animal (doi:10.1017/S1751731112000948).

Jansson, A., Nyman, S., Lindholm, A., et al., 2002. Effect of exercise metabolism of varying dietary starch and sugar proportions. Equine Veterinary Journal, Supplement 34, 17–21.

Julliand, V., de Fombelle, A., Drogoul, C., et al., 2001. Feeding and microbial disorders in horses: 3, Effects of three hay: grain ratios on microbial profile and activities. Journal of Equine Veterinary Science 21, 543–546.

Julliand, V., de Fombelle, A., Varloud, M., 2006. Starch digestion in horses: The impact of feed processing. Livestock Science 100, 44–52.

Julliand, V., Philippeau, C., Goachet, A.G., et al., 2008. Physiology of intake and digestion in equine animals. In: Saastamoinen, M.T., Martin-Rosset, W. (Eds.), Nutrition of the Exercising Horse, EAAP publication No 125. Wageningen Academic Publishers, The Netherlands, pp. 53–70.

Karren, B.J., Thorson, J.F., Cavinder, C.A., et al., 2010. Effect of selenium supplementation and plane of nutrition on mares and their foals: Selenium concentrations and glutathione peroxidase. Journal of Animal Science 88, 991–997.

Karr-Lilienthal, L.K., Kadzere, C.T., Grieshop, C.M., et al., 2005. Chemical and nutritional properties of soybean carbohydrates as related to nonruminants: a review. Livestock Production Sciences 97, 1–12.

Kienzle, E., 1994. Small intestinal digestion of starch in the horse. Revue Médicine Véterinaire 145, 199–204.

Kellems, R.O., Church, D.C., 2010. Livestock Feeds and Feeding, sixth ed. Prentice Hall, New Jersey, USA.

An, Le Van, Hong, Tran Thi Thu, Lindberg, J.E., 2004. Ileal and total tract digestibility in growing pigs fed cassava root meal with inclusion of fresh, dry and ensiled sweet potato (Ipomoea batats (L.) Lam) leaves. Animal Feed Science and Technology 114, 127–139.

Leonard, T.M., Baker, J.P., Willard, J., 1975. Influence of distillers feeds on digestion in the equine. Journal of Animal Science 40, 1086–1090.

Leskanich, C.O., Noble, R.C., 1999. Review article: The comparative role of polyunsaturated fatty acids in pig neonatal development. British Journal of Nutrition 81, 87–106.

Lindberg, J.E., 2005. Use of non-starch carbohydrate energy sources in performance horse feeds. In: Pagan, J.D. (Ed.), Advances in Equine Nutrition III. Nottingham University Press, Nottingham, UK, pp. 249–264.

Lindberg, J.E., 2008. Utfodring av unghästar med torkad vetedrank-tillväxt, kroppsmått och blodparametrar. Swedish University of Agricultural Sciences, Department of Animal Nutrition and Management, Uppsala, Report 269.

Lindberg, J.E., Jacobsson, K.G., 1992. Effects of barley and sugar-beet pulp on digestibility, purine excretion and blood parameters in horses. Pferdeheilkunde (Sonderdruck) 116–118.

Lindberg, J.E., Palmgren Karlsson, C., 2001. Effect of replacing oats with sugar beet pulp and maize oil on nutrient utilization in horses. Equine Veterinary Journal 33, 585–590.

Lindberg, J.E., Essén-Gustavsson, B., Dahlborn, K., et al., 2006. Exercise response, metabolism at rest and digestibility in athletic horses fed highfat oats. Equine Veterinary Journal, Supplement 36, 626–630.

Lindner, A., Gansen, S., 1995. Feeding of trotting racehorses in Germany: a survey among applicants for a trainer's license. Veterinary Clinical Nutrition 2, 29–35.

McDonald, P., Henderson, N., Heron, S., 1991. The Biochemistry of Silage, second ed. Chalcombe Publications, Canterbury, UK.

Meyer, H., 1992. Pferdefütterung, 2[e] Auflage. Verlag Paul Parey, Berlin und Hamburg.

Monsoor, M.A., 2005. Effect of drying methods on the functional properties of soy hull pectin. Carbohydrate Polymers 61, 362–367.

Moore-Colyer, M.J.S., Hyslop, J.J., Longland, A.C., et al., 2000. Intra-caecal fermentation parameters in ponies fed botanically diverse fibre-based diets. Animal Feed Science and Technology 84, 183–197.

Moore-Colyer, M.J.S., Hyslop, J.J., Longland, A.C., et al., 2002. The mobile bag technique as a method for determining the degradation of four botanically diverse fibrous feedstuffs in the small intestine and total digestive tract of ponies. British Journal of Nutrition 88, 729–740.

Muhonen, S., Julliand, V., Lindberg, J.E., et al., 2009. Effects of the equine colon ecosystem of grass silage and haylage diets after an abrupt feed change from hay. Journal of Animal Science 87, 2291–2298.

Müller, C.E., 2005. Fermentation pattern of small-bale silage and haylage as a feed for horses. Grass and Forage Science 60, 109–118.

Müller, C.E., 2009. Influence of harvest date of primary growth on microbial flora of grass herbages and haylage, and on fermentation and aerobic stability of haylage conserved in laboratory silos. Grass and Forage Science 64, 328–338.

Müller, C.E., Udén, P., 2007. Preference of horses for grass conserved as hay, haylage or silage. Animal Feed Science and Technology 132, 66–78.

Müller, C.E., Möller, J., Krogh Jensen, S., et al., 2007. Tocopherol and carotenoid levels in baled silage and haylage in relation to horse requirements. Animal Feed Science and Technology 137, 182–197.

Müller, C.E., von Rosen, D., Udén, P., 2008. Effect of forage conservation method on microbial flora and fermentation pattern in forage and in equine colon and faeces. Livestock Science 119, 116–128.

Nehra, R., Purohit, G.R., Sharma, T., et al., 2005. Common feeding stuffs of horses in arid zone-a survey. Veterinary Practitioner 6, 157–158.

NRC, 1998. Nutrient Requirements of Swine, 10th revised edition. National Academies Press, Washington D C, USA.

NRC, 2007. Nutrient Requirement of Horses, 6th revised edition. National Academies Press, Washington D C, USA.

O'Connor, C.I., Lawrence, L.M., Lawrence, A.C. St., et al., 2004. The effect of dietary fish oil supplementation on exercising horses. Journal of Animal Science 82, 2978–2984.

Olsson, N., Ruudvere, A., 1955. The nutrition of the horse. Nutrition Abstracts and Reviews 25, 1–18.

Ott, E.A., Asquith, R.L., 1986. Influence of level of feeding and nutrient content of the concentrate on growth and development of yearling horses. Journal of Animal Science 62, 290–299.

Ott, E.A., Asquith, R.L., 1994. Trace mineral supplementation of broodmares. Journal of Equine Veterinary Science 14, 93–101.

Ott, E.A., Johnson, E.L., 2001. Effect of trace mineral proteinates on growth and skeletal and hoof development in yearling horses. Journal of Equine Veterinary Science 21, 287–291.

Ott, E.A., Kivipelto, J., 2002. Growth and development of yearling horses fed either alfalfa or coastal bermudagrass: hay and a concentrate formulated for bermudagrass hay. Journal of Equine Veterinary Science 22, 311–319.

Ott, E.A., Feaster, J.P., Sandi, Lieb., 1979a. Acceptability and digestibility of dried citrus pulp by horses. Journal of Animal Science 49, 983–987.

Ott, E.A., Asquith, R.L., Feaster, R.L., et al., 1979b. Influence of protein level and quality on growth and development of yearling foals. Journal of Animal Science 49, 620–626.

Ott, E.A., Asquith, R.L., Feaster, R.L., 1981. Lysine supplementation of diets for yearling horses. Journal of Animal Science 53, 1496–1503.

Palmgren Karlsson, C., Jansson, A., Essén-Gustavsson, B., et al., 2002. Effect of molassed sugar beet pulp on nutrient utilization and metabolic parameters during exercise. Equine Veterinary Journal (Supplement) 34, 44–49.

Phuc, B.H.N., Lindberg, J.E., 2001. Ileal digestibility of amino acids in growing pigs given cassava root meal diets with inclusion of cassava leaves, leucaena leaves and groundnut foliage. Animal Science 72, 511–517.

Pettersson, D., Åman, P., 1987. The variation in chemical composition of triticales grown in Sweden. Acta Agriculturae Scandinavica 37, 20–26.

Potter, G.D., Arnold, F.F., Householder, D.D., et al., 1992a. Digestion of starch in the small or large intestine of the equine. Pferdeheilkunde (Sonderdruck) 3/4, 107–111.

Potter, G.D., Hughes, S.L., Julen, T.R., et al., 1992b. A review of research on digestion and utilization of fat by the equine. Pferdeheilkunde (Sonderdruck) 3/4, 119–123.

Ragnarsson, S., Lindberg, J.E., 2008. Nutritional value of timothy haylage in Icelandic horses. Livestock Science 113, 202–208.

Ragnarsson, S., Lindberg, J.E., 2010. Nutritional value of mixed grass haylage in Icelandic horses. Livestock Science 131, 83–87.

Reverter, M., Lundh, T., Lindberg, J.E., 1999. Ileal amino acid digistibilities in pigs of barley-based diets with inclusion of lucerne, white clover, red clover or perennial ryegrass. British Journal of Nutrition 82, 139–147.

Reverter, M., Lundh, T., Gonda, H.L., et al., 2000. Portal net appearance of amino acids in growing pigs fed a barley-based diet with inclusion of three different forage meals. British Journal of Nutrition 84, 483–494.

Richards, N., Hinch, G.N., Rowe, J.B., 2006. The effect of current grain feeding practices on hindgut starch fermentation and acidosis in the Australian racing Thoroughbred. Australian Veterinary Journal 84, 402–407.

Rodiek, A.V., Stull, C.L., 2007. Glycemic index of ten common horse feeds. Journal of Equine Veterinary Science 27, 205–211.

Saastamoinen, M.T., Koskinen, E., 1993. Influence of quality of dietary protein supplement and anabolic steroids on muscular and skeletal growth in foals. Animal Production 56, 135–144.

Särkijärvi, S., Saastamoinen, M., 2006. Feeding value of various processes oat grains in equine diets. Livestock Science 100, 3–9.

Sauvant, D., Perez, J.M., Tran, G., 2004. Tables of composition and nutritional value of feed materials. Wageningen Academic Publishers, The Netherlands.

Shurson, G.C., Whitney, M.H., Spiehs, M.J., et al., 2000. The value of distillers dried grains with solubles in pig diets. In: Lyons, T.P., Cole, D.J.A. (Eds.), Concepts in Pig Science 2000. Nottingham Nutrition International, Nottingham, UK, pp. 47–62.

Stein, H.H., Gibson, M.L., Pedersen, C., et al., 2006. Amino acid and energy digestibility in ten samples of distillers dried grain with solubles fed to growing pigs. Journal of Animal Science 84, 853–860.

Sunvold, G.D., Hussein, H.S., Fahey Jr., G.C., et al., 1995. In vitro fermentation of cellulose, beet pulp, citrus pulp and citrus pectin using fecal inoculum from cats, dogs, horses, humans, and pigs and ruminal fluid from cattle. Journal of Animal Science 73, 3639–3648.

Suttle, N.F., 2010. Mineral Nutrition of Livestock. CABI Publishing, Wallingford, UK.

Thomke, S., 1970. Über die Veränderung des Aminosäuregehaltes der Gerste mit steigendem Stickstoffgehalt. Zeitschrift für Tierphysiologie, Tierernährung und Futtermittelkunde 27, 23–31.

Thorson, J.F., Karren, B.J., Bauer, M.L., et al., 2010. Effect of selenium supplementation and plane of nutrition on mares and their foals: Foaling data. Journal of Animal Science 88, 982–990.

Thorvaldsson, G., Tremblay, G.F., Kunelius, H.T., 2007. The effects of growth temperature on digestibility and fibre concentration of seven temperate grass species. Acta Agriculturae Scandinavica, Section B, Soil and Plant Science, 57, 322–328.

Valberg, S.J., 1998. Exertional rhabdomolysis in the horse. In: Pagan, J.D. (Ed.), Advances in Equine Nutrition. Nottingham University Press, Nottingham, UK, pp. 507–512.

Van Soest, P.J., 1994. Nutritional Ecology of the Ruminant, second ed. Comstock, Ithaca, London.

Vervuert, I., Coenen, M., Bothe, C., 2003. Effect of oat processing on the glycaemic and insulin responses in horses. Journal of Animal Physiology and Animal Nutrition 87, 96–104.

Vervuert, I., Coenen, M., Bothe, C., 2004. Effect of corn processing on the glycaemic and insulinaemic responses in horses. Journal of Animal Physiology and Animal Nutrition 88, 348–355.

Vervuert, I., Bothe, C., Coenen, M., 2007. Glycaemic and insulinaemic responses to mechanical and thermal processed barley in horses. Journal of Animal Physiology and Animal Nutrition 91, 263–268.

Vervuert, I., Voigt, K., Hollands, T., et al., 2008. Effects of processing barley on its digestion by horses. The Veterinary Record, May 24, 54–58.

Vervuert, I., Voigt, K., Hollands, T., et al., 2009. Effect of feeding increasing quantities of starch on glycaemic and insulinaemic responses in healthy horses. Veterinary Journal 182, 67–72.

Waller, A.P., Geor, R.J., Spriet, L.L., et al., 2009. Oral acetate supplementation after prolonged moderate intensity exercise enhances early muscle glycogen re-synthesis in horses. Experimental Physiology 94, 888–898.

Willard, J.G., Willard, J.C., Wolfram, S.A., et al., 1977. Effect of diet on cecal pH and feeding behaviour of horses. Journal of Animal Science 45, 87–93.

Willing, B., Vörös, A., Roos, S., et al., 2009. Changes in faecal bacteria associated with concentrate and forage-only diets fed to horses in training. Equine Veterinary Journal 41, 908–914.

Wilkins, R.J., 1988. The preservation of forages. In: Ørskov, E.R. (Ed.), Feed Science, World Animal Science, B4. Elsevier Science Publishers B.V., Amsterdam, the Netherlands, pp. 231–255.

Woods, V.B., Fearon, A.M., 2009. Dietary sources of unsaturated fatty acids for animals and their transfer into meat, milk and eggs: A review. Livestock Science 126, 1–20.

18

Pastures and pasture management

Annette C. Longland

Introduction

Horses evolved as free-ranging animals with unrestricted access to grassland, and survived on a variety of forage species. These forages were often of low nutritional quality and included grasses, legumes, other forbs and various trees and shrubs. Wild horses and those extensively grazed on natural or semi-natural grasslands enjoy similar lifestyles to their wild ancestors. However, not so the majority of domestic horses today. Pressures on agricultural land dictate that most domestic horses have access to limited grazing areas, and these are frequently overstocked. Without appropriate management such paddocks deteriorate and can become little more than bare exercise areas of little nutritional value.

What is it we require from horse pastures? The ideal often encompasses all or some of the following: provision of: (a) sufficient grass to maintain the grazing horse; (b) sufficient grass for conservation for winter feed; (c) a mixture of forage species free from poisonous plants; and (d) a dense, well-cushioned turf on which horses can exercise safely.

In order for pastures to meet these criteria they need to be properly maintained and correctly stocked. Not only does appropriate pasture management benefit the horse, but it is also of financial advantage. Grazed grass is the most economical feed for grazing livestock (Mayne et al 2000) – on a dry matter basis, this equates to up to four times cheaper than hay/haylage and is 8–15 times cheaper than compound feeds at current UK feed prices.

Pastures

Pastures for horses usually contain a mixture of grasses, legumes and other forbs (herbaceous dicotyledonous species). Forage grasses are divided into two main categories, cool-season grasses that are found in temperate regions and warm-season species that are adapted to sub-tropical and tropical climates. Cool-season (C3) grasses start growth when temperatures reach 7°C with optimal growth between 16–24°C, whereas warm-season (C4) species start growth at around 15°C with optima between 32 and 35°C.

Grass (Family Poaceae)

There are more than 10 000 species of grass worldwide, and these have adapted to survive and proliferate in a wide range of environmental conditions including extremes of temperature, topography, soil types, osmotic stress (salinity) and water stress (flood or drought). Grasses may be annual, biennial, or perennial. Perennial grasses are commonly used in horse pastures.

Grass developmental stages

Grasses undergo a number of developmental stages. During the vegetative stage, grasses grow largely from the growing point located at the margin of the stem and roots, known as the crown. Shoots (tillers) arise from the crown, and consist of leaves, stem node, internode and a bud (Fig 18.1). During vegetative growth the stem remains compact within the crown, the internodes are short and the tillers consist almost entirely of leaf. Leaves are generally short lived (Lemaire 1988, Robson et al 1980), and are at their most productive in middle age. Soon after middle age they senesce (die slowly) from the tip of the leaf to the base. Once a certain number of leaves have formed on a tiller, the older, lower leaves die.

With increasing development, some tillers become reproductive, leaf production stops and the elongation (jointing) phase occurs, producing an upright stem with long upper internodes. The elongated stem then lifts the developing seedhead upwards, and the plant enters the reproductive phase where the seedhead becomes visible, pollen is shed (anthesis) and fertilization occurs. Thereafter, seeds develop, ripen and disperse. Once the seed is produced the reproductive tiller dies as does its associated root system. New tillers then arise from the crown as regrowth, and in this way the grass sward continues to grow after reproduction and can continue to do so year after year through the production of new tillers. Adventitious roots arise from buds at the base of the main shoot and from the daughter tillers producing a thick mat of roots.

If the growing point of a reproductive tiller is removed by cutting or grazing, the tiller will remain vegetative, and

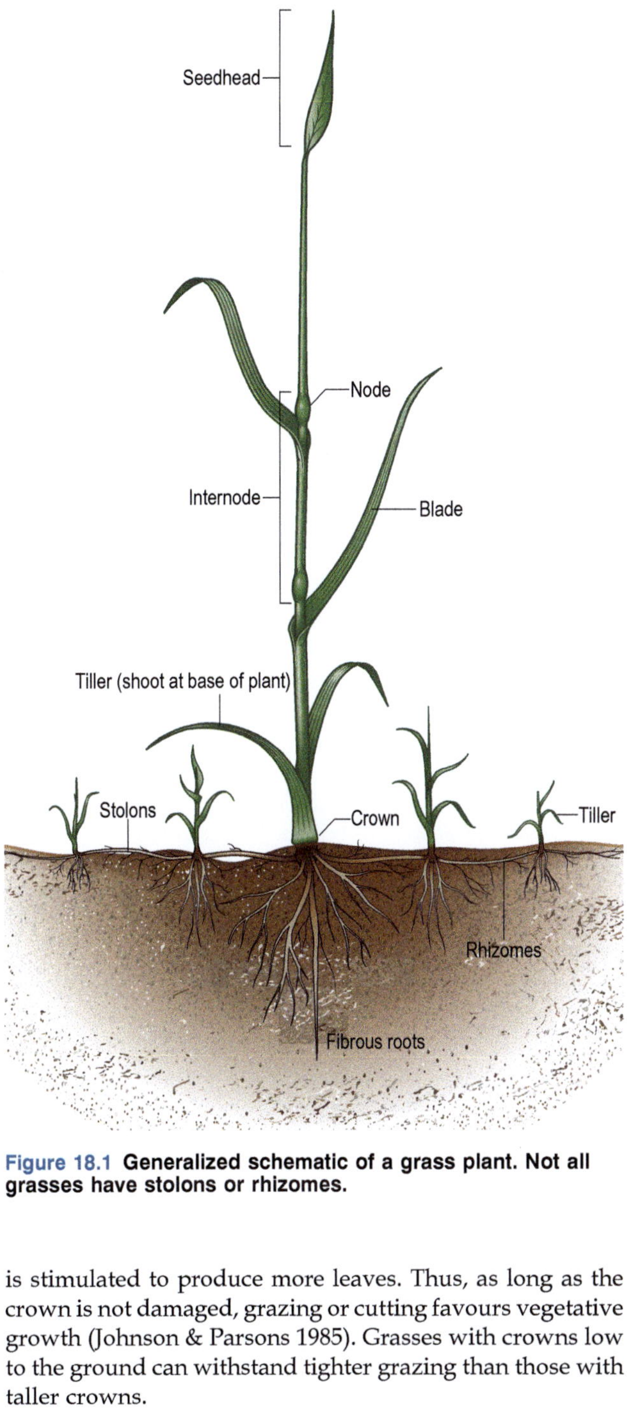

Figure 18.1 Generalized schematic of a grass plant. Not all grasses have stolons or rhizomes.

is stimulated to produce more leaves. Thus, as long as the crown is not damaged, grazing or cutting favours vegetative growth (Johnson & Parsons 1985). Grasses with crowns low to the ground can withstand tighter grazing than those with taller crowns.

Grass reproduction

Grasses can reproduce both sexually (i.e., by seed) and vegetatively (via leaf production). Seeds can be dispersed by wind, water, or by animals either by adhering to feathers or hair coats or passing, intact, through their digestive tracts. Such seed dispersal can result in seeds being transported considerable distances from the parent plant. Vegetative propagation, however, occurs more locally to the parent plant. There are three main growth habits that achieve this, the bunch (tussock) grasses, the stoloniferous grasses and the rhizomatous grasses. Each of these types of grasses produces tillers. The bunch grasses produce many tillers that originate from the crown and grow upwards from the base of the plant resulting in an ever thickening plant, giving it a bunched or tussock-type appearance. Examples of bunch grasses include perennial ryegrass, timothy, various fescues, meadow grasses, bluestems, and reed-canary grass. Stoloniferous grasses, such as the fescues, Rhodes grass and creeping bent, spread largely by means of lateral stems, stolons, which creep over the ground and give rise to new shoots periodically along its length. Rhizomatous grasses, such as Kentucky bluegrass spread by means of below ground stems known as rhizomes. The rhizomes terminate in a shoot that emerges some distance from the original plant, and as they mature these new shoots in turn produce rhizomes perpetuating the spread of the grass. As long as the crown of the plant is not damaged, such vegetative propagation allows plants to persist, despite grazing or cutting, without ever needing to produce seed.

Thus, swards with a high complement of stoloniferous or rhizomatous species result in complete ground cover, and tend to be relatively resistant to trampling and overgrazing. Swards that have been thinly sown with bunch grasses tend to be more open in structure, at least initially, with bare soil between plants, allowing ingress of weeds. However, if maintained in a vegetative state, properly sown bunch grasses will eventually produce sufficient tillers and adventitious roots to effect complete ground cover and crowd out weeds. Many pastures for horses contain a mixture of bunch and stoloniferous and/or rhizomatous species.

Legumes (family Fabaceae or Leguminosae)

Legumes are able to "fix" nitrogen from the atmosphere converting it into a form that can be used by the legume. Overall, legumes are higher in protein than grasses, and when incorporated in moderation, form a useful addition to horse pastures, as they provide biologically useful N for associated grasses.

Growth of legumes differs from that of grasses in that during the vegetative stage stems elongate immediately with leaves appearing alternately on either side of the stem, with branching occurring at leaf/stem junctions. The reproductive phase starts at the appearance of buds, arising on both the main stem and branches, that progress to the bloom (flowering) stages. Propagation of white clover and alfalfa is in many ways similar to that of perennial stoloniferous grasses, propagating vegetatively outwards. Many alfalfa varieties have an upright growth habit that is sensitive to grazing, and thus alfalfa varieties with low-set, crowns and thick stems are the more grazing tolerant types (Brummer & Bouton 1991). Red clover and bird's foot trefoil have intermediate growth habits. The growing points of white clover varieties, however, are located at the soil surface, and those that produce many branched stolons are particularly tolerant to continuous grazing (Brink et al 1988), although they may be damaged by trampling, particularly by shod hooves.

Key Points

- Pastures usually contain a mixture of grass, legumes, forbs and weeds
- Grasses are either cool-season (C3 metabolism) species that flourish in temperate regions or warm season (C4 metabolism) that grow in semi-tropical or tropical regions

Table 18-1 Effect of Growth Stage on Nutritive Value and Yield of Perennial Ryegrass (*L. perenne*)

Time	Developmental stage	Ruminant digestibility (g/kg DM)	CP (g/kg DM)	WSC (g/kg DM)	Dry matter yield (t/ha)
Early May	Vegetative	750	250	100	3
Late May	Elongation/early reproductive	660	160	150	6
Early June	Seed development	600	90	200	8

Data from Green et al 1971.

- Legumes "fix" nitrogen, increasing the protein content of the sward
- Grasses have either bunch or rhizomatous/stoloniferous growth habits
- Pasture species with low crowns are more resistant to grazing

Chemical composition of forages

All green plants derive their energy via the process of photosynthesis whereby they fix atmospheric carbon in the presence of light and water into glucose which is metabolized into various compounds. Leaves are the main photosynthetic tissues; they are at their most productive in middle age, when they produce more photosynthate (the products of photosynthesis) than they consume, transporting the unused assimilates to other plant parts. Photosynthate is distributed into the cell contents for use in metabolism, into reserves (as fructan or starch) for use in times of hardship (over wintering, drought, etc.), for storage in seeds (as starch), and incorporation into structural tissues (cell walls). The relative proportions of photosynthate that are partitioned for these various purposes differ throughout the growth cycle. As the plant matures, with an increase in the proportion of stem, the proportion of cell wall (cellulose, hemicellulose and lignin i.e. dietary fiber) increases, and that of cell contents (proteins, nonstructural carbohydrates (NSC), minerals and lipids) decreases (Beever, et al 2000). Cell contents are almost completely available to horses whereas cell walls are variably and incompletely degradable. Lignin is largely nondegradable in horses (Lewis 1994). Thus, the available nutrient content of forage changes markedly throughout the growing season.

It is clear from the above that the chemical composition, and as a consequence, nutritive value of grasses changes with growth stage. Thus, young leafy swards of perennial ryegrass contained nearly three times the crude protein (CP) and half the water-soluble carbohydrates (WSC) (WSC = sum of fructans and simple sugars: WSC + starch = NSC), and was 25% more digestible (as ascertained for ruminants) as the same sward a month later (Table 18-1). However, the dry matter (DM) yield of the young leafy sward was only ca. 0.38 of the one-month older sward. Therefore, there is a trade off between forage digestibility and DM yield. In addition to changes in CP and WSC content as the plant matures, the cell walls thicken and become lignified. As lignin is largely nondegradable in the equid gut, there is a concomitant decline in cell wall degradability with increasing lignification. During seed ripening there is a marked decline in CP and WSC content of the stem (Slepetys 2001) (Table 18-2).

Table 18-2 Effect of Stage of Seed Development on Water Soluble Carbohydrate (WSC) and Crude Protein (CP) Content of Stems

Grass species	Stem WSC content (g/kg DM)		Stem CP content (g/kg DM)	
	Seed setting	Fully ripe seed	Seed setting	Fully ripe seed
Poa pratensis	96	27	29	21
Festuca pratensis	155	25	41	22
Dactylis glomerata	83	2	51	29
Lolium perenne	212	76	31	26
Phleum pratense	95	13	44	28

Data from Slepetys 2001.

Although some of the WSC is transported to the developing seed, the majority is incorporated into cell walls (Gebbing et al 1999). Thus, when seeds have completed the ripening process, the stems are high in fiber and often highly lignified. Once the seed is dispersed, the residual stemmy material is normally of low nutritive value. Older leaves are also generally of lowered nutritional value, for when they senesce (age naturally and slowly) their cell contents are mobilized to other plant parts.

Swards maintained at a vegetative stage of growth through regular cutting still exhibit seasonal changes in chemical composition (Table 18-3). In eight varieties of perennial ryegrass, WSC levels increased in late spring, followed by a general decline during the summer, to rise again in early autumn, and then fall dramatically in late autumn. The fructan contents of four pasture grass monocultures over a growing season are shown in Table 18-4. Timothy and two perennial ryegrasses accrued high levels of fructan in early May, which had declined substantially by June to levels that varied slightly during the remainder of the growing season. The red fescue accumulated the most fructan in June, declining thereafter until the autumn when there was a further peak followed by a decline in fructan content. Proportions of cell walls (neutral detergent fiber, NDF), however, increased in summer, decreased briefly in early autumn and then rose again in late autumn. Protein contents declined as the season progressed to rise again in late autumn (Table 18-3). They then declined thereafter (Longland 2005). Likewise, eight varieties of perennial ryegrass managed for conservation as hay demonstrated changes in chemical composition, the first cut in May being

Table 18-3 Average Nutrient Composition of Eight Perennial Ryegrass Varieties When Managed for Grazing, Through Regular Cutting (Mean of Two Years) (Data from Longland, 2005)

Nutrient content (g/kg DM)	Harvest							
	Early April	End April	Mid-May	Early June	Early July	Early Aug	Early Sep	Early Oct
WSC	186	166	235	165	205	158	211	161
CP	262	231	175	212	175	181	187	243
NDF	419	471	443	499	466	535	457	473

Table 18-4 Fructan Contents (g/kg DM) of Three Species of Temperate Grass Commonly Found in Horse Pastures Determined on Seven Occasions Through the Growing Season (Mean of Four Replicate Field Plots), Harvested in 2006 (Data from Longland et al.)

Species/variety	Early April	Early May	Early June	Early July	Mid August	Mid September	Mid October
Red fescue	NS	110	129	92	102	121	102
Timothy	100	198	99	110	93	109	102
Perennial Ryegrass*	135	275	195	168	197	169	139

NS insufficient growth to sample.
Mean of four replicate field plots, harvested in 2006 (data from Longland et al in preparation).
*Mean of two varieties of perennial ryegrass.

Table 18-5 Effect of Harvest Date on WSC, CP and NDF Content (g/kg DM) of Eight Varieties of Ryegrass Managed for Conservation Harvested in Spring and Autumn (Mean of 2 Years) (Longland, 2005)

Nutrient	Spring	Autumn
WSC	339	143
CP	125	150
NDF	517	580

Table 18-6 Mineral Contents of Legume and Grass Pastures Sampled Between 2000 and 2010 (Dairy One)

Nutrient (g/kg)	Legume pasture	Grass pasture
Nitrogen (N)	4.32 (3.36–5.12)*	2.40 (1.12–3.52)
Phosphorus (P)	3.70 (2.9–4.5)	2.95 (0–8.63)
Potassium (K)	22.80 (20–35.4)	19.89 (8.6–31.2)
Calcium (Ca)	12.10 (8.4–15.9)	5.60 (2.73–8.37)
Sodium (Na)	2.40 (0.-5.4)	1.02 (0–4.3)
Zinc (mg/kg) (Zn)	40 (0–8.2)	30 (11–47)
Copper (mg/kg) (Cu)	9 (5–13)	9 (3–15)

*Average values and normal range in parenthesis. Sample numbers for legume pastures were 145 and for grass pastures >8000.

higher in WSC and protein and lower in cell walls (NDF) than the third cut taken in October (Table 18-5).

WSC contents of pastures can be particularly variable between years, with average values during the course of the grazing season of the same sward being 200, 240, and 104 g/kg DM in years 1, 2, and 3 after establishment (Longland 2005). Furthermore, there are considerable diurnal fluctuations in WSC content which may double over the course of a few hours under appropriate conditions (Longland 2005).

The mineral status of herbage is affected by a number of factors including forage type, soil mineral content/availability, growth stage and interactions with other minerals, and as a result the mineral content of pastures varies. Average contents of P, K, Ca, Na, Zn, and Cu for legume and grass pastures together with their normal ranges are given in Table 18-6. Legumes tend to be greater in N, and Ca than grass pastures, and may on average be higher in P and Na, but it is clear that there is considerable overlap between the mineral contents of the two pasture types. There are also seasonal fluctuations in mineral content, with P and K tending to decrease as the season progresses (Grace et al 2002, Kuusela 2006). Ca levels were found to be greatest in summer by Kuusela (2006) but not by Grace et al (2002) and Zn was found to increase at the end of the season by Cubitt et al (2004). The Ca:P ratio also varies with season, and in grass clover swards ranged from 1.11:1 at the beginning of the season to 1.94:1 mid-season declining to 1.65:1 at the end of the grazing season (Kuusela, 2006). However, reversed Ca:P (<1.1) ratios have also been reported in pastures (Coenen, personal communication and Lush 1934–see section on horse requirements below). Furthermore there were significant between-year variations in pasture mineral contents (Kuusela, 2006).

Nutrients, particularly the WSC are not evenly distributed within plants or indeed within a given organ, but show longitudinal variation reflecting "source-sink" fluxes. Thus, primary photosynthate is mobilized from areas of high photosynthetic activity to less active areas where it is elaborated into more complex molecules. Therefore, there is more total WSC and fructan at the base of leaves and sheaths than at the tip. The opposite tends to be true for protein (Table 18-7) (Pavis et al 2000).

Indeed, fructans only accumulate at the tips of leaf blades when the storage capacity of both leaf sheaths and elongation growth zones has already decreased (Guerrand et al 1996). Fructan contents are also greater in the stems than the leaves (Longland 2005) and greater in stem bases than apices (Smith 1967).

Table 18-7 Distribution of Protein, Total WSC, Simple Sugars and Fructan along The Length (Base to Tip) of Mature Leaf Sheaths, Mature Leaf Blades and Elongating Leaves, of 8-Week-Old *Lolium perenne* Plants (Data from Pavis et al., 2000)

Nutrient (g/kg fr matter)	Elongating leaf			Leaf sheath			Leaf blade		
Leaf section	base	mid	tip	base	mid	tip	base	mid	tip
Protein	4.5	3	6.5	1	1	1.5	2.5	4	4.5
Total WSC	17	12	8	12	7	8	12	11	5
Fructans	9	5	2	8	4	4	3	2	1.5

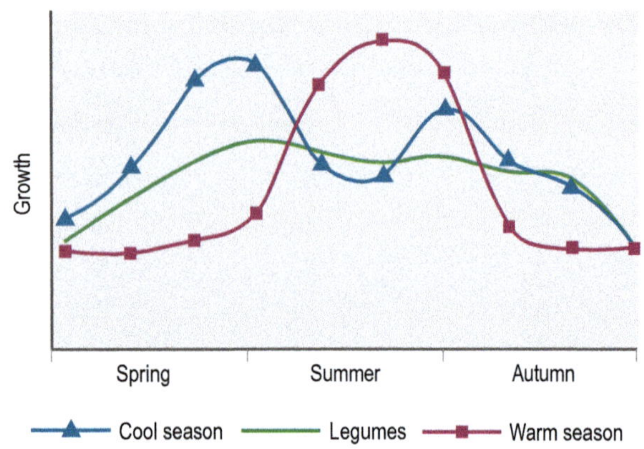

Figure 18.2 **Generalized seasonal growth patterns of cool-season grasses, warm-season grasses and forage legumes.**

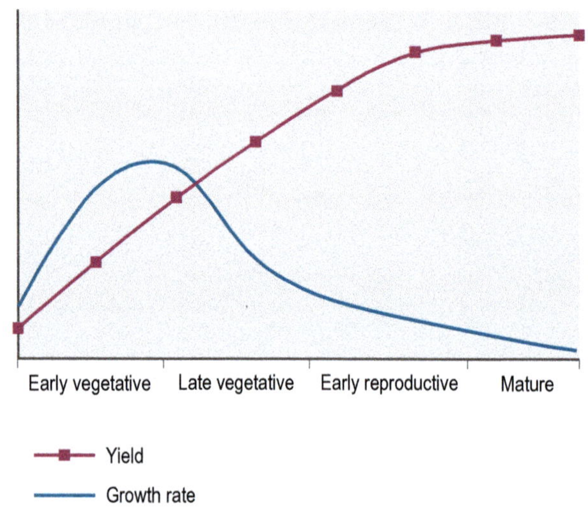

Figure 18.3 **Generalized growth rate and yield changes during grass development.**

It is important to note that irrespective of forage species and genetically predetermined developmental stages, forage growth and composition are greatly influenced by a number of environmental factors including precipitation, light intensity, temperature, soil fertility, salinity, herbivory and disease. Each factor, or a combination of these factors, can have a greater effect on composition content than stage of growth. (See section on pastures for laminitics.)

Key Points

- The chemical composition of pastures is highly variable and influenced by growth stage, season, and environmental conditions
- Early vegetative growth has the highest nutritive value, but low DM yield
- As plants mature, they become increasingly high in lignified cell wall content rendering them less degradable
- Pasture WSC content is particularly changeable with marked differences within hours, and the extent of such changes is hard to predict.

Seasonal growth

The rate of grass growth (i.e. dry matter accrual per unit time) is not uniform throughout the growing season. In early spring when leaf area is small, daily growth rate is slow. However, as the plant grows more leaf, the potential photosynthetic area increases rapidly and daily growth rate is greatest in the early and mid-vegetative stages in spring, declining during the late vegetative and reproductive phases and virtually ceases when the plant reaches maturity (Fig. 18.2), with cool season grasses undergoing a limited period of enhanced growth in the autumn (Fig. 18.3). Thus, cumulative plant yield increases very rapidly during the vegetative growth stages and plateaus during the reproductive and mature stages. Maintaining swards at a leafy vegetative stage will therefore generally increase overall DM yield.

Warm-season species grow during the summer months, and whereas the greatest growth of forage legumes is in spring, the subsequent decline in growth is much less than for grasses, resulting in more uniform yield throughout the growing season (Fig. 18.3). Areas that can support both warm and cool season species at different times of year can have substantially extended grazing seasons by using both types of grass to provide high quantities of quality pasture for much of the year. Additionally, yearly forage production can be further increased through seeding dormant warm season pastures with cool season annual grasses or small grain species.

Over-wintering of pasture species

Both grasses and legumes store carbohydrates in crowns and/or roots for over-wintering. The stored carbohydrates are used for plant respiration and to provide the energy source for the initiation of the new growth in the spring and following each harvest. If overgrazed, there will be insufficient reserves for strong re-growth and the plant will be weakened and may eventually die. Furthermore if overgrazing is so severe that the crowns are damaged the plant will die. Overgrazing eventually results in unproductive pastures of low vigor and sward density, allowing the ingress of weeds.

Key Points

- Maintaining swards at a leafy vegetative state can increase DM yield and quality
- Over-grazing will cause pasture deterioration

Pasture species for horses

There is a wide range of pasture species which are found in horse paddocks. Tables 18-8 and 18-9 show a number of cool and warm season grasses commonly used in horse pastures together with some of the advantages and disadvantages of each. Probably the most common legumes sown in horse pastures are white clover (*Trifolium repens*) and Alfalfa (*Medicago sativa*). Red clover (*Trifolium pretense*) may also be included in small amounts, but tends not to persist for more than a few years. Other species such as sanfoin (*Onobrychis viciifolia*), birds-foot trefoil (*Lotus corniculatus*) may also be sown but often require careful management if they are to establish and persist in the pasture (Sheldrick et al 1995). Both annual and perennial species of lespedeza (*Kummerowia* spp) may be used for horse pastures.

There are many more species of grasses, legumes and other species that are grazed by horses globally, that are of

Table 18-8 Some Common Cool-Season Grass Species Used in Horse Pastures

Species	Advantages	Disadvantages
Perennial ryegrass (*Lolium perenne*)	Establishes quickly, high yielding with N fertilizer, is highly digestible, and very palatable. Re-grows rapidly after even heavy grazing	Can produce high levels of water-soluble carbohydrates, so not suitable for laminitics. Endophyte infected species should not be fed to horses. Becomes stemmy and tillers poorly under dry or infertile conditions.
Timothy (*Phleum pretense*)	Traditional species for horses. Late flowering producing leafy forage in mid-season when such forage is scarce. Useful in cool wet conditions or heavy soils. Useful early growth on uplands. Easy to establish	Does not tolerate very close grazing, and late summer and autumn production can be low.
Cocksfoot/orchardgrass (*Dactylis glomerata*)	Can tolerate dryer and shadier conditions than many other grasses. Will grow on soils of mediocre fertility	May lack palatability. Clumpy growth habit if not defoliated regularly, can shade out other valuable species
Creeping red fescue (*Festuca rubra*)	Tillers well, Resistant to trampling – useful in areas of heavy traffic, e.g. gateways, water troughs. Tolerant to a wide range of conditions	Mediocre grazing value
Meadow fescue (*Festuca pratensis*)	Grows well on most soil types if moist and fertile. Cold-tolerant, useful in horse pasture mixes, good nutritive value	Susceptible to rust. Not as high yielding as orchard grass or tall fescue
Tall fescue (*Festuca arundinacea*)	Hardy, tolerant to drought, close grazing, heavy horse traffic, resistant to pests and pathogens, good yield	May contain the endophyte *Neotyphodium coenophialum*, produces alkaloids that particularly affect pregnant mares. Use of endophyte free varieties is recommended.
Kentucky bluegrass/smooth stalked-meadow grass (*Poa pratensis*)	Long-lived, useful on light & sandy soils since it is stoloniferous and resistant to severe drought. Leaves mainly near soil surface. Highly palatable	Low mid-season yield, aggressive, high fertility requirements
Crested dogstail (*Cynosurus cristatus*)	Palatable to horses, is a short grass that is leafy at the base helping to give a good 'bottom' to a sward. Winter hardy, tolerant to frequent defoliation, not dependent on fertilizer inputs	Can be mediocre in terms of nutritive value-which may be an asset for obese animals
Smooth bromegrass (*Bromus inermis*)	Palatable and nutritious in spring, early summer, late summer and autumn	Sensitive to close grazing and drought
Matua prairiegrass (*Bromus wildenowii*)	High quality, reasonably winter-hardy grass able to grow on sandy soils which may be limiting to other species. Nutritive value does not decline as rapidly with increasing maturity as many other species	Cannot withstand heavy grazing
Reed canary grass (*Phalaris arundinaceae*)	Well adapted to wet conditions, early spring growth palatable and nutritious	Old varieties may produce high levels of alkaloids in summer and become unpalatable

Table 18-9 Some Common Warm-Season Species Used in Horse Pastures

Species	Advantages	Disadvantages
Bermudagrass (*Cynodon dactylon*)	High yielding, acceptable nutritive value in many varieties, is grazing and trampling tolerant, forms almost solid turf	Some varieties may have poor cold-tolerance and moderate digestibility
Bahiagrass (*Paspulum notatum*)	Able to withstand heavy grazing and trampling-good general purpose species, grows on soils of mediocre fertility, relatively resistant to pests and pathogens	May be very high in fiber and unpalatable to horses so intakes may be reduced. Less cold tolerant than Bermuda grass
Dalllisgrass (*Paspulum dilatatum*)	Requires moist and reasonably fertile soil. Produces large amounts of basal leaf and can withstand close and frequent grazing. Has longer growing season than many perennial grasses	May suffer from ergot infestation at seed head stage–potentially toxic causing grass staggers
Big Bluestem (*Andropogon* spp.)	Adapted on soils that are at least moderately well drained. Complements cool-season grass-legume pastures in a rotational stocking system. Highly palatable, and makes good hay	Cannot withstand very tight grazing

varying and localized productivity and nutritive merit that are outside the scope of this article

Grazing behavior

Horses at pasture graze for an average of 12.5 hours out of 24, though this can occasionally rise to 16–17 hours grazing time at certain times of year (Ellis 2010). Feeding activity tends to be highest at dusk and dawn, and lowest immediately pre-dawn (Berger et al 1999, van Dierendonck et al 1996, Vulink 2001). Pasture intakes typically range from 2–2.5% of bodyweight (BW) as DM (reported in NRC 2007; equates to 95–118 g DM/kg$^{0.75}$ for a 500-kg horse) although intakes as high as 5.2% of BW (456 g DM/kg$^{0.75}$ for a 500-kg horse) have been reported (Smith et al 2007).

Horses confined to paddocks as opposed to those free-ranging in large areas, adopt a system of defecating in certain areas (latrines), that they will refuse to graze and over-grazing others which are free from manure, creating a system of "roughs" and "lawns" respectively (Odberg & Francis-Smith 1976). Thus, the manure fertilizes the roughs, resulting in areas of rank, overgrown and unpalatable herbage whilst at the same time, the lawns can become over-grazed with loss of preferred species accompanied by a decline in fertility by the continual transfer of nutrients from the lawns to the roughs. If left unattended, latrines have a habit of spreading outwards, further reducing the grazing area, so that considerable amounts of grazing can be lost to "roughs". As horses tend to graze more than 1 m away from dung patches (Fleurance et al 2007) it is easy to see how on small pastures in particular, that much of the grass (up to 90%) may be rendered unusable by latrine spread in very poorly managed paddocks (O'Beirne-Ranelagh 2005). If the situation is allowed to continue, the preferred species in overgrazed lawns decline and unpalatable, possibly poisonous, weeds can take their place.

Pasture intake

How much pasture do horses actually eat? There are a number of ways of measuring pasture intake by grazing livestock. These include both short- and long-term assessment of herbage intake. Short-term measurements (i.e. over a few hours) include weighing the animal before and after a set period of grazing time, after accounting for insensible water losses, excretory outputs and any water intake if drinking has been allowed (Longland et al 2011), through determining number of bites, and average herbage mass/bite over a set time period (Prache 1996) and from techniques involving the turnover of water or sodium (Silanikove et al 1987).

Longer-term measurements of pasture intake include: (a) calculations from pasture dry matter digestibility; (b) use of exclusion cages; (c) use of *n*-alkanes; (d) calculation from live weight change over several weeks from known requirements. Where the dry matter digestibility of a given pasture is known, collection of all fecal outputs allows intake to be back-calculated. Where exclusion cages are used, representative areas of evenly grown swards are excluded from grazing by use of cages, the pasture around the cages is then grazed, and intakes are calculated by the difference of total pasture mass (calculated from pasture in cages) and residual pasture herbage in the grazed areas. This method is probably the most practical for horse owners to use. Use of indigestible external markers such as *n*-alkanes are also used to determine intake in free grazing livestock (Mayes & Dove 2000). *n*-Alkanes are naturally occurring in plant waxes, but they are not found in mammals, nor are they digested by them. The animals are dosed regularly with synthetic alkanes, which together with the naturally occurring plant alkanes are determined in the feces, allowing intakes to be calculated. However, some values of intakes obtained from use of alkanes can seem very high. Changes in weight over a number of weeks can allow estimations of intake to be made from known DE requirements for maintenance, activity and gain (Longland et al 2011).

Reported DM intakes of pastures using a variety of the above techniques range from 1.5–5.2% of BW with 1.8–3.0% of BW being frequently reported (Edouard et al 2008, NRC 2007). Using the weight change method, Longland et al 2011, found that ponies grazing autumn pastures averaged intakes of 0.8% of BW as DM within 3 hours. Extrapolation of this data for animals grazing for 12–17 h suggests that if this rate of intake is maintained throughout the grazing period, daily intakes could be in the region of 3.2–4.5% of BW. Using *n*-alkanes, other studies have reported grazed pasture intakes of 5% or more of liveweight per day (Smith et al 2007, McMeniman 2003). Certainly ponies are able to consume ca. 5% of BW as DM of a pelleted chaff diet (Argo et al 2002)

Pasture palatability

There are relatively few well designed experiments on the palatability of various horse pasture species. However, from the studies that have been performed, the results have often been equivocal but the following general points have emerged.

1. Horses prefer to graze a mixed species pasture;
2. Palatability of a given species changes with growth stage and time of year, and thus a species that was untouched in summer may be favored in the winter months;
3. Individual horses have different preferences; and
4. Different varieties of the same species may vary in palatability.

Perennial ryegrass, a popular cool-season grass is not always highly palatable to horses (O'Beirne-Ranelagh 2005, Archer 1973). Palatable cool-season grasses include *Agrostis stolonoifera* (creeping bent), *A. capillaries* (common bent / browntop), *Bromus erecta* (upright brome), *Dactylis glomerata*, (orchardgrass/cocksfoot), *Cynosurus cristatus* (crested dogstail), *Festuca pratensis* (meadow fescue), *F. rubra* (red fescue), *F. ovina* (sheep's fescue), *F. arundinacea* (tall fescue), *Phleum pretense* (Timothy), *Poa pratensis* (smooth stalked meadow grass/Kentucky bluegrass), *Poa trivialis* (rough stalked meadow grass), *L.multiflorum* (perennial and Italian ryegrasses respectively). Palatable legumes include *Lotus corniculatus* (birdsfoot trefoil), *Medicago lupulina* (yellow trefoil/black medick), *Medicago sativa* (alfalfa), *Onobrychis viciofolia* (sainfoin) and *Trifolium repens* (white clover).

Horse requirements

The digestible energy (DE) contents of spring / summer pastures have been reported to range from 9.5–12 MJ/kg DM (Gallacher & McMeniman 1988), 7.05–11.2 MJ/kg DM in winter (Martin 1993) and 7.93 MJ/kg DM for stemmy, late summer ryegrass swards (Hunt 1995). These energy values are equivalent to those found in many compound feeds for horses, including those in work. According to NRC (2007), the maintenance energy requirements for a mature 500 kg horse range from 64–76 MJ /day, but heavily exercised horses or lactating mares and growing horses may require more than twice this amount (NRC 2007). Thus, ingestion of 10–12.5 kg DM (i.e. 2–2.5% of bodyweight as DM) of any of the pastures studied would meet or exceed the maintenance energy requirements of mature horses, but lactating mares or heavily exercised growing horses would require supplementation if grazing on pastures containing less than 11 MJ DE/kg DM (Table 18-10).

Crude protein (CP) contents of pastures in the UK average 156 g CP/kg DM, with reported ranges of 54–361 g CP/kg DM (MAFF 1992). The average CP maintenance requirement for a 500 kg horse is 630 g CP/day (NRC 2007). Thus, even pastures with the lowest reported CP contents would meet the maintenance requirement of a 500 kg horse consuming 2.5% of its bodyweight as DM, whereas the average CP content of pastures would exceed the CP requirement two- to threefold. However, lactating mares may not be able to ingest sufficient pasture to meet their protein requirements on very low protein pastures containing 54 g CP/kg DM, as this would necessitate ingesting some 5.6% BW as DM/day. Furthermore the quality of the protein, in terms of amino acid profiles, of such low protein pastures is unlikely to be ideal. However, "average" pastures containing 156 g CP/kg DM would meet the lactating mare CP requirements as well as those of growing horses ingesting pasture at 2% of BW/ day (Table 18-10).

The requirements for various minerals by various classes of horses of 500 kg at maturity are given in Table 18-10.

Table 18-10 Daily Requirements for Various Minerals by Horses of 500 kg at Maturity at Different Work Levels, Growth Stages or Physiological Status and Ability to Meet These Requirements on Grass Pastures of Average or Low Nutrient Content

Nutrient (g)	Level of work			Growth stage/physiological status				
	Maintenance[a]	Moderate	Heavy	Weanling	Yearling	2-year old	11 months gestation	1 month lactation
DE (MJ)*	70[b] + +	97 + –	146 – –	56 + –	78 – –	78 +–	90 + –	133 – –
Crude protein (CP)	630 + –	768 + –	1004 + –	669 – –	846 + –	770 + –	893 + –	1535 M –
Phosphorus (P)	14 + M	21 + –	29 + –	22 + –	21 + –	20 + –	26 + –	38 + –
Potassium (K)	25 + +	32 + –	53 + +	11 + +	17 + +	22 + +	26 + +	48 + +
Calcium (Ca)	20 + +	35 + –	40 + –	39 – –	38 – –	37 + –	36 + –	59 – –
Sodium (Na)	10 M –	18 – –	41 – –	4 – –	7 M –	9 M–	11 – –	13 – –
Zinc (mg) (Zn)	400 – –	450 – –	550 – –	169 – –	321 – –	430 – –	400 – –	500 – –
Copper (mg) (Cu)	100 – –	113 – –	125 – –	42 – –	80 – –	107 – –	125 – –	125 – –

*Requirements from NRC 2007, [a] average requirement for maintenance [b] +, –, M denote sufficient, insufficient or marginal supply of nutrients respectively in average or low quality grass pastures respectively, by growing and mature horses grazing 2 percent of BW/day (as DM). Ingestion by weanlings is estimated.

Mature horses, even those in heavy work grazing "average" pastures at 2% of BW/day would ingest sufficient P, Ca, and K to meet their requirements. However, if grazing pastures containing these minerals at the lower end of the normal range, only K would be in sufficient quantity to meet their needs for all types of level of work, whereas P and Ca would be deficient in horses performing moderate or heavy work. Likewise, K would generally be in excess for growing horses and mares in early lactation. Amounts of P and Ca ingested by lactating and pregnant mares grazing "average" pastures at 2–2.5% of BW/day (as DM) would be marginal for their requirements but would be deficient if grazing swards containing lower than average levels of these minerals. Although the Ca : P ratio in forages is often favorable for horses (Ca : P 2 : 1 or at least 1 : 1) there are occasions when such ratios have been found to be reversed (Lush 1934) and 30% of samples taken throughout the year from pastures in Germany had Ca : P ratios of <1.0 (M. Coenen, personal communication) but there was no apparent effect of seasonality. Such widespread inverted Ca : P ratios is a concern, particularly where such pastures constitute the entire diet for pregnant mares and young, growing horses, where correct bone formation could be severely compromised.

Na, Zn and Cu would all be deficient for all mature horses irrespective of their level of work grazing "average" pastures, as well as for growing horses pregnant and lactating mares. Indeed, Na, Zn, and Cu levels in north-central Virginia pastures were all found to be insufficient to meet the published requirements for growth and pregnancy, necessitating year-round supplementation, and Ca and P were deficient in the fall requiring targeted, seasonal supplementation with these nutrients (Cubitt et al 2004) (Table 18-10).

Key Points

- Providing there is sufficient herbage available, the energy content of most pastures should be sufficient to meet the maintenance energy requirements of mature horses. Mares in early lactation, growing horses and those that are heavily exercised may need energy supplementation when on pastures of low (less than 11–12 MJ DE/kg DM) DE content.
- Protein contents of average pastures should meet the needs of all classes of horse, but lactating mares, growing horses and heavily exercised horses grazing pastures of low protein content will require high quality protein supplementation.
- Pastures are nearly always deficient in sodium and often in zinc and copper, and these should be supplied as supplements. Extra calcium can be provided as a precaution against unfavorable Ca : P ratios.

Stocking density and grazing systems

Stocking density refers to the number of animals that are kept on a given unit of area. Over- and undergrazing both lead to deterioration of pastures. Overgrazing can be defined as when the level of grazing exceeds the recovery capacity of the herbage (~O' Beirne-Ranelagh 2005). Obvious signs of overgrazing include fields with visible horse droppings with horses grazing near them, bare soil patches, little grass and many weeds. Horses can graze down to 1 cm and horse pastures are frequently overstocked and overgrazed. Repeated and aggressive defoliation causes a concomitant reduction in the roots, as there is insufficient photosynthate being produced by the residual leaves to support a large root system (Weaver 1950). Likewise, a stunted root system cannot harvest sufficient nutrients from the soil to support a large growth of above ground tissues, and so a downward spiral of plant production can occur. Over time this results in a decrease in favorable, palatable species, which never have time to recover and these eventually disappear, with a concomitant ingress of weeds (Earl & Jones 1996). Continual, chronic overgrazing can eventually lead to the field becoming no more than an exercise area, with impoverished sward cover contributing little to the nutritional needs of the horse. Undergrazed fields will also deteriorate, as selective grazing of young, palatable herbage results in maturation and spread of less palatable species. Thus, mature, low quality forage accumulates and as the proportion of dead material increases, the pasture becomes unpalatable, reducing opportunities for selective grazing. Eventually, undergrazed pastures can revert to scrubland, and then woodland (Harper 1977, Jefferson & Robertson 2000).

To make best use of horse pastures, and maintain their desired productivity, it is important to stock them appropriately. Assuming that the annual forage requirements of the horse are to be met as grazed herbage and conserved as hay/haylage, the stocking density of a pasture is largely dictated by its average dry matter yield and the size of the horses therein. As the average yield of a pasture depends on the plant species it contains, soil type, pH and fertility, rainfall, temperature, light intensity etc., average yields may range from less than 1 t/ha annually for some extensive unimproved pastures to more than 25 tonnes DM/ha in highly productive, improved grassland (Hopkins et al 1990, Mayne et al 2000) and it is therefore impossible to give a precise, single stocking density for all pastures and horses. Therefore, some form of calculation needs to be made to estimate the correct stocking density for a given pasture. This can be accomplished most precisely in terms of calculating current and annual DM yield.

There are a number of ways to estimate DM yield. The first and probably most accurate method is to measure the DM content of the herbage cut at 5–6 cm above soil level, within a number (10–20) of 1 m^2 quadrats. The amount of DM from the different samples is averaged, and scaled up to give a value in terms of t/ha. The second commonly used method is to use a rising plate meter, that estimates both height and density of the sward and the resultant values converted to kg DM/ha. Measurements with the plate meter are taken every 5 m or so whilst walking a "W" through the field. A third, and possibly the most used but probably the least accurate method, is to measure sward height. This method takes no account of plant density. However, there are "rule of thumb" approximations of DM yield based on per inch of forage height. Thus an inch of the following grasses is estimated to equate to (in kg DM/ha), orchardgrass 202, tall fescue 235, bahiagrass 319, Bermuda grass 291 and alfalfa 252 (Lemus and Parish 2008).

Each of these methods as described above relates to forage DM yield at the time of sampling. The sum of values obtained when these methods are repeated throughout the growing season will give an estimate of annual yield for that pasture. To estimate annual forage DM yield under grazing conditions, cutting every 3–4 weeks, with four plots harvested weekly in rotation is widely used (Corrall & Fenlon

Table 18-11 Effect of Annual DM Yield on Area Required Per Horse to Meet the Annual DM Needs of Equids of Different Sizes

			Effect of annual DM yield on area (ha) required per horse to meet annual DM needs		
Body weight (kg) of horse	Daily DM *requirement (kg)	Annual DM requirement (t)	2.5 t DM/ha	5.0 t DM/ha	10.0 t DM/ha
250	5	1.8	0.73 (0.9–11.2)[a]	0.36 (0.45–0.63)	0.18 (0.23–0.32)
350	7	2.5	1.0 (1.25–1.75)	0.5 (0.63–0.88)	0.25 (0.31–0.44)
450	9	3.3	1.3 (1.63–2.27)	0.66 (0.77–1.2)	0.33 (0.41–0.58)
550	11	4.0	1.6 (2.0–2.8)	0.8 (1.0–1.4)	0.4 (0.5–0.7)
650	13	4.8	2.0 (2.5–3.5)	1.0 (1.25–1.75)	0.5 (0.63–0.89)

*Calculated at 2% BW/day.
[a]NB. The values in parenthesis are range of areas required assuming wastage of pasture due to defecation, urination and trampling. Such wastage can mount to 50–75% in continuous grazing systems and 25–30% in rotational grazing. The magnitude of such losses will vary greatly with the size of paddock, forage species, soil type, presence of trees, and prevailing weather.

1978). Although DM yield within a given pasture can vary considerably from year to year, estimates of DM yield may allow some broad pasture utilization strategies to be formulated for the following year. Table 18-11 gives estimates as to areas required to provide sufficient annual forage for different sizes of equidae from pastures of varying annual DM yield. Grazing is not an efficient process, and there can be considerable forage wastage during grazing, due to trampling, urination and defecation. It has been estimated that 50–75% may be wasted on continuously grazed pastures and 25–30% on those rotationally grazed (Mayne et al 2000). Thus when calculating the required area for a certain DM yield under grazing conditions then due account should be taken of such wastage.

If however, there is doubt as to the productivity of the pasture, and that it is accepted that some supplementary feed may be required by horses grazing poorly producing swards, and some means of controlling excess growth will be required at times of high production on more productive pastures, an allowance of 1 ha per 500 kg horse should provide sufficient grazing activity during the growing season (NRC 2007) and a suitable exercise area for the animals. If pastures are stocked more densely, then both the pastures and the horses will require more intensive management to keep both in good health (O'Beirne-Ranelagh 2005).

Grazing systems

Balancing changing pasture production on the one hand and animal forage requirements on the other, is key to efficient use of available grazing. This, together with maintaining pastures in a vegetative state stack the odds in favor of maximizing forage utilization during the growing season.

As grasses often grow some two to five times more quickly in spring (cool season grasses) or summer (warm season grasses) than in late autumn, there can be an early season oversupply of grass. If forage quality is to be maintained as a dense, leafy sward, this oversupply needs to be managed to prevent plant maturation and declines in digestibility. Adding extra horses, sheep or cattle to such pastures or in set stocking situations, closing up a proportion of the pasture for conservation as hay or haylage for winter feeding can address this problem. The aftermath of a hay/haylage crop can be re-grazed some 4–6 weeks post-harvest. If pasture productivity is to be maintained, the post-harvest stubble should be appropriately fertilized, to replace the nutrients removed in the crop.

Continuous grazing

Year-round continuous grazing in the truest sense only occurs on very extensive grazing systems such as hills and rangeland, where stocking density is low (Mayne et al 2000). Continuous grazing of smaller areas often results in the increasing dominance of less-desirable pasture species. When horses graze without restriction, they eat the most palatable species first. If grazed hard without being allowed time to recover, they will eventually die and roughs containing less preferred species spread, resulting in reduced pasture production and quality. For "good-doers", or those prone to laminitis, reduced pasture productivity may be considered an asset. However, for situations where productivity is to be maintained, the decline can be alleviated by co-grazing with other species such as sheep or cattle that have different herbage preferences, or if other livestock are not available, regular topping to prevent maturation and seeding of less preferred species will help. Harrowing of roughs will remove dead grass and help increase the fertility of overgrazed lawns. If the area is large enough, the deterioration will be gradual, but it is an inefficient system and if it carries a set number of animals and is not managed, it is likely to result in under-grazing in spring and early summer and overgrazing in winter. However, this system is low input in terms of labour and provision of temporary fencing.

Rotational grazing

Rotational grazing is where grassland is sequentially grazed and then rested to allow post-grazing recovery of the herbage. The length of grazing and rest periods differs depending on herbage yield. This system aims to maintain the sward at a leafy vegetative state during the growing season and therefore maximizes the nutritive value and productivity of the sward. Thus, comparisons of rotationally grazed pastures often show greater yield, digestibility and animal performance when compared with continuous grazing systems (Bryant et al 1962). Between three and six paddocks are usually required for each group of horses, either as permanently fenced fields or through temporary division of an existing pasture, often by electric fencing.

During the growing season in temperate regions, where cool-season grasses are used, if three paddocks are used, each paddock can be grazed for 3 weeks allowing the other paddocks to recover for 6 weeks (Fig 18.4A). As a general rule, for cool-season grasses in the UK, the height of the sward should not be allowed to fall below 2.5 cm, in winter and preferably 5 cm in summer to allow effective regrowth to 8–15 cm. In other locations with different pasture productivity and forage species, the grazing and rest heights of the swards may differ from those given above (see Table 18-12). Nevertheless, the aim in rotational grazing remains the same, i.e., to graze off all of the herbage evenly to a given height by the end of the allotted grazing time. If the paddock is under-stocked, visible "spot" grazing may occur resulting in areas of long, overly mature herbage. If this occurs, the long herbage should be mown to the same height as the rest of the sward at the end of the grazing period. The size of the paddocks can be adjusted to accommodate times of lower or greater pasture growth.

During the late autumn rotations are usually longer and larger areas are grazed to minimize the effect of poaching. During the winter if sufficient herbage and land area is available the entire area can be grazed. However, care must be taken to ensure over-grazing does not occur, with irreparable damage to over-wintering plant crowns.

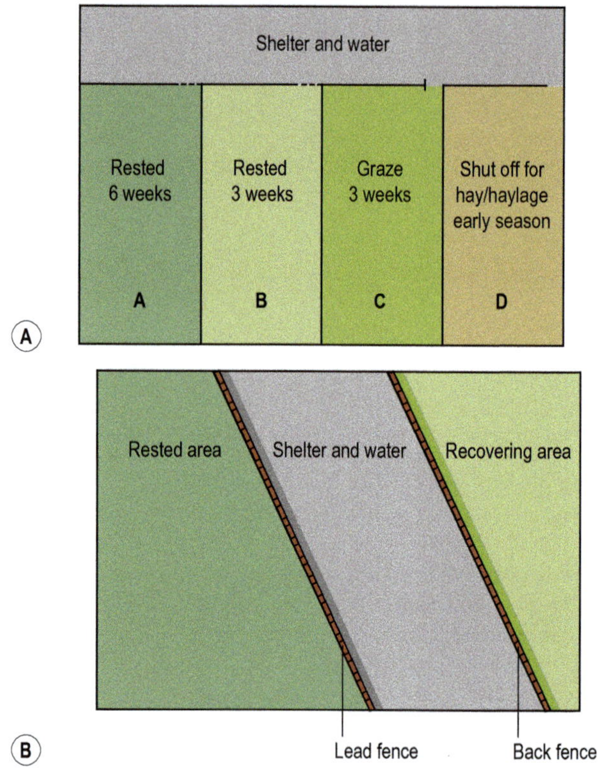

Figure 18.4 Schematic of rotational A) and strip B) grazing.

Table 18-12 Approximate 'Rule of Thumb' Sward Heights to Help Decision Making to Rest or Graze Pastures Containing Various Pasture Species, Together with Reported Annual Yields Achieved for Different Pasture Species

	Latin name	Minimum grazed height (cm)*	Grazing height (cm)	Yield (t/ha)
Cool season grasses				
Kentucky Bluegrass	*Poa pratensis*	5	8–20	5
Perennial Ryegrass	*Lolium perenne*	2.5–5	8–20	15
Smooth brome grass	*Bromus inermis*		10–15 or >22.5	12
Orchard grass	*Dactylis glomerata*	5–7.5	15–20	15
Tall fescue	*Festuca arundinacea*	5–7.5	10–15 or >22.5	12
Timothy	*Phleum pratense*	5	10–15	2–8
Creeping red fescue	*Festuca rubra*	2.5	5	2–5
Semi-improved grassland in Welsh uplands		5	5–10	2.8–4.0
White clover	*Trifolium repens*	2.5	<3	3–7
Alfalfa	*Medicago sativa*	10	20	2–16
Warm season grasses				
Bermuda grass	*Cynodon dactylis*	2.5–5	12.5	12
Small grains	*Avena sativa, Hordeum vulgare*	5–10	20	4–10
Big Bluestem	*Andropogon* sp.	15	22.5–50	17
Dallisgrass	*Paspalum dialtatum*	5	10–20	5–15
Bahiagrass	*Paspalum notatum*	5	15	6

*Height at which pastures should be rested to allow plant recovery.
Information from USDA NRCS (1997) and Williams, et al (2003).

Temporary division of existing fields requires that due attention be given to access to water and shelter (man-made or natural – trees, hedges, banks, etc.) for each of the paddocks. Water troughs can be moved, or a system of alleyways from side-by-side paddocks to permanently sited water troughs can be adopted. However, unless on hard standing this area can become very muddy if the weather is wet.

Strip grazing

A further type of rotational grazing is where strip-grazing is employed. Here electric fencing is used, the fence being moved forward a little every day or so to provide fresh grazing. A back fence in such systems is essential to allow the previously grazed grass to rest and recover without being over-grazed or trampled, and this can have droppings removed or harrowed, and be appropriately fertilized if necessary as it will not be grazed for some time (Fig 18.4B). Strip grazing provides the added advantage in that horses are never suddenly exposed to an entire paddock of fresh grass, and is also a useful way of restricting intake for animals predisposed to obesity and laminitis.

Sacrificial paddocks

Where the land area is insufficient to support grazing throughout the year, or the land is very wet, adopting a "sacrificial" paddock is a useful strategy. This is where a smaller area is used for turnout and the sward is allowed to be destroyed through poaching and overgrazing, and then is re-seeded and allowed to recover the following year. Sacrificial paddocks save the remaining fields from being damaged during the winter, periods of high precipitation or reduced growth due to drought.

Key Points

- Correct stocking density varies with time of year but can be managed for maximum herbage utilization
- Continuous stocking is the easiest system but may result in inefficient utilization of herbage
- Rotational or strip grazing allows better and targeted herbage utilization, but requires manpower to implement.
- Sacrificial paddocks can prevent the main grazing areas becoming damaged

Pasture manipulation

Pasture productivity and composition can be manipulated purely through grazing management. Different species start their growth at different times in spring, so a variety of species and cultivars is desirable to maximize productivity and to extend the grazing season (Baker et al 1965, Mayne et al 2000). The botanical composition of the sward may also be manipulated through different grazing strategies. Thus, productive ryegrasses benefit from being rested in winter and early spring and being grazed fairly hard throughout the late spring/summer and during the autumn "flush". However, their persistence can be reduced if grazed throughout the winter, and if not provided with sufficiently high N inputs. Conversely, other species such as crested dogstail, rough stalked meadow grass and white clover, that are resistant to cold and trampling and can thrive on less fertile soils may be grazed over the winter and rested at their peak growth period. This can allow them to compete with more productive, dominant species that require greater nutrient inputs that have been disadvantaged by winter grazing and reduced soil fertility (O'Beirne-Ranelagh 2005).

There are some situations where horse owners may wish to reduce the productivity of a sward by reducing the fertility of the soil. For example, improved pastures previously intended for maximizing outputs from highly productive ruminants need to be modified before they are grazed by horses if problems of obesity, laminitis, colic, etc. are to be averted. Taking a number of sequential hay or haylage crops without the addition of any fertilizer applied either by man or as excretory returns by grazing animals, will gradually reduce the fertility of the soil. As the N status of the soil declines, other pasture species will appear that are less reliant on high fertilizer inputs and the pasture will eventually return to a multi-species sward suitable for grazing horses. Alternatively, pastures that have been undergrazed during the spring and early summer that contain overly mature/stemmy, poor quality and relatively unpalatable herbage can provide grazing for "good-doers". Methods of changing pasture productivity and long-term botanical composition are described by O'Beirne-Ranelagh (2005).

Pastures for laminitis-prone equidae

It must be remembered that the nutrient requirements of horses differs between horses due to physiological status, age, size, workload and temperament (NRC 2007). The energy and protein requirements of mature animals which do little work are relatively modest, and can easily be met by moderate quality fresh or conserved pasture. In the wild, horses become fat in the summer which is utilized during the winter when herbage is scarce, and so at the beginning of spring are in lean condition. However, in domesticated equidae that are fed to maintain body weight year round and performing little work, such a cycle of "feast or famine" seen in wild equidae does not occur, with the domesticated "pasture pet" becoming increasingly rotund with each passing year. Obesity and overconsumption of NSC is associated with the onset of insulin resistance (IR) and laminitis (Treiber et al 2006). The NSC content of grasses can be substantial. Thus, cool-season species such as perennial and Italian ryegrass, cocksfoot and timothy can all accrue substantial levels of NSC, often above 200 g/kg DM, and perennial ryegrass varieties bred for high sugar content contained up to 330 g WSC/kg DM (Halling et al 2005) and more than 400 g WSC/kg DM was found in *Bromus* sp. (Chatterton et al 1989). Although the NSC contents of warm-season species are generally lower than those of cool-season grasses (warm season species accumulate starch as their storage carbohydrate whereas cool season species accrue fructan) leaves of warm-season grasses may contain 160 g starch/kg DM or more at peak periods (Wilson & Ford 1971).

Any factor that reduces growth, but maintains or increases photosynthesis will result in accumulation of reserve carbohydrates. Environmental factors that can encourage accumulation of high NSC contents include high light intensity, drought (Volaire and Lelievre, 1997), cool temperatures

(Chatterton et al 1989), nitrogen deficiency (McGrath et al 1997, Morvan-Bertrand et al 1999) and phosphorus deficiency (Wang & Tilberg 1997). Conversely, shade (Ciavarella et al 2000) warm temperatures (Chatterton et al 1989), fertilizer application (Jacobs et al 1989), and sufficient soil moisture can all decrease NSC content. Similarly, maintaining swards at an actively growing vegetative stage or those that have senesced will decrease NSC.

It should be noted that herbage NSC levels undergo diurnal fluctuations, reflecting photosynthetic activity on the one hand and utilization, translocation to and storage in distant organs on the other. Thus, on sunny days, particularly when conditions are cool, NSC accumulates during the day to be utilized and/or mobilized during the night to various sinks (Bowden et al 1968, Holt & Hilst 1969). WSC contents in perennial ryegrass on a sunny spring day rose from 250 g WSC/kg at 5 am to 310 g WSC/kg DM at 1–3pm declining to 180 g WSC/kg by 11pm (Longland 2005).

Conversely, on dull warm, damp days on fertile soils growth is rapid, there are fewer fluctuations in forage NSC content, as photosynthate production and utilization are more evenly balanced and NSC does not accumulate so readily. For example on a mild, October day with cloud cover and light rain, the same perennial ryegrass sward as sampled in the spring contained 150 gWSC/kg DM at 6 am, 1 pm and 8 pm, dipping to 120 g WSC/kg at 2 pm (Longland 2005). Thus grazing animals susceptible to laminitis should not be allowed access to pastures that have been subjected to environmental factors that encourage NSC accumulation in spring and autumn when NSC levels are highest or to those that have been overgrazed exposing plant crowns (i.e., NSC storage organs). Furthermore, laminitis-prone animals should not have unlimited access to very dense, healthy, leafy swards, which although per leaf may be low in NSC, the total amount consumed could be high (Watts & Pollitt, 2010).

Weed control

Plants that are growing where they are not wanted are regarded as weeds, and those that are toxic to horses should be eradicated. Weeds will appear on over-grazed, poached or bare land. The best form of weed control is to maintain a dense, vigorously growing sward. However, there will inevitably be occasions when weeds do appear. If there are just a few weeds, these can be removed mechanically by pulling or cutting, or being grazed off by other species (Popay & Field 1996), e.g. hard grazing by sheep will remove docks (*Rumex* sp.). Warm-season grass pastures can be cut down to 10 cm (4 inches) to remove or weaken weeds in early spring before the grasses have started to grow and again at 14 cm (6 inches) before the grasses have grown that high (Barnhart 1994). Otherwise, weeds may be treated by appropriate herbicide application. Blanket application of herbicide is not recommended, even those designed for use on grassland, as this can result in destruction of useful species of forbs, and reduction in species diversity. Instead, targeted application of herbicide is recommended. This can be achieved by "spot" treatment with a backpack sprayer, or if taller than the desired crop, weeds can be treated with a weed wiper, a device that can be passed over the entire field but herbicide is only applied to those standing proud of the sward (Lewis & Hopkins 2000). If herbicide is used, horses need to be removed from the pasture until the treated pasture is deemed safe for grazing. The length of time required may range from 24 hours or less to several weeks depending on the herbicide used and manufacturer's instructions.

Pasture toxicity

A number of pasture grasses and pasture weed species may be toxic to horses, usually either through production of toxins by the plants themselves or as a result of microbial parasitism or disease. More rarely some pasture species grown on heavily contaminated land may accrue toxic levels of heavy metals or other poisonous agents.

Inherent plant toxins

Various weeds are poisonous to horses, the most notorious include ragwort (*Seneccio* sp.), which produces hepatotoxic pyrrolizidine alkaloids that cause cumulative, irreversible liver damage, and if continued access is not prevented, death (Elcock & Oehme 1982, Gilles 1983). All parts of yew (*Taxus baccata*) are highly toxic to horses, containing the alkaloid taxane. The foliage remains toxic even when wilted or dried, death is rapid after consumption, with a lethal dose of 200–400 mg/kg body weight (Tiwary et al 2005). The roots of water hemlock (water dropwort, *Oenanthe crocata*), are highly toxic, containing oenanthotoxin, and death ensues soon after consumption. Other highly toxic weeds include *Solanum* species (the various nightshades and potato leaves/stems), bracken (*Pteridium aquilinum*), hemlock (*Conium maculatum*), horsetails (*Equisetum* sp), and *Rhododendron* sp.

In addition to weeds, various pasture species may also be toxic to horses. Various *Sorghums* species (e.g., Johnson hybrid grass and Sudan grass) all produce cyanogenic glycosides, which can accumulate to particularly high levels in young plants. Likewise, some varieties of white clover can be cyanogenic (Clarke et al 1990). All cyanogenic species/varieties should be avoided in horse pastures. Alsike clover (*Trifolium hybridum*) should be avoided as this contains hepatotoxic alkaloids (Cheeke & Schull 1985). Furthermore, varieties of Kikuyu grass (*Pennisetum clandestinum*) and some setaria species can contain high levels of oxalate as well as phytate causing calcium and phosphorus deficiencies (Williams 1987). All ragwort and other poisonous plants should be removed from paddocks, and paddock boundaries (e.g., hedges) should be checked for evidence of poisonous plants that might be within the reach of pastured horses. Poisonous plants can also appear in paddocks from unexpected sources. For example plants or plant parts may be deposited or blown into paddocks; clippings or branches of yew for example or water hemlock roots exposed in paddocks after receding river flooding or during ditch clearance etc. can all result in multiple and rapid fatalities of horses.

Microbial contamination

Contamination of pasture species by fungi either as pathogens or endophytes that produce mycotoxins can result in deterioration in equine health and performance, and pastures with high levels of fungal contamination should be avoided. *Claviceps* sp. produces sclerotia (ergots) causing ergot disease in a number of grass and small grain species including the ryegrasses, dalligrass, and canarygrass as well as various native species. Ergots produce a range of highly toxic alkaloids (e.g., ergotamine), which can cause death within hours of ingestion (Cheeke & Schull 1985). As ergots are found in seed heads, keeping pastures at a vegetative stage of growth will prevent contamination by ergots.

Endophytes are fungi which live inside a plant in a mutualistic or symbiotic relationship. The endophyte *Neotyphodium coenophialum* inhabits tall fescue, and produces the toxic alkaloid ergovaline, causing late abortion in broodmares, and impaired growth of youngstock (Lewis, et al 1997). *Neotyphodium lolii* infects perennial ryegrass and produces lolitrem B, an alkaloid that causes "ryegrass staggers" (Stynes & Bird 1983). However, there are endophyte-free, or non-toxic endophyte varieties of tall fescue and perennial ryegrass available; these are preferred for horse pastures.

Mineral contamination

Alfalfa grown in areas contaminated with high selenium levels, can accrue toxic levels of this micronutrient, leading to selenium toxicosis (Davies et al 2004). There is a view that high levels of nitrate ingestion can be poisonous to horses. Heavily fertilized pastures can lead to high levels of nitrate accumulating in the herbage (Allison 1998)

Key Points

- Weeds should be controlled
- Poisonous plants should be removed. If herbicides are used to kill poisonous plants, the dead material should be removed before allowing horses back onto the paddocks.
- Fields should be regularly checked for poisonous plants

Soil

The ideal horse pasture is on well-drained, fertile soils, yet most owners have to make the best of whatever soil is in their pastures. However, knowledge of the soil type and structure within pastures can aid in maximizing strategies for managing horse pastures effectively, as different soils have a significant impact on drainage, nutrient status and plant growth in horse paddocks.

Soil contains four main constituents, minerals, organic matter, water and air. There are three main types of soil, which are classified according to the size of the soil particles (soilnet.com). These are clay soils with a particle size of less than 0.002 mm in diameter, silts which range from 0.002–0.02 mm, and sandy soils which have particles from 0.02–2 mm in diameter. Soils are often referred to in terms of their texture, as being light, medium, or heavy. Light soils have a high sand content, are free draining resulting in rapid leaching of nutrients and a propensity to suffer in drought. Medium soils contain a significant amount of silt, and hold water and nutrients better than sandy soils, whereas heavy soils contain large amounts of clay, which hold nutrients well, but can become easily water logged due to slow movement of water through the small air spaces (Royal Horticultural Society UK website). Soil type/texture can be accurately determined in a laboratory, or more crudely by hand, following a series of questions in a key. Together with pH and nutrient analysis, laboratories should be able to advise, within the limitations of the soil type, on best management practice for that soil for horse pastures.

Soil structure refers to how soil particles associate with each other to form "crumbs" or larger structures. Soil structure is influenced by drying, wetting, microbial and animal (earthworm/insect) activity, root growth, organic matter and pH. Soils with favorable organic matter content will tend to be more stable in structure than those which are low in organic material. Soil structure can be determined by digging a hole and scraping the sides to see if the soil is a solid mass of individual soil particles or "crumbly", due to the presence of organic matter.

There are numerous soil types throughout the world, which support varying amounts of pasture growth. In general, however, digging a hole to about 1 m will allow the soil type to be assessed. Paddocks with "brown earth", often showing a gradual change in color or more discrete layers of color, with unrestricted root growth and invertebrate activity are likely to support good pasture growth, although the pH and drainage should be checked and amended as necessary. Soils which have a thin layer of brown soil covering a grayish colored wet soil, with little root growth or invertebrate activity in the gray soil will not encourage good plant growth, will be susceptible to poaching, and may need specialist assistance to rectify. Conversely, sandy soils where nutrients are easily leached from the upper layers, will not support good plant growth, but will be resistant to poaching.

Chalky soils (calcareous) are where brown soil covers chalk. This is a free-draining soil; resistant to deep poaching, but the degree of pasture growth will depend largely on the depth of the brown, top soil. Soils with a high content of organic material may be fertile and retain moisture reasonably well, but can become waterlogged if it overlies impermeable rock, but plants may succumb to drought in summer as soils very high in organic matter (e.g., peat) can dry out easily, and do not encourage deep rooting.

For soils to support proper plant growth they should be properly drained. Flooding occurs when water is unable to move away from the soil sufficiently quickly. Maintenance of existing ditches is important in this regard and can do much to alleviate localized and temporary flooding. Ditch sides should be shallower in sandy soils and can be deeper in heavier soils, which tend to be more stable. It is important that the ditch is deep enough to be below all drainage outlets and allow free drainage of surface run-off. If fields are very wet, it may be worth having a drainage system laid. This can consist of a series of underground pipes which then drain into a ditch or other waterway. Heavy soils may support "mole drains" where a "moler" opens up channels within the soil to allow drainage into ditches, and may remain patent for 10 years or more. However, the life expectancy of mole drains may be lengthened when used in conjunction with pipes (Thomasson 1975)

Key Points

- Soil type should be assessed for appropriate management strategies to be employed
- Good drainage is essential for good pasture productivity and should be maintained regularly

Seminatural grasslands

Many seminatural grasslands are frequently species rich, containing 30–40 species per m^2 (Wells 1975), and if stocked correctly can provide ideal extensive grazing grounds for maintaining horses, producing sustainable forage of mediocre nutritive value for both grazing and hay (Jefferson & Robertson 2000). However, all too often, fenced grazing areas are too small, resulting in overgrazing, reduction in species diversity, increase in bare ground and ingress of weeds such as ragwort, docks and thistles, resulting in horsesick pastures. However, if grazed lightly, with sward heights maintained at a minimum of 5 cm, horses can be used as conservation tools to maintain species diversity in neutral semi-natural grasslands.

Manure management

There are three main ways of controlling the development of spreading latrines: through harrowing, removal of droppings or managed latrines. Harrowing breaks up the droppings and spreads the manure more evenly across the field, helping prevent the highly localized, lush, rank growth of roughs. As harrowing spreads the manure, it also spreads internal parasites (e.g., worms) around the pasture. However, harrowing undertaken in warm, dry weather should result in desiccation of the droppings and the demise of the parasites. After harrowing, the pasture needs to be rested, often for 6 weeks or more, (a) to allow the manure dry out and kill the parasites and (b) for the manure to biodegrade and the surrounding pasture become palatable once again for horses. In addition to breaking up and spreading manure, harrowing also aerates the soil, pulls out dead grass, weeds etc. and through gently disturbing the soil surface can release minerals that can then be utilized by the growing plants.

Regular, ideally daily, removal of droppings ("poo-picking") from pastures allows the horses to continue to graze the paddock, without the build up of latrines. It is a labour intensive activity but will help maximize the use of available grazing, particularly in small paddocks. However, the problem then arises of what to do with the collected manure. A 500 kg horse will generally produce about 25 kg of manure per day which equates to ~9 tonnes per year. The manure typically contains ca. 5 kg N, 0.9 kg P, and 3.6 kg K per tonne (Westerndorf 2004) and thus is a valuable source of nutrients. The manure can be composted for spreading on fields at a later date, and if correctly composted, parasite eggs should be destroyed. If the manure is to be spread directly or before the composting process is complete, then it is better used on fields to be grazed by other species to prevent reinfection of horses. A review of composting manure from horse pastures is outside the scope of this article: instead the reader is directed to the various fact sheets provided by the extension centers by various universities.

A system of "managed" latrines has been proposed by O'Beirne-Ranelagh (2005), whereby two or three areas of pasture, containing less preferred species of herbage are chosen to become latrines. Droppings are picked up from elsewhere and deposited on these small and managed sites. Eventually, horses will learn to use these designated latrines, and droppings can be partially removed to stop the area of the latrines spreading. This system prevents the best parts of the pasture becoming latrines, and confines contamination by parasites to localized areas.

Each of these three systems has both advantages and disadvantages. Removal of droppings or creating artificial latrines still requires that the lawns be managed and fertilized to prevent their gradual decline, whereas harrowing is a seasonal activity and should not be carried out when the soil is wet and muddy.

Fertilization

As noted above, paddocks, and especially any lawns within them can become depleted of nutrients such as N, P, K, S, and Mg as well as other trace elements, through their continual transfer to roughs, through retention of minerals by the grazing animals, and loss to hay or haylage that is removed from the field. Therefore, in order to retain field fertility, it is necessary to replace these lost nutrients. However, the very rapid and lush growth that is encouraged by high fertilizer inputs to maximize meat and milk production by farm livestock are neither required nor desirable in pastures for horses. Instead, a more modest, even growth is preferable.

Fertilizers are classified as either inorganic (artificial fertilizers) or organic. Inorganic fertilizers are minerals that have been manufactured or mined, whereas organic fertilizers are of biological origin. These can be semiorganic (e.g., calcified seaweed) or wholly organic (e.g., farmyard manure). There is a perception by many horse owners that inorganic fertilizers are bad and semiorganic and organic fertilizers are good for horse pastures. However, this is not really the case; it is how the fertilizers are used that is important. Inorganic fertilizers are likely to be chemically purer and faster acting than their organic counterparts, whereas organic fertilizers act more slowly, making timing of application less critical and may not require split applications during the season.

Before fertilizing horse pastures, it is wise to have the soil pH and mineral status analyzed every 3–5 years to maximize the efficiency of the preferred fertilization program. The pH of the soil can greatly affect the availability of nutrients and a pH of around 6.5–7 is usually optimal for grass growth. In soils with a pH of 5 or lower most macrominerals e.g. N, P, K, Ca, and Mg are less available and with a pH much above 7 the availability of many micro minerals such as Fe, Mn, Zn, Cu, Co, and Al declines (Barker & Collins 2003). If the pasture pH is less than ca. 5–5.5 it should be raised via the application of lime. It takes considerable time (several months) for lime to raise soil pH and is most usefully applied at the end of the growing season. Lime can be obtained in a number of forms and may also contain other minerals such as magnesium or calcium to redress deficiencies known to be a problem in certain areas. There are usually one or two types of lime used within a given locality which the local contractor can advise upon. Correcting soil pH is essential as there is little point adding fertilizers to soils that render the fertilizer unavailable to the plants. The single most important nutrient required for herbage growth is nitrogen (N) (Younie 2000) followed by P and K. In addition to soil pH, many analytical laboratories will provide a report as to the mineral status (usually P, K and Mg levels) of the soil, and make recommendations as to how much of each element is required to redress deficiencies within a given field. Alternatively, the laboratory may convert the value to an index figure for ease of fertilizer application. If this index figure is above 2 for either P or K, then the soil contains enough of that mineral for grass growth. If the index is below 2, then addition of P and K is required, and can be applied annually.

As N is easily leached from soil and if applied as a single large dose gives rise to rapid, lush growth, which then declines; inorganic N fertilizer is usually applied in several smaller doses throughout the growing season. Frape (1998) suggests the following annual application rates for N, P, and K for horse pastures (Table 18-13). The suggested amounts of nitrogen fertilizer are very small by agricultural standards and will not produce rapid growth and large amounts of lush grass, but are designed to encourage more even, moderate growth when split into two or three separate applications. Thus, for horse paddocks application of some 20–35 kg N/ha 3–6 weeks prior to the grazing season is appropriate, with a further two to three applications to grazed fields later in the season as part of a rotation program, up to a total of ca. 50–60 kg N/ha per annum. Horses should not be allowed to graze fertilized paddocks until some 3 weeks have elapsed since the fertilizer was applied: longer may be necessary if lack of rain has prevented the fertilizer being completely washed into the soil (Frape 1998).

Many inorganic fertilizers on the market contain a mixture of N, P, and K at different ratios. Other macrominerals required by plants include Ca, Mg, and S which are also available, together with trace elements such as Fe, Mn, Zn, Cu, Co, Bo, Si, and Cl. Trace elements required by horses but not necessarily plants include Se, I, and Ch.

Farmyard manure (FYM) is a further source of fertilizer. It is bulky to handle and is of varying composition (Table 18-14). It is important to realize that table values can only be approximations, and will vary according to what the animal was fed and the amount and type of bedding that was used. Analysis of FYM can help in allowing more precisely targeted applications to pastures, to redress specific deficiencies, otherwise use of FYM can be a somewhat "hit or miss" process. FYM is normally applied in early spring or late summer so that it can be used by actively growing plants. Sheep and cattle manures are frequently used in horse pastures.

Application of FYM encourages invertebrate and microbial activity and results in improved soil structure (Edmeades 2003). Furthermore, FYM only needs to be applied once per year as the release of nutrients is slow as the manure is biodegraded and incorporated into the soil. It is essential that this process has been completed prior to harvesting for hay or haylage, otherwise the final product may become contaminated with manure rendering it unsuitable for feeding. Fields treated with FYM should be closed for some 6 weeks or so before horses are allowed to graze it.

A further means of supplying N to pasture is by incorporating legumes (e.g., white clover) as a minority species into the sward. Legumes can do much to improve the nitrogen status of the soil through their ability to "fix" atmospheric nitrogen, which is then available for utilization by other plants. Indeed, N fixation in pastures as an inorganic N fertilizer equivalent is suggested to range from 47–80 kg N/ha per annum for temperate European conditions where clover accounts for 10–29% of the ground cover (Kristensen et al 1995).

Table 18-13 Annual Fertilizer Application Rates (kg/ha) for Horse Pastures in Relation to the Analytical Laboratory Fertilizer Index (after Frape 1998)

P or K index	N	P	K
0	20–50	60	60
1	20–50	30	30
2	20–50	20	20
>2	20–50	0	0

Table 18-14 Typical Composition of Some Farmyard Manures (Available Nutrients kg/tonne)

Manure type	DM	Nitrogen	Phosphate P_2O_5	Potash K_2O	Magnesium Mg
Cattle[a]	25	6	3.5	8	0.7
Pig[a]	25	7	7	5	0.7
Horse[b]	21	5	4.4	9.2	Not reported

[a]From Agricultural Budgeting and Costings Book, 58, 2004.
[b]From Westerndorf 2004.

Renovation and reseeding

Complete reseeding is probably only necessary when converting fields from arable use to grassland. Otherwise, even degraded, overgrazed grasslands can be renovated, and should not need to be ploughed up and re-seeded. Pasture renovation involves both restoring grass cover in high traffic areas and the introduction or re-introduction of desired species at the expense of those that currently exist in the sward. In the latter case, it is essential to correct the conditions that led to deterioration of the pasture in the first place if the renovation process is to be successful in the long term (Hopkins 1986). This may involve attention to drainage and soil nutrient status, or to changes in grazing management. Areas that have become devoid of grass cover due to poaching should be harrowed and seeded with hardy species that are resistant to treading (e.g., red fescue). Where desired forage species are being introduced or re-introduced into existing sward the first step is to remove all weeds (see above) as they will prevent good establishment of sown species and will be more difficult to eradicate later. Oversowing is the easiest method of introducing new seed, whereby the existing sward is cut or grazed hard, to reduce competition for the new seedlings. The sward can then be harrowed to open up bare patches, and under preferably damp conditions, the seed can be broadcast, or directly drilled into the soil. Light harrowing followed by light rolling will press broadcast seed into contact with the soil encouraging germination. Oversown areas need to be allowed to establish for several months or even a year before being grazed by horses. Grazing with sheep, however, during the first year of renovation can reap benefits through

Box 18.1 Pasture Maintenance Calendar

Spring

1. In early spring, soil should be tested every 3–5 years, to allow targeted fertilizer and lime applications. Soils should be sampled to a depth of 10 cm from ca. 20 sites per area, which are then thoroughly mixed and subsampled prior to analysis.
2. When the ground is dry enough to prevent soil damage by machinery, pastures should be harrowed to remove dead grass and shallow weeds, aerate the soil, and even out uneven areas due to poaching.
3. Re-seed bare patches
4. Apply fertilizer to encourage vigorous but not excessive herbage growth. N.B. do not apply lime and fertilizer at the same time as lime can cause volatilization of fertilizer N.
5. When the ground is dry enough, the pasture can be rolled to consolidate loose soil, even out rough areas and encourage tillering.
6. Some of the pasture can be closed off for hay/haylage.
7. Weed control is important at this point and throughout the growing season, and topping should be implemented to remove seedheads and other overly long plant parts.

Late spring/summer

1. Control grazing through rotation or strip grazing.
2. Prevent overgrazing.
3. Continue the "war on weeds".
4. If inorganic fertilizer is used a second application may be given to hayfields and a third after the hay is harvested.
5. Remove droppings daily from small paddocks or spread by harrowing in hot weather.
6. Modest application of fertilizer after horses have been removed from grazed paddocks on one or two occasions during the grazing season to boost herbage production to meet the DM demands of the horses.

Top (cut) areas of long, rank rough grass regularly.

Autumn

1. Continue to control grazing by rotational or strip grazing, enlarge the allotted areas as DM yield declines.
2. Be mindful of rapid "flush" of growth and graze appropriately.
3. Remove animals from pastures with 2.5–5 cm remaining growth. Cut pasture to this level if necessary.
4. Remove horses from wet pastures.
5. Apply lime as appropriate at end of growing season.

Winter

1. Put horses on well drained, slightly sloping pastures with a dense sward to help guard against poaching. The larger the area the better to prevent localized poaching along field margins and gateways. If there is insufficient suitable land area available to allow grazing throughout the winter, consider using a sacrificial paddock and feeding conserved forage during this time.
2. Pastures that are not properly drained are unlikely to perform well, and can quickly become muddy quagmires. Ditch maintenance, through keeping clear of vegetation and silt can do much to improve the situation. Maintain ditches, hedges and other fencing in winter.

All operations should be carried out with due attention for the welfare of wildlife, especially ground-nesting birds.

their lightweight trampling encouraging tillering coupled with their even grazing habits in producing a well-established, secure, densely tillered, sward.

Cool season pasture mixes containing species such as red fescue (as it can be high yielding, is highly palatable and resists poaching) crested dogstail (highly palatable to horses and requires little in terms of fertilizer inputs), timothy and meadow grasses (nutritious and produce a thick turf), and varying amounts of perennial ryegrass varieties (to increase productivity), depending on the type of horse to be grazed, plus or minus small amounts of white clover (to fix N) are suitable for horse pastures. Although many commercially available horse pasture seed mixes are based on perennial ryegrass varieties, they may be less suitable as they yield indifferently with low fertilizer inputs, and some cultivars produce very high levels of NSC which is undesirable for most horses. Sowing rates vary from ca. 8–30 kg seed/ha. Warm season pastures are often sown with mixes containing some of the following: Bermudagrass, bahiagrass, dallisgrass, big bluestem and alfalfa, and clover mixes with sowing rates of 12–30 kg/ha.

Sorghum and Sudan grass should not be sown in horse pastures due to potentially toxic prussic acid contents.

Management practices – a yearly calendar and summary

From the foregoing it is clear that to maintain healthy and productive horse pastures they need to be managed. The exact management differs with the seasons and location but a generalized pattern of management activities is presented in Box 18.1.

Conclusion

From a nutritional standpoint, good quality pasture can be viewed as that which provides all or the majority of the nutrient requirements of the animal. These requirements will be quite different for lactating mares, young stock, competition horses and "pasture pets". Overstocking leading to overgrazing is probably the single most important factor leading to horse pasture deterioration.

High quality pastures for horses should:

- Be neither over- nor undergrazed
- Be species-rich including various grasses, legumes and some forbs that are appropriate for the class of equid grazing them
- Have a dense, closed sward that resists trampling and weed ingress, and provides a safe surface for exercise
- Be maintained in a vegetative state
- Be free from weed infestation
- Be free from significant latrine areas.

The addition of safe fencing, natural or man-made shelter and well-positioned water supply are important features of well-managed, high quality pastures.

References

Allison, C.D., 1998. Nitrate poisoning of livestock. New Mexico State University Guide. B-802.

Archer, M., 1973. The species preferences of grazing horses. Grass and Forage Science 28 (3), 123–128.

Argo, C.McG., Cox, J.E., Lockyer, C., et al., 2002. Adaptive changes in the appetite, growth and feeding behaviour of pony mares offered *ad libitum* access to a complete diet in either a pelleted or chaff-based form. Animal Science 74, 517–528.

Baker, H.K., Chard, J.R.A., Hughes, E., 1965. A comparison of cocksfoot and tall-fescue dominant swards for out-of-season production. Journal of the British Grassland Society 20, 84–90.

Barker, D.J., Collins, M., 2003. Forage fertilization and nutrient management. In: Barnes, R.F., Miller, D.A., Nelson, C.J. (Eds.), Forages, Vol. 2. Iowa State University, Ames IA.

Barnhart, S., 1994. Warm season grasses for hay and pasture. Iowa State University Extension Service. Ames IA, p. 569.

Beever, D.A., Offer, N., Gill, E.M., 2000. The feeding value of grass and grass products. In: Hopkins, A. (Ed.), Grass its Production and Utilisation, third ed. Blackwell Science, Oxford, pp. 140–190.

Berger, A.K., Scheibe, K., Eichhorn, A., 1999. Diurnal and ultradian rhythms of behaviour in a mare group of Przewalski horse (*Equus ferus przewalski*) measured through one year in semi-reserve conditions. Applied Animal Behaviour Science 64, 1–17.

Bowden, D.M., Taylor, D.K., Davis, W.E.P., 1968. Water-soluble carbohydrates in orchardgrass and mixed forages. Canadian Journal of Plant Science 48, 9–15.

Brink, G.E., Fairbrother, T.E., Rowe, D.E., 1988. Seasonal variation in morphology of continuously stocked white clover. Crop Science 38, 1224–1228.

Brummer, E.C., Bouton, J.H., 1991. Plant traits associated with grazing tolerant alfalfa. Agronomy Journal 83, 996–1000.

Bryant, H.T., Blaser, R.E., Hammes, Jr., R.C., et al., 1962. Method for Increased Milk Production with Rotational Grazing. Journal of Dairy Science 44 (9), 1731–1741.

Clarke, S., Taylor, J., Smith, K., 1990. Winter growth, seed production and cyanogenic potential of white clovers under irrigation at Neuapur, Victoria. Report no 2. Dept of Agriculture and Rural Affairs, Victoria, Australia.

Chatterton, N.P., Harrison, J.A., Bennet, J.H., et al., 1989. Carbohydrate partitioning in 185 accessions of gramineae grown under warm and cool conditions. Journal of Plant Physiology 143, 169–179.

Cheeke, P.R., Schull, L.R., 1985. Natural toxicant in feeds and poisonous plants. AVI Publishing, Westport CT.

Ciavarella, T.A., Dove, H., Leury, B.J., et al., 2000. Diet selection by sheep grazing *Phalaris aquatica* L pastures differing in water-soluble carbohydrate content. Australian Journal of Agricultural Research 51, 757–764.

Corrall, A.J., Fenlon, J.S., 1978. A comparative method for describing the season distribution of production from grasses. Journal of Agricultural Science, Cambridge 91, 61–67.

Cubitt, T.A., Staniar, B., Kronfeld, D.S., et al., 2004. Seasonal variation in nutrient composition of pastures in North Central Virginia. Journal of Animal Science 82 (suppl 1), 96.

Davies, J.G., Steffens, T.J., Engle, T.E., et al., 2004. Preventing selenium toxicity. Colorado State University extension services. Fact sheet No 6.110. Colorado University State Extension Service Publications.

Earl, J.M., Jones, C.E., 1996. The need for a new approach to grazing management – is cell grazing the answer? The Rangeland Journal 18, 327–350.

Edmeades, D.C., 2003. The long-term effects of manures and fertilisers on soil productivity and quality: a review. Nutrient Cycling in Agroecosystems 66, 165–180.

Edouard, N., Fleurance, G., Martin-Rosset, W., et al., 2008. Voluntary intake and digestibility in horses: effect of forage quality with emphasis on individual variability Animal 2 (10), 1526–1533.

Elcock, L., Oehme, F.W., 1982. Senecio poisoning in horses: a summary. Veterinary and Human Toxicology 24, 122.

Ellis, A., 2010. Biological basis of behaviour in relation to nutrition and feed intake in horses. In: Ellis, A.D., Longland, A.C., Coenen, M., et al. (Eds.), The Impact of Nutrition on the Health and Welfare of Horses. EAAP Publication No, 128. Wageningen Academic Publishers, Wageningen.

Fleurance, G., Duncan, P., Fritz, H., et al., 2007. Selection of feeding sites by horses at pasture: testing the antiparasite theory. Applied Animal Behaviour Science 108, 288–301.

Frape, D., 1998. Equine Nutrition and Feeding. Blackwell Scientific, Oxford.

Gallacher, R., McMeniman, N.P., 1988. The nutritional status of pregnant and non-pregnant mares grazing South East Queensland pastures. Equine Veterinary Journal 20, 414–419.

Gebbing, T., Shyderm, H., Kuhbauch, W., 1999. The utilization of pre-anthesis reserves in grain filling of wheat. Assessment by steady-state $^{13}CO_2/^{12}CO_2$ labelling. Plant Cell and Environment 22, 851–858.

Gilles, C.J., 1983. Outbreak of ragwort (*Senecio jacobea*) poisoning in horses. Equine Veterinary Journal 15 (3), 248–250.

Guerrand, D., Prud'homme, M.P., Boucaud, J., 1996. Fructan metabolism in expanding leaves, mature leaf sheaths and mature leaf blades of *Lolium perenne*. Fructan synthesis, fructosyltransferase and invertase activities. New Phytologist 134, 205–214.

Grace, N.D., Gee, E.K., Firth, E.C., et al., 2002. Digestible energy intake, dry matter digestibility and mineral status of grazing New Zealand Thoroughbred yearlings. New Zealand Veterinary Journal 50, 63–69.

Green, J.O., Corrall, A.J.,Terry, R.A., 1971. Grass species and varieties: Relationships between stage of growth yield and forage quality. GRI Technical report No 8. Grassland Research Institute, Hurley.

Halling, M.A., Longland, A.C., Martens, S., et al., 2005. Water soluble carbohydrates content of two varieties of perennial ryegrass (*Lolium perenne*) at eight European sites. In: O'Mara, F.P., Wilkins, R.J., L.'t Mannetje, D.K., et al. (Eds.), Proceedings of the XX International Grassland Congress, Dublin, Ireland. Wageningen Academic Publishers, Wageningen.

Harper, J.L., 1977. Population Biology of Plants. Academic Press, London.

Holt, D.A., Hilst, A.R., 1969. Daily variation in carbohydrate content of selected forage crops. Agronomy Journal 61, 239–242.

Hopkins, A., 1986. Botanical composition of permanent grassland in England and Wales, in relation to soil, environmental and management factors. Grass and Forage Science 41, 237–246.

Hopkins, A., Gilby, J., Dibb, et al., 1990. Response of permanent and re-seeded grassland to fertiliser nitrogen. 1. Herbage production and herbage quality. Grass and Forage Science 45, 43–55.

Hunt, W.F., 1995. Pastures for horses: a New Zealand perspective. In: Proceedings of the Equine Nutrition and Pastures for Horses Workshop. Richmond, pp. 17–19

Jacobs, J., Rigby, S., McKenzie, et al., 1989. Effect of nitrogen on pasture yield and quality for silage in western Victoria. In: Proceedings of the Australian Agronomy Conference. Australian Society of Agronomy, Australia, pp. 29–32. www.regional.org.au/au/asa/1998/6465jacobs.htm.

Jefferson, R.G., Roberston, H.J., 2000. Grassland management for natural landscapes and wildlife. In: Hopkins, A. (Ed.), Grass its Production and Utilisation, third ed. Blackwell Science, Oxford, pp. 292–312.

Johnson, I.R., Parsons, A.J., 1985. Use of a model to analyse the effects of continuous grazing management on seasonal patterns of grass production. Grass and Forage Science 40, 449–458.

Kristensen, E.S., Høgh-Jensen, H., Kristensen, I.S., 1995. A simple model for estimation of atmospherically derived nitrogen in grass-clover systems. Biological Agriculture and Horticulture 12, 263–276.

Kuusela, E., 2006. Annual and seasonal changes in mineral contents (Ca, Mg, P, K and Na) of grazed clover-grass mixtures in organic farming. Agricultural and Food Science 15 (1), 23–34.

Lemaire, G., 1988. Sward dynamics under different management programmes. In: Proceedings of the 12th General meeting of the European Grassland Federation, Dublin. Irish Grassland Association, Belcare, Ireland, pp. 7–23.

Lemus, R., Parish, J., 2008. Assessing needs and feed sources – how much forage do I have? Mississippi State University Extension Service, Publications: No 2458.

Lewis, L., 1994. Feeding and Care of the Horse, second ed. Blackwell Publishing, Oxford.

Lewis, G.C., Ravel, C., Naffaa, W., et al., 1997. Occurrence of *Acremonium* endophytes in wild populations of *Lolium* spp. in European countries and a relationship between level of infection and climate in France. Annals of Applied Biology 130, 227–238.

Lewis, G.C., Hopkins, A., 2000. Weeds, pests and diseases of grassland. In: Hopkins, A. (Ed.), Grass its Production and Utilisation, third ed. Blackwell Science, Oxford, pp. 119–133.

Longland, A.C., 2005. Seasonal changes in the WSC, N and fibre content of swards managed for conservation or grazing. In: Theodorou, M.K. (Eds.), Grazing and ensiling of energy-rich grasses with elevated sugar content for the sustainable production of ruminant livestock. EU Framework 5 publication.

Longland, A.C., Barfoot, C., Harris, P.A., 2011. The effect of wearing a grazing muzzle vs. not wearing a grazing muzzle on pasture dry matter intake by ponies. Journal of Equine Veterinary Science 31 (5), 282–283.

Lush, R.H., 1934. Calcium and phosphorus content of pasture grasses and legumes. American Society of Animal Producers 1934, 254–257.

MAFF, 1992. (UK Ministry of Agriculture Fisheries and Food) Feed Composition UK Tables of Feed Composition and Nutritive Value for Ruminants, second ed. Chalcombe Publications, Canterbury, UK.

Martin, R.G., 1993. The effects of nitrogen and energy supplementation on grazing broodmares and aspects of nitrogen metabolism in horses. PhD Thesis, University of Queensland, Brisbane.

McMeniman, 2003. Pasture intakes by young horses. A report for the Rural Industries Research and Development Corporation, RIDRC publication no. 00W03/005. RIDRC, Kingston, ACT, Australia.

Mayne, C.S., Wright, I.A., Fisher, G.E.J., 2000. Grassland management under grazing and animal response. In: Hopkins, A. (Ed.), Grass its Production and Utilisation, third ed. Blackwell Science, Oxford, pp. 247–291.

Mayes, R.W., Dove, H., 2000. Measurement of dietary nutrient intake in free-ranging mammalian herbivores. Nutrition Research Reviews 13, 107–138.

McGrath, V.B., Blakeney, A.B., Batten, G.D., 1997. Fructan to nitrogen ratio as an indicator of nutrient stress in wheat crops. New Phytologist 1361, 145–152.

Morvan-Bertrand, A., Boucaud, J., Prud'homme, M., 1999. Influence of initial levels of carbohydrates, fructans, nitrogen and soluble proteins on re-growth of *Lolium perenne* L. cv. Bravo following defoliation. Journal of Experimental Botany 50, 1817–1826.

NRC, 2007. Nutrient Requirements of Horses, sixth ed. National Academies Press, Washington DC.

O'Beirne-Ranelagh, E., 2005. Managing grass for horses, the responsible owners guide. JA Allen, London.

Odberg, F.O., Francis-Smith, K., 1976. A study on eliminative and grazing behaviour - the use of the field by captive horses. Equine Veterinary Journal 8, 147–149.

Pavis, N., Boucaud, J., Prud'homme, M.P., 2000. Fructans and fructan-metabolizing enzymes in leaves of *Lolium perenne*. New Phytologist. 150, 97–109.

Popay, I., Field, R., 1996. Grazing animals as weed control agents. Weed Technology 10, 217–231.

Prache, S., 1996. Intake rate, intake per bite and time per bite of lactating ewes on vegetative and reproductive swards. Applied Animal Behaviour 52 (1), 53–64.

Robson, M.J., Ryle, G.J.A., Woledge, J., 1980. The grass plant - its form and function. In: Jones, M.B., Lazenby, A. (Eds.), The Grass Crop - The Physiological Basis of Production. Chapman & Hall, London, pp. 25–83.

Royal Horticultural Society UK. apps.rhs.org.uk/advicesearch.

Sheldrick, R., Newman, G., Roberts, D., 1995. Legumes for Meat and Milk, second ed. Chalcombe Publications, Canterbury, UK, pp. 15–74.

Silanikove, N., Holzer, Z., Cohen, D., et al., 1987. Interrelationship between metabolism of tritiated water, 22sodium and dry matter intake by beef cattle consuming wheat straw and poultry litter in free choice. Comp Biochem Physiol A Comp Physiol 88 (1), 113–118.

Slepetys, J., 2001. Changes in the chemical composition of grass seed and stem during the period of ripening. Biolojica 2, 57–61.

Smith, D.G., Mayes, R.W., Hollands, T., et al., 2007. Validating the alkane pair technique to estimate dry matter intake by equids. The Journal of Agricultural Science 145, 273–281.

Smith, D., 1967. Carbohydrates in grasses. II. Sugar and fructosan composition of the stem bases of bromegrass and timothy at several growth stages and in different plant parts at anthesis. Crop Science 7, 62.

Stynes, B.A., Bird, A.F., 1983. Development of annual ryegrass toxicity. Australian Journal of Agricultural Research 34, 653–660.

Thomasson, A.J., 1975. Soils and Field Drainage. Soils Survey Technical Monograph No. 7, Harpenden, UK, p. 80.

Tiwary, A.W., Puschner, B., Kinde, H., et al., 2005. Diagnosis of *Taxus* (yew) poisoning in a horse. Journal of Veterinary Diagnostic Investigation 17 (3), 252–255.

Treiber, K.H., Kronfeld, D.S., Hess, T.M., et al., 2006. Evaluation of genetic and metabolic predispositions and nutritional risk factors for pasture-associated laminitis in ponies. Journal of the American Veterinary Medicine Association 228, 1538–1545.

USDA NRCS, 1997. Conservation practice standard prescribed grazing. University of Nebraska G1198.

Van Dierendonck, M.C., Bandi, N., Batdorj, D., et al., 1996. Behavioural observations of re-introduced Takhi or Przewalski horses (*Equus ferus przewalski*) in Mongolia. Applied Animal Behaviour Science 50, 95–114.

Vulink, J.T., Cornelissen, P., Drost, H.J., et al., 2001. Hindgut fermentation is not an evolutionary dead end :comparative feeding ecology of cattle and horses. In: Vulink, J.T. (Ed.), Hungry Herds, Management of Temperate Lowland Wetlands by Grazing. Proefschrift Rijksuniversiteit Groningen, PhD Thesis. Ministerie van Verkeer and Waterstaat, Lelystad, the Netherlands.

Volaire, F., Lelievre, F., 1997. Production, persistence, and water-soluble carbohydrate accumulation in 21 contrasting populations of *Dactylis glomerata* L subjected to severe drought in the South of France. Australian Journal of Agricultural Research 48, 933–944.

Wang, C., Tilberg, J.E., 1997. Effect of short term phosphoros deficiency on carbohydrate storage in sink and source leaves of barley (*Hordeum vulgare*). New Phytologist 136, 131–135.

Watts, K., Pollit, C., 2010. Equine laminitis - managing pasture to reduce the risk. RIRDC, nirdc.gov.au.

Weaver, J.E., 1950. Effect of different intensities of grazing on depth and quantity of roots in grasses. Journal of Range Management 3, 100–113.

Wells TCE, 1975. The floristic composition of chalk grassland in Wiltshire. In: Stern, L.F. (Ed.), Supplement to the Flora of Wiltshire. Natural History Section of Wiltshire Archaeological and Natural History Society, Devizes, pp. 99–125.

Westerndorf, W., 2004. Horses and manure. Rutgers Equine Science Center Publications: Factsheet 036, Rutgers, New Brunswick.

Williams, T.A., Evans, D.R., Rhodes, I., et al., 2003. Long-term performance of white clover varieties grown with perennial ryegrass under rotational grazing by sheep with different nitrogen applications. Journal of Agricultural Science 140, 151–159.

Williams, M.C., 1987. Nitrate and soluble oxalate accumulation in Kikuyu grass (*Pennisetum clandestinum*). Proceedings of the Western Society of Weed Science 40, 78–79.

Wilson, J.R., Ford, C.W., 1971. Temperature influences on the growth, digestibility, and carbohydrate compositions of two tropical grasses, *Panicum maximum* var *Trichoglume* and *Setaria sphacelata*, and two cultivars of the temperate grass *Lolium perenne*. Australian Journal of Agricultural Research 22 (4), 563–571.

Younie, D., 2000. The role and management of grassland in organic farming. In: Hopkins, A. (Ed.), Grass its Production and Utilisation, third ed. Blackwell Science, Oxford, pp. 365–387.

19

Specialized dietary supplements

Carey A. Williams

Introduction

The main component of any horse's diet should be forage, but forage frequently will not provide all the macro- and micronutrients required, even for maintenance. Forage alone may not provide sufficient energy for exercising animals, as well as pregnant/lactating mares and growing animals all of whom also tend to have increased macro- and micronutrient demands. In many situations, therefore, additional feeds or nutrients need to be added (or supplemented) to the core forage foundation. In other situations, targeted supplementation is employed to address a particular clinical issue or performance goal. When referring to diet supplementation, its definition therefore can change depending on the particular aim of the supplementation. Within this book when the additional nutrients and energy are being provided by proprietary feeds or cereal grains we have either referred to them by a generic term (complementary feeds or concentrates) or by the feed format (sweet feed, pelleted feed, compound feeds, etc.). In contrast, the term "specialized supplements" will be taken to refer to those ingredients or products that are not being added with the primary intention of providing increased energy intake or providing the recommended levels of micro or macronutrients but are being added with the specific goal of trying to improve performance, prevent a problem from occurring, and to combat or manage a problem after it arises.

There are various definitions in the published literature for a "dietary supplement". In a recent review for the National Research Council's (NRC 2009) *Safety of Dietary Supplements for Horses, Dogs and Cats*. The Committee on Examining the Safety of Dietary Supplements for Horses, Dogs and Cats defined an animal dietary supplement as:

> *A substance for oral consumption by horses, dogs, or cats, whether in/on feed or offered separately, intended for specific benefit to the animal by means other than provision of nutrients regarded as essential, or provision of essential nutrients for intended effect on the animal beyond normal nutritional needs, but not including legally defined drugs.*

Another definition from The Food and Drug Administration (FDA) defines a dietary supplement as:

> *A product taken by mouth that contains a "dietary ingredient" intended to supplement the diet. The "dietary ingredients" in these products may include: vitamins, minerals, herbs or other botanicals, amino acids, and substances such as enzymes, organ tissues, glandulars, and metabolites. Dietary supplements can also be extracts or concentrates, and may be found in many forms such as tablets, capsules, softgels, gelcaps, liquids, or powders. They can also be in other forms, such as a bar, but if they are, information on their label must not represent the product as a conventional food or a sole item of a meal or diet."*

The lack of a unified definition for supplement creates confusion. In the European Union, for example, there is no legal definition of a supplement and all such products or ingredients must be labeled as complementary feedstuffs, even though in practice owners and feeders clearly differentiate between traditional complementary feeds as described above and supplements.

The term "nutraceutical" also is commonly used to refer to specialized supplements. The word nutraceutical comes from the words "nutra" meaning nutrient and "ceutical" or "pharmaceutical" meaning a medical drug. Nutraceuticals have been defined as

> *any substance that may be considered a food or part of a food and provides medical or health benefits, including the prevention and treatment of disease*

by the Foundation for Innovation in Medicine (1991). Under such a description nutraceuticals could include nutrients (e.g., vitamin E), derivatives of nutrients (e.g., glucosamine), or herbs. Herbal medicine, also called "phytomedicine", is the use of therapeutic plants, plant parts or plant derived substances to aid in fighting against infections, diseases or enhancing overall health. However, in many countries, feed products with claims related to the prevention or treatment of disease are not legally allowed to be sold (exceptions include defined dietetic feeds).

The remainder of this chapter will focus on the mechanism of action and potential application of some "specialized supplements" used in horse diets.

Nutrients with established requirements (but fed in amounts far greater than minimal requirements, as defined by the NRC 2007)

Antioxidants including many vitamins (e.g., vitamins E and C), minerals (e.g., selenium), enzymes (e.g., superoxide dismutase and glutathione peroxidase) and nutrient derivatives (e.g. glutathione, lipoic acid) are often included as various mixes or cocktails within specialized supplements. The aim is to counter the negative effects of reactive oxygen species (ROS) or free radicals (see Figs 19.1 and 19.2 for an illustration of antioxidant action). Oxidative stress occurs when the antioxidant defense system in the body is overwhelmed with ROS (McBride & Kraemer 1999). ROS are primarily generated within the mitochondrial electron transport chain. An increase in ROS may occur due to a) increased exposure to oxidants from the environment, b) an imbalance in antioxidants, or c) increased production within the body from an increase in oxygen metabolism during exercise (Clarkson & Thompson 2000). Antioxidants are most effective when acting in combination with each other as some have the ability to recycle antioxidant radicals that are formed during the scavenging of ROS. For example, vitamin E forms a tocopherol radical that is inactive until glutathione or ascorbate reacts with the radical and returns it back to its active form. For detailed discussion on the mode of action of these antioxidants please refer to the relevant chapters in this book dealing with each nutrient.

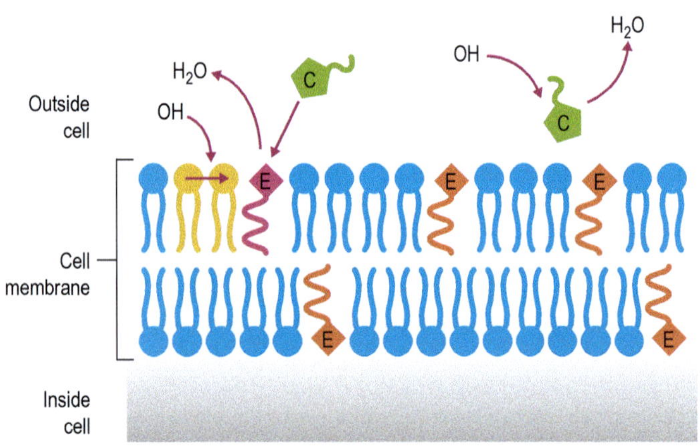

Figure 19.1 Illustration of a hydroxyl radical (OH) getting scavenged or converted to water (H_2O) by vitamin E (represented by the E within the diamonds) in the membrane and vitamin C (represented by the C within hexagons) in the space and fluid outside of the cell. The orange or solid colored parts of the cell membrane represent the dead or dying portion before they are regenerated after the action of vitamin E on the free radical.

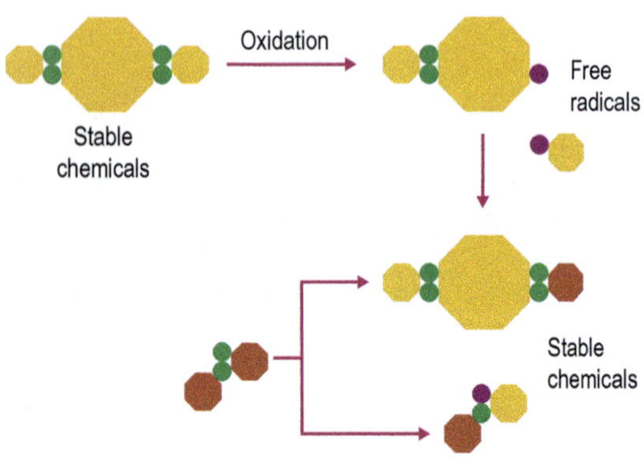

Figure 19.2 Illustration of how an antioxidant can scavenge a free radical or render them inactive by reforming two stable chemicals.

Vitamin E

Potential rationale for use

Vitamin E has strong antioxidant properties that are postulated to help support muscle and nerve as well as immune function (see also Chapter 17). Vitamin E is the major lipid-soluble, chain-breaking antioxidant of the body and provides antioxidant defence in cells, playing an important role in maintaining the integrity of cell membranes (see Chapter 9).

Data on efficacy

Vitamin E is the most commonly supplemented antioxidant in horses. One study found that a single bout of submaximal exercise did not affect plasma α-tocopherol concentration, but horses conditioned for several weeks may require higher levels of vitamin E supplementation than routinely recommended (Siciliano et al 1996). Also, humoral immune response to vaccination was improved by supplementing horses 50 IU/kg dry matter per day as compared to a basal diet containing 18 IU/kg dry matter (Baalsrud & Overnes 1986).

Vitamin E intake was calculated in competitive endurance horses via a pre-ride nutritional survey detailing intake 2 weeks prior to the 80-km endurance race (Williams et al 2005). Horses were estimated to consume 1150 to 4700 IU/day of vitamin E in their total diet during this time period. This level is 1.2 to five times higher than the recommended levels given by the NRC (2007); which, for these animals estimated intake, averages 1000 IU/day. In this particular study a negative correlation was found between vitamin E intake and the activities of creatine kinase (CK) and aspartate aminotransferase (AST), and a positive correlation was found with intake and plasma α-tocopherol activity during the endurance ride (Williams et al 2005). These findings suggested that vitamin E intake may affect muscle membrane permeability and/or injury in horses during endurance exercise.

Safety

High dietary intake may interfere with the absorption of other fat-soluble vitamins such as vitamins A, D and K, although this has not been proven. Measures of oxidative stress were unchanged in horses supplemented with vitamin E at nearly 10 times the NRC (2007) recommended amount, but were found to have lower plasma β-carotene levels than both the control or moderately (5000 IU/day) supplemented group, which may indicate that vitamin E, has an inhibitory effect on β-carotene metabolism (Williams & Carlucci 2006).

Recommended dosage

For antioxidant effects, supplementation at 5 times the NRC (2007) minimum dietary inclusion, or about 5000 IU/day for an average 500 kg horse, is recommended. The vitamin E content of vegetable oils is variable and the vitamin is included to help stabilize the oil itself. Additional vitamin E is recommended to be added to the diet when including increased levels of vegetable oil. The author recommends ~150 IU/100 ml of added oil.

Legal and ethical considerations

There are no legal or ethical considerations in vitamin E supplementation.

Vitamin C

Potential rationale for use

Vitamin C is another commonly added antioxidant, primarily included to help support respiratory health and immune function. Vitamin C scavenges antioxidant derived radicals and therefore can recycle or regenerate other components of the antioxidant system, particularly vitamin E (Chan 1993). Vitamin C is the primary antioxidant to neutrophil-derived oxidants in the lung and vitamin C concentrations in plasma as well as the epithelial lining fluid of the lungs have been shown to be reduced in horses with lung inflammation and in particular recurrent airway obstruction (RAO) (see Chapter 9). Under maintenance conditions horses have the ability to synthesize sufficient ascorbate, but the demand may increase as "stress" on the body is increased.

Data on efficacy

One study looking at the vitamin E and C interaction used 40 endurance horses competing in an 80-km race for the purpose of research (Williams et al 2004b). Plasma ascorbic acid concentrations were lower in the horses supplemented with vitamin E alone (5000 IU/day α-tocopheryl acetate) than those receiving the vitamin E plus C (same vitamin E dose, plus 7 g ascorbic acid/day) at rest. A study of polo ponies showed that throughout the polo season plasma α-tocopherol and ascorbic acid were higher in those given vitamin C in combination with vitamin E in the hard-working ponies, but this was not found with those in only light work or only supplemented with vitamin E (Hoffman et al 2001).

Safety

There are no proven safety concerns. However, there is the potential for excessive vitamin C to affect acid-base status, act as a pro-oxidant and cause gastrointestinal disturbances. There has also been a suggestion in horses that sudden cessation of vitamin C supplementation may decrease endogenous production and increase the risk of infection.

Recommended dosage

A recommended dosage for vitamin C is 10–20 mg/kg BW per day for high stress conditions, including prolonged transportation, exercise training, multiple days of competition, extreme climate changes, parturition, chronic separation from herd mates, or introduction to a new environment, where immune function may be decreased. For respiratory health, beneficial effects have been observed when vitamin C is provided at 9–10 mg/kg BW (Deaton et al 2004, Kirschvink et al 2002) as part of an antioxidant cocktail also including vitamin E (5 mg/kg BW; Deaton et al 2004).

Legal and ethical considerations

There are no legal or ethical considerations with vitamin C supplementation.

Substances with no known nutritional requirement

Carnitine

Potential rationale for use

Carnitine plays an important role in the utilization of fatty acids. As such, carnitine supplementation could potentially increase the contribution of fatty acids to oxidative metabolism and thus have a glycogen-sparing effect. It may also help in buffering the mitochondrial concentration of acetyl-CoA and in the regulation of pyruvate dehydrogenase activity, thereby providing a stimulatory effect on oxidative metabolism. Carnitine, specifically L-carnitine, is an important cofactor in the transport of long-chain fatty acids across the inner mitochondrial membrane. Accumulation of acetyl-carnitine provides a metabolic sink for the temporary storage of 2-carbon acetyl units formed from pyruvate and β-oxidation of FFAs, as well as preventing the local depletion of coenzyme A.

Data on efficacy

Studies in horses have not confirmed that carnitine availability is rate-limiting during exercise. Horse skeletal muscle contains high levels of L-carnitine. Foster and Harris (1992) reported muscle carnitine concentrations between 18.5 and 26.9 mmol/kg dry muscle, with highest values observed in trained horses. Although L-carnitine is poorly absorbed, supplementation with 10–60 g/day did increase plasma but not muscle concentrations (Foster et al 1988, Harris et al 1995). Similar levels of supplementation (10 g/day) to 2-year-old trotters for 5 weeks of training and 15 weeks of detraining, however, were reported to increase the carnitine concentration in the gluteal muscle by 50%. The exercise-induced decrease in muscle glycogen and increase in blood lactate tended to be lower in the L-carnitine-supplemented horses (Harmeyer et al 2001). Other studies have also reported an apparently beneficial effect of feeding L-carnitine on the blood lactate response to exercise (Zeyner & Harmeyer 1999) but this finding has not been consistent. For example, feeding 9 and 12 g/day L-carnitine to young thoroughbred horses had no effect on post-exercise lactic acid and ammonia concentrations, nor CK/AST activities, although a faster return to basal values of lactic acid was reported (Falaschini & Trombetta 2001).

L-carnitine supplementation of young Standardbred horses (10 g/day) during conditioning was reported to increase the proportion of type IIA fibers in middle gluteal muscle (Rivero et al 2002) suggesting possible metabolic advantages. In a later study, however, no affect on training induced changes in heart rate or lactate during exercise or recovery were seen following 10 weeks of L-carnitine supplementation (10 g L-carnitine) in two year olds (Niemeyer et al 2005).

More recent work in humans has suggested that although carnitine supplementation may not affect performance per se, it might modulate markers of metabolic stress and mitigate muscle soreness (Spiering et al 2007) according to the authors by attenuating the "hypoxic chain of events leading to muscle damage after exercise". This has not been explored to the author's knowledge in horses.

Safety

There are no known concerns with safety.

Recommended dosage

None. From the current literature, there is little evidence to support L-carnitine as an ergogenic aid and its use in horses for this purpose cannot be recommended until further information is available.

Legal and ethical considerations

There are no legal or ethical considerations in carnitine supplementation.

Creatine

Potential rationale for use

Creatine is marketed as an ergogenic aid for humans and horses. It is a key component of creatine phosphate (CP) and increased amounts of phosphocreatine (PCr) stored at the start of exercise may help to delay fatigue plus increased concentrations of free creatine may contribute to a faster resynthesis of PCr. This may be especially important in events requiring bouts of intensive but intermittent exercise. Elevation of the muscle creatine and PCr contents has been reported, in numerous studies in humans, to increase the capacity for sustained or intermittent hard exercise and may also exert an anabolic effect that increases peak strength.

Phosphocreatine provides a rapid but brief source of phosphate for the resynthesis of ATP during intensive exercise, acts as the "low ADP threshold sensor" as well as a buffer to ADP accumulation, and supports high-energy phosphate transfer. Recent reviews have concluded that creatine supplementation may exert benefits by: (1) influencing skeletal muscle directly through increasing muscle glycogen and phosphocreatine contents; (2) facilitating faster phosphocreatine resynthesis; (3) increasing expression of endocrine and growth factors mRNA; or (4) working indirectly through increased training volume (Rawson & Persky 2007, Safdar et al 2008).

Data on efficacy

Creatine is an amino acid derivative (methylguanidine-acetic acid) that occurs naturally in carnivorous diets. Horses, however, are likely reliant on synthesis from arginine, L-methionine and glycine. Creatine appears to be poorly absorbed from the intestinal tract in horses. A twofold increase in plasma concentration but no change in muscle content was observed when horses were fed 50 mg creatine/kg BW per day (Sewell & Harris 1995), a dose that results in a marked increase in muscle creatine content in man. Schuback et al (2000) also reported no change in muscle creatine content following creatine supplementation (100–120 mg/kg BW creatine monohydrate per day for 14 days), and observed no effect on performance parameters or muscle metabolic responses to exercise. A more recent study found no ultrasound changes in cross-sectional area and the thickness of the layer of fat of the longissimus dorsi muscle when 75 g of creatine monohydrate (about three-times that of the previous study by Sewel & Harris, 1995) was fed to Arabian horses for 90 days during aerobic training (Angelis et al 2007). Overall, there currently is no evidence to support the use of creatine as an ergogenic aid in horses.

Safety

There are no published safety concerns in horses. However, the effects of long-term use of large doses are unknown. Concerns have been expressed for example in humans with respect to the possible effects on renal function, especially in people with pre-existing renal insufficiency.

Recommended dosage

No effective dose known.

Legal and ethical considerations

There are no legal or ethical considerations in creatine supplementation.

Lipoic acid

Potential rationale for use

α-Lipoic acid (LA) and its reduced form, dihydrolipoic acid (DHLA), have received widespread attention as antioxidants with putative preventative and therapeutic implications for humans and experimental laboratory animals. α-Lipoic acid is an eight-carbon structure that contains a disulfide bond as a part of a dithiolane ring with a five-carbon tail. It is a cofactor in the conversion of pyruvate to acetyl CoA as part of the pyruvate dehydrogenase complex and also in α-ketoglutarate dehydrogenase (Reed et al 1951).

Lipoic acid is unique compared with other antioxidants because it is both water and fat soluble. It therefore can have activity in the cell membrane as well as in the cytoplasm. The carboxylic acid end allows it to be more water-soluble than tocopherol, and it contains more carbon atoms than ascorbic acid so it is more lipophilic (Biewenga et al 1997). Two sulfhydryl moieties allow for radical scavenging with both the reduced and oxidized form of LA (Dikalov et al 1997). Lipoic acid protects membranes by interacting with vitamin C and glutathione, which may also recycle vitamin E. Supplementing LA has found to be beneficial in a number of oxidative stress models, ischemia–reperfusion injury (Serbinova et al 1992), diabetes (Ziegler et al 1995), cataract formation (Maitra et al 1994), radiation injury (Ramakrishnan et al 1992), aging (Hagen et al 1999) and exercise (Khanna et al 1999).

Data on efficacy

Khanna et al (1999) compared rested and exercised rats supplemented with or without LA. The LA supplemented rats, both rested and exercised, had a higher glutathione (GSH) concentration, and a lower lipid peroxidation level measured by thiobarbituric acid reactive substances (TBARS) as compared to non-supplemented rats. Aged rats supplemented with LA had a higher mitochondrial membrane potential, ambulatory activity, GSH and ascorbate concentration; furthermore, the malondialdehyde concentration

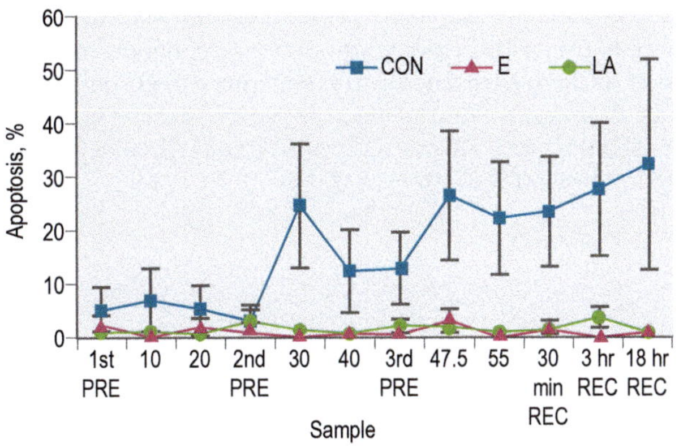

Figure 19.3 White blood cell apoptosis for the control (CON; *n* = 3), vitamin E (E; *n* = 3), and lipoic acid (LA; *n* = 3) groups. *Reprinted with permission from Williams et al 2004a.*

was five times higher in the non-supplemented rats (Hagen et al 1999).

In trained Arabian horses, supplementation with either lipoic acid or vitamin E mitigated measures of white blood cell apoptosis during a simulated endurance exercise test (Williams et al 2004a; Fig. 19.3); although it should be noted that this was not a crossover study. Lipoic acid supplemented horses also had increased whole blood total GSH concentrations when compared to the control group (Williams et al 2004a) and increased plasma levels of ascorbic acid and α-tocopherol. Both the vitamin E and lipoic acid supplemented groups had about 40% more total GSH, 30% more α-tocopherol, and 15% more ascorbic acid than the control group. This illustrates the collaborative nature of the recycling and scavenging of antioxidant radicals as such increases were found using either vitamin E or lipoic acid.

Safety

There are no reported safety concerns.

Recommended dosage

A dose of 10 mg/kg BW/day DL-α-lipoic acid is the dose typically used in research studies (Williams et al 2002) without evidence of any adverse effects but has never been put into a commercial antioxidant supplement at this concentration due to its high cost and bitter taste.

Legal and ethical considerations

There are no legal or ethical considerations in LA supplementation.

Probiotics

Potential rationale for use

Probiotics were first defined as, "substances secreted by one organism that stimulates the growth of another" (Lilley & Stillwell, 1965). Later, the US Office of Regulatory Affairs of the FDA and AAFCO defined probiotics as "a source of live, naturally occurring microorganisms" (Yoon & Stern 1995) and which are now called "direct-fed microbials" (DFM). In the EU within the category "zootechnical additives", the following functional group is included "'gut flora stabilizers': microorganisms or other chemically defined substances, which, when fed to animals, have a positive effect on the gut flora." This would include probiotic bacteria as well as yeasts. Their use is directed at maintaining, enhancing or re-establishing "beneficial" bacteria and other microflora within the gastrointestinal tract. However, there has been no evidence to prove that providing probiotics to animals with healthy thriving GI flora will have any beneficial effect.

Data on efficacy

Studies have investigated if bacteria will survive transit through a horse's GI system and shown that orally provided *Lactobacillus rhamnosus* bacteria will survive transit through a foal's GI system and colonize the hindgut when fed at extremely high doses (Weese et al 2003). This group also showed that provision of *Lactobacillus pentosus*, a strain of bacteria isolated from the equine intestine, actually increases the severity of foal diarrhea, which raises concerns over the choice of bacteria in probiotics and/or the quality control of the probiotic used (Weese & Rousseau 2005). However, another study showed that providing five strains of *Lactobacillus*, also isolated from the equine intestine, did decrease the incidence of foal diarrhea (Yuyama et al 2004).

Yeast cultures have also been evaluated for their probiotic properties. Specifically after feeding horses *Saccharomyces cerevisiae*, viable yeast cells were found in the large intestine (Medina et al 2002), which indicates that yeast can survive transit through the GI track. It is theorized that yeast supplementation will increase the pH of the GI track and help improve fiber digestion (e.g., Morgan et al 2007, Jouany et al 2009). However, not all studies show a significant beneficial effect (Hall et al 1990) and it is hard to make a recommendation for its use in aiding fiber digestion in horses provided typical forage based rations. Although the use of *Saccharomyces boulardi* has been reported to significantly reduce the duration and severity of acute enterocolitis in one study in hospitalized horses (Desrochers et al 2005), much more work is needed to evaluate the potential for live yeast supplementation to help in cases of colic, laminitis and diarrhea.

Safety

No safety concerns have been reported other than those associated with quality control (see above) and the potential lack of efficacy of certain strains of bacteria.

Recommended dosage

Optimal dosages have not been determined; however, Weese (2001) gives a starting point of 1×10^9 to 1×10^{11} colony-forming units (cfu) per 50 kg BW per day, which was determined by extrapolation from human research.

Legal and ethical considerations

No legal or ethical concerns at this time in the US; however, in Europe specific authorization is required to market probiotics for use in horses.

Superoxide dismutase

Potential rationale for use

Superoxide dismutase (SOD) is an enzymatic antioxidant, which catalyzes the dismutation of superoxide ions into oxygen and hydrogen peroxide. A number of reports have indicated that supplementation with SOD may be effective in reducing pro-inflammatory cytokines and inhibiting neutrophil infiltration to sites of tissue damage in several models of inflammation (Salvemini et al 1999, Masini et al 2002).

Data on efficacy

Although studies in rats (Radak et al 1995) and humans (Arent et al 2009, 2010a) have reported apparent beneficial effects with respect to exercise-associated oxidative stress and inflammation, limited research to date in horses has not demonstrated an effect of SOD supplementation on local (synovial fluid) or systemic markers of inflammation (Lamprecht & Williams 2012).

Safety

No safety issues have been reported.

Recommended dosage

No effective dose has been found for horses (Lamprecht 2009).

Legal and ethical considerations

There are no legal or ethical concerns at this time in the US.

Complex materials that contain a mixture of putative active ingredients

This group includes herbal supplements that contain active ingredients that are purported to affect the immune system among other various properties (antioxidant, anti-inflammatory, sedative, etc.). Some of these herbs can be classified as adaptogens, immunostimulants or both. Adaptogens increase resistance to stressors, physical, chemical or biological, whereas immunostimulants activate the nonspecific or innate defense mechanisms against viral, bacterial or cellular infections. Most of the studies to date in laboratory animals, humans and other species have determined that the immunologic effect of herbal supplements does not enhance normal immune response but may have beneficial effects if the immune system is compromised (Schulz et al 1998). A more recent reference suggests that very little scientific evidence is available for efficacy of herbal products use in humans, and only four of the top ten herbs in the United States have evidence based on randomized controlled trials (Bent & Ko 2004). Table 19-1 summarizes the active component, action, drug interactions, and equine research present for the major herbs described below.

Bee pollen

Potential rationale for use

Bee pollen and propolis are similar resinous substances collected from various plant sources by honeybees. Propolis contains polyphenols and flavonoids, as well as several specific antioxidant compounds including beta-carotene, caffeic acid and kaempferol (Ahn et al 2004, Gomez-Caravaca et al 2006, Christov et al 2006). Reported biological properties include antioxidant, antimicrobial, antifungal, anti-inflammatory, and immunoregulatory actions (Liebelt & Calcagnetti 1999). Propolis with strong antioxidant activity was also found to have high total polyphenol content (Ahn et al 2004). Antimicrobial effects have been observed against Gram-positive bacteria and yeasts (Uzel et al 2005). Anti-inflammatory effects of propolis may involve nitric oxide inhibition (Tan–No et al 2006).

Data on efficacy

Whilst there are numerous anecdotal reports of the benefits of supplemented bee pollen in horses including improved oxygen utilization, lower heart rates, and firmer muscle tone (Turner et al 2006), there has been little scientific research. In particular, the anti-inflammatory effects of bee pollen reported in other species require validation in the horse. A recent pilot study in horses examined the effects of bee-pollen based supplementation on physical fitness parameters, immunological status, and nutritional variables in 10 Arabian horses in training. Results indicated that supplementation with 118 g of a commercial 55% bee-pollen supplement for 42 days did not alter physical fitness or immunological variables. However, supplementation did significantly increase feed intake as well as nitrogen and phosphorus balance (Table 19-2; Turner et al 2006). The authors of the study theorized that the horses increased feed intake because of the high content of B vitamins, particularly thiamine, which was present in the supplement. Rats supplemented with propolis demonstrated increased weight gain, improved utilization of iron, increased calcium and phosphorus absorption, and improved regeneration efficiency of hemoglobin (Haro et al 2000). Whether this could be valuable in animals with a reduced appetite or poor nutrient digestibility is unknown and unproven.

Safety

A few adverse allergic reactions have been reported in humans and could potentially occur in horses.

Recommended dosage

No recommended effective dose is available at this time.

Legal and ethical considerations

There are no legal or ethical considerations using bee pollen.

Black tea

Potential rationale for use

Black tea (*Camilla sinensis*) contains several polyphenols, including aflavin, flavanols (in particular catechins and gallic acid), theaflavins, and phenolic acids (Sharma & Rao 2009). It is commonly marketed for its anti-inflammatory and antioxidant properties, but also for management of obesity and diabetes mellitus (Grove & Lambert 2010). Black tea theaflavins help to prevent cellular DNA damage by reducing oxidative stress and suppressing cytochrome P451A1 in rat liver (Sharma & Rao 2009). Black tea also prevents lipoprotein oxidation and production of both nitric oxide and superoxide in mice (Sharma & Rao 2009). In in vitro studies, anti-inflammatory effects have been associated with inhibition of gene expression for the inflammatory chemokine interleukin (IL)-8 (Benjamini et al 2000, Aneja et al 2004).

Table 19-1 Herbal Supplements and other Functional Foods

Common name	Scientific name	Active components[a]	Actions[a]	Potential toxicity or interaction[b]	Equine research
Bee pollen	Propolis	β-carotene, caffeic acid, kaempferol, phenethyl caffeate, *p*-hydroxyacetophenone, benzylhydroxybenzoate, coumaric, cinnamic acid	antioxidant, antimicrobial, antifungal, anti-inflammatory, immunoregulatory	None reported	Turner et al 2006
Devil's claw	*Harpagophytum procumbens*	Iridoid glycosides, acetylated phenolic glycosides, terpenoids	anti-inflammatory	Cause gastric ulcers, prolong bleeding time	Pearson et al 1999
Echinacea	*Echinacea purpurea, E. angustifolia, E. pallida*	Polysaccharides, glycoproteins, alkamides, cichoric acid	anti-inflammatory, antioxidant	May interfere with drugs processed by liver enzymes, not for use with a depleted immune system, or during pregnancy, possible allergic reactions	O'Neill et al 2002
Garlic	*Allium sativum*	sulfoxides, γ-glutamylcysteines	Antibacterial, antiviral, antifungal, antiparasitic	Heinz body anemia, uterine stimulant, prolong bleeding time, gastric ulcers, urticaria	Pearson et al 2005; Miyazawa et al 1991
Ginger	*Zingiber officinale*	paradol, gingerol, myoga	anti-inflammatory, antithrombotic, antioxidant, antibacterial	Cause gastric ulcers, prolong bleeding time	Liburt et al 2010; Smarsh et al 2010
Ginseng	*Panax ginseng, Panax quinquefolius, Eleutherococcus senticosus*	ginsenosides, essential oils, phytosterols	anti-inflammatory, antioxidant	May interfere with drugs processed by liver enzymes, potentate diuretics, decrease blood sugar, decrease coagulation	Pearson et al 2007
Valerian	*Valeriana fauriei, V. officinalis, V. edulis, V. wallichii*	valerenic acid, iridoid glycosides	Sedative, antispasmodic	May enhance effect of tranquilizers and anesthetics, may be prohibited substance, cause diarrhea and colic	N
Yucca	*Yucca schidigera*	saponins, resveratrol, yuccaols A–E	anti-inflammatory, antioxidant, antispasmodic, antiplatelet	May accelerate NSAIDs, cause diarrhea	N

[a]For references regarding ingredients or actions see text for the specific herb.
[b]Information compiled from Miller 1998, Poppenga 2001, Harman, 2002, Izzo et al 2005.
Reproduced with kind permission from Williams and Lamprecht (2008).

Data on efficacy

A significant decrease in the whole blood mRNA expression of tumor necrosis factor-α (TNF-α) and interferon-γ (IFN-γ) was observed in horses administered 28 g black tea extract diluted in 2 liters of water and administered via nasogastric tube vs. water placebo one hour prior to exhaustive treadmill exercise (Fig. 19.4; Streltsova et al 2006). Blood lactate concentrations, however, were higher in the black tea treatment throughout exercise. In a companion study, a single dose of black tea did not alter measures of antioxidant status, including GSH activity (Smarsh et al 2010). In contrast, college-age male athletes consuming 1760 mg/day of black tea extract for 9 days had increased total glutathione concentrations when compared to controls (Arent et al 2010b). The use of a single dose versus multiple doses may explain the difference in findings between studies. It may also explain why in the horse study black tea did not affect retinol concentrations, whereas studies in rats have shown significant increases in plasma vitamin A after a longer duration of supplementation (Wojciech et al 2010). More work using different doses and durations of supplementation is needed before any conclusions can be reached as to the benefits or otherwise of black tea administration in horses.

Table 19-2 Physical Fitness Variables at Rest and Recovery (1 hr Post–Exercise) in Horses Fed with and without Bee Pollen (BP and CO, Respectively)

Variable	Day 0		Day 42	
	Rest	Recovery	Rest	Recovery
Heart rate (bpm)*				
BP	40.2 ± 2.1	59.0 ± 2.7	45.4 ± 1.3	39.2 ± 2.0
CO	41.6 ± 1.6	54.8 ± 1.8	43.0 ± 2.2	43.6 ± 1.9
Hematocrit*				
BP	0.35 ± 0.01	0.38 ± 0.006	0.36 ± 0.006	0.30 ± 0.003
CO	0.37 ± 0.004	0.36 ± 0.01	0.38 ± 0.004	0.33 ± 0.008
Hemoglobin (g/dl)*				
BP	12.8 ± 0.3	13.5 ± 0.1	13.5 ± 0.3	12.3 ± 0.3
CO	14.3 ± 0.2	13.8 ± 0.3	15.1 ± 0.2	11.1 ± 0.1
Lactate (mmol/l)*				
BP	1.3 ± 0.2	3.3 ± 0.4	0.89 ± 0.08	0.67 ± 0.04
CO	1.2 ± 0.1	3.5 ± 0.3	0.59 ± 0.02	0.62 ± 0.02

*Overall decrease from day 0 to day 42 ($p \leq 0.0003$).
Reproduced with kind permission from Turner et al (2006).

Safety

No safety concerns have been reported for horses. However, concerns have been raised over potential adverse effects of high doses of green tea polyphenols including hepatotoxicity, vomiting and diarrhea (mechanism currently unknown) in other species (Grove & Lambert 2010).

Recommended dosage

Even though no toxicities or adverse effects have been reported, there has not been enough work to make a definitive dosage recommendation for the horse.

Legal and ethical considerations

There are no legal or ethical concerns at this time as long as the black tea supplement used is a theobromine and caffeine-free product. Theobromine and caffeine are banned substances in all types of racing and in some show organizations.

Cranberry

Potential rationale for use

Cranberry (*Vaccinium macrocarpon*) polyphenols have been shown to protect endothelial cells against stress-induced up-regulation of oxidant stress and inflammatory mediators (Youdim et al 2002). This compound has been commonly used for treatment of urinary tract infections in humans, but also more recently for its antioxidant capabilities although the evidence to date is limited especially for the latter (Cravotto et al 2010). Phenolics in cranberries, like quercetin and cyanidin, have highly effective radical scavenging structures and cranberries also contain anthocyanins, a type of flavonoid (Zheng & Wang 2003, Viskelis et al 2009).

Data on efficacy

A single pre-exercise dose of cranberry extract (30 g) did not alter antioxidant status or decrease oxidative stress in horses during exhaustive treadmill exercise in horses (Smarsh et al 2010). With respect to its anti-inflammatory properties, cranberry attenuated the TNF-α response in horses undergoing intense exercise, but not the appearance of IFN-γ (Liburt et al 2010). The effects of longer-term supplementation in horses have not been assessed. Dose–response studies are also yet to be performed.

Safety

No safety concerns reported. However, cranberry contains a number of phytochemicals that can modulate UDP-glucuronosyl transferase enzymes and therefore there is a potential for herb–drug interactions (Mohamed & Frye 2011).

Recommended dosage

No recommended effective dose is available at this time.

Legal and ethical considerations

There are no legal or ethical considerations in using cranberry.

Devils claw

Potential rationale for use

Devil's claw (*Harpagophytum procumbens*) is reported to have an anti-inflammatory effect in humans and laboratory animals. The active ingredients are various iridoid glycosides, acetylated phenolic glycosides, and terpenoids. Devil's Claw is primarily marketed for its painkilling and

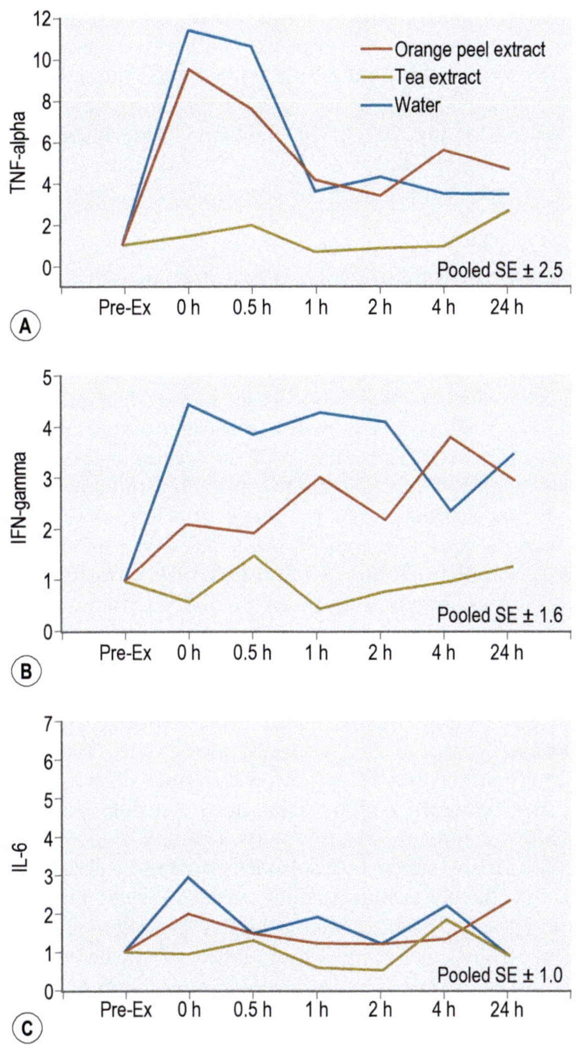

Figure 19.4 The graphs for TNF-α A), IFN-γ B), and IL-6 C) mRNA expression in whole blood of horses administered water, black tea and orange peel. There was a significant ($p<0.05$) effect of exercise on mRNA expression when horses were administered orange peel and water but no effect with black tea. There was no effect of treatment or exercise on IL-6.

Reproduced with kind permission from Streltsova et al 2006.

anti-inflammatory properties, and has many testimonials claiming relief from rheumatism and other joint disorders (Brien et al 2006). Some human clinical studies report a decrease in pain intensity and an increase in flexibility after supplementation with Devil's Claw extract. There is therefore potential cross over to the equine market.

Topical application of devil's claw decreased the expression of cyclooxygenase (COX)-2 in mouse skin (Kundu et al 2005). Harpagoside, a glycoside component of Devil's Claw, has been shown to suppress COX-2 and inducible nitric oxide synthase (iNOS) at both the mRNA and protein level in vitro (Huang et al 2006). Its effectiveness in reducing pain and inflammation associated with rheumatoid and osteoarthritis can be explained by its ability to block the production of inflammatory mediators like prostaglandin E_2 (PGE_2; Chantre et al 2000). A chondroprotective effect of Devil's Claw in rabbits was attributed to an increase in matrix metalloproteinase-2 (Chrubasik et al 2006).

Data on efficacy

Multiple studies have suggested that extracts with >50 mg of harpagoside per day may be helpful in alleviating lower back pain in humans (Chrubasik et al 2002) and a recent systematic review suggested some favorable effects on osteoarthritic pain (Cameron et al 2009). However, many of the studies carried out in humans to date have methodological flaws (Brien et al 2006) and therefore firm conclusions as to the efficacy of Devils Claw cannot be made (Cameron et al 2009).

A blinded, placebo controlled, cross-over designed study in horses with naturally occurring osteoarthritis examined the effect(s) of a proprietary polyherbal composite joint supplement containing Devil's Claw. An anti-inflammatory effect was observed in the horses due to a reduction in PGE_2 content of synovial fluid (Pearson et al 1999). However, all but one of the six horses used in this study had no change in lameness or flexion test score when examined by a veterinarian.

Safety

Potential to cause gastrointestinal upset linked to gastric ulcers (Izzo et al 2005). Acute, subacute and chronic toxicity studies did not show any adverse effects in a study in mice (Ibrahim et al 2010). Devil Claw preparations are unlikely to have clinically relevant effects on cytochrome P450 function (Modarai et al 2011) and drug interactions have not been reported in various species (Harman 2002) or, to the author's knowledge, in horses. Even so, caution should still be used when supplementing Devil's Claw as safe upper limits have not been determined.

Recommended dosage

No effective recommended dosage is available at this time.

Legal and ethical considerations in the horse

None at this time; however, caution is to be used when supplementing anything with anti-inflammatory properties. The International Federation for Equestrian Sports (FEI) prohibited substance list does not include Devil's Claw. However, there is a disclaimer at the end of the list stating, "And other substances with a similar chemical structure or similar biological effect(s)." This statement could potentially include Devil's Claw and other COX-2 inhibiting substances in this category.

Echinacea

Potential rationale for use

Echinacea (*Echinacea* sp.) has been reported to have anti-inflammatory and antioxidant properties (Colalto 2010) and as reviewed by Cravotto et al 2010. The three main species are *Echinacea purpurea*, *E. angustifolia*, and *E. pallida*. These species have a wide range of medicinal properties (Block & Mead 2003). An immunostimulatory effect is the most common rationale for use in horses. The active components of the echinacea species include polysaccharides, glycoproteins, alkamides and cichoric acid; the latter is a derivative of caffeic acid. However, it must be noted that depending on the species and commercial preparation of these products, the concentrations of these components will vary greatly.

Many research studies have looked at the biochemistry, immunopharmacology and clinical use of echinacea (Bauer et al 1998, Wagner & Jurcic 1991, Wildfeuer & Mayerhofer 1994, Parnham 1996, Gunning & Steele 1999). Some human studies have found that echinacea can enhance cytokine production, including TNF-α, IL-1, IL-6, and IL-10 by macrophages (Burger et al 1997). In humans (Wagner & Jurcic 1991) and mice (Roesler et al 1991), echinacea extracts have been shown to stimulate phagocytosis. Other studies have demonstrated a stimulating effect on lymphocyte function and proliferation in normal and diseased human mononuclear cells in vitro (See et al 1997). A meta-analysis study suggested some potential for Echinacea to reduce the incidence of the common cold in humans especially when co-administered with Vitamin C (Shah et al 2007). However Cravotto et al (2010) commented that "large scale randomized prospective studies are needed to take into account important variables such as plant species or variety, quality of preparation, dose, method of cold induction."

Data on efficacy

Only one placebo-controlled, randomized study has been reported in horses. This was carried out in eight horses supplemented with echinacea for 42 days at a level equivalent to 1000 mg standardized extract (O'Neill et al 2002). The authors concluded that the horses treated with echinacea were immune stimulated; however, results only showed a significant increase in lymphocyte count and a decrease in neutrophil count at day 35 of supplementation.

Safety

Echinacea interacts with various drugs in humans but more work is needed to clarify the risks (Colalto 2010). Persistent use has been associated with potential hepatotoxic effects and concurrent use with hepatotoxic drugs such as steroids is not recommended (Miller 1998, Barrett 2003). Other reported potential side effects include an IgE-mediated allergic reaction (Maskatia & Baker 2010). Drug interactions and safety in horses is unknown.

Recommended dosage

Due to the very limited research in horses, it is not possible to make dosage recommendations.

Legal and ethical considerations

There are no legal or ethical concerns at this time.

Garlic

Potential rationale for use

Garlic (*Allium sativum*) has been marketed for antimicrobial and antiparasitic properties. Garlic's putative active components include a number of organosulfur compounds (e.g., allicin) as well as a variety of nonsulfur compounds including steroid aponins and various organoselenium compounds (NRC 2009). The high sulfur content of garlic has been theorized to help cleanse the blood. In the horse industry, garlic is primarily fed for purported insect repellent effects. Respiratory health benefits (alterations in the physical properties of mucus) have also been claimed.

The intact garlic bulb of the garlic plant contains a complex mixture of cysteine sulfoxides, and γ-glutamylcysteines. When the bulb is disrupted the sulfoxidases are cleaved to the active form of thiosulfinate allicin (Munday & Munday, 2001). The chemistry underlying any potential biological activity of the putative active compounds in garlic is thought to be complex (NRC 2009).

Data on efficacy

A study conducted by Velerio and Maroli (2005), evaluated the repellent effect of garlic oil applied topically on human volunteers exposed to female sandflies and found that a 1% and a 0.005% garlic oil dilution provided 97 and 40% repellent effectiveness, respectively. Garlic has been shown to have a wide range of anti-parasitic properties that are effective against at least 12 human and non-human parasites (Anthony et al 2005). Crushed garlic preparations have been shown to have antibacterial properties. Certain strains of gram negative and gram positive bacteria have exhibited sensitivity to allicin (Ankri & Mirelman 1999, Chowdhury et al 1991). Another study found that a 57.1% w/v aqueous garlic extract containing 220 µg/ml allicin was effective in inhibiting the growth and killing several oral microorganisms including periodontal pathogens maintained on various agars supplemented with horse blood (Bakri & Douglas 2005).

Although garlic has been added to horse feed for its aroma, as a flavorant and/or palatant, to support respiratory health, or for antiparasitic or fly repellent properties, there is little if any research to support any of these potential benefits specifically in horses. Long term (83 days) supplementation of dried garlic at 32 mg/kg BW seemed to reduce respiratory signs, including accumulation of tracheal exudates and the number of neutrophils in a tracheobronchial aspirate, in horses in light work (Saastamoinen et al 2010).

Safety

Drug interactions with garlic have been reported in other species (NRC 2009). Toxicity with garlic is a possibility in all species with potential clinical signs including gastric irritation, decreased sperm production, Heinz body anemia, and occupational asthma (see NRC 2009). In dogs, 5 g/kg of fresh garlic increased oxidation of hemoglobin within red blood cells and decreased total hemoglobin concentration (Hu et al 2002). Garlic consumption also led to oxidation of red blood cells in sheep (Stevens 1984). Equine studies found that freeze dried garlic fed at >0.4 g/kg per day resulted in Heinz body anemia (Pearson et al 2005). In this study both horses fed garlic showed an increase in mean corpuscular volume, Heinz body score, platelet count, serum-free and total bilirubin concentration, and decreases in red blood cell count, blood and mean corpuscular hemoglobin concentration, and serum haptoglobin concentration. In a study by Saastamoinen et al (2010), supplemented animals showed a tendency for a decrease in Hb and RBC count over the 83 day period when fed garlic at 32 mg/kg BW. Another study has shown that some horses may develop urticaria in response to garlic administration (Miyazawa et al 1991).

Recommended dosage for the horse

The NRC (2009) reported that while more data are needed, intake levels of 15 mg/kg BW/day of dried garlic powder on a long-term basis were unlikely to result in a risk of an adverse event in horses under normal circumstances and that levels up to 90 mg/kg BW/day may not be associated with any adverse events in healthy, non exercising adult horses. However, the study of Saastamoinen et al (2010) suggests that long-term supplementation at 32 mg/kg BW might cause mild anemia.

Legal and ethical considerations

There are no legal or ethical considerations in garlic supplementation.

Ginger

Potential rationale for use

Ginger (*Zingiber officinale*) has been suggested to have anti-thrombotic, antioxidant, anti-inflammatory, and antibacterial properties. In the 1970s ginger was first shown to have anti-inflammatory properties including inhibition of prostaglandin synthesis (Kiuchi et al 1982) and more recently other anti-inflammatory activities have been reported (Grzanna et al 2005). The major constituents in ginger include paradol, gingerol and myoga (Grzanna et al 2005, Colalto 2010). In humans, ginger is often used in the treatment of nausea and dyspepsia (Colalto 2010). [8]-Paradol, a natural constituent of ginger, is a potent COX-1 inhibitor and also inhibits platelet aggregation in human whole blood.

Data on efficacy

A crossover study in nine horses evaluated the effects of a single 30 g dose of ginger extract diluted in 2 liters of water and administered via nasogastric tube on markers of inflammation and cardiovascular variables during recovery from exhaustive exercise (Liburt et al 2010). Ginger-treated horses had a significantly reduced recovery time in the fast phase of the VO_2 recovery curve, where the metabolic cost of exercise rapidly is replenished. However, ginger had a tendency to increase the pro-inflammatory cytokines TNF-α and IFN-γ as well as creatine kinase activity. It was speculated that the caustic ginger extract solution irritated the gastrointestinal tract after ingestion (Liburt et al 2010). In a companion study, ginger had no effect on markers of oxidative stress or antioxidant status in horses during exercise (Smarsh et al 2010). These findings are in contrast to reports from other species, where ginger supplementation has been shown to modulate antioxidant status. Ahmed et al (2000) reported a decrease in chemically-induced oxidative stress in rats fed a 1% ginger diet for 4 weeks. In another study, rats fed either 0.5%, 1% or 5% ginger for 1 month showed increases in activity of antioxidant enzymes (superoxide dismutase, glutathione peroxidase, and catalase) in the liver (Kota et al 2008). These studies suggest that the antioxidant effects of ginger extract may only occur after multiple administrations. This could account for the differences found between horse and rodent studies.

Safety

In humans it has been found that ginger can inhibit thromboxane synthetase and increase bleeding time, which could be detrimental if used with anticlotting drugs like warfarin (Backon 1986) although one study found no significant effects (see Colalto 2010). Although it has been suggested that ginger might cause gastric ulceration in horses, as shown in humans (Izzo et al 2005), many herbal supplements marketed for support of gastric health in horses contain ginger as a major ingredient. The author is not aware of any data to support or refute such an inclusion.

Recommended dosage

Given the lack of efficacy in horses there is no recommended dosage for use in horses. The lack of effect in most of the studies looking at the potential ergogenic effect of herbs/spices could be due to many factors including the fact that these compounds have no discernible clinical effect on performance or the studies conducted to date have not used the right form or dose of the material, or applied supplementation for an adequate length of time, etc.

Legal and ethical considerations

There are no legal or ethical considerations in ginger supplementation.

Ginseng

Potential rationale for use

Ginseng (*Panax* sp.) is commonly used for its immunostimulating properties; however, it is also used in humans for its potential to treat diabetes mellitus and to improve cognitive performance (Colalto 2010). In the equine industry, ginseng is marketed and sold for use in stimulating the immune system, decreasing stress during transport, competition or prolonged illness, and increasing optimal performance.

There are three primary species of interest: Asian ginseng (*Panax ginseng*), American ginseng (*Panax quinquefolius*), and Siberian ginseng (correctly called "eleuthero" or *Eleutherococcus senticosus*) (Block & Mead 2003). For all of these species, glycosidal saponins, also called ginsenosides, are a primary component. Other minor components include essential oils, phytosterols, amino acids, peptides, vitamins and minerals. Many of the ginsenosides have antioxidant properties that may help protect membranes of nerve and immune cells. Ginseng has been found to exert an inhibitory effect on IL-1β and IL-6 gene expression, decrease TNF-α production by macrophages, and decrease COX-2 expression, and suppress histamine and leukotriene release (Radad et al 2006). A recent review was also published as to ginseng's (among other herbs) possible mechanism in treating insulin resistance in horses and other species (Tinworth et al 2010); however, it is noted that any effects may vary depending on whether it is supplemented in a feeding or fasting state.

Data on efficacy

In vitro studies using human immune cells have demonstrated a stimulating effect on lymphocyte function and proliferation in vitro in normal and diseased human mononuclear cells (See et al 1997). The results from this study are consistent with other published research on its immune-stimulating properties in laboratory animals and humans. The immune response to 24 hours of road transport was apparently unaffected when a supplement that contained *Eleutherococcus senticosus* (Siberian Ginseng) with other ingredients was fed to horses (Stull et al 2004). Another study in horses found that ginseng might augment immune response to vaccination and help immune compromised animals (Pearson et al 2007). Horses were fed a low-dose of ginseng (~1.7 mg/kg body weight of total ginsenosides), with no adverse effects, for 28 days. The supplemented horses showed a greater antibody titre response by day 16 vs. the control group that peaked at day 21, and by day 28 the control group was at only 55% compared to the ginseng supplemented group. Supplemented horses also showed a greater percent of plasma T-lymphocytes compared to control horses (Pearson et al 2007).

Safety

The list of potential side effects for ginseng includes hypertension, insomnia, vomiting, headache, nervousness, sleeplessness, and epistaxis in humans. It has also been recommended to discontinue use of warfarin, heparin, aspirin, and other nonsteroidal anti-inflammatory drugs (NSAIDs) when taking ginseng (Block & Mead, 2003) although there is some controversy as not all studies have apparently reported a clinically relevant effect (Colalto 2010). These side effects have never been reported in horses; however, one should be careful when using ginseng in horses with long-term administration of NSAIDs (Miller 1998, Poppenga 2001).

Recommended dosage

There is no effective recommended dosage for horses at this time.

Legal and ethical considerations

There are no legal or ethical considerations in ginseng use.

Orange peel

Potential rationale for use

Orange peel, which is the primary waste fraction in the production of orange juice, contains flavonoids associated with antioxidant activity (Kanaze et al 2008). The glycosides hesperidin and naringin are mainly responsible for the purported antioxidant activity of citrus peel extracts (Kanaze et al 2008). Coniferin and phlorin are additional phenols in orange peels that have been found to aid in radical scavenging when administered in the form of orange peel molasses (Manthey 2004).

Data on efficacy

Orange peel extract contains citrus-derived polymethoxylated flavones that have an inhibitory effect on TNF-α expression in horses. One study in exercising horses reported that 30 g orange peel extract administered via nasogastric tube decreased IFN-γ expression at fatigue, and decreased the recovery time of cardiovascular parameters as compared to control (Fig. 19.4; Streltsova et al 2006). In a companion study, horses administered the orange peel extract one hour before exercise had significantly lower concentrations of plasma retinol compared to the control group (Smarsh et al 2010). Supplementation with hesperidin, a flavanone glycoside found in orange peel, may affect antioxidant status in animals undergoing physiological challenges. In rats, hesperidin (200 mg/kg/day) for 10 days significantly increased levels of superoxide dismutase (SOD), glutathione-*S*-transferase (GST), and GSH after chemical induction of oxidative stress (Arafa et al 2009). In the same study, healthy rats given the same amount of hesperidin had no changes in antioxidant concentrations. Naringin, another flavanone glycoside found in citrus peel, increased levels of SOD, CAT, and vitamin E in New Zealand White rabbits fed a high cholesterol diet compared to those without the naringin (0.5 g/kg diet) supplement (Jeon et al 2002).

Based on these studies supplementation with glycosides found in orange peel extract, may be beneficial only when the body is under severe oxidative stress, and when supplementation is given over time and not as a single administration. More work will need to be conducted to determine the appropriate effective dosage for horses.

Safety

No adverse effects have been reported.

Recommended dosage

There is no known recommended dose at this time.

Legal and ethical considerations in the horse

There are none.

Valerian

Potential rationale for use

Valerian (*Valeriana* sp.) contains valerenic acids, such as monoterpenes and sesquiterpenes, and iridoid glycosides that give the root a sedative and antispasmodic activity. In the volatile oil component of valerian, sesquiterpenes, are thought to be responsible for its biological effect (Houghton 1999). *Valeriana fauriei*, *V. officinalis*, *V. edulis*, and *V. wallichii* are more commonly studied species of valerian. The amount of active ingredient in each depends on the form and preparation of the product (e.g., capsule, tincture, tea, etc.). In one study, the highest concentration of valerenic acids were recovered in powder capsules, whereas the lowest amount was found in tinctures and teas (Lefebvre et al 2004). Valerian supplements are commonly sold for the treatment of insomnia, anxiety, and stress in humans (see Colalto 2010). There are no published data in the horse, although supplements are marketed with claims related to calming effects.

There is evidence that valerian decreases central nervous system activity in mice, with the effect equivalent to that of phenobarbital (Hendriks et al 1985). Valerian has also been suggested to be effective in treating insomnia and other sleep disorders in humans by reducing the breakdown of γ-aminobutyric acid resulting in sedation and a decrease in CNS activity (Riedel et al 1982, Houghton 1999, Colalto 2010). However, there does not appear to be sufficient evidence of efficacy in clinical trials with respect to insomnia or anxiety and Cravotto et al 2010 suggest that "more research is required into therapeutic dose, types of valerian preparation and the optimum period of use for therapeutic effect."

Data on efficacy

The suggestion that valerian can exert sedative effects in other species has resulted in a currently unproven assumption that it will produce the same effects in horses.

Safety

Valerian in humans and laboratory animals may prolong the action of barbiturates, interact with alcohol, and influence cytochrome P450 activities, and can modulate UDP-glucoronosyl transferase enzymes, although the in vivo consequences of these later two interactions are not well understood (Colalto 2010, Mohamed & Frye 2011). Nonetheless, there is potential for multiple drug interactions (Dunayev et al 1987, Miller 1998, Lefebvre et al 2004) and Cravotto et al (2010) report that the conclusions from a previous review were that there was insufficient evidence about the efficacy or safety of valerian.

Recommended dosage for the horse

There is no recommended dosage.

Legal and ethical considerations in the horse

Caution needs to be taken when supplementing valerian, as certain show organizations, such as the International Federation for Equestrian Sports (FEI), and the United States Equestrian Federation (USEF 2006) ban this product from use during competition.

Yucca

Potential rationale for use

Many oral equine joint supplements on the market today contain yucca, together with a variety of other ingredients. Many company testimonials and advertisements portray yucca as being able to reduce the risk of respiratory problems, such as RAO in horses; however, no scientific studies have been performed. Yucca (*Yucca schidigera*) contains steroid-like saponins, which have anti-inflammatory, antioxidant, and antispasmodic effects that may help to reduce pain associated with arthritis (Cheeke et al 2006). The saponins are natural detergents that form stable foams, which contain both fat- and water-soluble components. As much as 10% of the yucca stem contains saponins, making it one of the richest sources (Cheeke et al 2006). Yucca also contains other active components including polyphenols like resveratrol and yuccaols A–E (Oleszek et al 2001, Piacente et al 2004). These phenols are exclusively found in the bark and are not present in yucca extract (Oleszek et al 2001).

Data on efficacy

The potent antioxidant activity of the polyphenols has been postulated to be key to yucca's anti-arthritic properties (Oleszek et al 2001, Piacente et al 2004). It has been shown that yuccaols inhibit intrinsic nitric oxide synthetase (iNOS), an inflammatory agent that increases during inflammatory responses (Marzocco et al 2004). Resveratrol, as well as the yucca phenols, was found to inhibit nuclear factor κB, a transcription factor that controls the expression of iNOS (Tsai et al 1999).

Safety

There are no reported adverse effects.

Recommended dosage

The dosage is not known.

Legal and ethical considerations

There are no legal or ethical concerns for yucca at this time. However, as with Devil's Claw, caution is to be used when supplementing anything with anti-inflammatory properties. The International Federation for Equestrian Sports (FEI) prohibited substance list does not include yucca; however, there is a disclaimer at the end of the list stating, "And other substances with a similar chemical structure or similar biological effect(s)." This statement could potentially include yucca and other COX-2 inhibiting substances in this category.

Conclusion

Various supplements including herbs are being used in the equine industry. Despite many anecdotal reports of efficacy, most of the supplements have never been proven safe or effective in horses; therefore caution must be taken when selecting and using such supplements. The potential shown with in vitro studies does not always translate into the field situation for many potential reasons, including the effect of the digestive processes on active ingredients. The fact that certain herbs have been fed for centuries does not mean that they are always safe (e.g., garlic). There are also potential conflicts with certain medication rules within the equine industry, and the line between some herbs acting as calming agents or sedatives can be very fine. Cross-reactions and contraindications are known to occur between certain medicinal/drug therapies and herbal preparations. In animals currently being prescribed or about to be prescribed any medication, the veterinarian should be informed of the concurrent administration of any herbal preparation.

References

Ahmed, R.S., Seth, V., Pasha, S.T., et al., 2000. Influence of dietary ginger (*Zingiber officinales rocs*) on oxidative stress induced by malathion in rats. Food and Chemical Toxicology 38, 443–450.

Ahn, M.R., Kumazawa, S., Hamasaka, T., et al., 2004. Antioxidant activity and constituents of propolis collected in various areas of Korea. Journal of Agriculture and Food Chemistry 52, 7286–7292.

Aneja, R., Odoms, K., Denenberg, A.G., et al., 2004. Theaflavin, a black tea extract, is a novel anti-inflammatory compound. Critical Care Medicine 32, 2097–2103.

Angelis, F.H.F., Mota, M.D.S., Freitas, E.V.V., et al., 2007. Aerobic training, but not creatine, modifies longissimus dorsi muscle composition. Journal of Equine Veterinary Science 27, 118–122.

Ankri, S., Mirelman, D., 1999. Antimicrobial properties of allicin from garlic. Microbes and Infection 2, 125–129.

Anthony, J., Fyfe, L., Smith, H., 2005. Plant active components – a resource for antiparasitic agents?: A review. Trends in Parasitology 21, 462–468.

Arafa, H.M.M., Aly, H.A.A., Abd-Ellah, M.F., et al., 2009. Hesperidin attenuates benzol[α]pyrene-induced testicular toxicity in rats via regulation of oxidant/antioxidant balance. Toxicology and Industrial Health 25, 417–427.

Arent, S.M., Davitt, P., Golem, D.L., et al., 2009. The effects of a post-workout nutraceutical drink on body composition, performance, and hormonal and biochemical responses in Division 1 college football players. Comparative Exercise Physiology 6, 73–80.

Arent, S.M., Pellegrino, J.K., Williams, C.A., et al., 2010a. Nutritional supplementation, performance, and oxidative stress in college soccer players. Journal of Strength and Conditioning Research 24, 1117–1124.

Arent, S.M., Senso, M., Golem, D.L., et al., 2010b. The effects of theaflavin-enriched black tea extract on muscle soreness, oxidative stress, inflammation, and endocrine responses to acute anaerobic interval training: a randomized, double-blind, crossover study. Journal of the International Society of Sports Nutrition 7, 11.

Baalsrud, K.J., Overnes, G., 1986. Influence of vitamin E and selenium supplement on antibody production in horses. Equine Veterinary Journal 18, 472–474.

Backon, J., 1986. Ginger: inhibition of thromboxane synthetase and stimulation of prostacyclin: relevance for medicine and psychiatry. Medicine Hypothesis 20, 271-278.

Bakri, I., Couglas, C., 2005. Inhibitory effect of garlic extract on oral bacteria. Archives of Oral Biology 50, 645-651.

Barrett, B., 2003. Echinacea: A safety review. HerbalGram 57, 36-39.

Bauer, V.R., Jurcic, K., Puhlmann, J., et al., 1998. Immunologic in vivo and in vitro studies on Echinacea extracts. Arzneimittelforschung 38, 276-281.

Benjamini, E., Coico, R., Sunshine, G., 2000. Cytokines. In: Benjamini, E., Coico, R., Sunshine, E. (Eds.), Immunology: a Short Course, fourth ed. Wiley-Liss Inc, New York, pp. 229-251.

Bent, S., Ko, R., 2004. Commonly used herbal medicines in the United States: A review. American Journal of Medicine 116, 478-485.

Biewenga, G., Haenen, G.R.M.M., Bast, A., 1997. The pharmacology of the antioxidant lipoic acid. General Pharmacology 29, 315-331.

Block, K.I., Mead, M.N., 2003. Immune system effects of echinacea, ginseng, and astragalus: A review. Integrated Cancer Therapy 2, 247-267.

Brien, S., Lewith, G.T., McGregor, G., 2006. Devil's claw (*Harpagophytum procumbens*) as a treatment for osteoarthritis: A review of efficacy and safety. Journal of Alternative and Complementary Medicine 12, 981-993.

Burger, R.A., Torres, A.R., Warren, R.P., et al., 1997. Echinacea-induced cytokine production by human macrophages. International Journal of Immunopharmacology 19, 371-379.

Cameron, M., Gagnier, J.J., Little, C.V., et al., 2009. Evidence of effectiveness of herbal medicinal products in the treatment of arthritis - Part 1 osteoarthritis. Phytotherapy research 23, 1497-1515.

Chan, A.C., 1993. Partners in defense, vitamin E and vitamin C. Canadian Journal of Physiology and Pharmacology 71, 725-731.

Chantre, P., Cappelaere, A., Leblan, D., et al., 2000. Efficacy and tolerance of Harpagophytum procumbens versus diacerein in treatment of osteoarthritis. Phytomedicine 7, 177-183.

Cheeke, P.R., Piacente, S., Oleszek, W., 2006. Anti-inflammatory and anti-arthritic effects of yucca schidigera: a review. Journal of Inflammation 3, 6-13.

Chrubasik, S., Pollak, S., Black, A., 2002. Effectiveness of devil's claw for osteoarthritis. Rheumatology 41, 1332-1333.

Chrubasik, J.E., Faller-Marquardt, M., Chrubasik, S., et al., 2006. Potential molecular basis of the chondroprotective effect of *Harpagophytum procumbens*. Phytomedicine 13, 598-600.

Chowdhury, A., Ahsan, M., Islam, S., et al, 1991. Efficacy of aqueous extract of garlic and allicin in experimental shigellosis in rabbits. The Indian Journal of Medical Research 93, 33-36.

Christov, R., Trusheva, B., Popova, M., et al., 2006. Chemical composition of propolis from Canada, its antiradical activity and plant origin. Natural Product Research 20, 531-536.

Clarkson, P.M., Thompson, H.S., 2000. Antioxidants: what role do they play in physical activity and health? American Journal of Clinical Nutrition 72 (supplement), 637S-646S.

Colalto, C., 2010. Herbal interactions on absorption of drugs: Mechanisms of action and clinical risk assessment. Pharmacological research 62, 207-227.

Cravotto, G., Boffa, L., GEnzini, L., et al., 2010. Phytotherapeutics: an evaluation of the potential of 1000 plants. Journal of Clinical Pharmacy and Therapeutics 35, 11-48.

Deaton, C.M., Marlin, D.J., Smith, N.C., et al., 2004. Antioxidant supplementation in horses affected by recurrent airway obstruction. Journal of Nutrition 134, 2065S-2067S.

Desrochers, A.M., Dolente, B., Roy, M.F., et al., 2005. Efficacy of saccharomyces boulardii for treatment of horses with acute enteroclitis. JAVMA 227, 954-959.

Dikalov, S., Khamtsov, V.V., Zimmer, G., 1997. Reaction of lipoate and its derivatives with reactive oxygen species. In: Fuchs, J., Packer, L., Zimmer, G. (Eds.), Lipoic Acid in Health and Disease. Marcel Dekker, New York, NY, pp. 47-64.

Dunayev, V.V., Trzhetsinsky, S.D., Tishkin, V.S., et al., 1987. Biological activity of the sum of valepotriates isolated from Valalliariifolia Adams. Farmakologiia i Toksikologiia 50, 33-37.

Falaschini, A., Trombetta, M.F., 2001. Modifications induced by training and diet in some exercise related blood parameters in young trotters. Journal of Equine Veterinary Science 21, 601-604.

Foster, C.V.L., Harris, R.C., 1992. Total carnitine content of the middle gluteal muscle of Thoroughbred horses: normal values, variability and effect of acute exercise. Equine Veterinary Journal 24, 52-57.

Foster, C.V.L., Harris, R.C., Snow, D.H., 1988. The effect of oral L-carnitine supplementation on the muscle and plasma concentrations in the thoroughbred horse. Comparative Biochemistry and Physiology A 91, 827-835.

Foundation for Innovation in Medicine, 1991. The Nutraceutical Initiative: A proposal for economic and regulatory reform (white paper). Cranford, NJ.

Gomez-Caravaca, A.M., Gomez-Romero, R., Arraez-Roman, D., et al., 2006. Advances in the analysis of phenolic compounds in products derived from bees. Journal of Pharmaceutical and Biomedical Analysis 41, 1220-1234.

Grove, K.A., Lambert, J.D., 2010. Laboratory, epidemiological and human intervention studies show that tea (camellia sinensis) may be useful in the prevention of obesity. Journal of Nutrition 140, 446-453.

Grzanna, R., Lindmark, L., Frondoza, C.G., 2005. Ginger - An herbal medicinal product with broad anti-inflammatory actions. Journal of Medicinal Food 8, 125-132.

Gunning, K., Steele, P., 1999. Echinacea for the prevention of upper respiratory tract infections. Journal of Family Practice 48, 93.

Hagen, T.M., Ingersoll, R.T., Lykkesfeldt, J., et al., 1999. (R)-α-Lipoic acid-supplemented old rats have improved mitochondrial function, decreased oxidative damage, and increased metabolic rate. FASEB Journal. 13, 411-418.

Hall, R.R., Jackson, S.G., Baker, J.P., et al., 1990. Influence of yeast culture supplementation on ration digestion by horses. Journal of Equine Veterinary Science 10, 130-134.

Harman, J., 2002. The toxicology of herbs in equine practice. Clinical Techniques in Equine Practice 1, 74-80.

Harmeyer, J., Coenen, M., Vervuert, I., et al., 2001. Effect of L-carnitine (LC) supplementation during training on muscle carnitine and plasma biochemical values. Proceedings of the 17th Equine Nutrition and Physiology Symposium, Lexington, KY. Equine Nutrition and Physiology Society, Savoy, IL, p. 282.

Harris, R.C., Foster, C.V.L., Snow, D.H., 1995. Plasma carnitine concentration and uptake into muscle with oral and intravenous administration. Equine Veterinary Journal Supplement 18, 382-387.

Haro, A., Lopez-Aliaga, I., Lisbona, F., et al., 2000. Beneficial effect of pollen and/or propolis on the metabolism of iron, calcium, phosphorus, and magnesium in rats with nutritional ferropenic anemia. Journal of Agriculture and Food Chemistry 48, 5715-5722.

Hendriks, H., Bos, R., Woerdenbag, H.J., et al., 1985. Central nervous depressant activity of verenic acid in the mouse. Planta Medica 1, 28-31.

Hoffman, R.M., Morgan, K.L., Phillips, A., et al., 2001. Dietary vitamin E and ascorbic acid influence nutritional status of exercising polo ponies. Equine Nutrition and Physiology Symposium Proceedings 17, 129-130.

Houghton, P.J., 1999. The scientific basis for the reputed activity of valerian. Journal of Pharmacy and Pharmacology 51, 505-512.

Huang, T.H., Tran, V.H., Duke, R.K., et al., 2006. Harpagoside suppresses lipopolysaccharide-induced iNOS and COX-2 expression through inhibition of NF-κβ activation. Journal of Ethnopharmacology 104, 149-155.

Hu, Q., Yang, Q.,Yamato, O., et al., 2002. Isolation and identification of organosulfur compounds oxidizing canine erythrocytes from garlic (*Allium sativum*). Journal of Agriculture and Food Chemistry 50, 1059-1062.

Ibrahim, K.E., Al-Ashban, R.M., El-Sammani, S.A., 2010. Toxicity studies on devil's claw herbal medicine. Research Journal of Pharmacology 4, 69-73.

Izzo, A.A., Di Carlo, G., Borrelli, F., et al., 2005. Cardiovascular pharmacotherapy and herbal medicines: the risk of drug interaction. International Journal of Cardiology 98, 1-14.

Jeon, S.M., Bok, S.H., Jang, M.K., et al., 2002. Comparison of antioxidant effects of naringin and probucol in cholesterol-fed rabbits. Clinica Chimica Acta 317, 181-190.

Jouany, J.P., Gobert, J., Medina, B., et al., 2009. Effect of live yeast culture supplementation on apparent digestibility and rate of passage in horses fed a high-fiber or high-starch diet. Journal of Animal Science 87, 2844-2852.

Kanaze, F.I., Termentzi, A., Gabrieli, C., et al., 2008. The phytochemical analysis and antioxidant activity of orange peel (citrus sinensis) cultivated in Greece-crete indicates a new commercial source of hesperidin. Biomedical Chromatography 23, 239-249.

Khanna, S., Atalay, M., Laaksonen, D.E., et al., 1999. α-Lipoic acid supplementation: tissue glutathione homeostasis at rest and after exercise. Journal of Applied Physiology 86, 1191-1196.

Kirschvink, N., Fievez, L., Bougnet, V., et al., 2002. Efect of nutritional antioxidant supplementation on systemic and pulmonary antioxidant status, airway inflammation and lung function in heaves-affected horses. Equine Veterinary Journal 34, 705-712.

Kiuchi, F., Shibuya, M., Sankawa, U., 1982. Inhibitors of prostaglandin biosynthesis from ginger. Chemical and Pharmaceutical Bulletin (Tokyo) 30, 754-757.

Kota, N., Krishna, P., Polasa, K., 2008. Alterations in antioxidant status of rats following intake of ginger through diet. Food Chemistry 106, 991-996.

Kundu, J.K., Mossanda, K.S., Na, H.K., et al., 2005. Inhibitory effects of the extracts of Sutherlandia frutescens (L.) R. Br. and Harpagophytum procumbens DC. on phorbol ester-induced COX-2 expression in mice skin: AP-1 and CREB as potential upstream targets. Cancer Letters 218, 21-31.

Lamprecht, E.D., Williams, C.A., 2012. Biomarkers of antioxidant status, inflammation, and cartilage metabolism are affected by acute intense exercise but not superoxide dismutase supplementation in horses. Oxidative Medicine and Cellular Longevity, 2012:(E-pub) (in press).

Lefebvre, T., Foster, B.C., Drouin, C.E., et al., 2004. In vitro activity of commercial valerian root extracts against human cyotchrome P450 3A4. Journal of Pharmacy and Pharmaceutical Science 7, 265-273.

Liburt, N.R., McKeever, K.H., Streltsova, J.M., et al., 2010. Effects of ginger and cranberry extracts on the physiological response to exercise and

markers of inflammation in horses. Comparative Exercise Physiology 6, 157–169.
Liebelt, R.A., Calcagnetti, D., 1999. Effects of a bee pollen diet on the growth of the laboratory rat. American Bee Journal 139, 390–395.
Lilley, D.M., Stillwell, R.H., 1965. Probiotics: Growth promoting factors produced by microorganisms. Science 147, 747–748.
Maitra, I., Serbinova, E., Tritschler, H., et al., 1994. α-Lipoic acid prevents buthionine sulfoximine-induced cataract formation in newborn rats. Free Radical Biology and Medicine 18, 132–138.
Manthey, J.A., 2004. Fractionation of orange peel phenols in ultrafiltered molasses and mass balance studies of their antioxidant levels. Journal of Agricultural and Food Chemistry 52, 7586–7592.
Marzocco, S., Pacente, S., Pizza, C., et al., 2004. Inhibition of inducible nitric oxide synthase expression by yuccaol C from *Yucca schidigera roezl*. Life Science 75, 1491–1501.
Maskatia, Z.K., Baker, K., 2010. Hypereosinophilia associated with Echinacea use. Southern Medical Journal 103, 1173–1174.
Masini, E., Cuzzocrea, S., Mazzon, E., et al., 2002. Protective effects of M40403, a selective superoxide dismutase mimetic, in myocardial ischaemia and reperfusion injury in vivo. British Journal of Pharmacology. 136, 905–917.
McBride, J.M., Kraemer, W.J., 1999. Free radicals, exercise and antioxidants. Journal of Strength and Conditioning Research 13, 175–183.
Medina, B., Girad, I.D., Jacotot, E., et al., 2002. Effect of preparation of *Saccharomyces cerevisiae* on microbial profiles and fermentation patterns in the large intestine of horses fed a high fiber or starch diet. Journal of Animal Science 80, 2600–2609.
Miller, L.G., 1998. Herbal medicinals. Selected clinical considerations focusing on known or potential drub-herb interactions. Archives of Internal Medicine 158, 2200–2211.
Miyazawa, K., Ito, M., Ohsaki, K., 1991. An equine case of urticaria associated with dry garlic feeding. Journal of Veterinary Medicine and Science 53, 474–748.
Modarai, M., Suter, A., Kortenkamp, A., et al., 2011. The interaction potential of herbal medicinal products: A luminescence-based screening platform assessing effects on cytochrome P450 and its use with devil's claw (*Harpagophyti radix*) preparations. Journal of Pharmacy and Pharmacology 63, 429–438.
Mohamed, M.E., Frye, R.F., 2011. Effects of herbal supplements on drug glucronidation - review of clinical, animal and invitro studies. Planta Medica 77, 311–321.
Morgan, L.M., Coverdale, J.A., Froetschel, M.A., et al., 2007. Effect of yeast culture supplementation on digestibility of varying forage quality in mature horses. Journal of Equine Veterinary Science 27, 260–265.
Munday, R., Munday, C.M., 2001. Relative activities of organosulfur compounds derived from onions and garlic in increasing tissue activities of quinone reductase and glutathione transferase in rat tissues. Nutrition and Cancer-An International Journal 40, 205–210.
Niemeyer, A., Vervuert, I., Appelt, K., et al., 2005. Effects of L-carmitine supplementation on heart rate and selected metabolic responses in resting and exercising horses: a placebo-controlled double blind study. Pferdeheilkunde 21, 107–109.
NRC, 2007. Nutrient Requirements of Horses, sixth ed. National Academy Press, Washington, DC, USA.
NRC, 2009. Safety of Dietary Supplements for Horses Dogs and Cats. National Academy Press, Washington, DC, USA.
Oleszek, W., Sitek, M., Stochmal, A., et al., 2001. Resveratrol and other phenolics from the bark of Yucca schidigera Roezl. Journal of Agriculture and Food Chemistry 49, 747–752.
O'Neill, W., McKee, S., Clarke, A.F., 2002. Immunological and haematinic consequences of feeding a standardized Echinacea (Echinacea angustifolia) extract to healthy horses. Equine Veterinary Journal 34, 222–227.
Pearson, W., McKee, S., Clarke, A.F., 1999. The effect of a proprietary herbal product on equine joint disease. Journal of Nutraceuticals, Functional and Medicinal Foods 2, 31–46.
Pearson, W., Boermans, H.J., Bettger, W.J., et al., 2005. Association of maximum voluntary dietary intake of freeze-dried garlic with Heinz body anemia in horses. American Journal of Veterinary Research 66, 457–465.
Pearson, W., Omar, S., Clarke, A.F., 2007. Low-dose ginseng (*Panax quinquefolium*) modulates the course and magnitude of the antiobody response to vaccination against *Equid herpesvirus 1* in horses. The Canadian Journal of Veterinary Research 71, 213–217.
Parnham, M.J., 1996. Benefit-risk assessment of the squeezed sap of the purple coneflower (*Echinacea purpurea*) for long-term oral immunostimulation. Phytomedicine 3, 95–102.
Piacente, S., Montoro, P., Oleszek, W., et al., 2004. Yucca schidigera bark: phenolic constituents and antioxidant activity. Journal of Natural Products 67, 882–885.
Poppenga, R.H., 2001. Risks associated with the use of herbs and other dietary supplements. Veterinary Clinics of North America: Equine Practice 17, 455–477.
Radad, K., Gille, G., Linlin, L., et al., 2006. Use of ginseng in medicine with emphasis on neurodegenerative disorders. Journal of Pharmacological Sciences 100, 175–186.
Radak, Z., Asano, K., Inoue, M., et al., 1995. Superoxide dismutase derivative reduces oxidative damage in skeletal muscle of rats during exhaustive exercise. Journal of Applied Physiology 79, 129–135.
Ramakrishnan, N., Wolfe, W.W., Catravas, G.N., 1992. Radioprotection of hematopoietic tissues in mice by lipoic acid. Radiation Research. 130, 360–365.
Rawson, E.S., Persky, A.M., 2007. Mechanisms of muscular adaptations to creatine supplementation. International Sports Medicine Journal 8, 43–53.
Reed, L.J., DeBusk, B.G., Gunsalus, I.C., et al., 1951. Crystalline α-Lipoic acid: a catalytic agent associated with pyruvate dehydrogenase. Science (Wash DC). 114, 93–94.
Riedel, E., Hansel, R., Ehrke, G., 1982. Inhibition of gamma-amino butyric acid catabolism by valerenic acid derivatives. Planta Medica 46, 219–220.
Rivero, J., Sporleder, H.P., Quiroz-Rothe, E., et al., 2002. Oral L-carnitine combined with training promote changes in skeletal muscle. Equine Veterinary Journal Supplement 34, 269–274.
Roesler, J., Emmendorffer, A., Steinmuller, C., et al., 1991. Application of purified polysaccharides from cell cultures of the plant *Echinacea purpurea* to test subjects mediates activation of the phagocyte system. International Journal of Immunopharmacol 13, 931–941.
Saastamoinen, M.T., Hyyppä, S., Särkijärvi, S., 2010. Influence of garlic supplementation on respiratory health and incidence of anemia in horses. The impact of nutrition on the health and welfare of horses: 5th European Workshop on Equine Nutrition, Cirencester, UK 19–22 September 2010 (Ellis, A.D, Longland, A.C, Coenen, M, Miraglia, N. Eds). EAAP Publication 128, 280–282. DOI:10.3920/978-90-8686-711-0.
Safdar, A., Yardley, N.J., Snow, R., et al., 2008. Global and targeted gene expression and protein content in skeletal muscle of young men following short-term creatine monohydrate supplementation. Physiological Genomics 32, 219–228.
Salvemini, D., Riley, D.P., Lennon, P.J., et al., 1999. Protective effects of a superoxide dismutase mimetic and peroxynitrite decomposition catalysts in endotoxin-induced intestinal damage. British Journal of Pharmacology 127, 685–692.
Schuback, K., Gustavsson, B., Persson, S.G.B., 2000. Effect of creatine supplementation on muscle metabolic response to a maximal treadmill exercise test in Standardbred horses. Equine Veterinary Journal 32, 533–540.
Schulz, V., Hansel, R., Tyler, V.E., 1998. Agents that increase resistance to diseases. In: Mager, T. (Ed.), Rational Phytotherapy: A Reference Guide for Physicians and Pharmacists. Springer-Verlag, New York, NY, USA, pp. 269–285.
Serbinova, E., Khwaja, S., Rexnick, A.Z., et al., 1992. Thioctic acid protects against ischemia-reperfusion injury in the isolated perfused Langendorff heart. Free Radical Research Communications. 17, 49–58.
See, D.M., Broumand, N., Sahl, L., Tilles, J.G., 1997. In vitro effects of echinacea and ginseng on natural killer and antibody-dependant cell cytotoxicity in healthy subjects and chronic fatigue syndrome or acquired immunodeficiency syndrome patients. Immunopharmacology 35, 229–235.
Sewell, D., Harris, R.C., 1995. Effect of creatine supplementation in the Thoroughbred horse. Equine Veterinary Journal Supplement 32, 239–242.
Shah, S.A., Sander, S., White, C.M., et al., 2007. Evaluation of echinacea for the prevention and treatment of the common cold: a meta-analysis. Lancet Infectious Diseases 7, 473–480.
Sharma, V., Rao, L.J., 2009. A thought on the biological activities of black tea. Critical Review of Food Science and Nutrition 49, 379–404.
Siciliano, P.D., Parker, A.L., Lawrence, L.M., 1996. Effect of dietary vitamin E supplementation on the integrity of skeletal muscle in exercised horses. Journal of Animal Science 75, 1553–1560.
Smarsh, D., Liburt, N., Stretzalova, J., et al., 2010. Nutraceutical extracts affect oxidative stress and antioxidant status in intensely exercising horses. Equine Veterinary Journal 42 (Suppl. 38), 317–322.
Spiering, B.A., Kraemer, W.J., Vingren, J.L., et al., 2007. Responses of criterion variable to different supplemental doses of L-carnitine L-tartrate. Journal of Strength and Conditioning Research 21, 259–264.
Stevens, H., 1984. Suspected wild garlic poisoning in sheep. Veterinary Record 115, 363.
Streltsova, J.M., McKeever, K.H., Liburt, N.R., et al., 2006. Effect of orange peel and black tea extracts on markers of performance and cytokine markers of inflammation in horses. Equine and Comparative Exercise Physiology 3, 121–130.
Stull, C.L., Spier, S.J., Aldridge, B.M., et al., 2004. Immunological response to long term transport stress in mature horses and effects of adaptogenic dietary supplementation as an immunomodulator. Equine Veterinary Journal 36, 583–589.
Tan-No, K., Nakajima, T., Shoji, T., et al., 2006. Anti-inflammatory effect of propolis through inhibition of nitric oxide production on carrageenin-induced mouse paw edema. Biological and Pharmaceutical Bulletin 29, 96–99.
Tinworth, K.D., Harris, P.A., Sillence, M.N., et al., 2010. Potential treatments for insulin resistance in the horse: A comparative multi-species review. The Veterinary Journal 186, 282–291.

Tsai, S.H., Lin-Shiau, S.Y., Lin, J.K., 1999. Suppression of nitric oxide synthase and the down-regulation of the activation of NFkappaB in macrophages by reseratrol. British Journal of Pharmacology 126, 673–680.

Turner, K.K., Nielsen, B.D., O'Connor, C.I., et al., 2006. Bee pollen product supplementation to horses in training seems to improve feed intake: a pilot study. Journal of Animal Physiology and Animal Nutrition 90, 414–420.

United States Equestrian Federation (USEF), 2006. Drugs and Medications Guidelines. Hilliard, OH.

Uzel, A., Sorkun, K., Oncag, O., et al., 2005. Chemical compositions and antimicrobial activities of four different Anatolian propolis samples. Microbiology Research 160, 189–195.

Velerio, L., Maroli, M., 2005. Evaluation of repellent and anti-feeding effect of garlic oil (Allium sativum) against the bite of phlebotomine sandflies Diptera: Psychodidae. Annali dell'Istituto superiore di sanità 41, 253–256.

Viskelis, P., Rubinskiene, M., Jasutiene, I., et al., 2009. Anthocyanins, antioxidative, and antimicrobial properties of American cranberry (*Vaccinium macrocarpon* Ait.) and their press cakes. Journal of Food Science 74, C157–161.

Wagner, H., Jurcic, K., 1991. Immunological studies of plant extract combinations: in vitro and in vivo studies on the stimulation of phagocytosis. Arzneimittelforschung 41, 1072–1076.

Weese, J.S., 2001. A review of probiotics: Are they really "Functional Foods"? AAEP Proc 47, 27–31.

Weese, J.S., Rousseau, J., 2005. Evaluation of *Lactobacillus pentosus* WE7 for prevention of diarrhea in neonatal foals. Journal of the American Veterinary Medical Association 226, 2031–2034.

Weese, J.S., Anderson, M.E.C., Lowe, A., et al., 2003. Preliminary investigation of probiotic potential of *Lactobacillus rhamnosus* strain GG in horses: Fecal recovery following oral administration and safety. Canadian Veterinary Journal 44, 299–302.

Wildfeuer, A., Mayerhofer, D., 1994. The effects of plant preparations on cellular functions in body defense. Arzneimittelforschung 44, 361–366.

Williams, C.A., Carlucci, S., 2006. Oral vitamin E supplementation and oxidative stress, vitamin and antioxidant status in intensely exercising horses. Equine Veterinary Journal Supplement 36, 617–621.

Williams, C.A., Lamprecht, E.D., 2008. Some commonly fed herbs and other functional foods in equine nutrition: a review. The Veterinary Journal 178, 21–31.

Williams, C.A., Hoffman, R.M., Kronfeld, D.S., et al., 2002. Lipoic acid as an antioxidant in mature thoroughbred geldings: a preliminary study. Journal of Nutrition 132, 1628–1632.

Williams, C.A., Kronfeld, D.S., Hess, T.M., et al., 2004a. Lipoic acid and vitamin E supplementation to horses diminishes endurance exercise induced oxidative stress, muscle enzyme leakage, and apoptosis. In: Lindner, Arno (Ed.), The Elite Race and Endurance Horse. CESMAS, Oslo, Norway, pp. 105–119.

Williams, C.A., Kronfeld, D.S., Hess, T.M., et al., 2004b. Antioxidant supplementation and subsequent oxidative stress of horses during an 80-km endurance race. Journal of Animal Science 82, 588–594.

Williams, C.A., Kronfeld, D.S., Hess, T.M., et al., 2005. Vitamin E intake and systemic antioxidant status in competitive endurance horses. Equine and Comparative Exercise Physiology 2, 149–152.

Wojciech, L., Ewa, Z., Elzbieta, S., 2010. Influence of green tea on erythrocytes antioxidant status of different age rats intoxicated with ethanol. Phytotherapy Research 24, 424–428.

Yoon, I.K., Stern, M.D., 1995. Influence of direct-fed microbials on ruminal microbial fermentation and performance of ruminants: A review. Asian-Australasian Journal of Animal Science 8, 533–555.

Youdim, K.A., McDonald, J., Kalt, W., et al., 2002. Potential role of dietary flavonoids in reducing microvascular endothelium vulnerability to oxidative and inflammatory insults. Journal of Nutritional Biochemistry 13, 282–288.

Yuyama, T., Yusa, S., Takai, S., et al., 2004. Evaluation of a host-specific *Lactobacillus* probiotic in neonatal foals. International Journal of Applied Research in Veterinary Medicine 2, 26–33.

Zeyner, A., Harmeyer, J., 1999. Metabolic functions of L-carnitine and its effects as feed additive in horses. A review. Archives of Animal Nutrition 52, 115–138.

Zheng, W., Wang, S.Y., 2003. Oxygen radical absorbing capacity of phenolics in blueberries, cranberries, chokeberries and lingonberries. Journal of Agricultural Food Chemistry 51, 502–509.

Ziegler, D., Hanefeld, M., Ruhnau, K.J., et al., 1995. Treatment of symptomatic diabetic peripheral neuropathy with the anti-oxidant α-lipoic acid. Diabetologia 38, 1425–1433.

20

Feed hygiene and related disorders in horses

Josef Kamphues

Introduction

Energy, nutrient content, digestibility and palatability are the main parameters typically used to describe the nutritive value of ingredients intended for use in animal feeding. Nonetheless, factors related to "feed hygiene" are equally important and should be considered when choosing a feed. Feed hygiene is a very broad term that covers all the measures that are necessary to minimize health risks due to physical, chemical or biological contamination (as described in the EC Regulation on Feed Hygiene No 183/2005) of feeds and feedstuffs.

Worldwide there has been increased interest in the potential role feed contamination may play in horse health (Raymond et al 2000, Buckley et al 2007, Sacchi et al 2009). Recent epidemiological studies suggest that it is not uncommon for horse feedstuffs to be of moderate or poor "hygienic quality", which could predispose to various disorders (Germany: Wolf et al 2009, Austria: Kaya et al 2009, Switzerland: Wichert et al 2008). In 1996, the author developed the first systematic approach to characterize the hygienic status of equine feedstuffs. This was based on the evaluation of various hygiene problems encountered in equine feedstuffs. This work provides the core foundation for this chapter, which has been enriched by more recent published studies that have focused on more specific areas of contamination involving pathogenic fungi, endotoxins and mycotoxins.

Diversity/variety of contaminants in feeds for horses

To a greater or lesser extent all feedstuffs (and bedding/litter material) will be contaminated with a variety of substances and organisms. Depending on the conditions during growth, at harvest, during storage and mixing, etc., as well as the type of feeds and how they are provided to the horse, the level of contamination will vary between years, feed producers, and the people who take care of the horses. Whilst it is virtually impossible to eradicate contamination, it is important to minimize the load and eliminate those contaminants that are of high risk to the horse.

The different types of contaminants that may occur in feeds for horses (and sometimes also in litter and drinking water) are listed in Table 20-1 based on the EU directive, 183/2005. Contamination can occur at any point along the feed supply chain; production, harvesting and storage through to the point of ingestion. Unintentional contamination, for example, may arise from the use of fertilizers, herbicides and pesticides as well as from exposure to pollutants during production and harvesting. Due to adverse environmental or storage conditions in particular, the growth of bacteria, fungi and/or yeasts can result in the formation of a variety of chemical compounds that may cause health effects. Even processing itself can introduce unwanted and potentially toxic contaminants, for example dioxins within natural vitamin E products (Halbert & Archer 2007). Contaminants also can arise from the environment and possibly lead to unintended doping of the equine athlete (Barker 2008, Popot et al 2011). It is not always easy to determine the actual point of entry of certain contaminants and therefore on whom any responsibility should lie in the case of a dispute or adverse event. Good manufacturing, production and handling practices will help to reduce risk, as discussed later and in Chapter 21.

Key Points

- Most feedstuffs carry some form of unavoidable natural contamination; the challenge is to minimize any such contamination and the associated risks
- Contaminants can be biological (e.g. molds or pests), chemical (e.g. prohibited substances, heavy metals) or physical (e.g. stones, string) in nature;
- Contamination can also be present in forage and water, and occur at any point in the supply chain from primary growth to the feed room.
- Whilst the horse appears to be able to withstand a certain load (depending on the source), excessive contamination can affect health and performance and should be avoided.

Table 20-1 Contaminants in Feedstuffs and Bedding Materials for Horses: Examples of Their Occurrence and Veterinary Relevance (According to Kamphues 2007)

Categories and examples of contaminants	Examples in equine feeds and/or bedding material	Potential adverse effect	References
Biological contaminants			
Poisonous plants	1. Ragwort in roughage/hay 2. Autumn crocus in roughage/hay 3. Trisetum flavescens	1. Hepatotoxicity 2. Signs of colic (due to colchicin) 3. Calcinosis (blood vessels/kidney)	Kamphues & Meyer 1990; Wolf & Kamphues 2001
Dirt / "dust"	1. "Chaff" in uncleaned cereals, "fines" in concentrates 2. Soil/sand in/on hay, straw, beets, carrots 3. Feces and urine of rats, mice (uncovered forage and concentrates)	1. Impairment of respiratory tract (mechanical irritation) 2. Gastrointestinal disorders ("sand colic") 3. Exposure to pathogenic bacteria like *Salmonella, Leptospira, Listeria*	Clarke & Madelin 1987; Kirschvink et al 2002; Robinson et al 1996
Pests / insects	1. Moths in/on concentrates, cereals 2. Beetles in/on cereals, concentrates, hay, straw 3. Mites in cereals, hay, straw	1. Reduced feed palatability and lower feed intake 2. Allergic reactions, coughing 3. Signs of colic	Kamphues & Reichmuth 2000; Eder et al 2000; Rade et al 1998
Molds / yeasts	1. Epiphytic molds (like *Fusarium*) on cereals 2. Species indicating spoilage (*Aspergillus, Mucor*) 3. Yeasts on silages, cereals, (wet) concentrates	1. Gastrointestinal dysbiosis (altered flora composition) 2. Altered composition of intestinal flora/ respiratory problems 3. Mycosis (e.g. guttural pouch mycosis)	Gregory & Lacey 1963; Rade et al 1998; Wright et al 2009; Buckley et al 2007; Keller et al 2007; Blomme et al 1998
Bacteria	1. Epiphytic bacteria on cereals (like *Flavobacterium*) 2. Species indicating spoilage (like *Clostridia, Staph.*) 3. Pathogenic species like *Salmonella*, *Listeria Leptospira*, clostridia	1. Gastrointestinal dysbiosis (altered flora composition) 2. Gastrointestinal dysbiosis (altered flora composition and activity → gas formation) 3. Diarrhea, abortion (depending on species of bacteria)	Traub-Dargatz et al 2000; Sargison 1993; Raymond et al 2000
Toxins of microorganisms	1. Mycotoxins (cereals, grass, maize silage) 2. Endotoxins (from gram-negative bacteria) 3. Exotoxins such as botulism toxin	1. Mycotoxicosis (effects depending on kind of toxin) 2. Respiratory tract diseases (irritation, sensitization) 3. Intoxication	Liesener et al 2010; Raymond et al 2000, 2005; Sacchi et al 2009; Caloni & Cortinovis 2010, 2011 Snell 1966; Kamphues et al 1991; McGorum et al 1998; Pirie et al 2001, 2003
Chemical contaminants			
Fertilizer	Grass but also concentrates	Depends on kind of fertilizer	Kamphues et al 2009
Heavy metals	Roughage mainly	Depends on type of metal	
Rodenticides, insecticides	Use within the feed mill, confounding accidents, errors	Depends on type of substances	
Fluorine	Water	Teeth/bone alteration	
Ionophores	Cross-contamination of concentrates (coccidiostats)	Sudden death, cardiac and skeletal muscle degeneration, colic, myoglobinuria	Kamphues et al 1990; Aleman et al 2007; Hughes et al 2009; Dorne et al 2011
Physical contaminants			
Sand/soil	Concentration in roughage (paddocks without green fodder)	Colic (accumulation of sand)	Art et al 2002 Rollins & Clement 1979
Glass	Silage	Mechanical damage within the GIT	
Threads/ strings	Bales of hay/straw/silage	Impaired passage of ingesta, intestinal obstruction	

Practical evaluation of feed hygiene

In general, there are three main situations that warrant the initiation of a more detailed evaluation of the hygienic quality of a particular feedstuff or ration (Table 20-2). The first steps are to obtain the "history" of the feed through a detailed anamnesis, and then gather data through personal observations and diagnostic activities. Here, it should be emphasized that much of information can be obtained through an intensive and detailed visual appraisal of the feedstuffs in question. It may be necessary to take representative feed samples; these may be retained and appropriately stored as control baseline samples in case further evaluations are required, or directly subjected to chemical and/or microbiological analyses. Table 20-3 presents a summary of the systematic approach to assessment of feed hygiene status.

Visual examination enables detection of obvious abnormalities including contamination by dirt, pests and feces of rodents. Careful evaluation of the "fines" may show slight movements, indicating colonization by mites and/or insects (Kamphues 1996). Furthermore the proportion of "fines" in the feed provides an indication of the intensity of cereal cleaning or whether undesired abrasive processes may have occurred during the transport of pelleted concentrates (Kamphues et al 1989). The color of cereals may vary due to superficial contamination (molds/dirt/dust) but also due to genetic varieties (e.g., golden, yellow or black oats), which should not be confused with ergot contamination. In concentrates, the color should also reflect the type and nature of the ingredients (e.g., green due to grass/alfalfa meal) present in the feed. Understanding which feedstuffs are present in the feed can be valuable in other ways; for example, there can be higher risk of contamination by mycotoxins in oats when compared to other cereal grains (Edwards 2009). Two factors might explain this observation; oats are typically harvested later in the year (higher

Table 20-2 Typical Situations Requiring a More in-Depth Evaluation of Feed Hygiene

1. Questions from horse owners
   - based on observations regarding the quality of feed batches
   - regarding shelf-life and the suitability of feeds
   - regarding the treatment of feeds before feeding
2. Increased frequency of clinical disorders in horses, including
   - colic
   - respiratory disorders (e.g. recurrent airway obstruction or "heaves")
   - fertility problems (conception rate ↓ / abortions ↑)
   - poor performance
3. Prophylactic purposes/optimizing feed production and storage
   - feeding as a part of the whole management
   - recommendations concerning storage of feeds
   - control of feed quality before ingredients are used

Table 20-3 A Systematic Approach for Evaluation of the Hygiene Status of Equine Feeds (Progression Through All Steps Increases the Expenditure)

Step	Procedure	Relevance (examples)
1	Gather information on the feed by questioning the horse keeper on, e.g. - production/storing/treatment - observations after starting to use the feed - changes in defecation/feces quality	→ label of the feed? → weather at harvest? technical equipment? storing facilities? → reduced palatability? coughing? gastrointestinal disturbances? → watery feces
2	Conduct a thorough visual appraisal (appearance/odor/texture) - feed itself - feed circumstances/surrounding environment, e.g. cleanliness of utensils used, how long any soaked feed is left before feeding etc.	roughage: test DM content by feeling silages: test the smell (nuances of butyrate/alcohol); cereals: appearance of the surface(changes due to smell?) → compare to expected "normal qualities" for that feedstuff/feed: determine if there is an obvious smell of molds/yeasts or obvious presence of physical contaminants etc. → note air humidity/temperature/ storage conditions, etc.
3	Take appropriate samples of feeds (and bedding material) - from stored feedstuffs - from offered feedstuffs	ideally should represent the actually offered/ingested feed → may mean taking samples out of the trough! → time between delivery and sampling? → record history of the feed Always label feedstuffs with the batch or delivery number and date delivered.
3.1	Chemical analyses of: • dry matter content • acid content, pH-values (for haylage/silage)	generate objective values and compare to standards
3.2	Microbiological investigations type/kind and counts of bacteria type/kind and counts of molds and yeasts	Signs in horses specific for pathogenic bacteria? → indicative of spoilage/deterioration? see Table 20-6
3.3	Analysis for microbial toxins mycotoxins endotoxins (e.g. lipopolysaccharides)	In specialized laboratories only → related to clinical signs/molds detected → information regarding mass of Gram-negative bacteria

Table 20-4 Summary of the Main Differences between Silage and Haylage

Forage	Target species	Storage form	Date of 1st cut	Typical DM %	Preservation
Silage	Farmed ruminants	Clamp or large, round bales (300–500 kg)	Early May*	18–40	Fermentation (higher acid contents)
Haylage	Equines	Bales: small (25 kg); vacuum-packed large (180–250 kg); round or square, wrapped	Mid June*	55–70	Limited fermentation and preservation (due to higher DM content and pH-values)

*Northern hemisphere

frequency of bad weather) and the husk has a groove on the surface that predisposes it to contamination.

Assessment of dry matter (DM), temperature and the pH value of silage and haylage are important when considering suitability for feeding horses (Müller 2005, Müller et al 2011). The feeding of spoiled silages/haylages might result in excessive gas formation in the gastrointestinal tract of horses, resulting in colic. The main differences between silage (typically fed to farm livestock) and haylage (specifically made for horses) are their moisture content, extent of fermentation, date of harvest and nutrient content (Table 20-4). Low DM materials (<40%) require some form of fermentation of the plant sugars to form lactic acid that, in effect, "pickles" the grass. However in higher DM haylages, lower moisture and sugar contents restrict the opportunity for fermentation, and the main method of preservation is excluding air by wrapping or vacuum packing. If there are concerns with respect to the DM content of any feedstuff, it is recommended to send in samples for analysis (Table 20-5).

During the careful visual appraisal of hay, straw and silages there is also the need to be carefully checked for the presence of toxic plants or other potentially toxic contaminants (e.g., blister beetles in US-sourced alfalfa [lucerne] products). This chapter cannot do justice to the range of potential poisonous plants but over the last decade several published reports have underlined the clinical relevance of such contaminations (e.g., Kamphues & Meyer 1990, Wolf & Kamphues 2001). Important plant contaminants include *Equisetum palustre*, *Colchicum autumnale*, *Senecio jacobaea* and *Hypericum perforatum* in hay, as well as *Trisetum flavescens*, *Mercurialis annua* and *Senecio* spp. in silages, and *Apera spica venti* in straw (the latter is not a toxic plant but its ingestion has been associated with colic; Kamphues & Schad 1992).

Table 20-5 Suggested Quantitative Values Regarding the Dry Matter Content of Equine Feedstuffs Relating to Aerobic Spoilage

Oats/barley/maize	≥ 88% = very dry < 88 – > 85% = desirable	< 85% = unacceptable
Concentrates	≥ 86% required by feed legislation	< 85% = unacceptable
Hay/straw	≥ 86% = desirable 86 – 85% = insufficient	< 85% = unacceptable
Silages (wilted)	35–50% = normal range	< 30% = unacceptable
Haylage	55–70% = desirable	> 70% = risky

In earlier studies, for example, the cultural investigations were restricted to either thermophilic or thermotolerant species of moulds depending on the temperature used during incubation (Kirschvink et al 2002, Mair & Derksen 2000). Wright et al (2009) have emphasized that there is no correlation between the results (molds, fungal spores) obtained when the temperature during incubation was at either 22°C or 35°C. Accordingly, Raymond et al (2000) have recommended combining different incubation times and temperatures in order to obtain data on the wide spectrum of microorganisms present in feeds (7 days at 25°C: mesophile aerobic bacteria, molds, yeasts; 5 days at 40°C: thermotolerant fungi; 3 days at 55°C: thermophilic Actinomyces). The cost of such intensive analyses has prevented this approach being widely adopted in the field.

More than two decades ago, a standardized procedure for microbiological investigations was established for all "official" analyses of feedstuffs in Germany (Schmidt 1991). The intention was (and still is) to generate data on the extent of the "load" of mesophile aerobic microorganisms within feeds, including bacteria, molds and yeasts (divided into normal "epiphytic" and undesirable spoilage inducing organisms). This approach has facilitated the development of knowledge of what can be considered "normal" vs. "abnormal" microbiological contamination, and these parameters have been adopted for use in other countries (Switzerland and Austria). There is good agreement between the "upper normal values" used in Germany with data from other published studies (e.g., Raymond et al 2000, Wright et al 2009) when comparable analytical procedures have

Microbiological investigations to assess the hygiene status of feedstuffs and bedding material

There is variation in the methods used for microbiological examination of feedstuffs; in particular, methods can vary according to:

1. The pretreatment of the feed (diminution/dilution/incubation of feed-water suspension).
2. The temperature used for incubation (25 to 45°C).
3. The duration of incubation (2 to 7 days).

been used. It is also necessary to differentiate the results of microbiological analyses according to the reason for the investigation, e.g. some authors have focused on pathogenic fungi (*Aspergillus fumigatus*, *A. niger*, *A. flavus* and *Fusarium*), ignoring non-pathogenic species of molds, yeasts or bacteria (Buckley et al 2007).

As mentioned, all equine feedstuffs are contaminated (predominantly on their surface) by microorganisms that represent the so-called epiphytic flora; counts for bacteria and molds are typically ~10^6 colony-forming units (cfu)/g feed and ~10^3–10^4 cfu/g feed, respectively. Normally, the presence of these epiphytes neither harms the plant, seed or feed, nor impacts horse health. However, under certain circumstances (high humidity and temperature, physical damage; e.g., from insect or pest damage) there is opportunity for other undesirable microorganisms to multiply rapidly to the point that epiphytic flora no longer the predominant species (feed spoilage). During this spoilage process, the variety of species present decreases while the number of "spoilage-indicating bacteria (and molds)" increases, reaching values up to 10^9–10^{10} cfu/g feed. Concurrently, the smell of the feed changes (putrid/moldy/fusty/stuffy) and the feed begins to lose its original appearance. At this stage, microbiological analyses can provide useful information regarding the microbial species involved as well as their counts. With extreme spoilage, however, visual appraisal alone will reveal the impact of microbial contamination on the quality of the feed.

The contamination of the feed by distinct pathogenic species of bacteria such as *Salmonella* spp. or *Leptospira* spp. is a completely different scenario as these microorganisms are not normally present in feeds and these species do not result in typical feed spoilage. Nonetheless, even when present in relatively low levels these organisms can cause clinical illness (e.g., diarrhea and sepsis (*Salmonella*) or abortion (*Leptospira*)). Examination of feedstuffs for the presence of these pathogenic species is warranted when clinical disease occurs and feed is considered a possible source of the infection. It should also be noted that *Clostridium* spp. and *Listeria* spp. are common in the soil. Soil contamination therefore increases the risk of contamination. A visual check or rejection of material that feels "gritty" can help avoid such material. Ash analysis of forages can also provide information on above-average soil contamination.

Tables 20-6 and 20-7 provide information on microflora in feeds, including "normal" counts that have been detected in the absence of negative effects on animal health. Even when these values are exceeded, it is not possible to conclude that a particular feed has caused a problem. In general, however, when the "normal values" are exceeded by a factor of 5–10 there should be high suspicion that the feed has contributed to the observed problem.

Other methods for estimation of the potential microbiota load of the feed include measurement of structural constituents like ergosterol (from the cell wall of molds and yeasts) or the content of lipopolysaccharides (constituents of the cell wall of Gram-negative bacteria). The advantage of this approach is the detection of the entire cell mass of microorganisms (both dead and alive), and it can also be used for feeds that have been subjected to intensive heat treatment (which will destroy all alive microorganisms) or exposed to other treatments that prevent the use of the culture methods (for further details see Kamphues 1986).

Key Points

Systematic evaluation of feed hygiene involves

- History taking (including observations on horse health)
- Visual and organoleptic assessment of the feed
- Chemical analysis
- Microbiological analysis

Table 20-6 Characterization of Microorganisms Occurring on Feedstuffs (Analyzed by Microbiological Cultural Techniques: Bucher & Thalmann 2006)

Type of microorganisms	Classification	Group no.	Typical species that represent the group number (examples only)	Comments
Aerobic bacteria	"Epiphytic" (normal)	1	*Flavobacterium* *Pseudomonas*	
	Indication of spoilage / deterioration	2	*Bacillus* spp. *Staphylococcus*/ *Micrococcus*	Able to produce bacterial toxins
		3	*Streptomyces* spp.	
Aerobic molds	"Epiphytic" (normal)	4	*Verticillium* *Acremonium* *Fusarium* *Aureobasidium*	Mycotoxins[a]
	Indication of spoilage / deterioration	5	*Aspergillus* *Penicillium* *Scopulariopsis* *Wallemia*	Mycotoxins[a]
		6	*Mucor* spp.	Destruents
Yeasts	Indicating spoilage	7	All species	Gas producer

[a]Different types of mycotoxins are produced by the different mold species.

Table 20-7 Highest Acceptable Counts of Microorganisms in Typical Feedstuffs for Horses (VDLUFA 2011). The Group Numbers Correspond to Those in Table 20-6.

Microorganisms	Aerobic bacteria ×10⁶ cfu/g			Molds ×10³ cfu/g			Yeasts ×10³ cfu/g
Group number	1	2	3	4	5	6	7
Cereals							
- oats	50	1	0.05	200	50	2	200
- barley	20	1	0.05	40	30	2	100
- maize	2	0.5	0.05	20	30	5	60
By products							
- bran (wheat)	8	1	0.1	50	50	2	80
- soybean meal	1	1	0.1	10	20	1	30
Pelleted feed[a]	0.5	0.5	0.01	2	6	1	5
Mixed feed	5	0.5	0.1	3	20	5	50
Silages							
- maize/corn	0.4	0.2	0.03	5	5	5	1000
- grass	0.2	0.2	0.01	5	5	5	200
Roughages							
- hay	30	2	0.15	200	100	5	150
- straw	100	2	0.15	200	100	5	400

[a]The pelleting process should result in a reduced count of microorganisms.

Potential effects of poor feed hygiene on horse health

Feeds and feeding can adversely affect horse health in several ways, as summarized by Meyer & Coenen (2002):

- an oversupply or deficiency of energy and/or nutrients
- an unsuitable composition of the whole ration
- poor feeding methods
- the intake of toxic constituents from ingredients
- poor feed hygiene (specific ingredients or the whole ration).

Respiratory system

It has long been recognized that poor hygiene status of feed ingredients can adversely affect the health of the respiratory tract in horses. Exposure to dust and its constituents (fine particles of feeds, straw, feces, microorganisms, mites; toxins of microbial origin, chemically active substances like ammonia) is the most important challenge to the respiratory tract (McGorum 1994, McGorum et al 1998, Clarke & Madelin 1987, Kamphues et al 1991, Kamphues & Schulze Becking 1992, Robinson et al 1996, Mair & Derksen 2000, Raymond et al 2000, Pirie et al 2001, Rade & Kamphues 1999, Art et al 2002, Kirschvink et al 2002, Ward & Couetil 2005, Buckley et al 2007, Dunett 2009, Wolf et al 2009, Wichert et al 2008). The concentration and composition of airborne dust in horse stables differ markedly depending on the quality of feeds, method of feeding and type of bedding material (and its hygiene status), environmental conditions and other contributing factors (Fig. 20.1). There are several mechanisms underlying the development of respiratory disease associated with exposure to airborne dusts (Fig. 20.2).

Gastrointestinal tract

The role of poor feed hygiene in the etiology of colic and other gastrointestinal tract (GIT) problems has received very little attention. Raymond et al (2000) indicated that GIT disorders in horses could be caused by "moldy forage" but the main health risks were linked to the respiratory tract. In a field survey on feeding practices associated with colic in horses, Hudson et al (2001) observed that "feeding hay from round bales" increased the risk of colic. Nonetheless, more than 30 years ago Meyer (1979) emphasized the important role of feed hygiene in the occurrence of colic, for example:

- stimulated gas production in the GIT due to feed contamination by yeasts and other gas-producing microorganisms
- substances with antimicrobial properties in moldy feeds (especially roughages) that impair/suppress the GIT flora
- imbalances within the normal GIT flora enabling "exogenous microorganisms" (from feed/straw/litter) to colonize the alimentary tract
- improper physical form of ingredients due to fine cutting of roughage or ingestion without intensive chewing (for example the grass *Apera spica venti* as a contaminant in straw).

The results of some recent epidemiological studies provide support for the ideas expressed by Meyer (1979), for example Wichert et al (2008), Kaya et al (2009) and Wolf et al (2009). Kaya et al (2009), for example, observed an association between reduced hygiene quality of hay and the

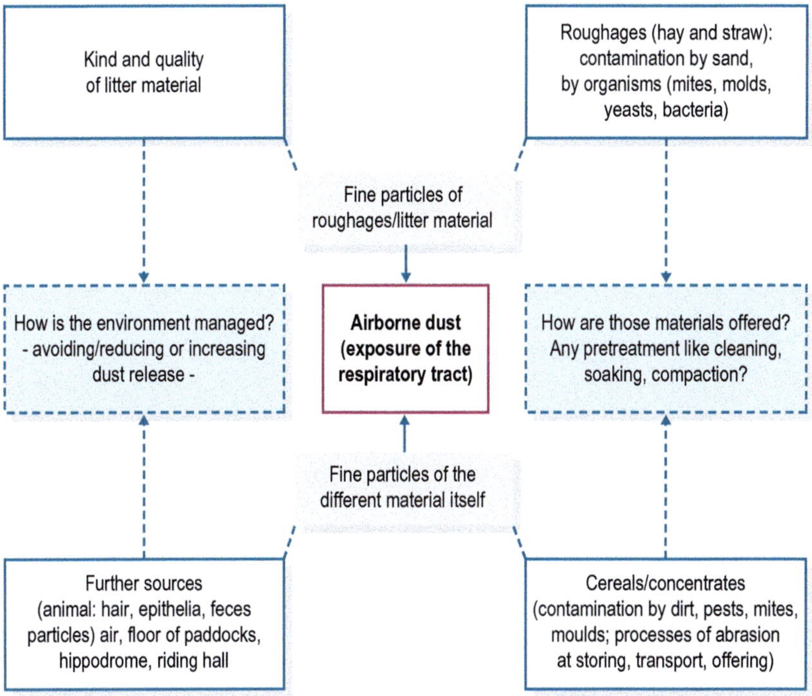

Figure 20.1 Sources of airborne dust that may result in exposure of the respiratory tract.

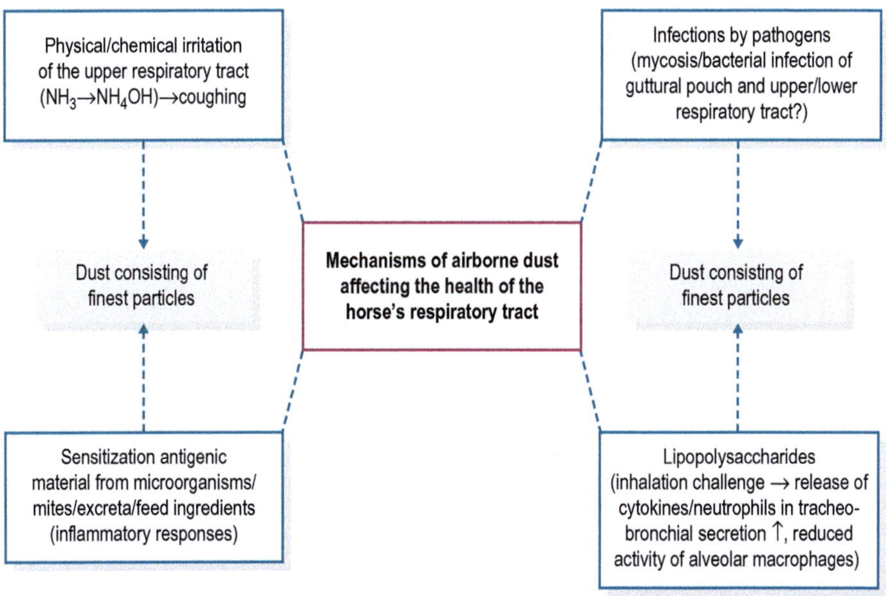

Figure 20.2 Mechanisms involved in the development of respiratory disease associated with exposure to airborne dusts.

incidence of colic in a population of horses in Austria. However, in general epidemiological studies on colic have not routinely included assessment of the hygienic quality of the feeds offered. Much more in-depth work is needed in this area.

Mycotoxins

Mycotoxins are undesirable substances that occur as secondary metabolites of fungal growth. They are produced by molds to aid their survival either as a defense mechanism or to help the mold colonize its host. Whilst viable molds have been associated with respiratory irritation and allergy in horses, more recently attention has turned to the potential for mycotoxins to cause adverse health effects. For some mycotoxins, such as fumonisins and aflatoxins, the effects on horses are well known, but for other mycotoxins the level at which any potential negative effect occurs are less clear.

As mentioned before, contamination of feeds by certain mycotoxins can be a risk for horses' health, depending on the mycotoxin and the amount present. Of special interest are fusariotoxins (Johnson et al 1997, Raymond et al 2000, Buckley et al 2004, Liesener et al 2010), but also mycotoxins from the ergot family produced by *Claviceps* spp. or by endophytic molds that occur in some species of grass worldwide (Riet-Correa et al 1988, Copetti et al 2002, Fayrer-Hosken et al 2008) leading to reduced fertility, especially to agalactia (due to prolactin antagonistic effects of the ergotamine-like substances). Table 20-8 gives a short overview on this class of contaminants.

Different genera/species of bacteria and molds are able to produce toxins and subsequently release these as contaminants in/on feeds. Today it is possible to detect various toxins that can either lead to general impaired health and wellbeing or to specific diseases which may be associated with fairly pathognomonic signs e.g. equine leukoencephalopathy (ELEM; due to fumonisins) or botulism (due to toxins of *Clostridium botulinum*). Table 20-8 lists some of the more important toxins. Here it has to be underlined that all *Fusarium* spp. produce their mycotoxins pre-harvest, while *Aspergillus* spp. and *Penicillium* spp. can also produce their toxins post-harvesting (e.g., when storing the feed).

For the mycotoxins summarized in Table 20-8 there are some data regarding the levels in feeds that are allowed (max. levels from feed legislation) or that could be tolerated (without adverse effects in horses) in the diet (with 88% DM).

- Aflatoxins = max. 0.02 resp. 0.01 mg/kg feed (ingredients/compound feeds)
- Ergovaline = 300–500 µg/kg diet lead to clinical symptoms
- Fumonisins = NOAEL: 10 µg/kg BW; max.: 5 mg/kg diet
- Zearalenone = safety margin: 5 µg/kg BW; max.: 2–3 mg/kg diet
- DON = tolerance in horses comparable to pigs (up to 1000 µg/kg diet; based on experiments of Schulz et al 2012).

As expected, the clinical signs that can occur after the ingestion of toxin contaminated feeds can affect the entire animal but there are also some relatively specific tropisms (aflatoxins → liver; fumonisins → white substance of the brain; endotoxins → exposure of the respiratory tract → COB/RAO like symptoms). These need to be taken into consideration by the veterinary practitioner. However, the fact that certain toxins are found in the feed does not necessarily mean that they are associated with the observed clinical signs.

Mycotoxin mitigation

Given that mycotoxins are often present in equine feedstuffs complete avoidance is difficult. Although once ingested mechanisms for at least partial detoxification and excretion of the mycotoxins exist, horses do not automatically self-protect by refusing mycotoxin-contaminated feeds. The use of sound practices in the production and storage of feedstuffs (see Table 20-9) is the main strategy for mitigation of mycotoxin load. Special attention leads to the following established methods:

- Rotation in crop production
- Selection of mold-resistant varieties
- Use of efficient fungicides
- Soil management (plowing instead of cultivating).

In the feed industry there are diverse measures to reduce the mycotoxin load of feeds. One of the most efficient is intensive cleaning of cereals and the prevention of mycotoxin formation during storage (sufficient dryness avoiding higher humidity). Last but not least the horse owner has to ensure suitable storage conditions (including well-known principles like first in – first out).

Table 20-8 Toxins Produced by Microorganisms That Belong to Feed Associated Microbial Contaminants

Toxin(s)	Produced by	Occurring in	Effects/remarks
Ergotalcaloids/ ergovaline	*Claviceps* spp. endophytic molds	Rye (bran), wheat grass (hay)	Prolactin antagonism, abortion (mare's health!)
Aflatoxins	*Aspergillus* spp. (*A. flavus!*)	Different feedstuffs (esp. imported ones[a])	Liver disease/dysfunction
Fumonisins	*Fusarium spp.* (*F. moniliforme*)	Cereals, especially in corn (byproducts)	Typical: equine leuko-encephalomalazia (ELEM)
Zearalenone	*Fusarium* spp. (*F. graminearum*)	Cereals, soybean corn byproducts	Estrogenic effects ("endocrine disruptor")
DON (type B-trichothecene)	*Fusarium* spp. (*F. graminearum*)	Wheat, barley; corn byproducts	Feed refusal (in other species: vomitus)
T2/HT2 (type A-trichothecene)[b]	*F. langsethiae* *F. sporotrichoides*	Oats, barley, corn byproducts	GIT: mucosal irritations/alterations
Satratoxine	*Stachybotrys* spp.	Roughages (straw/hay)	Central/nervous symptoms, salivation/tremor
Botulinum-toxin	*Clostridium botulinum*	Hay, wilted grass, silages, straw	Paralysis, salivation, sudden death
Endotoxines (lipopolysaccharides)	All Gram-negative bacteria (cell wall)	All feedstuffs (especially in "fines" of hay/ straw)	Changes in body temperature, respiratory diseases (→ COB/ RAO like changes)

[a]Feedstuffs imported from subtropical and tropical regions are especially prone to contamination with aflatoxin, but under certain circumstances (high temperature, changes in humidity) *Aspergillus* spp. may also produce toxins in Europe. See EFSA 2011
[b]There are also effects on immune system; loss of protection against oxidative damage is discussed too.

Table 20-9 A Guide to the Mitigation or Risk Management Activities That Should Take Place at All Stages of the Feed Supply Chain (See Also Chapter 21)

Stage	Activity
Supplier	Inhibition of fungi mitigates mycotoxin formation
Growth	Management of crop production chain (selection of varieties, plowing, residues of former crops, sequence of crops, use of fungicides, insect repelling programs, infection pressure from natural reservoirs, equipment cleaning and maintenance)
Harvest	Conditions at harvest; grain drying to DM content >86%
Storage	Protection against damage in the storage unit. Low moisture environment, controlled free water activity, insect and mite defense. Certain preservatives used in store (e.g. propionic acid) may prevent mold growth
Manufacturer	Good manufacturing practice and HACCP
Distributor of finished goods	Good finished product storage and stock management (e.g. 'first in first out', stock rotation). Ingress of moisture from leaks or vermin damage can cause mold growth and potentially lead to mycotoxin formation.
The end user or horse keeper	Correct storage of feedstuffs and stock management; Use by sell by date; Effective pest control and cleaning programs.

Currently, there is no routine procedure available for detoxification of feed; mycotoxin binders are available but they do not reduce the actual load of mycotoxins in feedstuffs. More work is needed to validate their use in the feed for horses.

Key Points – Mycotoxins

- Mycotoxins are undesirable substances that might occur in feedstuffs for horses, too.
- They occur as a consequence of the natural presence of molds.
- The presence of a mycotoxin or mycotoxins does not automatically indicate a problem but above certain limits clinical issues may occur.
- Valid analytical methods are essential for the evaluation of a feed that might contain a mycotoxin
- Limits and/or regulatory guidance are available for certain mycotoxins, although a lot more data is required with respect to the horse
- Effective risk reduction strategies exist for mycotoxins, and cover the whole process of sourcing feed, from initial crop growth and harvest to the final feed bucket (see Table 20-9)

Other potential contaminants

A number of chemical contaminants also may pose risk of feed-associated intoxication. These can be naturally occurring, such as morphine due to the inclusion of morphine-producing poppies (see Chapter 21), or due to cross-contamination. The most important substances with respect to cross-contamination are coccidiostats, which are used worldwide as feed additives in complete diets for poultry, rabbits and ruminants. Therefore special risk occur when such feeds are made in the same facilities as the equine feed. Similarly, several substances within the ionophore group are used as growth promoters in different species of food producing animals (not allowed in Europe). Therefore, it is not surprising that severe intoxications of horses have occurred globally due to accidental cross-contamination. Questions should always be asked when a typical equine concentrate is contaminated by pellets of a different color, size, diameter and/or texture. The typical effects of ionophore intoxication in horses are myodegeneration, pain, massive colic, ataxia, sweating, red colored urine and recumbency (Kamphues et al 1990, Aleman et al 2007, Hughes et al 2009). The toxicity of ionophores in horses varies in the order salinomycin > narasin > monensin > lasalocid.

The spectrum of contaminants also includes substances that can enter the feed (grass, silage, hay) through soil contamination. Worldwide, there are areas (and rivers) in which soils and sediments contain high levels of heavy metals (e.g., Pb, Cd, Hg, As). Horses at pasture or fed silages or hay produced in those regions therefore may be at risk for heavy metal intoxication (Casteel 2001, Palacios et al 2002, Liu 2003). Analyses of blood and further substrates (like hair) – in addition to feed analyses – are recommended to clarify suspicious cases, with some reference data available (Hoff et al 1998). Sporadic cases of clinical illness also may be encountered due to other less common contaminants (e.g., accidental contamination by fertilizers, rodenticides or pesticides).

A potential concern about alfalfa produced in parts of the US is the presence of blister beetles that contain the cytotoxin cantharidin. As little as 4–6 g of dried beetles may be fatal to a horse (Jones 2006). Blister beetles tend to swarm as they feed on alfalfa flowers and therefore large numbers may be sporadically incorporated in baled hay. First cut hay is almost always free of blister beetles because the insects overwinter as subadults and do not emerge until late May or early June in the south-western US. Similarly, the last cut of hay is often safe because it is harvested after the time during which the adult insects are active.

Water quality and hygiene

Drinking water should be clear, palatable and free of microorganisms and chemical contaminants. Changes in physical appearance of the water or a decrease in water intake are indications to evaluate of water quality. Contamination of the water source (e.g., parts of straw, feeds, feces and/or urine) is not uncommon and is usually obvious. However, reduced water intake or complete refusal may be caused by contaminants and/or constituents that are not detectable by visual appraisal. Under these circumstances it is recommended to take a sample of water for assessment of microbiological and physiochemical composition. For example, high iron content can result in lower palatability, while ground water with "naturally" high sulfate content may lead to watery feces (due to osmotic effects) and high concentrations of nitrite can result in methemoglobinemia. Under some environmental conditions hygienic deterioration of the water supply can occur, especially when a large supply is maintained for only a small number of horses, e.g. growth of algae (favored by light) and/or microorganisms (favored by temperature). This reiterates the need for water supplies to be checked daily and replenished on a regular basis.

Some recommended values (Kamphues et al 2007) regarding the physicochemical quality of drinking water are summarized in Table 20-10 (also see Chapter 4). These values are used as "official" data for the quality of water for food producing animals in Germany. Regarding the microbial contamination of drinking water for animals, the same quality criteria as for human beings should be applied:

- aerobic total viable count: max. 1000 cfu/ml (37°C)
- aerobic total viable count: max. 10000 cfu/ml (20°C)
- free from *E. coli* and coliform bacteria (in 10 ml)
- free from salmonellae and *Campylobacter* (in 100 ml)

Note that evaluation of the physicochemical parameters summarized in Table 20-10 is usually not necessary if horses are provided water from a public supply intended for human consumption. However, testing is indicated if the water comes from a "private" source (e.g., well, spring, creek or pond). In rare instances, microbial contamination may be caused by the formation of biofilms in water pipes.

Key Points – Water

- The quantity and quality of water supply should be evaluated regularly (in fields, header tanks in stables and water bowls)
- If concerned about water quality, both chemical and microbiological parameters should be assessed

Table 20-10 Recommended Physicochemical Composition of Drinking Water for Horses (Modified According to Kamphues et al 2007)

Parameter	Recommended values for drinking water	Comments (possible effects/dysfunctions due to divergent values)
pH-value	> 5 and < 9	Corrosions in the ductwork
electrical conductivity (µS/cm)	< 3000	Higher values: diarrhea might occur, palatability ↓
soluble salts, total (g/l)	< 2.5	
oxidability (mg/l)	< 15	Measurement of burden with oxidizable substances
Ca^{2+} (mg/l)	< 500	Calcination; technical dysfunctions
Fe (mg/l)	< 3	Palatability ↓, technical dysfunctions, biofilm formation possible
Na^+/ K^+/ Cl^- (mg/l)	< 500	Indicator for contamination (excreta, urine)
NO_3^- (mg/l)	< 200	Formation of methemoglobin; consider total intake (feed!)
NO_2^- (mg/l)	< 30	Methemo globinemia
SO_4^- (mg/l)	< 500	Laxative effect/diarrhea
NH_4^- (mg/l)	< 3	Indicator for contamination
As (mg/l)	< 0.05	Disturbance of health, performance ↓
Cd (mg/l)	< 0.02	Residues in the food chain
Cu (mg/l)	< 2	Consider total intake (feed!)
F (mg/l)	< 1.5	Teeth/bone disorders
Hg (mg/l)	< 0.003	General disorders (intoxication)
Mn (mg/l)	< 4	Precipitates in the distribution system, biofilm formation possible
Pb (mg/l)	< 0.1	Residues in the food chain
Zn (mg/l)	< 5	Mucosal alterations

Responsibilities of partners in the feed supply chain

The principles of feed legislation are to avoid any adverse effects on animal health; to minimize risk to feed quality; and to protect the consumer and the environment. The term "consumer protection" also includes aspects of economic interests (avoiding deception) and transparency (information on feed quality by labelling). With respect to animal health, it is not permissible to produce, sell or offer feeds that are capable of adversely affecting animal wellbeing. Based on the EC regulation no. 183/2005, however, the primary responsibility for feed safety rests with the feed business operator.

Table 20-11 summarizes the specific obligations for people who are engaged in feed production and feeding. The feed producer is responsible for feed quality (including hygiene) up until the point of delivery and/or until the "best before date" – providing the consumer has ensured appropriate conditions for feed storage. The consumer has the right to receive an "unspoiled feed" (and obviously massive infestation by mites or high counts of molds undeniably indicates spoilage). On the other hand, if the consumer has not stored the feed appropriately before feeding, the actual problem may be attributed to himself rather than to the producer. The gathering of objective data (e.g., mold counts, pictures, retained feed samples) is important when the hygienic quality of a feed

Table 20-11 Legislative Aspects in the Feed Supply Chain

Addressed to	Examples of obligations that are described in detail	European legislation
"Primary production" (= producing feeds on farms)	• measures of feed hygiene → minimizing biological, chemical and physical contamination Good Agricultural Practice – to protect against contamination arising from air, water, fertilizer, plant protection products, veterinary drugs, waste – to keep clean all things that will come in contact with feeds, use clean water – to control measures regarding mycotoxins/heavy metals/correct use of veterinary products	EC No. 183/2005 ANNEX II
"Feed business operators" (feed industry)	• continuous control of facilities/equipment, feed quality, storage and transport – Use of HACCP to identify and control hazards – ingredient and finished product quality specifications – in focus: cross-contamination – good storage conditions → to avoid spoilage/ deterioration – pest control system • regarding feed trading/marketing – labelling of feeds/diets – botanical purity (mostly 95 %) – moisture content (< 14 %) – composition (listed ingredients)	EC 183/2005 ANNEX II EC No. 767/2009
"Farmer/owner of animals" (people who feed horses)	• general obligations like "prohibited to offer feeds that could harm the animal" – clean feeding equipment/correct storage – feed/bedding material → not to become moldy – water: appropriate quality – person: ability, knowledge, competence	EC No. 183/2005 ANNEX III

Table 20-12 Main Hygiene Risks of Feedstuffs Frequently Used in Horse Nutrition

Feed type	Common problems	Evaluation
Cereals	1. mycotoxin development in the field 2. improper cleaning 3. infestation by mites 4. contamination of the cereal surface by molds/bacteria 5. delay of drying after the harvest	1. See Table 20-8 2. sieving: determine the "fraction of fines" 3. presence of mites: "honey like smell", "moving" dust, evaluation with a magnifier (10–20×) 4. appearance (gray), moldy smell, etc. 5. microbiological analyses (type and counts of microorganisms); mycotoxin testing.
Molassed products	Higher contamination by yeasts	Nuances of alcohol
Concentrates (pelleted products)	Prolonged storing leads to secondary spoilage due to increased moisture content (molds/ yeasts)	Texture (particles adhering together, swelling); the smell has moldy nuances
Hay/straw	Insufficient dry matter at harvesting[a]	Test the texture at harvesting/ storing → may feel clammy
	Storing → contamination by molds (spores), pests	Release of dust (mainly consisting of fungal spores) when "plumping up" the roughage
	Cross-contamination of prohibited substances/ drugs through ingestion of contaminated roughage (urine in particular)	Care and proper stable hygiene in particular for competing and racing animals
Haylage/Wilted grass silage	Aerobic deterioration via punctured or split packaging due to yeasts' activity → secondary: growth of molds/bacteria	May detect slightly increased temperature, also test the smell, issues if has moldy/dump nuances
Corn silage	Elevated counts of yeasts (aerobe deterioration) Vermin damage	Alcohol nuances in the smell

[a]High load of fungal spores mainly occurs when roughage is baled at a dry matter content of 75% or even lower (Séguin et al 2010).

Table 20-13 Examples of Key Circumstances and Conditions Enabling Spoilage of Feed and How They May Be Controlled

Factor/aspect	Relevance/effects	Comments
Harvesting		
- Moisture	Supports microbial growth	Promotes outdoor deterioration of feeds
- Cleaning	Reduces dirt/dust	Only dry cereals can be cleaned effectively
Storage		
- Time	Time related increase in risk of contamination	Weeks regarding pests, days for molds, hours regarding yeasts/bacteria
- Conditions	Risk level influenced by storage conditions including moisture and temperature (but also the presence of pests etc.)	Most problems occur with high temperature at a high air humidity
- Preserving agents	Use of propionic acid	Certain "mold inhibitors" can help to reduce the growth of molds but may not always be effective or without their own risks.
Feed processing		
- Intact/crushed	Crushing → substrate availability↑	Finely ground: highest susceptibility
- Pelleted/ unpelleted	Pressure/heat: microorganisms ↓	In general cooked products have the highest hygiene status – but can be contaminated for example during the production process if pipes etc. are not fully cleaned and pockets of old feed remain.
Offering the feed		
- Dry/wet[a]	Soaked feeds may help to avoid spread of dust but depending on environmental conditions need to be made and consumed quickly	Other potential ways to prevent a high content of fines/dust include choice of source material, techniques for separating dust prior to bagging or feeding etc.
- At the floor	Feeding from the floor may have some advantages regarding the respiratory tract but increases the risk of ingestion of sand/ earth	Avoid by using well maintained feeding utensils such as troughs.

[a]In horses with recurrent airway obstruction and other inflammatory airway diseases, the soaking or steaming of hay, use of hay cobs instead of hay, and pellets instead of grains is very important.

is in dispute. A clear understanding of expected norms for required quality parameters as well as "shelf life" is also paramount. The expiration date or best before date differs markedly between feedstuffs. Problems can occur in particular when ingredients have a moisture content >14% and simultaneously a high availability of sugar and starch due to cracking/grinding/cutting. Silage/haylage (where high moisture content will allow microbial growth and activity) can undergo a process of secondary fermentation within hours (at high external temperatures) or within 2–5 days (winter), thus the time that they need to be used after the opening of the package or bale is limited.

Finally Tables 20-12 and 20-13 summarize the key reasons why feed becomes contaminated and provide some suggestions how to prevent the occurrence of such contaminants.

Summary

In the feeding management of horses careful attention needs to be paid to the hygienic quality of feeds and bedding material. Infestation by mites and contamination by molds (hay, straw, cereals, and complete feeds) are relatively common, while contamination by yeasts (silage, haylage, molassed oats, sometimes concentrates) or bacteria (especially in oats) is less common. Aside from the adverse effects of these contaminants on nutritive value and palatability, there is a risk of provoking digestive disorders. As well as the potential adverse effects of the living microorganisms, the toxins produced by bacteria (e.g., *Clostridium botulinum*) or by different species of molds (mycotoxins produced by *Claviceps purpurea*, *Acremonium*, *Fusarium*, *Aspergillus*, and *Penicillium*) can cause adverse reactions in the horse. Dusty feedstuffs (especially roughage) expose the respiratory tract to mites, infectious microorganisms and toxins (e.g., lipopolysaccharides) and contribute to the pathogenesis of inflammatory airway diseases in horses. Chemical contaminants (e.g., coccidiostats, fertilizer, heavy metals) or physical contaminants (most commonly sand/soil) should not be ignored; similarly the quality of drinking water should be evaluated when feed-related problems are suspected.

Optimizing the conditions of feed production and storage (including straw as bedding material) is essential for horses health and performance. The application of sound hygiene practices in feed production and storage as well as feeding can help to minimize feed hygiene-related problems.

Acknowledgments

The author gratefully acknowledges the contributions of Ms. Ruth Bishop and Professor Manfred Coenen in the preparation of the mycotoxin part of this chapter.

References

Aleman, M., Magdesian, K.G., Peterson, T.S., et al., 2007. Salinomycin toxicosis in horses. JAVMA 230 (12), 1822–1826.

Art, T., McGorum, B.C., Lekeux, P., 2002. Environmental control of respiratory disease. In: Lekeux, P. (Ed.), Equine Respiratory Diseases. International Veterinary Information Service (www.ivis.org), Ithaca, NY.

Barker, S.A., 2008. Drug contamination of the equine racetrack environment: A preliminary examination. J Vet Pharmacol Therap 31 (5), 466–471.

Blomme, E., Del Piero, F., La Perle, K.M.D., et al., 1998. Aspergillosis in horses: a review. Equine Vet Educ 10 (2), 86–93.

Bucher, E., Thalmann, A., 2006. Mikrobiologische Untersuchung von Futtermitteln (Microbiological examination of feeds - orientation values to assess soundness). Feed Magazine/Kraftfutter, 2006 (6), 16–23.

Buckley, T., Pickard, J., Murphy, R., et al., 2004. Concentration of different mycotoxins in feed and straw on 6 Irish racehorse farms. Proc. International Society for Animal Hygiene, Saint Malo, 447, http://www.isah-soc.org/documents/2004/Buckley.pdf.

Buckley, T., Creighton, A., Fogarty, U., 2007. Analysis of Canadian and Irish forage, oats and commercially available equine concentrate feed for pathogenic fungi and mycotoxins. Irish Vet J 60 (4), 231–236.

Caloni, F., Cortinovis, C., 2010. Effects of fusariotoxins in the equine species. The Vet J 186, 157–161.

Caloni, F., Cortinovis, C., 2011. Toxicological effects of aflatoxins in horses. The Vet J 188, 270–273.

Casteel, S.W., 2001. Metal Toxicosis in Horses. In: The Veterinary Clinics of North America: Equine Pract 17 (3), 517–527.

Clarke, A.F., Madelin, T., 1987. Technique for assessing respiratory health hazards from hay and other source materials. Equine Vet J 19 (5), 442–447.

Copetti, M.V., Santurio, J.M., Boeck, A.A.P., et al., 2002. Agalactia in mares fed with grain contaminated with Claviceps purpurea. Mycopathologia 154, 199–200.

Dorne, J.L., Fernández-Cruz, M.L., Bertelsen, U., et al., 2011. Risk assessment of coccidostatics during feed cross-contamination: Animal and human health aspects. Toxicol Appl Pharmaco Jan 6. [Epub ahead of print].

Dunnett, C.E., 2009. The importance of diet and feeding practices in the development of common health issues in the horse. In: Briese, A., Clauß, M., Hartung, J., Springorum, A., Brno, T.E.U. (Eds.), Proceedings of the XIV ISAH Congress 2009, pp. 1063–1067.

Eder, C., Crameri, R., Mayer, C., et al., 2000. Allergen-specific IgE levels against crude mould and storage mite extracts and recombinant mould allergens in sera from horses affected with chronic bronchitis. Vet Immunol Immunopathol 73, 241–253.

Edwards, S., 2009. Investigation of *Fusarium* mycotoxins in UK barley and oat production. Report on Joint FSA/HGCA project, CO4033 and CO4034 HGCA 2706,UK.

EFSA, 2011. Scientific Opinion on the risks for animal and public health related to the presence of T-2 and HT-2 Toxin in food and feed. EFSA Panel on Contaminants in the Food Chain (CONTAM). EFSA Journal 2011 9 (12), 2481.

Fayrer-Hosken, R., Heusner, G., Hill, N., et al., 2008. Review on effects of fescue grass ergot alkaloids in the horse and preliminary study on effects of fescue grass ergot alkaloid in the stallion. J Equine Vet Sci 28 (11), 666–671.

Gregory, P.H., Lacey, M.E., 1963. Mycological examination of dust from mouldy hay associated with farmer's lung disease. J Gen Microbiol 30, 75–88.

Halbert, M.K., Archer, J.C., 2007. Dioxin and Furan contamination of deodorizer distillates and natural vitamin E supplements. J Food Comp Anal 20, 506–514.

Hoff, B., Boermans, H.J., Baird, J.D., 1998. Retrospective study of toxic metal analyses requested at a veterinary diagnostic toxicology laboratory in Ontario (1990–1995). Can Vet J 39, 39.

Hudson, J.M., Cohen, N.D., Gibbs, P.G., et al., 2001. Feeding practices associated with colic in horses. JAVMA 219, 1419–1425.

Hughes, K.J., Hoffmann, K.L., Hodgson, D.R., 2009. Long-term assessment of horses and ponies post exposure to monensin sodium in commercial feed. Equine Vet J 41 (1), 47–52.

Johnson, P.J., Casteel, S.W., Messer, N.T., 1997. Effect of feeding deoxynivalenol (vomitoxin)-contaminated barley to horses. J Vet Diagn Invest 9, 219–221.

Jones, S.L., 2006. Disorders of the large intestine causing diarrhoea. In: Proceedings of North American Veterinary Conference, Vol 20, pp. 124-127.

Kamphues, J., 1986. Lipopolysaccharides in feedstuffs - potential relevance, assessment and amounts. Übers Tierernährg 14, 131–156.

Kamphues, J., 1996. Risk of feedstuffs loaded by mites, moulds, bacteria and/or toxins in horses. Pferdeheilkd 12, 326–332.

Kamphues, J., 2007. Futtermittelhygiene: Charakterisierung, Einflüsse und Bedeutung (Hygiene of feeds and feeding - characterization, influences and relevance). Landbauforschung Völkenrode, Sonderheft 306, 41–55.

Kamphues, J., Meyer, H., 1990. Meadow saffron (*Colchicum autumnale*) in hay and colic in horses. Tierärztl Prax 18, 273–275.

Kamphues, J., Reichmuth, C., 2000. Vorratsschädlinge in Futtermitteln. Potentielle Schadorganismen und Stoffe in Futtermitteln sowie in tierischen Fäkalien. Sachstandsbericht, 4. Mitteilung, DFG, Wiley-VCH, Weinheim, pp. 238–284.

Kamphues, J., Schad, D., 1992. Verstopfungskoliken bei Pferden nach Fütterung von Windhalm-(Apera spica venti)-Heu. Proceedings of the 1st European Conference on Equine Nutrition, Pferdeheilkd (special edition) Hannover, pp. 213–215.

Kamphues, J., Schulze Becking, M., 1992. Milben in Futtermitteln - Vorkommen Effekte und Bewertung (mites in feedstuffs - prevalence, effects and judgement). Übers Tierernährg 20, 1–38.

Kamphues, J., Amtsberg, G., Klarmann, D., 1989. Feinanteile und Staub in Futtermitteln - quantitative und qualitative (Pilze, Bakterien und LPS) Aspekte. (Fines and dust in feedstuffs - quantitative and qualitative (moulds, bacteria and LPS) aspects. Berl Münch Tierärztl Wschr 102, 418–421.

Kamphues, J., Meyer, H., Liebler, E.M., et al., 1990. Clinical signs in horses after ingestion of feedstuffs containing ionophores. Dtsch tierärztl Wschr 97, 537–539.

Kamphues, J., Fimmen, H., Küstermann, S., et al., 1991. Lipopolysaccharides in feedstuffs for horses. Equine Vet Sci 11, 131–156.

Kamphues, J., Böhm, R., Flachowsky, G., et al., 2007. Empfehlungen zur Beurteilung der hygienischen Qualität von Tränkwasser für Lebensmittel liefernde Tiere unter Berücksichtigung der gegebenen rechtlichen Rahmenbedingungen (Recommendations for evaluating the hygienic quality of drinking water for food producing animals in accordance with current regulatory framework). Landbauforschung Völkenrode 3 (57), 255–272.

Kamphues, J., Coenen, M., Iben, C., et al., 2009. Supplemente zu Vorlesungen und Übungen in der Tierernährung, 11, überarbeitete Auflage. Verlag M.&H. Schaper, Hannover.

Kaya, G., Sommerfeld-Stur, I., Iben, C., 2009. Risk factors of colic in horses in Austria. J Anim Physiol Anim Nutr 93, 339–349.

Keller, K.M., Queiroz, B.D., Keller, L.A.M., et al., 2007. The Mycobiota and Toxicity of Equine Feeds. Vet Res Commun 31, 1037–1045.

Kirschvink, N., Di Silvestro, F., Sbaï, I., et al., 2002. The use of cardboard bedding material as part of an environmental control regime for heaves-affected horses: in vitro assessment of airborne dust and aeroallergen concentration and in vivo effects on lung function. Vet J 163, 319–325.

Liesener, K., Curtui, V., Dietrich, R., et al., 2010. Mycotoxins in horse feed. Mycotox Res 26, 23–30.

Liu, Z.P., 2003. Lead poisoning combined with cadmium in sheep and horses in the vincinity ferrous metal smelters. Sci Total Environ 309, 117–126.

Mair, T.S., Derksen, F.J., 2000. Chronic obstructive pulmonary disease: a review. Equine Vet Educ 12 (1), 35–44.

McGorum, B., 1994. Differential diagnosis of chronic coughing in the horse. In Practice 16, 55–60.

McGorum, B.C., Ellison, J., Cullen, R.T., 1998. Total and respirable airborne dust endotoxin concentrations in three equine management systems. Equine Vet J 30, 430–434.

Meyer, H., 1979. Bedeutung von Futter und Fütterung bei Koliken des Pferdes. Tierärztl Prax 7, 221–227.

Meyer, H, Coenen, M, 2002. Pferdefütterung 4. erw. und aktualisierte Aufl., Parey, Berlin.

Müller, C.E., 2005. Fermentation patterns of small-bale silage and haylage produced as a feed for horses. Grass and Forage Science 60 (2), 109–118.

Müller, C.E., Hultén, C., Gröndahl, G., 2011. Assessment of hygienic quality of haylage fed to healthy horses. Grass and Forage Sci 66 (4), 453–463.

Palacios, H., Iribarren, I., Olalla, M.J., et al., 2002. Lead poisoning of horses in the vincinty of a battery recycling plant. Sci. Total Environ 290, 81–89.

Pirie, R.S., Dixon, P.M., Collie, D.D.S., et al., 2001. Pulmonary and systemic effects of inhaled endotoxin in control and heaves horses. Equine Vet J 33 (3), 311–318.

Pirie, R.S., Collie, D.D.S., Dixon, P.M., et al., 2003. Inhaled endotoxin and organic dust particulates have synergetic proinflammatory effects in equine heaves (organic dust-induced asthma). Clin Exp Allergy 33, 676–683.

Popot, M.A., Garcia, P., Bonnaire, Y., 2011. Doping control in horses: housing conditions and oral recycling of flunixin by ingestion of contaminated straw. J Vet Pharmacol Therap 34, 612–614.

Rade, C., Kamphues, J., 1999. Zur Bedeutung von Futter und Fütterung für die Gesundheit des Atmungstraktes von Tieren sowie von Menschen in der Tierbetreuung (Effects of feeds and feeding on the health of the respiratory tract in animals and people handling animals). Übers Tierernährg 27, 65–121.

Rade, C., Koch, W., Leibold, W., et al., 1998. Antibodies against moulds and mites in sera of young horses experimentally exposed to those agents via oral and inhalative challenge. J Anim Physiol Anim Nutr 80, 239–245.
Raymond, S.L., Smith, T.K., Swamy, H.V.L.N., 2005. Effects of feeding a blend of grains naturally contaminated with *Fusarium* mycotoxins on feed intake, metabolism, and indices of athletic performance of exercised horses. J Anim Sci 83, 1267–1273.
Raymond, S.L., Heiskanen, M., Smith, T.K., et al., 2000. An investigation of the concentrations of selected Fusarium mycotoxins and the degree of mold contamination of field-dried hay. J Equine Vet Sci 20 (10), 618–621.
Riet-Correa, F., Mendez, M.C., Schild, A.L., et al., 1988. Agalactica, reproductive problems and neonatal mortality in horses associated with the investigation of Claviceps purpurea. Aust Vet J 65 (6), 192–193.
Robinson, N.E., Derksen, F.J., Olszewski, M.A., et al., 1996. The pathogenesis of chronic obstructive pulmonary disease of horses. Br Vet J 152, 283–306.
Rollins, J.B., Clement, T.H., 1979. Observations on incidence of equine colic in a private practice. Equine Pract 1, 39–43.
Sacchi, C., Gonzalez, H.H.L., Broggi, L.E., et al., 2009. Fungal contamination and mycotoxin natural occurrence in oats for race horses feeding in Argentina. Anim Feed Sci Technol 152, 330–335.
Sargison, N., 1993. Health hazards associated with the feeding of big sale silage. In Practice 15, 291–297.
Schmidt, H.L., 1991. Mikrobiologische Richtwerte für die Futtermittelbeurteilung. VII. Int. Kongr. Tierhygiene III, 923–928.
Schulz, A., Döll, S., Dänicke, S., et al., 2012. Effects of a deoxynivalenol (DON) contaminated wheat on feed intake and health status in horses. Proc Soc Nutr Physiol 21, 66.
Séguin, V., Lemauviel-Lavenant, S., Garon, D., et al., 2010. Effect of agricultural and environmental factors on the hay characteristics involved in equine respiratory disease. Agriculture, Ecosystems and Environment 135 (3), 206–215.
Snell, J.D., 1966. Effects of inhaled endotoxin. J Lab Clin Med 67, 624-632.
Traub-Dargatz, J.L., Garber, L.P., Fedorka-Cray, P.J., et al., 2000. Fecal shedding of Salmonella spp. by horses in the United States during 1998 and 1999 and detection of Salmonella spp. in grain and concentrate sources on equine operations. JAVMA 217 (2), 226–230.
VDLUFA, 2011. Verfahrensweise zur mikrobiologischen Qualitätsbeurteilung Methodenbuch III, 8. Erg. 2011, VDLUFA-Verlag, Darmstadt.
Ward, P., Couetil, L., 2005. Climatic and aeroallergen risk factors for chronic obstructive pulmonary disease in horses. AJVR 66 (5), 818–824.
Wichert, B., Nater, S., Wittenbrink, M.M., et al., 2008. Judgement of hygienic quality of roughage in horse stables in Switzerland. J Anim Physiol Anim Nutr 92 (4), 432–437.
Wolf, P., Kamphues, J., 2001. Vergiftungen beim Pferd (Horses - have they been poisoned?). Übers Tierernährg 29, 188–197.
Wolf, P., Kloetzer, P., Paulus, C., et al., 2009. A survey on the hygienic standard of feeds for horses and its implication for environmental conditions and animal health. In: Briese, A., Clauß, M., Hartung, J., Springorum, A. (Eds.), Proceedings of the XIV ISAH Congress 2009, 1087–1090, Publisher: Tribun EU, Gorkeho 41, Brno, CZ.
Wright, R.G., Bebbington, A.M., Boland, G.J., 2009. Assessment of methodologies to quantify respirable fungal spores in hay for horses. J Equine Vet Sci 29 (5), 402–403.

SECTION C Applied Nutrition – Feeds

The manufacturers' role in feed quality and safety

A discussion on methods used in feed manufacturing processes to assure feed hygiene and safety

21

Ruth Bishop

Introduction

Quality in equine feedingstuffs

Feed quality can mean different things to different people; for some it is the nutrient content or presence of certain ingredients, for others the consistent appearance and physical form and for others still it is the assured absence of undesirable substances.

All involved in the feed chain from suppliers of raw ingredients, manufacturers and distributors, to the end user, the horse owner/feeder, have a role to play in ensuring the horse receives a diet that is of appropriate quality and is safe to eat.

On its journey from individual ingredients to landing in the feed bucket, a feedstuff faces certain challenges to its inherent quality and safety that can arise through its harvest, storage and/or transport. Once in the feed room, the responsibility for quality and safety is with the owner or feeder of the horse, in ensuring that the feed has been stored appropriately, is the right product being fed at an appropriate level for the horse, and, if being fed in conjunction with other feedstuffs, no harmful deficiencies or excesses of nutrients are being administered.

The manufacturer's role is essentially to consistently make products that simultaneously contain those nutrients and ingredients which it holds out to be present, in the stated proportions and in its expected physical form, but that also *do not* contain levels or concentrations of substances that could affect the health or performance of horses, or the legal status of the feed. It is fundamentally illegal to knowingly manufacture or provide feed that is not safe. Manufacturers also have a commitment to ensure that appropriate recommendations for storage and use of their products are clearly visible for customer use.

Adverse quality can result not only in potential physical harm to the horse, but also seriously affect a feed business in several ways, including unwelcome media interest, loss of business, brand damage and prosecution. Therefore it is incumbent on feed producers to safeguard the safety, quality and integrity of feed products, to minimize the opportunity for product contamination and mis-manufacture.

There are many harmful or undesirable substances that can enter the equine diet, for example:

- Microbiological contaminants
- Pesticides
- Dioxins
- Mycotoxins
- Heavy metals
- Certain nutrients used at levels above those recognized as safe, for example selenium or rapidly digestible/fermentable carbohydrate.

Additionally to the list above, there is a further category of undesirable substance, those that are not considered harmful but are prohibited under the rules of racing and equestrian sport see Box 21.1 for recent examples of adverse feed product quality in the marketplace.

This chapter focuses on what the manufacturer's role in assuring feed quality and safety is, and outlines tools commonly used to help achieve this in practice.

The scope of this chapter is taken to apply to commercially manufactured and packaged products. However, the general principles may also apply to products where there is no required regulatory compliance, such as forage.

Box 21.1 Recent Examples of Adverse Feed Product Quality in the Marketplace

- April 2009: 21 polo ponies in Florida died of acute selenium toxicity, linked to a faulty manufacture of a supplement preparation (Anon 2009).
- May 2008: Nationwide product recall instigated after elevated Aflatoxin content found in equine and other feed products manufactured at three sites in the US (FDA 2008).
- Oct 2002 – Jan 2003: 43 horses, including 16 winners test positive for morphine in post race samples in UK and Ireland. The source was identified as racehorse feed (BHA 2004).

Characteristics of equine feeds

Whilst the equine diet is nominally described in terms of its forage and concentrate proportions, in practice a further degree of complexity exists due to the wide range of feed type, physical form, feeding rates, packaging and shelf life (Table 21-1) exhibited within the category of equine feedstuffs.

Table 21-1 Characteristics of Commonly Fed Equine Feedingstuffs with Typical Feeding Rates

Feedstuff	Forage	Chopped fibers	Cubes/ pellets	Sweet feeds/ coarse mixtures	Straights	Supplements	Treats
Feed form	Long, unprocessed fiber[a]	Blends of chopped forages +/– molasses or oil coatings	3–6 mm diameter extruded pellets	Mixtures of flakes, or other processed cereals, pellets and other ingredients coated in a molasses-type blend or oil coating	Single ingredients in unprocessed or processed form e.g. rolled oats, sugar beet pulp shreds	Mixtures of additives in powder, liquid, or granular form	Extruded pellet, baked biscuits
Typical feed rate	4–20 kg	0.5–4 kg	1–10 kg[b]	1–10 kg	0.5–10 kg	50–100 g	50–100 g
	8–44 lbs	1–6 lbs	2–22 lbs	2–22 lbs	2–22 lbs	1.5–4 oz	1.5–4 oz
Typical shelf life	1–2 years (not normally stated)	3–6 months	3–6 months	3–6 months	3–6 months	9 months–1 year	6–12 months
Packaging	None (hay) Plastic bags or wrap (haylage)	Plastic or paper sack or bag	Plastic or paper sack or bag	Plastic or paper sack or bag	Plastic or paper sack or bag	Plastic tubs	Plastic bag or tub

[a]In some countries, forage is presented in cube, pellet or wafer form.
[b]Where long forage is scarce or unavailable, complete pelleted fiber feeds, designed to provide the total daily diet, are available, with maximum feed rates therefore greater than the 10 kg described in the table.

It should also be noted that manufacturers can only directly influence the quality of their products up to the point of dispatch. With product shelf life extending from around 90 days to over one year, feed products have potential exposure to further risk of damage or contamination throughout the subsequent distribution chain right up to the point of consumption. Manufacturers should, however, offer guidance on the product packaging with respect to the optimum storage of feedstuffs to their customers.

Feed Ingredients

Whilst the main proportions of the equine diet are comprised of forage and cereal based ingredients, other components provide other essential nutrients (Table 21-2).

Manufacturing facilities

Given the variety in form of feed, it follows that there is a range of manufacturing processes, such as blending, pelleting, flaking and extrusion. It is not always the case that feed products for horses are manufactured in facilities that solely manufacture equine products; conversely it is more often the case that other animal feed products are manufactured in the same premises, especially feedstuffs for food producing animals.

In the EU, the Transmissible Spongiform Encephalopathy (TSE) Regulations (999/2001), which impose a Community-wide ban on the feeding of processed animal proteins to farmed animals, effectively exclude petfood manufacture in facilities manufacturing feed for equines. Although there are similar controls for certain bovine proteins in the US, horse feed can still be manufactured in facilities handling avian and porcine meat meals in the US, with their attendant risk of salmonella contamination.

Table 21-2 The Nature and Source of Common Feed Ingredients Used in Equine Diets

Ingredient source	Examples
Raw agricultural commodities	Oats, corn (maize), barley, peas, beans, lupins, naked oats, linseed, lucerne, straw, timothy hay, grass pellets, straw pellets
Human food by-products	Wheat bran, wheatfeed (wheat middlings), oatfeed (oat hull by-product), soy(a) hulls, rice bran, soy(a)bean meal, sunflower meal, linseed meal, sugar beet pulp, distillers grains, molasses.
Additives	Amino acids, vitamins, yeast products, mold inhibitors
Minerals	Limestone, calcium phosphates, salt, calcined magnesite (magnesium oxide)
Human grade ingredients	Vegetable oils (e.g. soya, corn), herbs

Key Points – The Manufacturer's Quality Challenge

- To make products that consistently contain what they should contain and do not contain that which they should not
- This challenge applies across a complex and variable mix of feed forms, ingredients, feed rate, packaging and shelf life
- The consequences of not doing so are in the least, adverse publicity and loss of business for a company, but in the worst case can result in a serious health concern for the horse itself

Drivers of feed assurance

The primary driver of feed quality and assurance is a fundamental desire to ensure both customer (the owner/feed purchaser) and consumer (the horse) satisfaction. It is also driven by individual manufacturers' own commitments to quality, by legislation, and by external factors such as requirements for due diligence, independent expert opinion and industry standards.

Regulatory requirements

In the EU, feed and food law are intrinsically linked and several pieces of legislation are in place designed to maximize food and feed safety. Furthermore, the horse is classed in the EU as a food-producing animal, such that manufacturers of equine products must follow legislation designed to ensure food safety throughout the food chain:

- EU Regulation (EC) No 178/2002 lays down the general principles governing food and feed in general, and food and feed safety in particular, at EU and member state level. Of particular note are articles 15 and 18 of the Regulation. Article 15 states that feed shall not be placed on the market or fed to any food-producing animal if it unsafe. Article 18 states that traceability of food, food-producing animals, and any other substance intended or expected to be incorporated into a food or feed, shall be established at all stages of production, processing and distribution.
- The European Regulation on Feed Hygiene (Regulation EC 183/2005) lays down general rules on feed hygiene, conditions and arrangements ensuring traceability of feed, and conditions and arrangements for registration and approval of feed establishments, applicable to the whole feed chain. It explicitly states that "Feed business operators shall put in place, implement and maintain, a permanent written procedure or procedures based on the HACCP principles." Industry guides to good practice were published in accordance with Article 22 of this Regulation, the European Feed Manufacturers Guide (2005) (http://www.fefac.org/code.aspx?EntryID=265, FEFAC) and the Feed Ingredients Standard (2007) (http://www.ifsa-info.net/lmbinaries/ifs.pdf. IFSA).
- EC regulation 1831/2003 on Feed Additives. Substances such as vitamins, trace elements and preservatives can only be used if they have undergone an assessment for safety, quality and efficacy.
- EC directive 2002/32 and Commission Regulation (EU) No. 744/2012 on Undesirable Substances and Products control contaminants such as heavy metals, certain mycotoxins, cyanogenic glycosides and dioxins. In addition, to listing maximum permitted levels for such substances, it prohibits the blending down of contaminated feeding stuffs (i.e., the mixing of a consignment in excess of a maximum permitted level for an undesirable substance, with another consignment of a lower contamination, to obtain a legal product).

In the US, the quality and safety of food for humans and animals is covered under one federal law, which is implemented by the Food and Drug Administration (FDA) and state agencies. Food for horses is considered to be "pet food", but there is no legal distinction for food consumed by companion animals versus livestock. As in the EU there is no separate distinction in the regulation for animal dietary supplements (see Chapter 19).

Legislative and regulatory requirements concerning animal feed in the US are governed by the Federal Food, Drug and Cosmetic Act (FFDCA) – the overarching law that gives the FDA the authority to oversee the hygiene and safety of feed and feed ingredients (see www.fda.gov/regulatoryinformation/legislation/federalfooddrugandcosmeticactfdcact/default.htm).

The FFDCA makes animal feed manufacturers responsible for ensuring that feed products:

- are pure and wholesome
- are produced under sanitary conditions
- contain no harmful substances
- are truthfully labelled.

Until recently there has been no legal requirement for Hazard Analysis Critical Control Point (HACCP), in the US but new legislation under the Food Safety Modernization Act will essentially require manufacturers to apply the principles of HACCP and provide the FDA with additional inspection and control authority.

Legally, under the FFDCA, any additive (as opposed to feed ingredient) that is added to or is expected to become a component of animal food, either directly or indirectly, must be approved by the FDA, unless it is generally recognized as safe for that use (GRAS).

Generally recognized as safe (GRAS) is an FDA designation that a chemical or substance added to food is considered safe by experts and so is exempted from the usual FFDCA food additive pre-market approvals.

A food substance may be GRAS either through scientific procedures or, for a substance used in food before 1958, through experience based on common use in food (see www.fda.gov/Food/FoodIngredientsPackaging/GenerallyRecognizedasSafeGRAS/default.htm).

GRAS status however does not necessarily provide a robust safety designation for additives used in equine products, as elegantly described in the recent NRC review of Safety of Dietary Supplements for Horses, Dogs and Cats (NRC 2009).

It should also be noted that most States also follow the Official Publication of the American Association of Feed Control Officials (AAFCO), commonly referred to as the AAFCO manual. This includes a list of all ingredients AAFCO has reviewed and found suitable for use in animal feeds. The Official Publication includes a list of approved food additives, the list of GRAS substances and the most up to date list of feed ingredients with their definitions.

The AAFCO Official Publication also characterizes and provides conditions of use for permitted feed ingredients, including limits on heavy metals and other commonly occurring contaminants.

Feed regulatory requirements may be similiar between different countries but may not be the same. For example Table 21-3 gives a comparison of the differences in regulatory limits in the US and EU in relation to mycotoxins.

For the category of equine supplements, conforming to the requirements of FFDCA/GRAS can prove challenging

Table 21-3 Comparison of EU* and FDA Regulatory Guidance on Key Mycotoxins (µg/kg in Feeds or Feed Ingredients with a Moisture Content of 12.5%)

Mycotoxin	US	EU	Material
Aflatoxin B1	–	5	Complementary feeds
Aflatoxin B1	–	10	Complete feeds
Aflatoxin B1, B2, G1, G2	20		Corn, peanut products, other animal feeds and feed ingredients excl. cottonseed for immature animals
DON (Vomitoxin)	–	8000	Cereals and cereal products except maize products
	–	12,000	Maize products
	5000		Grain and grain byproducts
Fumonisins B1 and B2	–	5000	Complementary feeds for pigs, horses, rabbits and pet animals
	–	60,000	Maize and maize products
	5000		Corn and corn by-products intended for equids and rabbits
Ochratoxin A	–	250	Cereals and cereal products
Zearalenone	–	2000	Cereals and cereal products except maize products
	–	3000	Maize products

*Commission Recommendation on the presence of deoxynivalenol, zearalenone, ochratoxin A, T2 and HT2, and fumonisins in products intended for animal feeding (2006/576/EC).

given that certain commonly used supplement ingredients or additives make not have GRAS status.

Finally, in the area of industry standards, in the absence of central regulation, and in notable cases, certain groups have developed their own standards, designed to generate industry credibility. A good example of this is, in the US, where the National Animal Supplement Council (NASC), a supplement industry association, has sought to address the apparent lack of specific regulation for equine supplements by both setting quality standards for the animal supplement industry and providing a forum for all those involved in the supply of such products from manufacturers to legislators. Further examples of industry self regulation can be seen in the various feed quality assurance schemes that operate in the US and EU (see section on demonstrating feed quality).

Key Points – Drivers of quality are both internal and external

- Internal: An individual company's desire to do its best for its customers, and to be able to demonstrate responsible behavior
- External
  - Independent expert opinion
  - Industry standards
  - Legislative requirements, e.g.:
    EU: (via EU 183/2005 – Feed hygiene regulations; EU 183/2003 Feed additives; EU 2002/32 – Undesirable substances)
    US: (via Federal Food Drug and Cosmetic Act (FFDCA), Food Safety and Modernization Act, GRAS, AAFCO Official Publication)

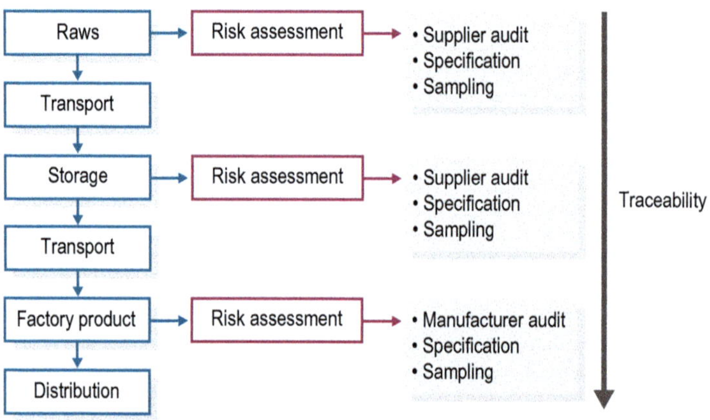

Figure 21.1 The manufacturers' approach to ensuring quality and safety in feed products.

Methods for achieving quality

General principles

The starting point for defining the quality required for a particular product or products is the product specification that both describes and quantifies both its desirable and undesirable characteristics. An individual company's quality assurance activities then act to ensure the specification is continuously delivered.

The general principles of assuring feed quality are:

- A co-ordinated supply chain providing well-defined (via specification) ingredients and products
- Traceability from the point of origin of the ingredient through to the use of the product
- Independently verified quality assurance activities.

This approach is summarized in Fig. 21.1, which shows that assurance of quality and feed safety in feed products should rigorously follow every step in the chain from field to point of dispatch.

This risk assessment process should be traceable and be based on supplier inspection and audit, appropriate product specification and sampling and testing, developed in line with any risks identified, that shows conformance to specification.

This is a preventative approach, based on identification of the hazards, assessment of the risk associated with the hazard (its significance, severity and likelihood of occurrence) and estimate of the effectiveness of potential control measures. This approach underlines many modern food safety systems.

It should be noted that no risk management options will provide absolute safety (i.e., there will always be some risk), the objective being to assess and manage the risk accordingly.

Table 21-4 shows examples of Feed Manufacturer QA and QC activities (see Box 21.2).

Box 21.2 Quality Assurance and Quality Control

These terms are often used interchangeably; however, they describe related but different approaches to quality.

Quality Assurance defines the standards to be followed in order to meet customer requirements, and is largely process driven. Quality Control ensures that these defined standards are followed at every step, through the conduct of various tests and checks.

They are interrelated in that quality control provides feedback to quality assurance to facilitate appropriate corrective and preventive actions to improve quality processes.

As a general principle, quality assurance is generally preventive, with activities focused on processes, whereas quality control is generally comprised of verification activities demonstrating that the quality standards set are continually being met.

Sampling and testing

A common perception is that sampling and testing alone will assure feed quality and safety, but this is not necessarily the case. Tests form an important component, but not the whole, of the assurance activity. Testing, particularly for microbiological contaminants, and mycotoxins, is time-consuming, often lacks sensitivity and specificity, and the levels of sampling routinely applied have a low probability of detecting defective lots if the proportion of defectives in the lot is low (ICMSF 2006).

In recognition of the limits of end-product testing, emphasis for verification of feed hygiene and safety has moved back up the supply chain into Good Manufacturing or Hygienic practice (GMP/GHP) and HACCP as a more reliable means of assuring product safety.

HACCP

The HACCP system is an internationally recognized methodology to help assure safe production for all foodstuffs. Essentially it provides a systematic approach to evaluation and reduction of risks.

It is comprised of three main parts:

1. The identification of hazards, determination of the severity of the hazard and an estimate of how likely it

Table 21-4 Quality Assurance and Quality Control

Examples of feed manufacturer Quality Assurance activities	
Action	**Outcome**
HACCP plan	Assesses potential food safety hazards (chemical, microbiological and physical) and identifies critical control points and monitoring systems for each.
Raw material risk assessment	Identified hazards inherent in the raw material or from its supply chain, and defines appropriate quality assurance and verification activities.
Raw material specification	Document issued by manufacturer to suppliers detailing the food safety, legal, quality and functional parameters to be adhered to.
Supplier audit	Regular (annual/biannual) assessment of supplier facilities, QA procedures, and performance against specification.
Finished product specification	Defines the parameters to be checked after manufacture – e.g. product appearance, nutrient profile, packaging quality.
Work instructions/standard operating procedures	Define how to conduct key operational processes.
Examples of feed manufacturer Quality Control procedures	
Action	**Outcome**
Incoming raw material assessment • Supplier check • Visual assessment • Nutritional check • Storage pests	Checks against defined specification – are the supplier and haulier approved, check no prohibited substances have been carried in the three previous loads Spear samples to check appearance – colour, grain- or pellet- size, absence of foreign bodies and insects Key nutrients checked vs. specification
Insect and vermin traps	Monitors background levels of storage pests in the manufacturing facility.
Finished product assessment • Visual assessment • Nutritional check • Undesirable substances check	Checks against defined specification: Colour, pellet size, mix components present in expected proportions Key nutrients checked to ensure present at specified levels, and to ensure legal conformance Monitoring checks for unwanted contaminants, such as naturally occurring prohibited substances, mycotoxins.

is that the hazard will occur. The risk level is affected by various factors including the growing, harvesting, processing, distributing and storing of any given feedstuff. Table 21-4 describes some hazards associated with equine feed manufacture and methods of control.

2. The determination of critical control points (CCP) required to control a given hazard. A CCP can be a location, practice, procedure or process, used to minimize or prevent unacceptable contamination, survival or growth of spoilage organisms (or pathogens), or the introduction of unwanted chemical substances or foreign objects.
3. The establishment and implementation of monitoring procedures to determine that each CCP is under control, with corrective actions defined for when a CCP result shows the system to be out of control.

Table 21-5 identifies common hazards found in equine feedingstuffs, their sources and effective control measures.

It can be seen from Table 21-5 that, for the ingredients used in equine feeds, many of the controls relate to preventing the intake of materials containing hazards into the manufacturing facility, as there can be limited opportunity to control them once part of a continuous flow manufacturing process.

Demonstrating feed quality

One way in which companies can demonstrate a commitment to quality is via external verification (auditing) of their systems. The most widely known and universal standard for quality in manufacturing is the International Organisation for Standardisation (ISO) standard 9001:2008 (Anon 2008)

This standard specifies requirements for a quality management system where an organization needs to demonstrate its ability to consistently provide product that meets customer and applicable statutory and regulatory requirements.

All requirements of ISO 9001:2008 are generic and are intended to be applicable to all manufacturing organizations, regardless of type, size and product provided.

In addition to the ISO standard, the animal feed sector internationally has adopted voluntary independent assurance schemes, specifically designed to demonstrate feed safety. These are usually administered by feed trade associations in individual countries and either exceed or meet regulatory standards for hygiene and feed safety in their country or region (Box 21.3).

Behind such labels and accreditation marks however, the hallmarks of a company committed to quality are:

- Leadership – a clearly defined commitment to quality from senior management.

Table 21-5 Examples of Potential Hazards, Their Sources and Controls in the Equine Feed Industry

Hazard	Source	Control of initial levels	Reducing levels	Prevention of increase in levels
Fungal spores	Air-dried forages	Monitor harvest and storage conditions; test when conditions indicate a suspected high risk; reject wet or visibly moldy material	–	Use of inhibitory factors e.g. preservatives
Salmonella	Protein-rich materials – primarily animal derived proteins, but also vegetable proteins Contaminated storage by pests carrying salmonella	Select suppliers with effective salmonella control systems	Cook, acidify, use of a_w, pH, preservatives	Use of inhibitory factors, e.g. preservatives, a_w, acidifiers; minimize cross-contamination
Monensin sodium	Contaminated vitamin and mineral premixes	Select suppliers with effective control systems or non-medicated lines; do not use Monensin on site	–	–
Fusarium mycotoxins	Cereals, cereal by-products	Monitor weather conditions through growth phase; test when conditions indicate high risk; reject high moisture (>15%) material; reject raw materials with levels above specification	Mycotoxins are stable – reduction difficult, however consider reformulation of diets to contain lower amounts of high risk materials.	Rapid drying and dry storage of cereals to prevent further growth of fungi/development of toxins
Morphine	Cross-contamination with morphine poppies (*Papaver somniferum*)	Source ingredients from sites neither growing nor processing *Papaver somniferum* spp. Do not use haulage that has previously carried *P. somniferum* or processed products thereof	–	Minimize cross-contamination risk in the supply chain

- Culture – quality is embedded in the company ethos and is lived and used each day by all company personnel.
- Well-Invested – People, equipment and expenditure are consistently resourced to deliver quality products.
- Simple – easy to understand systems and controls that all involved can follow.

Feed industry assurance schemes specific to equines

Technically, whilst not food safety hazards, contaminants that can cause a disqualification from competition or racing, are essentially hazardous to manufacturers and users of equine feedingstuffs. Whilst accidental contamination with such substances is rare, in the UK and Ireland there are two externally accredited quality assurance schemes allied to the UFAS and FEMAS feed assurance schemes, designed to minimize the risk of feed contamination with so called "prohibited substances". These feed assurance schemes are known as the "British Equestrian Trade Association (BETA) Naturally Occurring Prohibited Substances (NOPS) Appendices."

Examples of naturally occurring prohibited substances and sources of contamination are given in Table 21-6.

Box 21.3 Examples of Country-Specific Feed Assurance Schemes

- US and Canada: Safe Food, Safe Feed; NASC Quality Seal
- UK and Ireland: Universal Feed Assurance Scheme (UFAS) and Feed Materials Assurance Scheme (FEMAS)
- Holland: PDV GMP+
- Belgium: GMP
- Germany: QS
- Europe-wide:
  - FAMIQS for feed additive and premixtures
  - COCERAL GTP Scheme

Key Points – Achieving and Demonstrating Feed Quality

- Quality begins at the top of the company: leadership committed to quality, a culture of quality, and continued investment in quality operations, are prerequisites for a successful quality approach
- Quality is achieved through attention to detail across the whole supply chain from ingredient procurement to finished product distribution
- It is essential a recognized system for evaluation and reduction of risk (HACCP) is employed
- Focus is on both quality assurance and control activities; Quality control via testing alone will not reliably deliver feed quality and safety
- Accreditation to independently verified external quality assurance schemes is an indicator of commitment to quality

Challenges

Assurance of feed quality based on risk assessment implies defined limits of effect, methods of control and sampling procedures, and complete control throughout the supply chain. However, challenges exist in each of these areas.

Table 21-6 Key Naturally Occurring Prohibited Substances, the Nature of Contamination and Their Sources*

Nature of contamination	Prohibited substance	Source	Control measure
Naturally occurring in raw material	Hordenine	Germinating barley, Phalaris grasses (e.g. Reed canary grass).	High detection limits levels effectively set by regulators to allow for presence in barley.
	Bufotenine	Phalaris grasses	Do not use.
	Lupanine	Lupins	Do not (or restrict) use.
	Salicylic acid	Alfalfa (Lucerne)	High threshold levels set by regulators to allow for feed use.
	Valerenic acid	Valerian herb	Do not use in competition or racing diets.
	Caffeine, Theobromine Theophylline	Coffee and cocoa by-products used as feed materials (e.g., Cherco, biscuit meal)	Do not use raw material or ingredients containing these substances
Contaminants of crops	Atropine Hyoscine	Solanacae plant species as weeds in crops (e.g., *Atropa belladonna* – Deadly nightshade; *Datura stramonium* – Jimson weed, thorn apple)	Control via purchasing specification and via feed safety legislation e.g. EC Directive 2002/32 on Undesirable Substances and Products.
Manufacturing and shipping	Morphine Caffeine, theobromine	Cross contamination of feed ingredient via processing, haulage or storage.	Minimize cross contamination in the supply chain.

*There are some differences between sporting regulators in different countries/states and between equestrian sport and racing. Feed business operators and competitors alike should always check the rules for the country/state and competition discipline.

Appropriate sampling and testing for risk

One of the main challenges remains the difficulty associated with obtaining a precise and accurate estimate of the presence of certain hazards within such bulk lots - for many feed ingredients, more than 60% of the error associated with sampling and testing has been attributed to sampling alone (Casado et al 2009, Maxwell et al 2006).

This difficulty arises because contamination is often heterogeneous. For example, in the case of *Fusarium* mycotoxins, distribution can be nonuniform within a field, governed by the nature of the pathogen, local climatic conditions and crop/soil factors (Casado et al 2009). Salmonella is similarly considered heterogeneously distributed (CAC 1999, EFSA 2008).

Consequently, sampling plans for heterogeneously distributed materials require large numbers of samples and effective subsampling, as indicated in the EU sampling plans for *Fusarium* mycotoxins (Whitaker 2006; Table 21-7).

NB: Most grains delivered to manufacturers arrive in lots <50 t sourced from large stores containing >300 t.

These pose problems to manufacturers not only in terms of the practicality of taking this number of samples, but also in the inability to effectively test before an incoming load is allowed to enter the factory, due to the length of time required by current techniques.

In such situations, targeted sampling according to HACCP (i.e. sampling and testing to verify a CCP) is more sensitive and cost-effective than traditional sampling of finished products and feed materials (Box 21.4).

Lack of equine data

The principles of HACCP require, per hazard identified, an assessment of its significance, severity and likelihood of occurrence. However, there is often a lack of published data on the effect of certain hazards in the horse, not only in relation to health but also the effect of subacute or chronic loads on performance. Additionally, there is a need for more published assessment of normal concentrations of certain hazards in feed ingredients used in equine diets. This is especially true for certain microbiological contaminants and mycotoxins, and applies also to proposed mitigation strategies, for example mycotoxin binders.

Equally there is often little data on the safety of certain ingredients used in equine supplements. Whilst the effects of excesses of nutrients such as rapidly fermentable/digestible carbohydrates and selenium are well documented (see Chapters 8 and 10), similar data for certain additive ingredients is not routinely available (NRC 2009).

In drug and animal food additives reporting, it is the norm to report no observed adverse effect levels (NOAEL) or safe upper limits (SUL), however a recent report found that there was a lack of quality safety data in horses for three supplements, lutein, evening primrose oil and garlic that would satisfy such requirements (NRC 2009). This report however did provide benchmark historical safe intakes (HSI) and estimated presumed safe intakes (PSI) based on the limited data available. More classical safety data are required in this area, including more comprehensive adverse event reporting systems.

In such situations, research from other species can provide important signals as to safe or hazardous levels, but will not provide a guarantee of the same in equines.

Table 21-7 EU Sampling Plans (Commission Regulation EC 401/2006) for the Official Control of the Levels of Mycotoxins in Foodstuffs. General Sampling Procedure of Cereals and Cereal Products

Lot weight (t)	Sublots (t)	No. incremental samples	Aggregate sample (kg)
1500 or more	500	100	10
300–1500	3	100	10
50–300	100	100	10
<50	–	3–100	1–10

Box 21.4 Examples of HACCP-Based Sampling Points for the Monitoring of Salmonella in A Feed Mill (Adapted from EFSA 2008)

1. Samples of accumulated dust from the unloading pit for feed materials
2. Aggregate samples of dust from ingredient sieves
3. Aspirated dust from the production line
4. Dust emanating from pellet coolers
5. Dust within finished product bins

Feed quality and safety throughout the distribution chain

It is not always the case that feed is consumed by the horse soon after manufacture. With shelf life for equine feedingstuffs varying from 90 days to 2 years (see Table 21-1) there is a potential for spoilage throughout the distribution chain. It is usual for feed products to be distributed through a wholesale /retail distribution chain, meaning at least a one-step or two-step journey en route to the final destination, the feed room.

During this time, risks to equine feed products principally arise through poor handling and storage, of what for the most part is a relatively bulky, perishable commodity. Box 21.5 lists elements of good practice that can ensure feed arrives at its final destination close to the condition it left the manufacturer in, and are applicable to both commercial stores and private feed rooms.

Key Points – Challenges to a robust approach to Quality Assurance

- Taking and keeping appropriate samples: representative samples tested to a validated methodology underpin any quality assurance approach;
  - The use of HACCP will help determine where best to concentrate sampling and testing activities;
  - Testing methodology should be chosen according to the objective of the test;
- Interpreting data for the assessment of significance of results: assessment of significance underpins the risk assessment approach, but data may not always be available relative to the horse.
  - Using established methodologies from other species for risk assessment may be appropriate.

Box 21.5 Recommended Minimum Storage Standards

1. Buildings
   i. The store facility should be fit for the purpose: soundly constructed of durable materials, clean and dry, well lit and secure
   ii. Storage temperatures should be cool – a temperature of 12°C/54°F or below is recommended as insect activity is inhibited below this
   iii. The building should be proofed against birds, vermin and insects, with windows ventilation-netted
   iv. Glass lights must be covered or guarded, with any breakages cleaned up immediately and the lights replaced
   v. Eating, drinking and smoking should not be permitted in the feed storage area
2. Storage
   i. Good hygiene is the key – keep stores clean:
      - Immediately clean up any spillages
      - Vacuum the store weekly
      - A monthly deep clean is recommended (including floors, ledges and all surfaces that collect dust)
      - Fumigate the store annually
      - A regular (e.g. monthly) pest control program is recommended
   ii. Stock management
      - Check deliveries on entrance to the store to ensure that the correct product has been delivered in the right amount, that there are no damaged bags, and no build up of moisture or dirt on the bags
      - Remove any shrink wrap and hoods from pallets and individual bags before storing
      - Stock should be rotated on a first in first out basis i.e. the earliest codes being used or dispatched first
      - Bagged feed should be stored off the floor and away from walls, for instance on racking or a clean, dry pallet covered with a pallet liner, and with a 15 cm (6 in) gap between pallets to allow ventilation and inspection of product
      - Pallets of feed should not be stacked on top of each other for long periods of time
      - Stores should be checked at least weekly basis for damage to product, best before date, build up of dust and presence of insects
      - Potential contaminants (e.g. sanitizing agents, pesticides, medication) should be separately from bagged feed
   iii. In-store feed bins must be soundly constructed, hard wearing, cleaned after each use, dry and have sealed lids

  - Also, as more data on normal values for equine feedstuffs becomes available, acceptable daily exposures will be better defined.
- Product distribution – feed stuffs are perishable goods with finite shelf life that can be transported long distances, often across a number of distribution points before it reaches the final feed bucket. Thus product is exposed to a risk of damage after it has left the manufacturer until it is finally consumed.
  - Manufacturers can mitigate by printing storage information on pack and by issuing good storage guidance to their distribution chain at regular intervals (i.e., annually)

Conclusions

Ensuring feed quality is a complex task best approached systematically on the basis of risk assessment. There are well established systems that exist for this purpose that can be verified to a number of external standards.

That being said, it has to be remembered that assurance quality remains a risk management exercise, designed to minimize the risk of adverse quality incidents rather than guarantee their absence.

Quality however is not only achieved by completing a series of actions, but also describes a dynamic, continually evolving approach and determination by manufacturers to do the best for their customers.

References

Anon, 2009. Florida Department of Agriculture and Consumer Services http://www.doacs.state.fl.us/press/2009/04282009.html (accessed 2 February 2010).

Anon, 2008. European Standard EN ISO 9001:2008 Quality Management Systems: Requirements (English version).

BHA, 2004. http://w.com/resources/about/whatwedo/disciplinary/disciplinaryDetail.asp?item=083611 (accessed 2 February2010).

CAC (Codex Alimentarius Commission), 1999. Joint FAO/WHO Food standards program. Codex Committee on Food Hygiene. Principles and Guidelines for the Conduct of Microbiological Risk assessment. CAC/GL 30-1999. Secretariat of the joint FAO/WHO Food Standards programme. Food and Agriculture Organisation of the United Nations, Rome.

Casado, M., Rivas, D., Parsons, J., et al., 2009. Modelling a two-dimensional spatial distribution of mycotoxin concentration in bulk commodities to design effective and efficient sample selection strategies. Food Additives & Contaminants: Part A 26 (9), 1298–1305.

EFSA, 2008. Microbiological risk assessment in feeding stuffs for food-producing animals. The EFSA Journal 720, 28–84.

FDA, 2008. http://www.fda.gov/Safety/Recalls/EnforcementReports/2008/ucm120507.htm (accessed 2 February 2010).

ICMSF, 2006. Microorganisms in Foods 7. International Commission on Microbiological Specifications for Foods. In: Tompkins, R.B., et al. (Eds.), Microbiological Testing in Food Safety Management. Springer, Berlin.

Maxwell, C., Leung, K., Diaz-Llano, G., et al., 2006. Mycotoxins in pet food: a review on worldwide prevalence and preventative strategies. J Agric Food Chem 54 (26), 9623–9635.

NRC, 2009. Safety of Dietary Supplements for Horses, Dogs and Cats. National Academies Press, Washington DC.

Whitaker, T.B., 2006. Sampling Foods for mycotoxins. Food Additives and Contaminants 23 (1), 50–61.

Applied Nutrition

SECTION D

22 Assessment of body condition and bodyweight

Rebecca A. Carter, Alexandra H. A. Dugdale

Introduction

Assessment of a nutritional program is facilitated by measuring the outcome or end result of its application. When assessing the energy balance of a particular nutritional program, it is necessary to monitor an individual's alteration or stability of body mass. Excess consumption of digestible energy above what is required for maintenance, or a positive energy balance, is apparent by the accumulation of primarily adipose tissue in mature horses. Conversely, digestible energy intake below maintenance requirements, or a negative energy balance, would result in the loss of adipose and eventually muscle mass. Therefore, measurements of bodyweight and, if possible, lean and adipose tissue mass may be used to assess energy balance. The scoring of body condition, originally developed for production animals as an indicator of "flesh" (lean and adipose tissues) (Jeffries 1961), has become a commonly used tool for the assessment of body fat in horses and ponies (e.g., Henneke et al 1983). This method, however, has not been thoroughly validated for this purpose. Nevertheless, it offers a practical method for researchers and horse-owners alike to monitor overall nutritional status.

Bodyweight and body condition assessments are important tools for developing dietary rations that are appropriate for maintaining the optimal health of an individual horse. With these tools, it is possible to calculate digestible energy requirements, track changes in energy balance, and classify an animal's condition (e.g., underweight or overweight). This chapter discusses methods of assessing bodyweight and body condition in live equidae. A range of methods applicable to both clinical and research settings is provided, with the advantages and disadvantages of each outlined (Table 22-1). Additionally, appropriate methods for the assessment of regional fat distribution and considerations for choosing an appropriate assessment method are summarized.

Methods of assessing bodyweight

An accurate measurement of bodyweight is necessary for proper ration formulation and determining dosage of medications and anthelmintics. While bodyweight alone offers little information about body condition, it is often useful for monitoring changes within an individual, given that it reflects changes in energy balance over time. Bodyweight can either be directly measured with a scale, or indirectly estimated based on morphometric measurements of body size.

Direct measurement

Bodyweight is most accurately measured in horses by use of a calibrated weigh scale. Various scale designs are available, with some more portable models available. It is important that the scale is properly calibrated and leveled in order to obtain an accurate weight measurement. Fluctuations in bodyweight of up to approximately 5 kg may occur with feed and water intake, defecation, urination, and hydration status (Webb & Weaver 1979). Therefore, it is important to weigh at the same time of day with respect to feeding and exercise, in order to minimize the influence of normal daily variability on measurements.

Indirect measurement

Given that scales are relatively expensive to purchase, they are often only used at larger institutions and are usually not available in a small farm setting. Therefore, calculations have been developed for estimating bodyweight based on measurements of body size. The simplest and most practical application of estimating bodyweight is the use of commercially available weight tapes, which estimates bodyweight from girth circumference. Weight tapes are easily used by placing the tape at the base of the withers and running it around the girth circumference just behind the elbow and forelimb (Fig. 22.1). The measurement is taken while the horse is standing square and at the time of exhalation, so that additional lung volume is not included in the calculation. The accuracy of this technique is decreased for horses at the extreme ends of the scale, and may not be applicable for certain classes of horses, including pregnant mares, growing foals, and thin, fit horses (Gee & Harris 2005). Although accuracy of weight tapes is increased when height-specific tapes are used (Ellis & Hollands 2002), more accurate methods of estimating bodyweight include calculations that contain variables of height or length (Ellis & Hollands 1998).

Many formulas have been described for estimating bodyweight in horses (Table 22-2). In order to improve accuracy,

Table 22-1 Comparison of Methods for Assessment of Bodyweight and Body Condition in Horses

Method	Purpose	Applications	Materials	Advantages	Disadvantages
Direct bodyweight	Objective measurement of bodyweight	• Ration formulation • Medication dosage • Track changes in energy balance	• Equine-specific weigh scale	• Most accurate method of measuring bodyweight	• Expensive • Scales often difficult to transport
Indirect bodyweight	Estimation of bodyweight	• Ration formulation • Medication dosage • Track changes in energy balance	• Weight tape, or • Tape measure and calculator	• Inexpensive • Portable	• Less accurate than direct measurement • Less accurate for extreme body weights or compositions • Not applicable to pregnant mares
Morphometric measurements	Objective estimation of relative adiposity	• Comparison of relative adiposity within or between horses • Track changes in adiposity	• Weigh scale (BMI) • Tape measure • Calculator	• Easy to perform • Detects smaller increments of change than BCS • Measurements available for regional (neck) distribution	• Comparisons between horses of different body types inaccurate • Inter-evaluator bias may influence results • Extrapolates fatness of entire body from a single fat depot
Body condition score (BCS) Regional: Cresty neck score (CNS)	Subjective assessment of subcutaneous body fat	• Comparison of relative adiposity within or between horses	• Trained evaluator	• Can integrate all body areas • Easy to perform • Classify horses into underweight, overweight, or obese categories • Cutoff values available to imply risk for disease • Measurements available for regional (neck) distribution	• Only assesses subcutaneous fat • Inter-evaluator bias may influence results • May be influenced by coat length, gut fill, muscle mass, pregnancy, etc. • May not be comparable between different breeds or body types • Large measurement increments, cannot determine subtle differences
Ultrasonic fat depth	Objective measurement of subcutaneous body fat	• Estimation of body fat percentage • Track changes in fat depth	• Ultrasound instrument • Tape measure • Clippers • Conduction gel	• Less influenced by evaluator bias than BCS • Can depict small changes in subcutaneous fat depth • Can measure regional distribution	• Only measures subcutaneous fat • For body fat percentage, extrapolates fatness of entire body from a single fat depot; doesn't account for visceral or intramuscular fat depots
Total body water (TBW)	Objective measurement of TBW	• Calculation of total fat mass and fat-free mass • Calculation of body fat percentage	• Bioelectrical impedance device, or • Deuterium oxide, catheterization, blood collection • Equine-specific weigh scale	• Differentiates fat mass from fat-free mass • Measures all fat depots	• Does not differentiate contribution of different depots to total fat mass • Dependent on hydration status and gut fill • Calculations are dependent on accurate bodyweight measurement • Complex techniques more appropriate for research facilities

equations have been developed for specific types of horses, including Warmbloods (Kienzle & Schramme 2004) and Thoroughbred foals (Staniar et al 2004). When using weight formulas, it is important to make certain that measurements are taken according to the method from which the original equation was calculated. For example, girth circumference may be measured over the highest point of the withers (Carroll & Huntington 1988, Ensminger 1977), behind the slope of the withers (Fig. 22.1; Leighton-Hardman et al 1980, Milner & Hewitt 1969), one inch behind the highest point of the withers (Staniar et al 2004), or around the abdomen at the point of the umbilicus (Jones et al 1989). Additionally, some formulas use the body length from the point of buttock (tuber ischium) to the point of shoulder (head of humerus) (Fig. 22.1; Carroll & Huntington 1988, Leighton-Hardman et al 1980, Staniar et al 2004), while others use the length from the point of buttock to elbow (olecranon) (Ensminger 1977, Jones et al 1989), or from the point of shoulder to the point of hip (anterior part of trochanter major) (Milner & Hewitt 1969).

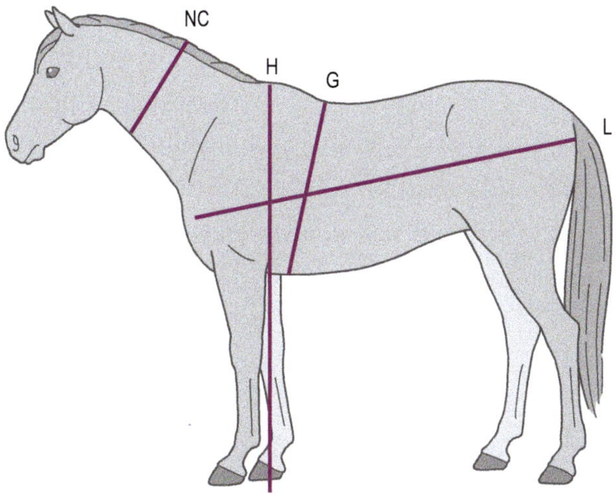

Figure 22.1 Location of common morphometric measurements used in body weight estimation and body condition assessment, with the horse in an appropriate square stance and neck position for measurments. NC, neck circumference; H, wither height; G, girth circumference; L, body length.

A widely used equation that has been evaluated in ponies and light breed horses (Reavell 1999) was developed by Carroll and Huntington (1988), and is applied as bodyweight=girth^2×length/y, where y=11877 for measurements in metric units (cm and kg) or y=330 for measurements in imperial units (in and lb). For larger horses, the equation of Jones et al (1989) was determined to be most accurate (Reavell 1999), although is awkward to use because of nonunity exponents: bodyweight (kg)=[umbilical girth (cm)$^{1.78}$×length (cm)$^{1.05}$]/3011.

Key Points

- Bodyweight can be monitored directly with a calibrated scale or indirectly using morphometric measurements
- A widely used equation evaluated in ponies and light breed horses for the estimation of bodyweight is: BW, kg = (girth^2, cm × length, cm)/11877.

Table 22-2 Formulas for Estimating Bodyweight (BW) from Morphometric Body Measures in Horses

Source	Units	Equation	Population
Traditional[a]	lb, in	BW = (Girth^2 × Length)/300	Adult
Marcenac & Aublet (1964)	kg, m	BW = Girth^3 × 80	Adult
Milner & Hewitt (1969)	lb, in	BW = (Girth^2 × Length)/228.1	Foal to Adult, Shetland to Shire
Willoughby (1975)	lb, in	BW = (0.14475 × Girth)^3 BW = (0.14341 × Girth)^3 BW = (0.1387 × Girth + 0.400)^3 BW = (0.1382 × Girth + 0.344)^3	Adult Males Adult Females Colts, 0–5 yr Fillies, 0–5 yr
Ensminger (1977)	kg, in	BW = (Girth^2 × Length + 22.7)/660	Adult
Leighton-Hardman (1980)	lb, in	BW = (Girth^2 × Length)/y (y = 276.9 to 332.7)[b]	Foal to Adult, Shetland to Shire
Carroll & Huntington (1988)	kg, cm	BW = (Girth^2 × Length)/11877 BW = (Girth^2 × Length) / 12265 BW = (Girth^2 × Length) / 11706	160 to 680 kg, 12 to 17 hh, BCS[c] 1 to 5, out of 5 BCS[c] < 2.5, out of 5 BCS[c] ≥ 3, out of 5
Jones et al (1989)	kg, cm	BW = (Girth$^{1.78}$ × Length$^{0.97}$) / 3011	>2 yr, 230 to 707 kg
Kienzle & Schramme (2004)	kg, cm	BW = −1160 + 2.594(Height) + 1.336(Girth) + 1.538(B) + 6.226(CB) + 1.487(N) + 13.63(BCS[d])	Adult Warmbloods
Staniar et al (2004)	kg, cm	M = ([Girth^2 × Length] + 4[C × C × F]) / 4π if M<0.27 m^3, BW = M × 1093 if M>=0.27 m^3, BW = M × 984 + 24	Thoroughbred foals, 0–17 mo.

[a]As referenced in Milner & Hewitt (1969)
[b]y-value dependent on body condition and breed
[c]Body condition score, scale 0–5 according to Leighton-Hardman (1980)
[d]Body condition score, scale 1–9 according to Kienzle & Schramme (2004)
B = body circumference; CB = cannon bone circumference; N = neck circumference; C = carpus circumference; F = left forelimb length.

Methods of assessing body condition

The objective of assessing body condition involves the estimation of body composition, or more specifically the differentiation between, and relative quantification of, fat (adipose tissue) mass and fat-free (lean) mass (e.g., bone and muscle). In humans, the "gold standard" for body composition assessment is hydrostatic weighing. This technique is based on Archimedes' principle and requires the subject to exhale completely and remain submerged underwater for ~10 seconds (Jensen 1992), which cannot be applied to horses for obvious technical reasons. Other accurate methods of body composition assessment used in humans and small animals include computed tomography and dual energy X-ray absorptiometry (DEXA). Due to size restrictions, these methods have not been applied in horses.

Dissection and carcass analysis have been used for validation of methods, such as estimation of body fat percentage from ultrasonic fat depth in horses (Westervelt et al 1976, Kane et al 1987), but their clinical usefulness is limited given that these techniques are not appropriate for live animals. Further, the estimation of body fat content from ultrasonic fat depths appears to be dependent upon the exact anatomical location of scanning and may also be dependent upon several factors including age, breed, sex, physiological status, previous nutritional history and season (Dugdale et al 2010). In reality, the more accurate methods of assessing adiposity are often substituted by less accurate, more practical methods.

Assessment of body condition score (BCS)

The most commonly used method for assessment of adiposity in horses is the rating of body condition based on a numerical scale with specific criteria for each category. This method is based on visual and physical (palpation) assessment of "superficial flesh" deposition in specified body regions. The term superficial flesh has been largely substituted by "subcutaneous fat" in description of BCS systems for horses.

Several BCS scales have been developed specifically for use in horses. The 0–5-point scale was first described by Leighton-Hardman (1980) and later adapted by Carroll and Huntington (1988). This BCS system assesses subcutaneous fat deposition in 3 body areas (neck, back and ribs, and pelvis) on a scale of 0 (very poor) to 5 (very fat). Each area is scored separately, then the pelvis score is adjusted by 0.5 point if it differs by 1 or more points from the back or neck scores to obtain the overall BCS.

A widely used BCS system, developed by Henneke et al (1983), has a broader range of numerical increments and encompasses more bodily areas for evaluation. This system involves scoring six areas of the horse's body (neck, withers, back, tailhead, ribs, and behind the shoulder) (Fig. 22.2) to categorize body condition on a scale from 1 (poor) to 9 (extremely fat) (Table 22-3, Fig. 22.3). Each body area is scored separately, and then scores are averaged to obtain the overall body condition score. The Henneke BCS system, originally developed for use in Quarter Horse broodmares, may be most appropriate for use in mature light breed horses (e.g., Quarter horses, Thoroughbreds and Arabians) that share similar body type and patterns of fat deposition.

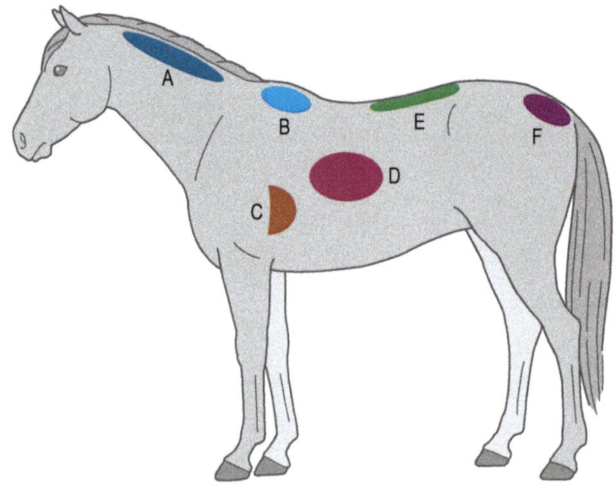

Figure 22.2 Location of subcutaneous adipose depots over the six bodily areas assessed by body condition scoring, according to Henneke et al (1983). A, neck; B, withers; C, behind the shoulder; D, ribs; E, topline; F, tailhead.

Application of the BCS system to Thoroughbred geldings has been described (Suagee et al 2008), and alterations in the BCS system have been developed to increase its suitability for Warmblood breeds (Kienzle & Schramme 2004). However, the application of the Henneke BCS system to classes of equidae with unique conformation or fat deposition patterns, such as ponies, draft breeds, or young horses needs to be performed and interpreted with caution.

Regardless, Kohnke's modification (1992) of the Henneke BCS system has been applied to pony breeds in research studies and clinical situations (Freestone et al 1992, Treiber et al 2006, Carter et al 2009c, Dugdale et al 2010). However, it is unknown whether the relationship between BCS and actual adiposity is similar between horses and ponies. Recent work on pony cadavers has shown an exponential association between BCS, as assessed using the Henneke or Carroll and Huntingdon systems, and body fat content (Dugdale et al 2011a). There was, however, a linear association between BCS (both systems) and overall "flesh" (total somatic soft tissues) content (Dugdale et al 2011a). This work supported the exponential relationship described between BCS (INRA system of 0 to 5) and body fat content in 20 French Sport horses (Martin-Rosset et al 2008). Once bony landmarks become obscured by superficial adipose tissue, adequate descriptors to differentiate "obese" from "super-obese" animals are lacking.

Many factors may influence the accuracy of condition scoring within an individual animal, including conformation, coat length, pregnancy, evaluator bias, gut fill, and muscle development. Ideally, the BCS systems would assess subcutaneous fat tissue independent of muscle mass. In reality, even with an experienced evaluator it is often difficult to differentiate adipose tissue from muscle, and in animals with relatively low muscle mass there can be underestimation of fat mass (e.g., aged horses).

Morphometric measurements

Bodyweight alone is uninformative for assessing relative adiposity or body condition, unless it is put into context by relating it to the size of the animal. For example, a

Table 22-3 Description of Individual Body Condition Scores

Score	Condition	Description
1	Poor	Animal is extremely emaciated. Spinous processes (part of vertebrae that projects upward), ribs, tailhead, hooks (tuber coxae; hip joints), and pins (tuber ischii; lower pelvic bones) projecting prominently. Bone structure of withers, shoulders, and neck easily noticeable. No fatty tissue can be felt.
2	Very thin	Animal is emaciated. Slight fat covering over base of the spinous processes, transverse processes (portion of vertebrae that projects outward) of lumbar (loin area) vertebrae feel rounded. Spinous processes, ribs, tailhead, hooks, and pins are prominent. Withers, shoulders, and neck structures are faintly discernible.
3	Thin	Fat is built up about halfway on spinous processes, transverse processes cannot be felt. Slight fat cover over ribs. Spinous processes and ribs are easily discernible. Tailhead is prominent, but individual vertebrae cannot be visually identified. Hook bones appear rounded, but are easily discernible. Pin bones are not distinguishable. Withers, shoulders and neck are accentuated.
4	Moderately thin	Negative crease along back (spinous processes of vertebrae protrude slightly above surrounding tissue). Faint outline of ribs is discernible. Fat can be felt around tailhead (prominence depends on conformation). Hook bones are not discernible. Withers, shoulders and neck are not obviously thin.
5	Moderate	Back is level. Ribs cannot be visually distinguished, but can be easily felt. Fat around tailhead begins to feel spongy. Withers appear rounded over spinous processes. Shoulders and neck blend smoothly into body.
6	Moderately fleshy	May have slight crease down back. Fat over ribs feels spongy. Fat around tailhead feels soft. Fat begins to be deposited along the sides of the withers, behind shoulders and along neck.
7	Fleshy	May have crease down back. Individual ribs can be felt, but with noticeable filling of fat between ribs. Fat around tailhead is soft. Fat is deposited along withers, behind shoulders and along neck.
8	Fat	Crease down back. Difficult to feel ribs. Fat around tailhead is very soft. Area along withers is filled with fat. Area behind shoulder is filled with fat and flush with rest of the body. Noticeable thickening of neck. Fat is deposited along inner thighs.
9	Extremely fat	Obvious crease down back. Patchy fat appears over ribs. Bulging fat around tailhead, along withers, behind shoulders and along neck. Fat along inner thighs may rub together. Flank is filled with fat and flush with rest of the body.

Adapted from Henneke et al (1983).

400 kg, 13 hh pony would have a drastically different body condition than a 400 kg, 16 hh horse. Body mass index (BMI) aims to adjust bodyweight for body size by dividing the weight of an individual by a measurement of body size. In humans, BMI is calculated as bodyweight/height^2. This index has been applied to horses with moderate correlations (r_s=0.35 to 0.60) between BMI and BCS (Carter et al 2009a, Donaldson et al 2004). In other animals including cats, a BMI has been applied where body length is integrated into the adjustment for body size, calculated as bodyweight/(height×body length) (Hoenig & Ferguson 2002). When this BMI was applied to horses, it similarly correlates with BCS (r_s=0.37 to 0.50). Additionally, a simple bodyweight to height ratio has been demonstrated to be correlated to BCS (r^2=0.58) and body fat percentage (calculated from rump fat thickness, see below) (r^2=0.43) (Henneke et al 1983). However, all of the above correlations are relatively weak, suggesting that one-off measures will not necessarily be accurate and precise predictors of actual body fat content.

Additional morphometric measurements that are useful for assessing relative body condition include the use of a body circumference in relation to body size. This assumes that an increase in circumference is mainly caused by an increase in fat mass. To support this assumption, a ratio of girth circumference to withers height was correlated to BCS (r^2=0.51) and body fat percentage (r^2=0.44) in Quarter horses (Henneke et al 1983). When girth and abdominal circumferences were adjusted by withers height, body length, or bodyweight, it was found that the girth to withers height ratio was the strongest predictor of BCS in horses and ponies (r_s=0.64 and 0.83, respectively), with a greater predictability than both calculations of BMI (Carter et al 2009a). Work in pony mares suggested similarly good prediction of body fat content when heart girth (r^2=0.91), belly girth (r^2=0.82), or mid-neck circumference (r^2=0.75), were adjusted for withers height (Dugdale et al 2011a). Further evaluation of these indices is clearly warranted.

Differences in body shape may inhibit direct comparison of morphometric ratios between different breeds or types of horses. For example, the relationship of girth to height ratio with BCS was different between horses and ponies, indicating that the girth to height ratio of a horse cannot be compared to the same measurement in a pony (Carter et al 2009a). Additionally, a single evaluator should perform multiple measurements to avoid slight variability in measurement techniques, especially for intra-horse comparisons of measurements over time.

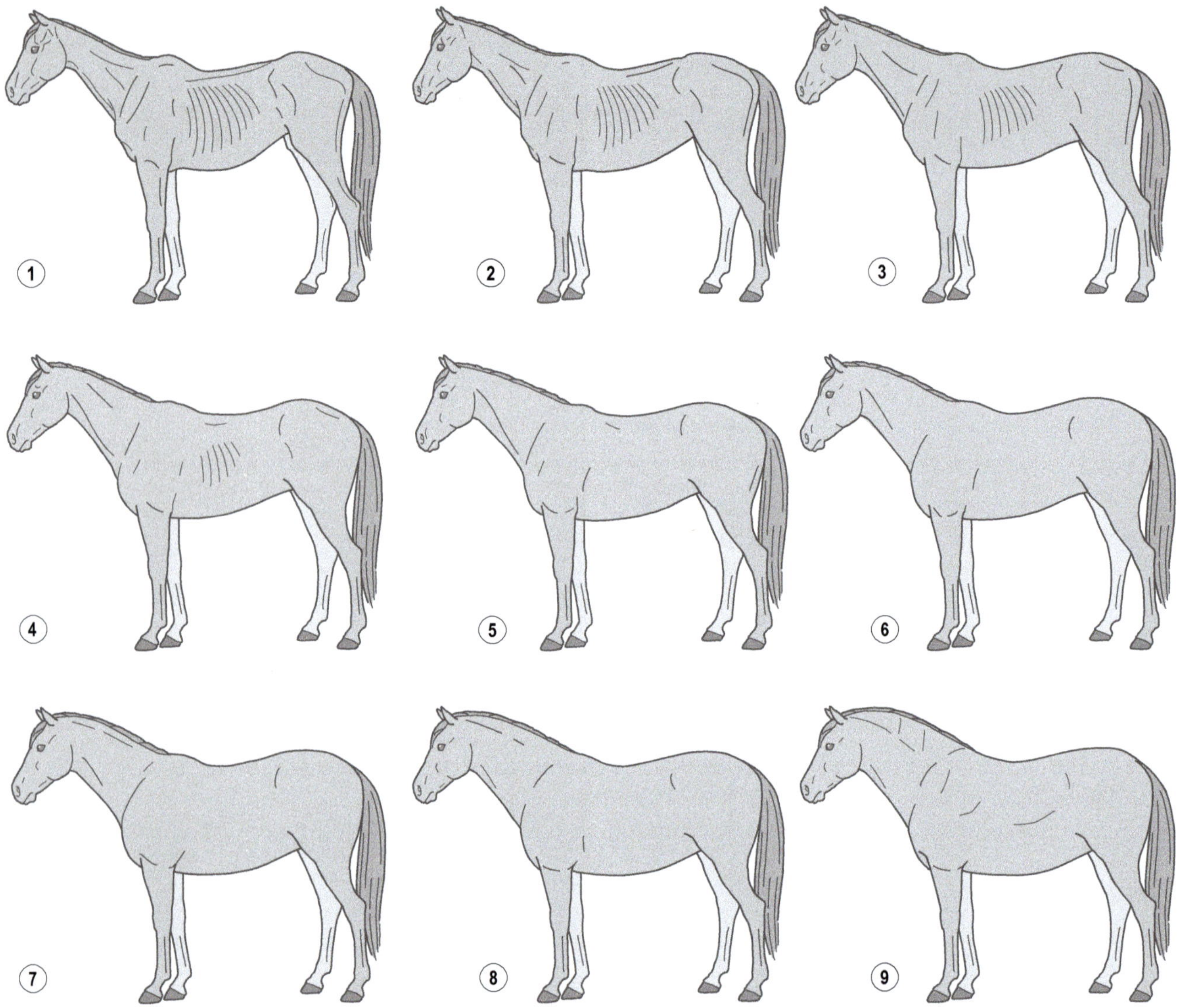

Figure 22.3 Illustrations of individual body condition scores as described by Henneke et al (1983).

Ultrasonic measurement of subcutaneous fat depth

Subcutaneous fat is visible via ultrasound assessment due to the difference in density between adipose and muscle tissue. The less dense adipose is visualized as a darker region above the relatively more dense skeletal muscle tissue (Fig. 22.4). The distance from the skin surface, at the top of the ultrasound screen, to the interface between adipose and muscle may be measured using the ultrasound calipers. Often times, it is necessary to prepare the area of skin where the measurement will be taken by clipping hair and using alcohol or gel to conduct the ultrasonic signal.

Percentage body fat may be calculated from subcutaneous fat thickness, with the assumption that fat depth at a specific body site (usually the rump) is proportional to generalized adiposity. By measuring ultrasonic subcutaneous fat thickness on the rump and comparing to carcass composition in horses and ponies, linear regression was used to develop predictive equations of percent body fat from rump fat thickness (Westervelt et al 1976). For horses, the equation of % body fat=4.70×(fat depth, cm)+8.64, was specific to a site of ultrasound fat depth over the rump 5 cm lateral from the midline at the center of the pelvic bone. The thickness of rump fat located in ponies according to the same definition (5 cm lateral from the midline at the center of the pelvic bone), but presumably at a slightly different anatomical site, was related to body fat content by a similar equation, where % body fat=5.58×(fat depth, cm)+3.83. Subsequently, a similar study in animals of body mass 281–474 kg evaluated five sites along the rump from the tailhead to the top of the croup, each site 10 cm from the midline (Kane et al 1987). Fat depth at the site second closest to the tailhead was most highly correlated with fat mass, and a predictive equation was calculated as % body fat=5.47×(fat depth, cm)+2.47. Kane and colleagues suggested that this near-tailhead site was anatomically most similar to the rump site used by Westervelt's group but cautioned that for ultrasonic fat depths to become a useful proxy for total body fat content, standardization of anatomical scanning site was a prerequisite.

Percent body fat calculated from subcutaneous fat thickness (from equations developed by Westervelt's group) has been used to calculate fat mass and fat-free mass based on

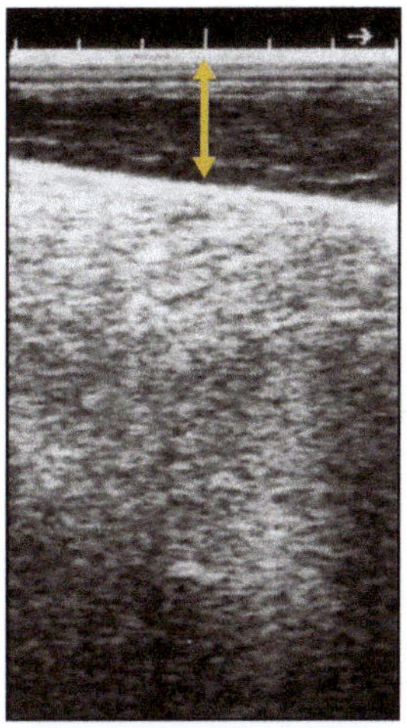

Figure 22.4 **Ultrasound image of subcutaneous fat when the probe is placed over the rump 5 cm lateral from the midline at the center of the pelvic bone. Subcutaneous fat depth is measured from the skin surface at the top of the screen to the interface between the adipose and muscle (double headed arrow).**

body weight (Henneke et al 1983, Kearns et al 2002, 2006). The indirect calculation of fat mass and fat-free mass with this method applies the assumption that subcutaneous fat thickness at the rump has a constant proportion to total fat mass, and that differences in body weight when fat depth remains constant are attributable to differences in fat-free mass. However, alternative fat depots in addition to subcutaneous fat, such as visceral or intramuscular adipose, also contribute to fat mass and are not accounted for in this calculation. In addition, it seems that different fat depots may behave differently during weight (fat) loss or gain and that nutritional history, physiological status and even season may affect the pattern of fat distribution (Gentry et al 2004, Dugdale et al. 2010 2011c).

The calculation of percent body fat from rump fat depth has several limitations. The current equations are based on data generated from a limited population of equidae: 8 horses and 11 ponies in one study (Westervelt et al 1976) or 6 horses in a second study (Kane et al 1987). Limited sample size and differences in methodology and results between studies warrant validation with future research. Additionally, differences between horses and ponies in the generated equations indicate that a larger proportion of total fat mass is comprised of subcutaneous fat mass for ponies compared to horses (Westervelt et al 1976). Therefore, equations may not be applicable across populations of equidae with differing patterns of fat distribution, which may include differences related to breed, age or sex. Regardless, monitoring changes in fat depths during changes in overall body condition may be a useful and objective adjunct to the subjective appraisal of BCS which is likely to change at a slower rate in fatter animals (Dugdale et al 2010).

Total body water (TBW)

A more accurate method of measuring fat mass and fat-free mass may be through the measurement of TBW, as these techniques account for multiple adipose depots. In horses, TBW has been assessed through deuterium oxide dilution, and bioelectrical impedance analysis (BIA).

In dilution techniques, deuterium oxide is administered via nasogastric tube (0.14 g/kg bodyweight) or intravenously (0.11–0.4 g/kg bodyweight) (Andrews et al 1997, Forro et al 2000, Fielding et al 2004, Carter et al 2010, Dugdale et al 2011b). Venous blood samples are collected before and 2–7 h after deuterium oxide dosing. The deuterium oxide content in plasma is analyzed by gas isotope ratio mass spectrometry following zinc reduction of the hydrogen isotopes present in plasma "water". The principle behind this method is that isotope equilibrates into all body water spaces and not into lipid compartments. Once equilibration occurs, plasma isotope concentration is representative of all body water spaces, and TBW is calculated according to the amount of isotope administered and its final concentration in plasma. Subsequent application of the fact that the triglyceride content of adipose tissue is anhydrous and the assumption that all lean tissues contain 73.2% water, allow calculation of lean (fat-free) body mass and body fat (fat-free mass=0.732/TBW; fat mass=bodyweight-fat-free mass) (Pace & Rathbun 1945, Wang et al 2000). Whether this latter assumption is necessarily always correct, at least at both ends of the body condition score spectrum where the inverse relationship between body water and fat contents is most extreme, remains to be determined. Although this hydration constant has not been determined specifically in horses, in other mammals it ranges between 0.71 and 0.77, with an overall average of 0.73 (Wang et al 1999). Dugdale and colleagues (2011b) determined near-perfect linear correlation between in vivo fat mass determined by deuterium oxide dilution and both dissected white adipose tissue mass and chemically-extracted lipid, the latter two determined from the cadavers, thus validating the technique at least in ponies. In this same study, total body fat content was again determined to be non-linearly related to BCS.

In BIA, electrode pairs are placed on the legs above the carpus and hock or at the poll and dock on the dorsal midline, and then electrical currents of different frequencies are transmitted through the body between the electrodes, allowing impedance (the vector between electrical resistance and reactance), to be measured (Forro et al 2000, Fielding et al 2004). This technique is based on the fact that low-frequency electric currents are conducted poorly by lipid-rich tissues, including cell membranes, so are conducted by extracellular water only. Conversely, currents of higher frequencies can penetrate cell membranes of tissues containing primarily water and electrolytes, such as skeletal muscle, but cannot penetrate stored triglycerides well, and thereby are conducted by both intra- and extra-cellular water, i.e. the TBW. Once again, lean tissues are assumed to contain 73.2% water to enable calculation of body fat content from the measurement of TBW.

In both dilution and BIA methods, horses need to be fasted prior to and during analysis and an accurate measurement of bodyweight is necessary for calculations of fat mass and fat-free mass. Additionally, some BIA systems require input of withers height and/or a BCS value.

The results of both D_2O dilution and BIA techniques depend upon the initial measurement of TBW. However, factors that influence TBW and contribute to variability in its measurement include changes in hydration status or gastrointestinal tract content. Of particular concern in equine studies, hydration status may change with exercise; although it has been reported that TBW re-equilibrates to pre-exercise values within 24 hours after an exercise session (McKeen & Lindinger 2004). Additionally, differences in transcellular fluid, including intraluminal gastrointestinal tract water and urine, and timing of urination and defecation with respect to bodyweight determination and TBW measurement could potentially influence calculations of TBW, fat mass, and fat-free mass. In horses, gastrointestinal tract content weight may vary from 5 to 20% of bodyweight depending on feeding status (Webb & Weaver 1979, Meyer 1996), potentially contributing to a large source of error in TBW and bodyweight measurement. In a pony cadaver study, ponies spanning BCS 1.3 to 7/9 had similar hydration of total gastrointestinal contents (ca. 89%) but total gut content, and therefore gut water, was inversely related to BCS (Dugdale et al 2011a). Gut contents accounted for 20% of body mass (~23% of TBW) in the thinnest pony, compared with 7% of body mass (~13% of TBW) in the fattest. The relatively greater tissue hydration in the thinnest animal and the greater gut water pool could both be sources of error when TBW measurement is used to derive body fat (Dugdale et al 2011b).

Although BIA has yet to be validated in equidae, some promising preliminary results using bioelectrical impedance spectroscopy (based on BIA but with extra mathematical modeling) have been presented (Van der Aa Kuhle et al 2008). This study used a poll-to-dock electrode configuration with needle electrodes that penetrated the skin, ensuring good contact and reducing stray current interference/shorting. This same study also determined total body water by D_2O dilution and extracellular fluid space by sodium bromide dilution, and reported good agreement with results obtained by BIA.

Key Points

- Ideal methods for assessment of body condition enable accurate estimation of body composition, specifically the differentiation between, and relative quantification of, fat (adipose tissue) mass and fat-free (lean) mass (e.g. bone and muscle)
- Generalized body condition can be assessed by body condition score, morphometric measurements, ultrasonic fat depth or total body water measurement

Assessment of regional fat distribution

Adipose tissue is regionally distributed among subcutaneous, visceral, body cavity, intermuscular and intramuscular depots. Complex, usually invasive methods are necessary to differentiate deposition among the different regions. However, more clinically applicable methods are available to discern regional fat distribution of subcutaneous adipose between some of the different body locations.

Regions of subcutaneous adipose accumulation during obesity, or where "bulges" of fat often develop, include the neck crest, behind the elbow, over the back and ribs, tailhead, sheath in males (udder in females), and supraorbitally (Fig. 22.5). Of particular interest has been characterization of the subcutaneous adipose depot along the crest of the neck, which contributes to the appearance of a "cresty neck" and has been implicated in risk for disease (Carter et al 2009c, Frank et al 2006, Johnson 2002).

The following methods have been applied to horses in order to assess regional accumulation of fat mass. Similar advantages and disadvantages are present when these methods are applied to a specific fat depot compared to their use for assessing overall body adiposity, as described in Table 22-1.

Morphometric measurements

Morphometric measurements that have been utilized specifically for the assessment of fat deposition along the neck include neck circumference midway between poll and withers (Fig. 22.1), mean neck circumference (average of neck circumferences 0.25, 0.50, and 0.75 the distance from the poll to withers), neck circumference to withers height ratio, neck crest thickness (measured with calipers) and neck crest height midway between the poll and withers (Bailey et al 2008, Carter et al 2009a, Frank et al 2006).

Cresty neck scoring (CNS)

While the BCS systems, especially the Warmblood BCS system (Kienzle & Schramme 2004), integrate the assessment of neck adiposity into the overall evaluation of body condition, a condition scoring system has been developed

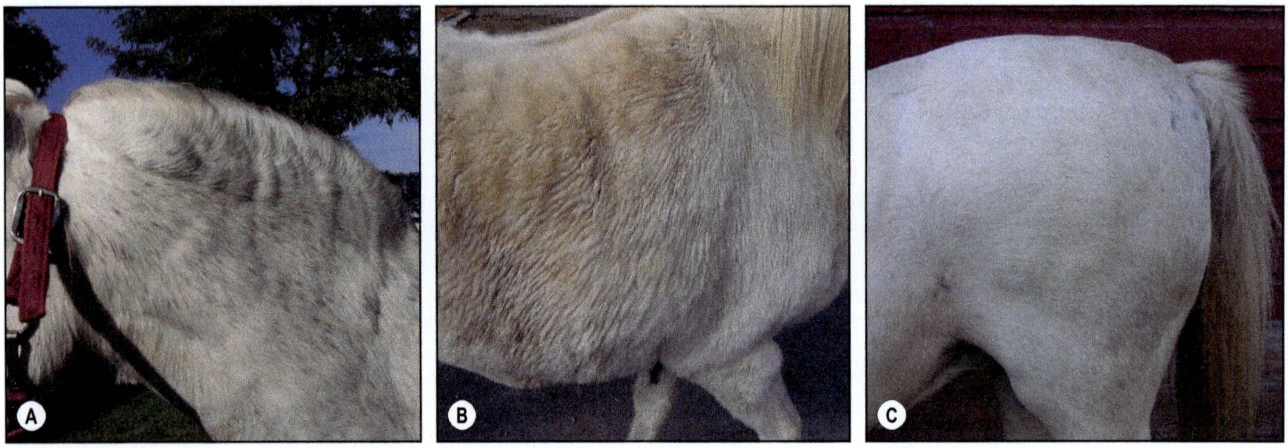

Figure 22.5 Body areas where regional subcutaneous fat accumulates during obesity, including along the crest of the neck A), over the back and ribs and behind the shoulder B), and over the rump C).

Table 22-4 Description of Individual Cresty Neck Scores

Score	Description
0	No visual appearance of a crest (tissue apparent above the ligamentum nuchae). No palpable crest.
1	No visual appearance of a crest, but slight filling felt with palpation.
2	Noticeable appearance of a crest, but fat deposited fairly evenly from poll to withers. Crest easily cupped in one hand and bent from side to side.
3	Crest enlarged and thickened, so fat is deposited more heavily in middle of the neck than toward poll and withers, giving a mounded appearance. Crest fills cupped hand and begins losing side to side flexibility.
4	Crest grossly enlarged and thickened, and can no longer be cupped in one hand or easily bent from side to side. Crest may have wrinkles/creases perpendicular to topline.
5	Crest is so large it permanently droops to one side.

Adapted from Carter et al (2009a).

specifically for assessing the neck crest depot (Table 22-4, Fig. 22.6) (Carter et al 2009a). By utilizing the CNS system in addition to a BCS system, the presence of a cresty neck can be differentiated from generalized obesity in an individual. This may be important in animals that have regional fat accumulation in the neck crest, but are not generally obese.

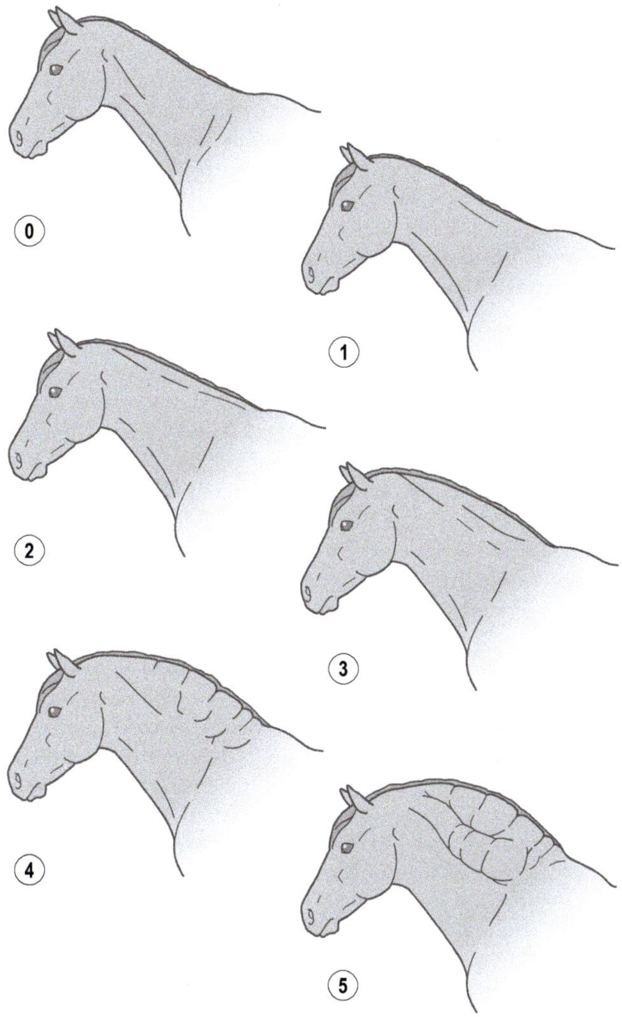

Figure 22.6 Illustrations of individual cresty neck scores as described by Carter et al (2009a).

Ultrasonic fat depth

Although ultrasound of fat depth at a single body site appears to have limited application for assessment of total body fat, it may have utility for monitoring regional fat distribution. In two studies weight gain resulted in increased fat depth along the back, rump and shoulder (Gentry et al 2004, Carter et al 2009b). However, although weight loss in ponies was accompanied by reductions in rib fat thickness, rump fat did not decrease consistently over the course of the study (Dugdale et al 2010). Conversely, exercise in ponies resulted in a decrease in shoulder and rump fat thickness, but no change in rib fat thickness (Westervelt et al 1976). Overall, it appears that changes in regional fat deposition are influenced by more than just nutrition and breed, such that season, exercise and other factors, such as recent nutritional history, may also be important.

Although ultrasonic measurement is the most accurate objective method for measuring subcutaneous fat distribution in live horses, the applicability of using this method in clinical situations across multiple body regions in a repeatable manner is limited. Additionally, this method is technically limited in areas containing greater amounts of connective tissue within the adipose tissue, such as the neck crest, because a discrete border between adipose and muscle is not easily discernable.

Key Points

- Regions of subcutaneous adipose accumulation during obesity, or where "bulges" of fat often develop, include the neck crest, behind the elbow, over the back and ribs, tailhead, the sheath in males (udder in females), and supraorbitally
- Methods that can differentiate regional subcutaneous fat distribution include morphometric measurements, cresty neck scoring or ultrasonic fat depth measurement

Implications for health and performance

Adipose tissue is important for maintaining good health because it provides an important energy source, it allows for storage of fat-soluble vitamins, insulates the body, protects organs, and contributes to glucose homeostasis. However, adipose tissue in excess may also cause problems because of its metabolic and endocrine effects, along with the potential effects of increased weight bearing. Therefore, an appropriate balance of fat mass is necessary to maintain good health.

Risk for disease

Although there is a lack of studies indicating a specific body fat amount under which a horse has increased risk for disease, it is well established in humans that malnourishment increases risk for contracting disease and severe malnutrition decreases survival rate (Schroeder & Brown 1994). It is often considered that a horse with BCS 1 or 2 is being neglected or abused when other factors of horse care and management are considered (Christie et al 2005).

Conversely, increased adiposity has associations with hyperinsulinemia, hyperleptinemia, dyslipidemia, relative insulin resistance, and increased inflammatory cytokine expression (Buff et al 2002, Frank et al 2006, Geor et al 2007, Vick et al 2007). Horses with BCS ≥ 7 had decreased insulin sensitivity (Hoffman et al 2003) and ponies with a BCS ≥ 7 had an increased risk of developing laminitis (Carter et al 2009c, Treiber et al 2006). It should be noted that the latter studies were performed in pony breeds, and it is unknown whether a similar BCS cutoff value is applicable to horse breeds in determining risk for obesity-associated laminitis.

Observations that equidae with cresty necks are prone to develop laminitis suggests that this depot may have physiological and metabolic implications in disease (Johnson 2002), but direct evidence is lacking. Measurements of neck circumference were correlated with glucose (r=0.71) and insulin (r=0.88) areas under the curve during combined glucose-insulin tests, indicating that horses with larger necks were more insulin resistant (Frank et al 2006). Additionally, ponies with a CNS ≥ 4 were at increased risk for developing obesity-associated laminitis (Carter et al 2009c). However, it often cannot be concluded that the effects of neck adiposity are independent of generalized adiposity, given that both usually increase or decrease simultaneously.

Reproductive performance

Low body condition has been associated with a decrease in reproductive performance. Mares with BCS 3 to 3.5 had an extended seasonal anestrous period compared to mares of BCS 7.5 to 8.5 (Gentry et al 2002), while mares with BCS < 4.5 had decreased pregnancy rates (Henneke et al 1984). Research indicates that high body condition may also negatively impact reproductive performance, given that mares with BCS > 7 exhibited longer inter-estrous intervals (36.7±4.8 vs. 26.0±0.5 days), prolonged luteal phases (30.0±5.6 vs. 17.7±0.2 days) and a higher incidence of anovulatory follicles compared to lean horses (Vick et al 2006, Fitzgerald et al 2008).

Athletic performance

There is evidence to suggest that either a high or extreme low body condition may negatively affect athletic performance in horses. Percentage body fat, calculated from ultrasonic fat depth, was inversely related to one-mile race performance in male Standardbred horses, but not females (Kearns et al 2002). In the same study, fat-free mass was positively related to race performance for both male and female horses. Additionally, the top finishers of a 150-mile race had lower BCS compared to horses that could not complete the race and horses that finished later in the race (BCS 4.4 vs. 4.8) (Lawrence et al 1992).

However, in separate studies of horses competing in the 100-mile Tevis Cup race, finishers had a higher BCS than horses disqualified for metabolic reasons (BCS 4.5 vs. < 3.5) (Garlinghouse et al 1999), and horses that did not complete due to metabolic reasons had lower BCS than horses excluded for non-metabolic reasons (BCS 2.9 vs. 4.3) (Garlinghouse & Burrill 1999). In these studies, no horses with a BCS < 3 completed the ride.

Excess fat reserves can contribute to decreased athletic performance due to the insulating effect of thicker fat cover and impairment of heat dissipation, or from the increased work effort required during exercise. For example, the addition of 10% load during treadmill exercise resulted in a 15% increase in oxygen consumption in exercising horses (Garlinghouse & Burrill 1999). Conversely, insufficient fat reserves can contribute to decreased athletic performance due to decreased substrate availability for energy transduction during exercise. Garlinghouse and colleagues (1999) suggested that an excessively low body condition can reflect a negative energy balance resulting from the energetic demands of an intense training program. A negative energy balance can result in not only a decrease in fat mass, but also a decrease in lean muscle mass, thereby limiting the force-generating components available to do the work.

Categorization of body condition

Given the results of previous research indicating decreased athletic and reproductive performance and increased risk of disease at the lower and upper end of the BCS scale, it is recommended that BCS ≤ 3 is considered underweight, BCS ≥ 7 is overweight, and BCS ≥ 8 is obese. Although differences may be apparent between individual horses, in general being underweight may affect overall health and athletic performance, being overweight may contribute to metabolic dysfunction (insulin resistance and laminitis) and obesity may additionally contribute to reproductive dysfunction in mares.

It is recommended that horses are maintained at a BCS of 4 to 6 (on the 1–9 scale), although more precise optimization within this narrow range may be further beneficial for success in various disciplines or for different classes of horses. Reproductive performance for broodmares may be optimal at BCS 5 or 6, whereas athletic performance may be optimal at BCS 4 or 5. For horses in which metabolic problems or obesity-associated laminitis is a problem, maintaining a BCS of 4 or 5 may decrease risk for metabolic disease.

Key Points

- High or excessively low body condition can affect risk for disease (e.g. laminitis), reproductive function and athletic performance
- Categorization of body condition as underweight (BCS ≤ 3, 1–9-point scale), moderate (BCS 4–6), overweight (BCS ≥ 7) or obese (BCS ≥ 8) can be used as an aid in the management of body condition for optimal health and performance

Choosing an assessment method

When deciding which method to use, it is important to consider the goals one intends to achieve by applying the method. In order to determine which method will suit your needs, the following questions may be helpful.

What resources are available?

Unavailability of a weigh scale, ultrasound instrument, or materials for TBW measurement, often necessitate the use of bodyweight estimation, condition scoring, or morphometric measurements which only need a tape measure and calculator to perform.

Is an assessment of bodyweight or body condition needed?

Bodyweight measurement is necessary for ration evaluation and determining dosage of medications, anthelmintics, etc., whereas body condition assessment informs decisions regarding disease risk/health status. Tracking changes in energy balance over time in an individual animal may be facilitated by either bodyweight or body condition measurements.

Is the method being used for inter-horse or intra-horse comparisons?

For intra-horse comparisons, a method with high precision and sensitivity is necessary, so that small changes can be repeatably detected. Methods best suited for this include direct measurement of bodyweight, morphometric measurements, ultrasonic subcutaneous fat thickness, and TBW. The scoring of body condition is often not sensitive enough to track small changes in body condition.

For inter-horse comparisons, a method with high accuracy is needed, so that differences can be detected across populations or so that horses can be classified for health implications. Methods best suited for this include morphometric measurements, BCS, ultrasonic fat depth, and TBW. Body weight is often not applicable to inter-horse comparisons because it does not adjust for body size.

Many times it is necessary to categorize an individual to determine health risks, then track changes in condition over time. For this situation, it may be necessary to start with one method (e.g. BCS) to determine health risks, and then switch to a more sensitive method (e.g., bodyweight or morphometrics) to track changes.

Which fat depots are of interest?

The assessment of subcutaneous fat, especially neck crest adipose, may be particularly helpful in determining risk for disease. Morphometric measurements, condition scoring, and ultrasonic fat depth have the ability to assess overall subcutaneous adipose deposition or a single subcutaneous adipose depot. Differentiation of total fat mass versus fat-free mass is only accurately measured in horses by TBW.

In nutritional research, it is often the intention to track changes in body composition in response to a treatment, such as exercise, feed restriction, or overfeeding. In these situations, it is important to assess as many fat depots as possible, given that depots are differentially regulated and changes in subcutaneous fat may not be parallel to changes in total fat mass (Carter et al 2010, Dugdale et al 2011c).

Conclusions

The assessment of bodyweight and body condition is important for the evaluation of a nutritional program and its impact on health and performance. In order to maximize the benefits of their use, it is important to consider the intended objective of their measurement (e.g. track intra-horse changes over time vs. make implications for disease risk) and apply methods that can best facilitate those objectives.

References

Andrews, F.M., Nadeau, J.A., Saabye, L., et al., 1997. Measurement of total body water content in horses, using deuterium oxide dilution. American Journal of Veterinary Research 58, 1060–1064.

Bailey, S.R., Habershon-Butcher, J.L., Ransom, K.J., et al., 2008. Hypertension and insulin resistance in a mixed-breed population of ponies predisposed to laminitis. American Journal of Veterinary Research 69, 122–129.

Buff, P.R., Dodds, A.C., Morrison, C.D., et al., 2002. Leptin in horses: Tissue localization and relationship between peripheral concentrations of leptin and body condition. Journal of Animal Science 80, 2942–2948.

Carroll, C.L., Huntington, P.J., 1988. Body condition scoring and weight estimation of horses. Equine Veterinary Journal 20, 41–45.

Carter, R.A., Geor, R.J., Staniar, W.B., et al., 2009a. Apparent adiposity assessed by standardised scoring systems and morphometric measurements in horses and ponies. The Veterinary Journal 179, 204–210.

Carter, R.A., McCutcheon, L.J., George, L.A., et al., 2009b. Effects of diet-induced weight gain on insulin sensitivity and plasma hormone and lipid concentrations in horses. American Journal of Veterinary Research 70, 1250–1258.

Carter, R.A., Treiber, K.H., Geor, R.J., et al., 2009c. Prediction of incipient pasture-associated laminitis from hyperinsulinaemia, hyperleptinaemia and generalized and localised obesity in a cohort of ponies. Equine Veterinary Journal 41, 171–178.

Carter, R.A., McCutcheon, L.J., Valle, E., et al., 2010. Effects of exercise training on adiposity, insulin sensitivity, and plasma hormone and lipid concentrations in overweight/obese, insulin resistant horses. American Journal of Veterinary Research 71 (3), 314–321.

Christie, J.L., Hewson, C.J., Riley, C.B., et al., 2005. A preliminary equine abuse policy with potential application to veterinary practice. Canadian Veterinary Journal 46, 250–252.

Donaldson, M.T., McFarlane, D., Jorgensen, A.J., et al., 2004. Correlation between plasma alpha-melanocyte-stimulating hormone concentration and body mass index in healthy horses. American Journal of Veterinary Research 65, 1469–1473.

Dugdale, A.H.A., Curtis, G.C., Cripps, P.J., et al., 2010. Effect of dietary restriction on body condition, composition and welfare of overweight and obese pony mares. Equine Veterinary Journal 42, 600–610.

Dugdale, A.H.A., Curtis, G.C., Harris, P.A., et al., 2011a. Assessment of body fat in the pony I: Relationships between the anatomical distribution of adipose tissue, body composition and body condition. Equine Veterinary Journal 43 (5), 552–561.

Dugdale, A.H.A., Curtis, G.C., Milne, E., et al., 2011b. Assessment of body fat in the pony II: validation of the deuterium oxide dilution technique. Equine Veterinary Journal 43 (5), 562–570.

Dugdale, A.H.A., Curtis, G.C., Cripps, P.J., et al., 2011c. Effects of season and body condition on appetite, body mass and body composition in *ad libitum* fed pony mares. The Veterinary Journal 190 (3), 329–337.

Ellis, J.M., Hollands, T., 1998. Accuracy of different methods of estimating the weight of horses. The Veterinary Record 143, 335–336.

Ellis, J.M., Hollands, T., 2002. Use of height-specific weigh tapes to estimate the bodyweight of horses. The Veterinary Record 150, 632–634.

Ensminger, M.E., 1977. Horses and Horsemanship, fifth ed. Interstate Printers and Publishers, Danville, p. 509.

Fielding, C.L., Magdesian, K.G., Elliott, D.A., et al., 2004. Use of multifrequency bioelectrical impedance analysis for estimation of total body water and extracellular and intracellular fluid volumes in horses. American Journal of Veterinary Research 65, 320–326.

Fitzgerald, B.P., Sessions, D.R., Vick, M.M., et al., 2008. Obesity and reproduction in the mare. In: The chronically infertile mare (Abstract book). The Havemeyer Foundation, p. 23.

Forro, M., Cieslar, S., Ecker, G.L., et al., 2000. Total body water and ecfv measured using bioelectrical impedance analysis and indicator dilution in horses. Journal of Applied Physiology 89, 663–671.

Frank, N., Elliott, S.B., Brandt, L.E., et al., 2006. Physical characteristics, blood hormone concentrations, and plasma lipid concentrations in obese horses with insulin resistance. Journal of the American Veterinary Medical Association 228, 1383–1390.

Freestone, J.F., Beadle, R., Shoemaker, K., et al., 1992. Improved insulin sensitivity in hyperinsulinaemic ponies through physical conditioning and controlled feed intake. Equine Veterinary Journal 24, 187–190.

Garlinghouse, S.E., Burrill, M.J., 1999. Relationship of body condition score to completion rate during 160 km endurance races. Equine Veterinary Journal 30 (Suppl.), 591–595

Garlinghouse, S.E., Bray, R.E., Cogger, E.A., et al., 1999. The influence of body measurements and condition score on performance results during the. 1998. Tevis Cup. In: Proceedings of the 16th Equine Nutrition and Physiology Society Symposium. Raleigh, NC, Equine Nutrition and Physiology Society, Savoy, IL.

Gee, H., Harris, P.A., 2005. Condition scoring and weight estimation: practical tools. In: Harris, P.A., Mair, T.S., Slater, J.D., et al (Eds.), Equine nutrition for all. Proceedings of the 1st British Equine Veterinary Association & WALTHAM Nutrition Symposia. Harrogate (UK), pp. 15–24.

Gentry, L.R., Thompson, D.L., Gentry, G.T., et al., 2002. The relationship between body condition, leptin, and reproductive and hormonal characteristics of mares during the seasonal anovulatory period. Journal of Animal Science 80, 2695–2703.

Gentry, L.R., Thompson, D.L., Gentry, G.T., et al., 2004. The relationship between body condition score and ultrasonic fat measurements in mares of high versus low body condition. Journal of Equine Veterinary Science 24, 198–203.

Geor, R.J., Thatcher, C.D., Pleasant, R.S., et al., 2007. Prevalence of hyperinsulinemia in mature horses: Relationship to adiposity. Journal of Veterinary Internal Medicine 21, 601.

Henneke, D.R., Potter, G.D., Kreider, J.L., et al., 1983. Relationship between condition score, physical measurements and body fat percentage in mares. Equine Veterinary Journal 15, 371–372.

Henneke, D.R., Potter, G.D., Kreider, T.L., 1984. Body condition during pregnancy and lactation and reproductive efficiency of mares. Theriogenology 21, 897–909.

Hoenig, M., Ferguson, D.C., 2002. Effects of neutering on hormonal concentrations and energy requirements in male and female cats. American Journal of Veterinary Research 63, 634–639.

Hoffman, R.M., Boston, R.C., Stefanovski, D., et al., 2003. Obesity and diet affect glucose dynamics and insulin sensitivity in Thoroughbred geldings. Journal of Animal Science 81, 2333–2342.

Jeffries, B.C., 1961. Body condition scoring and its use in management. Tasmanian Journal of Agriculture 32, 19–21.

Jensen, M.D., 1992. Research techniques for body composition assessment. Journal of the American Dietetic Association 92, 454–460.

Johnson, P.J., 2002. The equine metabolic syndrome peripheral Cushing's syndrome. Veterinary Clinics of North America Equine Practice 18, 271–293.

Jones, R.S., Lawrence, T.L., Veevers, A., et al., 1989. Accuracy of prediction of the liveweight of horses from body measurements. The Veterinary Record 125, 549–553.

Kane, R.A., Fisher, M., Parrett, D., et al., 1987. Estimating fatness in horses. In: Proceedings of the 10th Equine Nutrition and Physiology Society. Fort Collins, CO, pp. 127–131.

Kearns, C.F., McKeever, K.H., Kumagai, K., et al., 2002. Fat-free mass is related to one-mile race performance in elite standardbred horses. The Veterinary Journal 163, 260–266.

Kearns, C.F., McKeever, K.H., Roegner, V., et al., 2006. Adiponectin and leptin are related to fat mass in horses. The Veterinary Journal 172, 460–465.

Kienzle, E., Schramme, S., 2004. Body condition scoring and prediction of bodyweight in adult warm-blooded horses. Pferdeheilkunde 20, 517–524.

Kohnke, J., 1992. Feeding and Nutrition: the making of a champion. Birubi Pacific, Australia, pp. 163–166.

Lawrence, L., Jackson, S., Kline, K., et al., 1992. Observations on body weight and condition of horses in a 150 mile endurance ride. Equine Veterinary Science 12, 320–324.

Leighton-Hardman, A.C., 1980. Condition scoring and weight estimation. In: Equine Nutrition. Pelham Books, London. pp. 9–19.

McKeen, G., Lindinger, M.I., 2004. Prediction of hydration status using multi-frequency bioelectrical impedance analysis during exercise and recovery in horses. Equine and Comparative Exercise Physiology 1, 199–209.

Marcenac, L.N., Aublet, H., 1964. Encyclopedie du Cheval. Maloine, Paris.

Martin-Rosset, W., Vernet, J., Dubroeucq, H., et al., 2008. Variation of fatness and energy content with body condition score in sport horses and its prediction. In: Saasamoinene, M.T., Martin-Rosset, W. (Eds.), Nutrition of the exercising horse. European Association fot Animal Production Publication Number 125. Wageningen Academic Publishers, The Netherlands, pp. 167–176.

Meyer, H., 1996. Influence of feed intake and composition, feed and water restriction and exercise on gastrointestinal fill in horses. Equine Practice 18, 26–29.

Milner, J., Hewitt, D., 1969. Weight of horses: Improved estimates based on girth and length. Canadian Veterinary Journal 10, 314–316.

Pace, N., Rathbun, E.N., 1945. Studies on body composition III. The body water and chemically combined nitrogen content in relation to fat content. Journal of Biological Chemistry 158, 685–691.

Reavell, D.G., 1999. Measuring and estimating the weight of horses with tapes, formulae and by visual assessment. Equine Veterinary Education 11, 314–317.

Schroeder, D.G., Brown, K.H., 1994. Nutritional status as a predictor of child survival: summarizing the association and quantifying its global impact. Bulletin of the World Health Organization 72, 569–579.

Staniar, W.B., Kronfeld, D.S., Hoffman, R.M., et al., 2004. Weight prediction from linear measures of growing Thoroughbreds. Equine Veterinary Journal 36, 149–154.

Suagee, J.K., Burk, A.O., Quinn, R.W., et al., 2008. Effects of diet and weight gain on body condition scoring in Thoroughbred geldings. Journal of Equine Veterinary Science 28, 156–166.

Treiber, K.H., Kronfeld, D.S., Hess, T.M., et al., 2006. Evaluation of genetic and metabolic predispositions and nutritional risk factors for pasture-associated laminitis in ponies. Journal of the American Veterinary Medical Association 228, 1538–1545.

Van der Aa Kuhle, K., Cawdell-Smith, A.J., Ward, L.C., et al., 2008. Prediction of equine body composition with bioelectrical impedance spectroscopy. Proceedings of the Nutrition Society of Australia. Adelaide, Australia, December 2008.

Vick, M.M., Adams, A.A., Murphy, B.A., et al., 2007. Relationships among inflammatory cytokines, obesity, and insulin sensitivity in the horse. Journal of Animal Science 85, 1144–1155.

Vick, M.M., Sessions, D.R., Murphy, B.A., et al., 2006. Obesity is associated with altered metabolic and reproductive activity in the mare: Effects of metformin on insulin sensitivity and reproductive cyclicity. Reproduction, Fertility and Development 18, 609–617.

Wang, Z., Deurenberg, P., Wang, W., et al., 1999. Hydration of fat-free body mass: Review and critique of a classic body-composition constant. American Journal of Clinical Nutrition 69, 833–841.

Wang, Z., Deurenberg, P., Heymsfield, S.B., 2000. Cellular-level body composition model. A new approach to studying fat-free mass hydration. Annals of the New York Academy of Sciences 904, 306–311.

Webb, A.I., Weaver, B.M.Q., 1979. Body composition of the horse. Equine Veterinary Journal 11, 39–47.

Westervelt, R.G., Stouffer, J.R., Hintz, H.F., et al., 1976. Estimating fatness in horses and ponies. Journal of Animal Science 43, 781–785.

Willoughby, D.P., 1975. Growth and Nutrition in the Horse. A.S. Barnes and Co., London.

23

Ration evaluation and formulation

Catherine E. Dunnett

Feeding horses is often described as being a combination of art and science and the area of ration evaluation is probably the best illustration of this. Ration evaluation can provide a useful indicator of the appropriateness of a horse or ponies' diet, in terms of energy, macro- and micronutrient intake, as well as energy source. However, there are limitations to the accuracy of the information obtained from a ration evaluation and interpretation of the data should reflect this.

Practical ration evaluation invariably involves assessment of the suitability of a horse's current diet relative to its individual circumstances, with suggested changes being made where warranted. In most cases, a nutritionist will be presented with a dietary history of some kind, although there are notable exceptions to this where no dietary history is available, for example in acute welfare cases. Dietary history may also be scant where a radical change in circumstances, such as removal of a horse from pasture, or a recent purchase has occurred. Where available, a horse's current ration, as well as previous dietary history, is of immense value to a presiding nutritionist and will usually be the starting point for most evaluations.

Information needed for ration evaluation

There is a range of information that must be gathered in order to practically evaluate a current ration or indeed formulate a new ration, all of which will be discussed in this chapter including the factors mentioned in Box 23.1.

Integrity of the information

The integrity of the information regarding the current diet may be greater when it is gathered by the nutritionist themselves, or by another appropriate person. Being physically present during at least one feeding period is desirable and is likely to increase the accuracy of the dietary information obtained. The client or feeding manager can be questioned regarding the feeds used and their feeding habits and management. A nutritionist should also weigh all of the allocated quantities of feeds, supplements and forages. This presents a good opportunity to sample the components of the diet for any required laboratory analysis.

Information regarding a horse's current ration, as well as any other dietary history, can be unreliable and lack accuracy when provided by the owner, trainer or other third party. This can be due to:

- Lack of knowledge of the actual feeds used or feeding management in place by the owner or trainer, especially where they are not responsible for the feeding on a day to day basis.
- Lack of appreciation of differences in the quality or availability of grazing or variability of forage type or quality.
- Inaccurate assumptions regarding horse factors, e.g. the level of physical activity is often over-estimated.
- Inaccurate assumptions about the weight of feed fed and differences in density– this is reflected by the common reference to the proverbial "1 lb scoop" or coffee can.
- Inaccurate assumptions regarding the chemical composition of feeds.
- Poor reflection of forage intake including inaccurate statements such as ad libitum feeding of forage.
- Failure to account for wastage of either concentrate feeds or forage.

Remote ration evaluation

Remote ration evaluation through telephone, written or web-based questionnaires has become very common in recent years with many feed and supplement companies offering a free advice service. This type of evaluation allows clients to receive useful guidance on the appropriate use of particular products within a product range. However, remote ration evaluation also has the potential to be less robust, as there is reliance on the owner, trainer or other persons to provide accurate information regarding the individual horse, current ration and dietary history. However, the integrity of this information can be improved through

Box 23.1 Information Required for Ration Formulation Includes the Following

Factors associated with the horse	
Age	Young growing, mature, or aged
Physiological state	Pregnant, lactating, growing, body condition (overweight, ideal or underweight), presence of nutritionally related disease, behavior-related issues.
Activity	Maintenance, level of exercise, type of exercise
Preferences	Horses may have a preference for a particular feed type
Factors associated with the feed	
Dietary history	Nature, amount and analysis of current ration
Chemical composition	Sensory evaluation (e.g., indication of type of hay)
Laboratory analysis	e.g., protein, oil and fiber content and calculation of energy content
Hygienic quality	Sensory and/or laboratory analysis
Feedstuffs availability	There will be regional variation in the availability of different feedstuffs

skilled interview of the client by telephone and by ensuring that all feeds have been weighed.

Predicted versus actual analysis

The reliance on predicted or published nutrient content of feeds and forages as opposed to actual laboratory analysis may also affect the accuracy of the ration evaluation. With respect to end users, the use of predicted analysis is usually driven by economical constraints. The number of establishments that are prepared to undertake full nutritional laboratory analysis of feedstuffs, forages and grazing is relatively low.

Nutrient analysis of forage, for example alfalfa, can vary considerably depending on factors such as stage of growth at harvest, type of grass, fertility of the soil as well as the soil type and underlying geology of the land (Van Soest et al 1978). All of these factors will also affect the nutrient content of pasture. Whilst historical pasture analysis is sometimes available during ration evaluation, it is usually restricted to large professional establishments. It is therefore more common for a nutritionist to draw on published nutrient values for pasture and forage (NRC 2007), which introduces inherent inaccuracies. Localized regions of pasture inadequacy in trace minerals such as copper, for example in parts of Ireland, or extreme reductions in pasture quality (e.g., in UK moorland) may not be captured.

Proprietary feed and forage companies can usually provide analytical information regarding their feed or forage products, which is likely to be based at least in part on actual laboratory analysis, especially where the legally required declared analysis (e.g., protein, oil, ash and crude fiber) is concerned. Feed companies are also able to provide an accurate prediction of micronutrient content of proprietary feeds, where a vitamin and mineral premix has been used. It is, however, still relatively common for feed manufacturers to use published values for the prediction of other nutrients of importance such as starch, sugars, amino acids, etc.

Laboratory analysis of concentrate feed or forage can be carried out simply to confirm adherence to the declared analysis, or can offer more comprehensive information beyond this. Samples must be as representative of the feed or forage as possible, in order to avoid large discrepancies occurring between predicted and actual analysis due to sampling error.

Key Points

- Information pertaining to the horses' current physiological state is essential
- Previous dietary history is an extremely important part of ration evaluation
- Maintaining the integrity or accuracy of gathered information regarding the horse/horses, where ration is being evaluated, as well as the nature of the current ration will improve the evaluation process

Assessment of current ration

Energy content of feeds and forages

The energy content of feeds and forages must be obtained for accurate ration analysis, either through the use of predicted values or calculation from proximate analysis using published equations. The energy value of feeds can also be derived *in vivo* from feeding trials, although this would usually be beyond the scope of practical ration evaluation. Energy, which is usually described in terms of either joules (e.g. in Europe) or calories (e.g. in USA [1 kcal=4.184 kJ], is most often expressed as digestible energy (DE), although in Europe net energy (NE) or derivatives thereof as discussed in Chapter 4 are routinely used).

Feeds can also be described using the horse feed unit (HFU) or in French, *l'unite fouragire cheval* (UFC). The UFC corresponds to the NE value of 1 kg of standard barley (87% DM) in a horse at maintenance (2250 kcal). The UFC value of other feeds can be calculated by dividing their relative NE content in kcal by that of barley or from prediction from chemical analysis.

There are a number of published equations that can be used to calculate the DE or UFC content of feedstuffs from their chemical composition which have been previously reviewed (Harris 1999) and are summarized below. The energy value assigned to a feed, whether estimated or calculated, *must always be in the same format as the target energy requirements*, for example DE for NRC requirements (NRC 2007), UFC for INRA requirements. See Box 23.2.

Forage and feed sampling

Forage sampling

Forage samples should ideally be taken using a hay bore, which consists of a long metal cylinder that can be inserted to a given depth into a bale of hay, haylage or straw usually driven by an electric drill (Fig. 23.1). In this manner, several samples can be taken from many bales to build up a representative mixed sample of a particular batch of forage.

Box 23.2 Example of Equations Used to Determine DE and UFC from Feed Chemical Composition (see also Chapter 5)

Digestible energy

a) DE (kcal/kg DM) = 2118 +12.18 (CP) − 9.37(ADF) − 3.83(NDF − ADF) + 47.18(fat) + 0.35(NSc) − 26.3(Ash)

b) DE (MJ/kgDM) = DCP × 0.023 + DEE × 0.0381 + (DCF+DNFE) × 0.0172

c) DE (MJ/kg DM) = 11.1 + 0.0034 CP + 0.0158 CF − 0.00016 CF^2

l'unite fouragire cheval (UFC)

a) Forages

UFC = 0.0557 + 0.0006 CC + 0.2489 DE

UFC = 0.825 − 0.0011 CF + 0.0006 CP

b) Concentrates or raw materials

UFC = −0.134 + 0.0003 CF − 0.0004 CP + 0.0003 CC + 0.3160 DE

CC = cytoplasmic carbohydrate; CP = crude protein; DCP = digestible crude protein; ADF = acid detergent fiber; NDF = neutral detergent fiber; CF = crude fiber; DCF = digestible crude fiber; NSc = 100 − CP − EE − NDF − ash; DEE = digestible ether extract; DNFE = digestible nitrogen free extract.

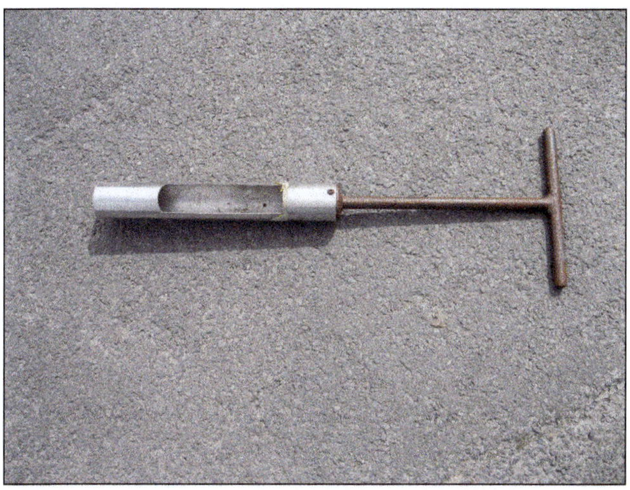

Figure 23.1 **Hay bale corer. Caution is required when sampling some very high DM bales that the friction does not present a fire risk.**
Photo courtesy Andrew Theodorou.

Where possible the sub-samples of hay should be mixed but there is also a reliance on the laboratory to resample for analysis in an appropriate way. Bales of haylage should be carefully re-sealed following sampling to avoid aerobic spoilage. Where a hay bore is not available, simple grab samples can be used to give an estimate of forage analysis, but again multiple samples should be taken from multiple bales from varying regions and depths within the bale where possible as this will require bales to be opened. In instances where forage is suspected of contributing to health issues such as colic or sporadic respiratory disease it may be necessary to establish the variability in nutritional value or quality of the forage. In this instance many single bales may need to be analyzed, with composite samples being taken from each individual bale.

For haylage, samples should be placed into sealed bags, expelling the air as far as possible prior to sealing. This is particularly important where fermentation characteristics or microbiological analysis of haylage is required. Due to the variable instability of haylage, once removed from their anaerobic environment (Cecilia 2009), samples of haylage should always be shipped to the laboratory immediately. Ideally, these should be sent on a next day delivery service, avoiding the possibility of haylage samples remaining in the post or being unprocessed over a weekend.

Complementary feed assessment and sampling

Complementary feed refers to any feed that is fed alongside forage or grazing to provide a balanced diet for the horse and in this context is synonymous with the term concentrate feed. Whilst legally within Europe the term complementary feed also incorporates feed supplements, these have not been included in this part of the discussion and will be addressed separately.

Proprietary complementary feed offers a certain amount of nutritional information as part of the legally required statutory statement. This usually consists of a guaranteed or typical nutritional analysis, plus a list of ingredients which may be expressed in percentage terms or simply in descending order of inclusion. The nutritional analysis may include reference to the content of moisture, crude protein, oil, crude fiber and ash. Additional information pertaining to the level of added fat soluble vitamins A, D, and E, as well as trace minerals such as copper may be provided. Whilst there may be some uniformity between countries (for example in Europe) we can expect a degree of variation in the information legally required across the world.

For complementary feeds, a similar approach to forage is required and multiple grab samples should be taken from several bags of feed. Ideally feed bags should be opened out on the floor, well mixed and then sampled accordingly. A simple protocol for concentrate feed sampling is described below.

- Open a bag of feed by cutting open down both sides and open up the bag completely.
- Using a clean scoop or shovel mix the contents of the bag thoroughly.
- Wearing latex gloves or using an inverted plastic bag take 10–12 samples of the feed bag covering all areas of the spread feed into a single clean sample bucket or bag to form a composite sample.
- Repeat this process with up to 10% of the total feed batch.
- Thoroughly mix the composite sample and then take two representative samples.
- Retain one sample and send the second to the laboratory.

Chain of custody for feed or forage samples

In instances where nutritional analysis of feed or forage forms part of a legal dispute which may require evidence being presented before a court or panel of arbitration, it is important to use established protocols for sampling and also to ensure a good chain of custody for the samples. This would ensure that sample integrity is maintained from the point of sampling to the time of analysis. It can therefore be established that the analysis results presented within a legal setting refer to the actual samples taken from a particular feed on a particular day and that these have not been contaminated or adulterated in any way. This process can be simplified by the use of public service individuals with expertise in sample collection who may be called upon by a farmer or owner in situations of a suspected nutritional problem. This may be required during the investigation of potential feed contamination (e.g. following a positive post race or competition urine sample for prohibited substances), as defined by a sport's governing body. Equally this type of sampling protocol may also be required by trading standards in order to establish conformity to statutory declaration.

Assessment of vitamin–mineral and specialized supplements

Feed supplements can also be analyzed for adherence to their specification, in order to ensure that they contain the declared level of active ingredients. This is particularly important where a product is reputed to help maintain an aspect of health e.g. the reputed ability of a product to support joint health may depend on the level of particular active ingredients being present. Previously glucosamine-containing oral joint supplements have been shown to have poor adherence to their declared specification in terms of the amount of this active ingredient they contained (Oke et al 2006). In this study, of the products analyzed, 39% were shown to contain less glucosamine than claimed by the manufacturer and 17% had less than 30% of the amount claimed. It is also not uncommon for specialized supplement ingredients to exhibit a reduced or even absent level of the bioactive substance, (e.g., harpagosides, which are the active ingredient in Devils claw; Dunnett 2010).

Assessment of pasture

Pasture sampling should be carried out using an established format, which may include walking a large "W" or "M" within each paddock and cutting representative samples of grass at numerous points. Areas of heavy contamination with urine or dung should be avoided and in order to minimize soil contamination samples should not be cut too close to the ground or pulled rather than cut (Fig. 23.2). Additionally samples should ideally be taken on dry days to avoid soil contamination from splash back. Further details on pasture sampling procedures and precautions have been previously provided (MacNaeidhe 1995).

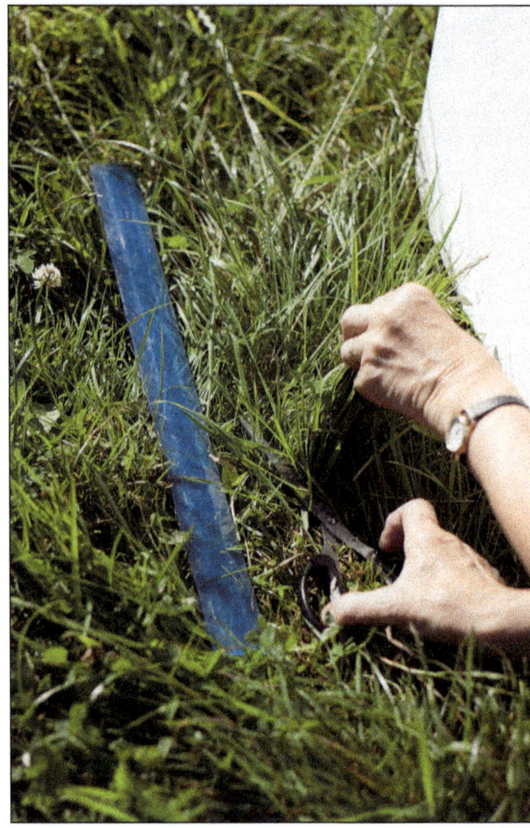

Figure 23.2 Example of collecting grass for analysis – avoiding soil contaminated herbage. Sample along the length of meter rule, cut at grazing height, and place samples into ice-box immediately.
Photo courtesy of Andrew Theodorou.

Laboratory analysis of feed and forage samples

Appropriate sample preparation, extraction and analysis of the analytes requested is then required, ideally using an established, experienced laboratory with appropriate external accreditation. Where laboratory results show any unexpected deviation from declared analysis or established levels, repeat analysis should always be requested.

The analysis requested from the laboratory will depend on what information is required and the specific ration evaluation questions being asked. For example, analysis may be undertaken in order to assess the suitability and/or quality of a particular batch of forage, or a feed mix may be analyzed to enable calculation of a DE value. Alternatively laboratory analysis of a proprietary feed may be required to check for adherence to the declared analysis or typical analysis provided by the manufacturer. Individual raw materials may be analyzed so that they can be added to a database enabling the formulation of proprietary feeds or a ration of straights. "Straights" are a colloquial term that refers to a mixture of straight feeding stuffs such as oats, barley, alfalfa, sugar beet, etc. that can be mixed to provide a complementary or concentrate feed for horses. Table 23-1 gives examples of some of the analytical profiles that could be requested for different situations.

Assessment of forage consumption

Assessment of forage intake requires a record of both the weight of forage offered, which can be easily achieved when horses are fed individually, but is more problematic in group fed animals. Wastage of forage should also be recorded in order to increase accuracy. Wastage of forage can be particularly high in performance horses (Geor 2005), that may self-limit forage intake when a high level of energy rich concentrate feed is fed. Where hay is soaked or steamed, the weight offered should be recorded prior to such treatment.

An indication of the dry matter of forage is advantageous and is a necessity where haylage is considered. The dry matter content of haylage can vary considerably both between suppliers and to a lesser extent from batch to batch from the same supplier. A moisture probe can be used to provide an estimate of the dry matter content of haylage by

Table 23-1 Examples of Analysis Requested for Different Feed Types for Specific Purposes

Analysis justification	Sample	Analysis	Further useful analysis
Nutritional contribution of pasture to overall ration or identification of issue such as low Cu or high heavy metals	Pasture	Full macro & micro mineral screen	DM, CP, O, CF, Ash
Nutritional contribution of hay to overall ration or fitness to feed (respiratory)	Hay	DM, CP, O, CF, Ash, Total molds & yeasts at 25 and 37°C	Mycotoxin screen Characterization of molds
Nutritional contribution of hay to overall ration or fitness to feed (respiratory) and or stability	Haylage	DM, CP, O, CF, Ash, Total molds & yeasts at 25 and 37°	Fermentation parameters pH, VFA, Lactic acid etc.
Calculation of DE and/or adherence to declared analysis	Complementary feed	DM, CP, O, CF, Ash, Cu, Vit E	Full macro & micro mineral screen plus vitamins A and D
Assessment of suitability for individuals with laminitis	Complementary feed Hay haylage	Starch and total sugars	Full macro & micro mineral screen plus vitamins A and D
Calculation of DE and or assessment of Ca:P ratio of overall ration	Cereal grains e.g. oats	Ca and P, DM, CP, O, CF, Ash (or other parameters required for calculation of DE	Mycotoxin screen
Stability and indication of oxidation	High oil feed vegetable oil	Peroxide value	Fatty acid profile or omega 6 to omega 3 ratio
Assessment supplement being fit for purpose, or adherence to declaration	Probiotic supplement e.g. live yeast	Total viable count CFU/kg	

DM = dry matter; CP = crude protein; O = oil.

sampling at multiple sites. This enables increased accuracy of a ration assessment that is carried out on a yard. In addition it will provide important information for the horse owner or trainer to help ensure a more consistent intake of forage dry matter. This is essential information during ration evaluation as large differences in the dry matter content of haylage between batches will affect the delivery of energy and nutrients to the horse. Dry matter analysis is also relevant when soaked feeds such as sugar beet are used.

Assessment of grazing consumption

For horses or ponies that spend time at pasture, an assessment of grass intake must be made. This is often problematic and represents a significant area for inaccuracy within the overall ration evaluation, both in terms of energy and macro- and micronutrient intake. However, if the animal is maintaining bodyweight when out at pasture (or being fed conserved forages) this reflects adequate energy intake. In contrast, animals increasing or losing bodyweight in such circumstances may have access to too much or too little pasture or forage, respectively. This may be due to factors such as herbage yield, stocking density, etc. or may reflect a clinical issue. This is of course more significant in animals where grass represents a significant portion of their diet including brood mares, leisure horses or ponies and endurance horses. Voluntary dry matter intake (VDMI) will be influenced by grazing behavior, which can be affected by a number of factors such as quality and quantity of grazing, gender, age, breed, breeding status and also whether the animals are at grass in isolation or with a group. This has been reviewed extensively in Chapters 3 and 18, and also previously (NRC 2007). The effect of forage quality on voluntary intake is not simple in horses and appears to vary between individuals with some increasing and others decreasing their voluntary intake in response to a reduction in forage quality and dry matter digestibility (Edouard et al 2008). The effect of sward height was more straightforward, with horses choosing grass with a higher sward when patches are of an equal quality (Edouard et al 2009), presumably to maximize intake.

Whilst it is recognized that the rate of intake of pasture is commonly affected by body size and mouth morphology in other mammals, the effect in horses and ponies has only recently been reported to conform to this model. Ponies appear to be able to increase their rate of consumption by increasing bite size; however, their overall intake seems to be limited by the maximum achievable processing speed (the time taken to bite and masticate), which is greater in larger horses as it increases with body size (Fleurance et al 2009).

Ultimately, dry matter intake of horses and ponies at grass, which is discussed in greater depth in Chapter 18, can vary widely between individuals and most estimates suggest a range of between 1.6–3.6% of bodyweight (NRC 2007) with lactating mares typically at the higher end of this range for VDMI (2.6–3.1%). Ponies are estimated to have a high VDMI in comparison to horses, which may approach 5% of body weight when stabled and provided with ad-libitum fiber based complete feed. Ponies also appear to have the capability to consume a high proportion of their predicted VDMI in a relatively short period of time when grazing time is restricted (Dugdale et al 2011). It has been reported that ponies are capable of ingesting nearly 50% of their total daily dry matter intake during only 3 hours of grazing (Ince et al 2011).

In young horses (yearlings and 2-year-old Salle Francais breed), intake relative to metabolic bodyweight was 82 g OM/kg $LW^{0.75}$/day and did not vary with age. However, the 2-year-old horses exhibited a reduced foraging time and a higher rate of intake (Pascal et al 2000).

When using ration evaluation software programs, the contribution of grass to total daily dry matter intake can either be indicated manually by the user, or in some instances will be predicted by the software. This is often achieved simply by subtraction of the dry matter contribution of other feeds from a predicted total dry matter intake. Time spent at grass is also sometimes used to predict grass intake by ration evaluation programs, although the derivation of the calculations used for this practice is questionable given the paucity of data in this area.

An estimate or assumption of VDMI of grass must be made and used to assess the contribution of grass to energy, protein and macro- and micronutrient intake. Information regarding the nutrient analysis of grazing is also therefore required. For horses or ponies at grass that exhibit optimal body condition, maintenance requirements for energy and protein can be assumed to be satisfied. However, comparable assumptions cannot be made for broodmares or youngstock.

Grass intake will obviously be affected by factors such as availability, palatability and digestibility of the grazing. This in turn will be affected by the stocking density and also the pasture maintenance program including use of fertilizer, overseeding and the removal of droppings. A common sense approach needs to be taken to adjust the likely VDMI upwards or downwards based on at least the availability of grass and stocking density. For example, overgrazed or drought stricken pasture and/or a high stocking density will severely reduce the VDMI compared to well managed grazing with a low stocking density.

Key Points

- Assessment of grazing intake is problematic but an appreciation of those factors that impact pasture forage consumption is essential
- In practical terms, estimation of the contribution of grazing to total feed intake using assumptions on total dry matter intake is sometimes necessary

Matching intake to requirements

Assessment of energy and micronutrient intake

Once all of the information regarding feed intake and analysis of feeds and forage has been gathered, the task of assessing the ability of the ration to satisfy daily requirements for a particular horse or group of horses begins. Other information such as age, body condition and level of exercise undertaken as well as breeding or growth status must of course also be established. Whilst difficult to quantify, environmental influences on energy requirement should not be ignored (Cymbaluk & Christison 1990).

In harsh weather conditions a regular assessment of bodyweight and/or condition is required, in order to react to any early indication of change in bodyweight through small adjustments to the ration. The assessment of body condition and determination of the level of exercise per day represents a further area for potential inaccuracy. Preferentially such information should be obtained directly by the nutritionist.

Bodyweight and condition

There is a lack of awareness of body condition and also some resistance amongst horse owners to accept that horses or ponies are overweight, leading to inaccuracy of owner assessment (Wyse et al 2008). Body weight can be assessed easily where there is access to a weighbridge, or alternatively an estimation of bodyweight can be made using measurements of heart girth, length, and wither height (Carroll & Huntington 1988). A number of commercially available weigh tapes are also available, which simplifies this process. A good correlation exists between bodyweight calculated using a weight tape in comparison to that measured on a weighbridge (Ellis & and Hollands 1998). However, weigh tapes may be more useful for determining differences in bodyweigh over time for individual animals as their accuracy can be variable. In addition, this method is less useful in pregnant mares, growing horses, very fit as well as extremely thin or fat animals, as discussed in Chapter 22.

Body condition score should also be assessed and there are a number of scoring systems available. A condition score system can involve an overall assessment of the whole body according to an arbitrary scale of, for example, 1–5. Alternatively, condition score of different regions of the body, such as neck, withers, loin, tail head and ribs can be assessed in isolation and a mean condition score calculated accordingly. The latter method may be more robust where horses are not of a standard shape such as broodmares and horses in race training. However, in obese animals that require caloric restriction, changes in body condition may not always be apparent with initial weight loss as shown previously in ponies (Dugdale et al 2010, Henneke et al 1983). Body condition score should not be relied upon in isolation to trigger further caloric restriction and is therefore ideally used in conjunction with actual bodyweight. (Further recommendations can be found in Chapter 28.)

Physiological state of the horse

There are a number of calculation systems that seek to accurately estimate the energy and nutrient requirements of exercising horses and those that are pregnant or lactating including those defined by the NRC and also Institut Scientifique de Recherche Agronomique (INRA), SCAN, and GEH (Coenen 1999).

With respect to exercise, all of these systems for estimation of energy and nutrient requirements require an assessment of the level of daily exercise, which is open to considerable personal interpretation. Horse owners often overestimate the volume and intensity of exercise undertaken by their horses, with the result that energy and nutrient requirement can also be misjudged (Coenen & Vervuert 2001). Assessment of the level of exercise needs to consider both the duration of exercise per day and also the intensity of exercise. The intensity and duration of the exercise will influence where the emphasis should be placed in terms of energy source within the diet.

Breeding animals require special consideration as their energy and nutrient requirements will vary during pregnancy as well as lactation. These represent a very nutritionally demanding life stage. Growing animals should be considered in the context of their breed or type, as differences in rate of growth and potential susceptibility to growth related skeletal problems including developmental orthopedic disease may influence the choice of feed. For breeds where there appears to be a higher prevalence of DOD (see Chapter 32) and slower growing types such as ponies, there may be some benefit from a relatively greater reliance on forage within the ration. In addition, further consideration should be given to the key energy sources within any complementary feeds. Balancer feeds are feeds that are fed at a much lower level than conventional concentrate feeds (typically 100 g/100 kg bodyweight) and which have a high nutrient density and often low starch and sugar content. Such balancer feeds can be fed in isolation with grazing or other forages and therefore may be worth considering in such cases.

In pony and miniature breeds, where the prevalence of obesity and laminitis is increased, careful consideration of grazing management in terms of paddock size, hours at grass and stocking rate should be made. Restriction of grazing may be required to maintain normal body condition and to reduce the risk of laminitis in other animals. This is also true during pregnancy, lactation as well as growth to avoid excess weight gain or growth rate and to ensure adequate provision of quality protein and other macro- and micronutrients through the provision of complementary feeds.

Establishing forage intake and a suitable forage to concentrate ratio

It is well established that forage remains a very important component of the diet for all horses and ponies irrespective of their life stage or level of exercise. Nutritionists agree that forage should always provide the foundation upon which the diet is based. Forage not only contributes to the overall energy and nutrient content of a horses' ration but also helps to maintain digestive health through a physical effect on the movement of food through the gut, retention of fluid within the digestive tract and a protective effect on the microbial balance within the hindgut, especially in horses fed a high starch ration. It is therefore advisable to maintain a minimum level of forage in the diet, which for hay the authors suggest should be 1% of bodyweight per day 'as fed' as an absolute minimum, although for most leisure horses this should be nearer to 1.5% of bodyweight 'as fed' per day. For haylage, where dry matter may range from 60–75%, a higher intake of 1.25% 'as fed' is recommended by the author as being the minimum quantity advised. Whilst the author agrees that in the strictest terms, forage intake should be evaluated on a dry matter basis, this is not always practical due to the absence of analysis of the hay or haylage concerned. The author also agrees that in most circumstances, a higher intake of forage should be encouraged. In leisure horses particularly a diet consisting of almost 100% forage, combined with a low-intake nutrient-dense concentrate feed such as a balancer, can be advised. In addition, a higher intake of forage should also be encouraged in performance horses, on the basis that digestive health and psychological wellbeing can be maintained. In this instance, owners or trainers should be encouraged to use forage with a higher digestibility, in order to increase the contribution made to energy intake and reduce the appearance of "hay belly". However, in reality there is considerable resistance to a high forage intake in some performance sectors such as racing. This is largely due to the potential or perceived reduction in energy intake as well as the disadvantage of increased gut-fill. The author believes that a pragmatic approach is often needed to ensure that at least the minimum advised quantity of forage is fed under these circumstances.

The suitability of the ratio of forage to concentrate in the daily ration should also be assessed. The main determinants for assessing its suitability are likely to be dietary energy requirement, appetite and the relevance of gut fill. Additionally, where it is desirable to limit starch and sugar intake (e.g., due to a specific condition a higher forage to concentrate ratio can be used).

Forage to concentrate ratio is usually high and may be near to 100% in leisure horses and other animals with a relatively low energy requirement. In horses with a high energy requirement (e.g., mares in early lactation, or racehorses where appetite may be limiting), a lower forage to concentrate ratio is usually perceived to be necessary in order to achieve the desired overall daily energy intake. A higher intake of forage relative to concentrate feed is associated with a greater gut fill or weight due to the presence of fiber and associated water in the hindgut. This may be a disadvantage in horses undertaking short periods of fast exercise where speed may be impeded by the extra weight, whereas for long slower exercise such as endurance racing the presence of fiber and associated water in the gut can be a significant advantage (Harris 2009). However, even for racehorses a minimum amount of forage in the diet is essential for health and this is generally regarded to be 1% of bodyweight (DM basis) (Geor 2005) but the author would recommend this practically on an 'as fed' basis as an acceptable minimum whilst encouraging a higher intake. Recently it has been suggested that a higher forage to concentrate ratio can be used in diets for performance diets where a period of forage reduction prior to racing or competition is undertaken (Connysson et al 2010). A lower forage to concentrate ratio can be necessary when forage intake is reduced due to physiological state, for example in last trimester broodmares, where the developing foal occupies a greater space within the abdomen. Equally in old horses with poor dentition intake of traditional sources of forage may be reduced and so alternatives such as chaffs or high-fiber cubes may need to be considered. The forage to concentrate ratio may be reduced in reality where digestibility of forage is low (e.g., in mature forage), or where quality is reduced (e.g., as a result of mold or mycotoxin contamination). Normalization of forage to concentrate ratio in this instance can be re-established by sourcing an improved forage source.

Calculated versus actual energy intake

Given the inherent inaccuracies involved in the calculation of daily energy requirement, dietary history in conjunction with assessment of bodyweight and condition can be invaluable in allowing comparison of the effectiveness of current estimated intakes against predicted energy requirements. Studies have suggested that calculated energy requirements determined using previous NRC recommendations (NRC 1989) were overestimated in growing horses (Lawrence 2009), and the most recent edition has made adjustments accordingly (NRC 2007). Assuming that an individual horse or pony is in energy balance and in appropriate body condition then in practical terms their current feed intake (and the estimated energy provided by their forage and complementary feed), provides a good representation of their actual energy requirement, as it already factors in elements such as age, level of exercise, environmental influences etc.

Sensitivity analysis

Describing the traditional ration evaluation process leads us to conclude that it is subject to significant inherent variation or error, largely as a result of the difficulty in accurately defining energy and nutrient intake as well as requirements. It has been previously suggested that the cumulative error in the estimation of feed intake alone may be 10% in stabled horses, but much higher at 20–40% in animals with access to pasture (Kronfeld 2001). Other potential sources of error include differences in the actual (analysis) vs. estimated (via tables) feed nutrient content as well as individual differences in energy and nutrient requirements due to between-horse variation. Sensitivity analysis has been described and utilized by researchers in an attempt to limit the impact of such variability on nutritional outcome (Kronfeld 2001). The aim of such analysis is to test the robustness of a ration by exploring the effect of using a range in key variables (such as intake and requirements) rather than using simply a mean value. For example, looking at overall dry matter intake in a horse fed a mixed ration of hay, cereals and grass, sensitivity analysis may consider the impact on energy and nutrient intake over a range of dry matter intakes of perhaps 2–3% of bodyweight as opposed to only a single average intake of 2.5% of bodyweight. Whilst carrying out such analysis manually is time consuming, it is feasible that in the future sensitivity analysis could be incorporated as a feature within ration evaluation software to improve the probability of detecting a weakness within a given ration.

Key Points

- Calculation of the energy requirement is problematic due to the many variables involved and inherent variation between individuals
- Current ration, together with bodyweight and condition, is valuable in determining true energy requirement
- Forage intake should always be maximized for a given horse. However, a degree of pragmatism may be required to achieve owner or trainer compliance due to either real or perceived constraints on forage intake by the owner or trainer

Other considerations

Meal size and/or frequency

Meal size and frequency is an area of feeding management that should always be investigated and addressed, as it has a significant impact on digestive physiology (Metayer et al 2004) and health (Bell et al 2007, White 2005). As horses evolved as grazing animals, their digestive system is adapted to an almost constant intake of grazed food material. Meal feeding, wherever possible, should be sympathetic to this aspect of their evolution. During any ration evaluation a note of the frequency of feeding as well as the actual feeding times (both forage and complementary feed) should be made and then assessed. The number of feeds recommended per day will depend on the total feed intake in order to maintain each feed below a maximum meal size, as discussed below. Changes to the feeding times can be suggested, especially when horses are left for prolonged periods without feed or forage, or where feeding times are skewed towards one part of the day. Ideally horses will not be left for more than 2–3 hours without forage or feed, in the context of the likely rate of gastric emptying and passage of feed through the small intestine. When making such suggestions practical issues such as staffing needs to be considered, as well as reference to when, in practical terms, exercise can be undertaken or the effect of impending competition. Where relevant the impact of weekends and also days of racing or competition on feeding times, frequency and meal size should also be assessed.

Meal size (kg) both for the total feed and for the individual ingredients is important information to be recorded and commented upon. Meal size and frequency has an impact on pre-cecal transit time for example (De Fombelle et al 2004) and may therefore affect the digestibility of nutrients that are digested enzymatically in the small intestine. This includes protein, starch and sugars, oil as well as some minerals and vitamins.

It is also important to calculate the starch and simple sugar intake or load (4 g/kg) per meal. The prececal digestion of starch is reported to be compromised when meal size is large, and where starch intake exceeds 0.4% of bodyweight (NRC 2007).

In order to minimize starch overload to the hindgut, meal size should be limited to a level that will maintain starch intake per meal below 2 g/kg BW, although some researchers suggest that should be no more than 1 g/kg BW (Harris et al 2006). As the starch content of feed varies considerably, maximum meal size should always be calculated on a case by case basis (Table 23-2). However, other factors, such as the potential effect of meal size on digestibility, should be taken into consideration when addressing meal size. For complementary feeds recommendations of a maximum meal size of 2–3 kg (for a 500-kg horse) has been advocated previously, however, the validity of this will depend on the starch content of the feed in order to remain below 1 g/kg BW starch per meal.

Within the professional sector practical issues including staffing and horse management have a significant influence on feeding practice. In race training yards in the UK the first meal of the day, which is given shortly before exercise, is traditionally small, typically 1 kg or less, whilst the evening

Table 23-2 Estimated Meal Size to Deliver Starch at 1 g/kg BW or 2 g/kg BW per Meal Using Feeds with Varying Starch Content in a 500 kg Horse

Starch content of feed (%)	Size of meal (excluding chaff)	
	Delivery of 1 g/kg BW	Delivery of 2 g/kg BW
20	2.5 kg	5 kg
30	1.7 kg	3.4 kg
40	1.25 kg	2.5 kg
50	1 kg	2 kg

meal is most often the largest and the lunchtime feed being intermediate. This can also be true in breeding establishments, where a small early feed is desired to enable mares be turned out to grass early in the morning and consequentially the evening feed may be oversized. Owners or trainers should be encouraged to reduce meal size by increasing the number of meals per day, or redistributing feed into the smaller feeds. Where this is not possible for practical reasons a lower starch feed should be considered. The owner or trainer should always be made aware of the potential implication of exceeding the guidance on starch intake in terms of prececal starch digestibility and digestive health.

Whilst the correlation between fecal and cecal pH is not straightforward and depends largely on sampling technique, there is some potential for the use of fecal pH during ration evaluation as an indicator of hindgut acidosis (Santos et al 2009, Williamson et al 2007).

Feed refusals

Horses that repeatedly leave a proportion of their hay or other feeds, especially where body condition is compromised should be evaluated more closely in conjunction with the client's veterinarian in order to investigate more thoroughly any nutritional causes of apparent reduced appetite. Once this has been established appropriate veterinary treatment, or changes in feed management should be applied. Poor dentition (Ralston 2005), gastric ulceration (Bell et al 2007), feed contamination or instability (Raymond et al 2003), as well as ill health, pain or stress can all reduce voluntary feed intake.

In addition, a high intake of complementary/cereal based feed can lead to reduced forage consumption, as horses may self limit their forage intake. This is largely due to the increased palatability of cereal based feeds in comparison to forage. In performance horses, a healthy intake of forage should be established at the start of the training season (1–1.5% of bodyweight 'as fed') but should not be allowed to reduce below the previously discussed minimum of 1% of bodyweight 'as fed'. Performance horses should always be fed to maintain an appropriate level of body condition (4 to 5 out of 9, dependent on exercise discipline) and preconceived ideas of how much a horse that is ready to race should be fed must be avoided.

Feed safety

During a ration and feed management evaluation process, the question of feed safety needs to be addressed. Mite infestation of feed, rancidity and gross molding or yeast contamination of feed or forage can be assessed visually or by smell. Samples of feed and/or forage may be required for laboratory analysis in order to assess this. Aspects to consider include:

- Microbiological cleanliness of feed or forage – molds and yeasts
- Mycotoxin contamination of feed, forage or the stable environment
- Instability including rancidity of oil or high oil feeds or supplements
- Mite infestation of feed or feed bins
- Over supplementation
- Non-nutritive and antinutritive factors.

Molds such as *Aspergillus* sp. and actinomycetes pose a significant risk for respiratory health in horse (Raymond et al 1997, 2000). The microbiological cleanliness of forage should ideally be established prior to purchase, especially in large commercial yards. This can be achieved through analysis of a total mold and yeast count, together with characterization of molds present. However, limited room for storage of forage makes this practically difficult in many instances.

Mycotoxin contamination of feed has been shown in horses, for example, to have the potential to reduce feed intake and result in an increase in the blood concentrations of the liver enzyme gamma glutamyl transferase (Raymond et al 2003, 2005). However, although mycotoxins are reported to adversely affect health in other species, their practical relevance to equine health, with the exception of specific diseases such as aflatoxicosis and "rye grass staggers", has not as yet been fully evaluated and to a certain extent mycotoxins are inherent to our environment. Guidance may need to be given regarding forage and feed storage, including cleanliness of preparation equipment, buckets, scoops, bins and hay barns. Further discussion can be found in Chapters 20 and 25.

When evaluating supplement use as part of the overall ration, risk of over supplementation in particular should be assessed, especially where multiple feeds and supplements have the potential to contain common ingredients. Oversupplementation of micronutrients should be avoided not only because of direct toxicity through the specific micronutrient but also because of potential adverse effects on other nutrients. Oversupply of one nutrient can for example result in undesirable interactions within the gastrointestinal tract so that an excess of one mineral can potentially induce a secondary deficiency in another as a result of decreased absorption; for example, high phosphorus intake may affect calcium absorption (NRC 2007). Particular care also needs to be used when evaluating the use of supplement products containing selenium or fat-soluble vitamins where the maximum tolerable level is relatively low (NRC 2007).

The ration should also be evaluated for the possible presence of non-nutritive or antinutritive factors, which are undesirable and can represent a potential health hazard. Antinutritive factors are compounds found naturally in particular plants and ingredients that have an impact on physiological function. Lectins, trypsin inhibitors and phytoestrogens, which can be found in soybean, cyanogens found in linseed and sorghum, quinolizidine alkaloids found in lupin, glucosinolates found in rapeseed, gossypol found in cottonseed, and saponins found in alfalfa are all examples of antinutritive factors that potentially can have a negative impact on an aspect of animal health (D'Mello 2000). Although many antinutritive factors are destroyed by the heat treatment involved in feed processing, their potential contributory effect on health issues should always be considered during ration evaluation. European feed legislation incorporates measures to limit the presence of undesirable substances such as dioxins, mycotoxins in feed requiring due diligence on the part of feed manufacturers in order to comply.

Prohibited substances

For horses that compete, either under the rules of racing or other jurisdictions such as the FEI, guidance should be given on measures that can be put in place to reduce the risk of exposure to feed contamination with substances considered by these authorities to be prohibited, whether these are naturally occurring or not. Unlike many horse racing authorities, the FEI maintains a definitive list of prohibited substances including feed additives (FEI 2011).

Owners or trainers, for example, should be made aware of the ingredients provided by their whole ration. Particular attention should be drawn to specialized feed supplements containing nutraceutical type additives, especially those that have been implicated in previous doping offenses. Recent examples of such ingredients include chilli pepper (capsaicin), devils claw (harpagosides), and valerian (valerenic acid). Avoidance of products containing these ingredients is obviously prudent unless the manufacturer is able to offer clearly defined withdrawal times for their product prior to competition or racing. In addition, increased familiarity with the measures taken by manufacturers to reduce the risk of contamination of their products with prohibited substances should be encouraged. Particularly owners or trainers should be aware of the potential risk areas for contamination with high risk ingredients and consider using feeds that adhere to industry best practice (see chapter re quality of feeds). This is equally relevant for feed supplements despite the usually low level of intake in comparison to feed. Previous cases have shown that supplements are a major risk as potential sources of contamination, particularly for substances where no threshold exists for their analysis in post race or competition urine samples. The use of communal buckets and stirrers also needs to be highlighted as a potential risk for contamination with medications etc.

In very "competitive establishments" samples of all batches of feeds and supplements should ideally be taken before feeding and appropriately stored for a suitable period, until the window for post race or event sampling by the authorities has passed. Further information concerning the risks associated with prohibited substances in feed and feeding and management measures that can be taken to reduce these risks is available from the BETA website (www.BETA-uk.org).

Consideration of health status

When conducting a ration evaluation, the appropriateness of the current diet should always be appraised in terms of any relevant feed related health issues indicated by the horses' past history. As discussed in other chapters within this book, diet has been implicated in the etiology or management of many clinical conditions including laminitis, certain muscle disorders, gastric ulceration, renal insufficiency and developmental orthopedic issues. Key areas to consider, when providing nutritional advice in these circumstances, over and above meeting the energy and nutrient requirements, include energy source, meal size, antioxidant provision, and non-nutrient additives.

The use of supplements

The use of feed supplements is widespread amongst horse owners and trainers world-wide and the type of supplement fed varies considerably. The author regards a supplement as a complementary feed that contains ingredients of nutritional benefit but that do not contribute to energy intake in any significant way (Table 23-3).

The use of feed supplements within a ration can be quite irrational and lack justification in some instances. However, owners or trainers may be reluctant to stop using particular supplements, even when they have no valid scientific basis, especially where the owner or trainer has experienced a recent good competitive season. Ideally feed supplements, whether for specific nutritional purposes or to help with the maintenance of health, should only be used when there is

Table 23-3 Examples of Supplement Types Commonly Used in Horse Rations

Examples of supplements	Likely ingredients
Broad spectrum vitamin & mineral	Full range of vitamins, macro and micro minerals
Specific micronutrient	Calcium, phosphorus, copper, selenium
Amino acid	Branch chain amino acids (BCAA), lysine, beta alanine
Additional vitamin	Vitamin C or vitamin E
Digestive support	Live yeasts, prebiotic, mycotoxin binders, antacids
Oral joint supplements	Glucosamine and/or derivatives, chondroitin, hyaluronic acid, collagen, rosehip
Immune support	Antioxidants, omega 3 fatty acids, glutamine
Health maintenance	Antioxidants for respiratory function Antigastric–duodenal ulcerogenic ingredients
Ergogenic aids	Dimethyl glycine, creatine, BCAA, Ribose

Inclusion in this table does not infer efficacy nor endorsement for use in feed rations.

good justification for their use in the horse in general, or in a specific individual. For example, a specific vitamin or mineral containing supplement may be used to address a sub-optimal level of a particular micronutrient or vitamin in the basal diet. Alternatively, a nutraceutical containing supplement may be used to help maintain health and optimal function of a particular body system such as the joint or digestive function.

Efficacy of any supplement should ideally be supported by some research in the target species, in this case in the horse. For nutritional supplements that include micronutrients with established requirements, supplementation must be justifiable based on these requirements. NRC nutrient requirements are regarded as being minimal and supplementation may attempt to achieve an optimal intake of certain nutrients based on available additional published work or accepted opinion. For nutraceuticals, some proven benefit or effect on the target physiological system should have been demonstrated as well as overall safety.

Unfortunately a large number of nutraceutical supplements are either not supported by research in horses, or may only have preliminary supporting data. In this context, a pragmatic approach may be required, as in some instances the ingredients may simply not have been investigated sufficiently for beneficial effects to be proven or disproven unequivocally. High quality published research in other species, in the absence of data in horses, can be a sufficient impetus for a nutritionist to support the use of a particular nutraceutical supplement. However, the nutritionist must have considered whether the benefit of a supplement in another species is likely to confer a benefit in the horse, despite any potential variances including absorption from the gut or uptake into target tissue. In addition, the safety of the product in horses must also be considered carefully. The manufacturer may be able provide to get data from formal or informal feeding trials to establish both palatability and safety. In this instance, an owner or trainer should be encouraged to feed the product in such a way that some form of evaluation of its benefits may be made.

Other factors that need to be considered when evaluating the use of a particular feed supplement include:

- Identification of included nutrients from objective data provided on label/package.
- Evaluation of the level and delivery of active ingredients for which information is not provided on the label/package.
- Consideration of any negative effects on palatability.
- Additive or associative effects with respect to the core diet.
- Over supply of micronutrients from multiple sources should be avoided, especially where narrow safety margins exists e.g. selenium.
- Ensure owners/trainers/veterinarians are aware of any possible interactions with drug treatments and any heightened risk from prohibited substance with respect to the rules of racing or competition.

Key Points

- The little research carried out on new and novel ingredients in horses necessitates an informed but pragmatic approach to supplement use by the nutritionist or nutrition expert
- Where nutrition of an individual impinges on health it will be necessary to liaise and collaborate with the owner's or trainer's veterinary surgeon

Ration evaluation software

Once all of the relevant information has been collected during a ration evaluation the suitability of the actual current ration or the proposed future ration must be determined. This will involve comparison against published requirements with respect to energy, protein and micronutrient intake as well as consideration of other aspects such as amount of fiber/sugar and starch provided by the diet. This can, of course, be carried out manually or simply by developing an excel spreadsheet to compare the energy and nutrient intake with published daily requirements. There are also a number of software packages available for this purpose. Ration evaluation software for horses is frequently used by nutritionists, feed advisers, veterinarians and horse owners as well as trainers for this purpose. These programs significantly simplify the ration evaluation process through automation, although great care must be taken in interpretation of their output.

Many of the ration evaluation softwares programs available will use the minimum NRC (1989, 2007) requirements as their basis for evaluating a horses' energy, protein, and micronutrient needs. However, especially within Europe, some also only use those published by INRA, SCAN or GEH. In some instances, there is also the option for the user to modify the requirements for individual micronutrients according to their own knowledge, or research information.

Input data

The input information required by these software programs includes details about the horses and feeds used. A database of feeds including comprehensive nutrient analysis is often provided and updated by the software developer, although the facility for the nutritionist to add their own feed or forage analysis is also usually available. Other details concerning the horse in question such as age, bodyweight, level of exercise, and growth or breeding status of the animals must be provided as well as the weight of individual feeds and forages fed daily. Arbitrary adjustments for likely differences in energy requirements are also incorporated in some instances to account for differences between "metabolic type" (e.g., Thoroughbreds, Warmbloods, and ponies). Other useful features that may be included allow for example the user to alter the ration according to body condition so that the daily energy intake can be adjusted without affecting the required intake of micronutrients or protein. There is also usually a facility for comparison of cost between alternative rations. This can be useful for where feed costs are an important factor in feed management.

Data output

The comparison of a ration against requirements can be viewed in a tabular or graphical format (see Fig. 23.3 and Table 23-4). Graphical presentation, with color-coded keys allows the user to easily appreciate the benefits and

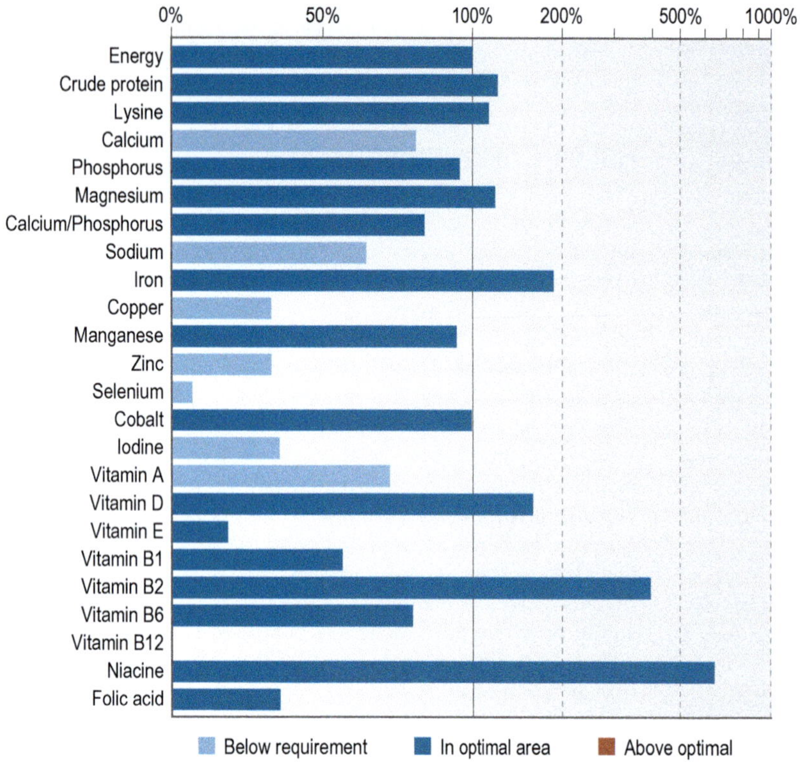

Figure 23.3 Graphical representation of ration and requirements.

limitations of a particular ration. Software functionality also often allows integration with other software programs. Copy and paste functions make their inclusion in reports or visual presentations easy.

Advantages and disadvantages

The main advantage of these software programs is that they simplify the ration evaluation process greatly, by automating the mathematical calculations required. The programs are also a very useful educational tool for students to help them to evaluate horse rations in a practical/applied way. However, it is important especially within a teaching environment that the basis of ration evaluation and derivation of the calculations involved are robustly understood.

The main disadvantage of ration evaluation software is that most products do not attempt to account for the usually imprecise input data and the variability in energy and nutrient requirements between individual animals. Most software packages as described by Kronfeld (2001) use mean values for nutritional requirements, as well as the analytical compositions of ingredients, and the intakes of forages plus feeds to yield a single evaluation. Additionally, there may be a failure by the user to appreciate the limitations of (or caveats around) the output, which is sometimes due to a lack of appreciation of the derivation of the calculations used. Such interpretation is the "added value" a trained, experienced equine nutrition expert brings. Other disadvantages include:

- If a database of nutritional analysis of ingredients, feeds and forage is not provided (and ideally constantly updated) by the software manufacturer, it can be laborious and time consuming to develop and maintain the accuracy of such a database.
- The accuracy and reliability of the output data from ration evaluation software remains very reliant on the integrity of both the horse and feed input data.
- Emphasis can be erroneously placed on the requirements in terms of absolute values, especially for micronutrient requirement, where the reality is often that an optimum range for intake may exist (Kronfeld 2001).
- To date, most programs do not offer an evaluation of energy intake beyond absolute requirement. In other words, no provision is made for the suitability of the source of energy, in terms of the balance between hydrolyzable carbohydrate, fiber and oil, which has great relevance for many individuals in terms of clinical need or performance.
- Software programs do not generally discriminate between the type of exercise, for example between horseracing and endurance racing, which have very different practical requirements.
- The suitability of the diet in terms of "fitness to feed" or the quality of ingredients cannot be determined simply through using a ration evaluation program.

Ration evaluation software can be used successfully to assess the potential suitability of an existing ration in terms of meeting guideline macro- and micronutrient requirements, or can be used to create a new ration in a similar manner. In terms of energy intake the author feels that the horse's current diet, taking into consideration its body condition, can be the best indicator of daily energy requirement. Notwithstanding this ration evaluation software is a very useful tool, especially where used to complement other methods of ration evaluation. This combined or holistic approach to ration evaluation helps ensure that the potential

Table 23-4 Example Horse – Ration 1. This is a Representative "Traditional Diet" Illustrating the Potential for Inadequate Micro Nutrient Intake when Rations are Based on Hay and Cereals without Vitamin and Mineral Fortification

Feeds and allowances in ration		
Meadow hay, average	7.00	kg
Unmolassed sugar beet pulp	0.50	kg
Oats	3.00	kg
Calcium/phosphorus ratio 1.4 Crude protein 9.78 g/MJ Zinc/copper ratio 3.97		

Further information	
Horse type	**Training – Competition**
Body weight	500 kg
Further information	Moderate work (1.50 × maintenance) Roughage allocation acceptable

Provision of nutrients

Nutrients	Unit	Requirements	Intake	Balance	%
Energy	MJ	96.67	97.51	0.83	101
Crude protein	g	767.88	953.50	185.63	124
Lysine	g	33.02	37.50	4.48	114
Calcium*	g	42.00	34.10	−7.90	81
Phosphorus	g	25.20	24.25	−0.95	96
Magnesium	g	14.38	17.45	3.07	121
Sodium*	g	22.19	14.40	−7.79	65
Iron	mg	562.50	1070.00	507.50	190
Copper*	mg	146.25	48.40	−97.85	33
Manganese	mg	562.50	537.00	−25.50	95
Zinc*	mg	585.00	192.00	−393.00	33
Selenium*	mg	1.46	0.10	−1.36	7
Cobalt	mg	0.73	0.73	0.00	100
Iodine*	mg	4.53	1.64	−2.89	36
Vitamin A*	IU	29250.00	21000.00	−8250.00	72
Vitamin D	IU	4290.00	7000.00	2710.00	163
Vitamin E*	mg	1080.00	205.00	−875.00	19
Vitamin B1*	mg	56.25	32.00	−24.25	57
Vitamin B2	mg	22.50	90.00	67.50	400
Vitamin B6	mg	11.25	9.00	−2.25	80
Vitamin B12	mg	0.11	0.00	−0.11	0
Niacin	mg	112.50	745.00	632.50	662
Folic acid	mg	11.25	4.10	−7.15	36

*Requirements are written into the software based on (~125% of NRC).

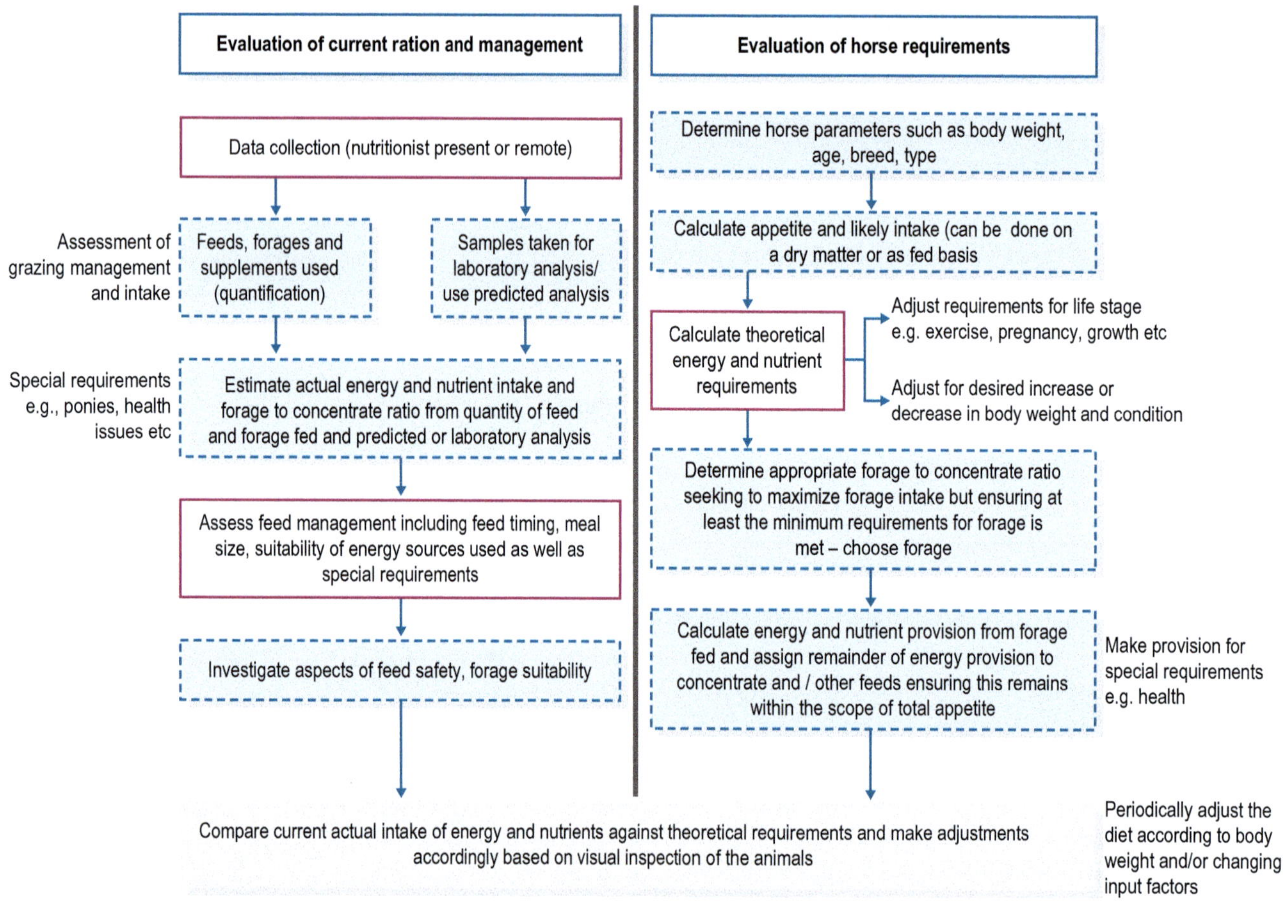

Figure 23.4 Flow diagram of stages during a ration evaluation scheme.

limitations of any software output are taken into consideration.

There is of course more than one strategy to ration evaluation and a number of stages are required to reach an optimal end point (see Fig. 23.4).

> **Key Points**
>
> - Ration evaluation software is a useful tool for the nutrition expert. However, care is required in the interpretation of the output and the limitations of such software should be fully appreciated
> - There may be more than one way to achieve a suitable ration end point for an individual horse or pony that allows flexibility to incorporate practicalities and preferences of the owner, trainer and/or horse

Examples of ration evaluation

Example 1: Recommending a ration (Table 23-5)

Calculate a feed ration for a 500 kg horse, housed in a stable on shavings, exercised at the weekends only (light work). The horse is an 8-year-old Anglo Arab at normal body condition (score 5 out of 9). Grass hay is the forage of choice and has been estimated (through analysis) to have an energy content of 7.5 MJ/kg on an 'as fed' basis. The horse undertakes pleasure riding of low intensity but has a tendency to be excitable. The horse is exercised daily, either through light hacking or on a horse walker, with more work undertaken at the weekends, which may include a low level showjumping or dressage competition.

Example 2: Evaluating current ration (Table 23-6)

A 3-year-old Thoroughbred racehorse in full training (bodyweight 415 kg) is fed with 3 kg of hay (10 MJ/kg) and 7 kg of concentrate feed with high oat inclusion (DE 13 MJ/kg). Three meals are fed per day, the first of 1 kg and then 3 kg and 3 kg respectively. The horse is considered to be in hard work but in moderate to poor body condition but not showing any indication of poor performance. A basic evaluation of this ration is shown in Table 23-6.

Advantages, disadvantages/limitations of various manufacturing processes

Successful ration evaluation requires a thorough understanding of the range of feed type options available in order to build a ration. This in turn requires a good understanding of the various manufacturing processes together with their advantages and limitations.

Traditionally proprietary manufactured feed has been available in pelleted form, or as a coarse mix (sweet feed or muesli) or chaff, but extruded feed has also emerged as an alternative in recent years. Additionally, there are a growing number of fiber-based feeds that combine a traditional

Table 23-5 Example 1: Recommending a Ration

Rationing (predictive method)	
Estimate bodyweight	Weighbridge bodyweight confirms 500 kg
Predict voluntary feed intake (influenced by appetite)	Intake set at 2% of bodyweight 'as fed', although this may vary between individuals = (2/100) × 500 kg = 10 kg feed per day
Calculation of energy requirement	Energy requirement for maintenance (NRC 2007) DE (MCal/day) = 1.4 + (0.03 x BW in kg) = 1.4 + (0.03 × 500) = 16.4 MCal/day To convert to MJ/day × 4.183 = 69 MJ per day. (round to nearest 0.5) Account for exercise factors NRC multiplication factor for light work Maintenance × 1.25 = 20.5 MCal /day = 86 MJ/day
Adjust energy requirements to take account of condition score	No adjustment to be made
Determine appropriate forage to concentrate ratio	Set forage to concentrate ratio at 70:30 70% of appetite = (70/100) × 10 kg = 7 kg of forage 1.4% of bodyweight provided as forage therefore ration meets minimum forage requirements. Assess type and quality of hay and ensure ration evaluation reflects this
Determine proportion of total feed intake for concentrates & choose appropriate feed	= 10 kg – 7 kg = 3 kg
Calculate contribution of forage to total energy intake	= 7 kg × 7.5 = 52.5 MJ/day
Calculate contribution of concentrates to energy contribution by subtraction	= total energy requirement – contribution from forage = 86 – 52.5 MJ = 33.5 MJ
Determine energy level of concentrate feed	Divide energy contribution required from concentrate feed by feed required daily to satisfy appetite =33.5 MJ/3 kg = ~11 MJ/kg Traditional leisure cube for example can be fed
Determine concentrate feed type	Horse is in light work doing low intensity exercise and has a tendency to be excitable – nutritionist recommends a concentrate feed that is low in starch and sugars but high in digestible fiber and oil.
Evaluate nutrient delivery & balance the ration	Input data into ration evaluation software to ensure that the requirement for protein/key amino acids, macro and micro minerals and vitamins is met; calcium to phosphorus balance of the diet is within acceptable limits. Recommend an appropriate supplement to correct any imbalance is fed if required.
ALTERNATIVE Feeding strategies that could provide the same nutrient provision	Whilst this particular horse was stabled all the time, it is not unusual for similar horses to be kept at grass permanently where simply some form of vitamin and mineral supplementation could be provided. Equally the horse may have been fed a near to 100% forage diet whilst stabled with a low intake balancer feed

Table 23-6 Example 2: Evaluating Current Ration

Rationing (assessment method)	
Estimate bodyweight	Weighbridge bodyweight confirms 415 kg
Calculate total feed intake	Hay fed at 3 kg per day Concentrate feed fed at 7 kg per day Total intake = 10 kg per day As a percentage of bodyweight = 2.4% 'as fed' This is acceptable for total feed intake for a horse in full training
Calculation of energy intake	Energy requirement for maintenance (NRC) Forage (DE = 10) fed at 3 kg = 3 kg × 10 MJ = 30 MJ Concentrate feed (DE 13 MJ/kg) fed at 7 kg = 7 kg × 13 MJ = 91 MJ/day Total daily energy intake = 121 MJ/day This compares against a theoretical requirement of 27.8 MCal or 116 MJ/day for horse in hard work – horse's body condition confirms that current feed intake is inadequate to maintain condition, which in the absence of health issues suggests that the energy intake for hard work is applicable. Ration therefore slightly exceeds the energy required for this horse in hard work although condition is described as poor by trainer
Adjust energy requirements to take account of condition score	Horse in suboptimal condition and requires condition may be related to low forage to concentrate ratio and large meal size – adjust and re assess. Collaboration with the trainer's veterinary surgeon is required to rule out any health issue that may be contributing to the horse's poor condition.
Determine current forage to concentrate ratio	Forage to concentrate ratio = 3 kg: 7 kg = 30:70 Forage to concentrate ratio is too low and forage intake only represents 0.7% of bodyweight on an 'as fed' basis and therefore ration does not meet minimum forage requirements to maintain health and digestive function.
Adjustments recommended	Consider sourcing a forage of higher feed value Increase forage intake to at least 1% of bodyweight 'as fed'. A higher forage intake can be suggested but owner or trainer compliance may not be achieved. Adjust concentrate feed intake to improve forage to concentrate ratio Adjust forage to concentrate ratio to 50:50
Calculate contribution of forage to total energy intake	= 5 kg × 10 MJ/kg = 50 MJ/day
Calculate contribution of concentrates to energy contribution by subtraction	= total energy requirement – contribution from forage = 116 – 50 MJ = 66 MJ
Determine energy level of concentrate feed	Divide energy contribution required from concentrate feed by feed required daily to satisfy appetite To maintain a forage to concentrate ratio of at least 50:50 Ration requires 5 kg of forage and 5 kg of concentrate feed to be fed as 3–4 meals depending on starch content of feed (see Table 23-4). = 66 MJ/5 kg = ~13 MJ/kg concentrate
Determine concentrate feed type	Horse is in hard work doing high intensity exercise – nutritionist recommends a concentrate feed that has a moderate to high low starch and sugars content with adequate digestible fiber and some oil. Remainder of energy required (66 MJ) can be satisfied by 5 kg of a 13 MJ/kg Racing Cube.
Evaluate nutrient delivery & balance the ration	Input data into ration evaluation software to ensure that the requirement for protein, macro and micro minerals and vitamins is met and that calcium to phosphorus balance of the diet is within acceptable limits.
Further recommendations	Nutritionist recommends monitoring bodyweight for a period of 1 month following dietary change to ensure body condition score improves (10–20 kg per month). If improvement is not apparent further investigation for loss of condition will be required. Horse can additionally be supplemented with some vegetable based oil 100 ml per day to help improve condition. Additional vitamin E may be required.

coarse mix with chop such as grass, straw, or alfalfa. There are several feed technology processes involved in the preparation of feed ingredients many of which, such as micronizing, steam flaking, and extrusion include a cooking phase. Heat is also a feature in the high temperature drying process that can be used for the preparation of both grass and alfalfa in both pellets as well as chaff format.

Mechanical treatment of cereals

The most basic preparation of cereal ingredients involves mechanical treatment such as grinding, rolling or crimping. This process serves to break the hard outer seed coat or hull of cereal grains thus making them theoretically more accessible to the horse's digestive enzymes. Grinding also significantly increases the surface area for the digestive enzymes and is reputed to have the greatest effect on pre-cecal starch digestibility compared to other mechanical treatments where the effect is limited. The effect of mechanical treatment on oat starch however, is limited due to its naturally high prececal digestibility (Hoffman 2003). One of the main disadvantages of mechanical processing of grain is that once the seed coat is penetrated the stability of the grain is reduced. This leaves it vulnerable to increased oxidation and nutrient breakdown as well as increasing the risk of mold and mycotoxin contamination.

Pelleting

Pelleting was one of the first technologies to be introduced into the horse feed sector. During the process a number of discrete ingredients, which are ground or milled, are mixed and then combined with small amounts of liquid before being pressed through a die to form a pellet, which is then cut to size. In some instances, steam is used during a conditioning phase, which will gelatinize some of the starch present. Gelatinization effectively breaks down the tertiary structure of starch helping to make it more accessible to the horse's digestive enzymes. However, aggressive cooking can result in an increase in the formation of less digestible or retrograde or resistant starch. Starch gelatinization not only improves digestibility, but also helps to bind the materials together. Temperatures reaching 65.5–93.3°C (150–200°F) can be achieved during the pelleting process. Pellets can also be produced where the heating phase is absent. Here, the heat is produced as a result of physically forcing the ingredients through the pelleting die. Pellets that contain a large amount of fiber and a limited level of starch for example are often produced in this way. However, in some instances pellets produced in such a way require the addition of binders such as lignosulfate to help form a good pellet and to maintain its integrity during handling and storage. Pellets where the ingredients have a significant levels of starch (20% or above) should ideally be manufactured with a conditioning phase.

Advantages and disadvantages

One of the main advantages of pellets is that they allow a more uniform feed to be produced and they facilitate the even distribution of additives such as vitamins and minerals or yeast. Additionally, pellets allow the incorporation of high levels of certain milled ingredients such as oatfeed, wheatfeed, soya hulls, linseed meal, soya meal, or dried sugar beet pulp. Whilst some of these ingredients can be byproducts from other industries, this does not detract from their nutritional value and their beneficial properties when producing feeds with diverse energy and functional requirements.

Pellets also generally have a low moisture content (9–15%) and are therefore microbiologically relatively stable with a low dust content. In addition, as they are compacted they are denser than other feeds, which improves storage efficiency and transport costs.

On the practical side pellets are easy to feed and are relatively economical. They are usually palatable and prevent horses from sorting and then leaving certain ingredients, which may happen with mixed feeds. Pellets can also often have a slightly lower starch content than coarse mixes or sweet feeds of a similar specification, due to the nature of the ingredients used. In pellet formulation there is a tendency to use less whole cereal ingredients (e.g., maize and peas) and more milled ingredients, which often have a lower integral starch content. Pellets can also be soaked, which softens them allowing easier intake by geriatric or other horses where dental health severely limits feed intake (Ralston 2007).

Consumption of pellets, however, can be faster compared to other feeds (Argo et al 2002), which in greedy feeders can increase the risk of choke (Ralston 2005) and also may affect transit time through the small intestine affecting digestibility. Pellets can also be perceived by the consumer as being bland and do not offer the same visual appeal as coarse mixes or chop based feeds.

Balancer feeds

So-called "balancer feeds" are a relatively new form of pelleted product that are designed to be fed at a lower intake per day (typically 100–200 g per 100 kg bodyweight). These are generally sold as small pellets, typically 4 mm in diameter, but can also be produced as a coarse mix. They usually have a higher energy density (typically 12–14 MJ/kgDE) and offer a more concentrated source of vitamins and minerals than conventional feeds. They characteristically have a higher inclusion of ingredients such as soya or milk based ingredients that are regarded as providing protein of a higher biological value/quality.

Advantages and disadvantages

The main advantage of balancers is that they can provide the desired intake of vitamins, minerals and quality protein within a relatively small amount of feed. Balancers are particularly suited to animals on a high forage-based diet, such as those whose bodyweight/condition precludes the need for a high concentrate feed intake. Specific balancers to complement a ration of cereal straights such as oats are also available and the formulation may differ in specific aspects such as calcium and phosphorus content.

Micronization and steam flaking

Whilst the ingredients in a pellet are effectively heat processed during the pelleting process, there are other more thorough cooking processes that are now widely used in the feed industry.

Micronization is a method of cooking ingredients using dry heat through infra red rays. Micronization reputedly achieves the gelatinization of starches at a lower temperature and with a reduced cooking time in comparison to other cooking methods. The ingredients pass along moving belts at variable speeds under gas burners, which create the infrared heat. Once cooked, the ingredients are then usually rolled, which serves to increase their surface area. A diverse range of ingredients can be micronized including cereals such as barley, pulses including soya, vegetables (e.g., peas), and oilseeds such as linseed. More recently even sugar beet has been micronized effectively to produce a flaked product that has a reduced requirement for soaking prior to feeding.

Advantages and disadvantages

There is evidence that micronization has a positive effect on prececal starch digestibility but also on the digestion of protein in the small intestine (Rosenfeld & Austbo 2009). The major disadvantage of the micronization process is that it is relatively expensive and so increases the cost of cereals per tonne. It also reduces the stability of cereal and thus potentially increases its vulnerability to mold or mycotoxin contamination. However, the beneficial effects of micronization on starch digestibility of cereals such as barley and maize outweighs any disadvantages and hence it is a very widely used process within the feed industry.

Steam flaking is an alternative method of cooking cereal that as the name suggests uses wet heat during the steaming process. The cereal grain is subjected to steam in a closed steam chest at various pressures and times during which the grain absorbs moisture from the steam. The grain is then passed between pressure rollers to provide thin flakes. Again the cooking process facilitates the gelatinization of starch in a similar way to that of micronization.

Extrusion

Extrusion technology is a relative newcomer to the equine feed industry, although it has been used within the pet and human sector for a long time. The ingredients usually including cereal are ground and then placed into a sealed barrel or conditioner and, exposed to hot steam and pressure, albeit for a brief but intense time. The nature of the ingredients in terms of starch content and the type of extruder (twin or single screw) can influence the extrusion temperature. Typically if using super heated steam then the ground slurry of ingredients would be subjected to temperatures of around 120°C for up to 60 s, although the temp can range between 115–160°C and the time between 20–30 s and 1 min. When the extrusion temperature is too hot there is a greater risk of denaturing proteins.

The aim of the extrusion cooking process is to soften the mixture and break down the tertiary or complex structure of starches present via a gelatinization process. The doughy mixture is then forced through an extruder (essentially a steel tube with a rotating auger or screw), which serves to increase the pressure, in the presence of more water and steam. Finally, the mixture is forced through the narrow end of a die with cone-shaped holes, which allows the mixture to expand as it emerges through the wider end. The kibbles as they are known are formed by the action of rotating knives. The kibbles are then cooled and dried. The extrusion conditions, in terms of temperature, pressure and time can be altered and this has an effect on the degree of expansion, as well as on the nutritional properties of the finished product both in terms of starch gelatinization and also other interactions between nutritional components.

Advantages and disadvantages

Due to the nature of the extrusion process and the physical nature of the final kibble produced, it is very easy to add high levels of ingredients such as oil. This can either be added to the pre cooked mixture but can also be spray dried onto the cooling kibbles. This allows a high oil addition approaching 20%.

The moisture content of extruded kibble is usually very low and so mold formation during storage can be less of an issue. In addition, the kibbles also tend to have low dust content, which is advantageous for respiratory health. Extrusion has a beneficial effect on feed digestibility through the gelatinization of starch (Vervuert et al 2008) and it also has been shown to have a beneficial effect on protein digestibility (Rosenfeld & Austbo 2009).

Extruded feeds are also light and therefore have a reduced energy density, allowing an increase in meal volume for greedy feeders and those that are overweight. It has also been reported that eating time is extended compared to other feeds, although this is not supported in a recent study comparing extruded and pelleted feeds (Mary et al 2008). However, the high temperature involved in the extrusion process has a negative effect on vitamin stability and between 5–40% of some vitamin activity may be lost depending on the temperature and cooking time (Anderson & Sunderland 2002). Manufacturers will usually add an overage or extra vitamins to compensate for the predicted loss during the extrusion process.

Extrusion can also have an adverse effect on starch digestibility when the extrusion conditions are not optimized. This occurs through the formation of increased quantities of retrograde starch, a form of starch that is resistant to digestion prececally (Tran et al 2008). In addition, the formation of Maillard reaction products, which are complexes between free amino acids and reducing sugars, whilst contributing to improved palatability may actually reduce the availability of free amino acids (Tran et al 2008). Extrusion is also a relatively expensive process in comparison to other technology and storage and transport costs can be increased due to the low energy density of the kibbles.

High temperature drying

High temperature drying is a technique used mainly in Europe to dry forages such as alfalfa and grass. The alfalfa or grass is harvested and then wilted for a period of about 12 hours before being flash dried by placing it in a large drum that is exposed to heat ranging from 800–1000°C for a relatively short period of time. The purpose of the drying process is to stabilize the forage by reducing the moisture content from about 75–80% down to about 12–15%. The high-temperature dried material may then be combined with other forages such as straw or hay before being coated with a coating such as molasses to suppress dust and increase palatability. Vegetable oil is also sometimes used as an alternative coating which increases the energy density.

High temperature dried alfalfa or grass are most often marketed in isolation as chaff (short chopped alfalfa, typically with a chop length around 2 cm), which may be used to generally slow down the rate of eating and prevent greedy horses or ponies from bolting their feed. These products are also beneficial in providing bulk for horses and ponies with a reduced energy requirement. In addition, feeding chaff at 20% of meal size, can extend eating time, increase time spent chewing and so presumably the production of saliva when compared to pelleted feeds (Ellis et al 2005).

Advantages and disadvantages

The main advantage of high temperature dried forage is that it reduces the risk of mold contamination due to the fast drying conditions used (compared to forage that is harvested and dried naturally, especially in a very unpredictable European climate). High-temperature drying of forages is reputed to preserve more of the nutrients that are reduced during the traditional field or barn drying process. Certainly, the content of vitamin A, in the form of β-carotene was found to be significantly higher in high temperature dried alfalfa when compared to field dried forage (Hauge & Aitkenhead 1931). This was thought to be due to the rapid denaturing of enzymes involved in the destruction of β-carotene, as well as a rapid reduction in the moisture content.

High temperature drying also retains the green color of forage compared to natural drying, which reflects the overall carotenoid content and is preferable from a consumer perspective.

The high-temperature drying process, again however, is a relatively expensive process but the industry in Europe has enjoyed subsidies under the green crop fodder scheme that provides a financial subsidy based on dry matter produced.

Another potential disadvantage of the high temperature drying process is the nature of the volatile organic compounds omitted during the drying process. Certainly emissions of sulfur based compounds, which are present in the alfalfa stem have been suggested to potentially be an issue for human health (Adapa et al 2007). However the extent of such emissions may depend on drying conditions.

References

Adapa, P.K., Schoenau, G.J., Tabil, L.G., et al., 2007. Customized and value-added high quality alfalfa products: A new concept. Agricultural Engineering International: the CIGR Ejournal 9, 1–28.

Anderson, J.S., Sunderland, R., 2002. Effect of extruder moisture and dryer processing temperature on vitamin C and E and astaxanthin stability. Aquaculture 207, 137–149.

Argo, C.M., Fuller, G.Z., Lockyer, C., et al., 2002. Adaptive changes in appetite, growth and feeding behaviour of pony mares offered ad libitum access to a complete diet in either a pelleted or chaff-based form. Animal Science 74, 517–528.

Bell, R.J.W., Mogg, T.D., Kingston, J.K., 2007. Equine gastric ulcer syndrome in adult horses: A review. New Zealand Veterinary Journal 55, 1–12.

Carroll, C.L., Huntington, P.J., 1988. Body condition scoring and weight estimation of horses. Equine Veterinary Journal 20, 41–45.

Cecilia, E.M., 2009. Long-stemmed vs. cut haylage in bales: Effects on fermentation, aerobic storage stability, equine eating behaviour and characteristics of equine faeces. Animal Feed Science and Technology 152, 307–321.

Coenen, M., 1999. German feeding standards. In: Pagan, J.D., Geor, R.J. (Eds.), Advances in equine nutrition II. Nottingham University Press, Kentucky, USA, pp. 365–378.

Coenen, M., Vervuert, I., 2001. Hinweise zur Rationsberechnung fur Pferde. In: Coenen, M., Vervuert I. (Eds.), Dem Pferd auf's Maul geschaut. ausgewählte Themen zur Futtermittelkunde Band II, Hannover, ISBN 3-00-008728-1, pp. 97–100.

Connysson, M., Essen-Gustavsson, B., Lindberg, J.E., et al., 2010. Effects of feed deprivation on Standardbred horses fed a forage-only diet and a 50:50 forage-oats diet. Equine Veterinary Journal 42, 335–340.

Cymbaluk, N., Christison, G., 1990. Environmental effect on thermoregulation and nutrition of horses. Veterinary Clinics of North America Equine Practice 6 (2), 355–372.

D'Mello, J.P.F., 2000. Antinutritional factors and mycotoxins. In: D'Mello, J.P.F. (Ed.), Farm Animal Metabolism and Nutrition. CAB International, Wallingford, UK.

De Fombelle, A., Veiga, L., Drogoult, C., et al., 2004. Effect of diet composition and feeding pattern on the prececal digestibility of starches from diverse botanical origins measured with the mobile nylon bag technique in horses. Journal of Animal Science 82, 3625–3634.

Dugdale, A., Curtis, G.C., Cripps, P., et al., 2010. Effect of dietary restriction on body condition, composition and welfare of overweight and obese pony mares. Equine Veterinary Journal 42, 600–610.

Dugdale, A., Curtis, G.C., Cripps, P., et al., 2011. Effects of season and body condition on appetite, body mass and body composition in ad libitum fed pony mares. Veterinary Journal 190 (3), 329–337.

Dunnett, M. 2010. The level of harpagosides analysed in samples of raw material by LCMSMS, Ed: Dunnett, C.E, Unpublished.

Edouard, N., Fleurance, G., Martin-Rosset, W., et al., 2008. Voluntary intake and digestibility in horses: effect of forage quality with emphasis on individual variability. Animal 2, 1526–1533.

Edouard, N.G., Fleurance, G.R., Dumont, B., et al., 2009. Does sward height affect feeding patch choice and voluntary intake in horses? Applied Animal Behaviour Science 119 (3), 219–228.

Ellis, J.M., Hollands, T., 1998. Accuracy of different methods of estimating the weight of horses. Vet Rec 143, 335–336.

Ellis, A.D., Thomas, S., Arkell, K., et al., 2005. Adding chopped straw to concentrate feed: The effect of inclusion rate and particle length on intake behaviour of horses. Equine Nutrition Conference, Hannover, Germany. Pferdeheilkunde 31, 35–36.

FEI, 2011. http://www.feicleansport.org/.

Fleurance, G.R., Fritz, H., Duncan, P., et al., 2009. Instantaneous intake rate in horses of different body sizes: Influence of sward biomass and fibrousness. Applied Animal Behaviour Science 117 (1), 84–92.

Geor, R.J., 2005. Nutritional management of the equine athlete. In: Hinchcliff, K.W, Geor, R.J., Kaneps, A.J. (Eds.), Equine exercise physiology. The science of exercise in the athletic horse. Saunders Elsevier, New York, pp. 301–325.

Harris, P., 2009. Feeding management of elite endurance horses. Veterinary Clinics of North America: Equine Practice 25, 137–153.

Harris, P., Bailey, S.R., Elliott, J., et al., 2006. Countermeasures for pasture-associated laminitis in ponies and horses. Journal of Nutrition 136 (7 Suppl.), 2114S–2121S.

Harris, P.A., 1999. Comparison of the digestible energy and net energy systems for the horse. In: Pagan, J.D., Geor, R.J. (Eds.), Advances in Equine Nutrition II. Nottingham University Press, Kentucky, USA, pp. 199–215.

Hauge, S.M., Aitkenhead, W., 1931. The effect of artificial drying upon the vitamin A content of alfalfa. Journal of Biological Chemistry 93, 657–665.

Henneke, D.R., Potter, G.D., Kreider, J.L., et al., 1983. Relationship between condition score, physical measurements and body fat percentage in mares. Equine Veterinary Journal Supplement 15, 371–382.

Hoffman, R.M., 2003. Carbohydrate metabolism in horses. In: Ralston, S.L., Hintz, H.F. (Eds.), Recent Advances in Equine Nutrition. International Veterinary Information Service (www.ivis.org), Ithaca, NY.

Ince, J., Longland, A., Moore-Colyer, M., et al., 2011. Changes in proportion of dry matter intake by ponies with access to pasture and haylage for 3 and 20-hours per day respectively for 3 weeks. Journal of Equine Veterinary Science 31, 230–356.

Kronfeld, D.S., 2001. A practical method for ration evaluation and diet formulation: an introduction to sensitivity analysis. In: Pagan, J.D., Geor, R. (Eds.), Advances in Equine Nutrition II. Nottingham University Press, Nottingham, pp. 1–12.

Lawrence, L.M., 2009. The New NRC: updated requirements for pregnancy and growth. In: Pagan, J.D. (Ed.), Advances in Equine Nutrition IV. Nottingham University Press, Nottingham, pp. 123–132.

MacNaeidhe, F., 1995. Procedures and precautions used in sampling techniques and analysis of trace elements in plant matrices. Science of the Total Environment 176, 25–31.

Mary, E.G., Michael, L.J., Randel, H.R., et al., 2008. The effects of feed form on consumption time and glucose and insulin response to a concentrate meal in equines. Journal of Equine Veterinary Science 28 (5), 289–294.

Metayer, N., Lhote, M., Bahr, A., et al., 2004. Meal size and starch content affect gastric emptying in horses. Equine Veterinary Journal 36, 436–440.

NRC, 1989. Nutrient requirements of horses, 5th revised edition. National Academy Press, Washington DC.

NRC, 2007. Nutrient Requirements of Horses, 6th ed. The National Academies Press, Washington DC.

Oke, S., Aghazadeh-Habashi, A., Weese, J.S., et al., 2006. Evaluation of glucosamine levels in commercial equine oral supplements for joints. Equine Veterinary Journal 38, 93–95.

Pascal, M., Jean-Louis, P., Patrick, D., et al., 2000. Ingestion d'herbe au paturage par le cheval de selle en croissance : effet de l'age des poulains et de la biomasse d'herbe. Annales de Zootechnie 49, 505–515.

Ralston, S.L., 2005. Feeding dentally challenged horses. Clinical Techniques in Equine Practice 4, 117–119.

Ralston, S.L., 2007. Evidence-based equine nutrition. Veterinary Clinics of North America – Equine Practice 23, 365–384.

Raymond, S.L., Curtis, E.F., Winfield, L.M., et al., 1997. A comparison of respirable particles associated with various forage products for horses. Equine Practice 19, 23–26.

Raymond, S.L., Heiskanen, M., Smith, T.K., et al., 2000. An investigation of the concentrations of selected *Fusarium* mycotoxins and the degree of mold contamination of field-dried hay. Journal of Equine Veterinary Science 20, 616–621.

Raymond, S.L., Smith, T.K., Swamy, H.V.L.N., 2003. Effects of feeding a blend of grains naturally contaminated with *Fusarium* mycotoxins on feed intake, serum chemistry, and hematology of horses, and the efficacy of a polymeric glucomannan mycotoxin adsorbent. Journal of Animal Science 81, 2123–2130.

Raymond, S.L., Smith, T.K., Swamy, H.V.L.N., 2005. Effects of feeding a blend of grains naturally contaminated with Fusarium mycotoxins on feed intake, metabolism, and indices of athletic performance of exercised horses. Journal of Animal Science 83, 1267–1273.

Rosenfeld, I., Austbo, D., 2009. Digestion of cereals in the equine gastrointestinal tract measured by the mobile bag technique on caecally cannulated horses. Animal Feed Science and Technology 150 (3), 249–258.

Santos, T., Almeida, F., Godoi, F., et al., 2009. Buffer capacity, pH and faeces consistency in horses submitted to dietetic starch overload. Cienc. Rural 39, 1782–1788.

Tran, Q.D., Hendriks, W.H., van der Poel, A.F.B., 2008. Effects of extrusion processing on nutrients in dry pet food. Journal of the Science of Food and Agriculture 88, 1487–1493.

Van Soest, P.J., Mertens, D.R., Deinum, B., 1978. Pre-harvest factors influencing quality of conserved forage. Journal of Animal Science 47, 712–720.

Vervuert, I., Voigt, K., Hollands, T., et al., 2008. Effects of processing barley on its digestion by horses. Veterinary Record 162, 684–688.

White, N.A., 2005. Prevalence, Demographics, and risk factors for colic prognosis and strategies for prevention. In: AAEP focus meeting on Colic. Quebec, Canada.

Williamson, A., Rogers, C.W., Firth, E.C., 2007. A survey of feeding, management and faecal pH of Thoroughbred racehorses in the North Island of New Zealand. New Zealand Veterinary Journal 55, 337–341.

Wyse, C.A., McNie, K.A., Tannahil, V.J., et al., 2008. Prevalence of obesity in riding horses in Scotland. Veterinary Record 162, 590–591.

24 Assessment of nutritional status from analysis of blood and other tissue samples

Ingrid Vervuert, Ellen Kienzle

In theory, feed analysis and ration calculation is the method of choice to evaluate adequate nutrient intake or to detect nutrient deficiencies or excesses (see Chapter 23). There are, however, certain obstacles in the path of those who want to use this method. Feed analysis may be costly and time consuming and quite often it is difficult or impossible to obtain an accurate nutritional history, which is a condition sine qua non. Owners may just forget or disregard the supplement, which is the culprit in cases of excess, or, in cases of deficiency they may not know that the horse does not eat its supplements. In forensic cases, an inaccurate nutrition history may even be given deliberately. There may be situations where the ration is well known but still additional information on the nutritional status of the horse may be helpful. Also, horse owners and trainers often assume that analysis of a blood sample is a fool proof and highly efficient method for the assessment of a horse's nutritional status, and ask their veterinarian to perform such analyses. A prime example is that in practice any decline in red cell indices is often misinterpreted to be due to an insufficient iron intake. The hematocrit and blood hemoglobin are commonly used to evaluate iron status in horses; however these parameters does not provide information on iron status. In reality, iron deficiency anemia is very rare in horses and most often arises secondary to severe (external) blood loss (Hinchcliff et al 2008).

Sample preparation and handling can be a source of considerable error in the analysis of nutrient status. Hemolysis can confound serum or plasma analyses due to the mixing of red cell contents with the serum/plasma. Hemolysis for example may increase the concentrations of nutrients with high content in red blood cells such as iron and potassium, resulting in composite values sometimes far above the reference range for the serum/plasma alone. For some parameters there may be considerable differences between the values expected in plasma and serum, and for some laboratory methods one or the other is required. Using particular anticoagulants such as EDTA can be an issue for some determinations and therefore it is critical that samples are collected in the appropriate medium for the evaluations required. Vitamins, metabolites and enzymes may not be stable and may require special preparations or very short time lag between sampling and analysis. Some variables may be affected by feeding, fasting and/or physical activity, so the timing of sampling and the condition of the horse before sampling can be an important consideration. It is therefore strongly recommended to seek information on sample preparation and handling before taking action. The home page of professional laboratories usually provides information relevant to sample collection and handling.

Tables 24-1–24-4 provide the authors' summary recommendations on sample types and parameters which may be helpful in assessing nutritional status in horses, specifically protein, macrominerals, trace elements, and vitamins (further discussion on the use of urine, hair, hoof horn, or liver samples for nutrient analysis is presented below). This nonexhaustive list also mentions certain parameters that the authors believe are not very useful, but which are nevertheless analysed quite often. The typical practical situations for the respective nutrient excess or deficiency are described. Important interferences and sources of errors are given, as well as reference ranges. According to different methods of analyses, a certain variation is possible, and it is recommended to check with the chosen laboratory. Comments are also made on the informative value of the selected parameter. The informative value of analytical findings can differ when comparing results from a single animal vs. a number of animals in a herd. Thyroid hormone concentrations, for instance, are not a good indicator of iodine nutrition in a single animal as hormone concentrations can be below reference values for reasons unrelated to iodine intake (Wehr et al 2002). On the other hand, low hormone concentrations in a large number of animals from a single herd may indicate iodine deficiency.

Urine

Blood, plasma and serum values of various nutrients are strictly regulated by various hormones, e.g. blood calcium by parathyroid hormone (Weisrock et al 2011). Significant changes from the reference range will therefore not occur unless there is a severe deficiency or excess, often in association with severe clinical problems. However, changes in blood values especially for some minerals may not always be present even when there are clinical signs indicative of deficiency or excess. For example, plasma or serum calcium concentration can be within the reference range in animals with skeletal disease due to calcium deficiency (McDowell 2003). It is therefore important to use alternative substrates for those nutrients where nutritional status cannot be detected reliably by blood analysis. Analysis

Table 24-1 Factors in Nutritional Assessment of Protein

Nutrient	Feeding situation	Preferred sample type for assessment of nutritional status	Analyte, unit	Reference range[a]	Informative value of selected parameter	Interference factor	Explanatory notes	Key references
Protein	*Excessive protein intake:* Excessive protein intake is frequently observed especially when high amounts of protein-rich feedstuffs such as alfalfa, grass or protein concentrates are included in the diet. Under maintenance conditions an excessive protein intake is usually not critical. In exercising horses performing under hot conditions, excessive protein intake should be avoided.	Plasma	Urea, mmol/l	3–5 mmol/l	In otherwise healthy performance horses, high urea concentrations in the plasma (>8.3 mmol/l) reflect an excessive protein intake. If such concentrations are found please check the ration.	Renal insufficiency may impair urea excretion by the kidneys, resulting in an accumulation of plasma urea. To evaluate renal function in more depth plasma creatinine is frequently used to diagnose and monitor kidney diseases.		Meyer 1983, Graham-Thiers et al 1999, 2005, Meyer & Coenen 2002, Kohn et al 2005, Connysson et al 2006, Hackl et al 2006, Riond et al 2009, Frape 2010, van den Hoven et al, in press
	Deficient protein intake: A severe protein deficiency is a rare situation in the equine feeding practice other than in cases of general malnutrition when encountered in combination with an energy deficiency or in cases of a severe intestinal parasitosis. However, a deficient intake of certain essential amino acids such as lysine in the growing foal or in the lactating mare is a more common feeding situation. In horses with chronic diseases there can be an increased protein turnover resulting in a marginal protein status.		Urea, mmol/l Urea-nitrogen, mmol/l Protein, g/l Albumin, g/l	3–5 mmol/l 3.56–8.5 mmol/l 55–75 g/l 26–37 g/l	In general, a long lasting deficient protein intake causes a fall in the concentration of plasma urea (<2 mmol/l), plasma total protein (<55 g/l) and plasma albumin (<25 g/l). If such concentrations are found please check the ration.	Plasma urea may increase due to mobilization of lean body mass or by an impaired kidney function (false negative results). Total plasma protein increases in combination with a reduced extracellular fluid volume which frequently occurs during heavy exercise through sweating or by an impaired water intake or other conditions of dehydration. The decrease in plasma albumin can be linked to either protein deficiency, a failure of albumin synthesis in liver diseases, albumin losses in renal or gastrointestinal diseases, or in intestinal parasitism.	In cases where a specific essential amino acid deficiency is suspected, changes in plasma concentrations may be used for assessment, however reference ranges have not been validated in the horse.	

[a]Reference ranges: Most labs have specific reference ranges which have to be considered.

Table 24-2 Factors in Nutritional Assessment of Minerals

Nutrient	Feeding situation	Preferred sample type for assessment of nutritional status	Analyte, unit	Reference range[a]	Informative value of selected parameter	Interference factor	Explanatory notes	Key references
Calcium (Ca)	*Excessive Ca intake*: Excessive Ca intake is frequently observed when high amounts of Ca-containing minerals are supplemented in the equine diet, especially in combination with Ca-rich feedstuffs like alfalfa, molassed sugar beet pulp or clover hay. *Deficient Ca intake*: A deficient Ca intake can be observed when grain based diets without any Ca supplementation are fed to horses, especially in lactating mares and growing horses. A combined Ca deficiency and P excess will result in nutritional secondary hyperparathyroidism. Occasionally, oxalate containing plants like *Rumex* species have the potential to bind Ca hereby impairing Ca absorption with the highest severity in lactating mares and growing horses. Additionally, acidifying diets (grain-based diets supplemented with ammonium chloride or sodium chloride) to prevent bladder stones might cause Ca deficiency as Ca elimination is increased via the kidneys.	No suitable substrate available, ration formulation is recommended!	Total plasma or serum Ca, mmol/l Calculation of fractional excretion (FE[b]) by the following formula: Ca urine ÷ Ca plasma or serum × creatinine plasma or serum ÷ creatinine urine, expressed in %. Using plasma Ca without FEp is not valid!	Total Ca: 2.4–3.4 mmol/l FE_{Ca}: 5.3–40 %	The plasma or serum total Ca concentration (2.4–3.4 mmol/l) does not reflect Ca intake as Ca in blood is tightly regulated by certain hormones like calcitonin or parathyroid hormone. Urine is strongly limited by a wide range of Ca elimination by the kidneys even under identical Ca intake, the rapid precipitation of Ca in the urine and diurnal fluctuations of Ca elimination depending on feed intake or other influencing factors like exercise. Analysis of Ca in urine is strongly limited by Ca precipitation. The Ca intake leads to an almost linear intestinal absorption of Ca and in the following, Ca is eliminated predominately by the kidneys. A low FE_{Ca} reflects Ca deficiency and a high FE_{Ca} reflects Ca excess. However, FE_{Ca} is very limited as a wide range of FE_{Ca} is regularly observed.	The acidification (e.g., by hydrochloric acid) of urine to solubilize Ca in urine is essential to avoid Ca precipitation. A high fluctuation of FE is observed during the day depending on feed intake or exercise.	Total plasma or serum Ca consist of ionized Ca^{2+} (~50%), protein-bound Ca (~41%, bound mainly to albumin) and complexed to organic and inorganic acids (~9%, e.g., lactate). For diagnosis of clinical stages like hypocalcemia in colics, ionized Ca^{2+} is the preferred sample type. *Hypercalcemia*: Useful tool to diagnose certain disease stages like chronic renal failure or toxicosis induced by vitamin D misapplication or plant induced calcinosis by *Trisetum flavescens*. *Hypocalcemia*: Can be observed in periparturient mares, in severe cases of colics, and after surgery.	Gray et al 1988, Harris 1988, Bickhardt et al 1996, Lewis 1994, McKenzie et al 2002, McDowell 2003, van Doorn et al 2004, Smith 2009, Toribio et al 2005, 2007, Vervuert et al 2006, Berlin & Aroch 2009, Frape 2010, Weisrock et al 2011

Table 24-2 *Continued*

Nutrient	Feeding situation	Preferred sample type for assessment of nutritional status	Analyte, unit	Reference range[a]	Informative value of selected parameter	Interference factor	Explanatory notes	Key references
Phosphorus (P)	*Excessive P intake*: Excessive P intake is observed when bran is the major component in the diet. A high P intake and a low Ca intake or a P/Ca ratio >3/1 can cause secondary nutritional hyperparathyroidism. *Deficient P intake*: Milk-based diets in suckling foals >2 months are low in P. Late stages of plant growth and an inadequate fertilization management lead to a low P content in pastures and forages.	Plasma, serum Plasma, serum + urine	Calculation of fractional excretion (FE) by the following formula: Inorganic P, mmol/l P urine ÷ P plasma or serum x creatinine plasma or serum ÷ creatinine urine, expressed in %	Inorganic P: 0.7–1.7 mmol/l FE_P: 0.05–4.1 %	P values decrease with increasing age. An excessive P intake is reflected by hyperphosphatemia, a deficient P intake is associated by hypophosphatemia. FE_P reflects an excessive P intake, but a P-deficient diet can induce bone demineralization which may also increase FE_P.		*Hyperphosphatemia*: acute renal failure, cell lysis, rhabdomyolysis, strenuous exercise, vitamin D toxicity or enterocolitis are also linked with hyperphosphatemia. *Hypophosphatemia*: A chronic renal failure may be associated with hypophosphatemia.	
Magnesium (Mg)	*Excessive Mg intake*: Horses have a high tolerance against an excessive Mg intake. Excessive Mg intake is frequently observed in rations (2–3-fold above requirement) through the addition of Mg-containing supplements or by adding Mg sulfate as a laxative into the diet to treat intestinal impaction. *Deficient Mg intake*: Mg deficiency may occasionally occur on intensively fertilized pasures in lactating mares and in horses during stress.	Plasma, serum Plasma, serum + urine	Calculation of fractional excretion (FE) by the following formula: Total Mg, mmol/l Mg urine ÷ Mg plasma or serum x creatinine plasma or serum ÷ creatinine urine, expressed in %	Total Mg: 0.5–1.2 mmol/l FE_{Mg}: 14–21%	Mg values decrease with increasing age. Plasma/serum values and FE_{Mg} are good indicators to assess Mg intake. A high or low plasma/serum Mg value or FE_{Mg} reflect Mg excess or Mg deficiency, respectively.		Total plasma or serum Mg consists of ionized Mg^{2+}, protein-bound Mg (bound mainly to albumin) and complexed to organic and inorganic acids (e.g., lactate). For diagnosis of clinical stages like hypomagnesemia in endotoxemia, ionized Mg^{2+} is the preferred sample type. *Hypomagnesemia*: Gastrointestinal diseases like colic or diarrhea are also linked with hypomagnesemia.	

Sodium (Na)	Excessive Na intake: Horses can tolerate a high salt intake (NaCl, e.g. by salt brine or salt supplements) providing they have adequate water available. *Deficient Na intake*: Forages and grains contain relatively low amounts of Na, resulting in a deficient Na intake, especially in exercising horses (sweat losses) unless Na is added by salt supplements.	Plasma, serum Plasma, serum + urine	Na, mmol/l Calculation of fractional excretion (FE) by the following formula: Na urine ÷ Na plasma or serum × creatinine plasma or serum ÷ creatinine urine, expressed in %	Na: 132–146 mmol/l Fe_{Na}: 0.04–0.52%	Serum or plasma Na values are only suitable to detect Na toxicity. FE_{Na} is a suitable parameter to assess Na deficiency.		*Hypernatremia*: Water deprivation and excessive use of mineralcorticoids or Cushing's disease will cause hypernatremia. Salt poisoning occurs in combination with water restriction. *Hyponatremia*: Several diseases like diarrhea, ascites, ruptured bladder, renal failure, or gut torsion may result in hyponatremia.	
Chloride (Cl)	*Excessive Cl intake*: See Na intake *Deficient Cl intake*: Roughage and grain based diets in exercising horses with intensive sweat losses result in Cl deficiency unless salt (NaCl) is added to the diet.	Plasma, serum Plasma, serum + urine	Cl, mmol/l Calculation of fractional excretion (FE) by the following formula: Cl urine ÷ Cl plasma or serum x creatinine plasma or serum ÷ creatinine urine, expressed in %	Cl: 99–109 mmol/l	Serum or plasma Cl values are only suitable to detect Cl toxicity. FE_{Cl} is a suitable parameter to assess Cl deficiency.		*Hyperchloremia*: Water deprivation will cause hyperchloremia. Salt poisoning occurs in combination with water restriction. *Hypochloremia*: Several diseases like diarrhea, ascites, ruptured bladder, renal failure, or gut torsion may result in hypochloremia.	

Table 24-2 *Continued*

Nutrient	Feeding situation	Preferred sample type for assessment of nutritional status	Analyte, unit	Reference range[a]	Informative value of selected parameter	Interference factor	Explanatory notes	Key references
Potas sium (K)	*Excessive K intake*: High K intake is frequently observed as forages are rich in K, especially after K fertilization. Horses have a high tolerance against high K intake. *Deficient K intake*: Severe sweat losses without K supplementation may occur in exercising horses fed grain based diets.	Plasma, serum	K, mmol/l	2.8–4.8 mmol/l	Serum or plasma K are suitable parameters to assess K intake.	Hemolysis and prolonged storage of whole blood (> 6 hours) without separation of plasma or serum will falsify results.	*Hyperkalemia*: Hyperkalemia induced by a high K intake (e.g., forages) is unlikely. A transient increase in plasma/serum K is observed during strenuous exercise. Several diseases like acute renal failure or muscle disorders will cause hyperkalemia. *Hypokalemia*: Marginal K intake or excessive sweat losses cause low K concentrations in plasma or serum. A transient decrease in plasma/serum K is observed after strenuous exercise and during intensive chewing and ingestion of forages. Several diseases like anorexia, diarrhea, gut torsion or peritonitis may result in hypokalemia.	

[a]Referance ranges: Most labs have specific reference ranges which have to be considered.
[b]FE: Fractional excretion describes the percentage of the respective filtered electrolyte by the kidneys (e.g., Ca, P, Na) which is excreted in the urine. Recommendation for urine sampling: Constant diet for at least 14 days; use freely voided urine sample, preferential 8 h after feed withheld and pre-exercise. Urine creatine >9 mmol/l and urine pH > 7. A standardized protocol according to Harris (1988) is recommended for scientific purposes.

Table 24-3 Nutritional Assessment of Metal Ions

Nutrient	Feeding situation	Preferred sample type for assessment of nutritional status	Analyte, unit	Reference range[a]	Informative value of selected parameter	Interference factor	Explanatory notes	Key references
Copper (Cu)	*Excessive Cu intake*: Excessive Cu intake is frequently observed when high amounts of Cu-containing minerals are supplemented in the equine diet. Environmental pollution (e.g., fertilization with swine manure) may cause high Cu concentrations in forages. Horses are quite resistant to an excessive Cu intake. *Deficient Cu intake*: A deficient Cu intake may occur feeding exclusively plants with a very low Cu concentration. A very high Ca or Zn intake may interfere with Cu absorption (see Chapter 32).	Plasma Hair Liver	Cu, µmol/l Cu, mg/kg dry matter (DM) Cu, mg/kg DM	19–21 µmol/l 4–10 mg/kg DM 10–100 mg/kg DM	*Plasma*: Plasma Cu is not a very sensitive parameter as plasma Cu may remain within reference ranges despite excessive Cu intake. Very low or very high plasma Cu concentrations may occur for various reasons other than dietary Cu intake (e.g. injury, inflammation). Higher plasma Cu values are observed in pregnant mares and stallions. Furthermore, breed related differences are observed. *Hair*: Higher Cu concentrations in hair are observed in draft horses. High Cu concentrations in hair may reflect long term Cu excess, low Cu concentrations may assess long term Cu deficiency. *Liver*: Newborn foals have higher liver Cu concentrations as Cu is transferred to the fetal liver in dependency of the dam's Cu intake. High Cu concentrations may reflect a high Cu intake a long time before Cu analysis. High Cu concentrations are observed in different liver diseases in horses with normal Cu intake.	*Serum*: Serum values are lower than plasma values. *Plasma*: Hemolysis will falsify the results. *Hair*: Contamination of hair will falsify the results. Mane and tail may have different Cu concentrations than other hair sources. Cu concentration in hair is not influenced by natural hair color.		Grace et al 1999, Gee et al 2000, Vervuert et al 2000, Casteel 2001, Hyyppä et al 2002, Wehr et al 2002, Wichert et al 2002a, b, McDowell 2003, van Weeren et al 2003, Vervuert 2008, Frape 2010

Table 24-3 *Continued*

Nutrient	Feeding situation	Preferred sample type for assessment of nutritional status	Analyte, unit	Reference range[a]	Informative value of selected parameter	Interference factor	Explanatory notes	Key references
Zinc (Zn)	*Excessive Zn intake*: Excessive Zn intake is frequently observed when high amounts of Zn-containing minerals are supplemented in the equine diet. Zinc toxicosis has been reported by airborne pollution from Zn processing industries or by mixing errors in commercial compound feeds. *Deficient Zn intake*: A deficient Zn intake may occur feeding exclusively feeds with a very low Zn concentration. A very high Ca intake may interfere with Zn absorption.	Plasma Hair	Zn, µmol/l Zn, mg/kg DM	15–29 µmol/L 70–500 mg/kg DM	*Plasma*: Plasma Zn is not a very sensitive parameter as plasma Zn may remain within the reference ranges despite a moderate excessive Zn intake. Very low plasma Zn concentrations may occur for various reasons despite dietary Zn intake (e.g., chronic inflammation or uremia). In the first weeks of Zn supplementation, frequently a drop in plasma Zn is observed. *Hair*: High or low Zn concentrations in hair may reflect long term Zn excess or Zn deficiency, respectively.	Zn contamination of blood sampling tubes. Zn contamination of hair sample (e.g., by Zn ointment).		

Selenium (Se)	*Excessive Se intake*: Excessive Se intake is frequently related to an uncritical handling with Se-containing supplements. Occasionally, mixing errors result in Se acute Se intoxication. In North America, the intake of Se-accumulator plants like *Astragalus* species may result in excessive Se intake. *Deficient Se intake*: A deficient Se status is observed in newborn or suckling foals (white muscle disease) due to a low Se intake by forages and grain based diets without Se supplementation of the dam.	Mine hairlinea Plasm Guard hair Heparinized whole plasma	Se, mg/kg DM Se, mg/kg DM Se, µmol/l GPx activity, U/g Hb (GPx = Glutathione peroxidase, Hb = hemoglobin)	Adult horses: 0.5–2.5 µmol/l Foals: 0.6–1.2 µmol/l Mane hairline: <0.3 mg/kg DM Guard hair: <0.7 mg/kg DM Whole blood GPx: 30–150 (200) U/g Hb	*Plasma*: Plasma Se reflects the extremes of Se intake, the plasma Se responds very quickly to the removal of Se sources, herby declining to normal Se ranges. *Hair*: Se in hair is a sensitive indicator to assess Se poisoning. *Whole blood GPx*: Reflects long-term Se intake as Se-containing GPx is incorporated in the red cells during erythropoiesis.	Whole blood GPx: Susceptible to adverse effects of transportation as hemolysis may occur.	Plasma Se levels reach a plateau >3.7 µmol/l. Whole blood GPx: GPx is a Se-containing enzyme. Same labs transform GPx activities into Se concentrations which is not reliable.	
Manganese (Mn)	*Excessive Mn intake*: Horses have a high tolerance against excessive Mn intake. *Deficient Mn intake*: Mn deficiency has not been reported in horses.	Plasma, serum	Mn, µmol/l	0.3–0.9 µmol/l	Avoid Mn contamination of blood sampling tubes.	Reference ranges are based on a very limited data pool. Information about reliability are lacking in the horse.	There is a lack of knowledge about Mn metabolism in horses.	

Table 24-3 *Continued*

Nutrient	Feeding situation	Preferred sample type for assessment of nutritional status	Analyte, unit	Reference range[a]	Informative value of selected parameter	Interference factor	Explanatory notes	Key references
Iron (Fe)	*Excessive Fe intake*: Excessive Fe intake occurs usually iatrogenically (e.g., parenteral application of Fe-containing drugs). Excessive Fe intake is observed when high amounts of Fe-containing minerals are supplemented in the equine diet. Foals in particular are very sensitive to an Fe overload. *Deficient Fe intake*: A deficient Fe intake is unlikely in adult horses. Only severe blood losses may induce a Fe deficiency in adult horses. A deficient Fe intake may occur in foals without access to soil contaminated forages in milk-based diets (milk is low in Fe).	Serum	Ferritin, µg/l Iron, µmol/l Total iron binding capacity, mg/l Transferrin saturation index, %	Adult horses: 70–300 µg/l Foals (2–6 weeks old): 50–100 µg/l 14–25 µmol/l 230–470 mg/l 25–45%	Serum ferritin: This parameter is not very sensitive to assess an excessive Fe intake. But low ferritin values may indicate a low Fe intake or low iron stores. Serum Fe: The serum Fe concentration is not suitable to estimate Fe intake.	*Serum ferritin*: Species specific assays are recommended. Serum needs to be refrigerated or frozen for transportation. *Serum Fe*: Hemolysis will falsify the results.	The use of all four parameters in combination with clinical conditions (e.g., exclusion of liver diseases) improves diagnostic assessment of Fe status. High ferritin concentrations may occur due to inflammation (acute phase protein), liver diseases or various infections and exercise. High serum Fe values are observed in patients with liver diseases regardless of the level of Fe intake.	

Iodine (I)	*Excessive I intake*: Excessive I intake is related to an uncritical handling with I-containing supplements and excessive algae/ seaweed intake. *Deficient I intake*: A deficient I intake is observed due to a low I intake by forages and grain based diets in I deficient areas.	Serum Urine	I, μmol/l Total T3 (total triiodothyronine), nmol/l Total T4 (total iodothyronine = thyroxine), nmol/l Free T3, pmol/l Free T4, pmol/l I, μmol/l I: creatinine, μmol/g	0.6–0.85 μmol/l 0.3–2 nmol/l 3–56 nmol/l 4.6–5.4 pmol/l 0.6–1.9 pmol/l 0.16–11.8 μmol/l 0.09–23.6 μmol/g	Serum I: This parameter is not recommended to assess I status. Serum I values are higher in newborn foals. Serum total T3 and T4, free T3 and free T4: These parameter are not very sensitive to assess I intake. Lower values are observed in adult horses. Low values may occur in I excess and I deficiency. *Urine I or ratio urine I:creatinine*: Very sensitive parameter of I intake.	Iodine content is difficult to analyze in organic material. Analysis of specific weight of the urine is necessary to exclude errors resulted by an extreme urine dilution or extreme urine concentration.	Hypothyroidism may occur regardless of the level of I intake.	
Cobalt (Co)	*Excessive Co intake*: Horses have a high tolerance against excessive Co intake. Deficient Co intake: A Co deficiency has not been reported in horses.	Plasma, serum Serum	Co, μmol/l Vitamin B12, pmol/l	0.32–1.21 μmol/l 517–1314 pmol/l	There is no information about the value of serum/plasma Co or vitamin B12 analysis.		Co is an integral part of vitamin B12. The hindgut microflora use Co to synthesize vitamin B12, other functions of Co are unknown.	

[a]Reference ranges: Most labs have specific reference ranges which have to be considered.

Table 24-4 Nutritional Assessment of Vitamins

Nutrient	Feeding situation	Preferred sample type for assessment of nutritional status	Analyte, unit	Reference range[a]	Informative value of selected parameter	Interference factor	Explanatory notes	Key references
Vitamin A	*Excessive vitamin A intake*: Excessive vitamin A intake is frequently observed in rations by vitamin A-containing supplements. Deficient Vitamin A intake: The intake of overstored forages is associated with a deficient vitamin A intake. Long-term storage of forages can lead to an extensive destruction of provitamin A carotenoids, mainly β-carotene. Under average storage conditions there is a decrease in provitamin A carotenoids about 6–7% per month.	Plasma, serum Liver	Retinol, μmol/l Retinyl ester % of total retinol Retinyl ester (e.g. retinyl palmitate), mg/kg DM	0.5–1.1 μmol/l <50% 100–500 mg/kg DM Adult horses in the upper range.	Relative sensitive indicators of long term deficient Vitamin A intake. Excessive Vitamin A intake: Plasma/serum Vitamin A levels tend to be maintained until liver exceed the capacity for storage.		See β-carotene	Sklan & Donoghue 1982, Mäenpää et al 1988, Jeroch et al 1993, Greiwe-Crandell et al 1997, Peltier et al 1997, Breidenbach et al 1998, Schweigert & Gottwald 1999, Kienzle et al 2003, Harmeyer & Schlumbohm 2004, Combs 2008, Frape 2010

β-carotene	*Excessive β-carotene intake*: Horses have a high tolerance against excessive β-carotene intake. *Deficient β-carotene intake*: see vitamin A deficiency	Serum	β-carotene, μmol/l	>0.2 μmol/l Horses on pasture have values in the upper range. Around parturition serum β-carotene levels tend to increase in the mare.	Relative sensitive indicator of β-carotene intake.		β-carotene content in the roughage may be adequate to maintain vitamin A requirements in adult horses. β-carotene content may not be sufficient to maintain β-carotene functions independent of vitamin A-like ovarian activity, improved conception rates or reduction in embryonic mortality. The degree of the green color in forages is a reliable indicator of its carotene content. β-carotene content in grass Before spike: 250–500 mg/kg DM After blossom: 50 mg/kg DM β-carotene losses during harvesting: Drying process on the ground: up to 70% losses β-carotene losses during storage 4–6 months: up to 60 % losses Bleached hay: complete β-carotene losses	

Table 24-4 *Continued*

Nutrient	Feeding situation	Preferred sample type for assessment of nutritional status	Analyte, unit	Reference range[a]	Informative value of selected parameter	Interference factor	Explanatory notes	Key references
Vitamin D	*Excessive vitamin D intake*: Excessive vitamin D intake is frequently observed by the uncritical handling with vitamin D-containing supplements. Occasionally the intake of toxic plants causes vitamin D intoxication. In general, horses have a low tolerance to high vitamin D intake. *Deficient vitamin D intake*: Horses are relatively independent of exogenous vitamin D intake as long as they have access to sunlight (formation of vitamin D by the action of ultraviolet light in the skin).	Plasma, serum	Calcidiol, nmol/l Calcitriol, pmol/l Ca, P (only for excess)	<10 nmol/l 20–40 pmol/l See above	Plasma calcidiol: Relative sensitive indicator to asses vitamin D intake. Plasma calcitriol: Plasma calcitriol is not suitable to assess vitamin D intake. Vitamin D excess may cause hypercalcemia and/or hyperphosphatemia, useful as a first check method, interference see Ca and P		Vitamin D intoxication may result from the intake of toxic plants (plant-induced calcinosis, see also Ca) like *Trisetum flavescens*, *Solanum malacoxylon* or parenteral application of vitamin D. Vitamin D intoxication leads to a cumulative storage of Ca in tissues like kidneys, liver, lungs, aorta and heart. Vitamin D nomenclature: Vitamin D2 = ergocalciferol Vitamin D3 = cholecalciferol 25-OH-D3 (25-hydroxyvitamin D3 = calcidiol); 1,25-(OH)2-D3 (1,25 dihydroxyvitamin D3 = calcitriol).	

Vitamin E	*Excessive vitamin E intake*: Horses have a high tolerance against excessive vitamin E intake. For example, the vitamin E intake on pasture may vary in the range of 10–12 mg/kg BW (recommendation: 1–2 mg/kg BW). *Deficient Vitamin E intake*: The intake of overstored forages is associated with a deficient Vitamin E intake. Vitamin E deficiency is frequently associated with Se deficiency especially in newborn foals.	Plasma	α-tocopherol, mg/l	1.0–3.0 mg/l	Plasma vitamin E is a sensitive indicator of vitamin E intake.			

Table 24-4 *Continued*

Nutrient	Feeding situation	Preferred sample type for assessment of nutritional status	Analyte, unit	Reference range[a]	Informative value of selected parameter	Interference factor	Explanatory notes	Key references
Vitamin B1 (thiamin)	*Excessive vitamin B1 intake*: Horses have a high tolerance against excessive vitamin B1 intake. *Deficient vitamin B1 intake*: Feed processing and long-term storage can lead to an extensive destruction of thiamin in grains or forages, intake of thiaminase containing plants (e.g., horsetail (*Equisetum* spp.), bracken fern (*Pteridium aquilinum*), sensitive fern (*Onoclea senibilis*)).	Heparinized or EDTA whole blood h Erythrocytes	Thiamin, nmol/l Transketolase, %	8.0–11.8 nmol/l Foals have values in the lower range <16 (20)%	Whole blood thiamin: Description of actual intake, not reliable to describe tissues stores. Erythrocyte transketolase: Very sensitive indicator detecting thiamin deficiency, but the reference ranges are adapted from humans, data for horses are not established yet.		Erythrocyte transketolase activity: Any enhancement in enzyme activity resulting from the added thiamin. A stimulation of >16% has been taken as a thiamin deficiency, e.g., by intake of thiaminase containing plants, disturbances in the intestinal microflora, loss of appetite or intestinal parasitism.	

[a]Reference ranges: Most labs have specific reference ranges which have to be considered.
Other water-soluble B-vitamins: In general, biosynthesis of the gut flora is adequate to meet requirements. A low forage intake, diarrhea or antimicrobial treatment may impact synthesis.

of urine is a good alternative for most of the major macrominerals provided the sample is not extremely diluted or concentrated (see Tables 24-1–24-4). This can be excluded through concurrent measurement of the specific gravity and creatinine concentration. However, parameters in urine, even if they are related to specific gravity or creatinine, may still vary to a large extent. Furthermore, postprandial and post exercise fluctuations have to be considered. The calculation of the fractional excretion (FE) for electrolytes such as Ca, P, or Na is the author's recommended method to assess their status. FE values describe the percentage of the respective filtered electrolyte by the kidneys (e.g. Ca, P, or Na) that is excreted in the urine (Smith 2009). In order to perform the FE calculation, measurement of urine and plasma concentrations of the respective electrolyte and creatinine is required (see Tables 24-1–24-4).

Hair

The authors consider that hair is a reliable tool to assess the extremes of Cu and Se status and to some extent Zn intake (Lowe et al 2009, McDowell 2003). Nutrient composition of hair (Cu, Zn, Se) reflects long term dietary supply but the validity and interpretation of results can be confounded by environmental contamination. Hair (tail, mane, and/or body hair) may have been treated with products containing trace elements, with consequent alteration in the apparent mineral composition of the sample. Zn ointment used shortly before a hair sample is taken for example might result in a hair Zn content which is unrelated to zinc intake. The authors therefore recommend that for other major minerals or trace elements horse hair analysis is not a reliable tool to assess nutrient intake.

Hoof horn

Hoof horn has been suggested to be valuable in the assessment of trace element status. Sample contamination, however, can be a serious confounder. The hooves are in direct contact with the ground (including feces and urine) and/or with shoes made of various metallic alloys. They also may have been treated with various chemicals such as copper sulfate or formalin. For obvious reasons, in a live horse samples of hoof horn should only be obtained from the most distal parts of the hoof. This, however, means that any results will reflect the nutrient intake of the period in which this horn was growing (i.e., 6 to 12 months before sampling). In addition, the location (wall, sole, toe, heel) and the sampling procedure (metal tools, contamination) can affect values. It goes without saying that horn shavings from hoof trimming with a rasp are absolutely unsuitable for analysis.

Liver

The liver is involved in the storage and metabolism of many micronutrients and therefore the informative value of liver samples can be quite high. The collection of biopsy samples, however, is not without potential risk and is rarely a good choice in the live animal because of the high risk to benefit ratio. In addition, it should be recognized that only a very small quantity of tissue from a very restricted area of the liver will be available for analysis; such a sample may not be representative of the liver as a whole. On the other hand, analysis of liver samples obtained at post mortem is highly recommended. Although preserving a liver sample in formalin is an excellent method for preservation for future histological examinations it is not suitable for micronutrient analysis. For nutrient analysis, in most cases the liver samples should simply be frozen at –20°C until analysis can be undertaken.

References

Berlin, D., Aroch, I., 2009. Concentrations of ionized and total magnesium and calcium in healthy horses: effects of age, pregnancy, lactation, pH and sample type. Veterinary Journal 181 (3), 305–311.

Breidenbach, A., Schlumbohm, C., Harmeyer, J., 1998. Peculiarities of vitamin D and of the calcium and phosphate homeostatic system in horses. Veterinary Research 29 (2), 173–186.

Bickhardt, K., Deegen, E., Espelage, W., 1996. Kidney function tests in horses – methods and reference values in healthy animals. Deutsche Tierärztliche Wochenschrift 103 (4), 117–122.

Casteel, S.W., 2001. Metal toxicosis in horses. Veterinary Clinics North American Equine Practice 17 (3), 517–527.

Combs, G.F., 2008. The vitamins. Fundamental Aspects in Nutrition and Health, third ed. Elsevier, USA, pp. 95–180.

Connysson, M., Muhonen, S., Lindberg, J.E., et al., 2006. Effects on exercise response, fluid and acid-base balance of protein intake from forage-only diets in standardbred horses. Equine Veterinary Journal 36 (Suppl.), 648–653.

Frape, D., 2010. Equine Nutrition and feeding, fourth ed. Wiley-Blackwell, Oxford, pp. 37–89.

Gee, E.K., Grace, N.D., Firth, E.C., et al., 2000. Changes in liver copper concentration of thoroughbred foals from birth to 160 days of age and the effect of prenatal copper supplementation of their dams. Australian Veterinary Journal 78 (5), 347–353.

Grace, N.D., Pearce, S.G., Firth, E.C., et al., 1999. Concentrations of macro- and micro-elements in the milk of pasture-fed thoroughbred mares. Australian Veterinary Journal 77 (3), 177–180.

Graham-Thiers, P.M., Kronfeld, D.S., Kline, K.A., 1999. Dietary protein influences acid-base responses to repeated sprints. Equine Veterinary Journal 30 (Suppl.), 463–467.

Graham-Thiers, P.M., Kronfeld, D.S., 2005. Amino acid supplementation improves muscle mass in aged and young horses. Journal Animal Science 83 (12), 2783–2788.

Gray, J., Harris, P.A., Snow, D.H., 1988. Preliminary investigations into the calcium, magnesium status of the horse. In: Blackmore, D.J. (Ed.), Animal Clinical Biochemistry. Cambridge University Press, Cambridge, pp. 307–317.

Greiwe-Crandell, K.M., Kronfeld, D.S., Gay, L.S., et al., 1997. Vitamin A repletion in thoroughbred mares with retinyl palmitate or beta-carotene. Journal of Animal Science 75 (10), 2684–2690.

Hackl, S., van den Hoven, R., Zickl, M., et al., 2006. Individual differences and repeatability of post-prandial changes of plasma-free amino acids in young horses. Journal Veterinary Medicine Series A Physiology Pathology Clinical Medicine 53 (9), 439–444.

Harmeyer, J., Schlumbohm, C., 2004. Effects of pharmacological doses of Vitamin D3 on mineral balance and profiles of plasma Vitamin D3 metabolites in horses. Journal Steroid Biochemistry Molecular Biology 89–90 (1–5), 595–600.

Harris, P.A., 1988. Collection of urine. Equine Veterinary Journal 20, 86–88.

Hinchcliff, K.W., Geor, R.J., Kaneps, A.J., 2008. Equine Exercise Physiology. Saunders Elsevier, Philadelphia, p. 307.

Hyyppä, S., Höyhtyä, M., Nevalainen, M., et al., 2002. Effect of exercise on plasma ferritin concentrations: implications for the measurement of iron status. Equine Veterinary Journal 34 (Suppl.), 186–190.

Jeroch, H., Flachowsky, G., Weißbach, S., 1993. Futtermittelkunde. Gustav Fischer Verlag Jena, Stuttgart.

Kienzle, E., Kaden, C., Hoppe, P.P., et al., 2003. Serum beta-carotene and alpha-tocopherol in horses fed beta-carotene via grass-meal or a synthetic beadlet preparation with and without added dietary fat. Journal Animal Physiology Animal Nutrition (Berl) 87 (3–4), 174–180.

Kohn, R.A., Dinneen, M.M., Russek-Cohen, E., 2005. Using blood urea nitrogen to predict nitrogen excretion and efficiency of nitrogen utilization in cattle, sheep, goats, horses, pigs, and rats. Journal Animal Science 83 (4), 879–889.

Lewis, L.D., 1994. Feeding and Care of the Horse, second ed. Lippincott Williams & Wilkins Philadelphia, pp. 19–61.

Lowe, N.M., Fekete, K., Decsi, T., 2009. Methods of assessment of zinc status in humans: a systematic review. American Journal of Clinical Nutrition 89 (Suppl), 2040S–2051S.

Mäenpää, P.H., Koskinen, T., Koskinen, E., 1988. Serum profiles of vitamins A, E and D in mares and foals during different seasons. Journal of Animal Science 66 (6), 1418–1423.

McDowell, L.R., 2003. Minerals in animal and human nutrition, first ed. Elsevier Science BV, Amsterdam Netherlands, pp. 33–100.

McKenzie, E.C., Valberg, S.J., Godden, S.M., et al., 2002. Plasma and urine electrolyte and mineral concentrations in Thoroughbred horses with recurrent exertional rhabdomyolysis after consumption of diets varying in cation-anion balance. American Journal of Veterinary Research 63 (7), 1053–1060.

Meyer, H., 1983. Protein metabolism and protein requirement in horses. 4th International Symposium. Clermont Ferrand, pp. 343–364.

Meyer, H., Coenen, M., 2002. Pferdefütterung. Parey Buchverlag Berlin 39–52.

Peltier, M.M., Peltier, M.R., Sharp, D.C., et al., 1997. Effect of beta-carotene administration on reproductive function of horse and pony mares. Theriogenology 48 (6), 893–906.

Riond, B., Wenger-Riggenbach, B., Hofmann-Lehmann, R., et al., 2009. Serum protein concentrations from clinically healthy horses determined by agarose gel electrophoresis. Veterinary Clinical Pathology 38 (1), 73–77.

Schweigert, F.J., Gottwald, C., 1999. Effect of parturition on levels of vitamins A and E and of beta-carotene in plasma and milk of mares. Equine Veterinary Journal 31 (4), 319–323.

Sklan, D., Donoghue, S., 1982. Serum and intracellular retinol in the equine. British Journal Nutrition 47 (2), 273–280.

Smith, B.P., 2009. Large animal internal medicine. Mosby Elsevier, St. Louis MO, p. 1390.

Toribio, R.E., Kohn, C.W., Hardy, J., et al., 2005. Alterations in serum parathyroid hormone and electrolyte concentrations and urinary excretion of electrolytes in horses with induced endotoxemia. Journal Veterinary Internal Medicine 19 (2), 223–231.

Toribio, R.E., Kohn, C.W., Rourke, K.M., et al., 2007. Effects of hypercalcemia on serum concentrations of magnesium, potassium, and phosphate and urinary excretion of electrolytes in horses. American Journal of Veterinary Research 68 (5), 543–554.

van Den Hoven, R., Bauer, A., Hackl, S., et al., epub. 2010. A preliminary study on the changes in some potential markers of muscle-cell degradation in sub-maximally exercised horses supplemented with a protein and amino acid mixture. Journal of Animal Physiology Animal Nutrition (Berl). doi: 10.1111/j.1439-0396.2010.01097.x.

van Doorn, D.A., van der Spek, M.E., Everts, H., et al., 2004. The influence of calcium intake on phosphorus digestibility in mature ponies. Journal of Animal Physiology Animal Nutrition (Berl) 88 (11–12), 412–418.

van Weeren, P.R., Knaap, J., Firth, E.C., 2003. Influence of liver copper status of mare and newborn foal on the development of osteochondrotic lesions. Equine Veterinary Journal 35 (1), 67–71.

Vervuert, I., 2008. Major mineral and trace element requirements and functions in exercising horses. In: Saastamoinen, M.T., Martin-Rosset, W. (Eds.), Nutrition of the exercising horse. EAAP Publication No. 125, pp. 207–218, ISBN 978-90-8686-071-5.

Vervuert, I., Coenen, M., Höltershinken, M., et al., 2000. Aktuelle Befunde zur Beurteilung der Selenversorgung beim Pferd. Tierärztliche Praxis 3, 172–177.

Vervuert, I., Stanik, K., Coenen, M., 2006. Effects of different levels of calcium and phosphorus intake on calcium homeostasis in exercising horses. Equine Veterinary Journal 36 (Suppl.), 659–663.

Wehr, U., Englschalk, B., Kienzle, E., et al., 2002. Iodine balance in relation to iodine intake in ponies. Journal of Nutrition 132 (6 Suppl 2), 1767S–1768S.

Weisrock, K., Winkelsett, S., Martin-Rosset, W., et al., epub. 2011. Long-term effects of intermittent equine parathyroid hormone fragment (ePTH-1-37) administration on bone metabolism in healthy horses. Veterinary Journal doi: 10.1016/j.tvjl.2010.12.032.

Wichert, B., Kreyenberg, K., Kienzle, E., 2002a. Serum response after oral supplementation of different zinc compounds in horses. Journal of Nutrition 132 (6 Suppl 2), 1769S–1770S.

Wichert, B., Frank, T., Kienzle, E., 2002b. Zinc, copper and selenium intake and status of horses in Bavaria. Journal of Nutrition 132 (6 Suppl 2), 1776S–1777S.

25 Effects of diet on behavior – normal and abnormal

Becky Hothersall, Christine J. Nicol

Abnormal oral behaviors like crib-biting are undesirable for many reasons. They are widely thought to indicate sub-optimal welfare and high proportions of owners perceive such behaviors to lower the economic value of a horse and adversely affect performance (McBride & Long 2001). A combination of welfare concerns and pragmatic economic considerations has inspired a considerable body of research into the role of diet and feeding in the etiology of abnormal oral behavior. In contrast, diet's influence on normal behavior, reactivity and response to stressful stimuli has been little studied, despite the potential benefits to performance, the human–horse relationship and safety. The results of the small number of studies in this area converge to suggest that diet may affect behavior through the alteration of digestive function. Where the underlying processes have been revealed, they are generally consistent with the mechanisms that have been hypothesized to influence stereotypy development. Dietary influences on normal and abnormal behavior may therefore be governed by the same processes. These findings may help both to improve understanding of the development of stereotypies and to design dietary regimens that are beneficial in terms of horses' physical and mental well-being.

This chapter therefore considers evidence that modern management and feeding practices influence aspects of normal behavior such as foraging, and may contribute to the development of redirected or stereotypic behavior. It then describes mechanisms by which digestive processes might exert an influence on behavior and examples of where this has been observed. Recent studies are reviewed that may provide ways to alter diet to optimize behavior or performance. Where possible, suggestions are also made for how these might be applied to reducing the risks of stereotypies. Finally, examination of other potential methods of modifying behavior through dietary supplements or foraging enrichment are considered.

Abnormal oral behavior associated with diet and feeding

Crib-biting, wind-sucking and wood-chewing are abnormal, apparently functionless behaviors whose initiation is thought by many to be associated with diet and feeding management. Crib-biting occurs when a fixed object is grasped by the incisor teeth, the lower neck muscles contract to retract the larynx caudally and air is drawn into the cranial esophagus, producing a characteristic grunt (McGreevy et al 1995). Wind-sucking involves the same suite of movements, except that the horse does not actually grasp a fixed object. Once developed by an individual horse, crib-biting (used here to include wind-sucking) tends to become increasingly fixed and rigid in form and orientation over time and is usually performed repetitively. Wood-chewing is sometimes called crib-biting by horse owners but is a more varied and flexible behavior pattern lacking the invariant, repetitive movements that define a true stereotypy (Mason, 1991) so is perhaps best described as a redirected behavior. Wood-chewing is a behavior worthy of study, however, as it often precedes or is associated with crib-biting. In a four-year prospective study, Waters et al (2002) recorded the onset of stereotypic behavior in young horses. Some 30.3% of young horses showed wood-chewing and 10.5% showed crib-biting, but notably, 74% of the horses that developed crib-biting had previously shown wood-chewing.

Locomotor stereotypies such as weaving, box walking and nodding will not be considered here as there is little evidence to suggest they are associated directly with diet. For example, weaving (a stereotyped lateral movement of the head and neck) peaks in frequency just *prior* to feeding (Clegg et al 2008, Ninomiya 2007) and appears to represent anticipation of an exciting or stressful event combined with frustration at the horse's inability to leave the confined area. Factors that reduce the general aversiveness of the confined environment, particularly providing increased visual access to other horses, can significantly reduce the incidence of weaving (Cooper et al 2000, McAfee et al 2002). In contrast, such enrichment of the stabled environment appears to have little effect on the incidence of crib-biting where it is an established habit (Nicol 1999a), but foraging enrichment appears to have at least short term benefits (see 'Foraging Enrichment' page 451)

Cross-sectional surveys estimating the prevalence of abnormal oral behaviors have spanned various countries, breeds and management conditions. Not surprisingly, their estimates have varied considerably but summarizing early surveys from the UK, Italy, Sweden, and Canada on a range of breeds and uses, Nicol (1999a) described an overall mean prevalence of 4.13% crib-biting and 11.78% wood-chewing. Recent reports have reported similar values. A survey of 312 nonracing horses in Prince Edward Island yielded an owner-declared prevalence of 3.8% crib-biting and 3.8% wood chewing (Christie et al 2006). Albright et al (2009) reported an overall prevalence of 4.4% crib-biting in a study of 3574 American horses, though only 3.5% of a Swiss population of horses showed either locomotor or oral stereotypies (Bachmann et al 2003). In contrast, a 4-year longitudinal study of 225 foals revealed substantially higher rates: crib-biting was initiated by 10.5% of horses at a median age of 20 weeks, and wood-chewing by 30.3% of horses at a median age of 30 weeks (Waters et al 2002). It is not clear whether some young horses cease wood-chewing and crib-biting as they mature, or whether the lower levels reported in adults reflect a differential loss of these individuals to the adult population. Even if the former is the case, stereotypic oral behaviors affect a considerable number of horses and can come to dominate the behavioral repertoire of some individuals. Nicol et al (2002) reported one foal that performed crib-biting for nearly 50% of the time. Using a sample of 5 Thoroughbred geldings with an established crib-biting habit, Clegg et al (2008) recorded all incidences of crib-biting for 30 s of every 5 min period for 22 h per day. By extrapolation, they estimated that the horses in their study performed an average of 1470 crib-bites during each 22-h stabled period.

Key Points

- Abnormal oral behaviors such as crib-biting and wood-chewing appear to be associated with diet and feeding management whereas locomotor stereotypies are more closely linked with frustration, anticipation and aversive confined environments
- Crib-biting and wood-chewing habits are often initiated early in life
- Estimates vary but these behaviors are observed in a few percent of horses across various breeds and uses (and can come to dominate the behavioral repertoire of some individuals)

Time budgets and feeding patterns in the wild and in modern husbandry

Grazing is the predominant activity of the free-living horse's day. Studies of feral horses and primitive Przewalski's horses under near-natural conditions generally yield observations that at least 50% of daylight is spent feeding (van Dierendonck et al (1994, Przewalski's horse): 30–68%; Lamoot and Hoffman (2004): 68%, Mayes and Duncan (1986): 57–75% of daylight, 49–53% of nocturnal hours; Boyd (1988): 48–59%). Berger et al (1999) expressed time grazing as 52% of all activity.

Przewalski's horses reintroduced into the wild were mostly active during daylight (Berger et al 1999) tending to graze at dawn and in the afternoon and rest during the morning (van Dierendonck et al 1994). Mayes and Duncan (1986) also describe predominant daytime grazing by Camargue horses but with significant periods also occurring before dawn and after dusk. Feeding activity too varies with season. It constituted a smaller proportion of the time budget in summer of Przewalski's horses (Berger et al 1999) and of feral Haflinger mares (Lamoot & Hoffman 2004) and Camargue mares (Mayes & Duncan 1986). This probably reflects the lower nutritional quality of forage during the colder months, when body condition (Berger et al 1999, Kuntz et al 2006) and activity levels have both been observed to drop (Berger et al 1999) in Przewalski's horses. Ransom et al (2010) similarly found that feral female horses in low body condition spent more time feeding and less time resting and in maintenance and social behavior than high condition females.

Studies of equine time budgets have used different observation methods but some estimates of other activities have been made. Lying time has been estimated at between 0.4% (Boyd 1988, Przewalski's horses) and 5% (Salter & Hudson 1979, feral horses) of daytime hours and time standing resting between 11% and 23% in feral horses (Duncan 1980, 1985, Salter & Hudson 1979). Locomotion occurs at a low level while grazing and otherwise seems to occur between around 5% and 15% of observed time (Boyd 1988, Duncan 1980, 1985).

The eating habits of stabled horses tend to be more limited by the timing of meals and forage provision, but very little information is available on feeding behavior or indeed time budgets of such animals. Stabled mares fed hay ad libitum spent an average of 60% of a 24-hour period eating (Elia et al 2010). In a group of stabled horses fed concentrate and forage meals in the morning and evening, with additional forage at midday, scan sampling showed more foraging occurred at night than during the day (though this may have been influenced by providing most of the forage ration in the evening). Forage eating took up over 30% of the horses' time across the 24-hour period. Lying behavior took up 16.1% of scans and occurred almost entirely during the night (Cooper et al 2007). When seven Welsh mountain pony mares were offered ad lib access to a complete diet, they spent approximately 50% of the day feeding in summer, and 44% in winter and consumed feed in discrete meals of around 40 minutes. The rate of food consumption was inversely associated with body condition score (Dugdale et al 2011).

Crib-biting has not been reported in studies of feral or free-living domestic horses, but it has been observed when Przewalski horses are kept in captivity (Boyd 1986), suggesting that domestic management practices are a necessary cause of the behavior. Modern horse management is associated with substantial changes in the nature, quantity and frequency of food consumption in horses that are often confounded with other aspects of management. For example, horses receiving a substantial proportion of their energy requirements as discrete meals of concentrate feeds are likely to be those that are regularly stabled. Stabling curtails opportunities for a range of behaviors in the horse's normal repertoire such as foraging, locomotion and social contact. Separating the behavioral consequences of diet from those of frustration, excess energy reserves or lack of stimulation is therefore likely to be difficult. Controlled experiments comparing groups of horses, or the same individuals over varying treatments, suggest that even if the provision of concentrate feeds removes the physiological need to forage throughout the day, the motivation may remain. Through a series of experimental manipulations using fistulae and injection of nutrients, Ralston and colleagues concluded that oropharyngeal stimuli (taste, chewing, smell), nutrient feedback, and changes in energy availability (measured as glucose and insulin levels) all exert some degree of control over feeding behavior in horses (reviewed in Ralston 1984). Horses given ad libitum access to concentrate feed ate around 10 meals per day and engaged in multiple "nibbling" bouts (less than 150 g) in between meals, which were rarely separated by more than 3 hours (Ralston et al 1979). More recently, Dugdale et al (2010) reported that ponies provided with ad libitum access to a short chopped forage based meal ate an average of 16 meals per day and had a slower rate of intake than when food was limited. A patch choice experiment indicated that when grazing, horses forage so as to maximize energy intake rate (Edouard et al 2009). This will have been an adaptive strategy for a species that evolved to survive on grasses, and may contribute to horses' tendency to consume even large, energy-dense meals quickly.

Behaviors such as coprophagy (ingestion of feces), wood-chewing and bed-eating are often considered to be aberrant but may simply reflect motivation to feed outside of meal-times due to cues from gut fill, time since the last meal, or a drop in blood glucose. These behaviors may specifically represent attempts to ingest fiber as they are often ameliorated by greater provision of roughage. Horses fed an all-concentrate diet spent significantly more time engaged in wood-chewing and coprophagy than horses fed only hay (Willard et al 1977) and Redbo et al (1998) reported that the risk of wood-chewing correlated negatively with the amount of roughage available. Bed-eating is most common in horses bedded on straw and those lacking access to fibrous feed (Mills et al 2000). When Zeyner et al (2004) varied the amount of hay provided in addition to oats, they observed restless and nervous behavior in the horses with the lowest intake. Behavior was "quieter" and both aggressive behavior at feeding time and coprophagy were eliminated when the diet contained more hay. In this particular study, total caloric intake was lower in horses fed less hay so hunger may also have been an important determinant of behavior. Mares offered ad-lib orchard grass hay or a complete pelleted feed in a counterbalanced order had a higher motivation for hay – measured by an operant response – when fed the pelleted diet. Time spent in food searching behavior was also an order of magnitude lower when fed hay (Elia et al 2010).

Crib-biting is similarly increased by a low forage or high-grain diet (Bachmann et al 2003, McGreevy et al 1995, Redbo et al 1998, Waters et al 2002) and decreased by the use of straw bedding, possibly because this may function as an additional source of dietary fiber (McGreevy et al 1995, Christie et al 2006). Most of these studies have been cross-sectional in nature so conclusions about cause and effect must be drawn with great care. However, a longitudinal study has shown that feeding practices have a significant effect on the relative rate of development of oral stereotypies. Waters et al (2002) found that feeding grain-based feeds immediately after weaning resulted in a four-fold increase in risk. A prospective study of foal behavior suggested that individual differences in feeding patterns or feeding motivation of foals may also have an influence. Foals that developed abnormal oral behavior (wood chewing, crib-biting or both) after weaning had, prior to weaning, spent more time suckling and twice as much time teat nuzzling as other foals (Nicol & Badnell-Waters 2005). It is possible that foals with the greatest suckling motivation may be most affected by sudden weaning methods that instantly prevent suckling.

Key Points

- Crib-biting has only been observed in domesticated or captive equids
- Free-living horses evolved to spend a large proportion of their time grazing on fibrous food
- The diets of many domesticated horses include infrequent, large and energy dense meals with limited forage.
- Undesirable oral behaviors are likely to reflect a motivation to graze and/or ingest additional fiber

Digestive processes and links with behavior

A closer look at digestive processes reveals plausible mechanisms by which both abnormal and undesirable normal behavior might result from concentrate-heavy feeding practices. There is a common perception that excess energy from concentrate feeds causes "fizzy" or unwanted excitable behavior (Jansson et al 2002). Large, high starch meals result in large fluctuations in plasma glucose and insulin after feeding (Harris 2005, Stull & Rodiek 1988, Pagan et al 1999), which are indeed likely to cause peaks and troughs of energy. Low fiber, high starch diets are also associated with a number of digestive and metabolic disorders (Hoffman 2003, Kronfeld & Harris 2003). Many problems seem to stem from the horse being unable to regulate gut acidity during digestion and absorption (Mills & Clarke 2002) and excitable, irritable or abnormal oral behavior may plausibly stem from visceral discomfort in either the fore- or hind-gut, or from its sequalae.

The foregut

After ingesting large cereal-based meals, the higher proportion of dry matter in the stomach contents slows the mixing of feed and gastric juice, leading to the potential for dysfermentation in the stomach (Harris et al 2006). Wild horses would have historically eaten wild cereals that they encountered and so ingestion of cereals is not an "unnatural" modern phenomenon; it is more that their proportions in modern diets lead to a vastly decreased time spent chewing compared with a grazing lifestyle. For example, the average horse eating a kilo of hay would chew 3400 times, taking 40 minutes while the same weight of oats could be consumed in 10 minutes with only 850 jaw movements (see Harris & Arkell 2005). Elia et al (2010) found that horses chewed over 43,000 times a day when eating ad-lib hay, and only around 10 000 times a day when fed a pelleted diet. This exacerbates matters by reducing opportunities to moisten food with alkaline saliva. As a consequence, large starchy meals may result in discomfort and even gastric colic (Harris & Arkell 2005). Ralston (2007) states that feeding large grain meals is strongly correlated with ulceration but notes that careful verification through controlled studies is still needed. Estimated starch intakes of more than 2 g/kg bodyweight per day or 1 g/kg per meal were both found to be risk factors for the development of equine gastric ulceration syndrome (EGUS) in a study of Danish horses not in active race training (Luthersson et al 2009). Stall housing was previously reported as a risk factor for ulceration of the squamous epithelium (Murray & Eichorn 1996). Luthersson et al (2009) suggested that the free movement associated with grazing may help to move stomach contents through the gastrointestinal tract, but gut pH did not decrease over a 24-hour period when horses were stall-housed rather than grazing in paddocks (Husted et al 2008). As subjects had unrestricted access to hay in that study, perhaps stall housing as a risk factor reflects its tendency to co-occur with intermittent feeding rather than a direct effect of confinement per se. Fecal pH was observed to be lower in horses fed a pelleted diet compared with when the same horses ate ad-lib hay (Elia et al 2010).

The fact that crib-biting horses are similarly at increased risk of digestive upset including certain types of colic (Archer et al 2004, 2008, Hillyer et al 2002), gastric ulceration (Nicol et al 2002) and altered gut-transit time (McGreevy & Nicol 1998, McGreevy et al 2001) hints at an involvement of digestive processes in stereotypy. Interestingly, Waters et al (2002) found that sudden weaning methods that involve the isolation of foals also significantly increase risk of developing crib-biting. They suggest that this may reflect upset eating patterns in the young foal, stressed by the sudden removal of its mother and access to milk. Even short periods of not eating lead to stomach acidity, early onset of ulceration (Murray & Eichorn 1996, Nieto et al 2009) and an increased risk of some colics (Archer et al 2008). The newly isolated foal will therefore be particularly at risk of gut-related problems. Any of these digestive imbalances are likely to impair the welfare of affected horses but evidence is emerging that they may have economic consequences as well. Experimentally-induced gastric ulceration adversely affected physiologic indices of performance (Nieto et al 2009) and a case study reported that treatment of existing EGUS with the proton pump inhibitor omeprazole resulted in improved race earnings in 4 racehorses (Franklin et al 2008). This presents financial corroboration of previous findings that moderate to severe gastric ulceration in racehorses improved significantly faster with omeprazole versus treatment using the same compound minus the drug component (Murray et al 1997).

Because horses only produce saliva when chewing (Alexander 1966) but secrete acid into the stomach continuously, it has been proposed that horses suffering from foregut acidity problems may wood-chew or crib-bite in an attempt to stimulate additional saliva production (Nicol 1999b). In support of this hypothesis, crib-biting foals showed significantly greater evidence of stomach inflammation and early ulceration than normal foals (Nicol et al 2002). Feeding antacids reduces these clinical signs, and also tends to result in a reduction in crib-biting behavior (Nicol et al 2002, Mills & Macleod 2002). Measurement of saliva production from the submandibular gland indicated that crib-biting horses produced smaller quantities of saliva than non-stereotypic horses but that this difference was compensated for by the action of crib-biting (Moeller et al 2008). This study measured behavior over a short period and it would be interesting to explore how substantially crib-biting might mitigate the effects of low saliva production in the long term. Associations between crib-biting and gastrointestinal disturbance would seem to indicate that it is not wholly successful, but it is equally possible that such disturbance would be worse in the absence of crib-biting. This highlights the potential welfare consequences of simply treating the outward symptoms of stereotypies (such as the use of anti-cribbing collars) without understanding their underlying causes. If crib-biting becomes an anticipatory or habitual behavior, the initiating cause may also not be immediately apparent and this further complicates both diagnosis and treatment.

The hindgut

Large meals can overwhelm the capacity of the stomach and small intestine and increase transit rates of digesta. Potter et al (1992, cited in Delobel & Cuvelier 2008) concluded that more than 3.5–4 g/kg body weight starch per meal (about 3 kg of barley for a 500 kg horse) exceeded capacity for enzymatic digestion and increased the amount of starch reaching the posterior ileum. Luthersson et al (2009) recently advised a lower limit, 2 g starch/kg body weight per day or 1 g/kg per meal, as they found that higher starch levels were a risk factor for EGUS. Intense episodes of hydrolyzable carbohydrate fermentation in the hindgut and a resulting drop in pH can occur, as measured in the caecum (Willard et al 1977) or feces (Rowe et al 1994, dos Santos et al 2009). Correspondingly, feeding more than 4 kg grains (usually oats in this study) was recently identified as a risk factor for low fecal pH in New Zealand racehorses (Williamson et al 2007). This finding was not general to commercial pre-mixed feeds, possibly because cereal grains within such mixes tend to undergo a greater degree of processing, which in turn facilitates fermentation earlier in digestion (Harris & Arkell 2005). Tinker et al (1997) did report an increased colic risk associated with levels of concentrate feeding greater than 2.5 kg per day. Interestingly, in Williamson's study, fecal pH was slightly but significantly higher in the very small sample of only six horses recorded as displaying stereotpyies. However, interpretation of this finding is difficult as these included both oral and locomotor stereotypies.

Discomfort caused by the overflow of readily fermentable carbohydrates into the hindgut has been linked with increased anxiety and aggression in rats (Hanstock et al 2004) and with undesirable oral behaviors including bed eating and wood chewing in horses. These were reduced by dietary supplementation with virginiamycin, an antibiotic which altered fecal pH (Johnson et al 1998). Presumably selective bacterial proliferation was halted, preventing rapid fermentation of sugar and starch. The study did not include any crib-biting horses. Willard et al (1977) also reported that cecal pH was lower in three horses fed a sweet concentrate feed compared with when the same individuals were fed only hay. Relative proportions of specific volatile fatty acids (VFAs) in the cecum were also altered, and infusions of disodium carbonate both increased cecal pH in concentrate-fed horses and reversed the pattern of VFA proportions. It was also noted that the infusions reduced the time spent wood chewing and engaging in coprophagy but the finding did not reach statistical significance in this very small sample.

Increased total gut transit time has been recorded in crib-biters (McGreevy et al 2001), and when both crib-biting and eating hay were prevented, orocecal transit time was significantly longer than in non-stereotypic horses (McGreevy & Nicol 1998). Freire et al (2008) later suggested that crib-biting and weaving are not influenced by hindgut acidosis. This conclusion was based on the failure of virginiamycin supplementation to reduce performance of these stereotypic behaviors but seems speculative in light of interpretational difficulties presented by the study design. For example, no mention was made of an increase in the amount of grain in the subjects' diet partway through the study, revealed by examination of a companion paper (Freire et al 2009). Virginiamycin reduced exploratory behavior and altered water intake but similar results were attributed to the change in diet in the other study. Measurements were averaged across two time periods and this nominally accounted for the horses consuming different diets in each period, but the completely separate analyses permit no consideration of interactions or carry-over between periods.

Virginiamycin supplementation was apparently successful in mitigating the moderate to severe lameness due to laminitis that was otherwise induced by feeding 8 kg of maize-based pellets per day (Rowe et al 1994). It has been suggested that hindgut acidosis in racehorses may commonly lead to low-level laminitis that can limit the horse's performance potential (Linford et al 1993). As with foregut processes, deleterious effects may therefore extend to performance as well as behavior. In some cases, the very pain or discomfort associated with riding may itself go on to alter behavior. Horses assessed by chiropractic examination to have back problems, that were likely to cause pain, demonstrated increased aggression and a reduction in positive responses in interactions with humans (Fureix et al 2010).

Further evidence linking stereotypy with digestion and potential confounding factors

A temporal association between crib-biting and the delivery of concentrated feed provides another indicator to its causation. In horses fed concentrates once daily, the rate of crib-biting rose dramatically in the period immediately after feeding, peaking some 4 to 8 hours after meal delivery (Clegg et al 2008). This is consistent with a function in attempting to buffer the stomach. Providing concentrates in smaller, more frequent, meals might be expected to ameliorate some of the problems associated with starch overload. Indeed, splitting concentrate rations into smaller meals has been shown to reduce the overall incidence of crib-biting (Cooper et al 2005). It is worth bearing in mind that changes to the feeding regimen may have unintended consequences for other individuals stabled nearby. In the above study, weaving, nodding and oral stereotypies all increased significantly in horses in the control group when they observed the experimental horses being fed extra meals.

On the other hand, crib-biting may also in part be a learnt response in anticipation of discomfort because when Gillham et al (1994) measured cribbing in the 30 minutes after providing various types of feed, responses peaked only 10 minutes after ingestion. A 200 g meal of a sweetened grain ration or of a high protein pelleted feed increased crib-biting 14–16-fold after 10 minutes and even alfalfa pellets increased cribbing by a factor of around 7.

Experimental and epidemiological studies of stereotypy tend to be cross-sectional, making it very difficult to separate confounded factors. For example, several surveys have reported breed differences in the prevalence of crib-biting. Risk appears to be higher in thoroughbred and warmblood horses (Tinker et al 1997, Bachmann et al 2003) but breed is likely to be confounded with various management factors such as the type of activity for which they are used, extent of stabling and amount of concentrate feed given. Because the physiological status of the control horses and the stereotypic horses in the period before the onset of stereotypy is unknown, it is also impossible to assess whether horses with a predisposition to develop stereotypy are perhaps more reactive, or have different digestive physiology than horses with no such predisposition. A lack of differences in plasma cortisol concentrations or average heart rates has been reported between crib-biting, weaving and control horses (Clegg et al 2008) and comparisons of plasma beta-endorphin have proved inconsistent (Gillham et al 1994, McGreevy & Nicol 1998, Pell & McGreevy 1999). But the onset and performance of stereotypy may alter the physiology of stereotypic horses, perhaps to levels that no longer differ significantly from normal horses. Nicol (1999b) called for longitudinal studies of individual horses to understand causality of stereotypies but these are expensive, time consuming and logistically difficult and so are still disappointingly rare.

Key Points

- Excitable, irritable or abnormal behavior may stem from visceral discomfort or its consequences in the fore- or hindgut
- *Foregut*: Meal feeding of concentrates may increase gastric acidity, discomfort, ulceration and even some forms of colic by limiting opportunities for saliva production and increasing the proportion of the time during which the stomach is empty
- Crib-biting horses are at greater risk of such digestive problems and the behavior may serve to increase saliva production
- *Hindgut*: large starchy meals may also overwhelm the stomach's capacity and result in acidity due to hydrolysable carbohydrate fermentation occurring in the hindgut

Effects of dietary carbohydrate, fiber and oil on behavior

Problems associated with digestion of concentrates would ideally be avoided by mimicking the natural eating patterns of the ancestral horse, providing prolonged access to a low-calorie ration comprising predominantly fiber (e.g., hay or pasture). Horses in heavy work, though, may not be able to sustain requirements for energy or specific nutrients through forage alone and another approach is needed to easing problems caused by intermittent meal feeding, plus limited roughage and high dietary starch. The replacement of some carbohydrates with fiber and oil as an energy source may be beneficial in minimizing glycemic and insulinemic fluctuations (Williams et al 2001), with more energy coming from gradual and sustained hindgut digestion of fermentable carbohydrates from fiber (Harris et al 2006). In human children, breakfast foods with a lower glycemic index are associated with improved performance in attention tasks (Mahoney et al 2005, Benton et al 2007); a comparable response in horses might result in calmer or less distractible behavior. The slowing of feed intake (Harris & Arkell 2005) and possibly of gastric emptying rates (Geor et al 2001, but see Lorenzo-Figuera et al 2005) caused by the addition of fiber and oil, may decrease the behavioral need to forage by extending satiety as well as potentially reducing fermentation- or acidosis-related discomfort. Frank et al (2005) concluded that supplementation with corn oil, refined rice bran oil or crude rice bran oil did not counteract the ulcerogenic effects of a high starch diet but fiber provision was the same (unrestricted) for supplemented and control diets.

In pig farming, sows are commonly subject to feed restriction during gestation, creating a persistent behavioral need to forage. In a review, Meunier-Salaun et al (2001) concluded that incorporating fiber in diets without changing overall energy intake substantially increased eating time, reduced feeding rate and feed motivation (in operant tests). Stereotypic behavior, restlessness and aggression were also reduced. There may, therefore, be a role for such an approach in the management of stereotypies in horses but so far this remains untested. In contrast, a number of small scale studies have produced preliminary results indicating that normal behavior can be influenced by oil and/or fiber supplementation, though the mechanisms have rarely been pinpointed and Ralston (2007) notes the confounding influence of a simple reduction in dietary starch in most studies. Coprophagy and aggressive behavior observed by Zeyner et al (2002, cited in Zeyner et al 2004) in horses fed a high-starch diet (despite high hay intake) was not seen if starch was partially replaced by fat. MacLeay et al (1999) interpreted lower packed cell volume and heart rate before a standardized exercise test as meaning horses fed a fat-rich diet were less excitable than horses fed a high carbohydrate diet. It should be noted here that these were Thoroughbred horses genetically predisposed to exertional rhabdomyolysis. These horses were also observed informally as being more docile and willing to exercise but the diets were not isocaloric and no differences were reported between the fat diet and low carbohydrate diet providing the same energy.

Horses fed test diets containing additional fats displayed reduced spontaneous locomotion and reactivity to sudden visual stimuli and similar trends were seen in reactivity towards acoustic and pressure stimuli (Holland et al 1996b). The same group of authors reported that foals given access to a "fat and fiber" (FF) dietary supplement performed more grazing behavior and appeared to be less stressed than foals provided with a starch and sugar (SS)-based supplement, in at least some of the weaning groups observed (Holland et al 1996a). The FF foals also had lower cortisol levels both before and after weaning and it was suggested that this diet helped foals to cope with the stress of weaning. In a pair of related trials, foals given an FF supplement fed more (Ordakowski et al 2003) and tended to be more "relaxed" (Redgate et al 2004) during a feed preference test than foals fed an SS supplement.

A larger sample was used by Nicol et al (2005) who examined the behavior at weaning, and subsequently during validated behavioral tests (Visser et al 2001) of 17 foals raised under identical conditions except for being fed on either an FF or SS diet. Weaning is widely accepted to be a stressful time for foals and heart rates recorded by Visser et al (2002) indicated that their novel object and handling tests – replicated here – were likely to have induced a state of mild fear. Under these conditions, FF foals demonstrated consistently reduced reactivity and increased investigation. Behavior at weaning depended somewhat on whether foals were barn- or paddock-weaned but in both cases locomotion was reduced in FF foals. In behavioral tests at 9–10 months, FF foals spent more time investigating and less time looking at a novel object (a slowly twirling golf umbrella). They also spent less time walking away from a novel person and completed a handling test in a shorter time than SS foals. A related study at the same stud farm by researchers at the University of Bristol found complementary results in 17 unweaned 3 month old foals. Subjects were born to mares fed an FF or SS diet in the last trimester of pregnancy. In a similar novel object test, FF foals spent a greater proportion of time walking towards the umbrella and investigating the environment than SS foals; SS foals spent longer looking at the umbrella without approaching. Latency to approach the umbrella was shorter in FF foals, and only individuals from this group touched it (Hothersall et al 2008). While fearfulness and investigative behavior appeared to be affected in challenging situations, very few differences were observed in the normal behavioral profiles of the groups at pasture in either of these studies.

Corroboration of these effects comes from a study of 28 adult horses on isocaloric diets differing in fat content, though in this case both diets were high in starch. Redondo et al (2009) fed horses both diets in a cross-over design and exposed them to a startling visual stimulus (Redondo et al 2009). Feeding horses an increased proportion of dietary fat (10% rather than 3%) for the 2 months preceding testing diminished their startle response when exposed to a moving jack-in-the-box with the holder on the end of a rope some distance away in an otherwise empty arena. Oil-supplemented horses moved from the object over a shorter time and distance. Their heart rate also increased less and heart rate variability was greater; reaction time did not differ between groups. Resting blood cortisol was again significantly lower in the period during which horses were fed the high oil diet.

Evidence for diet-mediated physiological changes

The attenuation of startle responses in ridden horses could prove beneficial in the prevention of accidents caused by horses "spooking" but the findings of Redondo et al (2009)'s study are particularly intriguing given that the authors offer no explanation of how the diets might have influenced behavior or cortisol. To avoid extraneous disturbances, testing took place in the middle of the night. Neither the timing nor the quantity of the twice-daily food provision was stated, but presumably testing occurred many hours after the last feed. This effectively rules out the involvement of short-term glycemic fluctuations or foregut (but not necessarily hindgut) discomfort in the greater startle response of the horses.

In general, little information is available on mechanisms by which diet may mediate behavior. A companion study to that of Nicol et al (2005) examined the effects of the two diets on various physiological parameters in their study foals (Wilson et al 2007). Fecal pH was not altered by diet and the visual appearance of the gastric mucosa did not differ between diet groups. When tested at 40 weeks of age, blood glucose rose more sharply following a meal in SS foals, which had significantly higher total blood glucose and lower total blood gastrin than FF foals during the 6-hour period following a meal. Insulin levels also appeared to rise faster in SS foals but the difference did not reach significance. Since gastrin stimulates the secretion of gastric acid, the lack of difference in gastric mucosa condition despite increased gastrin production in FF foals was slightly unexpected. But additional gastrin production may have been balanced by increased eating time, and therefore saliva production, in the FF foals, increasing the water content of the swallowed bolus. Both this and potentially slower gastric emptying of the oily, fibrous food could buffer the stomach from acid secretion and enhance mixing with gastric juices, reducing the risk of dysfermentation by stomach flora. However, foals in Nicol et al's study were not fed a standardized time before tests and the 3-month-old foals (Hothersall et al 2008) ate very small quantities of feed in proportion to their body weight. This again reduces the likelihood that the findings can be explained by glycemic response or digestive processes. As gastric conditions also did not differ between the groups studied by Nicol and Wilson (a possible but unexplored explanation for the results found by Redondo et al (2009)), longer-term mechanisms may underlie the behavioral differences observed.

Glucoregulation and the serotonergic system

Recent studies on insulin resistance (Treiber et al 2005) suggest that over a period of many months, FF diets may facilitate more stable glucoregulatory patterns, with smaller fluctuations in glucose and insulin. This could have consequent effects on brain function. The serotonergic system modulates mood and emotion and low levels of serotonin are reliably associated with depression in laboratory animals and humans (Schloss & Williams 1998). Serotonin synthesis is dependent on the availability of its precursor amino acid, tryptophan, in the brain (Schaechter & Wurtman 1990). Increased insulin decreases plasma concentrations of most amino acids but raises levels of tryptophan. This also influences the extent to which free tryptophan is taken up by a transporter protein by reducing the availability of competing large neutral amino acids (LNAAs). The best proxy measure of CNS serotonin level is therefore the ratio of tryptophan to LNAA (Fernstrom 2005, Markus et al 2005). Although the groups did not differ overall in Try:LNAA ratios, changes over the testing period suggest that FF foals in Wilson et al (2007)'s study may have had a higher resting Try:LNAA ratio levels. In a recent study, blood plasma serotonin was higher in Dutch warmblood horses fed a high fiber versus a high starch diet, when sampled 3 hours after feeding. Plasma tryptophan itself did not differ significantly, though further investigation is warranted as there was an interaction between sex and diet (Alberghina et al 2010).

It is also possible that gluco-regulation may be further influenced by mare diet in gestation. Mares in late pregnancy undergo changes in insulin sensitivity that function to reserve glucose for fetal requirements (Hoffman 2003), and these were more evident in FF than SS mares (Hoffman et al 2003). Finally, there is preliminary evidence that mare diet in pregnancy can affect insulin sensitivity in foals: up to the age of 80 days, basal plasma glucose concentrations were higher in foals born to mares fed a high starch compared with a low starch diet during the last trimester. Foals born to mares fed the high starch diet during pregnancy also tended to have lower insulin sensitivity at 160 days. Notably, these results were seen despite all mares being fed the low starch diet post-partum (George et al 2009).

Key Points

- Replacement of some carbohydrates with fiber and/or oil can provide more stable and sustained gradual release of energy
- An increasing number of studies suggest that oil and fiber content can influence behavioral and physiological responses to challenge or novelty. The mechanisms for this are not yet clear but one possibility is alteration of mood or emotion through the serotonergic system

Behavior modification by feed supplements

Tryptophan depletion can cause anxious and depressive behavior in rats (Blokland et al 2002). Conversely, enhanced Try:LNAA ratios increased alertness and attention in humans (Markus et al 2005). On the basis of such results, tryptophan is sold commercially as a calmative for horses, either alone or in a mixture of vitamins, minerals and or herbs. A recent review concluded that while calming effects of supplementation have been demonstrated in some species, there is currently no scientific evidence for tryptophan's efficacy in horses; indeed some studies indicate that at low doses it may cause excitability (Grimmett & Sillence 2005). Two studies subsequently confirmed that a commercial dose of tryptophan did not affect any behavioral parameters in response to social isolation, a novel person or object, or to a handling test (Malmkvist & Christensen 2007, Noble et al 2008) even though plasma tryptophan levels were raised (Noble et al 2008). However, evidence from other species suggests effects may be more apparent on aggression rather than fear or reactivity (Grimmett & Sillence 2005) and comparable tests have not yet been applied to the horse.

Other than tryptophan, "calming supplements" commonly include magnesium, complexes of B-vitamins including thiamine, lecithins, essential amino acids, probiotics and herbs or herbal extracts. The basis for including many of these ingredients appears to be that deficiencies can cause clinical problems; for example severe thiamine deficiency can cause convulsions (Read & Harrington 1981). There is an absence of controlled trials indicating that high intake of these substances will have a calming effect, besides which, commercial concentrate feed formulations usually provide adequate levels of such nutrients. A study in laboratory mice demonstrated antidepressant- and anxiolytic-like effects of magnesium at doses of 20 and 30 mg/kg (Poleszak et al 2004) but no comparable data are available for horses. The inclusion of lecithins, probiotics and in some cases "gastric herbs" indicates a growing recognition that digestive processes may contribute to excitable behavior. Only one study (Holland et al 1996b) has examined the effects of probiotic/lecithin supplements on behavior and these results were confounded with dietary fat content. Spontaneous activity and reactivity to some sudden stimuli were lower in horses supplemented with soy lecithin *and* corn or soy oil but parallel reductions were seen in the group supplemented with corn oil alone.

It is plausible that supplements improving digestive comfort might result in changes similar to those seen in FF versus SS feeds. Indeed, many high-starch cereal feeds now include a live yeast supplement with the purpose of limiting undesirable changes within the intestinal environment associated with grain feeding. A supplement of *Saccharomyces cerevisiae* increased the concentration of viable yeast cells in the cecum and colon (with minimal effect on microbial counts) and modified pH, lactic acid, ammonia, acetate and butyrate concentrations in horses fed a diet causing starch overload of the hindgut (Medina et al 2002). Conversely, in a recent study of Thoroughbred geldings, direct-fed lactic acid bacteria supplements had limited effects in preventing acidosis induced by increased starch intake (Swyers et al 2008). However, a trend was noted towards an increase in fecal pH in horses fed a *Lactobacillus acidophilus* (but not a mixed *Lactobacillus*) supplement, and the authors suggest that significant effects might be observed under more severely acidotic conditions. If such supplements were able to ameliorate gut conditions they might potentially have value in the treatment of stereotypic oral behavior but to date, this does not appear to have been tested directly.

Ralston (2007) outlined the paucity of evidence for health benefits of equine herbal supplements. The capacity for herbal ingredients to modify behavior in horses has been subject to even less validation and claims for calming effects are at best likely to be extrapolations from humans or other species. Common ingredients include valerian, vervain, *Withania somnifera* (Indian ginseng), passion flower, hops, chamomile, lemon balm, and peppermint. Some of these may have potent effects and should be considered as medicines rather than food additives. For example, valerian is used as a sedative in humans and contains a number of active compounds. These include valerenic acid 5a, which exerts pentobarbital-like central depressant activity; valtrate and isovaltrate which have antidepressant properties, and didrovaltrate whose tranquilizing effects are similar to those of benzodiazepines (Klepser & Klepser, 1999). A valerian-based supplement significantly diminished increases in heart rate variables in response to vibration stress (Peeters et al 2004) in pigs but effects on horses have not been studied. Given that humans using benzodiazepines would be cautioned against tasks such as driving, it seems reasonable to be concerned that valerian might affect co-ordination or performance in horses. Owners should also be aware that valerenic acid is banned during competition under International Federation for Equine Sport (FEI) rules (FEI 2010). Bioactive glycowithanolides, isolated from the roots of *Withania somnifera*, produced anxiolytic and antidepressant effects in rats similar to the benzodiazepine lorazepam and the tricyclic antidepressant imipramine, respectively (Bhattacharya et al 2000). Again, it is not known whether comparable effects would be seen in the horse but presumably few owners would willingly dose their animals with prescription medications that had undergone no testing for that species.

Whole plants may contain a range of active compounds and unlike synthetic drugs, the active ingredients of herbs are affected by unpredictable parameters including growing conditions, harvesting and storage procedures, and contamination (Davidson 1999). Given the pharmaceutical properties of some of their constituents, there is a great deal of scope for herbal preparations to modify behavior; the concern is that it may be impossible to assess the dosage or even identify what active ingredients are responsible for any behavioral changes observed. This obviously creates difficulties in predicting their effects and assessing their safety. In the absence of supporting data, supplement manufacturers tend to keep their claims vague and none explicitly purport to influence stereotypy. Anecdotal reports from recent experimental studies point to an intriguing possibility that may merit exploration. With a view to manipulating palatability or even digestibility of feedstuffs, Brøkner et al (2008) examined the effect of an unspecified blend of essential oils on chewing, eating and fecal composition in Icelandic horses. The essential oils had little influence on any parameters measured but did significantly increase the frequency with which visible saliva was observed during concentrate meals. Meanwhile, Moeller et al (2008) observed that horses often visibly lose saliva from the mouth while crib-biting. If the goal of crib-biting is to increase saliva production, the development of supplements or ingredients capable of stimulating saliva without affecting feeding behavior might conceivably be of benefit; clearly further and more formal testing would be required to verify whether such effects can be achieved.

Another area ripe for exploitation is the supplementation of feeds with polyunsaturated fatty acids (PUFAs). Dietary supplementation of the omega-3 fatty acid docosahexaenoic acid (DHA) and its pre-cursor eicosapentaenoic acid (EPA) has been found to improve cognitive function in humans – DHA is essential to brain development, both pre- and post-natally, and EPA influences mood and behavior (for review, see Kidd 2007). Advertising of many food products – such as oily fish – now capitalizes on these links by emphasizing their omega-3 oil content. PUFA supplementation in rats has been shown in some studies to increase learning ability (Lim & Suzuki 2001, but see Wainwright et al 1999) and to replicate the behavioral effects of antidepressants in a number of stressful situations (Venna et al 2009). Again in rats, dietary deficiencies in DHA are cumulative and appear to retard cognitive function: second generation rats had significantly lower brain DHA and fared worse on an olfactory discrimination task (Greiner et al 2001). Maternal sources of polyunsaturated acids also appear to affect fetal and neonatal development in pigs (Leskanich & Noble, 1999). In horses too, there is some suggestion that the influence of PUFA supplementation could span generations, either in utero or if milk composition affected subsequent development. Long-chain fatty acid composition in milk is expected to be directly related to that of dietary fats in hind-gut fermenting species such as the horse because unsaturated fatty acids will not undergo significant hydrogenation by gut flora prior to absorption. Hoffman et al (1998) detected differences in the colostrum and milk composition of horses fed FF and SS diets. These included levels of various unsaturated fatty acids (though not specifically EPA and DHA). The authors discuss the potentially protective effects of linoleic acid – found at increased levels in the milk of fat supplemented mares, both by them and by Zeyner et al (1996, cited by Hoffman et al 1998) – in the prevention of gastric ulcers in foals through production of prostaglandins. Formulations of fiber- and oil-supplemented concentrate feeds do not currently appear to be marketed as providing enhanced levels of beneficial PUFAs or their precursors, but Delobel and Cuvelier (2008) recently collated published information on the fatty acid composition of various oils that have been used in dietary supplementation for horses. Given the apparent potential for effects on behavior and cognition, and perhaps the scope for broodmares' diets to influence the long term health of their offspring, it seems likely that this will be an area of future research interest.

Key Points

- There is no published evidence supporting the use of calming or herbal supplements in horses
- Certain ingredients contained in some herbal supplements have the potential to cause potent and poorly-studied pharmacological effects that may affect horses' performance or coordination
- Some preliminary evidence does suggest beneficial digestive effects of supplements containing live yeast or lactic acid bacteria

Foraging enrichment

Implementing simple techniques of foraging enrichment could potentially provide an alternative method for beneficially altering patterns of behavior in stabled horses where meal feeding is necessary or access to pasture is limited. Horses provided with a feed-dispensing foraging device filled with high-fiber pelleted feed spent around 14% of their time engaged in using it. When the device was present they spent significantly less time moving, ingesting concentrates, standing and nosing their bedding (Winskill et al 1996). Concerns have been voiced, however, that frustration behavior may be directed toward such devices when they become empty (Henderson & Waran 2001, Goodwin et al 2007b). Horses fed more frequently and for longer in total during trials where multiple rather than single types of feed were available. Similar patterns were seen whether concentrates or forages were used (Goodwin et al 2002, 2005, Thorne et al 2005), and with concentrates, provision of multiple feeds also resulted in horses spending less time standing (Goodwin et al 2005). Horses offered a choice between stables containing multiple or single forages generally entered the closest stable but then moved to the one offering multiple forages (Goodwin et al 2007a). Overall, there appears to be promise in using foraging enrichments to replicate patterns of more natural patch foraging behavior. Particularly where these interventions result in prolonged roughage intake, they are likely to promote good welfare by combining digestive benefits with provision of stimulation and opportunities for activity. Studies examining how well these effects persist over longer periods are needed.

Key Points

- Foraging devices or provision of multiple forage types can alter time budgets and increase feeding time in the short term
- Longer term studies are needed to assess the persistence of the enrichment value of such modifications

Conclusions

There is an accumulation of evidence to suggest that modern diet and feeding practices have substantial effects on the behavior of horses and most evidence seems to suggest that emulating horses' natural eating patterns by lowering starch, increasing roughage and feeding little and often is beneficial to their health and welfare. Links between diet and the development of abnormal oral behavior are well established but by no means uncontroversial. More controlled studies are required to understand the mechanisms underlying effects of diet on both normal and abnormal behavior. In particular, future studies that examine the role of different dietary components separately would help to clarify the routes by which diet appears to influence reactivity in horses and how these might relate to the development and maintenance of stereotypic oral behavior. Further longitudinal studies will be particularly valuable to fill in current gaps in knowledge. Well-designed, peer-reviewed clinical trials are needed to assess clinical evidence of efficacy, side-effects and interactions with drugs before any feed supplements can be recommended for behavioral modification. Even if they prove effective, supplements may simply treat the symptoms and not the cause. In order to ensure good welfare, attempts to relieve behavioral problems should begin by examining whether aspects of management such as diet, exercise and the social environment can be improved.

References

Alberghina, D., Giannetto, C., Visser, E.K., et al., 2010. Effect of diet on plasma tryptophan and serotonin in trained mares and geldings. Veterinary Record 166, 133–136.

Albright, J.D., Mohammed, H.O., Heleski, C.R., et al., 2009. Crib-biting in US horses: Breed predispositions and owner perceptions of aetiology. Equine Veterinary Journal 41, 455–458.

Alexander, F., 1966. A study of parotid salivation in the horse. Journal of Physiology 184, 646–656.

Archer, D.C., Pinchbeck, G.L., French, N.P., et al., 2008. Risk factors for epiploic foramen entrapment colic: An international study. Equine Veterinary Journal 40, 224–230.

Archer, D.C., Proudman, C.J., Pinchbeck, G., et al., 2004. Entrapment of the small intestine in the epiploic foramen in horses: a retrospective analysis of 71 cases recorded between 1991 and 2001. Veterinary Record 155, 793–797.

Bachmann, I., Audige, L., Stauffacher, M., 2003. Risk factors associated with behavioral disorders of crib-biting, weaving and box-walking in Swiss horses. Equine Veterinary Journal 35, 158–163.

Benton, D., Maconie, A., Williams, C., 2007. The influence of the glycaemic load of breakfast on the behavior of children in school. Physiology & Behavior 92, 717–724.

Berger, A., Scheibe, K.M., Eichhorn, K., et al., 1999. Diurnal and ultradian rhythms of behavior in a mare group of Przewalski horse (*Equus ferus przewalskii*), measured through one year under semi-reserve conditions. Applied Animal Behavior Science 64, 1–17.

Bhattacharya, S.K., Bhattacharya, A., Sairam, K., et al., 2000. Anxiolytic-antidepressant activity of *Withania somnifera* glycowithanolides: an experimental study. Phytomedicine 7, 463–469.

Blokland, A., Lieben, C., Deutz, N.E., 2002. Anxiogenic and depressive-like effects, but no cognitive deficits, after repeated moderate tryptophan depletion in the rat. Journal of Psychopharmacology 16, 39–49.

Boyd, L., 1986. Behavior problems of equids in zoos. Veterinary Clinics of North America 2, 653–663.

Boyd, L.E., 1988. Time budgets of adult Przewalski horses: effects of sex, reproductive status and enclosure. Applied Animal Behavior Science 21, 19–39.

Brøkner, C., Norgaard, P., Hansen, H.H., 2008. Effect of feed type and essential oil product on equine chewing activity. Journal of Animal Physiology and Animal Nutrition 92, 621–630.

Christie, J.L., Hewson, C.J., Riley, C.B., et al., 2006. Management factors affecting stereotypies and body condition score in nonracing horses in Prince Edward Island. Canadian Veterinary Journal-Revue Veterinaire Canadienne 47, 136–143.

Clegg, H.A., Buckley, P., Friend, M.A., et al., 2008. The ethological and physiological characteristics of cribbing and weaving horses. Applied Animal Behavior Science 109, 68–76.

Cooper, J.J., McDonald, L., Mills, D.S., 2000. The effect of increasing visual horizons on stereotypic weaving: implications for the social housing of stabled horses. Applied Animal Behavior Science 69, 67–83.

Cooper, J.J., MCall, N., Johnson, S., et al., 2005. The short-term effects of increasing meal frequency on stereotypic behavior of stabled horses. Applied Animal Behavior Science 90, 351–364.

Cooper, J.J., Campbell, J., Harris, P., 2007. Observations on the 24 hour activity patterns of stabled horses. Proceedings of the British Society of Animal Science. p. 34.

Davidson, H.P.B., 1999. Herbs – a sage of all wisdom or a waste of thyme? Proceedings of the British Equine Veterinary Association Specialist Days on Behavior and Nutrition. Newmarket, UK.

Delobel, A., Cuvelier, C., 2008. Fat-supplemented diets for horses: characteristics, palatability and digestibility. Annales De Medecine Veterinaire 152, 34–46.

Duncan, P., 1980. Time-budgets of Camargue horses. II. Time-budgets of adult horses and weaned sub-adults. Behavior 72, 26–49.

Duncan, P., 1985. Time-budgets of Camargue horses. III. Environmental influences. Behavior 92, 186–208.

Dos Santos, T.M., De Almeida, F.Q., De Godoi, F.N., et al., 2009. Buffer capacity, pH and faeces consistency in horses submitted to dietetic starch overload. Ciencia Rural 39, 1782–1788.

Dugdale, A.H.A., Curtis, G.C., Cripps, P., et al., 2010. Effect of dietary restriction on body condition, composition and welfare of overweight and obese pony mares. Equine Veterinary Journal 42 (7), 600–610.

Dugdale, A.H.A., Curtis, G.C., Cripps, P.J., et al., 2011. Effects of season and body condition on appetite, body mass and body composition in ad libitum fed pony mares. The Veterinary Journal 190 (3), 329–337.

Edouard, N., Fleurance, G., Dumont, B., et al., 2009. Does sward height affect feeding patch choice and voluntary intake in horses? Applied Animal Behavior Science 119, 219–228.

Elia, J.B., Erb, H.N., Houpt, K.A., 2010. Motivation for hay: Effects of a pelleted diet on behavior and physiology of horses. Physiology and Behavior 101, 623–627.

FEI, 2010. http://www.feicleansport.org/ProhibitedSubstancesList_Jan2010.pdf.

Fernstrom, J.D., 2005. Branched-chain amino acids and brain function. Journal of Nutrition 135, 1539S–1546S.

Frank, N., Andrews, F.M., Elliott, S.B., et al., 2005. Effects of dietary oils on the development of gastric ulcers in mares. American Journal of Veterinary Research 66, 2006–2011.

Franklin, S.H., Brazil, T.J., Allen, K.J., 2008. Poor performance associated with equine gastric ulceration syndrome in four Thoroughbred racehorses. Equine Veterinary Education 20, 119–124.

Freire, R., Clegg, H.A., Buckley, P., et al., 2008. Behavioral and physiological effects of virginiamycin in the diets of horses with stereotypies. Veterinary Record 163, 413–417.

Freire, R., Clegg, H.A., Buckley, P., et al., 2009. The effects of two different amounts of dietary grain on the digestibility of the diet and behavior of intensively managed horses. Applied Animal Behavior Science 117, 69–73.

Fureix, C., Menguy, H., Hausberger, M., 2010. Partners with bad temper: reject or cure? A study of chronic pain and aggression in horses. PLoS ONE 5 (8), e12434. doi:10.1371/journal.pone.0012434.

Geor, R.J., Harris, P.A., Hoekstra, K.E., et al., 2001. Effect of corn oil on solid phase gastric emptying in horses. Proceedings of the American College of Veterinary Internal Medicine. Denver, Colorado, p. 288.

George, L.A., Staniar, W.B., Treiber, K., et al., 2009. Insulin sensitivity and glucose dynamics during pre-weaning foal development and in response to maternal diet composition. Domestic Animal Endocrinology 37, 23–29.

Gillham, S.B., Dodman, N.H., Shuster, L., et al., 1994. The effect of diet on cribbing behavior and plasma beta-endorphin in horses. Applied Animal Behavior Science 41, 147–153.

Goodwin, D., Davidson, H.P.B., Harris, P., 2002. Foraging enrichment for stabled horses: effects on behavior and selection. Equine Veterinary Journal 34, 686–691.

Goodwin, D., Davidson, H.P.B., Harris, P., 2005. Sensory varieties in concentrate diets for stabled horses: effects on behavior and selection. Applied Animal Behavior Science 90, 337–349.

Goodwin, D., Davidson, H.P.B., Harris, P., 2007a. Foraging enrichment for individually housed horses: practicality and effects on behavior. Vet Record 160, 548–551.

Goodwin, D., Davidson, H.P.B., Harris, P., 2007b. A note on behavior of stabled horses with foraging devices in mangers and buckets. Applied Animal Behavior Science 105, 238–243.

Greiner, R.S., Moriguchi, T., Slotnick, B.M., et al., 2001. Olfactory discrimination deficits in n-3 fatty acid-deficient rats. Physiology & Behavior 72, 379–385.

Grimmett, A., Sillence, M.N., 2005. Calmatives for the excitable horse: A review of L-tryptophan. Veterinary Journal 170, 24–32.

Hanstock, T.L., Clayton, E.H., Li, K.M., et al., 2004. Anxiety and aggression associated with the fermentation of carbohydrates in the hindgut of rats. Physiology & Behavior 82, 357–368.

Harris, P.A., 2005. Hints on nutrition for optimal growth. Proceedings of the 1st BEVA & Waltham Nutrition Symposia "Equine Nutrition for All". Harrogate, United Kingdom.

Harris, P.A., Arkell, K., 2005. How understanding the digestive process can help minimise digestive disturbances due to diet and feeding practices. Proceedings of the 1st BEVA & Waltham Nutrition Symposia "Equine Nutrition for All". Harrogate, United Kingdom.

Harris, P.A., Coenen, M., Frape, D.L., et al., 2006. Equine nutrition and metabolic disease. In: Higgins, A., Snyder, J. (Eds.), Equine Manual. Elsevier Saunders, London.

Henderson, J.V., Waran, N.C., 2001. Reducing equine stereotypies using an Equiball. Animal Welfare 10, 73–80.

Hillyer, M.H., Taylor, F.G.R., Proudman, C.J., et al., 2002. Case control study to identify risk factors for simple colonic obstruction and distension colic in horses. Equine Veterinary Journal 34, 455–463.

Hoffman, R.M., 2003. Carbohydrate metabolism in horses. In: Ralston, S.L., Hintz, H.F. (Eds.), Recent Advances in Equine Nutrition 1. International Veterinary Information Service (www.ivis.org), Ithaca, New York.

Hoffman, R.M., Kronfeld, D.S., Cooper, W.L., et al., 2003. Glucose clearance in grazing mares is affected by diet, pregnancy, and lactation. Journal of Animal Science 81, 1764–1771.

Hoffman, R.M., Kronfeld, D.S., Herbein, J.H., et al., 1998. Dietary carbohydrates and fat influence milk composition and fatty acid profile of mare's milk. Journal of Nutrition 128 (Suppl.), 2708S–2711S.

Holland, J.L., Kronfeld, D.S., Hoffman, R.M., et al., 1996a. Weaning stress is affected by nutrition and weaning methods. Pferdeheilkunde 12, 257–260.

Holland, J.L., Kronfeld, D.S., Meacham, T.N., 1996b. Behavior of horses is affected by soy lecithin and corn oil in the diet. Journal of Animal Science 74, 1252–1255.

Hothersall, B., Nicol, C.J., Kelland, A., et al., 2008. Effects of diet on learning and responsive behavior of young foals. Proceedings of the International Society for Equitation Science. Dublin, Ireland, p. 82.

Husted, L., Sanchez, L.C., Olsen, S.N., et al., 2008. Effect of paddock vs. stall housing on 24 hour gastric pH within the proximal and ventral equine stomach. Equine Veterinary Journal 40, 337–341.

Jansson, A., Nyman, S., Lindholm, A., et al., 2002. Effects of dietary starch and sugar on exercise metabolism. Equine Veterinary Journal 34 (Suppl.), 17–21.

Johnson, K.G., Tyrrell, J., Rowe, J.B., et al., 1998. Behavioral changes in stabled horses given nontherapeutic levels of virginiamycin. Equine Veterinary Journal 30, 139–143.

Kidd, P.M., 2007. Clinical findings and structural-functional synergies with cell membrane phospholipids. Alternative Medicine Review 12, 207–227.

Klepser, T.B., Klepser, M.E., 1999. Unsafe and potentially safe herbal therapies. American Journal of Health-System Pharmacy 56, 125–138.

Kronfeld, D.S., Harris, P., 2003. Equine grain associated disorders. Compendium on Continuing Education for the Practicing Veterinarian 25, 974–983.

Kuntz, R., Kubalek, C., Ruf, T., et al., 2006. Seasonal adjustment of energy budget in a large wild mammal, the Przewalski horse (*Equus ferus przewalskii*) I. Energy intake. Journal of Experimental Biology 209, 4557–4565.

Lamoot, I., Hoffmann, M., 2004. Do season and habitat influence the behavior of Haffinger mares in a coastal dune area? Belgian Journal of Zoology 134, 97–103.

Leskanich, C.O., Noble, R.C., 1999. The comparative roles of polyunsaturated fatty acids in pig neonatal development. British Journal of Nutrition 81, 87–106.

Lim, S.Y., Suzuki, H., 2001. Changes in maze behavior of mice occur after sufficient accumulation of docosahexaenoic acid in brain. Journal of Nutrition 131, 319–324.

Linford, R.L., Obrien, T.R., Trout, D.R., 1993. Qualitative and morphometric radiographic findings in the distal phalanx and digital soft-tissues of sound thoroughbred racehorses. American Journal of Veterinary Research 54, 38–51.

Lorenzo-Figuera, M., Preston, T., Ott, E.A., et al., 2005. Meal-induced gastric relaxation and emptying in horses after ingestion of high-fat versus high-carbohydrate diets. American Journal of Veterinary Research 66, 897–906.

Luthersson, N., Nielsen, K.H., Harris, P., et al., 2009. Risk factors associated with equine gastric ulceration syndrome (EGUS) in 201 horses in Denmark. Equine Veterinary Journal 41, 625–630.

Mayes, E., Duncan, P., 1986. Temporal patterns of feeding in free-ranging horses. Behavior 96,105–129.

Macleay, J.M., Valberg, S.J., Pagan, J.D., et al., 1999. Effect of diet on thoroughbred horses with recurrent exertional rhabdomyolysis performing a standardised exercise test. Equine Vet J Suppl 30, 458–462.

Mahoney, C.R., Taylor, H.A., Kanarek, R.B., et al., 2005. Effect of breakfast composition on cognitive processes in elementary school children. Physiology & Behavior 85, 635–645.

Malmkvist, J., Christensen, J.W., 2007. A note on the effects of a commercial tryptophan product on horse reactivity. Applied Animal Behavior Science 107, 361–366.

Markus, C.R., Jonkman, L.M., Lammers, J.H.C.M., et al., 2005. Evening intake of alpha-lactalbumin increases plasma tryptophan availability and improves morning alertness and brain measures of attention. American Journal of Clinical Nutrition 81, 1026–1033.

Mason, G., 1991. Stereotypies – a critical review. Animal Behavior 41, 1015–1037.

McAfee, L.M., Mills, D.S., Cooper, J.J., 2002. The use of mirrors for the control of stereotypic weaving behavior in the stabled horse. Applied Animal Behavior Science 78, 159–173.

McBride, S.D., Long, L., 2001. Management of horses showing stereotypic behavior, owner perception and the implications for welfare. Veterinary Record 148, 799–802.

McGreevy, P., Nicol, C., 1998. Physiological and behavioral consequences associated with short-term prevention of crib-biting in horses. Physiology & Behavior 65, 15–23.

McGreevy, P.D., Cripps, P.J., French, N.P., et al., 1995. Management factors associated with stereotypic and redirected behavior in the thoroughbred horse. Equine Veterinary Journal 27, 86–91.

McGreevy, P.D., Webster, A.J.F., Nicol, C.J., 2001. Study of the behavior, digestive efficiency and gut transit times of crib-biting horses. Veterinary Record 148, 592–596.

Medina, B., Girard, I.D., Jacotot, E., et al., 2002. Effect of a preparation of Saccharomyces cerevisiae on microbial profiles and fermentation patterns in the large intestine of horses fed a high fiber or a high starch diet. Journal of Animal Science 80, 2600–2609.

Meunier-Salaun, M.C., Edwards, S.A., Robert, S., 2001. Effect of dietary fibre on the behavior and health of the restricted fed sow. Animal Feed Science and Technology 90, 53–69.

Mills, D.S., Clarke, A., 2002. Housing, management and welfare. In: Waran, N. (Ed.), The Welfare of Horses. Kluwer Academic Publishers, Dordrecht.

Mills, D.S., Eckley, S., Cooper, J.J., 2000. Thoroughbred bedding preferences, associated behavior differences and their implications for equine welfare. Animal Science 70, 95–106.

Mills, D.S., Macleod, C.A., 2002. The response of crib-biting and windsucking in horses to dietary supplementation with an antacid mixture. Ippologia 13, 33–41.

Moeller, B.A., Mccall, C.A., Silverman, S.J., et al., 2008. Estimation of saliva production in crib-biting and normal horses. Journal of Equine Veterinary Science 28, 85–90.

Murray, M.J., Eichorn, E.S., 1996. Effects of intermittent feed deprivation, intermittent feed deprivation with ranitidine administration, and stall confinement with ad libitum access to hay on gastric ulceration in horses. American Journal of Veterinary Research 57, 1599–1603.

Murray, M.J., Haven, M.L., Eichorn, E.S., et al., 1997. Effects of omeprazole on healing of naturally-occurring gastric ulcers in Thoroughbred racehorses. Equine Veterinary Journal 29, 425–429.

Nicol, C.J., 1999a. Stereotypies and their relationship to management. In: Harris, P.G., Davidson, H.P.B., Green, R. (Eds.), British Equine Veterinary Association Specialist Day on Behavior and Nutrition. Equine Veterinary Journal, Harrogate.

Nicol, C.J., 1999b. Understanding equine stereotypies. Equine Veterinary Journal 28 (Suppl.), 20–25.

Nicol, C.J., Badnell-Waters, A.J., 2005. Suckling behavior in domestic foals and the development of abnormal oral behavior. Animal Behavior 70, 21–29.

Nicol, C.J., Badnell-Waters, A.J., et al., 2005. The effects of diet and weaning method on the behavior of young horses. Applied Animal Behavior Science 95, 205–221.

Nicol, C.J., Davidson, H.P.B., Harris, P.A., et al., 2002. Study of crib-biting and gastric inflammation and ulceration in young horses. Veterinary Record 151, 658–662.

Nieto, J.E., Snyder, J.R., Vatistas, N.J., et al., 2009. Effect of gastric ulceration on physiologic responses to exercise in horses. American Journal of Veterinary Research 70, 787–795.

Ninomiya, S., 2007. Social leaning and stereotypy in horses. Behavioral Processes 76, 22–23.

Noble, G.K., Brockwell, Y.M., Munn, K.J., et al., 2008. Effects of a commercial dose of L-tryptophan on plasma tryptophan concentrations and behavior in horses. Equine Veterinary Journal 40, 51–56.

Ordakowski, A.L., Davidson, H.P.B., Redgate, S.E., et al., 2003. Characteristics of foal feeding behavior. Proceedings of the WALTHAM International Symposium. Bangkok.

Pagan, J.D., Harris, P.A., Kennedy, M.A.P., et al., 1999. Feed type and intake affects glycaemic response in Thoroughbred horses. Proceedings of the Equine Nutrition & Physiology Symposium. Raleigh, North Carolina, USA.

Peeters, E., Driessen, B., Steegmans, R., et al., 2004. Effect of supplemental tryptophan, vitamin E, and a herbal product on responses by pigs to vibration. Journal of Animal Science 82, 2410–2420.

Pell, S.M., McGreevy, P.D., 1999. A study of cortisol and beta-endorphin levels in stereotypic and normal Thoroughbreds. Applied Animal Behavior Science 64, 81–90.

Poleszak, E., Szewczyk, B., Kedzierska, E., et al., 2004. Antidepressant- and anxiolytic-like activity of magnesium in mice. Pharmacology Biochemistry and Behavior 78, 7–12.

Ralston, S.L., 1984. Controls of feeding in horses. Journal of Animal Science 59, 1354–1361.

Ralston, S.L., 2007. Evidence-based equine nutrition. Veterinary Clinics of North America: Equine Practice 23, 365–384.

Ralston, S.L., Vandenbroek, G., Baile, C.A., 1979. Feed-intake patterns and associated blood-glucose, free fatty-acid and insulin changes in ponies. Journal of Animal Science 49, 838–845.

Ransom, J.I., Cade, B.S., Hobbs, N.T., 2010. Influences of immunocontraception on time budgets, social behavior, and body condition in feral horses. Applied Animal Behavior Science 124, 51–60.

Read, D.H., Harrington, D.D., 1981. Experimentally induced thiamine-deficiency in beagle dogs – clinical observations. American Journal of Veterinary Research 42, 984–991.

Redbo, I., Redbo-Torstensson, P., Odberg, F.O., et al., 1998. Factors affecting behavioral disturbances in race-horses. Animal Science 66, 475–481.

Redgate, S.E., Ordakowski-Burk, A.L., Davidson, H.P.B., et al., 2004. A preliminary study to investigate the effect of diet on the behavior of weanling horses. Proceedings of the International Society for Applied Ethology. Helsinki, Finland.

Redondo, A.J., Carranza, J., Trigo, P., 2009. Fat diet reduces stress and intensity of startle reaction in horses. Applied Animal Behavior Science 118, 69–75.

Rowe, J.B., Lees, M.J., Pethick, D.W., 1994. Prevention of acidosis and laminitis associated with grain feeding in horses. Journal of Nutrition 124, 2742S–2744S.

Salter, R.E., Hudson, R.J., 1979. Feeding ecology of feral horses in Western Alberta. Journal of Range Management 32, 221–225.

Schaechter, J.D., Wurtman, R.J., 1990. Serotonin release varies with brain tryptophan levels. Brain Research 532, 203–210.

Schloss, P., Williams, D.C., 1998. The serotonin transporter: a primary target for anti-depressant drugs. Journal of Psychopharmacology 12, 115–121.

Stull, C.L., Rodiek, A.V., 1988. Responses of Blood Glucose, Insulin and Cortisol Concentrations to Common Equine Diets. Journal of Nutrition 118, 206–213.

Swyers, K.L., Burk, A.O., Hartsock, T.G., et al., 2008. Effects of direct-fed microbial supplementation on digestibility and fermentation end-products in horses fed low- and high-starch concentrates. Journal of Animal Science 86, 2596–2608.

Thorne, J.B., Goodwin, D., Kennedy, M.J., et al., 2005. Foraging enrichment for individually housed horses: practicality and effects on behavior. Applied Animal Behavior Science 94, 149–164.

Tinker, M.K., White, N.A., Lessard, P., et al., 1997. Prospective study of equine colic risk factors. Equine Veterinary Journal 29, 454–458.

Treiber, K.H., Boston, R.C., Kronfeld, D.S., et al., 2005. Insulin resistance and compensation in Thoroughbred weanlings adapted to high-glycemic meals. Journal Of Animal Science 83, 2357–2364.

van Dierendonck, M.C., Bandi, N., Batdorj, D., et al., 1994. Behavioral observations of reintroduced Takhi or Przewalski horses (*Equus ferus przewalskii*) in Mongolia. Applied Animal Behavior Science 50, 95–114.

Venna, V.R., Deplanque, D., Allet, C., et al., 2009. PUFA induce antidepressant-like effects in parallel to structural and molecular changes in the hippocampus. Psychoneuroendocrinology 34, 199–211.

Visser, E.K., Van Reenen, C.G., Hopster, H., et al., 2001. Quantifying aspects of young horses' temperament: consistency of behavioral variables. Applied Animal Behavior Science 74, 241–258.

Visser, E.K., Van Reenen, C.G., Van Der Werf, J.T.N., et al., 2002. Heart rate and heart rate variability during a novel object test and a handling test in young horses. Physiology & Behavior 76, 289–296.

Wainwright, P.E., Xing, H.C., Ward, G.R., et al., 1999. Water maze performance is unaffected in artificially reared rats fed diets supplemented with arachidonic acid and docosahexaenoic acid. Journal of Nutrition 129, 1079–1089.

Waters, A.J., Nicol, C.J., French, N.P., 2002. Factors influencing the development of stereotypic and redirected behaviors in young horses: findings of a four year prospective epidemiological study. Equine Veterinary Journal 34, 572–579.

Willard, J.G., Willard, J.C., Wolfram, S.A., et al., 1977. Effects of diet on cecal pH and feeding behavior of horses. Journal of Animal Science 45, 87–93.

Williams, C.A., Kronfeld, D.S., Staniar, W.B., et al., 2001. Plasma glucose and insulin responses of Thoroughbred mares fed a meal high in starch and sugar or fat and fiber. Journal of Animal Science 79, 2196–2201.

Williamson, A., Rogers, C.W., Firth, E.C., 2007. A survey of feeding, management and faecal pH of Thoroughbred racehorses in the North Island of New Zealand. New Zealand Veterinary Journal 55, 337–341.

Wilson, A.D., Badnell-Waters, A.J., Bice, R., et al., 2007. The effects of diet on blood glucose, insulin, gastrin and the serum tryptophan: Large neutral amino acid ratio in foals. Veterinary Journal 174, 139–146.

Winskill, L.C., Waran, N.K., Young, R.J., 1996. The effect of a foraging device (a modified 'Edinburgh foodball') on the behavior of the stabled horse. Applied Animal Behavior Science 48, 25–35.

Zeyner, A., Geißler, C., Dittrich, A., 2004. Effects of hay intake and feeding sequence on variables in faeces and faecal water (dry matter, pH value, organic acids, ammonia, buffering capacity) of horses. Journal of Animal Physiology and Animal Nutrition 88, 7–19.

26 Controversial areas in equine nutrition and feeding management

The Editors' views

Patricia A. Harris, Manfred Coenen, Raymond J. Geor

Practical feeding of horses is both an art and a science – the science provides foundation knowledge for the formulation of a ration and the art is adjusting this ration to best fit the circumstances of an individual horse, taking into account the needs and beliefs of the owner as well as the availability of feedstuffs, environmental influences etc. There is not one correct way to feed any horse, providing some flexibility to individualize rations but also enabling the development of myths and feeding traditions that become established practice and yet are based on little or no objective evidence.

This chapter looks at some of the arguments commonly put forward for and against a range of nutritional and feeding management practices/beliefs. Wherever possible, our comments are based on scientific evidence and refer to the state-of-the-art as we perceive it; however, where scientific evidence is not available or is inconclusive our comments will of necessity be derived from individual personal experiences and even beliefs. Even when scientific evidence is available, conclusions often vary according to the circumstances and the individual. In this chapter, therefore, we have tried to highlight some of these controversial areas and provide *our* current opinion. For this reason, reference citations have been kept to a minimum.

Questions concerning feed intake

Can a healthy horse lose condition due to its biological limitation in feed intake?

The answer to this important question is simply NO, even for horses with high energy requirements (e.g. lactation or heavy athletic training and competition). In healthy horses, weight loss will reflect problems with feed quality and/or adequacy of supply.

Should dry matter intake be expressed as a percentage of bodyweight (BW) rather than metabolic BW (kg$^{0.75}$ BW)?

Here, the answer is less straightforward – some of the key arguments for and against are given below:

Yes: The determination of metabolic body weight is an allometric scaling procedure that provides an across species term for energy requirements at maintenance level. The scaling factor commonly used (0.75) is not necessarily optimal for the horse (and certainly is not always valid for other biological aspects, e.g. heart size). Perhaps more importantly from a practical viewpoint, the expression of dry matter (DM) intake as a % of actual BW is much easier to apply in the field, e.g. DM intake = 2% of BW is much more applicable than the artificial term of 120 g DM/kg$^{0.75}$ BW.

No: Over a wide range of BW (e.g., 100 to 1000 kg) DM intake cannot be a simple linear function of BW. Ponies show different chewing and swallowing characteristics than horses; the ratio of feed mass to dental surface area differs between small and large equids and the ingesta transit time will also vary.

Our opinion: Several biological phenomena related to intake, such as oropharyngeal feed processing, are not linearly related to BW i.e. they are scaled by a factor <1. Although 0.75 may not be optimal, given the biological relationship between DM intake and energy requirement there is rationale for use of metabolic BW (i.e., DM kg$^{0.75}$ BW). Even so, further adjustments may be needed for certain breeds/individuals and circumstances. For example, ponies maintained on pasture may have proportionally a higher DM intake than a horse even when expressed on a metabolic BW basis; thin ponies in the summer with ad libitum access to feed may have much higher intake than an obese animal of the same breed and size offered the same feed (see Dugdale et al 2011). Expressing the requirements for other nutrients as a percentage of BW or DM intake is similarly problematical and currently not recommended (see also Chapter 9).

Has the limit of dry matter intake in horses been determined?

Much of the relevant literature is discussed in Chapter 3.

Yes: We have sufficient information available for most practical purposes but recent work has suggested that average intakes are likely to be higher than previously suggested (e.g., up to 12 kg DM for a 250 kg nonobese pony or 4.8% of BW - Dugdale et al 2011). It seems unlikely that there is much more flexibility for higher intakes considering the time required for ingestion of 1 kg DM.

No: Not in all circumstances and for all types of feed. Complex interactions between type of feed, available time and physiological status are likely to impact maximal DM intake.

Our opinion: We have sufficient information to define limits of DM intake by a healthy horse/pony with free access to typical feedstuffs and with no restriction in time budget. It is important to understand that, from evolutionary, physiological and behavioral viewpoints; the horse is adapted to spend long periods of time engaged in foraging/feed ingestion activity. Management practices that encourage prolonged feeding activity are beneficial to health and welfare as long as energy overconsumption is avoided.

Should we be using minimal requirements (RQ) or basic recommendations (RC) or "optimal" recommendations (OR)?

The adequacy of energy intake can be readily assessed by repeated evaluation of body condition; however, it is not possible to visually determine whether or not the horse is being fed a balanced diet providing recommended levels of amino acids, macro- or micronutrients - unless the intakes are sufficiently low or high to cause overt signs of deficiency/toxicity. Overt deficiency or toxicity is rare in the developed world although conditions such as big head disease (nutritional secondary hyperparathyroidism due to a marked imbalance in the Ca:P ratio of a diet through excessive phosphorus intake) are still reported in some countries. Animals may appear to be fit and healthy, yet their diet at the time of examination may not meet one or more nutritional requirements.

In discussions on how to feed horses, it is frequently stated that "they have had horses for years, never ensured that they were receiving adequate micronutrients and never had any problems"; and therefore: "the recommendations must be wrong". This reflects a common misunderstanding of RQ and RCs which is discussed below. For the purpose of the following discussions, we have used the following definitions:

- Minimum requirement (RQ) is taken to be representative of the minimal intakes to sustain life in an average healthy horse within the population;
- Basic recommendations (RC) include a "safety margin" so that they should cover the minimal needs for the majority of healthy animals in a population; and
- Optimal recommendations (OR) enable the needs of particular individuals or groups of individuals with specific needs to be met (e.g. those animals with certain clinical conditions or experiencing increased "stress"). By necessity, ORs tend to be more opinion based.

Many nutrition texts and feeding standard publications (e.g., National Research Council: 2007) present RCs or a mixture of both RQs and RCs. The main rationale for RCs is to include safety margins or to compensate for absence of complete data on strict RQs. Although it may seem pedantic, it is very important to differentiate between RQ and RC. Feeding below RC is not in conflict with sound nutritional practice, but feeding below RQ is in conflict with scientific evidence and often problematic from a legal standpoint (not of minor importance).

However, it is still possible to feed below the RQ without clinically apparent adverse effects. Conversely, problems related to nutrition may become apparent when horses are fed at or above the RQ. In part, these divergent scenarios can occur because the system used to define requirement data assumes that all horses are the same and therefore, for example, the needs of a Clydesdale are identical to those of a Thoroughbred. Unless a diet is obviously imbalanced, it can often be difficult to practically determine whether the ration is adequate or not unless a full nutritional evaluation is carried out. Full nutritional evaluations are expensive, can only represent a snapshot in time, and can be difficult to achieve especially if pasture forage is part of the ration. Day-to-day variability in nutrient profile in feedstuffs (pasture, preserved forages, even commercial feeds) coupled with individual differences in intake make it impossible to achieve complete accuracy. That said, as an initial step it is possible to use generic tables of analytical data to get an indication of whether the diet is likely to be limiting in one or more nutrients.

Published nutritional surveys in which in-depth nutritional analyses were used have reported that many categories of horse, even elite performance animals, are often not being fed the RQ intakes of several key nutrients - let alone more "optimal levels" recommended by some. Yet, these animals are still competing and, according to their owners, apparently healthy. There are several possible interpretations: (1) the recommended RQ intakes are not valid in general or for those individuals specifically; (2) the imbalance is being masked by an oversupply of a complementary nutrient; or (3) the imbalance has not been present for long enough to manifest as a clinical problem. Alternatively, the horse may have a problem associated with the diet but this link has not been made by the owner/trainer. As many horses change owners relatively frequently - and young thoroughbred racehorses rarely stay with the same trainer until they are geriatric - it is very difficult to determine the long-term chronic effects on health, etc. of suboptimal nutrient intakes at various times within an animal's life. There has been little or no work on the concept of epigenetics in the horse but perhaps we should consider this more seriously in the future. Ideally, it would be great to raise, train, compete and retire large number of animals on diets that provide all the nutrients at the level we consider to be suboptimal, at recommended levels and at optimal levels. This, however, remains an unrealistic goal.

Do we know what the true RQ is? There are differences in RQ data published by the various authorities. Although the concept of an RQ is not debatable, in reality *there is a range of values that represent RQ for any nutrient* and there are differences in what can be considered an RQ because of the following:

1. *Dimensions*: It is usual to standardize RQ data by referring to BW or metabolic BW (i.e. $BW^{0.75}$). As discussed above, the use of actual BW implies a linear change in requirements e.g. from a 100-kg pony to an 800-kg draft horse. Many of the published RQ values were derived from studies that used animals in the middle of this BW range and consequently the RQs may not be applicable to animals at the extremes of BW. This is why some authorities apply allometric scaling, such as $BW^{0.75}$ (or another exponent number), in the development of RQ values. Another issue is the use of unit per day or unit per kg DMI for expression of RQs. The latter is traditionally used for trace elements and is very convenient in daily use; however, this dimension fixes the nutrient requirement to another nutritional factor (feed intake) that has its own flexibility – as discussed above.
2. *Basic method for defining RQ:* The basic principle is to calculate RQ = endogenous losses/utilization + product/utilization. This is commonly referred to as the *factorial approach.* In many instances, RQ values have been derived from data for other species rather than the equid, and this approach may not be valid. The utilization rate must be evaluated in animals in different physiologic states across a range of intakes. Variance in the applied utilization rate has a significant impact on the calculated RQs.
3. The method for defining RQ described above ignores the *interaction between different metabolic systems*, as it takes a nutrient in isolation and then balances input with minimal output to reach the point of equilibrium. Individual nutrients, however, have important impacts on other systems e.g. feeding at the RQ for protein may limit the capability of the immune system. Calculating RQs based on purely the factorial approach may have adverse effects on body homeostatic mechanisms. Chloride is a simple example; feeding Cl strictly according to the RQ derived from the factorial approach may result in lowered Cl concentration in blood and an alkalemic shift in acid-base balance.
4. *Experimental data*: Differences arise in transforming experimental data, especially if results across different studies are inconsistent. A good example is milk yield in mares. The published data show a very wide range even when they are standardized to BW or $BW^{0.75}$. As a result, there is no single universal model that can be used for incorporation of milk yield into RQ calculations.
5. *How to quantify other biological effects such as the impact of exercise?* Exercise effort should be readily quantifiable; a horse of known BW moves from A to B in a certain time. In contrast to daily gain or milk yield, however, exercise is difficult to quantify in terms of additional requirements for energy and nutrients. There are several external factors that contribute to marked variation in the metabolic cost of converting chemical energy into kinetic energy, including fitness, dietary regimen, environmental conditions, terrain etc.

Our opinion:

1. A primary goal in the development of requirement data is to define the energy and nutrient provision that drives any metabolic process without activating compensatory strategies in the animal in order to cope with either limited or excess availability of that nutrient. In some situations, health and performance, at least in the short term, will be maintained in the face of limited nutrient supply due to the impact of compensatory mechanisms (e.g., enhanced absorption efficiency and/or reduced excretion). This does not imply that nutrient provision below the guidelines provided in this book and elsewhere is recommended.
2. Clarity is needed in recommendations on the amount of any nutrient that should be provided in the ration. It should be made clear whether the value is a *requirement* and therefore should be considered (practically) as a minimal level to sustain life (with the provisos above) vs. a *recommendation*, which implies that a safety margin has been built-in. There also may be justification for developing rations on the basis of *optimal intakes*, especially when a particular system (such as the immune system) may benefit from increased intakes (e.g. horses in stressful circumstances such as intense physical activity and travel for athletic competition). Nonetheless, at present most *optimal* recommendations are based on personal experiences or beliefs and have little or no scientific basis.
3. For most end-users (nutritionists, veterinarians, etc.), we recommend the selection and use of one reference publication (NRC, GEH or INRA). Tables 1-5 in Appendix show energy and nutrient recommendations as published by the NRC and GEH and as suggested in this book for a 500-kg horse at various life stages (together with values used by one of the editors (P.H.) that represent a mix of recommended and optimal requirements).

The dilemma of "supplementation"

Even the term supplement is controversial as it can be taken to include products that: (1) restore nutritional balance to a ration, e.g., forage or cereal balancer feeds; or (2) provide a safety margin when the nutrient quality of a ration is not known (see Chapter 19). The utility of such supplements is clear and is not further discussed here. Instead, this discussion focuses on compounds or plant material that are used to provide one or more nutrients in a specific preparation (e.g., amino acids in gelatin) or one or more non-nutritional factors (e.g., flavonoids) in order to support metabolic processes (e.g. antioxidative capacity) or provide some other purported benefit. This type of supplementation is one of the most hotly debated topics in equine nutrition. The challenge for science and practice is to find the balance – on the one hand, not immediately dismissing the possible advantages of a given supplement (even if there is a dearth of efficacy and safety data), while on the other hand, not accepting all "claims" that lack any supporting evidence.

Do we need supplements?

Many arguments for and against the use of supplements have been given over the years - examples are given below:

No: Supplements are unnecessary because a balanced diet will provide all the nutrients required.

Yes: One of the tenets of good feeding is to feed the horse as an individual, and supplements are a means by which the diet can be tailored. A supplement enables one to consider specific individual conditions (e.g. a horse with a nervous temperament or poor hooves) or environmental risks (e.g. the effect of housing on lung health; the impact of travel on the immune system). Supplementation in such circumstances may work to counteract the imbalance between nutrient supply and demand and help to restore "normality". In other situations supplementation may help to provide additional boost or support to enable enhanced performance or reduce the risk of certain clinical conditions developing.

Do they work?

No: While there has been a marked increase in the number of specialized dietary supplements on the market, this has not been matched by a concomitant increase in research on the safety, efficacy etc. of these products. Many substances are marketed without adequate understanding of their function *in the horse*. Too often there is little or no evidence regarding the effect of a supplement on a particular metabolic or physiological mechanism, nor data to suggest that this process is of any relevance to the health, behavior or athletic performance of a horse. For most supplements, there is little scientific evidence derived *from the horse* to support marketing claims. Reported positive effects can reflect owner perceptions (placebo effect).

Yes/some: There is increasingly evidence that nutrition can play a very important role in the management of certain disease conditions in man and other animals - nutritional requirements may change or the affected individual may respond to the inclusion of particular nutrients or feedstuffs in the diet. In the equine field too, there is prior and emerging scientific evidence for a few products/supplements (e.g. high doses of biotin and certain hoof problems; antioxidant supplement and lung health; Kirschvink et al 2002). Even if scientific support is currently lacking, this should not be taken as indication that a given supplement is not of benefit to the horse.

Our opinion:

- There can be considerable misinformation and hype associated with some supplements, and this makes it very difficult for owners/feeders to make informed decisions regarding the "value" of a particular supplement.
- Some form of tailoring of the diet may be of benefit in some horses. For some animals, such tailoring may occur through the appropriate choice of the feedstuffs that make up the core ration but for many the addition of one or more supplements is the primary method. It is important to realize that horses are *individuals* and they do not always respond in the same way and so what might work for one individual may not for another. The underlying cause of a particular problem may also differ between individuals, which again may affect their response to the supplement. For example, although an adequate and balanced diet will in most cases support good quality hoof horn and growth, under certain circumstances additional supplementation of biotin (e.g., 3–4 mg/100 kg BW/day for a minimum of 6–9 months) will enhance hoof quality. However, some types of hoof horn defects will not respond to biotin alone and other nutrients in adequate or perhaps higher than normally recommended levels may be needed for benefits to occur. Some problems with hoof wall quality and growth may not respond to any form of nutritional manipulation and, unfortunately, clinical evaluation does not enable prediction of these different outcomes.
- In an ideal scenario, the following information would be available to guide selection of an ingredient for inclusion in a ration:
  1. Identification of a target metabolic process known to be "limiting" to one or more physiological function
  2. Knowledge of how this process might be beneficially influenced
  3. Identification of an ingredient or compound that might have such effects
  4. Definition of the active ingredient(s)
  5. Information on potential side effects
  6. Verification that use of the product does not violate legal and regulatory mandates
  7. Evidence that the product can be absorbed from the gastrointestinal tract
  8. Evidence that there is a positive impact on the target process in the horse
  9. Data on the source and formulation of the ingredient that is linked to the evidence above
  10. Effective dosage or dose range for a particular source and formulation in the horse
  11. Safety data based on both experimental studies and when fed in the field – using indicators appropriate to the particular compound and its postulated effects.

Consider a Thoroughbred horse that has begun a rigorous breaking and training program that results in recurrent muscle pain. The goal of decreasing oxidative and inflammatory damage to muscle may initiate the search for plant or plant extracts (points 1 and 2 above). Such a search could lead one to consider "ginger" and, based on work in other species (point 3), use of a ginger supplement might be explored. Data related to points 4–6 could be gathered from the literature as well as the various regulatory authorities. The NRC safety of dietary supplements for horses, dogs and cats provides useful guidance in particular with respect to historical safe intakes and presumed safe intakes (NRC 2009). Information from points 1–6 should be the absolute minimum basis for a decision on the inclusion of an ingredient in the diet of a horse. Ideally, however, data from points 7–11 will be evaluated prior to making this decision. The key point here is that, in most circumstances, it is unlikely that each point (especially points 7–10) can be supported by equine-specific information

Safety is an important consideration that is often forgotten with respect to supplements. One argument is that the "only thing hurt by trying a product that doesn't work is your wallet" – but this is not always true. The importance of proven efficacy with respect to safety may in fact depend on the nature of the supplement and its intended use. Consider the feeding of a "calming agent" – if this has a placebo effect on the rider so that they ride more positively and confidently this may result in a better behaved horse even if the agent itself has no direct effect on the behavior of the animal. This could be considered a positive outcome even if the product does not work – on the other hand, if a product is marketed to reduce the risk of a certain condition such as laminitis and it does not work, the animal will be placed at clinical risk. Utilising a supplement in the absence of a diagnosis may delay pursuit of a thorough clinical workup (e.g., feeding an iron supplement to a horse with anemia due to a chronic inflammatory condition). A supplement can also result directly in an adverse effect through toxicity, interaction with other components of the ration or medications etc. The nature of the supplement, how it was made or processed, what it is being fed with, the status of the horse, etc. all may influence whether a particular supplement is safe or not. Depending on the material, there may be a risk of contamination by unwanted and/or potentially toxic materials (NRC 2009). Cross-reactions and contraindications are known to occur between certain medicinal/drug therapies and herbal/spice preparations. Taking into consideration all sources of a particular nutrient in the ration can be very important when considering adding a supplement or a mixture of different supplements, all of which contain that nutrient. For selenium, the differences between adequate, optimum and potential toxic levels of intake are fairly small, and toxic levels can be reached if multiple selenium-containing supplements are used. Safety can be difficult to determine under all circumstances, for example the fact that certain herbs have been fed for centuries does not mean that they are always safe to be fed at <u>any</u> intake level and in any form as has been demonstrated for garlic (see NRC 2009).

Conflict between athletic performance and optimal digestive health and behavior

In general terms, provision of too little energy will result in weight loss, loss of performance and possibly illness, whereas the feeding of excess energy may result in weight gain, hyperactivity and other adverse effects. Therefore, the feeding of an appropriate supply of energy is critical to health, vitality and performance of any horse. Additionally, there is evidence that the source of energy can impact health and performance, for example, the potential adverse effects of starch-rich diets on gastrointestinal health and the current recommendation of no more than 2 g starch/kg BW/day. However, it can be difficult to convince trainers to feed a racehorse within this guideline, highlighting a discrepancy between what is recommended by "theoretical" nutritionists and what is likely to be adopted in the field.

What is the minimum forage requirement?

Bodyweight and gut fill are important considerations for the performance horse. For every kilogram of average dry hay, around 2.5–3.5 kg of water may be consumed; this will add to the weight of the horse and may adversely affect performance. Therefore, many trainers believe that forage should be restricted to reduce gut fill and therefore body weight in high performance horses. An additional concern raised is that "filling" a horse with forage reduces appetite for cereals and therefore reduces daily energy intake.

Our opinion:

- Discussion of this issue often ignores the important role of roughage/forage in digestion, metabolism and health. Consider the feeding of 10 kg DM hay with either low (40%) or high (70%) DM digestibility. Simplistically, this will result in 6 and 3 kg of undigested DM, respectively. Assuming a consistent fecal water content (20% DM in feces), the low and high digestibility hays will require 24 and 12 liters of water, respectively. In other words, the lower digestibility hay will result in a doubling of gut fill at the same level of intake. In other words, the actual feeding value or quality of the forage can have as much of an effect on gut fill and water turnover as the amount of forage being fed. Therefore, high performance horses should be fed high quality forage to minimize the impact on gut fill.
- There is an additional and essential benefit to good quality forage with high amounts of fermentable nonhydrolyzable carbohydrates such as cellulose or pectins. The water trapped within these materials results in an enforced water transfer from the small intestine into the hindgut. These carbohydrates are well fermented and decomposed in the hindgut, so most of the bound water is released and available for absorption; this may help to offset sweat fluid losses in horses performing endurance exercise and/or work in hot conditions. Less well fermented

forages retain more water and so less water is available for absorption.

- There are perhaps two main reasons for considering that there is a minimum requirement for forage (and fermentable fiber):
  - *Support of gastrointestinal function and health,* as discussed in several chapters (see Chapter 34).
  - *Benefit to behavior* – in a discussion on requirements this is perhaps a revolutionary idea. The nutrition–behavior interaction in horses is simple but difficult to accept in traditional feeding practice. The natural time budget of the horse can be split into: (a) feeding (12–15 h per day), (b) social contacts, (c) standing and walking, and (d) sleep. If we use the horse for work (e.g., transportation of tourists in cities), it will be necessary to reduce the time available for activities a, b and c. To ensure adequate energy intake in the face of this time constraint, the feeding of a higher energy, less bulky ration can be practiced. If we use the same diet without the time commitment to work, the horse will not double sleep time, may not be able to increase time in social activity, and is not able to forage for its "hotwired" 12–15 h period. Several studies have reported an unacceptable increase in abnormal behaviors with low forage intakes (see Chapter 25). The most promising strategy for prevention of such behaviors is to enable the horse to spend as much time as possible in feed intake-related behavior. Environmental enrichment devices and mechanisms to prolong intake time are especially helpful when forage intakes have to be reduced in horses or ponies on a weight loss regimen.

Conclusion: To ensure gastrointestinal and behavioral health, the following is provided as a recommendation – feed forage (grass and preserved forages) at 15 g DM/kg BW/day to all animals, including those with high energy requirements (in which case young less mature high energy providing forages should be considered). For many animals, forage should represent the majority of the ration (a forage balancer feed should be added to ensure a balanced diet). The absolute minimum level of forage provision for animals undergoing feed restriction for weight loss purposes is 10 g DM/kg BW/day. A target minimum for other animals, including race horses, is 12.5 g DM/kg BW/day.

Is there a minimum dietary starch (and/or simple sugar requirement?

It is well recognized that muscle glycogen is an important source of energy for ATP synthesis in muscle during intensive exercise (see Chapter 2). Both short-term, intense exercise and longer-duration, submaximal exercise is associated with a substantial decrease in muscle glycogen stores. Furthermore, low muscle glycogen content can contribute to skeletal muscle fatigue and poor performance. Therefore, provision of feedstuffs that support muscle glycogen synthesis is an important consideration in the development of rations for athletic horses. For human athletes, a diet that provides at least 65–70% of energy as hydrolyzable carbohydrates (starches and sugars) appears to be optimal for ongoing restoration of muscle glycogen stores. Similarly, there is a common belief that the diet of athletic horses must contain a certain quantity of starch (and sugar) to support adequate muscle glycogen concentrations. Nonetheless, knowledge of the relationship between diet composition and muscle glycogen storage in the horse remains incomplete. As discussed in Chapter 2, there are marked differences in carbohydrate (CHO) metabolism between horses and humans. The horse has a limited ability to digest hydrolyzable CHO and its main source of energy is derived from fermentation of cellulose, hemicellulose and other fermentable fibers. As well, the rate of post-exercise muscle glycogen synthesis is two- to threefold slower in the horse when compared to man and, in contrast to the outcome in human athletes, feeding strategies involving diets high in hydrolyzable CHO do not substantially alter the rate of muscle glycogen replenishment (see next section). So, is there a minimum dietary starch (and simple sugar) requirement?

No (in many situations): It can be argued that for many (if not most) horses engaged in regular exercise training and competition, there is no requirement for dietary starch. Several factors need to be taken into consideration with respect to the impact of dietary management on energy metabolism and performance in animals used for athletic activities, including the intensity of exercise (which influences the mix of energy substrates used for ATP synthesis and the extent of muscle glycogen utilization) and the interval between hard exercise bouts (and therefore the time available for replenishment of muscle glycogen stores).

During light and moderate intensity exercise, a mix of different substrates (long-chain fatty acids, blood glucose, VFAs and muscle glycogen) will be used for ATP synthesis in muscle. At high-intensity exercise, there is increased reliance on muscle glycogen but even during racing (1600–2000 m) in Thoroughbred or Standardbred horses muscle glycogen concentrations decrease by no more than 25–30%. Providing the interval between hard exercise bouts is no shorter than 2–3 days, muscle glycogen stores will be replenished regardless of diet composition (see next section). Interestingly, the muscle (gluteus medius) glycogen concentrations of Standardbred trotters in exercise training that were fed forage-only diets ranged between 550 and 630 mmol/kg dry weight, comparable to values reported for horses maintained on conventional forage/grain rations (Essén-Gustavsson et al 2010). In this study, horses were fed forages with either "high" (16.6%) or "low" (12.5%) crude protein. Muscle glycogen concentrations were ~13% higher with the high CP forage, perhaps due to higher dietary supply of amino acids and/or water-soluble carbohydrates (WSC; high: ~160 g/100 kg BW/day vs. low: ~105 g/100 kg BW/day). Whether this difference in muscle glycogen content was due to the higher CP, WSC, or some other factor remains to be determined.

Yes (in some circumstances): Anecdotally, racehorses appear to perform better when the ration contains some starch (and simple sugar), with the suspicion that muscle glycogen concentrations are suboptimal when the diet provides <10% DE from starch and simple sugar. These anecdotal observations require confirmation by well-designed studies.

Our opinion: On balance, there is not an absolute requirement for dietary starch and sugar. Although further work is needed to establish the effect of diet composition on muscle glycogen metabolism in horses performing different levels of exercise, current information suggests that the feeding of diets rich in starch and simple sugars is not essential for the maintenance of muscle glycogen concentrations within the expected range of ~500–700 mmol/kg dry weight.

Is there a maximum in starch (+ simple sugars) intake for horses?

To clarify, the term water soluble carbohydrate (WSC) is used to describe the combination of simple (primarily glucose, sucrose, and fructose) and more complex (oligosaccharides and fructans) sugars. Starch, which is formed by polymers of glucose, is not water soluble and therefore is not a component of the WSC fraction. The simple sugars and starch can be digested in the small intestine providing digestive capacity has not been exceeded (with glucose and fructose as the primary products of this small intestinal digestion). Alternatively, they can be fermented resulting in the production of volatile fatty acids and, specifically if rapidly fermented by Gram-positive bacteria, lactic acid. This fermentation starts in the stomach, and depending on the transit time may continue in the small intestine, but the main site of fermentation is the hindgut (see Chapter 8). Whether there is a maximum simple sugar and starch (SS) intake for horses (on a per meal basis) needs to be evaluated from a number of different viewpoints.

1. *Gastric function*: When large cereal-based (SS) meals are fed, the swallowed bolus has a higher DM content than for a forage or pasture based meal and the stomach contents, therefore, have a higher DM content; there is slower and/or reduced mixing of the feed with the gastric juices, and therefore an increased risk of dysfermentation. Whether this results in a clinical or subclinical problem may depend on factors such as the amount of available sugars and starches plus the individual animal's microbial population. The products of gastric fermentation likely influence the risk of gastric ulceration and there appears to be an increased risk of gastric ulceration with high starch intakes – in one study, risk of grade 2 nonglandular ulceration was significant at starch intake >1 g/kg BW per meal and >2 g/kg BW/day estimated starch (see Chapter 34). Finally, high-starch meals (e.g., cereal grains, sweet feeds) also produce a temporary enforced gastric fill as the rate of input of swallowed feed exceeds the rate of emptying. With such rations therefore exists the risk for gastric discomfort and rupture at the greater curvature. Although such conditions are not induced typically by the ingestion of normal diets, depending on the size of the meal there can be a temporary gastric overload and possibly gastric discomfort.
2. *Intestinal microbiota*: It is generally accepted that very high starch/sugar intakes can result in disturbances to gut function and adverse clinical sequelae such as laminitis and colic (see Chapters 27 and 29). However, more moderate starch intakes can still significantly influence the intestinal microbiota. A ration of 50% hay and 50% grain (compared with a hay only ration) has been shown to promote the proliferation of lactic acid producers and to depress lactic acid consumers and cellulose utilizing bacteria in all segments of the equine gastrointestinal tract. Similar changes in the hindgut microbial community were observed even at low levels of starch feeding (oat starch, ~1.2 g/kg BW/day), emphasizing the sensitivity of the microbiota to diet composition (Willing et al 2009). The question arises, is lactic acid production within the intestinal tract good or bad? Data from pigs suggests that even a little starch fermentation in the gut, in particular in the hindgut, will reduce the prevalence of Salmonella shedding (Betscher et al 2010). Perhaps there is similar benefit to the horse associated with a certain amount of starch fermentation in the intestinal tract but this remains to be determined.
3. *Endocrine/metabolic responses and risk of certain disease conditions*: Associations between dietary starch/simple sugar (SS) content and risk of clinical disease have been proposed for at least two conditions – polysaccharide storage myopathy (PSSM) and endocrinopathic laminitis (see Chapter 27 Chapter 31). A profound and/or sustained increase in circulating insulin concentrations appears to be a risk factor for laminitis in some horses and ponies, especially those with a metabolic syndrome phenotype. Similarly, diets that result in pronounced post-feeding glycemic and insulinemic responses appear to increase risk of subclinical or clinical myopathy in horses with PSSM. In both situations, dietary recommendations include severe restriction of SS intake especially in the form of concentrate meals that can be ingested quickly and therefore can result in substantial increases in blood insulin and glucose concentrations (i.e., no or very limited quantities of starch/sugar-based feeds). The upper limit of SS intake in these animals (i.e., the threshold beyond which risk of clinical disease increases) is not well defined but it seems likely that their tolerance for SS is lower when compared to healthy animals. Of course, supply of simple sugars from forages (pasture or preserved) is another concern in the feeding management of laminitis-prone or PSSM horses (see Chapter 26).

Our opinion: The question of what constitutes maximal SS intake per meal remains a contentious issue and recommendations are likely to change over time as new information becomes available regarding the effect of SS load on various aspects of health. For the last 15–20 years, the most common recommendation (specifically pertaining to starch intake) has been a maximum of 2 g/kg BW per meal with use of starches with high prececal digestibility (e.g., oat starch, corn or barley starch providing they have been subjected to heat treatment). This recommendation was based on studies examining "starch by-pass" to the hindgut in relation to intake. More recent work that has characterized the effect of starch load on for example fermentation in the proximal gut, risk of gastric ulceration and hindgut microbial community have provoked a rethink on "what a safe amount of SS" is in an individual meal. Based on this work, there is rationale for setting an upper limit of ~1 g/kg BW per meal at least for starch - whether this limit should include simple sugars is not currently confirmed; our recommendation is that sugars should be included. We recognize that these recommendations are at odds with common feeding practice, especially amongst racehorse trainers.

Pre- and post-exercise feeding management of athletic horses

This is an important area of interest to many owners/trainers and three of the key areas are considered here.

Is it possible to speed up muscle glycogen replenishment rate through starch and sugar provision?

As mentioned above, the rate of muscle glycogen replenishment in horses is slow relative to other mammalian species. Following exercise that severely depletes muscle glycogen content (by >50–60% of pre-exercise value), as long as 48–72 h is required for complete restoration of glycogen stores. In horses competing on consecutive days (e.g. three-day event horses; multi-day endurance rides), multiple heats in a single day (e.g., show jumpers) or subject to frequent (every 48 h) hard training/competitive events, nutritional strategies that enhance the rate of muscle glycogen synthesis may be beneficial to training response and athletic performance. So the question is whether this can be achieved in the horse safely.

Yes: Intravenous infusion of large amounts of glucose (~2.5 kg over a 12-h period) will restore muscle glycogen concentration to pre-depletion levels within 24 h. Diets of only grain-mix (corn, oats, and barley) or corn fed immediately after glycogen-depleting exercise resulted in a modest increase in the rate of glycogen synthesis (~12 mmol/kg DW/h vs. ~8 mmol/kg DW/h for isocaloric hay only or hay-grain diets), and muscle glycogen concentration was modestly (but significantly) higher at 48 h post-exercise in the high-grain feeding scenario (see Lacombe et al 2004, Jose-Cunilleras et al 2006).

No: Setting aside the effect of intravenous glucose administration, the type of post-exercise feeding strategy has minimal influence on glycogen synthesis rate and therefore the time required for restoration of muscle glycogen stores. The high starch (cereal grain) feeding used in experimental studies yields only a modest gain in glycogen synthesis rate and this apparent benefit must be weighed against the potential health risks. Other nutritional treatments that have been shown to enhance glycogen restoration in man do not appear to affect glycogen synthesis rate in horses. For example, the addition of leucine to post-exercise oral glucose feedings appears to augment insulin response when compared to glucose administration alone but this treatment is without effect on post-exercise muscle glycogen synthesis (see Chapter 2 for further discussion).

Our opinion: The feeding of rations with high starch (and sugar) content is neither particularly effective nor safe when the impact of this approach on muscle glycogen synthesis and risk of gastrointestinal disturbance is considered. The interval between very hard exercise bouts is the most important consideration with respect to the optimization of pre-exercise muscle glycogen stores; this interval should be at least 48–72 hours. Recently published work has shown that the restoration of hydration and electrolyte/acid-base balance may be more important to the enhancement of glycogen synthesis than additional glucose load (Waller et al 2009).

When to feed before performance-type exercise?

There is evidence from several studies that the timing and composition of a meal consumed before exercise can influence the metabolic response in horses. In particular, the hyperglycemia and insulinemia associated with the digestion and absorption of grain or SS-rich meals affects the mix of substrates utilized during a bout of exercise. The rise in insulin concentrations promotes fuel storage while inhibiting lipolysis and therefore the mobilization of fatty acids. As such, this endocrine response is in conflict with the need to mobilize fuel stores for ATP synthesis in contracting skeletal muscle. In general, insulin concentrations peak between 120 and 180 min after a SS-rich meal; and insulin may not return to baseline for 3–4 h after a meal with >1 g starch/kg per meal. Therefore, pre-exercise meal feeding should be completed 3–4 h before the start of exercise, and the SS content of these meals should be no more than 1 g/kg per meal.

The size/volume of a pre-exercise meal is another consideration. Large meals (hay or grain/concentrate or mixtures) should not be fed in the 3–4 hour period before exercise because they may result in a decrease in plasma volume due to fluid shifts into the gastrointestinal tract. A large full stomach may restrict the space available for lung expansion although there is no published data on this subject. Gastrointestinal tract discomfort due to inappropriate rations or feeding practices may have an effect on performance. In addition, following a meal blood flow is diverted to the gut to enable the products of digestion to be efficiently utilized – this may reduce the blood flow to contracting muscle and other tissues (e.g., the skin for thermoregulation). However, when fed animals were exercised at ~75% of maximum heart rate, the increase in heart rate and cardiac output was sufficient to meet the increased demands of both working muscle and the digestive tract (Duren et al 1992). Whether the same is true during higher intensity exercise is not known.

Strategies for pre-exercise "loading" of water and electrolytes in healthy hydrated horses are sometimes advocated, (e.g., endurance horses) as a means to offset anticipated sweat fluid losses during exercise. It must be emphasized, however, that body fluid and electrolyte content should be viewed as a barrel of fixed volume – there is no capacity to add to this volume, with any excess excreted via the renal route. After consumption of a meal, there is overflow from the "barrel" into urine over the following 3–6 h period. However, the imposition of exercise during this window of time will reduce the magnitude of this overflow and the "gain" in water and electrolytes from the meal may help to offset sweat fluid losses during exertion. Sodium will start to appear in the sweat within 30–60 min post administration. The administration of relatively large quantities of electrolyte (e.g., 50–60 g NaCl) either as a paste or top-dressed on feed will result in (short-term) positive electrolyte as well as water balance providing the horse responds to the expected stimulation of thirst. The time lag between electrolyte feeding and drinking response, however, is more than 1 h, and this lag must be taken into consideration when recommending pre-exercise electrolyte "loading". Furthermore, the horse should be adapted to this strategy during training as opposed to a sudden introduction of this strategy on race day. Even then, the horse's drinking response may be inhibited by exposure to new surroundings, water source, etc. Different strategies are required during and after the ride (see Chapter 14).

Our opinion:

- It is generally accepted that competition-like (non-racing) bouts of exercise should be delayed for a period of time post-feeding; however, there is still considerable debate regarding the length of this interval, i.e., 2, 3, 4 or 6 h. Feed withholding for 12 h or longer before exercise is certainly not recommended for several reasons – potential increase in risk for gastric ulceration, behavioral abnormalities, tendency to ingest poorly digestible fiber if bedded on straw during feed withholding, etc.
- Our current recommendation is to allow consumption of small forage meals (1–2 kg, as fed basis) in the 1–3 h period before competition-like (non-racing) exercise. Grain-based meals that promote a substantial insulin response are not recommended within this time period.
- Insufficient information is available to formulate clear recommendations for feeding management of racehorses before races. As a guide, we recommend restricting the size of pre-race meals (<1 kg) and feeding no later than 2–3 h before the race. In addition, ~1 kg of forage should be available to the horse during the 2–3 h period pre-race to promote chewing and salivation without excessive gut fill (e.g., hay in a "double" haylage net). Due to the observation that alfalfa hay may decrease the incidence and severity of gastric ulcers in horses in training, it may be helpful if this forage is alfalfa or 50:50 grass:alfalfa.
- With respect to water and electrolyte balance during exercise, the preferential timing of exercise may be around 2 h after any electrolyte loading (to a healthy hydrated animal with access to clean water) but this may need to be adjusted to the individual animal.

Is excessive dietary protein a problem?

During a program of physical conditioning (exercise training) there is a substantial change in protein metabolism, including increased turnover of muscle proteins and an increase in endogenous losses in association with increased feed ingestion and sweat production. Dietary protein requirements of exercising horses are higher when compared to animals at maintenance – but is it possible to feed too much protein? Table 26-1 presents a point and counterpoint regarding this question.

Nutrition and skin health

We would like to thank Professors Knottenbelt (University of Liverpool) and Sloet van Oldruitenborgh-Oosterbaan (Utrecht University) for their invaluable contribution to the following section.

A wide variety of nutritional factors may play a role in equine dermatology. However, only very limited evidence-based medicine is available on this subject and hardly any scientific research has been focused on the relationship between nutrition and skin health of the horse. Most information is empirical or anecdotal and is largely based on the experiences of equine clinicians and dermatologists.

It is easy to forget that the skin, like other organs, requires essential nutrients to support normal function. Almost any inappropriate food material and any gross deficiency of the basic requirements can affect the skin to some extent. However, even prolonged malnutrition may have surprisingly little effect on the skin and hair; animals maintained in very harsh environments seldom have any evidence of deficiency diseases and indeed may have remarkably good skin condition. Energy deficits are reported to cause a dry, scurfy, moth-eaten coat with poor skin elasticity. In addition, normal hair shedding and re-growth can be impaired significantly with long coats and patchy molting. Nonetheless, it is remarkable that even in the face of such severe deprivation the skin is often normal. Concurrent ectoparasites and other bacterial and fungal skin infections often complicate these cases. Nevertheless, there are defined dermatological problems specifically related to nutrition which include:

Table 26-1 Pros and Cons of Protein Feeding

Area	Yes	No	Editors' conclusions
Acid–base balance	Oxidation of the phosphorus and sulfur in protein adds to the acid load on the body	These effects are small and there is no evidence of clinically important alterations in acid–base balance due to variations in protein intake	Restriction of protein intake is not justified on the basis of effects on acid–base balance.
Thermal load	Protein is inefficiently converted to useable energy with proportionally higher amounts of waste energy (heat) produced	Not an issue unless working hard for long periods of time in adverse environmental conditions	Probably not an issue for most horses; possible exception is an endurance horse in hot/humid conditions
Water requirements	Excess nitrogen must be removed from the body, resulting in increased water requirements (the excess protein is lost primarily as urea in the urine)	Not an issue if plenty of water available	Probably not an issue for most horses; possible exception is an endurance horse in hot/humid conditions
Respiratory challenge	May lead to higher environmental ammonia – the excreted urea is converted to ammonia by bacteria	Not an issue if kept in a well ventilated environment	Not likely to be a major issue with good stable management – Could be a concern if respiratory system already compromised
Is there an upper limit?	Recommend <2 g digestible protein (DP)/kg/day for an athletic horse	Horses will often ingest far more than this (e.g., when out on good quality pasture) without apparent ill effects.	Absolute protein intake probably not a major concern. An exception is a horse with chronic respiratory problems kept in confinement. In these circumstances, a limit between 2–2.5 g DP/kg BW is advisable.

- *Direct nutritional factors*: too much of a nutrient (e.g., selenium toxicosis), too little of a nutrient (e.g., copper deficiency, zinc deficiency), or toxic nutrients (phototoxic problems). These problems often have pathognomonic clinical signs.
- *Indirect nutritional factors*: food allergy/food related hypersensitivities that may present as well-recognized skin disorders such as urticaria.

Nowadays, horses in most parts of the world are fed good quality diets and this makes disorders caused by nutritional deficiencies or toxicities very rare. Although cases of copper and zinc deficiency are mentioned in many text books, the authors (Knottenbelt, Sloet van Oldruitenborgh-Oosterbaan and the editors) have never encountered cases. On the other hand, the addition of excessive supplements to the horse's diet may be now a greater risk as owners take on ill-advised supplementary feeding and in particular mineral supplements (e.g. selenium toxicosis; see Chapter 10).

Do feed allergies occur?

By far the most common allergic disorder of the skin in horses is insect bite hypersensitivity (sweet itch). Food hypersensitivity or food allergy is rare and not well scientifically supported in horses although Professor Knottenbelt has reported personal experience of cases. Food hypersensitivity is associated with the ingestion of a substance in the horse's diet and is most likely a hypersensitivity reaction to an allergic ingredient. Whether food intolerance (a toxic reaction to food) exists in the horse is unclear. So, all skin reactions to food substances in the horse are considered to be food hypersensitivity and this disorder is itself rare. No age, breed, or gender predilection has been reported. The most common clinical signs are pruritus (seasonal or non-seasonal), urticaria (seasonal or non-seasonal and with or without pruritus). The pruritus can be so severe that self-mutilation occurs.

The diagnosis "food hypersensitivity" can only be made on the basis of a positive result after application of an elimination diet and then a reoccurrence of the clinical signs after provocative exposure. A suggested approach is to move the horse to a completely new surrounding (on another bedding and another roughage source, preferably away from home), and provide no concentrates and no supplements. The clinical signs should disappear within 2–6 weeks. If this is the case, then different feed items can be reintroduced one by one and in general the causative ingredient should provoke a reoccurrence of the clinical signs within 1–14 days. Although the general feeling is that the underlying cause is often protein-related, there have been anecdotal reports of horses that react to the sugar derived from cane (but have no reaction to beet sugar). Some horses will recover if the amount of the cereal being fed is reduced but there are many that continue to show recurrent or sometimes persistent urticaria in the face of continued exposure. In some cases this continues until the feed responsible is completely withdrawn. Reintroduction of even a small amount (usually ~200 g is enough) results in a complete recurrence of the typical syndrome. Such a response suggests that the horse has an inappropriate hypersensitivity to some component of the feed material.

Biopsies of the dermis are not very useful for diagnosis. Often the secondary lesions resulting from the pruritus are more serious.

Our opinion: Food allergies may occur in a few individuals but it appears to be very rare and individual in nature. The use of serological tests and intradermal testing with food ingredients is not recommended as there is very limited scientific support for either testing procedure.

What are protein bumps?

A specific form of food reaction is "protein bumps" (sweet feed bumps). This widely recognized condition is manifest as small 1–3 mm skin "bumps", often with a little crust (Fig. 26.1). These lesions can easily be mistaken for some forms of dermatophilosis. Histology is rarely done as "horsemen" recognize the problem and simply decrease the amount of protein in the diet of the horse. Whether this represents some form of hypersensitivity or a specific response to "excessive protein" is not known. There is limited scientific description of this condition (Hallebeek et al 1995)

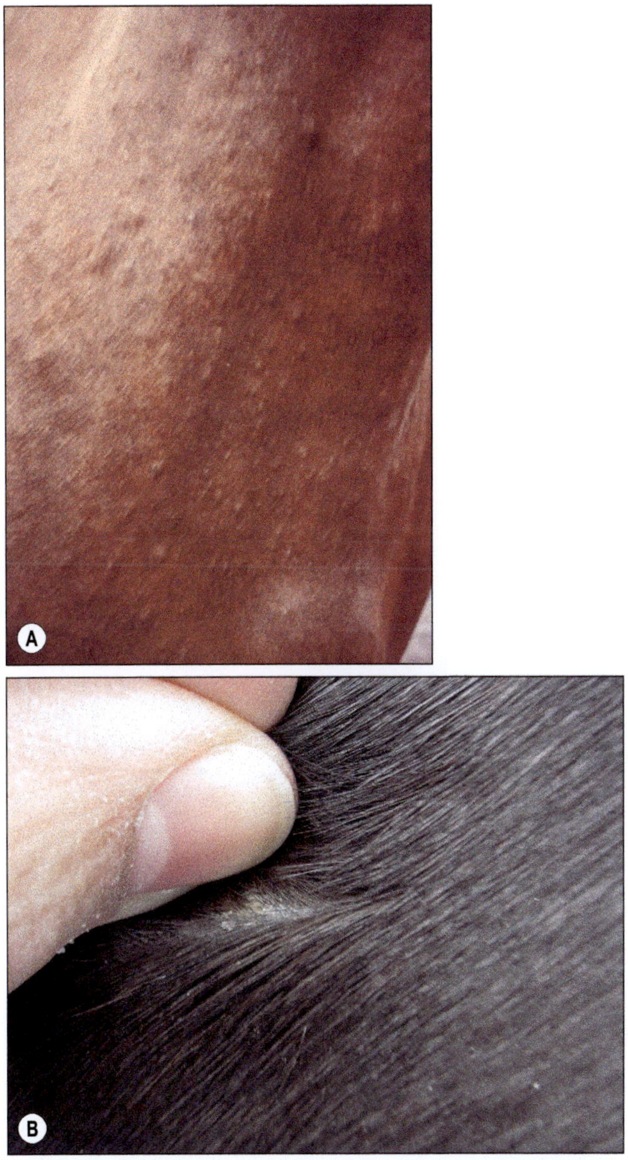

Figure 26.1 An adult Warmblood horse with "protein bumps". **A)** Raised nodules are especially evident along the dorsal thoracic region; **B)** A close-up view of a nodule demonstrating typical scaling and flaking of the skin.
Photographs courtesy of Professor Marianne Sloet van Oldruitenborgh-Oosterbaan (Utrecht University).

Conclusion

Feeding recommendations vary based on an individual's interpretation of the published literature as well as personal experience. In addition, published nutrient requirements vary, in part because different "expert" groups place different value on particular publications and may have access to different pieces of information (e.g., unpublished data or data that has been published in a language that is accessible by that particular expert group). They may also have different experiences and expertise with use of certain systems, feeding practices, and even types of horses. In this chapter, we have pooled the thoughts of the three editors from different countries with a diversity of approaches to equine nutrition and feeding management. It is acknowledged that answers to many of the questions posed in this chapter remain incomplete. Furthermore, there are many other areas of horse nutrition that could have been included in this - controversial - chapter.

References

Betscher, S., Beineke, A., Schonfeld, L., et al., 2010. Effects of diet's physical form (grinding intensity; meal/pellets) on morphological and histological parameters (e.g. ratio of neutral to acid mucins) of the gastrointestinal tract in weaned piglets. Livestock Science 134, 149–151.

Dugdale, A., Curtis, G.C., Cripps, P., et al., 2011. Effects of season and body condition on appetite, body mass and body composition in ad libitum fed pony mares. The Veterinary Journal 190, 329–337.

Duren, S.E., Manohar, M., Sikkes, B., et al., 1992. Influence of feeding and exercise on the distribution of intestinal and muscle blood flow in horses. Pferedeheilkunde 9, 24–28.

Essén-Gustavsson, B., Connysson, M., Jansson, A., 2010. Effects of crude protein intake from forage-only diets on muscle amino acids and glycogen levels in horses during training. Equine Veterinary Journal 42 (Suppl. 38), 341–346.

Hallebeek, A.J.M., Sloet van Oldruitenborgh-Oosterbaan, M.M., 1995. "Oat bumps" in horses, differential diagnosis and nutritional aspects. Tijdschr Diergeneesk 120, 588–591.

Jose-Cunilleras, E., Hinchcliff, K.W., Lacombe, V.A., et al., 2006. Ingestion of starch-rich meals after exercise increases glucose kinetics but fails to enhance muscle glycogen replenishment in horses. The Veterinary Journal 171, 468–477.

Kirschvink, N., Fievez, L., Bougnet, V., et al., 2002. Effect of nutritional antioxidant supplementation on systemic and pulmonary antioxidant status, airway inflammation and lung function in heaves affected horses. Equine Veterinary Journal 34, 705–712.

Lacombe, V.A., Hinchcliff, K.W., Kohn, C.W., et al., 2004. Effects of feeding meals with various soluble carbohydrate content on muscle glycogen synthesis after exercise in horses. American Journal of Veterinary Research 65, 916–923.

National Research Council., 2007. Nutrient Requirements of Horses, 6th revised edition. National Academies Press, Washington DC.

National Research Council. Safety of Dietary Supplements for Horses, Dogs, and Cats. Animal Nutrition Series., 2009. National Research Council of the National Academies. National Academies Press, Washington, DC.

Waller, A.P., Heigenhauser, G.J.F., Geor, R.J., et al., 2009. Fluid and electrolyte supplementation after prolonged moderate-intensity exercise enhances muscle glycogen resynthesis in horses. Journal of Applied Physiology 106, 91–100.

Willing, B., Vörös, A., Roos, S., et al., 2009. Changes in faecal bacteria associated with concentrate and forage-only diets fed to horses in training. Equine Veterinary Journal 41, 908–914.

SECTION E

Clinical Nutrition

27 Laminitis

Raymond J. Geor, Patricia A. Harris

Laminitis is a systemic condition that manifests in the foot and results in varying degrees of pain, lameness and debilitation. The most straightforward definition of laminitis is failure of the bond between the inner hoof wall and the distal phalanx. When the connection between the distal phalanx and the hoof wall lamellae is compromised, the weight of the horse and the forces of locomotion can result in structural collapse of the foot with rotation or sinking of the distal phalanx and injury to other structures within the hoof capsule. This pathology and associated unrelenting pain can necessitate euthanasia on humane grounds. Accordingly, laminitis is a major animal welfare concern. Research to unravel its pathogenesis and develop improved treatment as well as control strategies, is a very high priority for the equine industry.

Laminitis may best be regarded as a syndrome rather than a single disease entity because there are multiple inciting causes and possibly pathophysiological pathways (Harris 2011), which can be summarized into three primary categories (Table 27-1): (1) sepsis/systemic inflammatory conditions (e.g., gastrointestinal disease, septic metritis, pneumonia, carbohydrate overload); (2) endocrine/metabolic (e.g., associated with insulin resistance, obesity &/or pituitary pars intermedia dysfunction); and (3) mechanical overload (supporting limb laminitis). Nutrition has long been linked to laminitis. Indeed, around 350 BCE Aristotle used the term "barley disease" in obvious reference to the development of laminitis after consumption of excessive cereal grains (grain overload) and, since the 1970s, carbohydrate overload (the bolus administration of large quantities of a starch gruel) has been one of the primary experimental models of laminitis (Harris & Geor 2010). Over the last 20 years, survey studies have indicated that many cases of laminitis occur in horses and ponies kept at pasture, giving rise to the term *pasture-associated laminitis* (Hinckley & Henderson 1996, USDA 2000, Treiber et al 2006, Menzies-Gow et al 2010a).

Clinical cases of pasture laminitis often occur under conditions that favor accumulation of rapidly fermentable non-structural carbohydrates (fructans, simple sugars and/or starches) in grass and clover. It has been argued, therefore, that pasture laminitis is triggered by carbohydrate overload of the hindgut and the systemic absorption of substances that initiate lamellar failure (Bailey et al 2004a). This hypothesis is supported by experimental studies in which the administration of oligofructose, a commercial fructan, induces laminitis in healthy horses (van Eps and Pollitt 2006). However, the extent to which this model reflects events during development of naturally-occurring laminitis is unknown, particularly in view of the fact that only a very small proportion of any population develops pasture laminitis even during periods of theoretical highest risk. This observation has stimulated research on possible reasons for the apparent increased susceptibility of certain horses and ponies. Relatively recently, evidence has emerged that animals with an insulin resistant phenotype are at an increased risk for pasture-associated laminitis (Treiber et al 2005, 2006, Bailey et al 2008, Carter et al 2009). Additionally, the discovery that prolonged intravenous infusion of insulin induces laminitis in healthy animals has widened the perspective on potential pathophysiologic mechanisms of laminitis (Asplin et al 2007, De Laat et al 2010) and raised the possibility that diet (including pasture grazing) might provoke episodes of laminitis via effects on insulin dynamics, particularly in insulin resistant animals. The term *equine metabolic syndrome* (EMS) is currently used to describe horses and ponies with an insulin-resistant phenotype linked with laminitis susceptibility (Geor & Frank 2009, Frank et al 2010), while *endocrinopathic laminitis* is sometimes used to describe the EMS-associated laminitis as well as that associated with pituitary pars intermedia dysfunction (PPID, equine Cushing's disease; McGowan 2010).

This chapter focuses on nutritionally-associated laminitis (grain overload, pasture laminitis) as well as the laminitis that occurs in horses and ponies with underlying endocrine and metabolic disturbances that are impacted by diet and feeding management (i.e., EMS and PPID).

Epidemiology and risk factors

Recent systematic reviews have highlighted the lack of quality information with respect to the epidemiology of equine laminitis, including data on prevalence, inciting causes and risk factors (Wylie et al 2011a,b). The reported disease frequency has ranged from 1.5% to 34% in different studies, with factors such as sample size and type (e.g. ponies vs. horses), underlying laminitis etiology, case definition, modes of diagnosis, climate, and feeding/management practices likely contributing to this wide variation in

Table 27-1 Conditions Associated with an Increased Risk of Laminitis (Eades 2010, Harris & Geor 2010)

1. **Sepsis/septic inflammatory conditions**
   - Gastrointestinal diseases, e.g. strangulating small or large intestinal obstructions; duodenitis-proximal jejunitis; acute typhlocolitis; Potomac Horse Fever
   - Retained fetal membranes/septic metritis
   - Pneumonia/pleuropneumonia (especially due to Gram-negative bacteria)
2. **Nutrition**
   - Grain (starch) overload (alimentary carbohydrate overload)
   - Pasture grazing (pasture-associated laminitis)
3. **Endocrine and metabolic disorders**
   - Obesity and insulin resistance (equine metabolic syndrome)
   - Pituitary pars intermedia dysfunction (equine Cushing's disease)
4. **Miscellaneous**
   - Mechanical overload (supporting limb laminitis)
   - Ingestion of black walnut shavings
   - Corticosteroid administration (although evidence is *very* weak)

frequency of laminitis (Wylie et al. 20011a). Hinckley and Henderson (1996) surveyed veterinarians and horse owners to estimate the number of acute and chronic laminitis cases in a population of approximately 113 000 horses and reported about 1700 cases of both acute and chronic laminitis with an overall prevalence of 3%. Approximately 61% of the laminitis cases occurred in horses kept at pasture (Hinckley & Henderson 1996). The United States Department of Agriculture (USDA) survey reported that 13% of horse operations had had at least one case of laminitis during the previous 12 months with 1% of horses affected at any one time (based on owner responses). Laminitis was identified as the most common cause of foot lameness, accounting for up to 16% of all lameness cases. Additionally, nutritionally-associated laminitis accounted for more than 50% of the cases, with 46% attributed to pasture grazing and 7% to grain overload (Kane et al 2000, USDA 2000).

A retrospective study in the south of England reported the prevalence, incidence and seasonality of laminitis in a population of about 1000 horses/ponies kept on a single farm and maintained at pasture (Menzies-Gow et al 2010a). Over a 6-year period, 23.5% of the population had at least one episode of veterinary diagnosed laminitis; the highest prevalence (2.6%) and incidence (16 cases/1000 animals) of laminitis occurred in May. A positive association was found between hours of sunshine and the prevalence and incidence of laminitis, but there were no associations with rainfall or monthly temperature. The association between hours of sunshine and incident laminitis was presumed to reflect altered nutritional intake (i.e., increased consumption of nonstructural carbohydrates during periods of bright sunshine that promote plant photosynthesis and carbohydrate accumulation) rather than the direct effect of exposure of horses to sunlight. Other studies have reported an increased risk of laminitis during the spring and summer months (Dorn et al 1975, Hinckley & Henderson 1996, USDA 2000) although evidence of seasonality is inconsistent (Polzer & Slater 1997, Wyllie et al 2011b).

Menzies-Gow et al (2010a) also observed that approximately one-third of animals diagnosed with laminitis had at least one more episode during the study period. Moreover, about 24% of these animals had a repeated episode in the same year as the original diagnosis. These observations confirm the clinical impression that some animals are prone to repeated episodes of laminitis (Buckley et al 2007) and focus attention on the possibility that there are phenotypic or genetic factors associated with susceptibility. With regards to genetic factors, laminitis in a foal attributable to disruption of a single molecule of the hemidesmosome adhesion complex was believed to be the result of an inherited recessive defect that lead to failure in expression of the protein plectin (French & Pollitt 2004). Additionally, Belgian foals with mechanobullous disease (epidermolysis bullosa) are at an increased risk of laminitis (Frame et al 1988).

In the study by Menzies-Gow et al (2010a), univariate analysis revealed that animals ≥14.3 hands in height were at reduced risk of laminitis while females, light animals (<400 kg) and animals with a weight-to-height ratio <7.51 kg/in were at higher risk. Female gender also was a significant risk factor in multivariate analysis, a finding in agreement with several other studies (Dorn et al 1975, Alford et al 2001, Slater et al 1995). The reason for the apparent increased laminitis risk in mares is not known. The height and weight associations with laminitis lend support to the clinical impression that ponies are at higher risk as compared to horses, although in multivariate analysis weight but not height was revealed as a significant risk factor (Menzies-Gow et al 2010a). In a prospective study of pasture-associated laminitis, the majority of affected animals (89 of 107 cases) were overweight/obese (Menzies-Gow et al 2010b). Additionally, overweight animals were at increased risk of severe clinical signs and were less likely to survive. These findings are consistent with earlier reports that identified obesity as a risk factor for laminitis (Alford et al 2001). Increased load bearing by the feet is one potential explanation for the increased risk of laminitis in overweight/obese animals.

Several studies have characterized metabolic risk factors for pasture-associated laminitis in ponies (Treiber et al 2005, 2006, Bailey et al 2007, 2008, Carter et al 2009). In an inbred herd of Welsh and Dartmoor ponies, laminitis risk was associated with the clustering of hyperinsulinemia, obesity and hypertriglyceridemia – this phenotype was termed "prelaminitic metabolic syndrome (PLMS)" (Treiber et al 2006). The PLMS criteria predicted 11 of 13 cases of clinical laminitis observed in May of the same year, with an odds ratio of 10.4 (i.e. ponies with this phenotype were at approximately 10-times higher risk for laminitis). Pedigree analysis suggested a dominant mode of inheritance of the PLMS phenotype, supporting the possibility of a genetic basis for laminitis predisposition (Treiber et al 2006). A subsequent study of this pony population demonstrated that the presence of obesity (generalized or regional, i.e., cresty neck), hyperinsulinemia (insulin >32 mU/l when sampled on winter pasture) or hyperleptinemia (>7.3 ng/ml) were useful predictors of laminitis episodes when ponies were exposed to high carbohydrate pasture (Carter et al 2009). A study of out-bred ponies in the UK also revealed an association between apparent insulin resistance (IR) and predisposition to pasture laminitis, and provided evidence of hypertension in the high risk ponies (Bailey et al 2008). Interestingly, expression of this metabolic phenotype was only noted in summer but not winter, suggesting interaction with environmental factors such as consumption of summer pasture forage (Bailey et al 2008). As mentioned, EMS rather than PLMS has been broadly adopted to describe horses and ponies with an insulin resistant phenotype and associated predisposition to laminitis. These animals are often overweight or obese (or have localized large fat deposits, e.g., a "cresty neck") and exhibit abnormal insulin dynamics, either resting hyperinsulinemia or an exaggerated increase in insulin concentration in response to oral or intravenous glucose challenges (Frank et al 2010, Frank 2011). In addition to pony breeds, Morgan Horses, domesticated Spanish mustangs, European warmbloods and American saddlebreds are thought to be at increased risk for development of EMS; however, currently there is insufficient evidence to support or refute this belief. It should be emphasized that non-obese animals that may or may not show IR also can experience recurrent laminitis.

Laminitis is a common occurrence in horses with PPID (equine Cushing's disease), with prevalence between 50% and 80% in some reports (Schott et al 2001, Donaldson et al 2002, 2004, McGowan 2010). Donaldson et al (2004) reported that 28 of 40 cases of laminitis (70%) seen in primary veterinary practice were associated with high plasma adrenocorticotropic hormone (ACTH) concentrations and a presumptive diagnosis of PPID.

Key Points – Risk factors for laminitis

- Pasture turnout can be a trigger factor for laminitis, even in lean, non-obese animals that do not have increased basal plasma insulin concentrations
- Horses and ponies with an obese, insulin-resistant phenotype are at an increased risk of laminitis when turned out to pasture with high nonstructural carbohydrate content (simple sugars, fructans, and starch)
- Animals with pituitary pars intermedia dysfunction (PPID) are at increased risk of laminitis
- Predisposing events and risk factors for laminitis may be additive in nature.

Pathogenesis

Most of our current knowledge of the pathogenesis of laminitis has been derived from four experimental models of the condition, specifically: (1) carbohydrate overload (high starch); (2) black walnut extract administration; (3) oligofructose (fructan) overload; and (4) insulin-induced laminitis (Eades 2010). Findings from studies using these models have given rise to several interlinking hypotheses regarding key mechanisms of lamellar failure and laminitis development, including inflammation, activation of degradative matrix metalloproteinases, hemodynamic alterations within the digital microvasculature, and disruption of lamellar epithelial cell function by hyperinsulinemia (Belknap et al 2009, Harris & Geor 2010, Eades, 2010). Although much progress has been made in describing cellular and molecular events in lamellar tissue during the development of laminitis, understanding of the pathophysiology of the condition remains incomplete. Moreover, as mentioned, questions remain regarding the relevance of these experimental models to the pathogenesis of naturally-occurring laminitis. The following subsections briefly discuss these models in the context of nutritionally associated and endocrinopathic laminitis.

Carbohydrate overload

Alimentary carbohydrate overload and associated risk for development of laminitis can occur when horses and ponies ingest excessive quantities of simple sugars, starches and/or fructans. Circumstances for carbohydrate overload include the ingestion of large amounts of starch-rich cereal grains (accidental access or inappropriate feeding management) or pasture forage that, under certain conditions, may have high content of these nonstructural carbohydrate (NSC) fractions (especially fructans). Experimentally, carbohydrate overload-induced laminitis has been created by the bolus administration (via gastric gavage) of a mixture of cornstarch and wood flour (~17 g/kg bodyweight (BW); Obel 1948, Garner et al 1975, Pollitt & Visser 2010) or oligofructose (OF, 5.0–12.5 g/kg BW; van Eps & Pollitt 2006, Kalck et al 2009). It is thought that most of the consequences of carbohydrate overload occur after passage of undigested starch or fructan to the hindgut and stem from the rapid fermentation of this substrate within the cecum and large intestine. Horses have a limited capacity for prececal digestion of starch; the exact limit varies between horses and is also affected by grain type and meal size but in general there is some "by-pass" of undigested starch to the hindgut especially when more than 2 g starch/kg BW is consumed as a single meal or unprocessed corn/barley is fed (see Chapter 8). Fructans are not degraded by mammalian enzymes (Nilsson et al 1988). Some ingested fructan (in particular the short chain inulin-type fructans) may undergo acid hydrolysis in the stomach or microbial fermentation in the foregut (Coenen et al 2005); however the bulk of the ingested material will pass unaltered to the large intestine where it will undergo fermentation (Longland et al 2012a).

Carbohydrate overload with starch or oligofructose elicits similar digestive and systemic disturbances. The possible sequence of events that leads to the development of laminitis is shown in Fig. 27.1. The rapid fermentation of starch or oligofructose in the hindgut induces profound changes in the hindgut microbiome, with disappearance of *Escherichia coli* and rapid proliferation of Gram-positive bacteria that preferentially ferment these substrates and produce lactic acid as an end-product of fermentation, particularly the equine hindgut streptococcal species (EHSS; *Streptococcus bovis* and *Streptococcus lutetiensis*; Milinovich et al 2006, 2010). D- and L-lactate are produced by bacterial fermentation, contributing to a sharp increase in hindgut acidity; the pH of intestinal contents may decrease to values as low as 4 (Milinovich et al 2010). D-lactate is not produced by mammalian metabolism and therefore its presence in blood is an indicator of hindgut bacterial fermentation. In the oligofructose model, blood D-lactate concentrations peaked at approximately 20 hours after dosing, coinciding with the nadir in fecal pH (van Eps & Pollitt 2006).

Hindgut acidity triggers death and lysis of large numbers of bacteria and release of endotoxins, exotoxins and other microbial components into the intestinal milieu (Milinovich et al 2010, Pollitt & Visser 2010). There is also evidence of an increase in the synthesis of vasoactive amines within the

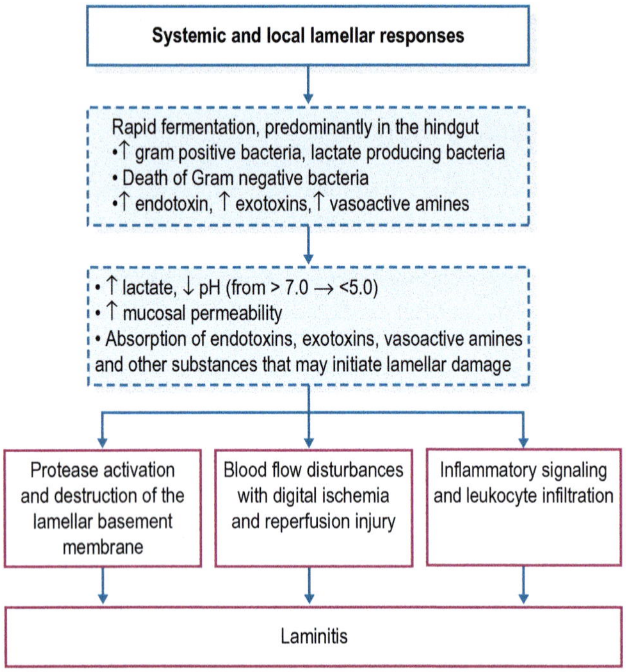

Figure 27.1 Schematic overview of events that may lead to development of laminitis after consumption of excessive quantities of rapidly fermentable carbohydrate. See text for detailed description.

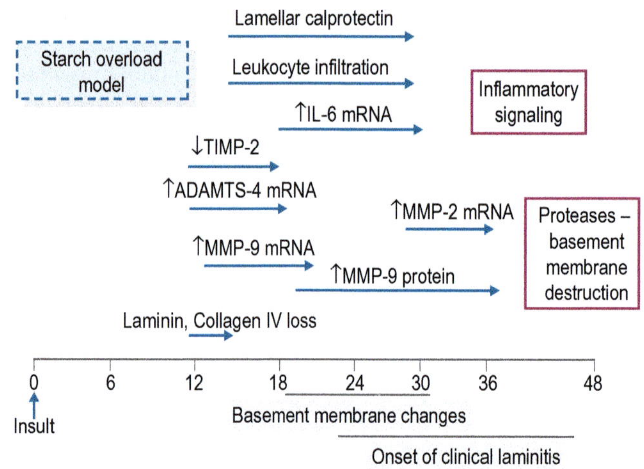

Figure 27.2 A time line of some of the molecular and cellular events that have been documented during the developmental phase of carbohydrate overload laminitis (IL-6, interleukin-6; TIMP, tissue inhibitor of matrix metalloprotease; MMP, matrix metalloprotease; ADAMTS-4, aggrecanase).
Adapted from Orsini 2010 (with permission).

hindgut under conditions of carbohydrate overload (Bailey et al 2003, Elliott & Bailey 2006, Crawford et al 2007). Within 24 h of carbohydrate overload, there is compromise of the intestinal mucosal barrier with degeneration and sloughing of epithelial cells, submucosal inflammation, and an increase in intestinal permeability (Sprouse et al 1987, Weiss et al 1998). The increase in intestinal permeability presumably favors absorption of exotoxins, endotoxins, other bacterial components, and vasoactive amines into the circulation. In both models, increased plasma endotoxin concentration has been detected between 8 and 12 h after starch/fructan overload (Sprouse et al 1987, Bailey et al 2009) and is associated with clinical signs of illness including tachycardia, tachypnea and pyrexia. There also is evidence of systemic inflammation with increased cytokine mRNA expression in blood, platelet activation, and activation of leukocytes (Eades et al 2007, Bailey et al 2009, Pollitt & Visser 2010). Diarrhea and clinical signs of moderate-to-severe hypovolemic shock, which may be life-threatening, are additional features of the carbohydrate overload (especially starch) models that generally occur prior to onset of lameness (Pollitt & Visser 2010).

The precise role of endotoxemia in the pathogenesis of laminitis is unclear. Intravenous infusion of endotoxin (lipopolysaccharide, LPS) does not induce development of laminitis in healthy horses (Menzies-Gow et al 2004, Tóth et al 2009). On the other hand, a clinical study has identified endotoxemia as a risk factor for laminitis in hospitalized horses although in these cases laminitis was associated with severe illness (Gram-negative sepsis) rather than nutritional factors and the diagnosis of endotoxemia was based on clinical parameters rather than direct measurement of plasma endotoxin (Parsons et al 2007). It is possible that endotoxin absorbed from the intestinal tract plays a role during the developmental phase of carbohydrate overload laminitis, perhaps by "priming" inflammatory and hemodynamic mechanisms involved in lamellar injury and failure. In support of this hypothesis, Tóth et al (2009) reported that pretreatment of horses with lipopolysaccharide (i.e., endotoxin) might increase the incidence and severity of laminitis induced by the administration of OF (5 g/kg BW). Other bacterial and non bacterial products absorbed from the gastrointestinal tract also may contribute.

In the starch and OF overload models, clinical signs of laminitis develop 24–48 hours after bolus dosing (Pollitt & Visser 2010). Despite intensive study, the mechanism(s) that links the rapid fermentation of carbohydrate in the intestine and associated systemic responses with development of acute laminitis remains to be identified. A schematic overview of the timeline of some of the molecular and cellular events occurring during the developmental phase of starch overload laminitis is shown in Fig. 27.2. The information has been drawn from several studies in which measurements were made in laminar biopsy samples obtained at discrete time points (most often up until the onset of Obel Grade [OG] 1 laminitis; see Orsini 2010). Current evidence for the roles of inflammation, oxidant stress, matrix degradation, and venous/endothelial dysfunction is summarized below.

Lamellar leukocyte infiltration and inflammatory signaling

In both the starch and oligofructose models, there is evidence of systemic inflammation, increased expression of chemokines in lamellar tissue, plus infiltration and activation of leukocytes in lamellae (Belknap et al 2007, Falerios et al 2011a, b, Visser & Pollitt 2011a). These observations have led to the suggestion that the lamellar failure of laminitis is analogous to the organ injury and failure that occurs as a result of sepsis (Belknap et al 2007). In the starch model, there was an eightfold increase in calprotectin-positive leukocytes in laminar tissue harvested at the developmental phase (onset of fever, 10–20 hours post-dosing) with a more marked increase at the onset of OG1 lameness together with a moderate increase in CD163-positive (monocyte-macrophage) cells (Faleiros et al 2011a). Maximal leukocyte infiltration preceded development of epithelial stress and basement membrane (BM) degradation, raising the possibility that leukocyte infiltration may contribute to BM breakdown and structural failure in these models (Faleiros et al 2011b). In the oligofructose model, calprotectin-positive leukocytes also were detected in laminar tissue 18–24 hours post-dosing, although it was suggested that leukocyte infiltration and activation may be a reaction to, rather than a cause of, the lamellar pathology in this model (Visser & Pollitt 2011a, b). Increased inflammatory signaling has been detected in laminar tissue after starch or OF overload with, for example, several-fold increases in the mRNA concentrations for cytokines (interleukin (IL)-6, IL-1β), chemokines (CXCL1, CXCL8) and cell adhesion molecules (ICAM-1, E-selectin; Belknap et al 2007, Leise et al 2011). However, the majority of these inflammatory events occur at or near the onset of lameness rather than in the early developmental stages (Leise et al 2011), suggesting that other events may contribute to the initiation of lamellar pathology.

Oxidative tissue injury

Oxidant stress-associated lamellar damage may develop when there is excessive production of reactive oxygen species (ROS) and reactive nitrogen species (RNS), a reduced antioxidant capacity, or both (Roberts et al 2009). As equine laminar tissue is devoid of superoxide dismutase (SOD) it may be highly susceptible to damage by the superoxide anions (Loftus et al 2007). Increased lipid (increased 4-hydroxynonenal [4-HNE]) and protein (increased 3-nitrotyrosine) oxidant stress has been observed in laminar tissue after BWE administration but not in tissues harvested during the developmental and OGI phases of starch overload laminitis (Loftus et al 2007, Burns et al 2011). More work is needed to elucidate the role of oxidative stress in the pathogenesis of laminitis; however current evidence indicates that tissue oxidative stress is not central to the development of starch overload laminitis (Burns et al 2011).

Enzymatic dysregulation

Disruption of the lamellar BM is a primary lesion in carbohydrate overload laminitis. Some studies have concluded that up-regulation of matrix metalloproteases (MMPs), in particular MMP-2 and MMP-9, is responsible for the BM damage (as reviewed by Clutterbuck et al 2010) but other work has indicated that degradation of the lamellar BM occurs prior to changes in MMP (2 and 9) expression and activation (Visser & Pollitt 2012). The protease aggrecanase-1 (ADAMTS-4) is upregulated very early in the developmental phase and its role in BM degradation merits further investigation (Kyaw-Tanner et al 2008).

Alterations in vascular and endothelial function

The role of altered digital hemodynamics in laminitis is controversial with both increased and decreased perfusion detected in experimental models (see Robertson et al 2009). Nonetheless, venous dysfunction may contribute to lamellar injury in concert with other mechanisms. Laminar edema due to venous constriction has been observed during the developmental phase of carbohydrate overload laminitis (Allen et al 1990). Concurrently, there is an increase in digital venous endothelin-1 (Eades et al 2007) which has been shown to induce intense constriction of laminar veins (Keen et al 2008). The increased venous resistance during the prodromal phase can be inhibited by administration of an endothelin-1 antagonist (Eades et al 2006). Other mechanisms contributing to vasoconstriction might include localized platelet activation (with release of serotonin and thromboxane) and the formation of platelet–neutrophil aggregates, which has been demonstrated in carbohydrate overload laminitis (Weiss et al 1997). Vasoactive amines formed by bacteria in the intestinal tract, such as tyramine, tryptamine and phenylethylamine, also may contribute to altered digital hemodynamics although direct evidence is lacking (Elliott & Bailey 2006). Horses and ponies with IR and pre-existing endothelial cell dysfunction may be more susceptible to digital vasoconstriction under conditions of carbohydrate challenge and/or hyperinsulinemia (Geor & Frank 2009, Robertson et al 2009, Berhane et al 2009a,b).

Clinical relevance

The starch overload model is relevant to the laminitis that develops in animals subsequent to the ingestion of excessive grain or other starch-rich feedstuff (e.g., bread). Anecdotally, the risk for development of laminitis is very high when horses consume more than 1.2–1.5 kg/100 kg BW (i.e., 6 to 7.5 kg for a 500-kg horse) over a 1–2 hour period, especially grains with poor prececal starch digestibility such as unprocessed wheat, corn, barley or sorghum. However, susceptibility likely varies between individuals and smaller quantities of grain may induce laminitis in some animals. Conversely, overt laminitis appears to be rare in Thoroughbred racehorses fed large quantities of cereal grain. Clinical signs of depression, pyrexia, hypovolemia, and profuse, watery diarrhea may manifest prior to the onset of laminitis. Recognition of grain engorgement and/or its consequences constitutes a medical emergency (see Case Management).

The relevance of the OF model to pasture-associated laminitis is less certain. The fructans in grasses are very different in structure to the simple oligofructoses used in the experimental studies and even if similar "triggering" amounts of fructan can be ingested whilst out on pasture this occurs over several hours rather than as a bolus. Nonetheless, clinical observations have suggested that risk of laminitis is highest when horses or ponies are grazing lush (i.e., green, actively photosynthetic) or stressed (i.e., environmental conditions that restrict forage growth) pastures with high NSC content – fructans, simple sugars and/or starch (Longland & Byrd 2006). In Northern European countries, the fructan content of perennial ryegrass varies between <100 g and >400 g/kg of dry matter (DM) depending on the season and growing conditions. Myriad factors impact pasture NSC/water-soluble carbohydrate (WSC) contents but, in general, it is highest in spring, lowest in mid-summer and intermediate in the fall. In a recent study, analysis of 245 samples of pasture grasses (perennial ryegrass, timothy and fescue) harvested throughout a growing season showed that ~20% of samples contained >20% WSC (fructans + simple sugars) on a DM basis, ~5% of samples with >25% WSC, and ~3% with >30% WSC (Annette Longland, personal communication). The average fructan content of ryegrass samples harvested in May was 27% of DM. There also can be marked daily fluctuations in forage NSC that coincide with patterns of energy storage (photosynthetic activity) and utilization.

Table 27-2 Estimated Intakes of Fructan and Simple Sugars by a 250-kg Pony Grazing Upon Pasture with Moderate (200 g/kg Dry Matter [DM]) or High (350 g/kg DM) Water-Soluble Carbohydrates (WSC = Fructan + Simple Sugars)

		Intakes (g/kg BW/day)			
		Fructan		Simple sugars	
% BW (DM basis)	*DM Intake (kg)*	*Moderate*	*High*	*Moderate*	*High*
3.0	7.5	4.8	6.0	1.2	2.1
4.0	10.0	6.4	11.2	1.6	2.8
5.0	12.5	8.0	14.0	2.0	3.5

Fructan and simple sugars (the sum of glucose, fructose and sucrose) are assumed to comprise, respectively, 80% and 20% of the total WSC in the moderate and high concentration scenarios.

During periods of growth and intense photosynthetic activity, pasture WSC tends to rise during the morning, reaching maxima in the afternoon and then declining overnight. In one study of spring pasture in northern Virginia, the nadir in forage WSC occurred between 0400 h and 0500 h (~15% WSC, DM basis), with peak values between 1600 h and 1700 h (~22–24% WSC) (Byrd et al 2006).

Under some conditions the intake of pasture WSC by grazing equids may approach the amount (as OF) known to induce laminitis when administered as a single dose (Longland & Byrd 2006; Table 27-2). Dry matter intake of horses with free access to pasture may exceed 3% of BW per day (i.e., 15 kg DM intake for a 500-kg horse), while ponies may consume as much as 5% of BW (Longland et al 2011a). A 250-kg pony at pasture with a WSC content of 35% DM (with 80:20 ratio of fructan to simple sugars) would need to consume only about 4.7 kg DM forage (1.9% of BW) to achieve a fructan dose of 5 g/kg BW, which is equivalent to the dose of OF used by Kalck et al (2009) to induce laminitis in some healthy animals. This amount of forage could be ingested in as little as 5–6 h; over a 24-h period in which total forage consumption might approach 5% of BW (12.5 kg DM) fructan intake would approach 14 g/kg BW. It is possible that the WSC dosage required to trigger digestive and metabolic disturbances in susceptible animals (i.e. animals with the EMS phenotype) is lower than that needed to reliably induce disease in healthy experimental animals. Another possibility is that "sub-threshold" doses of WSC consumed over several days induce multiple subclinical insults, with cumulative damage to the lamellae that ultimately manifests as clinical laminitis.

Insulin-induced laminitis

In healthy ponies and horses, the administration of a prolonged (~48 h) euglycemic hyperinsulinemic clamp (EHC) via simultaneous infusions of insulin and glucose induces Obel grade 1–2 laminitis (Asplin et al 2007, De Laat et al 2010). In this model, the induction of supraphysiological hyperinsulinemia (serum insulin ~1000–1100 mU/l) is accompanied by pronounced digital pulses and a significant increase in hoof wall surface temperature (De Laat et al 2010). Pathological features are similar to those described in the OF overload model, although marked leukocyte infiltration and inflammation do not appear to be features of the insulin model (Asplin et al 2010, De Laat et al 2012). The mechanism by which high circulating insulin concentrations (and perhaps also increased glucose flux) induce laminitis has not been elucidated and is the subject of current research. The involvement of increased matrix metalloproteinase activity is unlikely (De Laat et al 2011a). Insulin-like growth factor (IGF)-1 receptor has been identified on lamellar epithelial cells (Bailey & Chockalingham 2009) and it has been proposed that insulin signaling via these receptors may be involved in the pathogenesis of insulin-induced laminitis.

Clinical relevance

Findings from the insulin model have implications for nutritionally associated laminitis, providing a potential explanation for episodes of disease following consumption of feeds and forages that elicit pronounced insulinemic responses. Indeed, it has been argued that hyperinsulinemia is the unifying factor in endocrinopathic and pasture-associated laminitis (McGowan, 2010). Studies of grazing horses have shown a positive relationship between pasture NSC content and circulating insulin concentrations (Byrd et al 2006), and marked exacerbation of hyperinsulinemia has been observed in ponies with an insulin-resistant (EMS) phenotype when they are grazing spring pasture (NSC ~15–18% DM; Treiber et al 2006, 2008). In healthy, nonobese Thoroughbred mares grazing spring (April) pasture, serum insulin concentrations followed a circadian pattern that mirrored changes in forage NSC content, with peak insulin concentrations approaching 100–110 mU/l (Byrd et al 2006). Serum insulin concentrations in Welsh and Dartmoor ponies kept at pasture, some of which were insulin resistant and prone to recurrent pasture laminitis, increased markedly during the months of April and May (values as high as 600–700 mU/l). This occurrence coincided with an increase in pasture grass NSC content and the incidence of laminitis (Treiber et al 2008). Additionally, feeding inulin (to simulate intake of fructan from spring grass) to ponies can elicit an exaggerated insulin response in insulin resistant ponies that are predisposed to laminitis (Bailey et al 2007). Seasonal influences on insulin dynamics also may influence risk of pasture laminitis. A recent study demonstrated exaggerated post-dexamethasone insulin responses in previously laminitic ponies in April and July when compared to responses in December. As well, the increase in serum insulin concentrations in response to dexamethasone administration was significantly higher in previously laminitic than in normal ponies (Bailey et al 2007, Borer et al 2009). It is therefore possible that episodes of laminitis in pasture kept animals, especially those with an EMS phenotype, are directly linked to increases in circulating insulin associated with the consumption of NSC-rich forage.

Whether or not hyperinsulinemia plays an essential or exclusive role in the development of endocrinopathic laminitis remains to be determined. Although high (>750–1000 mU/l) serum insulin concentrations have been detected (Treiber et al 2008) in ponies with clinical laminitis, the authors also have observed similar high or even higher insulin concentrations in ponies without evidence of clinical laminitis. Conversely, some laminitis-prone animals do not exhibit abnormal insulin dynamics. It is possible that other factors contribute to lamellar pathology in the insulin model, for example the effects of an increase in glucose flux during the prolonged EHC. To try and address this question, healthy horses were recently subjected to a 48-h IV glucose infusion that delivered an amount of glucose equivalent to that administered in the EHC experiments (De Laat et al 2011b). This protocol resulted in marked hyperglycemia (~11–12 mmol/l), moderate endogenous hyperinsulinemia (~200 mU/l), and histological evidence of mild lamellar pathology in at least one foot of all treated horses (but not clinical laminitis). When these findings were interpreted in light of previous studies, De Laat et al concluded that: "laminitis may be induced by either insulin alone or a combination of insulin and glucose, but likely not by glucose alone". The authors also suggested that a potential threshold for development of insulin-induced lamellar pathology may be at or below a serum concentration of ~200 mU/l (De Laat et al 2011b). However, in our view these conclusions should be interpreted with considerable caution pending further research. First, the experimental design precluded definitive conclusions regarding cause of the observed lamellar lesions. For example, a protocol that involved suppression of endogenous insulin secretion (e.g., by simultaneous infusion of somatostatin) would be needed to specifically address the hypothesis that laminitis is induced by increased glucose flux. Second, and as mentioned above, the clinical observation of profound hyperinsulinemia in animals without evidence of clinical laminitis raises several questions regarding the cause-and-effect relationship between circulating insulin and laminitis. For example, it is possible that some animals develop tolerance to the effects of high circulating insulin; if so, it will be impossible to determine a threshold of hyperinsulinemia that portends development of laminitis in all animals. It must also be recognized that recurrent laminitis can occur in some animals with no apparent background of high insulin concentrations. As well, it is possible, even likely that another mechanism(s) contributes to laminitis susceptibility in high-risk animals with an insulin resistant (EMS) phenotype – see below.

Other factors potentially increasing susceptibility to laminitis

Aside from hyperinsulinemia, there may be other factors that render certain individuals more susceptible to laminitis (Fig. 27.3). Insulin resistance in humans and animal models of metabolic syndrome is characterized by vascular endothelial dysfunction that contributes to development of hypertension. Insulin is a vasoregulatory hormone, invoking vasodilatation through pathways similar to those of insulin-mediated glucose metabolism (Kim et al 2006). In insulin resistant states, insulin's ability to counteract endothelin-1 associated vasoconstriction may be compromised due to decreased nitric oxide synthesis, while compensatory hyperinsulinemia might stimulate increased endothelin-1 production (Kim et al 2006). The resulting imbalance between the production of nitric oxide and secretion of endothelin-1 favors vasoconstriction and also contributes to platelet activation and leukocyte adhesion, all of which have been

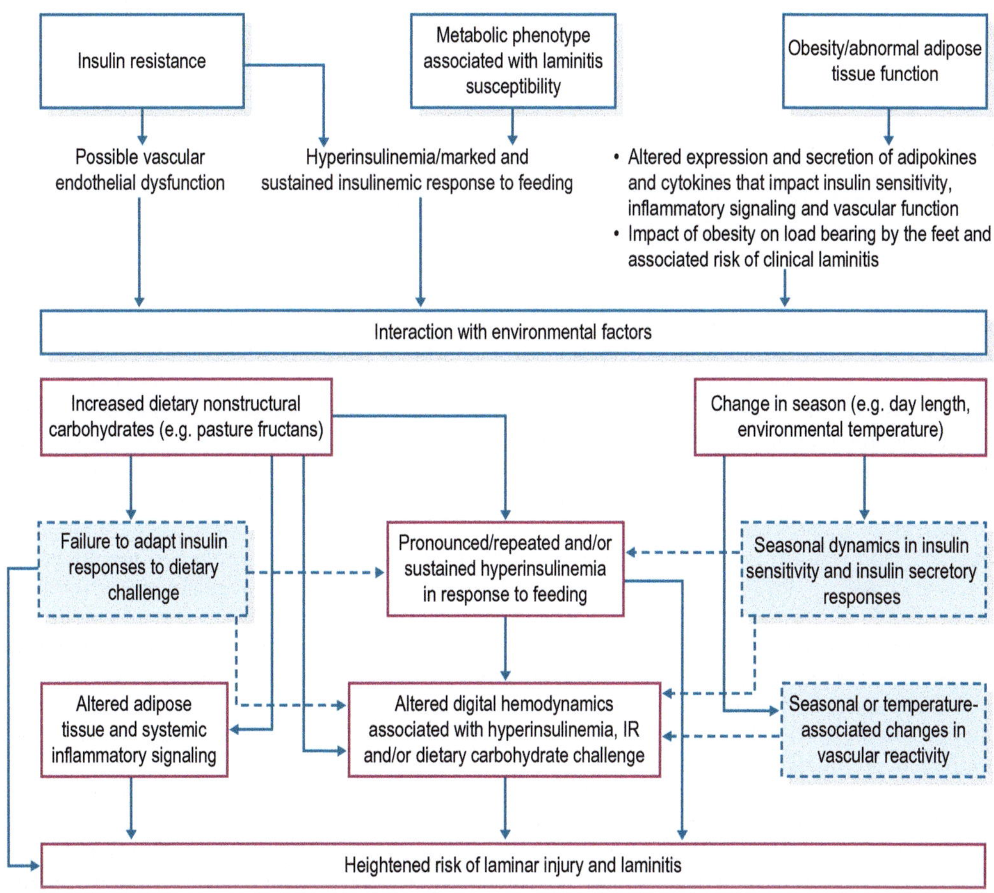

Figure 27.3 Potential interactions between metabolic phenotypic and environmental factors that alter risk for the development of laminitis.

proposed as pathophysiological mechanisms in the development of carbohydrate overload-induced laminitis (Bailey et al 2004a,b, Eades et al 2007). Bailey et al (2008) documented hypertension in insulin resistant, laminitis prone ponies at summer pasture, suggesting that vascular endothelial dysfunction also is a component of the metabolic syndrome phenotype in equids. EMS animals may therefore be more susceptible to digital vasoconstriction, platelet aggregation, and neutrophil adherence and emigration into lamellar tissues under conditions of alimentary carbohydrate overload (Geor & Frank 2009).

A pro-inflammatory state in EMS could amplify lamellar inflammation and destruction associated with carbohydrate overload. Similar to findings in other species (Wild & Byrne 2006) there is some evidence linking obesity in horses and ponies with a proinflammatory state. Blood tumor necrosis factor-α (TNF-α) and IL-1β mRNA expression was higher in obese horses and identified as an independent risk for IR (Vick et al 2007), while increased serum TNF-α concentrations have been observed in a well characterized population of laminitis-prone ponies (Treiber et al 2009). Given the possibility that inflammatory mechanisms contribute to the development of carbohydrate overload-induced laminitis, it is conceivable that EMS animals are more susceptible because of their pre-existing pro-inflammatory state (or the quantity of carbohydrate required to trigger events that result in clinical laminitis may be lower in EMS vs. normal animals). However, recent studies have not supported the inflammatory hypothesis. Groups of lean, insulin sensitive and obese, insulin-resistant ponies were fed a low or high NSC diet for 7 days prior to harvest of lamellar and adipose tissues for evaluation of inflammatory events. The high NSC challenge mimicked exposure to spring pasture. Although some of the obese, insulin resistant and one of the lean ponies fed the high NSC diet developed clinical laminitis toward the end of the feeding period, there was no evidence of induction or exacerbation of inflammatory signaling in adipose or lamellar tissues (Burns et al 2012). These findings suggest that other mechanisms contributed to the development of laminitis under these carbohydrate challenge conditions.

Another possibility is that laminitis-prone horses or ponies have differences in their gut flora compared with animals less prone to laminitis, with heightened hindgut fermentative responses to a given load of NSC and increased production of substances that may be involved in the triggering of laminitis, including vasoactive amines (Elliott & Bailey 2006). Coenen et al (2005) observed marked interhorse variation in apparent fermentative activity after consumption of Jerusalem artichoke (a source of inulin, a fructan), as assessed by the rise in breath hydrogen and methane. Although Crawford et al (2007) did not detect differences in fecal pH or amine concentrations when healthy and laminitis-predisposed ponies were fed supplementary inulin (3 g/kg BW daily) there were differences in the responses of fecal bacterial populations with a marked increase in the numbers of streptococci in the laminitis-prone but not healthy ponies (Newbold et al 2009).

As mentioned, it is possible that animals with an EMS phenotype are more prone to digital vasoconstriction as a result of IR and associated vascular endothelial cell dysfunction. Finally, chronic oxidative stress has also been suggested as a mechanism of lamellar injury in laminitis-prone animals with an EMS phenotype. Higher concentrations of urinary TBARS (thiobarbituric acid reactive substances) were reported in chronic laminitic ponies when compared to ponies who did not suffer from laminitis (Neville et al 2004). However, a study that examined measures of inflammation and redox status in pastured ponies with and without a prior history of laminitis found no differences in markers of antioxidant function (Treiber et al 2009).

The pathophysiology of laminitis in PPID is poorly understood. Possible mechanisms include the adverse effects of high endogenous glucocorticoids, IR or hyperinsulinemia. It warrants mention, however, that hypercortisolemia is an inconsistent finding in PPID (van der Kolk et al 1995, Schott 2006) and, similarly, not all horses with PPID have evidence of IR or hyperinsulinemia (Reeves et al 2001).

Key Points – Pathogenesis

- The various experimental models used to induce laminitis may provide some insight into the naturally occurring condition but they are unlikely to mirror all clinical manifestations precisely
- Pasture associated laminitis is likely to have a complex etiology potentially involving hyperinsulinemia in association with or independent of hindgut carbohydrate overloading
- The development of laminitis in horses or ponies without evidence of systemic illness (i.e. sepsis-related laminitis) should alert veterinarians to the possibility of underlying metabolic and endocrine disturbances (i.e., EMS or PPID).

Management of cases

A detailed discussion on the medical management of acute and chronic laminitis is beyond the scope of this chapter and the reader is referred elsewhere for more information (van Eps 2010, Morrison 2010). In brief, the general principles of management comprise: (1) identification and treatment of the underlying or predisposing primary condition (e.g., treatment of grain overload) and/or removal of inciting cause (e.g., removal from pasture or access to grain-based feeds); (2) evaluation of the severity of laminitis, including lateromedial hoof radiographs that will provide information on structural integrity of the hoof (e.g., rotation or sinking of the distal phalanx) and also provide baseline data for the purposes of monitoring responses to treatment and determining prognosis; and (3) prompt institution of treatments targeting pain relief and minimization of progression of laminitis. The latter will include strategies intended to promote stability of the distal phalanx and the hoof–lamellar interface, including removal of shoes, housing on deeply littered bedding, and application of sole support (e.g., pads or silicone rubber inserts positioned against the sole or application of tape-on shoes used in conjunction with silicone putty applied over the palmar/plantar aspect of the sole).

Affected animals should be evaluated for evidence of prior episodes of laminitis as well as underlying metabolic and endocrine abnormalities (i.e., EMS and PPID). There may be history of prior episodes of pasture-associated laminitis and/or evidence of hoof wall "founder lines" indicative of previous episodes. Evaluation of insulin sensitivity is indicated but testing should be delayed until after resolution of the acute laminitic episode because laminitis-associated pain and stress will confound test results. Dietary management including a decision on whether or not affected animals should be allowed to return to pasture after resolution of the laminitis episode is another important consideration. These aspects are discussed below.

Emergency treatment of grain overload

Horse owners or caregivers may request evaluation and treatment of animals that have recently ingested a large amount of grain but are yet to exhibit clinical signs indicative of grain overload, including laminitis. Alternatively, grain overload is recognized or suspected based on clinical signs such as colic, abdominal distension, tachycardia, sweating and trembling as well as laminitis (bounding digital pulses, weight shifting, lameness and reluctance to move). Aggressive treatment is indicated in both situations. In general, the prognosis is fair to good for horses without clinical signs of grain overload and laminitis at the time of initial evaluation. On the other hand, prognosis is guarded to poor for horses with clinical signs at the time of presentation; affected animals may succumb to hypovolemic and/or septic shock or require humane euthanasia due to the progression and severity of the laminitis.

Gastric lavage for removal of grain/feed material is indicated if the horse is evaluated in the first 4 to 6 hours after grain ingestion or if substantial feed material is present in the stomach on evaluation. The presence of substantial gas or fluid in the stomach may indicate gastric dilatation; a nasogastric tube should be left in place for 12 to 24 hours to maintain gastric decompression. In the absence of gastric reflux, substances that bind toxins and/or promote transit of ingesta should be administered, for example mineral oil (2 to 4 liters once daily for 1 to 3 days) and/or activated charcoal (0.25 kg in 1 to 2 liters of water, single dose). Marked colonic and/or cecal distension can develop in some affected animals; cecal trocharization may be required for relief of distension.

Intravenous fluid therapy is indicated to restore circulating volume and correct dehydration; isotonic crystalloid fluids (25–50 ml/kg IV) with or without hypertonic saline (2–4 ml/kg IV bolus, once) or a colloid plasma volume expander (e.g. 6% Hetastarch, 5–10 ml/kg IV bolus, once) are recommended for resuscitation. After initial resuscitative therapy, IV polyionic crystalloid fluids should be administered for rehydration (100 to 200 ml/kg as needed) and maintenance (50 to 75 ml/kg per day). Anti-inflammatory and analgesic therapy is indicated for management of the systemic effects of grain overload as well as laminitis; several drug treatment regimens have been described (see Belknap 2010). Treatments that target mitigation of endotoxemia include the administration of plasma (regular plasma or hyperimmune plasma with anti-LPS antibodies) or polymyxin-B (2000 to 6000 IU/kg, diluted in 500–1000 ml of 0.9% NaCl solution, IV every 12 h for 1 to 3 days). Polymyxin-B should not be administered until after correction of fluid deficits and is contraindicated in patients with compromised renal function.

Research has demonstrated that digital hypothermia induced by continuous immersion of the distal limb in ice and water inhibits early lamellar inflammatory signaling and reduces the severity of laminitis when treatment is initiated at the time of experimental carbohydrate (oligofructose) overload (van Eps et al 2012). There is rationale, therefore, for prompt instigation of continuous distal limb cryotherapy (maintaining water temperature at 3–5°C) especially in animals that have consumed excessive grain but are not showing clinical signs. Cryotherapy boots for horses are now commercially available.

Dietary management

Evidence-based recommendations for feeding management of horses with acute or chronic laminitis are lacking. The following are the authors' recommendations; these may require modification as more data becomes available.

Complete removal of feeds that may have been involved in the development of laminitis (and have the potential to exacerbate severity of current laminitis) is essential. In horses that have consumed excessive grain but do not have clinical signs of grain overload, all feed should be withheld for 24 h followed by a gradual introduction to hay (or alternate preserved forage) feeding over the next 24–48 h. Restriction of NSC intake (i.e., use of hay with NSC content <10–12% DM) is recommended to minimize post-feeding increases in circulating insulin that may increase risk for development of laminitis. For horses with clinical signs of grain overload, feed should be withheld until resolution of signs of colic, gastric/large intestinal distension, and gastric reflux. If laminitis does not develop, a gradual return to normal diet can be initiated 48–72 h post grain engorgement. Conversely, a longer period of special dietary management is indicated for animals that develop laminitis – hay with low NSC content (<10–12% DM) should be fed at 1.5% to 2% of BW until resolution of laminitis. An appropriate "ration balancer" feed (0.5 to 1.0 kg/day for a 400–600 kg horse) should be added to the diet to provide amino acids, vitamins and minerals lacking in the hay ration. Alternatively, a complete diet appropriately fortified and shown to produce a low glycemic/insulinemic response can be fed.

Similar principles apply in the dietary management of horses and ponies that develop pasture-associated laminitis. Affected animals must be removed from pasture, housed either in a dry lot (mild laminitis) or a box stall with deep bedding (more severe laminitis), and introduced to a low NSC, preserved forage-based ration with an appropriate forage balancer. The duration of confinement and restricted diet as well as decisions regarding a return to pasture grazing will depend on the severity and time course of the laminitis and the presence of underlying endocrine and metabolic problems. In general:

- The horse or pony should be held off pasture until there has been complete resolution of the acute laminitis episode and, where indicated, diagnostic testing for EMS and PPID. If there is no evidence of EMS or PPID, a gradual reintroduction to pasture may be considered. Start with 1 to 2 hours of grazing, once or twice per day, or turnout for longer periods if the horse is fitted with a grazing muzzle (fitted appropriately and which allows limited grazing but access to water; see Chapter 28). More caution may be required under a number of circumstances, i.e., when pasture is green and growing rapidly (e.g., in spring) or is stressed (through drought/inappropriate management, etc.) or where clover has become dominant.

- Obese, insulin resistant animals should be held off pasture for a longer period (e.g., 2–3 months), allowing time for implementation of management changes (i.e., dietary restriction, increased physical activity) that result in weight loss and improved insulin sensitivity. Similarly, horses with PPID should be held off pasture pending improvement in clinical signs, e.g. treatment with pergolide.
- Some EMS and PPID affected animals with history of repeated episodes of laminitis require permanent housing in a dry lot because they appear to be susceptible to further episodes of laminitis in the face of even small variations in pasture availability and nutrient content.
- Whilst there are no specific data to support the increased provision of certain vitamins and trace elements, it may be helpful to provide additional biotin (with total biotin intake of 3–5 mg/100 kg BW) in a ration providing sufficient amino acids, zinc and calcium etc. in order to help support optimal hoof growth and quality.
- The use of bran mashes (particularly when fed solus with forage) is likely to be contraindicated, especially in animals unaccustomed to bran within their diet. Apart from being potentially an irritant to the gastrointestinal tract, bran has an unbalanced Ca:P ratio and is deficient in many key nutrients such as lysine.
- As discussed above, the relevance of oxidative stress in the pathophysiology of laminitis is unclear - however, the authors recommend that laminitic animals are provided with higher than maintenance intake of vitamin E (e.g. 150–200 IU/kg diet DM).

Key Points – Management of acute cases

- Prompt veterinary treatment is essential
- Remove potential initiating cause(s) and initiate where relevant (e.g., EMS or PPID associated cases) appropriate long-term treatment and management strategies
- In the short to medium term, laminitic animals should be fed a forage-based diet which typically will require supplementation with a forage balancer to ensure adequate protein, amino acid, vitamin and mineral intake for an animal under stress

Countermeasures to nutritionally associated laminitis

Countermeasures for avoidance of nutritionally-associated laminitis are focused on two areas: (1) countering potential metabolic and endocrine predisposing factors in high-risk horses and ponies; and (2) strategies for limiting intake of rapidly fermentable carbohydrates from pasture and other feedstuffs. Horses and ponies with a history of laminitis or physical characteristics suggestive of EMS or PPID should be carefully evaluated, including assessment of body condition and the presence of abnormal fat deposits, plus screening tests for IR. We currently recommend that horses with IR and/or hyperinsulinemia undergo interventions to help improve insulin sensitivity, including strategies for induction of weight loss (restriction in dietary energy intake, increased physical activity), control of dietary NSC intake, and possibly use of pharmacologic agents purported to increase insulin sensitivity and/or promote weight loss.

Identification of high-risk animals

Endocrinopathic laminitis occurs in association with PPID (equine Cushing's disease) and EMS. Animals with these conditions are therefore at an increased risk of laminitis and consequently early recognition may enable instigation of countermeasures (dietary and exercise management, pharmacologic treatment) that lower risk for development of further episodes of laminitis. Definitive diagnosis of both PPID and EMS is challenging. Clinical presentation of PPID and EMS can be similar and one view, albeit controversial is that the clinical features of EMS and PPID represent a continuum of the same condition (Frank et al 2010). Importantly, disturbances in insulin regulation (IR and exaggerated insulin responses to IV or oral glucose challenge) are a feature of both conditions and given the postulated association between hyperinsulinemia and laminitis, laboratory screening for IR is critical in the identification and management of laminitis risk (see below).

Classical clinical signs of PPID include abnormalities of the hair coat (ranging from failure to completely shed the winter coat in spring to hypertrichiasis), loss of muscle mass/tone, abnormal subcutaneous fat deposition, polyuria-polydipsia (PUPD), and recurrent infections. Testing methods used in the diagnosis of PPID include the overnight dexamethasone suppression test (ODST), a combined dexamethasone suppression-thyrotropin-releasing hormone stimulation test, and measurement of baseline plasma ACTH concentrations (Schott 2006). Results of these tests can be affected by pain, so testing should not be performed during acute episodes of laminitis nor at certain times of the year depending on the geographical location. Although the actual risk is probably very low, owners may decline the ODST due to a concern that the administration of dexamethasone may precipitate an episode of laminitis; measurement of ACTH concentrations is the recommended approach in these situations.

Current criteria for a diagnosis of EMS (also see Chapter 28) include: (1) generalized (body condition score, BCS $\geq$ 7/9) or regional (e.g. neck crest fat accumulation) obesity; (2) resting hyperinsulinemia (>20 mU/l) or exaggerated insulin dynamics in response to oral or IV glucose challenge; and (3) evidence of current or historical laminitis (e.g., divergent growth rings or "founder lines" on the hoof wall) (Frank et al 2010). Plasma ACTH concentrations and results of the DST are normal in EMS animals. The obesity criterion is somewhat controversial because some horses and ponies with an insulin resistant phenotype linked to laminitis susceptibility are not obese (Bailey et al 2007, 2008). Conversely, some overweight/obese animals are not insulin resistant and do not appear to be at increased risk of laminitis. Accordingly, screening for IR and/or abnormal insulin dynamics is critical in the diagnosis of EMS. Measurement of serum leptin concentration also may be of value in the assessment of laminitis risk. Higher leptin concentrations have been detected in insulin resistant horses and ponies

(Gentry et al 2002, Frank et al 2006, Carter et al 2009) and in a group of inbred ponies with a high incidence of laminitis, hyperleptinemia (>7.3 ng/ml) was a useful predictor of the development of laminitis when ponies were subsequently exposed to spring pasture (Carter et al 2009). One author has suggested that a "fasting" leptin concentration >7 ng/ml is supportive of a diagnosis of EMS (Frank 2011). Hypertriglyceridemia (>50 mg/dl) has been detected in ponies with an EMS phenotype (Treiber et al 2006, Bailey et al 2008) but further studies are needed to determine the utility of serum triglyceride concentrations in the diagnosis of EMS.

Current research seeks to characterize the genetic basis for the equine metabolic syndrome phenotype and associated laminitis risk. The identification of a particular gene or set of genes associated with laminitis susceptibility and/or the metabolic syndrome phenotype may lead to the development of more sensitive and specific laboratory screening tests.

Evaluation of insulin sensitivity and dynamics

Insulin resistance in horses and ponies is often characterized by hyperinsulinemia and normoglycemia, indicative of compensated IR wherein the glucose homeostasis is maintained by increased insulin secretion from the pancreas. Although more work is needed to determine appropriate cutoffs (e.g. accounting for variation due to season or habitual diet), serum insulin concentrations of >20 mU/l or >30 mU/l (where 1 mU/l = 1 μU/ml = ~7 pmol/l) have been used to define hyperinsulinemia and diagnose IR (Frank et al 2010, Frank 2011). These somewhat arbitrary cutoff values are primarily based on measurements using the Siemens Coat-A-Count insulin radioimmunoassay. Recent studies have shown that this assay is the most accurate of the currently available commercial assays; however, samples with an insulin concentration that exceeds the highest standard should be diluted with insulin-depleted equine serum rather than the manufacturer's diluent (Tinworth et al 2011, Borer et al 2012b). It also is important to recognize that within an individual animal there can be marked inter-day variation in serum insulin concentrations, and this is a major limitation in the use of resting insulin concentrations for diagnosis of IR.

When measuring resting insulin concentrations, standardization of sampling and analytical procedures is critical for interpretation, as results can be affected by a number of animal and environmental factors. Stress associated with a change in housing, feeding or sampling procedures may affect results. Most importantly, diet composition, particularly the NSC content of feeds and forages (Borgia et al 2009), can impact insulin concentration. Marked fluctuations in insulin concentrations (values rising from 10–20 mU/l to >80–100 mU/l) have been observed in horses and ponies grazing pasture with high NSC content (Byrd et al 2006, Treiber et al 2008). Similarly, grain, concentrate and even hay feeding is associated with variable hyperinsulinemia that may persist for several hours.

A suggested sampling protocol is as follows: All feed and forage should be withheld for 6–8 hours prior to sampling (from late evening), with blood drawn before 10 am. For animals maintained at pasture, removal from pasture the day prior to sampling is recommended, especially during periods of active forage growth (e.g., spring) when the high sugar content of pasture forage can affect resting blood glucose and insulin concentrations. In laminitic animals testing should be delayed until after resolution of the acute laminitic episode because the associated pain and stress may exacerbate hyperinsulinemia.

Proxy estimates of insulin sensitivity derived from single measurements of blood insulin and glucose have been used for diagnosis of IR and abnormal insulin secretory response in horses (Treiber et al 2006, Borer et al 2012a). The most commonly used proxies are RISQI (insulin$^{-0.5}$), QUICKI (1/(log[fasting insulin] + log[fasting glucose])) and MIRG (modified insulin-to-glucose ratio: 800 − 0.3 × [insulin − 50]^2)/[glucose − 30]). Separate studies have shown that these proxies can distinguish between groups of laminitis-prone and control ponies (Treiber et al 2006, Borer et al 2012a), but they cannot accurately predict predisposition to laminitis in individual animals (Borer et al 2012a). Seasonal variation in the proxy measurements of insulin sensitivity and insulin secretory response also has been observed (Borer et al 2012a).

Repeat evaluation of resting insulin concentration or application of a dynamic test of glucose tolerance or insulin sensitivity is warranted for evaluation of IR in animals with borderline initial results (e.g. resting insulin <20 mU/l) but other clinical or historical findings indicative of EMS or PPID. The gold standard methods for assessment of insulin sensitivity (i.e., euglycemic-hyperinsulinemic clamp; Minimal Model analysis of a frequently sampled intravenous glucose tolerance test) are impractical in clinical settings. Alternate dynamic testing procedures that can be performed in field settings are a combined glucose-insulin test (CGIT) and an oral sugar test (OST; Frank 2011) – see Box 27.1 for details. With the CGIT, a diagnosis of IR is rendered when blood glucose does not return to baseline (pre-infusion) values within 45 min or when serum insulin concentration is >100 mU/l at this time point (Frank 2011). However, it is important to note that there can be considerable variability in the results even in the same animal.

The OST involves oral administration of 15 ml corn syrup (Karo Light Syrup, Ach Food Companies Inc., Cordova, TN, USA) per 100 kg BW (about 75 ml for a 500-kg horse, providing ~75 g of sugars). Preliminary studies have indicated that serum insulin concentrations exceed 50 mU/l between 60 and 90 min post-dosing in insulin resistant animals whereas serum insulin remains <30 mU/l in healthy horses. Further validation studies, including evaluation of the effects of season (time of year), are required however.

Decreasing intake of rapidly fermentable carbohydrates

Complete elimination of pasture access is not always necessary and many horses or ponies that have had one or more episodes of pasture laminitis can return to grazing activity providing there has been successful implementation of countermeasures to obesity and IR. Even in such cases, restriction at certain times of the year may be necessary (e.g., spring and autumn; on bright sunny but frosty days). Although restriction of grazing to 1–2 hours at a time seems a reasonable strategy to limit NSC intake, in reality there is minimal information on the quantity of pasture a horse or pony may be able to ingest during these short periods of grazing activity. Recent work looking at the effect of grazing muzzles has shown that whilst there can be considerable

Box 27.1 Methods for Dynamic Assessment of Glucose Tolerance and Insulin Dynamics in Horses (See Eiler et al 2005, Frank 2011)

Principle: Laminitis-prone animals with a metabolic syndrome phenotype are insulin resistant and exhibit (1) exaggerated insulinemic responses to oral carbohydrate challenge; and (2) reduced rate of decay in blood glucose and insulin concentrations after intravenous administration of glucose and insulin.

Oral sugar test

Method:

- Feed is withheld for at least 10 hours prior to testing (e.g., no feed after 7–8 pm leave one flake or biscuit of hay for late evening consumption, administer the test at ~7 or 8 am the next day).
- Corn syrup* at a dosage of 15 ml per 100 kg BW (75 ml for a 500-kg horse) is administered *per os* by use of 60-ml catheter-tip syringes. *Corn syrup administration can be performed by owner or caregiver.*
- A blood sample (plain vacutainer tube) is collected 75–90 min after dosing for measurement of serum insulin concentration.

Interpretation: Serum insulin concentration >50 mU/l (>350 pmol/l) indicates an abnormal insulin response. Note that more work is required to establish appropriate cutoff values. As well, it must be emphasized that an abnormal insulin value is not a specific indicator of laminitis risk.

Combined glucose-insulin test

Method:

- Feed is withheld for at least 10 hours prior to testing (e.g., no feed after 7–8 pm, leave one flake or biscuit of hay for late evening consumption, administer the test at ~7 or 8 am the next day).
- Insert and secure a catheter into a jugular vein for blood sampling.
- Obtain a baseline blood sample for measurement of blood glucose concentration by use of a handheld glucometer.
- Administer 150 mg/kg BW 50% dextrose intravenously (into contralateral jugular vein), followed immediately by 0.10 U/kg BW regular insulin.
- Collect additional blood samples at 1, 5, 15, 25, 35, 45, 60, 90, 105, 120, 135 and 150 minutes after glucose-insulin injection. Measure blood glucose concentrations.
- Preferred – measure serum insulin concentrations in 0 and 45 min samples.

Interpretation: Insulin resistance is evidenced by a blood glucose concentration that remains above the baseline value at 45 min (and/or an insulin concentration >100 mU/l [>690 pmol/l] at this time point).

*In the USA, Karo Light Corn Syrup™ is preferred.

individual and day-to-day variability in intake, ponies can ingest up to 1% of their BW in DM of grass within 3 hours (Longland et al 2011a). Another study showed that ponies can consume from 22 to 49% of their daily DM intake within a 3 hour turnout period and that they adapt to short turnout periods by increasing DM intake (Ince et al 2011). Therefore, restricted grazing may not adequately limit daily intake of NSC and rapidly fermentable carbohydrates, particularly at times of the year when pasture forage sugar and/or fructan content is high.

As mentioned, on sunny days the NSC content of temperate grasses in the Northern Hemisphere tends to rise during the morning, reaching maxima in the afternoon and declining overnight. In one study of spring pasture in Northern Virginia (Byrd et al 2006), the nadir in forage NSC occurred between 0400 h and 0500 h (~15% NSC, DM basis), with highest values between 1600 h and 1700 h (~22–24% NSC). Furthermore, serum insulin concentrations in mares grazing upon this pasture displayed a similar circadian pattern that was strongly related to the NSC content. These observations support the common recommendation, at least with respect to temperate grasses in the Northern Hemisphere, to turn susceptible animals out very late at night or very early in the morning with removal from pasture by mid-morning. Again, this approach may not be foolproof in spring because the NSC content of early morning pasture, while lower when compared to the same pasture in the afternoon, may not be safe for susceptible animals.

Specific recommendations regarding pasture turnout for laminitis-prone animals is provided in Box 27.2.

Countering endocrine-metabolic risk factors

Obesity has been associated with IR and risk of laminitis although, as mentioned previously, not all obese horses are insulin resistant or apparently at increased risk for laminitis. Nonetheless, in obese animals with a history of endocrinopathic laminitis, weight loss via dietary restriction and, if possible, increased physical activity should help to minimize risk of future episodes of laminitis. Strategies for promotion of weight loss are discussed in Chapter 28. Control of dietary NSC intake, use of specialized dietary supplements, and pharmacologic treatments for PPID and enhancement of insulin sensitivity are discussed here.

Restriction of dietary nonstructural carbohydrates

The primary goal in the feeding management of insulin resistant horses and ponies (obese or non-obese) is avoidance of feeds rich in NSC (starches, sugars, and/or fructans) that may increase risk of laminitis, either by exacerbation of hyperinsulinemia or via disturbances to the hindgut microbial community that may trigger events that lead to laminitis. This requires knowledge of the carbohydrate composition of feedstuffs for horses. The reader is referred to another chapter in this book (Chapter 8) for a review of methods used for analysis and reporting of carbohydrate fractions in feeds. The general guidelines for feeding management of insulin resistant horses include:

1. *No grain or sweet feeds* (i.e., feedstuffs rich in starch and/or sugars). The starch content of oats, barley and corn are, approximately 45–55%, 60–65% and 65–75% of DM respectively. Sweet feeds contain grains plus molasses and the NSC content of some of these feeds can approach 45–50% DM. Provision of these feeds to insulin resistant equids is likely to exacerbate hyperinsulinemia.
2. *Restricted or no access to pasture.* At certain times of the year, pasture forage NSC content may approach 40% DM. In susceptible animals, ingestion of this NSC-rich forage will increase risk for development of laminitis. (Even with moderate NSC content, if there is a plentiful supply of grass overall NSC intake over a relatively short period of time can be quite high, as discussed above).

Box 27.2 Advice Regarding Pasture Turnout for Laminitis-Prone Horses and Ponies

- Consider zero grazing (whilst providing the horse with a suitable forage alternative as well as options for activity and socializing) in situations where it is considered essential to severely restrict intake of sugars, starches and fructans, or when caloric restriction is needed for management of body weight. A dirt paddock that accommodates exercise and group housing is recommended in these circumstances.
- Turn horses out to pasture when forage nonstructural carbohydrate (NSC) concentrations are likely to be at the lowest, such as very late at night through until early morning, removing horses from the pasture by mid-morning in Northern hemisphere.
- Do not allow horses to graze pastures that have not been properly managed by regular grazing or cutting. Good management is indicated by maintenance of a young, leafy sward rather than mature, stemmy herbage that contains higher stored fructans. Another important consideration is herbage yield – high intake of pasture forage with moderate NSC may be as problematical as smaller quantities of high NSC forage.
- Avoid/restrict pasture turnout in spring (before flower development) and autumn as well as during the period of flowering and early seeding.
- Do not allow horses to graze on pastures that have been exposed to low temperatures (e.g. frosts) with warm, bright sunny weather or pastures that have been "stressed" through drought or poor management.
- Consider maintaining turnout by:
  - Use of grazing muzzles (ensure the animal can obtain sufficient water intake; be aware of possible behavioral changes; ensure that the muzzle is fitted correctly and animals are provided with substantial time without the muzzles).
  - Strip grazing behind other horses or sheep;
  - Cutting (by mower) the pasture and removing clippings;
  - Putting a deep layer of wood chips over a small paddock or using dry lots/indoor schools etc. Note that animals housed on sandy soils may be at increased risk of sand-associated colic, especially when on restricted rations.
- Rotate use of paddocks regularly (preferably with other species such as sheep or cattle) to keep grass at an appropriate height and prevent the pasture from becoming "stressed" through either under or over-grazing.

3. *A diet based on grass hay (or hay substitute) with low (<10–12% DM) NSC content.*
4. *Feeding for maintenance of bodyweight and BCS.* Weight gain will typically exacerbate IR, so it is important to avoid overfeeding. Regular evaluation of bodyweight and/or BCS is the best way to assess the adequacy or otherwise of energy provision.

Horses and ponies that have had recent episodes of laminitis and are insulin resistant should be denied access to pasture until there is improvement in insulin sensitivity. After improvement in insulin sensitivity (e.g., evidenced by correction of resting hyperinsulinemia and/or reduced insulinemic response to a standardized glucose challenge) there can be a gradual reintroduction to pasture, e.g. restricted grazing time (1–2 hours per day), strip grazing, or turnout with a grazing muzzle. Even after improvement in insulin sensitivity, it is advisable to restrict or avoid any grazing during periods when pasture forage NSC is likely to be high – during spring and early summer; after summer or fall rains that cause the grass to turn green; and when pastures have been subjected to drought or frost stress, conditions that favor fructan accumulation). Some equids remain persistently hyperinsulinemic despite weight loss and use of other dietary approaches to improve insulin sensitivity, and/or appear to be intolerant of even small fluctuations in pasture or preserved forage nutrient composition. These animals may have to be permanently housed off pasture and fed preserved forage known to be low in NSC (and produce a low insulin/glucose response upon ingestion).

The core diet for animals at high-risk of laminitis should be based on grass hay. Mature hay is preferred due to lower digestible energy and NSC content when compared to less mature hay. Alfalfa hay or other legumes such as clover are less preferred because, on average, these forages have higher energy and NSC content when compared to grass hay. Ensiled forages generally have lower NSC contents than hay made from the same crop. However, despite the generally lower NSC content of haylage compared to hay, the high palatability of some haylages may result in higher total NSC/energy intake. Ideally, the results of proximate nutrient analysis, including direct measurement of starch and sugars (i.e., NSC), should be reviewed before selection of the hay. A NSC content of less than 10–12% DM is currently recommended. In the absence of data on hay NSC content, some nutritionists have recommended soaking hay in water for 30 to 60 min before feeding to leach water soluble carbohydrates (WSC; sugars and fructans). However, recent work has suggested that under typical management conditions this practice is variable in outcome and may not result in substantial change in the WSC content of some hays (Longland et al 2011b). Soaking hay should therefore be used as an adjunct to choosing low NSC-containing hay. Whilst sufficient scientific evidence is not currently available to determine whether the 10–12% DM upper limit of NSC content is optimal, clinical experience suggests that this recommendation is reasonable. Additionally, in a small study of healthy Quarter horses vs. horses affected by polysaccharide storage myopathy, hay with a NSC content of <10.8% did not impact glycemic and insulinemic responses whereas a moderate increase in serum insulin concentration was observed after consumption of hay with NSC >16% (Borgia et al 2009).

Caution is required in using the ethanol-soluble carbohydrate (ESC) fraction as a measure of the simple sugar fraction of the feed in question (and based on this, the assumption that WSC – ESC estimates the fructan content) as some smaller molecular weight fructans and other carbohydrate oligomers may also be soluble in 80% ethanol. It is also important to note that the McLeary colorimetric method ("megazyme") for fructan determination results in variable and substantially underestimated values for the fructan content of certain feeds and forages including timothy (Longland et al 2012).

Forage only diets are very unlikely to provide adequate protein, minerals or vitamins. Supplementing the forage diet with a low-calorie commercial ration balancer product that contains sources of high-quality protein and a mixture of vitamins and minerals to balance in particular the low vitamin E, copper, zinc, selenium and other minerals typically found in mature grass hays is therefore recommended. These products can be fiber based or may be designed to be fed in small quantities (e.g., 0.5–1.0 kg/day fed as is or mixed with hay chop [chaff]). Such fiber-based, low energy feeds can help to extend chewing and feeding time especially in animals provided a restricted diet.

Not all insulin resistant horses and ponies are obese and, in some of these animals, a ration of mostly hay may not meet energy requirements particularly when some weight gain is desired or the animal is competing in athletic events. One approach is to add non-molassed sugar beet pulp to the ration, e.g. 1–2 kg (0.5 to 1.5 lb)/day. Beet pulp is rich in highly-digestible fibers, provides more digestible energy when compared to most hay types, and does not elicit a marked glycemic or insulinemic response unless molasses is added at the time of processing. Beet pulp shreds should be soaked (in a volume of water three- to fourfold higher than that of the beet pulp) prior to feeding. The energy density of the ration also can be increased by feeding vegetable oil, for example mixed with sugar beet pulp shreds or with hay cubes that have been softened in water. Corn and soy oils are commonly used in equine rations, but need to be fresh, non-rancid and introduced gradually to the ration. One standard cup (about 225 ml or 210 g) of vegetable oil provides 1.7 Mcal of digestible energy. Depending on energy requirements, ½ to 1 cup of oil can be fed once or twice daily (up to a maximum of ~1 ml oil/1 kg BW). Smaller amounts (e.g. ¼ cup once daily) should initially be fed, with a gradual increase over a 7–10 day period. Supplemental antioxidant (1–2 IU vitamin E per 1 ml of added oil) should be provided. Stabilized rice bran (~20% fat) is another option for increasing the energy density of the diet, providing the calcium:phosphorus ratio of the final ration is considered.

Another approach to dietary management of the lean or working insulin-resistant horse is to provide a commercial feed along with hay. Most feed companies now offer products with lower starch and sugar content (<20–25% NSC, DM basis) when compared to traditional sweet feeds (40–50% NSC) or cereal grains. Digestible fibers (sugar beet pulp and/or soy hulls) and vegetable oils are included in place of starch-rich ingredients and energy density is similar or even higher when compared to sweet feeds. In theory, these lower NSC feeds result in lower post-feeding glycemic and insulinemic responses and carry lower risk for disturbances in hindgut function associated with the rapid fermentation of starch and/or sugars. However, glycemic/insulinemic responses cannot be reliably predicted from the formulation (or assessment of NSC content) and actual measurement of post-feeding glucose and insulin concentrations in horses is currently required to verify that the feed is "low-glycemic" (Geor & Harris 2009, Vuervert et al 2009). These products are often marketed for use in horses and ponies at high risk for laminitis, including those with IR or PPID, although minimal published data is available to support or refute these medical claims. Nonetheless, these feeds are convenient for clients, the principle is sound, and providing these feeds do actually result in low post-feeding glucose and insulin responses they are likely to be useful when fed according to manufacturer's recommendations.

Dietary supplements

A number of supplements are marketed with claims for improved insulin sensitivity or reduced risk of laminitis but evidence of efficacy is scant (Tinworth et al 2010a). Many products contain magnesium, chromium and/or cinnamon. Daily feeding of the streptogramin antibiotic virginiamycin has been recommended for prevention of pasture-associated laminitis, purportedly by preventing the overgrowth of Gram-positive cecal bacteria (Bailey et al 2004a). However, this product has only limited availability (e.g., not available in the US) and anecdotally is not effective in all cases. The feeding of a protected hindgut buffer product (sodium bicarbonate) mitigated decreases in the fecal pH associated with significant amounts of grain feeding and pasture grazing (Pagan et al 2007) but data on efficacy for prevention of laminitis are not available.

Chromium is thought to potentiate insulin action via activation of insulin-receptor kinase and/or inhibition of insulin receptor tyrosine phosphatase (Lau et al 2008). Studies in people have shown that suboptimal intake of chromium (trivalent form) contributes to IR in type 2 diabetes and metabolic syndrome. Moreover, some but not all studies have shown improvement in glucose tolerance in insulin resistant human patients (Anderson 2000). Supplemental chromium (2.5 to 5.0 mg/day) has been fed to insulin-resistant horses and ponies (Vervuert et al 2008, Chameroy et al 2011). In one preliminary report, overweight (BCS 7.6 ± 0.8) hyperinsulinemic ponies were fed a yeast product with or without chromium together with hay for 4 weeks. An oral starch tolerance test (STT) was performed at the beginning and end of the supplementation period, and peak insulin responses were modestly lower in the supplemented animals at the end of the study period (Vervuert et al 2008). In contrast, the feeding of a supplement containing 5 mg/day chromium (as yeast), 8.8 g/day magnesium and other unspecified nutraceuticals for 16 weeks did not alter morphometric measurements, resting serum glucose and insulin concentrations, or insulin sensitivity in obese horses with a history of laminitis (Chameroy et al 2011). Additional research is required to determine the efficacy of chromium supplements in the management of IR in horses.

There also is interest in the effects of magnesium nutrition on insulin sensitivity and other aspects of metabolism. Some studies in humans have demonstrated an association between magnesium status and IR in type 2 diabetes (Barbagallo et al 2003, Song et al 2006). A review of randomized double-blind controlled trials that evaluated the effects of magnesium supplementation in patients with type 2 diabetes concluded that supplementation may be effective in reducing fasting plasma fasting concentrations and increasing high-density lipoprotein cholesterol but only in patients with actual magnesium deficiency which was determined by measurement of intraerythrocytic concentrations (Song et al 2006). There are no published data on the magnesium status of obese and/or insulin resistant horses or ponies. The aforementioned study by Chameroy et al. (2011) reported that magnesium supplementation at 8.8 g/day (an amount which exceeds daily requirements) did not impact insulin sensitivity in obese laminitic horses.

There are no published studies on the effects of cinnamon supplementation in horses. Studies in humans patients with type 2 diabetes and IR have yielded conflicting results perhaps related in part to the source of cinnamon used (Khan et al 2003, Vanschoonbeek et al 2006), although a review of all randomized controlled clinical trials concluded that cinnamon is effective in reducing postprandial glucose concentrations (Kirkham et al 2009)

Daily supplementation with 45 g short-chain fructo-oligosaccharide (scFOS) for 6 weeks resulted in a modest improvement in insulin sensitivity and decrease in resting serum insulin concentrations of obese Arabian horses fed a 50:50 grass hay and sweet feed diet (Respondek et al 2011). The mechanism of this apparent improvement in insulin sensitivity is unknown although it warrants mention that scFOS supplementation has also been shown to improve insulin sensitivity and modulate the transcription of genes involved in adipose tissue glucose and lipid metabolism in obese dogs (Respondek et al 2008).

Medical treatment

Although diet and other conservative measures are front-line strategies for avoidance of endocrinopathic laminitis, there are indications for medical treatment in PPID and perhaps also EMS. Drug therapy is important in the long-term management of PPID and has been reported to limit the recurrence of laminitis in affected animals (Walsh 2010). The combined D1/D2 dopamine receptor antagonist pergolide mesylate is the drug of choice for treatment of PPID (Durham 2010). Doses between 0.001 and 0.003 mg/kg (PO, once daily) are effective in alleviating clinical signs of PPID and decreasing plasma ACTH concentrations (Schott 2006, Walsh 2010). Inappetance has been observed in 5% to 10% of horses after initiation of treatment; in some horses temporary cessation of pergolide therapy with reintroduction at a lower dose is necessary to overcome this reduction in appetite.

There is developing interest in the pharmacologic treatment of EMS that might reduce risk of laminitis (Durham 2010). Levothyroxine sodium and metformin have been used in the treatment of EMS (Durham et al 2008, Frank et al 2008, Frank 2011), while the thiazolidinedione drug pioglitazone hydrochloride has undergone preliminary investigation in healthy horses (Suagee et al 2011, Wearn et al 2011). Levothyroxine sodium has been recommended as a short-term treatment (e.g., 3 months) while the effects of dietary restriction and increased physical activity take effect, and in circumstances where these management changes have failed to effect adequate weight loss and control of laminitic episodes (Frank 2011). In healthy horses, a 6-month period of levothyroxine treatment resulted in weight loss and increased insulin sensitivity although there was wide individual variability in response (Frank et al 2008). Weight loss is thought to be due to the effects of increased thyroxine on basal metabolic rate. Clinical experience has indicated variable (and sometimes limited) beneficial response to levothyroxine in EMS animals. The recommended dosage for weight loss in mature horses is 48 mg/day (about 4 teaspoons, administered in feed) for 3 to 6 months depending on clinical response. Treated animals should be gradually weaned from the drug when treatment goals have been attained; a recommended protocol involves decreasing the dosage from 48 mg/day to 24 mg/day for 2 weeks, then 12 mg/day for a further 2 weeks. Dietary restriction (including restricted access to pasture) is recommended during treatment due to a concern that levothyroxine will induce hyperphagia and therefore offset beneficial effects on body weight.

The biguanide drug metformin is widely used for control of hyperglycemia and improvement in insulin sensitivity in humans with diabetes mellitus (Musi et al 2002, Durham 2010). The primary mechanism of action appears to be activation of AMP-activated protein kinase (AMPK); in liver this results in suppression of hepatic gluconeogenesis while in skeletal muscle activation of AMPK enhances glucose uptake via GLUT4 transport proteins (Musi et al 2002). Equine studies have demonstrated poor oral bioavailability of metformin in horses (Hustace et al 2009) and ponies (Tinworth et al 2010b), while studies to date have reported no effect of metformin (at doses up to 15 mg/kg, orally two or three times daily for 2 to 3 weeks) on insulin sensitivity in healthy (Firshman et al 2009) or obese, insulin-resistant animals (Tinworth et al 2012). On the other hand, two studies have shown that metformin moderates hyperglycemia and hyperinsulinemia in horses. Metformin at 15 mg/kg PO twice daily (q12) resulted in decreases in the plasma glucose and insulin concentrations of insulin-resistant horses and ponies within 2 weeks of the start of treatment (Durham et al 2008), while Rendle et al (2013) have reported moderation of plasma glucose and insulin responses when metformin was administered at a dose of 30 mg/kg prior to oral glucose dosing. It is thought that these effects of metformin are mediated via a decrease in enteric glucose absorption (Sakar et al 2010). The observation that metformin lowers glucose and insulin responses in horses suggests that this drug may be useful in the management of insulin resistant animals that are provided access to pasture that contains significant NSC. However, further studies are needed to examine the effect of metformin treatment on glycemic and insulinemic responses in grazing horses

Monitoring

Regular monitoring of plasma ACTH and serum insulin concentrations, bodyweight and BCS is recommended in horses at risk for endocrinopathic laminitis. Pergolide treatment of horses with PPID should result in a decrease in plasma ACTH; concentrations often decrease below 70 pg/ml although may remain above the diagnostic cutoff (35 pg/ml, during the November - July period; Cornell University Animal Health Diagnostic Laboratory). Regular monitoring of resting serum insulin concentrations may provide some indication of the effectiveness of management changes (e.g. sample 2–3 weeks after a change in diet or reintroduction to pasture). However, due to the individual variability in insulin concentrations and the possibility that other factors contribute to risk of laminitis, low insulin concentrations cannot be taken to mean no ongoing risk.

Key Points – Nutritional countermeasures in laminitis-prone animals

- The identification of laminitis-prone animals (e.g., horses or ponies with EMS or PPID) enables instigation of nutritional countermeasures that may help to limit further episodes
- Dietary management focuses on restricted intake of rapidly fermentable carbohydrates (sugars, starches and fructans) that may increase risk of laminitis via disturbances to the hindgut environment or induction of hyperinsulinemia.

Strategies include restricted access to pasture and the feeding of forage with NSC <10–12% DM
- A number of dietary supplements are marketed with claims for improved insulin sensitivity or reduced risk of endocrinopathic laminitis but evidence of efficacy is scant

Summary

The consumption of excessive quantities of NSC can induce laminitis in any horse and pony, as evidenced by the experimental starch or oligofructose overload models that induce laminitis in the majority of animals. In field settings, however, risk of laminitis appears to be highest in animals with underlying metabolic and endocrine abnormalities (EMS and PPID), with episodes of laminitis most likely reflecting an interplay between animal genotypic/phenotypic (e.g., insulin resistance, hyperinsulinemia and/or obesity) and environmental (especially dietary NSC content) factors. Strategies to reduce the risk of laminitis therefore focus on the identification of high-risk animals as well as diet and exercise interventions that correct obesity and control intake of NSC. There is interest in the use of insulin-sensitizing drugs for treatment of laminitis-prone animals, although more research is needed to examine efficacy.

References

Alford, P., Geller, S., Richardson, B., et al., 2001. A multicenter, matched case-control study of risk factors for equine laminitis. Preventive Veterinary Medicine 49, 209–222.

Allen, D., Clark, E.S., Moore, J.N., et al., 1990. Evaluation of equine digital Starling force and hemodynamics during early laminitis. American Journal of Veterinary Research 51, 1930–1934.

Anderson, R.A., 2000. Chromium in the prevention and control of diabetes. Diabetes Metabolism (Paris) 26, 22–27.

Asplin, K.E., Sillence, M.N., Pollitt, C.C., et al., 2007. Induction of laminitis by prolonged hyperinsulinaemia in clinically normal ponies. Veterinary Journal 174, 530–535.

Asplin, K.E., Patterson-Kane, J.C., Sillence, M.N., et al., 2010. Histopathology of insulin-induced laminitis in ponies. Equine Veterinary Journal 42, 700–706.

Bailey, S.R., Chockalingham, S., 2009. Proliferative effects of insulin on equine lamellar epithelial cells medicated by the IGF-1 receptor. In: Proceedings of 2nd AAEP Foundation Equine Laminitis Research Workshop, West Plam Beach, Florida, p. 26.

Bailey, S.R., Baillon, M.L., Rycroft, A.N., et al., 2003. Identification of equine cecal bacteria producing amines in an *in vitro* model of carbohydrate overload. Applied Environmental Microbiology 69, 2087–2093.

Bailey, S.R., Marr, C.M., Elliott, J., 2004a. Current research and theories on the pathogenesis of acute laminitis in the horse. Veterinary Journal 167, 129–142.

Bailey, S.R., Menzies-Gow, N.J., Marr, C.M., et al., 2004b. The effects of vasoactive amines found in the equine hindgut on digital blood flow in the normal horse. Equine Veterinary Journal 36, 267–272.

Bailey, S.R., Menzies-Gow, N.J., Harris, P.A., et al., 2007. Effect of dietary fructan and dexamethasone on the insulin response of ponies predisposed to laminitis. Journal of the American Veterinary Medical Association 231, 1365–1373.

Bailey, S.R., Habershon-Butcher, J.L., Ransom, K.J., et al., 2008. Hypertension and insulin resistance in a mixed-breed population of ponies predisposed to laminitis. American Journal of Veterinary Research 69, 122–129.

Bailey, S.R., Adair, H.S., Reinemeyer, C.R., et al., 2009. Plasma concentrations of endotoxin and platelet activation in the developmental stage of oligofructose-induced laminitis. Veterinary Immunology and Immunopathology 129, 167–173.

Barbagallo, M., Dominguez, A., Galioto, A., et al., 2003. Role of magnesium in insulin action, diabetes and cardiovascular syndrome X. Molecular Aspects of Medicine 24, 39–52.

Belknap, K.J., 2010. The pharmacologic basis for the treatment of developmental and acute laminitis. Veterinary Clinics of North America Equine Practice 26, 115–124.

Belknap, J.K., Giguère, S., Pettigrew, A., et al., 2007. Lamellar proinflammatory cytokine expression patterns in laminitis at the developmental stage and at the onset of lameness: Innate versus adaptive immune response. Equine Veterinary Journal 39, 42–47.

Belknap, J.K., Moore, J.N., Crouser, E.C., 2009. Sepsis – from human organ failure to laminar failure. Veterinary Immunology and Imunopathology 129, 155–157.

Berhane, Y., Jordan, H., Bailey, S.R., et al., 2009a. Modulation of endothelium-dependent relaxation of equine digital arteries by insulin and hypoxia. In: Proceedings of the 2nd AAEP Foundation Equine Laminitis Research Workshop, Palm Beach, Florida, American Association of Equine Practitioners, Lexington, KY, p. 36.

Berhane, Y., Putignano, C., Bailey, S.R., et al., 2009b. Effect of amine metabolism by SSAO on endothelium – dependent vasodilatory responses of Krebs perfused equine digits. In: Proceedings of the 2nd AAEP Foundation Equine Laminitis Research Workshop, Palm Beach, Florida, American Association of Equine Practitioners, Lexington, KY, p. 37.

Borer, K.E., Menzies-Gow, N.J., Berhane, Y., et al., 2009. Seasonal influence on insulin and cortisol results from overnight dexamethasone suppression tests in normal and previously laminitic ponies. In: Proceedings of the 2nd AAEP Foundation Equine Laminitis Research Workshop, Palm Beach, Florida, American Association of Equine Practitioners, Lexington, KY, p. 38.

Borer, K.E., Bailey, S.R., Menzies-Gow, N.J., et al., 2012a. Use of proxy measurements of insulin sensitivity and insulin secretory response to distinguish between normal and previously laminitic ponies. Equine Vet J (in press).

Borer, K.E., Bailey, S.R., Menzies-Gow, N.J., et al., 2012b. Evaluation of a commercially available radioimmunoassay and species-specific ELISA to measure high concentrations of insulin in equine serum. American Journal of Veterinary Research (in press).

Borgia, L., Valberg, S., Watts, K., et al., 2009. Glycemic/insulinemic response to feeding hay with different water soluble carbohydrate content in healthy and polysaccharide storage myopathy-affected horses. Journal of Equine Veterinary Science 29, 355–357.

Buckley, P., Morton, J., Coleman, G., 2007. Repeated observation of naturally occurring laminitis in pony club horses in regional Australia. In: Proceedings of the Australian College of Veterinary Scientists, College of Science Week Scientific Meeting, Gold Coast, Australia, pp. 10–11.

Burns, T.A., Westerman, T., Nuovo, G.J., et al., 2011. Role of oxidative tissue injury in the pathophysiology of experimentally induced equine laminitis: a comparison of 2 models. Journal of Veterinary Internal Medicine 25, 540–548.

Burns, T.A., Watts, M.R., Geor, R.J., et al., 2012. Laminar inflammatory events in lean and obese ponies subjected to high carbohydrate feeding: Implications for pasture-associated laminitis. Forum of the American College of Veterinary Internal Medicine 26, 732.

Byrd, B.M., Treiber, K.H., Staniar, W.B., et al., 2006. Circadian and seasonal variation on pasture NSC and circulating insulin concentrations in grazing horses. Journal of Animal Science 84 (Suppl 1), 330–331 (abstract).

Carter, R.A., Treiber, K.H., Geor, R.J., et al., 2009. Prediction of incipient pasture-associated laminitis from hyperinsulinemia, hyperleptinemia and generalized and localized obesity in a cohort of ponies. Equine Veterinary Journal 40, 171–178.

Chameroy, K.A., Frank, N., Elliott, S.B., et al., 2011. Effects of a supplement containing chromium and magnesium on morphometric measurements, resting glucose, insulin concentrations, and insulin sensitivity in laminitic obese horses. Equine Veterinary Journal 43, 494–499.

Clutterbuck, A.L., Harris, P., Allaway, D., et al., 2010. Matrix metalloproteinases in inflammatory pathologies of the horse. Veterinary Journal 183, 27–38.

Coenen, M., Vervuert, I., Moessler, A., 2005. Hydrogen and methane exhalation profiles of horses after consumption of grassmeal (cellulose), sugar beet pulp (pectin), oats (starch) and Jerusalem artichoke (fructan). In: Proceedings of the 19th Equine Science Symposium, Tuscon, Arizona, Equine Science Society, Champaign, IL, pp. 158–160.

Crawford, C., Sepulveda, M.F., Elliott, J., et al., 2007. Dietary fructan carbohydrate increases amine production in the equine large intestine: implications for pasture-associated laminitis. Journal of Animal Science 85, 2949–2958.

De Laat, M.A., McGowan, C.M., Sillence, M.N., et al., 2010. Equine laminitis: induced by 48 h hyperinsulinaemia in Standardbred horses. Equine Veterinary Journal 42, 129–135.

De Laat, M.A., Kyaw-Tanner, M.T., Nourian, A.R., et al., 2011a. The developmental and acute phases of insulin-induced laminitis involve minimal metalloprotease activity. Veterinary Immunology and Immunopathology 140, 275–281.

De Laat, M.A., van Eps, A.W., McGowan, C.M., et al., 2011b. Equine laminitis: Comparative histopathology 48 hours after experimental induction with insulin or alimentary oligofructose in Standardbred horses. Journal of Comparative Pathology 145, 399–409.

De Laat, M.A., Sillence, M.N., McGowan, C.M., et al., 2012. Continuous intravenous infusion of glucose induces endogenous hyperinsulinaemia and lamellar histopathology in Standardbred horses. Veterinary Journal 191 (3), 317–322.

Donaldson, M.T., Lamonte, B.H., Morresey, P., et al., 2002. Treatment with pergolide or cyproheptadine of pituitary pars intermedia dysfunction (equine Cushing's disease). Journal of Veterinary Internal Medicine 16, 742–746.

Donaldson, M.T., Jorgensen, A.J., Beech, J., 2004. Evaluation of suspected pituitary pars intermedia dysfunction in horses with laminitis. Journal of the American Veterinary Medical Association 224, 1123–1127.

Dorn, C.R., Garner, H.E., Coffman, J.R., et al., 1975. Castration and other factors affecting the risk of equine laminitis. Cornell Veterinarian 65, 57–64.

Durham, A., 2010. The pharmacologic basis for the treatment of endocrinopathic laminitis. Veterinary Clinics of North America Equine Practice 26, 303–314.

Durham, A.E., Rendle, D.I., Newton, J.E., 2008. The effect of metformin on measurements of insulin sensitivity and beta cell response in 18 horses and ponies with insulin resistance. Equine Veterinary Journal 40, 493–500.

Eades, S.C., 2010. Overview of current laminitis research. Veterinary Clinics of North America: Equine Practice, Advances in Laminitis, Part 1 26, 51–63.

Eades, S.C., Stokes, A.M., Moore, R.M., et al., 2006. Effects of an endothelin receptor antagonist and nitrogelycerin on digital vascular function in horses during the prodromal stages of carbohydrate overload-induced laminitis. American Journal of Veterinary Research 67, 1204–1211.

Eades, S.C., Stokes, A.M., Johnson, P.J., et al., 2007. Serial alterations in digital hemodynamics and endothelin-1 immunoreactivity, platelet-neutrophil aggregation, and concentrations of nitric oxide, insulin and glucose in blood obtained from horses following carbohydrate overload. American Journal of Veterinary Research 68, 87–94.

Eiler, H., Frank, N., Andres, F.M., et al., 2005. Physiologic assessment of blood glucose homeostasis via combined intravenous glucose and insulin testing in horses. American Journal of Veterinary Research 66, 1598–1604.

Elliott, J., Bailey, S.R., 2006. Gastrointestinal derived factors are potential triggers for the development of acute equine laminitis. Journal of Nutrition 136, 2103S–2107S.

Faleiros, R.R., Johnson, P.J., Nuovo, G.J., et al., 2011a. Laminar leukocyte accumulation in horses with carbohydrate overload-induced laminitis. Journal of Veterinary Internal Medicine 25, 107–115.

Faleiros, R.R., Leise, B.S., Watts, M., et al., 2011b. Laminar chemokine mRNA concentrations in horses with carbohydrate overload-induced laminitis. Veterinary Immunology and Immunopathology 144, 45–51.

Firshman, A., Hustace, J., Peterson, K., et al., 2009. The effect of metformin on insulin sensitivity in horses. In: Proceedings of the American College of Veterinary Internal Medicine Annual Forum, Montreal, Canada

Frame, S.R., Harrington, D.D., Fessler, J., et al., 1988. Hereditary junctional mechanobullous disease in a foal. Journal of the American Veterinary Medical Association 193, 1420–1424.

French, K.R., Pollitt, C.C., 2004. Equine laminitis: congenital, hemidesmosomal plectin deficiency in a Quarter Horse foal. Equine Veterinary Journal 36, 299–303.

Frank, N., 2011. Equine metabolic syndrome. Veterinary Clinics of North America: Equine Practice 27, 73–92.

Frank, N., Elliott, S.B., Brandt, L.E., et al., 2006. Physical characteristics, blood hormone concentrations, and plasma lipid concentrations in obese horses with insulin resistance. Journal of the American Veterinary Medical Association 228, 1383–1390.

Frank, N., Elliott, S.B., Boston, R.C., 2008. Effects of long-term oral administration of levothyroxine sodium on glucose dynamics in healthy adult horses. American Journal of Veterinary Research 69, 76–81.

Frank, N., Geor, R.J., Bailey, S.R., et al., 2010. Equine metabolic syndrome. Journal of Veterinary Internal Medicine 24, 467–475.

Garner, H.E., Coffman, J.R., Hahn, A.W., et al., 1975. Equine laminitis of alimentary origin: an experimental model. American Journal of Veterinary Research 36, 441–444.

Gentry, L.R., Thompson, D.L., Gentry, G.T., et al., 2002. The relationship between body condition, leptin, and reproductive and hormonal chracteristics of mares during the seasonal anovulatory period. Journal of Animal Science 80, 2695–2703.

Geor, R., Frank, N., 2009. Metabolic syndrome – From human organ disease to laminar failure in equids. Veterinary Immunology and Immunopathology 129, 151–154.

Geor, R.J., Harris, P.A., 2009. Dietary management of obesity and insulin resistance: Countering risk for laminitis. Veterinary Clinics of North America Equine Practice 25, 51–65.

Harris, P., 2011. Laminitis after 2000 years: Adding bricks to our wall of knowledge. Veterinary Journal (in press): doi:10.1016/j.tvjl.2011.09.014.

Harris, P.A., Geor, R.J., 2010. Recent advances in the understanding of laminitis and obesity. In: Ellis, A.D., Longland, A.C., Coenen, M., Miraglia, N. (Eds.), The Impact of Nutrition on the Health and Welfare of Horses. Wageningen Academic Publishers, Wageningen, pp. 215–233 (EAAP Publication 128).

Hinckley, K., Henderson, I., 1996. The epidemiology of equine laminitis in the UK. In: Proceedings of the 35th Congress of the British Equine Veterinary Association, Warwick, UK, British Equine Veterinary Association Fordham, UK, pp. 62–63.

Hustace, J.L., Firshman, A.M., Mata, J.E., 2009. Pharmacokinetics and bioavailability of metformin in horses. American Journal of Veterinary Research 70, 665–668.

Ince, J., Longland, A.C., Newbold, J.C., et al., 2011. Changes in proportions of dry matter intakes by ponies with access to pasture and haylage for 3 and 20 hours per day respectively for six weeks. Journal of Equine Veterinary Science 31, 283–284.

Kalck, K.A., Frank, N., Elliott, S.B., et al., 2009. Effects of low-dose oligofructose treatment administered via nasogastric intubation on induction of laminitis and associated alterations in glucose and insulin dynamics. American Journal of Veterinary Research 70, 624–632.

Kane, A.J., Traub-Dargatz, J.L., Losinger, W.C., et al., 2000. The occurrence and causes of lameness and laminitis in the US horse population. In: Proceedings of the 46th American Association of Equine Practitioners Annual Meeting, San Antonio, Texas, pp. 277–280.

Keen, J.A., Hillier, C., McGorum, B.C., et al., 2008. Endothelin mediated contraction of equine laminar veins. Equine Veterinary Journal 40, 488–492.

Khan, A., Safdar, M., Ali Khan, M.M., et al., 2003. Cinnamon improves glucose and lipids of people with type 2 diabetes. Diabetes Care 23, 3215–3218.

Kim, J.K., Montagnani, M., Koh, K.K., et al., 2006. Reciprocal relationships between insulin resistance and endothelial dysfunction: Molecular and pathophysiological mechanisms. Circulation 113, 1888–1904.

Kirkham, S., Akilen, R., Sharma, S., et al., 2009. The potential of cinnamon to reduce blood glucose levels in patients with type 2 diabetes and insulin resistance. Diabetes Obesity Metabolism 11, 1100–1113.

Kyaw-Tanner, M.T., Wattle, O., van Eps, A.W., et al., 2008. Equine laminitis: membrane type matrix metalloproteinase-14 (MMP-14) is involved in acute phase onset. Equine Veterinary Journal 40, 482–487.

Lau, F.C., Bagchi, M., Sen, C.K., et al., 2008. Nutrigenomic basis of beneficial effects of chromium(III) on obesity and diabetes. Molecular and Cellular Biochemistry 317, 1–10.

Leise, B.S., Faleiros, R.R., Watts, M., et al., 2011. Laminar inflammatory gene expression in the carbohydrate overload model of equine laminitis. Equine Veterinary Journal 43, 54–61.

Loftus, J.P., Belknap, J.K., Stankiewicz, K.M., et al., 2007. Laminar xanthine oxidase, superoxide dismutase and catalase activities in the prodromal stage of black walnut induced equine laminitis. Equine Veterinary Journal 39, 48–53.

Longland, A.C., Byrd, B.M., 2006. The importance of pasture nonstructural carbohydrates in equine laminitis. Journal of Nutrition 136, 2099S–2102S.

Longland, A.C., Barfoot, C., Harris, P.A., 2011a. The effect of wearing a grazing muzzle vs. not wearing a grazing muzzle on pasture dry matter intake by ponies. Journal of Equine Veterinary Science 31, 282–283.

Longland, A.C., Barfoot, C., Harris, P.A., 2011b. Effects of soaking on the water-soluble carbohydrate and crude protein content of hay. Veterinary Record 168, 618–622.

Longland, A.C., Ince, J.C., Moore-Colyer, M.J.S., et al., 2012a. Degradation of grass and grass fructan by equine gastrointestinal digesta in vitro. Journal of the Science of Food and Agriculture (submitted).

Longland, A.C., Dhanoa, M.S., Harris, P.A., 2012. Comparison of a colorimetric and a high performance liquid chromatography method for the determination of fructan in pasture grasses for horses. Journal of the Science of Food and Agriculture 92, 1878–1885.

McGowan, C., 2010. Endocrinopathic laminitis. Veterinary Clinics of North America Equine Practice 26, 233–237.

Menzies-Gow, N.J., Bailey, S.R., Katz, L.M., et al., 2004. Endotoxin-induced digital vasoconstriction in horses: associated changes in plasma concentrations of vasoconstrictor mediators. Equine Veterinary Journal 36, 273–278.

Menzies-Gow, N.J., Katz, L.M., Barker, K.J., et al., 2010a. Epidemiological study of pasture-associated laminitis and concurrent risk factors in the South of England. Veterinary Record 167, 690–694.

Menzies-Gow, N.J., Stevens, K., Barr, A., et al., 2010b. Severity and outcome of equine pasture-associated laminitis managed in first opinion practice in the UK. Veterinary Record 167, 364–369.

Milinovich, G.J., Trott, D.J., Burrell, P.C., et al., 2006. Changes in equine hindgut bacterial populations during oligofructose-induced laminitis. Environmental Microbiology 8, 885–898.

Milinovich, G.J., Klieve, A.V., Pollitt, C.C., et al., 2010. Microbial events in the hindgut during carbohydrate-induced equine laminitis. Veterinary Clinics of North America: Equine Practice, Advances in Laminitis, Part 1 26, 79–94.

Morrison, S., 2010. Chronic laminitis: Foot management. Veterinary Clinics of North America Equine Practice 26, 425–446.

Musi, N., Hirshman, M.F., Nygren, J., et al., 2002. Metformin increases AMP-activated protein kinase activity in skeletal muscle of subjects with type 2 diabetes. Diabetes 51, 2074–2081.

Neville, R.F., Hollands, T., Collins, S.N., et al., 2004. Evaluation of urinary TBARS in normal and chronic laminitic ponies. Equine Veterinary Journal 36, 292–294.

Newbold, C.J., Macias, B., Crawford, C., et al., 2009. Changes in the bacterial populations in the equine hindgut following the addition of inulin to the diet. In: Proceedings of the British Society of Animal Science: Advances in Animal Biosciences. Cambridge University Press, Cambridge, UK, p. 16.

Nilsson, U., Oste, R., Jagerstad, M., et al., 1988. Cereal fructans: In vitro and in vivo studies in availability in rats and humans. Journal of Nutrition 118, 1325–1330.

Obel, N., 1948. Studies on the histopathology of acute laminitis. Almqvist & Wiksells Boktryckeri AB, Uppsala.

Orsini, J.A., 2010. Cutting edge research updates. Journal of Equine Veterinary Science 30, 449–454.

Pagan, J.D., Lawrence, T.J., Lawrence, L.A., 2007. Feeding protected sodium bicarbonate attenuates hindgut acidosis in horses fed a high-grain ration. In: Proceedings of 54th Annual Convention of the American Association of Equine Practitioners. American Association of Equine Practitioners, Lexington, KY, pp. 530–533.

Parsons, T.S., Orsini, J.A., Krafty, R., et al., 2007. Risk factors for development of acute laminitis in horses during hospitalization: 73 cases (1997–2004). Journal of the American Veterinary Medical Association 230, 885–889.

Pollitt, C.C., Visser, M.B., 2010. Carbohydrate alimentary overload laminitis. Veterinary Clinics of North America: Equine Practice, Advances in Laminitis, Part 1 26, 65–78.

Polzer, J., Slater, M.R., 1997. Age, breed, sex and seasonality as risk factors for equine laminitis. Preventive Veterinary Medicine 179–184.

Reeves, H.J., Lees, R., McGowan, C.M., 2001. Measurement of basal serum insulin concentration in the diagnosis of Cushing's disease in ponies. Veterinary Record 149, 449–452.

Rendle, D.I., Rutledge, F., Hughes, K.J., et al., 2013. Effects of metformin hydrochloride on glucose and insulin responses in horses. Equine Veterinary Journal (in press).

Respondek, F., Swanson, K.S., Belsito, K.R., et al., 2008. Short-chain fructo-oligosaccharides influence insulin sensitivity and gene expression of fat tissue in obese dogs. Journal of Nutrition 138, 1712–1718.

Respondek, F., Myers, K., Smith, T.L., et al., 2011. Dietary supplementation with short-chain fructo-oligosaccharides improves insulin sensitivity in obese horses. Journal of Animal Science 89, 77–83.

Robertson, T.P., Bailey, S.R., Peroni, J.F., 2009. Equine laminitis: a journey to the dark side of venous. Veterinary Immunology and Immunopathology 129, 1930–1934.

Roberts, R.A., Laskin, D.L., Smith, C.V., et al., 2009. Nitrative and oxidative stress in toxicology and disease. Toxicological Science 112, 4–16.

Sakar, Y., Meddah, B., Faouz, M.A., et al., 2010. Metformin-induced regulation of the intestinal D-glucose transporters. Journal of Physiology and Pharmacology 61, 301–307.

Schott, H.C., 2006. Pituitary pars intermedia dysfunction: challenges of diagnosis and treatment. In: Proceedings of the 52nd American Association of Equine Practitioners Annual Convention. San Antonio, Texas, American Association of Equine Practitioners, Lexington, KY, pp. 60–73.

Schott, H.C., Coursen, C.L., Eberhart, S.W., et al., 2001. The Michigan Cushing's project. In: Proceedings of the 47th Annual Convention of the American Association of Equine Practitioners. American Association of Equine Practitioners, Lexington, KY, pp. 22–24.

Slater, M.R., Hood, D.M., Carter, G.K., 1995. Descriptive epidemiological study of equine laminitis. Equine Veterinary Journal 27, 364–367.

Song, Y., He, Y., Levitan, E.B., et al., 2006. Effects of oral magnesium supplementation on glycaemic control in Type 2 diabetes: a meta-analysis of randomized double blind controlled trials. Diabetes Medicine 23, 1050–1056.

Sprouse, R.F., Garner, H.E., Green, E.M., 1987. Plasma endotoxin levels in horses subjected to carbohydrate overload induced laminitis. Equine Veterinary Journal 19, 25–28.

Suagee, J.K., Corl, B.A., Wearn, J.G., et al., 2011. Effects of the insulin-sensitizing drug pioglitazone and lipopolysaccharide administration on insulin sensitivity in horses. Journal of Veterinary Internal Medicine 25, 356–364.

Tinworth, K.D., Harris, P.A., Sillence, M.N., et al., 2010a. Potential treatments for insulin resistance in the horse: A comparative multi-species review. Veterinary Journal 186, 282–291.

Tinworth, K.D., Edwards, S., Harris, P.A., et al., 2010b. Pharmacokinetics of metformin after enteral administration in insulin-resistant ponies. American Journal of Veterinary Research 71, 1201–1206.

Tinworth, K.D., Wynn, P.C., Boston, R.C., et al., 2011. Evaluation of commercially available assays for the measurement of equine insulin. Domestic Animal Endocrinology 41, 81–90.

Tinworth, K.D., Boston, R.C., Harris, P.A., et al., 2012. The effect of oral metformin on insulin sensitivity in insulin-resistant ponies. Veterinary Journal 191, 79–84.

Toth, F., Frank, N., Chameroy, K.A., et al., 2009. Effects of endotoxaemia and carbohydrate overload on glucose and insulin dynamics and the development of laminitis in horses. Equine Veterinary Journal 41, 852–858.

Treiber, K.H., Hess, T.M., Kronfeld, D.S., et al., 2005. Insulin resistance and compensation in laminitis-predisposed ponies characterized by the Minimal Model. Pferdeheilkunde 21, 91–92.

Treiber, K.H., Kronfeld, D.S., Hess, T.M., et al., 2006. Evaluation of genetic and metabolic predispositions and nutritional risk factors for pasture-associated laminitis in ponies. Journal of the American Veterinary Medical Association 228, 1538–1545.

Treiber, K.H., Carter, R.A., Harris, P.A., et al., 2008. Seasonal changes in energy metabolism of ponies coincides with changes in pasture carbohydrates: Implications for laminitis. Journal of Veterinary Internal Medicine 22, 735–736 (abstract).

Treiber, K., Carter, R., Gay, L., et al., 2009. Inflammatory and redox status of ponies with a history of pasture-associated laminitis. Vet Immunol Immunopathol 129, 216–220.

USDA. 2000. Lameness and laminitis in US horses. USDA:APHIS:US, CEAH, National Animal Health Monitoring System. US Department of Agriculture, Washington DC.

van der Kolk, J.H., Wensing, T., Kalsbeek, H.C., et al., 1995. Laboratory diagnosis of equine pituitary pars intermedia adenoma. Domestic Animal Endocrinology 12, 35–39.

van Eps, A.W., Pollitt, C.C., 2006. Equine laminitis induced with oligofructose. Equine Veterinary Journal 38, 203–208.

van Eps, A.W., 2010. Acute laminitis: Medical and supportive therapy. Veterinary Clinics of North America Equine Practice 26, 103–114.

van Eps, A.W., Leise, B.S., Watts, M., et al., 2012. Digital hypothermia inhibits early lamellar inflammatory signaling in the oligofrucotse laminitis model. Equine Veterinary Journal 44, 230–237.

Vanschoonbeek, K., Thomassen, B.J., Senden, J.M., et al., 2006. Cinnamon supplementation does not improve glycemic control in postmenopausal type 2 diabetic patients. Journal of Nutrition 136, 977–980.

Verveurt, I., Obwald, B., Coenen, M., 2008. Effects of chromium supplementation on metabolic profile in insulin resistant ponies. In: Proceedings of the 12th Congress of the European Society for Veterinary Clinical Nutrition, Vienna, Austria, European Society for Veterinary Clinical Nutrition, p. 40 (abstract).

Vervuert, I., Voigt, K., Hollands, D., et al., 2009. Effect of feeding increasing quantities of starch on glycaemic and insulinaemic responses in healthy horses. Veterinary Journal 182, 67–72.

Vick, M.M., Adams, A.A., Murphy, B.A., et al., 2007. Relationships among inflammatory cytokines, obesity, and insulin sensitivity in the horse. Journal of Animal Science 85, 1144–1155.

Visser, M.B., Pollitt, C.C., 2011a. The timeline of lamellar basement membrane changes during equine laminitis development. Equine Veterinary Journal 43, 471–477.

Visser, M.B., Pollitt, C.C., 2011b. Lamellar leukocyte infiltration and involvement of IL-6 during oligofructose-induced equine laminitis development. Veterinary Immunology and Immunopathology 144, 120–128.

Visser, M.B., Pollitt, C.C., 2012. The timeline of metalloprotease events during oligofructose induced equine laminitis development. Equine Veterinary Journal 44, 88–93.

Walsh, D.M., 2010. Field treatment and management of endocrinopathic laminitis in horses and ponies. Veterinary Clinics of North America Equine Practice 26, 379–390.

Wearn, J.G., Suagee, J.K., Crisman, M.V., et al., 2011. Effects of the insulin-sensitizing drug, pioglitazone and lipopolysaccharide administration on markers of systemic inflammation and clinical parameters in horses. Veterinary Immunology and Immunopathology (Epub ahead of print).

Weiss, D.J., Evanson, O.A., McClenahan, D., et al., 1997. Evaluation of platelet activation and platelet-neutrophil aggregates in ponies with alimentary laminitis. American Journal of Veterinary Research 58, 1376–1380.

Weiss, D., Evanson, O., MacLeay, J., et al., 1998. Transient alteration in intestinal permeability to technectium Tc99m diethylenetriaaminopentaacetate during the prodromal stages of alimentary laminitis in ponies. American Journal of Veterinary Research 59, 1431–1434.

Wild, S.H., Byrne, C.D., 2006. ABC of obesity: Risk factors for diabetes and coronary heart disease. British Medical Journal 333, 1009–1011.

Wylie, C.E., Collins, S.N., Verheyen, L.P., et al., 2011. Frequency of equine laminitis: A systematic review with quality appraisal of published evidence. The Veterinary Journal 189, 248–256.

Wylie, C.E., Collins, S.N., Verheyen, L.P., et al., 2011. Risk factors for laminitis: A systematic review with quality appraisal of published evidence. The Veterinary Journal. doi:10.1016/j.tvjl.2011.10.020.

Obesity

Raymond J. Geor, Patricia A. Harris

Obesity is an emergent problem in domestic horse and pony populations that has health and welfare implications. Equine obesity, in particular, has been associated with insulin resistance and hyperinsulinemia, which are risk factors for laminitis, particularly the pasture-associated form of this condition. Recognition of these adverse consequences of obesity has prompted research on the epidemiology and pathophysiology of obesity in equids as well as strategies for weight loss and other aspects of management that may mitigate risk of obesity-associated health problems. This chapter reviews current knowledge of the prevalence, causes and consequences of obesity in horses and ponies. It also provides recommendations for dietary and exercise management of obesity based on current knowledge and understanding.

Definition of obesity

Obesity can be simply defined as an expanded mass of adipose tissue in the body (Figs 28.1 and 28.2). Obesity also can be defined as a disease in which excess body fat has accumulated to such an extent that health may be adversely affected. In human populations, obesity has been defined by either direct (e.g., magnetic resonance imaging (MRI) or dual-energy X-ray absorptiometry (DEXA) imaging) or indirect (e.g., bioelectrical impedance) quantitative assessment of body fat content, or has been based on anthropometric approaches that utilize simple clinical measures such as body mass index (BMI; weight/height^2, kg/m^2) or waist circumference (WC; Bosy-Westphal et al 2006). At the population level, measurement of body fat mass has no advantage over BMI or WC in the prediction of obesity-related metabolic risk (Bosy-Westphal et al 2006, Tulloch-Reid et al 2003), and BMI is the most widely used index for evaluation of being overweight or obese in human patients (Romero-Corral et al 2008). BMI categorizes people as normal or "healthy" weight (BMI 18.5 to 24.9), overweight (BMI 25 to 29.9), obese (BMI 30 to 34.9), or severely obese (BMI ≥ 35). In large-scale population studies there is a close relationship between BMI and incidence of several chronic conditions associated with excess fat (e.g., diabetes mellitus, hypertension, cardiovascular disease; Kopelman 2000). The underlying assumption is that most variation in weight for persons of the same height is due to fat mass. However, BMI may not reflect the same degree of fatness (adiposity) across different populations due to differences in race/ethnicity, age and body proportions. BMI does not differentiate between elevated body fat content and preserved or increased lean mass (e.g., in athletic individuals). As well, BMI is insensitive to variations in body fat distribution (e.g., central obesity) that are important predictors of metabolic and cardiovascular risk (Romero-Corral et al 2008, Shea et al 2011).

There is no universal definition of obesity in horses and ponies. As described in Chapter 22, horses or ponies with a body condition score (BCS) 7 (using the Henneke 9-point system; Henneke et al 1983) are considered overweight while animals with BCS of 8 or 9 are obese. Minimal data are available on body fat mass in horses and ponies, although recently the deuterium oxide dilution technique has been validated for the measurement of body fat in the Welsh mountain pony (Dugdale et al 2011a). In general, it appears that body fat is likely to be greater than 20–25% of body mass in animals with BCS ≥ 7, and values of up to 47% have been measured in ponies (Dugdale et al 2011a). It is important, however, to note limitations of BCS for assessment of adiposity (Dugdale et al 2012). Fundamentally, the BCS system provides a measure of "superficial flesh" but it does not assess subcutaneous fat independent of muscle mass. The current BCS systems also do not evaluate fat within the abdominal cavity, nor do they allow differentiation between obese (i.e., Henneke BCS 9) and "super obese" individuals. Studies in French sport horses and Welsh ponies have demonstrated an exponential relationship between BCS and body fat content (Martin-Rosset et al 2008, Dugdale et al 2011a) although recent work has suggested that the relationship may be more appropriately explained by a power function (body fat % K_{ave}^2). Whereas there is a linear relationship between BCS and total fat mass in animals with BCS < 7, BCS is a very insensitive indicator of fat mass at BCS ≥ 7. Ultrasound determinations and the use of BIA (see Chapter 22) have the potential to provide some useful information as to fat content and distribution but much more work is needed to develop simple yet accurate methods for estimation of adiposity (including the distribution of fat mass) in horses and ponies. The availability of such methods will facilitate the development of breed-specific definitions of obesity and improve knowledge of the relationship between adiposity and disease risk.

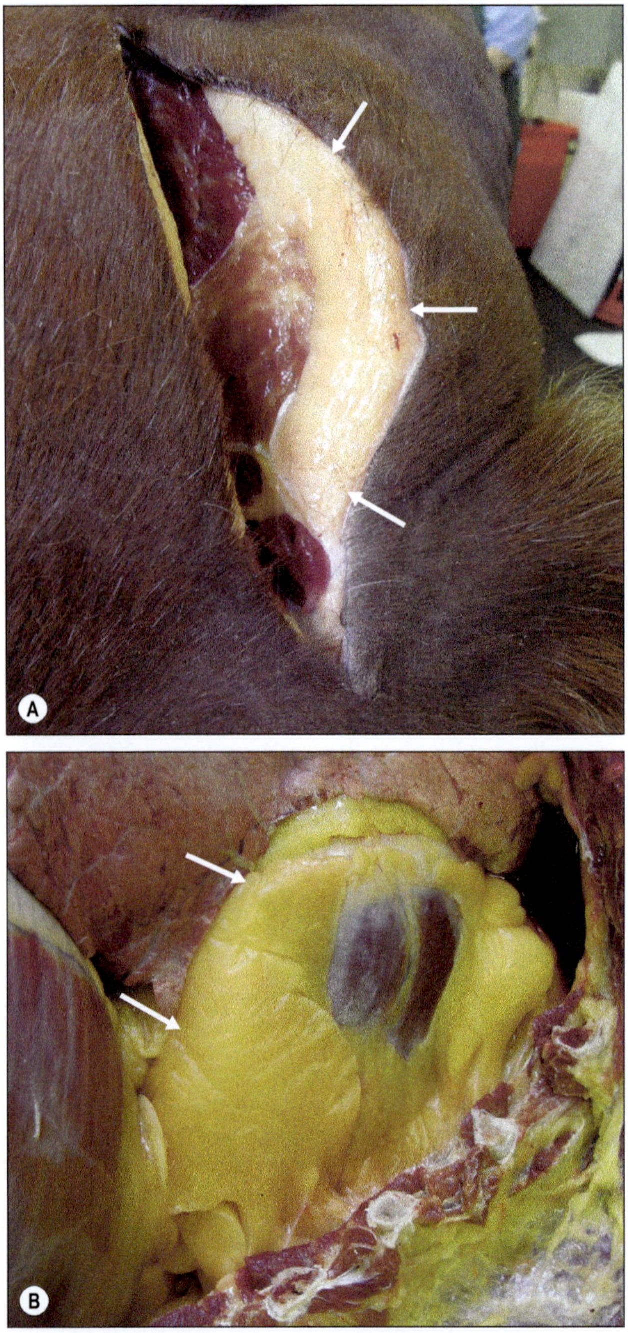

Figure 28.1 Postmortem images from an obese horse demonstrating substantial subcutaneous tailhead region A) and internal (pericardial) B) fat deposition.
Images courtesy of Dr. Caroline Argo, University of Liverpool.

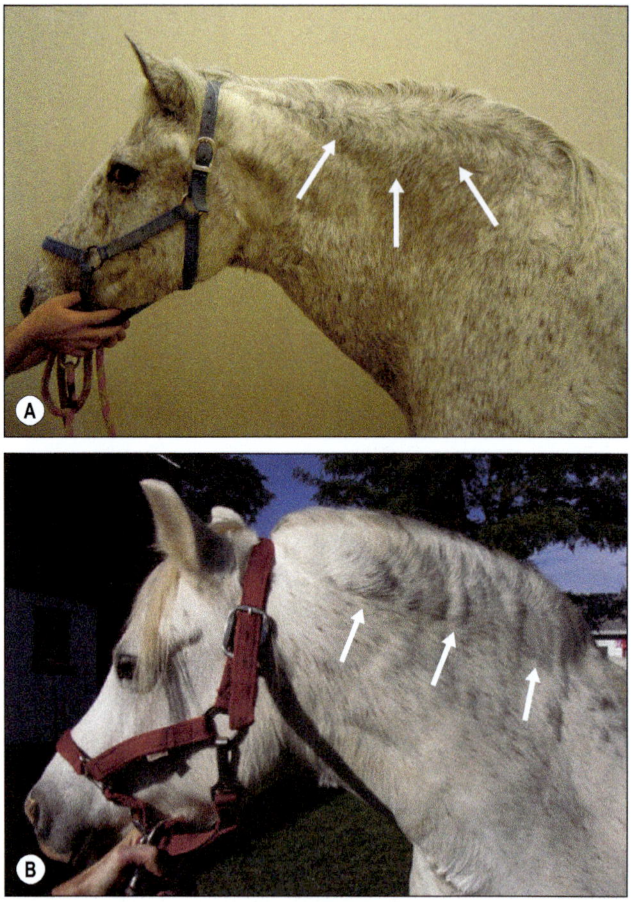

Figure 28.2 Images of a horse A) and pony B) with prominent nuchal crest subcutaneous fat deposition ("cresty neck").

Recently, there have been several reports of different subtypes of obesity in human populations including individuals that are obese but metabolically healthy ("healthy obesity") and those that are metabolically obese but normal weight (MONW) (Wildman et al 2008, Romero-Corral et al 2010). Although they have normal BMI, people with MONW have a clustering of metabolic and cardiovascular risk factors normally associated with obesity, including increased triglyceride and cholesterol concentrations and systemic inflammation. In US populations, 32% of phenotypically obese people are metabolically normal, whereas 23% of subjects with BMI in the healthy range (<25 kg/m^2) exhibit clustering of cardiometabolic abnormalities (Wildman et al 2008). Although mechanisms underlying differences in these phenotypes have not been fully elucidated, it is apparent that people with "metabolically benign" obesity have lower visceral, liver and muscle fat content when compared to normal weight or obese individuals with insulin resistance and other metabolic abnormalities (Karelis 2008, Stefan et al 2008). These observations highlight the need for more sensitive measures of body fat mass and distribution (e.g., DEXA, MRI) as well as measurement of various metabolic variables when assessing risk for chronic diseases. Similarly, it is likely that different obesity phenotypes exist in horse and pony populations. For example, whereas there is a negative association between BCS and measures of insulin sensitivity in horses (Hoffman et al 2003, Vick et al 2007), not all obese horses are insulin resistant. In addition, insulin resistance and hyperinsulinemia have been detected in horses and ponies with lean or moderate body condition (Bailey et al 2007).

Prevalence

The 1998 USDA National Animal Health Monitoring System (NAHMS) study estimated that approximately 1.5% of the horse population in the United States was overweight or obese (Anon 1998). However, these estimates were based on owner assessment of body condition rather than standardized methods for assessment of body fatness (e.g., BCS). Indeed, the results of recent prospective studies in which standardized methods were used for physical assessment have demonstrated that the prevalence of overweight/obesity in pleasure horse populations is far higher than the NAHMS estimates. Wyse et al (2008) examined 319 pleasure riding horses kept at 22 horse operations in south-west Scotland and found that 112 animals (35%) were fat (defined as BCS 5/6) and 32 horses (10%) were obese (BCS 6/6). In a study of 366 horses in North Carolina, 48% were considered to be overweight or obese (BCS >6/9, Henneke scale) (Pratt-Phillips et al 2010), while a cross-sectional study of 300 mature horses in south-western Virginia reported that 97 horses (32.3%) were over conditioned (BCS 7) and 56 (18.7%) were obese (BCS 8–9) (Thatcher et al 2012).

It should be noted that the above studies were conducted during the summer months when horses may be more predisposed to weight gain due to increased availability of pasture forage and seasonal changes in feed intake and metabolism (Arnold et al 2006, Kuntz et al 2006). Nonetheless, in a small survey study (127 horses and ponies in north Somerset, England) the incidence of obesity was high (~28%) when animals were evaluated at the end of winter although prevalence was even higher at the end of summer (~35.5%; Giles et al 2012). More studies are needed to establish the prevalence of and risk factors for obesity in different populations of horses across the globe. Two recent studies have reported poor agreement between the owners' perception of whether their horses were overweight / obese or not and the actual body condition score; less than 50% of owner estimates for fat horses agreed with the BCS (Stephenson et al 2011, Wyse et al 2008). These observations suggest that horse owners tend to underestimate body fatness in their horses and this may be a risk factor for obesity in horses, as has been reported in cats (Allen et al 2000).

Key Points

- Available data indicate that obesity is far more common than previously recognized, with the prevalence of overweight/obesity up to 50% in some subpopulations
- Current systems used to estimate body condition enable categorization of animals as thin, moderate or overweight. However, they cannot accurately predict body fat content or distribution, especially in thin (BCS<2–3/9) or fat (BCS≥7/9) animals

Potential contributing factors

The causes of obesity are likely to be multifactorial, with the involvement of genetic and environmental factors, especially overfeeding in combination with minimal physical activity. Very few studies have looked at the risk factors for obesity in horses and ponies (Thatcher et al 2012, Giles et al 2011). In the study by Thatcher and colleagues (2012), the feeding of hay reduced the odds of being over-conditioned or obese, while the feeding of up to 1.4 kg/day of complementary feed (concentrate) increased odds of being over-conditioned /obese. In the UK study (Giles et al 2011), the final logistic regression model for prediction of BCS, coming out of the winter, included breed, age, worming frequency and minutes in trot per hour of ridden exercise but not the estimated amount of feed provided; interestingly however, this model only explained 33% of the variation in BCS.

The following discussion on potential contributing factors for overweight/obesity mostly reflects the authors' opinion and should be interpreted with caution pending the results of further study on risk factors and mechanisms.

Overfeeding

Weight gain and obesity reflect an imbalance between energy intake and expenditure, although genetics may play a strong role in the face of excess caloric intake. An individual's energy requirement is affected by several external factors such as environmental conditions and the level of exercise being undertaken (including activity during turnout) as well as innate factors such as life stage and genetics. Although no study has reported a direct correlation between the prevalence of obesity and excess energy intake, anecdotal observations point to overfeeding as a major contributing factor. Many domesticated horses and ponies spend much of the day in confinement housing (stalls or small drylots) with occasional use in riding activities – two to three times a week. In these circumstances, daily energy requirements are often no higher than maintenance levels and easily met by provision of a moderate-to-good quality forage. Yet many of these animals are also fed grains, sweet feeds and other feeds with high caloric density and/or turned out for several hours a day on energy rich pastures, such that energy intake can greatly exceed requirements. Multivariable logistic regression analysis of data from 300 pleasure horses demonstrated that the feeding of grain-concentrate (1.4 kg/day vs. none) increased the odds for horses to be overweight or obese (odds ratio 2.2) (Thatcher et al 2012). The potential for weight gain to occur with overfeeding was highlighted by the results of an experimental study in which the bodyweight of Arabian geldings was increased by 20% when they were fed 200% of maintenance energy needs over a 3-month period (with 65% of calories from sweet feed; Carter et al 2009b). In the study by Giles et al (2011), however, very little of the observed variation in BCS, in animals spending >6 h per day out at pasture, could be explained by traditional management factors such as feeding level, feed type and amount of structured exercise.

The caloric intake of animals turned out to pasture may greatly exceed requirements and contribute to weight gain, especially at times of the year when there is an abundant supply of nutrient-rich forage (e.g., during spring and early summer when environmental conditions favor forage growth and nutrient storage). Ponies provided 24-hour access to pasture may consume up to 5% of bodyweight per day as dry matter and up to 1% BW in only 3 h of pasture turnout, highlighting the potential for weight gain in pastured animals (Longland et al 2011a, b).

Disruption of seasonal patterns of feed intake and body weight regulation

Wild animals adapted to temperate climates demonstrate seasonal fluctuation of body mass in concert with a number of other physiological adaptations that are entrained to photoperiod and result in fairly stable body weight over a number of seasons (Fuller et al 2001, Arnold et al 2006, Kuntz et al 2006). Appetite is highest during spring and summer, coinciding with a plentiful supply of forages and promoting growth (young stock) and deposition of adipose tissue and weight gain (mature animals). During winter when feed is less plentiful, appetite and metabolic rate decrease and energy stored in white adipose tissue is mobilized to compensate for energy deficits due to reduced feed intake (Fuller et al 2001). These seasonal adaptations are also apparent in domesticated ponies. For example, thin and moderately conditioned Welsh Mountain pony mares provided ad libitum access to a complete feed consumed more in summer (maximal 4.6±0.3% of body mass [BM] as dry matter intake [DMI] per day) than in winter (maximal 3.5±0.1% BM as DM intake/day) (Dugdale et al 2011b). Interestingly, peak DMI by obese (BCS >8) ponies in this study was half that reported for non-obese ponies and the body weight remained constant in the obese ponies regardless of the season. These observations raise questions about the effect of obesity on energy requirements and appetite.

Several factors may disrupt these seasonal patterns in appetite as well as metabolism and therefore promote development of obesity. First, many modern horses and ponies are provided access to pastures with "improved" forages that have been selected for the promotion of growth and fattening in cattle and sheep. Across the seasons, these forages likely have much higher nutritional value when compared to the forages available to animals in "non-domestic" conditions. Even in circumstances where pasture availability and nutritional quality decline during winter, conventional husbandry dictates that horses are provided supplemental hay and, in many situations, also energy-dense complementary feeds. Additionally, horses and ponies are usually provided shelter from the cold of winter and/or a rug is applied to assist with thermoregulation. Taken together, these factors mitigate winter-associated weight loss and over time such management practices likely favor progressive weight gain.

Genetics

Genetics may be another factor in the predisposition to obesity. Horse owners and veterinarians often use the term "easy keeper" to describe a horse or pony with a tendency to be overweight and that appears to require fewer calories than most horses to maintain condition. Ponies and certain horse breeds (e.g., Morgans, Arabs, Paso Finos) appear to fit this description, whereas other breeds (e.g., Thoroughbreds) fit the description of "hard keepers" that often have difficulty in maintaining bodyweight and condition. One hypothesis, as yet unproven, is that certain lines of horses and ponies have inherited genetic traits that have facilitated survival on poor quality forages and/or in the face of limited feed availability – the so-called "thrifty genotype" (Treiber et al 2006). This strategy may fail when these animals are supplied with abundant feed, particularly grains or pasture forage rich in NSC, resulting in weight gain, obesity and difficulty in sustaining weight loss once obese.

Altered hormonal regulation of appetite and energy balance

Studies in humans and laboratory animal species indicate complex regulation of appetite, body weight and adipose tissue mass. The hormones leptin and ghrelin are recognized to have a major influence on energy balance, and alterations in the leptin and ghrelin systems have been implicated in the development and/or maintenance of obesity (Klok et al 2007). Ghrelin, which is primarily produced in the stomach, appears to function as an appetite-stimulatory signal and short-term mediator of energy balance. In humans, plasma ghrelin concentrations increase during the preprandial period and the magnitude of the increase is correlated with hunger scores (Cummings et al 2004). As well, intravenous infusion of ghrelin induces hunger and food intake in people (Wren et al 2001). For this reason, ghrelin is sometimes referred to as the "hunger hormone". In addition to its orexigenic effect in humans, ghrelin stimulates gastrointestinal motility, gastric acid secretion and pancreatic exocrine secretion, all of which increase in anticipation of meals (Delzenne et al 2011). Interestingly, ghrelin concentrations are lower in obese compared to normal weight humans, consistent with observations that appetite is reduced in the obese state (Klok et al 2007). Ghrelin concentrations and appetite increase after weight loss and persistent elevations in ghrelin may, in part, contribute to poor weight loss maintenance (Adams et al 2010). In horses, plasma ghrelin decreases in response to oral and intravenous glucose administration (Gordon and McKeever 2006), while feed intake and plasma ghrelin concentrations were higher in horses subjected to interval exercise vs. the control (no exercise) condition (Gordon et al 2006). These observations suggest that plasma ghrelin responds to nutritional signals and may play a role in appetite regulation in horses. To date, however, there have been no reports of ghrelin concentrations in obese equids before or after weight loss.

Leptin, the product of the *ob* gene, provides information to the brain regarding availability of body fat stores, promoting satiety and reduction in food intake when energy balance is positive or fat stores are plentiful (Spiegelman & Flier 2001). Leptin is primarily produced by adipocytes and circulating concentrations are generally in direct proportion to the amount of adipose tissue (Schwartz et al 1996). One study in horses has shown a positive association between circulating leptin concentrations and BCS (Buff et al 2002). However, other studies have shown a wide range of leptin concentrations in horses with similar apparent adiposity (Gentry et al 2002), suggesting that factors other than adipose tissue mass affect leptin production and secretion.

Leptin regulates feeding behavior by binding to central nervous system receptors (primarily in the hypothalamus) and modulating the activity of neurons in appetite control centers (Meister 2000). Leptin causes an increase in the expression of melanocortins, such as alpha-melanocyte-stimulating hormone (α-MSH), which help to regulate energy homeostasis by inducing satiety and increasing fat metabolism. In other species, it has been suggested that α-MSH is very important in the integration of metabolism and appetite. A weak positive correlation has been shown between this hormone and BMI in horses (Donaldson et al 2004). However, further work is needed to determine whether a melanocortin receptor defect contributes to the pathophysiology of obesity or alternatively whether plasma α-MSH concentration is simply a correlate of adiposity (Donaldson et al 2004).

Leptin increases energy expenditure in rodents and humans via activation of the sympathetic nervous system (Enriori et al 2006). In obese, leptin-deficient mice (*ob/ob*), exogenous administration of leptin reduces hyperphagia and obesity (Halaas et al 1995). However, most obese people have greater leptin concentrations than lean individuals and obesity is associated with a disturbed diurnal variation in circulating leptin (Enriori et al 2006). It remains unclear whether these abnormalities in the leptin system are a cause or consequence of obesity, but one view is that chronic overfeeding can lead to development of leptin resistance with a sustained hyperleptinemia associated with a failure of leptin to suppress appetite and increase energy expenditure. In this context, leptin resistance may contribute to the maintenance of obesity.

Plasma leptin concentration in horses is affected by energy balance and feeding state (McManus & Fitzgerald 2000, Cartmill et al 2005, Buff et al 2006). Higher plasma leptin concentrations were reported in fed horses compared with fasted horses, with higher values in the afternoon than the morning only in the fed horses (Buff et al 2006). Plasma leptin concentration decreases in response to short-term feed restriction (McManus & Fitzgerald 2000, Van Weyenberg et al 2008a) and increases following meal feeding (Cartmill et al 2005). The insulin increase associated with meal feeding appears to drive the postprandial increase in plasma leptin (Cartmill et al 2005). Dexamethasone administration has also been shown to be a potent stimulator of leptin secretion in horses, whereas physiological elevation of cortisol concentrations following ACTH administration produced only minor increases in leptin (Cartmill et al 2005).

Hyperleptinemia, defined as a serum leptin concentration >10–12 ng/ml, has been identified in obese horses and ponies (Cartmill et al 2003, Frank et al 2006). One research group has categorized horses with high BCS (i.e. overweight/obese) by low (<5 ng/ml) and high (>12 ng/ml) resting leptin concentrations (Cartmill et al 2003), and have reported that horses from the high leptin group also have decreased insulin sensitivity and exaggerated insulin responses to glucose infusion when compared to "low leptin" horses of similar body condition (Cartmill et al 2003, Caltabilota et al 2010). The authors hypothesized that the hyperleptinemic condition is a result of reduced insulin sensitivity, associated with a chronic increase in circulating insulin and hence long-term stimulation of adipose tissue output of leptin (Caltabilota et al 2010).

Lack of physical activity

Decreased need and/or opportunity for physical activity are considered to be primary drivers in the still growing epidemic of obesity and associated metabolic disorders in human populations (Booth et al 2008). It is well established that even short-term physical inactivity (or decreased daily ambulatory activity) increases fat mass, reduces lean body mass and impairs systemic as well as skeletal muscle insulin sensitivity in both rodents and humans (Booth et al 2008, Laye et al 2007). Although the role of physical activity in development of obesity in horses and ponies is unknown, it is likely that a lack of exercise – in combination with excess feeding – is a contributing factor.

Key Points

- Obesity occurs when calorie (energy) intake exceeds requirements over a period of time
- Genetic and environmental factors particularly diet and exercise management, likely contribute to the risk for development of obesity

Disease associations

There is mounting evidence, in humans and other companion animals (dogs, cats), linking obesity with increased risk of multiple chronic diseases including diabetes mellitus, cancer and cardiovascular disease (Kopelman 2000, Laflamme 2011). Studies in humans have indicated that obesity increases all-cause mortality rates (Seidell 2010), while one study in dogs reported that even moderately overweight animals were at greater risk for earlier morbidity. In addition, median lifespan was reduced when compared to lean dogs (Kealy et al 2002). Box 28.1 lists diseases and disorders that have been associated with obesity in horses and ponies.

Obesity has been proposed as a risk factor for laminitis in horses and ponies, especially the pasture-associated form of this condition (Frank et al 2006, Treiber et al 2006). Obesity and/or the regional accumulation of fat deposits (e.g., "cresty neck") are a feature of the equine metabolic syndrome, a recently described condition that is associated with increased susceptibility to laminitis (Johnson 2002, Frank et al 2010). A recent study in the UK reported that the majority of animals with pasture-associated laminitis were overweight or obese. Moreover, BMI was positively associated with severity of laminitis and negatively associated with outcome (survival) (Menzies-Gow et al 2010). It remains to be established whether obesity directly increases the risk and severity of laminitis (e.g., due to mechanical forces exerted on the lamellar tissue associated with increased load bearing) or whether the increased risk is due to other factors

Box 28.1 Conditions of Horses for Which Risk May Be Increased by Obesity

- Orthopedic disorders
  - Laminitis
  - Osteoarthritis
- Endocrine and metabolic disorders
  - Equine metabolic syndrome
  - Insulin resistance
  - Glucose intolerance
  - Hyperinsulinemia
  - Dyslipidemia
  - Hyperlipemia and hepatic lipidosis
- Abdominal/intestinal disorders
  - Pedunculated lipomas and increased risk of small intestinal strangulation
- Miscellaneous
  - Heat intolerance
  - Exercise intolerance
  - Exacerbation of an aging-related pro-inflammatory state

associated with obesity, such as insulin resistance (IR) and inflammation (see Chapter 27 and Box 28.2 for further discussion on risk factors and mechanisms of laminitis).

In horses, as in other species, obesity has been associated with IR (Powell et al 2002, Hoffman et al 2003, Frank et al 2006, Vick et al 2007). In a cross-sectional study of Thoroughbred mares, insulin sensitivity assessed by use of the euglycemic-hyperinsulinemic clamp technique was negatively correlated with BCS and estimated fat mass (Vick et al 2007). Evidence of a cause-and-effect relationship between body condition (fatness) and insulin sensitivity has come from weight gain and loss studies. In Arabian geldings, insulin sensitivity was decreased to one-quarter of the baseline value after a 20% weight gain (with an increase in mean BCS from 6/9 to 8/9; Carter et al 2009a), while weight loss of 10% to 15% in obese ponies resulted in improved glucose tolerance (Van Weyenberg et al 2008b) or mitigation of resting hyperinsulinemia (Dugdale et al 2010). Conversely, Quinn et al (2009) did not detect a change in insulin sensitivity associated with moderate (~15% of starting body weight) weight gain in Thoroughbred geldings. More recently, an increase in adiposity alone did not cause IR in horses and ponies that gained weight on a high fat, low glycaemic diet. The addition of a single daily glucose meal in fact appeared to improve insulin sensitivity despite the increased adiposity (Bamford et al 2012). In this context, it is important to emphasize therefore that not all obese horses are insulin resistant - and that IR can occur in nonobese horses. Similarly, up to 40% of obese adult humans remain metabolically healthy and insulin-sensitive (Bluher 2010), supporting the hypothesis that not all excess body weight (adiposity) carries equal risk. As discussed below, adipose tissue inflammation may be central to the link between obesity and IR. Other factors such as aerobic fitness (enhances insulin sensitivity), the presence of ectopic fat in the liver and skeletal muscle (associated with IR independent of total adipose tissue mass) and the duration of obesity also impact the relationship between adipose tissue mass and insulin sensitivity (Bluher 2010, Klöting et al 2010).

In addition to laminitis, IR has been implicated in the pathogenesis of pituitary pars intermedia dysfunction (equine Cushing's disease; Johnson et al 2004) and hyperlipemia (Jeffcott & Field 1985, Reid & Mohammed 1996). Obesity, therefore, may contribute to the pathogenesis of these conditions via exacerbation of IR. In broodmares, obesity and IR have been associated with prolonged luteal phase and lengthened interovulatory intervals (Vick et al 2006), but the impact of these alterations in the estrous cycle on reproductive performance requires further study.

Other proposed effects of obesity in horses include impaired thermoregulation, exercise intolerance, and the development of benign lipomas in mesenteric adipose tissue with associated increased risk of colic due to small intestinal strangulation ("pedunculated lipomas"; Garcia-Seco et al 2005). It also warrants mention that aging may modulate risk of obesity-associated disorders. While peripheral blood mononuclear cells from old horses have increased inflammatory cytokine production compared with those from young animals, obese old horses have even greater frequencies of lymphocytes and monocytes producing inflammatory cytokines than do thin old horses (Adams et al 2009). This suggests that obesity may play an important role in the apparent age-related dysregulation of inflammatory cytokine production (Adams et al 2009). Reduction of body weight and body condition in fat old horses significantly reduced the percent of interferon-γ (IFN-γ) and tumor necrosis factor-α (TNF-α) positive lymphocytes and monocytes as well as circulating concentrations of TNFα (Adams et al 2009).

Box 28.2 Equine Metabolic Syndrome

In human medicine, the metabolic syndrome is a set of diagnostic criteria that identifies individuals at high risk for morbidity associated with IR, primarily type 2 diabetes and cardiovascular disease (Alberti et al 2006). Although the criteria for diagnosis of metabolic syndrome vary, the core components are obesity (especially visceral), IR, dyslipidemia and hypertension. In horses and ponies susceptible to recurrent laminitis, an insulin resistant phenotype resembling the human metabolic syndrome has been described (Johnson 2002, Treiber et al 2006, Bailey et al 2008, Frank et al 2010). Descriptions of this laminitis-predisposed phenotype have varied but have included a clustering of obesity (generalized and/or regional), IR, hyperinsulinemia, hyperleptinemia, mild hypertriglyceridemia and current or historical (e.g., founder lines) evidence of laminitis. Johnson (2002) proposed use of the term *equine metabolic syndrome* (EMS) to describe horses and ponies with this phenotype, while Treiber et al (2006) coined *prelaminitic metabolic syndrome* (PLMS) for identification of a set of risk factors in Welsh and Dartmoor ponies that predict increased risk of pasture-associated laminitis.

A diagnosis of EMS is based upon clinical examination and evaluation of basal insulin concentrations and/or glucose and insulin dynamics in response to oral or intravenous glucose challenge (Frank 2011). Affected animals may be hyperinsulinemic at rest (insulin >20 mU/l) or exhibit an exaggerated increase in serum insulin in response to glucose administration. Recently, an oral sugar test has been developed to enable simple assessment of insulin dynamics (Frank 2011). This test involves the oral administration of 15 ml corn syrup per 100 kg BW (about 75 ml for a 500 kg horse, providing 75 g of sugars). Preliminary studies have indicated insulin concentration exceeds 50 mU/l between 60 and 90 min post-dosing in insulin resistant animals whereas serum insulin remains <30 mU/l in healthy horses. Further validation studies are required, however. Dietary restriction and increased physical activity are cornerstones of the management of EMS. For EMS animals that do not respond to conservative management, the administration of levothyroxine sodium has been recommended to promote weight loss and improve insulin sensitivity but responses can be individually variable. The biguanide drug metformin has also been used for treatment of IR but efficacy is uncertain (Tinworth et al 2011).

Pathophysiology of obesity

Adipose tissue

Adipose tissue is now recognized as the largest endocrine organ in the body and plays a major role in regulation of immune, metabolic and vascular physiology (Hutley & Prins 2005, Balistreri et al. 2010). Two types of adipose tissue are present in mammals: white adipose tissue (WAT) and brown adipose tissue (BAT). The WAT is the predominant type, located in the subcutaneous region and also in discrete visceral regions surrounding internal organs (e.g., heart,

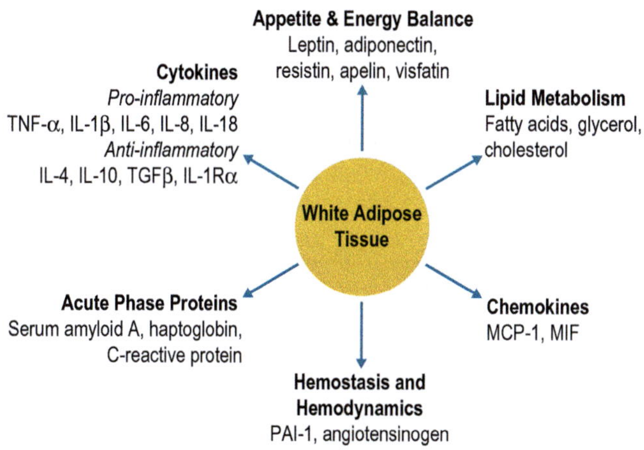

Figure 28.3 An illustration highlighting the secretory and endocrine function of white adipose tissue (based on studies in humans and other species). IL = interleukin; TNF = tumor necrosis factor; MCP = monocyte chemoattractant protein; MIF = macrophage migration inhibitory factor; PAI-1 = plasminogen activator inhibitor-1; TGF = transforming growth factor.

kidneys, gastrointestinal tract, uterus) and also against the internal walls of the abdomen and thorax. The major function of WAT is storage of triglycerides within lipid droplets, providing energy to the body during periods of energy restriction. Adipokines and other proteins synthesized and secreted by adipocytes in WAT also contribute to the regulation of energy balance (e.g., leptin, adiponectin), inflammation and vascular function (Fig. 28.3). The WAT contains several cell types including mature adipocytes, preadipocytes, multipotent mesenchymal stem cells, fibroblasts, endothelial cells, nerve cells and macrophages. The presence of stem cells and preadipocytes is thought to enable expansion of adipose tissue in obesity (Tan & Vidal-Puig, 2008).

The primary function of BAT is thermogenesis. Although primarily found in neonates (located mainly around the neck and large blood vessels of the thorax) recent studies have identified BAT depots in adult humans (Virtanen et al 2009). BAT's role in heat generation is facilitated by uncoupled oxidative phosphorylation due to the presence of uncoupling protein-1 on the inner mitochondrial membrane (Rousset et al 2004). The presence and location of BAT in mature horses has not been described.

Adipose tissue dysfunction in obesity

The mechanisms of metabolic complications (e.g., insulin resistance) arising from obesity remain unclear. Two primary theories have been proposed based upon experimental evidence in laboratory animal species and, to a lesser extent, humans: (1) *lipotoxicity*, where excess lipids spillover from a dysfunctional adipose tissue promoting fat deposition in the liver and skeletal muscle that, in turn, contribute to impairment in insulin sensitivity in these tissues (Cusi 2010); and (2) *adipose tissue inflammation*, with release of proinflammatory cytokines and other hormone-like proteins (collectively termed "adipokines") from dysfunctional adipose tissue that impact insulin sensitivity (Trayhurn 2005, Gauthier & Ruderman, 2010).

Constraints in adipose tissue expandability in the face of chronic caloric excess may trigger the cascade of events that lead to development of obesity-associated metabolic complications (Tan & Vidal-Puig 2008). As adipocytes achieve their maximum storage capacity, they alter their secretion profile towards one that promotes insulin resistance (Balistreri et al 2010). In rodent models of diet-induced obesity, the initial response to a positive caloric balance is a rise in both adiponectin and leptin, a profile that favors adipogenesis and insulin sensitivity. Subsequently, there is increased secretion of pro-inflammatory cytokines, including TNF-α, C-reactive protein (CRP), interleukin-6 (IL-6) and monocyte chemoattractant protein (MCP)-1, and a decline in adiponectin; a profile that favors insulin resistance and other co-morbidities such as hypertension (Tan & Vidal-Puig 2008). Adipocyte size is linked to adipokine-secretory profile and insulin sensitivity; specifically, hypertrophic adipocytes with high triglyceride stores exhibit enhanced expression and secretion of proinflammatory cytokines (Maffeis et al 2007, Kabir et al 2011). This observation supports the idea that there is a limit in adipocyte storage capacity, beyond which there are alterations in metabolic profile.

Increased recruitment of monocyte/macrophage cells into fat and enhanced cross-talk between adipocytes and macrophages that amplifies the production and secretion of adipokines are thought to contribute to obesity-associated adipose inflammation in humans. Decreased tissue perfusion during expansion of WAT with increased expression of hypoxia inducible factor-1α (HIF-1α) and signaling of Toll-like receptors (especially TLR4) by free fatty acids also may contribute to the development and maintenance of an inflammatory state (Trayburn & Wood 2004).

Cross-sectional studies of morbidly obese human subjects with an insulin-resistant or insulin-sensitive metabolic profile have provided additional insight into the interrelationships between obesity, adipose tissue inflammation and IR. Insulin resistant subjects had significantly higher mRNA levels of TNF-α, IL-6 and IL-1β, increased adipocyte size, higher macrophage infiltration into fat, and lower circulating adiponectin when compared to noninsulin-resistant obese patients (Barbarroja et al 2010, Klöting et al 2010). These observations reinforce the concept that inflammation of adipose tissue is a major contributor to the development of obesity-associated IR, at least in humans and other species. It is also evident that some obese individuals have adipose tissue that is better equipped to deal with caloric excess, perhaps due to a greater capacity for fat (triglyceride) storage before development of adipose tissue dysfunction.

In horses, associations between BCS, blood mRNA levels of TNF-α as well as IL-1β, and IR have been reported, suggesting that systemic inflammation also may play a role in the IR of obesity in horses (Vick et al 2007), although age may have been a confounding factor. There was increased expression of genes encoding for chemokines (IL-8 and MCP-1) but not pro-inflammatory cytokines in the nuchal crest adipose tissue of horses in association with diet-induced weight gain and development of IR (Carter et al. 2008). In contrast to observations in rodents and humans, there also was no detectable change in the macrophage content of adipose tissue after weight gain. The role of inflammation in the pathophysiology of obesity in horses is therefore uncertain.

Is location of fat deposition important?

In humans, the anatomic distribution of adipose tissue (especially excessive visceral fat) impacts risk of obesity-associated adverse outcomes such as IR, diabetes mellitus and cardiovascular disease (Montague & O'Rahilly 2000, Kuk et al 2006). For example, in obese human subjects visceral fat mass is a strong and independent predictor of IR (Klöting et al 2010). The deleterious effects associated with an enlarged visceral fat depot are thought to result from its secretions entering the portal venous drainage, enabling direct access of pro-inflammatory adipokines and free-fatty acids (FFAs) from visceral adipocytes to insulin-sensitive hepatocytes. In this "portal hypothesis", chronic exposure of the liver to elevated FFAs increases hepatic lipogenesis and liver triglyceride content, both of which contribute to systemic hyperinsulinemia and consequent IR (Montague & O'Rahilly 2000). The observation that removal of intra-abdominal visceral adipose tissue improves glucose tolerance in rats, in association with decreased hepatic triglyceride storage, provides support for this hypothesis (Foster et al 2011).

There may be a similar association between regional adiposity and disease risk in horses and ponies. In healthy horses on a hay only diet, the mRNA concentrations of IL-1β and IL-6 were significantly higher in nuchal crest AT than in other subcutaneous and visceral depots (Burns et al 2010). Another study in mature geldings (breed and diet information not provided) reported higher leptin and lower CCL5 and IL-10 mRNA expression in nuchal adipose tissue compared to other depots, while adiponectin expression was lower in the tail head when compared to nuchal crest and kidney depots (Bruynsteen et al 2011). The differences in expression of inflammation-related genes in nuchal adipose tissue is an interesting finding in light of clinical observations associating neck fat accumulation (i.e. a "cresty neck") with risk of laminitis (Carter et al 2009a). Additionally, a strong correlation between mean neck circumference and the magnitude of IR has been reported (Frank et al 2006) although other reports have not identified an association between neck circumference and IR independent of overall body condition (Carter et al 2009c, Dugdale et al 2010). Other equine studies have shown that visceral fat has higher lipogenic activity when compared to adipose tissue from the nuchal crest region (Suagee et al 2010) and highest content of GLUT-4 in mesenteric and omental fat when compared to samples from the retroperitoneal, tailhead and nuchal crest depots (Waller et al 2011). Further research is needed to characterize the metabolic properties of different adipose depots in horses and determine the role of adipose tissue dysfunction (e.g., inflammation) in obesity.

Key Points

- Obesity is associated with increased risk of several conditions including laminitis, insulin resistance and a chronic pro-inflammatory state
- Not all obese animals show alterations in physiological or metabolic status and further research is needed to elucidate factors that may protect against the development of metabolic dysfunction in these individuals

Management of obesity

Most cases of obesity are associated with an imbalance between energy intake and expenditure – and, as in humans, "eating less" and "exercising more" are the key strategies to achieve a more ideal bodyweight and condition in horses and ponies.

Important steps in the development of weight loss and management programs include –

1. A thorough history and clinical examination that will include the recording of relevant medical history (e.g., previous episodes of laminitis), body weight (BW; preferably via direct measurement on a calibrated scale/weigh bridge or indirect assessment by use of a weigh tape), BCS, and other morphometric measurements e.g., neck circumference, abdominal circumference. The hooves should be examined for evidence of "founder lines." These baseline data are important for subsequent assessments of the effectiveness of any weight loss program.
2. Owner/trainer recognition that the horse or pony is overweight or obese – different equestrian disciplines and breeds have adopted different accepted "norms" in body condition. Nonetheless, the effectiveness of any weight loss program is critically dependent upon the willingness of the owner or caregiver to comply with the plan. Current or historical evidence of laminitis provides a strong argument for the prompt institution of a weight loss and maintenance program. Achieving weight loss and maintaining a more ideal BW and BCS is a long term commitment.
3. Evaluation of the current feeding program and housing – this will include a thorough evaluation of what feed is being provided (including supplementary feed, hay, pasture quality and time allowed for grazing) and in what quantities. Proximate analysis of feeds and forage will enable estimation of true DE and nutrient intake. Note that some animals, when allowed free access to pasture, preserved forage or forage replacer feeds, may ingest up to 5% of BW per day (Dugdale et al 2011a, Longland et al 2011a, b). Ration components (including haynets) should be weighed for accurate assessment of feed intake. Maintenance energy requirements for horses typically range between 30 and 35 kcal digestible energy (DE) per kg BW per day, i.e. 15.0 to 17.5 Mcal DE/day for a 500-kg horse – the low end of this range has been used to estimate maintenance needs of "easy keeper" horses or ponies with a tendency to be overweight or obese. However, the amount and type of feed actually needed to maintain bodyweight varies between individuals and depends on several factors, including age, temperament, environmental conditions, level of physical activity and metabolic efficiency.
4. Assessment of the weekly workload and soundness for exercise – how many hours per week is the horse or pony engaged in structured physical activity e.g., riding? There is a tendency for horse owners and caregivers to overestimate the DE needs of horses performing structured riding activities, with resultant overfeeding and weight gain. The impact of exercise level on DE requirements varies between animals and adjustments in feeding should be based on regular monitoring of BCS and BW over time. Information on current activity level and soundness for exercise will form the basis for development of recommendations for physical activity (see below).

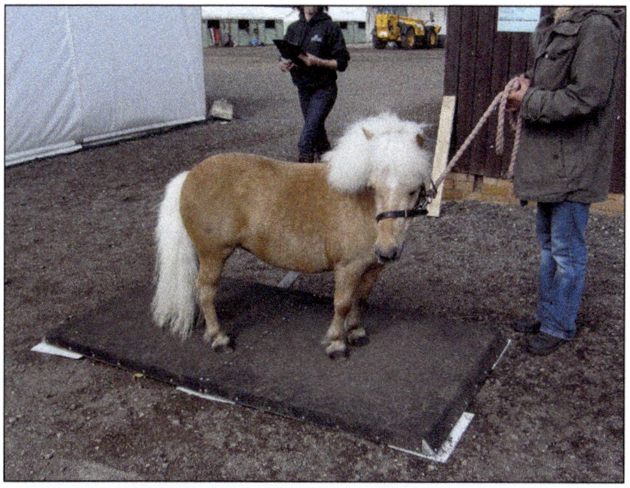

Figure 28.4 **Direct measurement of bodyweight on a calibrated weighbridge (walk-on platform scale) is recommended for assessment of the effectiveness of a weight loss program.**
Image courtesy of Isabel Harker, Mars Horsecare.

5. Set realistic goals for weight loss and regularly monitor progress – in the authors' experience there can be wide variation in the response of obese horses and ponies to weight loss treatment programs. In some, there is a substantial loss of body weight and adiposity after 2–3 months of diet restriction and increased physical activity. In others, progress can be frustratingly slow and further adjustments to diet and the level of physical activity may be needed for satisfactory improvement. However, a target weight loss of up to 0.5% per week (relative to BW after the first week of dietary restriction) is reasonable based upon data from studies in ponies and other species. Bodyweight and BCS should be monitored regularly (i.e. every 2–4 weeks) under standardized conditions (Fig. 28.4); note *that appropriate levels of weight loss may not always be accompanied by a detectable change in BCS in the first few months* (Dugdale et al, 2010).
6. Make all dietary changes gradually and avoid prolonged periods of feed withholding. Abrupt starvation in obese ponies, donkeys and miniature horses (especially pregnant animals) carries the risk of hyperlipemia and is not recommended. In addition, severely restricting access to forage may increase risk of gastric ulceration and stereotypic behaviors.
7. Develop, and continually update, an appropriate *weight maintenance* program once the target weight and body condition have been achieved. This will include monthly assessment of BW and BCS to ensure that the feeding program is appropriate to the current level of physical activity and other environmental influences on energy requirements (e.g., ambient conditions).

Controlled weight loss programs

Several recent studies have examined the effects of nutritional restriction and/or increased physical activity on weight loss and other measures of health in overweight/obese horses or ponies; findings from these studies are summarized here.

Rate of weight loss

Van Weyenberg et al (2008b) aimed to achieve a weekly weight loss of 1.0% relative to ideal BW during an 18 week trial in nine obese Shetland ponies. Interestingly, it was observed that the initial level of energy restriction (70% of maintenance energy requirements based on ideal BW [not defined fully] during weeks 1–5) failed to achieve this target rate of weight loss (total of 3.2% or about 0.6% of BW per week). Subsequently, the ponies were restricted to 50% (weeks 6–13) and 35% (weeks 14–18) of estimated energy requirements and by the end of the 18-week trial the ponies had lost 18% of initial BW, while BCS had decreased from 8–9/9 to 4–5/9. Ponies were fed a mixture of alfalfa hay and straw (two meals per day) in an amount equivalent to 0.9% (1.7±0.3 kg), 0.65% (1.2±0.2 kg) and 0.5% (0.8±0.1 kg) of BW (as fed) for the 70%, 50% and 35% energy restriction periods, respectively (Van Weyenberg et al 2008b). In horses and ponies, as in other species, decreased caloric intake is likely to result in lowered basal metabolic rate, making it difficult to maintain a constant rate of weight loss.

A more recent study has indicated that weekly weight loss of about 0.7% can be achieved with less severe energy restriction (Dugdale et al 2010). Five Welsh Mountain pony mares (10±2 years of age; BW 257±20 kg; BCS 6.8/9±0.5) were individually housed and were initially provided ad libitum access to a chaff-based complete diet (average intake of 2.6% BW per day) and then restricted to 1.0% BW (providing 67% of estimated maintenance energy requirements based on obese BW) for 12 weeks. Mean BW decreased by 4.3±1.1% during the first week and then at a rate of 0.7±0.1% per week, resulting in an overall rate of weight loss of 1.0% weekly over the 12 week study. Fat (adipose tissue) accounted for 47±20% of the body mass loss, and fatter ponies lost relatively more fat. The same research group compared the effects of two dietary restriction protocols on weight loss in 12 mixed breed (Shetland pony to Warmblood), overweight/obese (BCS 7.0 to 8.8/9) ponies and horses (Curtis et al 2010). The animals were offered feed at 1.25% BW as DM daily for 16 weeks. Group 1 (n=6) was provided grass hay (DE, 7.5 MJ/kg DM) at 1.15% BW and 0.1% BW as a ration balancer feed (DE, 13.8 MJ/kg DM), while Group 2 (n=6) received 0.8% BW as a chaff-based complete feed (DE, 8.5 MJ/kg DM) and 0.45% BW of the grass hay. Hay was fed from nets with small mesh openings. The rate of weight loss was similar between treatments with a mean weekly loss (relative to outset BW) of 0.49±0.06%. Mean BCS decreased by 0.07/9±0.02 units per week. However, minimal weight loss occurred in 4 of the 12 animals, emphasizing that there can be wide variation in individual responses to dietary restriction.

Gordon and coworkers (Gordon et al 2009) examined weight loss in overweight Quarter Horse and Thoroughbred horses provided hay (1% BW) and low calorie feed (0.5% BW) with and without exercise for a 12-week period when compared to horses fed a control diet without exercise. The authors reported greater weight loss with the restricted diet (about 60% of DE requirements) and exercise regimen. However, the study was confounded because the amount of feed provided to the restricted diet/exercise group was reduced to 0.3% BW after 6 weeks. After 12 weeks, weight loss in the control group was not significantly different from the restricted diet/exercise group despite an approximately

40% higher daily DE intake. The restricted diet/exercise group was housed indoors whereas the control animals were kept outdoors. The authors hypothesized that the harsher winter climate along with the opportunity for greater voluntary activity may have contributed to weight loss in the control horses (Gordon et al 2009).

Overall, it is apparent that weight loss of 0.5–0.7% of BW per week can be achieved in overweight/obese horses and ponies when energy intake is limited to ~70% of maintenance requirements. However, wide individual variation in weight loss response to dietary restriction can be expected and more severe restriction may be needed to achieve weight loss in some animals. Much more work is needed to evaluate effective strategies for promotion of safe weight loss in obese horses and ponies.

Effect of dietary restriction on metabolic variables and overall health

The desired metabolic response to energy restriction is increased mobilization and utilization of stored triglycerides (TG) with an associated decrease in fat mass. As mentioned, one concern is that severe restriction in obese animals, especially ponies and donkeys, may precipitate profound hypertriglyceridemia and hyperlipemia. Dugdale et al (2010) observed a slight increase in mean serum NEFA concentrations during 12 weeks of dietary restriction while plasma TG and total cholesterol concentrations were unchanged. Similarly, Van Weyenberg et al (2008b) reported that plasma non-esterified fatty acids (NEFA) and TG concentrations were minimally changed after dietary restriction at 70% and 50% of estimated requirements. However, plasma NEFA and TG concentrations were, respectively, threefold and fourfold higher after the more severe period of energy restriction (35% of requirements). Although no clinical problems were observed in this study, the marked increase in plasma TG concentration with severe energy restriction highlights the need for close monitoring during application of weight loss protocols.

Especially in confinement housing, the decrease in feeding time due to dietary restriction may give rise to undesirable behaviors in some animals. Dugdale et al (2010) reported no abnormal behaviors in ponies fed 1.0% of BW per day for 12 weeks but did observe that the time spent in "play" activity and rest increased by 36±11% and 438±95%, respectively. These authors suggested that daily feed rations should be offered as several meals; if hay is fed it should be offered in doubled, small mesh nets that prolong feeding time. Other forms of environmental enrichment (e.g., housing with a companion) are also recommended.

Another goal of weight loss is improvement in insulin sensitivity and mitigation of hyperinsulinemia. In their study of obese Shetland ponies, Van Weyenberg et al (2008b) reported that weight loss (mean decrease 18% of initial BW) was associated with a reduced glucose peak, decreased baseline insulin values and a decreased area under the curve for glucose and insulin in response to the oral glucose tolerance test. Basal insulin concentration decreased from 39.6±29.1 mU/l to 13.2±1.6 mU/l in a mixed group of overweight/obese horses and ponies that lost about 8% BW over 16 weeks (Curtis et al 2010), while a 12% BW decrease in obese ponies also resulted in a marked reduction or correction of initial hyperinsulinemia (Dugdale et al (2010). Taken together, these findings are indicative of improved insulin sensitivity and glucose tolerance after weight loss. In ponies, weight loss also resulted in a marked decrease in plasma leptin concentrations (Van Weyenberg et al 2008b).

Feeding recommendations for weight loss

Caloric restriction is of paramount importance in the management of obese equids – creation of a state of negative energy balance is needed to achieve loss of BW. Several different dietary strategies can be applied depending on the present and desired body condition as well as other individual circumstances. In some situations, the removal of calorie-dense manufactured feeds from the diet, restriction from access to "lush" pasture, and an increase in structured physical activity may be sufficient to promote weight loss (e.g., overweight but not obese animals). For obese animals, however, more severe energy restriction may be needed for effective weight loss.

Initial approach

1. Decrease or eliminate grain and manufactured, calorie-dense feeds from the diet (e.g., commercial sweet feeds, feeds containing added fats). Excessive feeding of other "treats" such as carrots and apples also should be curtailed.
2. Evaluate the quality of the current forage, ideally by proximate analysis. Early maturity hay with a high leaf-to-stem ration should be replaced by later maturity hay with lower energy content. Forage-based, low-calorie feeds complete with vitamins and minerals are now available commercially. This type of feed offers convenience and may be used as a substitute for hay or fed as a component of the ration along with hay. This forage or substitute can be fed at 1.5% to 2.0% of BW depending on previous level of feeding and current body condition. When mature grass hays are fed, intake of vitamin E, copper, zinc, selenium and other minerals etc. may not meet requirements and provision of a vitamin–mineral supplement is therefore recommended. Many feed companies sell a low calorie "ration balancer" feed for this purpose. In addition, to vitamins and minerals, these products contain sources of high-quality protein and are usually designed to be fed in small quantities (e.g., 0.5 to 1.0 kg/day, fed as is or mixed with hay chop). Studies in humans and other species have indicated that maintaining adequate indispensable amino acid is important for mitigation of loss of lean (muscle) body mass during severe energy restriction (Arathuzik & Goebel-Fabbri 2011). Table 28-1 shows example weight loss diets.
3. Restrict access to pasture grazing, especially pastures that have abundant, rapidly growing forage (lush pastures). It is preferable to maintain turnout, either in a large dry-lot or at pasture with the horse wearing a grazing muzzle that restricts but does not eliminate grazing (Fig. 28.5). Longland et al (2011b) have shown that grazing muzzles will significantly reduce the rate of DM intake on autumn pasture (sward height 8–15 cm). Without muzzles ponies consumed an average of 0.08 BW in a 3 h period (vs. 0.014 BW with muzzles). It is important to ensure that horses wearing grazing muzzles are able to consume adequate water. Some horses do not tolerate grazing muzzles, and they

Table 28-1 Three Weight Loss Diets for a 400-kg Pony

	Scenario 1	Scenario 2	Scenario 3	Nutrients requirement for maintenance (NRC 2007)
% Bodyweight DMI (%)	1.5	1.5	1.25	
Total intake (as fed, kg)	6.6	6.6	5.5	
Grass hay (kg)	6.6	6.1	4.8	
Low calorie feed balancer (kg)		0.5	0.7	
Total estimated DE (MJ)	53.5	54.7	46.2	56
% DE requirement	95.5	97.6	66.8	
Crude protein (g)	535	619	564	504
Lysine (g)	17.8	24.5	24.2	21.7
Calcium (g)	37.5	45.2	44.8	16
Phosphorus (g)	17.8	22.5	21.4	11.2
Magnesium (g)	10.1	12.3	11.5	6
Copper (mg)	44.6	121	144	80
Zinc (mg)	178	365	410	320
Selenium (mg)	0.6	1.5	1.8	0.8
Manganese (mg)	505	547	479	320
Vitamin E (IU)	297	1274	1616	400 IU
Comments	Deficient in lysine, copper, zinc, selenium and vitamin E	Fully balanced	Fully balanced	

DMI = dry matter intake; DE = digestible energy; MJ = megajoule
In scenarios 1 and 2, it assumed that the current diet far exceeds DE requirements and that overfeeding has contributed to weight gain/obesity. In this situation, a recommended initial feeding strategy is to provide DE intake at or slightly below NRC requirements. This can be achieved by feeding 1.5% BW of average quality grass hay (Scenario 1) although this diet is deficient in several nutrients. The addition of 0.5 kg of a low calorie feed balancer feed corrects these deficiencies (Scenario 2). Scenario 3 is applicable to situations requiring restriction of DE intake below NRC maintenance recommendations, starting at a DMI of 1.25% of bodyweight. Daily DMI can be further reduced to 1.0% bodyweight if more severe restriction is needed to effect weight loss (approximately 3.5 kg grass hay and 0.9 kg feed balancer; note that a larger amount of the feed balancer is needed to meet nutrient requirements in this scenario).
The authors acknowledge the input of Ms. Clare Barfoot, Mars Horsecare (UK) Ltd., in the preparation of this table.

Nutrient Composition of the Hay and Balancer Feed Used in the Weight Loss Diets

Nutrient DM	Hay	Low calorie balancer
Estimated DE/kg	8.9	11.5
Crude protein (%)	9	27.8
Lysine (%)	0.3	1.8
Calcium (%)	0.55	3.3
Phosphorus (%)	0.3	1.3
Magnesium (%)	0.16	0.66
Copper mg/kg	7.5	178
Zinc (mg/kg)	30	444
Selenium (mg/kg)	0.1	2.2
Manganese (mg/kg)	85	178
Vitamin E (IU/kg)	50	2220

can alter herd dynamics. Alternate approaches that may restrict pasture forage intake include strip grazing behind other livestock; mowing and removal of clippings before grazing activity is permitted; and application of a deep layer of woodchips over a small paddock.

4. Increase structured physical activity, e.g., increased frequency and duration of riding or other forms of exercise.

It should be noted that simply restricting the time allowed for grazing may not be an effective strategy for weight loss.

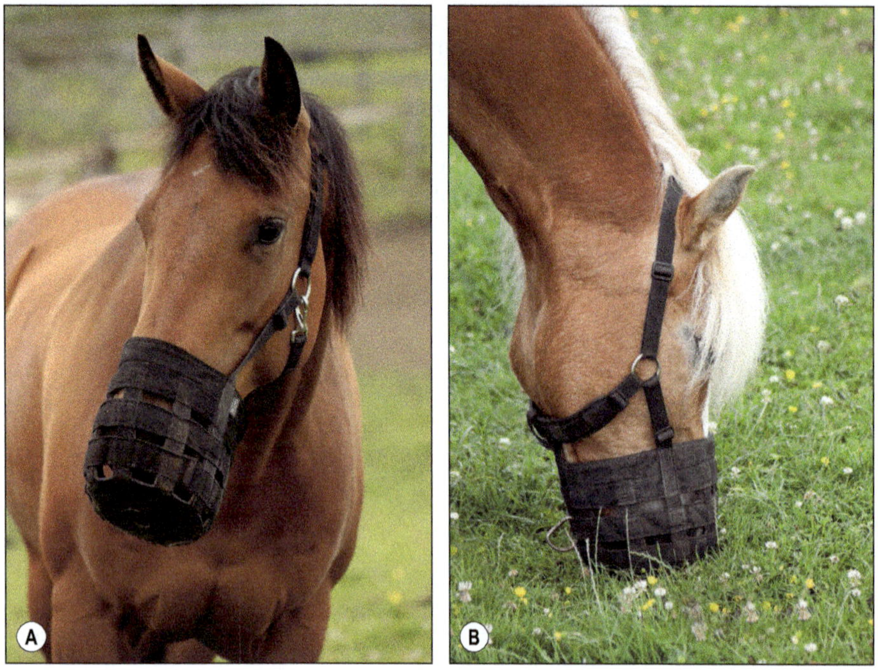

Figure 28.5 Grazing muzzles substantially restrict pasture forage dry matter intake.
Images courtesy of Hannah Briars, Mars Horsecare.

A study in obese pony mares reported no change in body weight when ponies were provided 12 h/day of access to pasture (during daytime or night time), perhaps due to increased forage consumption during the restricted grazing period (Buff et al 2006). Ponies have been observed to consume 40% of their daily DM intake during 3 hours of pasture turnout (Ince et al 2005) and can ingest up to 1% of BW as DM within 3 h of pasture turnout (Longland et al 2011a).

More severe restriction

A more severe reduction in feed (caloric intake) is indicated for more obese animals or when the above approaches prove ineffective.

1. Grain and commercial, energy-dense feeds should be removed from the diet.
2. Pasture intake should be severely limited and in many cases eliminated. Forage with low-to-medium energy content (≤8 MJ [~2 Mcal] per kg DM) should be the primary energy-providing component of the ration. In a study of obese ponies provided a free choice forage (chaff) diet during winter and summer, voluntary intake (DM basis) was about 2% of bodyweight and BCS was unchanged during the study period (Dugdale et al 2011a). As a general guide, therefore, hay or hay substitute should initially be provided at no more than 1.5% of current BW per day (DM basis, with most hays around 90% DM), i.e. 3.7 kg for a 250 kg pony; 7.5 kg for a 500 kg horse. Horse owners/clients should be instructed to weigh the ration. If there has been minimal weight loss after 6–8 weeks, the feeding rate should be decreased to 1.25% BW and then to 1.0% BW. The authors do not recommend feeding lower amounts of forage (<1.0% BW on DM basis) as this may increase risk of hindgut dysfunction, gastric ulcers, stereotypical behaviors such as wood chewing, and coprophagy. Substituting straw for up to 50% of the hay ration is one way to lower the energy density diet and maintain a reasonable level of DM intake. On average, the energy content of straw is lower than that of grass hay. Straw that is clean and with minimal cereal head should be selected; thoroughly shaking the straw prior to feeding will remove any loose cereal. There may be increased risk of gastric ulceration and impaction colic with straw feeding. As with any change in feeding, the straw should be gradually introduced into the ration, which helps to reduce the risk of impaction – although this remains a significant risk with certain breeds (e.g., Thoroughbreds) and individuals. The risk of gastric ulceration also increased when straw is the main forage.
3. As above, provide a ration balancer or vitamin–mineral-protein product along with forage.
4. The ration should be divided into three or four feedings per day. Strategies to prolong feed intake time should also be considered, such as the use of hay nets with multiple small holes.

Feed non-structural carbohydrate content

Avoidance of feedstuffs rich in NSC (starches, sugars and/or fructans) is recommended for obese, insulin-resistant horses or ponies due to concerns that provision of such feeds will increase of risk of laminitis via exacerbation of hyperinsulinemia (see Chapter 27). A common recommendation is to feed hay with an NSC content of less than 10–12% DM. Ideally, the hay is selected after direct measurement of starch and sugar contents. In the absence of data on hay NSC content, soaking hay in water for 30 to 60 min before feeding to leach water soluble carbohydrates (WSC; sugars and fructans) has been recommended. However, recent work has suggested that this strategy has a variable and unpredictable effect on hay WSC content (Longland et al 2011c) and if used as an adjunct management measure the soaking should be done using water around 16°C or more.

Physical activity

In humans, prescriptive exercise is widely used in the management of obesity (Hawley 2004) and physical activity also should be a cornerstone of weight loss and weight maintenance programs for horses and ponies. The combination of caloric restriction and regular physical activity can result in more substantial weight loss when compared to either strategy alone, and the addition of physical activity to dietary intervention is considered essential for successful long-term weight-loss maintenance (Catenacci & Wyatt 2007). One study of obese Thoroughbred mares (n=3) demonstrated improvements in insulin sensitivity without a change in BW following 7 days of round pen (15–20 min/day) exercise (Powell et al 2002). A more recent study of overweight or obese Arabian horses did not detect an effect of longer term (8 weeks, four sessions per week) exercise on insulin sensitivity or basal insulin concentration, although BW and total body fat mass (estimated by the deuterium dilution method) were significantly decreased by, respectively, 4% and 34% after the 8-week period of exercise training (Carter et al 2010). Importantly, the horses of the study by Carter et al (2010) were not subjected to dietary restriction. The combination of physical activity and dietary restriction may have resulted in more substantial reductions in BW and fat mass.

For overweight/obese horses or ponies already in work, an increase in the number, duration and/or intensity of exercise events is recommended. For sedentary animals, a general recommendation is to start with 2–3 sessions per week (walking, riding or lungeing), averaging around 20–30 min per session. Subsequently, there should be a gradual, stepwise increase in the intensity and duration of exercise. Veterinary advice should be obtained before initiating an exercise program in animals that have had recent episodes of laminitis or any history of lameness. The combination of increased physical activity and dietary restriction should be applied until goal BW and/or BCS is obtained. Thereafter, feeding rate should be adjusted on the basis of work demands and regular assessments of BW and BCS.

Additional considerations

In group housing situations it may be necessary to separate the obese horse or pony to allow strict control of feed intake. For animals housed in stalls, dietary restriction can promote intake of bedding. Straw should not be used for bedding because its ingestion can substantially increase daily caloric intake. Similarly, it has been reported that obese ponies and horses under dietary restriction can ingest as much as 3.5 kg wood shavings per day when this material is used as bedding (Curtis et al 2011). Where consumption of wood shavings is observed, consideration should be given to use of rubber matting alone or an alternative such as peat moss. Allowing horses to remain outdoors during winter (and without the application of rugs/blankets) may facilitate weight loss by increasing energy expenditure for thermoregulation.

Treatment with levothyroxine sodium has been recommended for obese, insulin resistant horses or ponies in which more conservative approaches (i.e., dietary restriction, exercise) have failed to effect adequate weight loss. In healthy horses, a 16-week period of levothyroxine treatment resulted in a 10% reduction in BW and 1.8-fold increase in mean insulin sensitivity (Frank et al 2008). However, clinical experience has indicated variable (and sometimes limited) beneficial response to levothyroxine in EMS animals. The recommended dosage for weight loss in mature horses is 48 mg/day (about 4 teaspoons, administered in feed) for 3 to 6 months depending on clinical response. Treated animals should be gradually weaned from the drug when treatment goals have been attained; a recommended protocol involves decreasing the dosage from 48 mg/day to 24 mg/day for 2 weeks, then 12 mg/day for a further 2 weeks (Frank 2011). More work is needed to evaluate the true efficacy, optimal dose and dosing regimen for levothyroxine and other medications such as metformin (Tinworth et al 2011).

A number of supplements (e.g., chromium, betaine, soy protein) have been marketed with claims for enhanced weight loss but evidence of efficacy in equids is lacking (see Tinworth et al 2010).

Monitoring weight loss

The BCS system is useful for estimation of subcutaneous fat mass in equids but may not be a sensitive indicator of weight loss, at least during the early phase. Dugdale et al (2010) recorded BCS, heart and belly girth and ultrasound-derived measures of subcutaneous fat depth in obese ponies during weight loss over a 12-week period. Mean BW decreased by approximately 12% and was associated with significant decreases in heart and belly girth measurements as well as rump width and rib subcutaneous fat depth. However, a change in BCS was not detected. Similarly, neck circumference – a measure of neck crest adiposity – did not change during the study. Other studies of longer duration and with a greater magnitude of weight loss (18%) when compared to the study of Dugdale et al (2010) have reported a significant decrease in BCS in association with weight loss (Van Weyenberg et al 2008b). It is therefore recommended that, in addition to BCS, heart and belly girth (and, if feasible, ultrasound fat depth) be recorded during a weight loss program. These measures should be recorded at monthly intervals during the weight loss program, and every 6–8 weeks during weight maintenance.

Key Points

- Prevention is the best medicine – feeding programs for horses and ponies should be designed and monitored to prevent development of obesity
- Weight loss programs must be targeted to the individual animal. **Strategies for management of overweight/obese animals include:**
  - Promotion of weight loss and improved insulin sensitivity via dietary restriction and, when possible, an increase in physical activity
  - Avoidance of feeds that may exacerbate insulin resistance and hyperinsulinemia (feeds rich in non-structural carbohydrates such as grains, grain-based commercial feeds, and "lush" or stressed pasture forages)
  - In some animals, treatment with levothyroxine sodium may be indicated for promotion of weight loss if appropriate dietary restriction and exercise regimens are not effective
- Regular monitoring and adjustments in feeding and physical activity are required – individual animals will lose weight at different rates and will require different levels of feed restriction
- **Once target weight has been achieved, an ongoing program of weight maintenance is needed**

Conclusion

Obesity is an emergent problem in domestic horse and pony populations. Obesity is caused by an imbalance between energy intake and energy expenditure although a number of innate (e.g., genetics) and environmental factors influence this balance. The expansion of adipose tissue mass in obesity may be associated with development of insulin resistance, a chronic pro-inflammatory state and increased risk of health problems. Increased recognition of the health risks associated with obesity has focused attention on the development of safe and effective strategies for promotion of weight loss. Dietary restriction, ideally combined with increased physical activity, is paramount in the management of obesity. Medical treatment with levothyroxine sodium may be an additional option for obese animals that do not respond to conservative measures such as dietary restriction and increased physical activity.

References

Adams, A.A., Katepalli, M.P., Kohler, K., et al., 2009. Effect of body condition, body weight and adiposity on inflammatory responses in old horses. Veterinary Immunology and Immunopathology 127, 286–294.

Adams, C.E., Greenway, F.L., Brantley, P.J., 2010. Lifestyle factors and ghrelin: critical review and implications for weight loss maintenance. Obesity Reviews 12, e211–e218.

Alberti, K.G., Zimmet, P., Shaw, J., 2006. Metabolic syndrome – a new world-wide definition. A consensus statement from the International Diabetes Federation. Diabetes Medicine 23, 469–480.

Allen, F.J., Pfeiffer, D.U., Jones, B.R., et al., 2000. A cross-sectional study of risk factors for obesity in cats in New Zealand. Preventive Veterinary Medicine 46, 183–196.

Anon, 1998. Baseline Reference of 1998 Equine Health and Management, Part 1. National Animal Health Monitoring System, United States Department of Agriculture (http://www.aphis.usda.gov/animal_health/nahms/equine/downloads/equine98/Equine98_dr_PartI.pdf).

Arathuzik, G.G., Goebel-Fabbri, A.E., 2011. Nutrition therapy and the management of obesity and diabetes: An Update. Current Diabetes Reports 11, 106–110.

Arnold, W., Ruf, T., Kuntz, R., 2006. Seasonal adjustment of energy budget in a large wild mammal, the Przewalski horse (*Equus ferus przewalksi*). II. Energy expenditure. Journal of Experimental Biology 209, 4566–4573.

Bailey, S.R., Menzies-Gow, N.J., Harris, P.A., et al., 2007. Effect of dietary fructans and dexamethasone administration on the insulin response of ponies predisposed to laminitis. Journal of the American Veterinary Medical Association 231, 1365–1373.

Bailey, S.R., Habsershon-Butcher, J.L., Ransom, K.J., et al., 2008. Hypertension and insulin resistance in a mixed-breed population of ponies predisposed to laminitis. American Journal of Veterinary Research 69, 122–129.

Balistreri, C.R., Caruso, C., Candore, G., 2010. The role of adipose tissue and adipokines in obesity-related inflammatory diseases. Mediators of Inflammation. doi:10.1155/2010/802078.

Bamford, N.J., Potter, S.J., Harris, P.A., et al., 2012. Effect of increasing adiposity, induced by high fat low glycaemic diet or similar diet with once daily glucose, on insulin sensitivity in horses and ponies. In: Proceedings of the Australian Equine Science Symposium 4, 19.

Barbarroja, N., Lopez-Pedrera, R., Mayas, M.D., et al., 2010. The obese healthy paradox: is inflammation the answer? Biochemical Journal 430, 141–149.

Bluher, M., 2010. The distinction of metabolically "healthy" from "unhealthy" obese individuals. Current Opinion in Lipidology 21, 38–43.

Booth, F.W., Laye, M.J., Leese, S.J., et al., 2008. Reduced physical activity and risk of chronic disease: the biology behind consequences. European Journal of Applied Physiology 102, 381–390.

Bosy-Westphal, A., Geisler, G., Onur, S., et al., 2006. Value of body fat mass vs anthropometric obesity indices in the assessment of metabolic risk factors. International Journal of Obesity 30, 475–483.

Bruynsteen, L., Erkens, T., Peelman, L.J., et al., 2011. Depot-specific mRNA expression by equine adipocytes. In: Proceedings 15th Congress European Society of Veterinary and Comparative Nutrition. p. 63.

Buff, P.R., Dodds, A.C., Morrison, C.D., et al., 2002. Leptin in horses: tissue localization and relationship between peripheral concentrations of leptin and body condition. Journal of Animal Science 80, 2942–2948.

Buff, P.R., Spader, B.R., Morrison, C.D., et al., 2006. Endocrine responses in mares undergoing abrupt changes in nutritional management. Journal of Animal Science 84, 2700–2707.

Buff, P.R., Johnson, P.J., Wiedmeyer, C.E., et al., 2006. Modulation of leptin, insulin and growth hormone in obese pony mares under chronic nutritional restriction and supplementation with ractopamine hydrochloride. Veterinary Therapeutics 7, 64–72.

Burns, T.A., Geor, R.J., Mudge, M.A., et al., 2010. Proinflammatory cytokine and chemokine gene expression profiles in subcutaneous and visceral adipose tissue depots of insulin-resistant and insulin-sensitive light breed horses. Journal of Veterinary Internal Medicine 24, 932–939.

Caltabilota, T.J., Earl, L.R., Thompson, Jr., D.L., et al., 2010. Hyperleptinemia in mares and geldings: Assessment of insulin sensitivity from glucose responses to insulin injection. Journal of Animal Science 88, 2940–2949.

Carter, R.A., McCutcheon, L.J., Burns, T.A., et al., 2008. Increased adiposity in horses is associated with decreased insulin sensitivity but unchanged inflammatory cytokine expression in subcutaneous adipose tissue. Journal of Veterinary Internal Medicine 22, 735 (abstract).

Carter, R.A., Treiber, K.H., Geor, R.J., et al., 2009a. Prediction of incipient pasture-associated laminitis from hyperinsulinemia, hyperleptinemia, and generalized and localized obesity in a cohort of ponies. Equine Veterinary Journal 41, 171–178.

Carter, R.A., McCutcheon, L.J., George, L.A., et al., 2009b. Effects of diet-induced weight gain on insulin sensitivity and plasma hormone and lipid concentrations in horses. American Journal of Veterinary Research 70, 1250–1258.

Carter, R.A., Staniar, W.B., Cubitt, T.A., et al., 2009c. Apparent adiposity assessed by standardized scoring systems and morphometric measurements in horses and ponies. Veterinary Journal 179, 204–210.

Carter, R.A., McCutcheon, L.J., Valle, E., et al., 2010. Effects of exercise training on adiposity, insulin sensitivity, and plasma hormone and lipid concentrations in overweight or obese, insulin-resistant horses. American Journal of Veterinary Research 71, 314–321.

Cartmill, J.A., Thompson, D.L., Storer, W.A., et al., 2003. Endocrine responses in mares and geldings with high body condition scores grouped by high vs. low resting leptin concentrations. Journal of Animal Science 81, 2311–2321.

Cartmill, J.A., Thompson, D.L., Storer, W.A., et al., 2005. Effect of dexamethasone, feeding time, and insulin infusion on leptin concentrations in stallions. Journal of Animal Science 83, 1875–1881.

Catenacci, V.A., Wyatt, H.R., 2007. The role of physical activity in producing and maintaining weight loss. Nature Clinical Practice. Endocrinology & Metabolism 3, 518–529.

Cummings, D.E., Frayo, R.S., Marmonier, C., et al., 2004. Plasma ghrelin levels and hunger scores in humans initiating meals voluntarily without time- and food-related cues. American Journal of Physiology: Endocrinology and Metabolism 287, E297–E304.

Curtis, G.C., Barfott, C.F., Dugdale, A.H., et al., 2010. Comparison of two practical weight loss protocols for the management of overweight and obese horses and ponies. In: Ellis, A.D., Longland, A.C., Coenen, M., et al. (Eds.), The impact of nutrition on the health and welfare of horses. European Association for Animal Production Publication Number 128. Wageningen Academic Publishers, Wageningen, The Netherlands, p. 237.

Curtis, G.C., Barfoot, C.F., Dugdale, A.H., et al., 2011. Voluntary ingestion of wood shavings by obese horses under dietary restriction. British Journal of Nutrition 106 (Suppl. 1), S178–S182.

Cusi, K., 2010. The role of adipose tissue and lipotoxicity in the pathogenesis of type 2 diabetes. Current Diabetes Reports 10, 306–315.

Delzenne, N., Blundell, J., Brouns, F., et al., 2010. Gastrointestinal targets of appetite regulation in humans. Obesity Reviews 11, 234–250.

Donaldson, M.T., McFarlane, D., Jorgensen, A.J., et al., 2004. Correlation between alpha-melanocyte-stimulating hormone concentration and body mass index in healthy horses. American Journal of Veterinary Research 65, 1469–1473.

Dugdale, A.H., Curtis, G.C., Cripps, P., et al., 2010. Effect of dietary restriction on body condition, composition and welfare of overweight and obese pony mares. Equine Veterinary Journal 42, 600–610.

Dugdale, A.H., Curtis, G.C., Harris, P.A., et al., 2011a. Assessment of body fat in the pony: Part I. Relationship between the anatomical distribution of adipose tissue, body composition and body condition. Equine Veterinary Journal 43, 552–561.

Dugdale, A.H., Curtis, G.C., Cripps, P., et al., 2011b. Effects of season and body condition on appetite, body mass and body composition in ad libitum fed pony mares. Veterinary Journal 190, 329–337.

Dugdale, A.H., Grove-White, D., Curtis, G.C., et al., 2012. Body condition scoring as a predictor of body fat in horses and ponies. Veterinary Journal (http://10.1016/t.tvjl.2012.03.024).

Enriori, P.J., Evans, A.E., Sinnayah, P., et al., 2006. Leptin resistance and obesity. Obesity 14 (Suppl. 5), 254S–258S.

Foster, M.T., Shi, H., Seeley, R.J., et al., 2011. Removal of intra-abdominal visceral adipose tissue improves glucose tolerance in rats: Role of hepatic triglyceride storage. Physiology & Behavior 104, 845–854.

Fuller, Z., Cox, J.E., Argo, C.M.C.G., 2001. Phtoperiodic entrainment of seasonal changes in the appetite, feeding behavior, growth rate and pelage of pony colts. Animal Science 72, 65–74.

Frank, N., 2011. Equine metabolic syndrome. Veterinary Clinics of North America: Equine Practice 27, 73–92.

Frank, N., Elliott, S.B., Brandt, L.E., et al., 2006. Physical characteristics, blood hormone concentrations, and plasma lipid concentrations in obese horses with insulin resistance. Journal of the American Veterinary Medical Association 228, 1383–1390.

Frank, N., Elliott, S.B., Boston, R.C., 2008. Effects of long-term oral administration of levothyroxine sodium on glucose dynamics in healthy adult horses. American Journal of Veterinary Research 69, 76–81.

Frank, N., Geor, R.J., Bailey, S.R., et al., 2010. Equine metabolic syndrome. Journal of Veterinary Internal Medicine 24, 467–475.

Garcia-Seco, E., Wilson, D.A., Kramer, J., et al., 2005. Prevalence and risk factors associated with outcome of surgical removal of pedunculated liomas in horses: 102 cases (1987–2002). Journal of the American Veterinary Medical Association 226, 1529–1537.

Gauthier, M.-S., Ruderman, N.B., 2010. Adipose tissue inflammation and insulin resistance: all obese humans are not created equal. Biochemical Journal 430, e1–e4.

Gentry, L.R., Thompson, D.L., Gentry, G.T., et al., 2002. The relationship between body condition, leptin, and reproductive and hormonal characteristics of mares during the seasonal anovulatory period. Journal of Animal Science 80, 2695–2703.

Giles, S., Harris, P.A., Nicol, C.J., et al., 2011. Variation in body condition in small groups of horses. In: Proceedings of ISES: principles and practices - science at work. p. 101.

Giles, S., Nicol, C.J., Rands, S.A., et al., 2012. Fat all year round - The welfare consequences of continuous equine obesity. In: Proceedings of the UFAW conference (in press).

Gordon, M.E., McKeever, K.H., 2006. Oral and intravenous carbohydrate challenges decrease active ghrelin concentrations and alter hormones related to control of energy metabolism in horses. Journal of Animal Science 86, 1682–1690.

Gordon, M.E., McKeever, K.H., Bokman, S., et al., 2006. Interval exercise alters feed intake as well as leptin and ghrelin concentrations in standardbred mares. Equine Veterinary Journal Supplement 36, 596–605.

Gordon, M.E., Jerina, M.L., Raub, R.H., et al., 2009. The effects of dietary manipulation and exercise on weight loss and related indices of health in horses. Comparative Exercise Physiology 6, 33–42.

Halaas, J.L., Gajiwala, K.S., Maffei, M., et al., 1995. Weight-reducing effects of the protein encoded by the obese gene. Science 269, 543–546.

Hawley, J.A., 2004. Exercise as a therapeutic intervention for the prevention and treatment of insulin resistance. Diabetes Metabolism Research Reviews 20, 383–393.

Henneke, D.R., Potter, G.D., Kreider, J.L., et al., 1983. Relationship between condition score, physical measurements and body fat percentage in mares. Equine Veterinary Journal 15, 371–372.

Hoffman, R.M., Boston, R.C., Stefanovski, D., et al., 2003. Obesity and diet affect glucose dynamics and insulin sensitivity in Thoroughbred geldings. Journal of Animal Science 81, 2333–2342.

Hutley, L., Prins, J.B., 2005. Fat as an endocrine organ: Relationship to the metabolic syndrome. American Journal of Medical Science 330, 280–289.

Ince, J.C., Longland, A.C., Moore-Colyer, M., et al., 2005. A pilot study to estimate the intake of grass by ponies with restricted access to pasture. Proceedings of the British Society of Animal Science, p. 109 (abstract).

Jeffcott, L.B., Field, J.R., 1985. Epidemiological aspects of hyperlipaemia in ponies in south eastern Australia. Australian Veterinary Journal 62, 140–141.

Johnson, P.J., 2002. The equine metabolic syndrome: Peripheral Cushing's Syndrome. Veterinary Clinics of North America: Equine Practice 18, 271–293.

Johnson, P.J., Messer, N.T., Ganjam, V.K., 2004. Cushing's syndromes. insulin resistance and endocrinopathic laminitis. Equine Veterinary Journal 36, 194–198.

Kabir, M., Stefanoski, D., Hsu, I.R., et al., 2011. Large size cells in the visceral adipose depot predict insulin resistance in the canine model. Obesity 19, 2121–2129.

Karelis, A.D., 2008. Metabolically healthy but obese individuals. Lancet 372, 1281–1283.

Kealy, R.D., Lawler, D.F., Ballam, S.L., et al., 2002. Effects of diet restriction on life span and age-related changes in dogs. Journal of the American Veterinary Medical Association 220, 1315–1320.

Klok, M.D., Jakobsdottir, S., Drent, M.L., 2007. The role of leptin and ghrelin in the regulation of food intake and body weight in humans: a review. Obesity Reviews 8, 21–34.

Klöting, N., Fasshauer, M., Dietrich, A., et al., 2010. Insulin sensitive obesity. American Journal of Physiology: Endocrinology and Metabolism 299, E506–E515.

Kopelman, P.G., 2000. Obesity as a medical problem. Nature 404, 635–643.

Kuk, J.L., Katzmarzyk, P.T., Nichaman, M.Z., et al., 2006. Visceral fat is an important predictor of all-cause mortality in mean. Obesity (Silver Spring) 14, 336–341.

Kuntz, R., Kubalek, C., Ruf, T., et al., 2006. Seasonal adjustment of energy budget in a large wild mammal, the Przewalski horse (*Equus ferus przewalksi*). I. Energy intake. Journal of Experimental Biology 209, 4557–4565.

Laye, M.J., Thyfault, J.P., Stump, C.S., et al., 2007. Inactivity induces increases in abdominal fat. Journal of Applied Physiology 102, 1341–1347.

Laflamme, D.P., 2011. Obesity in dogs and cats: What is wrong with being fat? Journal of Animal Science 90, 1653–1662.

Longland, A.C., Ince, J., Harris, P.A., 2011a. Estimation of pasture intake by ponies from liveweight change during six weeks at pasture. Journal of Equine Veterinary Science 31, 275–276.

Longland, A.C., Barfoot, C., Harris, P.A., 2011b. The effect of wearing a grazing muzzle vs not wearing a grazing muzzle on pasture dry matter intake by ponies. Journal of Equine Veterinary Science 31, 282–283.

Longland, A.C., Barfoot, C., Harris, P.A., 2011c. Effects of soaking on the water-soluble carbohydrate and crude protein content of hay. Veterinary Record 168, 618–622.

Maffeis, C., Silvagni, D., Bonadonna, R., et al., 2007. Fat cell size, insulin sensitivity and inflammation in obese children. Journal of Pediatrics 151, 647–652.

Martin-Rosset, W., Vernet, J., Dubroeucq, H., et al., 2008. Variation of fatness and energy content of the body with body condition score in sport horses and its prediction. In: Saastomoinen, M.T., Martin-Rosset, W. (Eds.), Nutrition of the Exercising Horse. European Association for Animal Production Publication Number 125. Wageningen Academic Publishers, Wageningen, The Netherlands, pp. 167–176.

McManus, C.J., Fitzgerald, B.P., 2000. Effects of a single day of feed restriction on changes in serum leptin, gonadotropins, prolactin, and metabolites in aged and young mares. Domestic Animal Endocrinology 19, 1–13.

Meister, B., 2000. Control of food intake via leptin receptors in the hupothalamus. Vitamins & Hormones 59, 265–304.

Menzies-Gow, N.J., Stevens, K., Barr, A., et al., 2010. Severity and outcome of equine pasture-associated laminitis managed in first opinion practice in the UK. Veterinary Record 167, 364–369.

Montague, C.T., O'Rahilly, S., 2000. The perils of portliness: causes and consequences of visceral adiposity. Diabetes 49, 883–888.

National Research Council, 2007. Nutrient Requirements of Horses, 6th revised edition. National Academies Press, Washington, DC.

Powell, D.M., Reedy, S.E., Sessions, D.R., et al., 2002. Effect of short-term exercise training on insulin sensitivity in obese and lean mares. Equine Veterinary Journal (Suppl. 34), 81–84.

Pratt-Phillips, S.E., Owens, K.M., Dowler, L.E., et al., 2010. Assessment of resting insulin and leptin concentrations and their association with managerial and innate factors in horses. Journal of Equine Veterinary Science 30, 127–133.

Quinn, R.W., Burk, A.O., Hartsock, T.G., et al., 2009. Insulin sensitivity in Thoroughbred geldings: effect of weight gain, diet and exercise. Journal of Equine Veterinary Science 28, 728–738.

Reid, S.W., Mohammed, H.O., 1996. Survival analysis approach to risk factors associated with hyperlipemia in donkeys. Journal of American Veterinary Medical Association 209, 1449–1452.

Romero-Corral, A., Somers, V.K., Sierra-Johnson, J., et al., 2008. Accuracy of body mass index in diagnosing obesity in the adult general population. International Journal of Obesity (London) 32, 959–966.

Romero-Corral, A., Somers, V.K., Sierra-Johnson, J., et al., 2010. Normal weight obesity: a risk factor for cardiometabolic dysregulation and cardiovascular mortality. European Heart Journal 31, 737–746.

Rousset, S., Alves-Guerra, M.C., Mozo, J., et al., 2004. The biology of uncoupling proteins. Diabetes 53, S130–S135.

Schwartz, M.W., Peskind, E., Raskind, M., et al., 1996. Cerebrospinal fluid leptin levels: relationship to plasma levels and to adiposity in humans. Nature Medicine 2, 589–593.

Seidell, J.C., 2010. Waist circumference and waist/hip ratio in relation to all-cause mortality, cancer and sleep apnea. European Journal of Clinical Nutrition 64, 25–42.

Shea, J.L., King, M.T.C., Yi, Y., et al., 2011. Body fat percentage is associated with cardiometabolic dysregulation in BMI-defined normal weight subjects. Nutrition, Metabolism and Cardiovascular Diseases. doi:10.1016/j.numecd.2010.11.009.

Spiegelman, B.M., Flier, J.S., 2001. Obesity and its regulation of energy balance. Cell 104, 531–543.

Stefan, N., Kantartzis, K., Machann, J., et al., 2008. Identification and characterization of metabolically benign obesity in humans. Archives of Internal Medicine 168, 1609–1616.

Stephenson, H.M., Green, M.J., Freeman, S.L., 2011. Prevalence of obesity in a population of horses in the UK. Veterinary Record 168, 131.

Suagee, J.K., Corl, B.A., Crisman, M.V., et al., 2010. De novo fatty acid synthesis and NADPH generation in equine adipose and liver tissue. Comparative Biochemistry and Physiology. Part B, Biochemistry and Molecular Biology 155, 322–326.

Tan, C.Y., Vidal-Puig, A., 2008. Adipose tissue expandibility: the metabolic problems of obesity may arise from the inability to become more obese. Biochemical Society Transactions 36, 935–940.

Tinworth, K.D., Harris, P.A., Sillence, M.N., et al., 2010. Potential treatments for insulin resistance in the horse: A comparative multi-species review. Veterinary Journal 186, 282–291.

Tinworth, K.D., Boston, R.C., Harris, P.A., et al., 2011. The effect of oral metformin on insulin sensitivity in insulin-resistant ponies. Veterinary Journal Feb 22 (Epub ahead of print).

Thatcher, C.D., Pleasant, R.S., Geor, R.J., et al., 2012. Prevalence of over conditioning in mature horses: in Southwest Virginia during the summer. Journal of the Veterinary Internal Medicine 26, 1413–1418.

Trayhurn, P., 2005. Adipose tissue in obesity – an inflammatory issue. Endocrinology 146, 1003–1005.

Trayburn, P., Wood, I.S., 2004. Adipokines: inflammation and the pleiotropic role of white adipose tissue. British Journal of Nutrition 92, 347–355.

Treiber, K.H., Kronfeld, D.S., Hess, T.M., et al., 2006. Evaluation of genetic and metabolic predispositions and nutritional risk factors for pasture-associated laminitis in ponies. Journal of the American Veterinary Medical Association 228, 1538–1545.

Tulloch-Reid, M.K., Williams, D.E., Looker, H.C., et al., 2003. Do measures of body fat distribution provide information on the risk of type 2 diabetes in addition to measures of general obesity? – Comparison of anthropometric predictors of type 2 diabetes in Pima Indians. Diabetes Care 26, 2556–2561.

Van Weyenberg, S., Hesta, M., Buyse, J., et al., 2008a. Short-term effects of energy changes on plasma leptin concentrations and glucose tolerance in healthy ponies. Veterinary Journal 178, 233–237.

Van Weyenberg, S., Hesta, M., Buyse, J., et al., 2008b. The effect of weight loss by energy restriction on metabolic profile and glucose tolerance in ponies. Journal of Animal Physiology and Animal Nutrition 92, 538–545.

Vick, M.M., Sessions, D.R., Murphy, B.A., et al., 2006. Obesity is associated with altered metabolic and reproductive activity in the mare: effects of metformin on insulin sensitivity and reproductive cyclicity. Reproduction, Fertility and Development 18, 609–617.

Vick, M.M., Adams, A.A., Murphy, B.A., et al., 2007. Relationships among inflammatory cytokines, obesity, and insulin sensitivity in the horse. Journal of Animal Science 85, 1144–1155.

Virtanen, K.A., Lidell, M.E., Orava, J., et al., 2009. Functional brown adipose tissue in healthy adults. New England Journal of Medicine 360, 1518–1525.

Waller, A.P., Kohler, K., Burns, T.A., et al., 2011. Naturally-occurring compensated insulin resistance selectively alters glucose transporters in visceral and subcutaneous adipose tissues without change in AS160 activation. Biochimica et Biophysica Acta 1812, 1098–1103.

Wildman, R.P., Muntner, P., Reynolds, K., et al., 2008. The obese without cardiovascular risk factoring clustering and the normal weight with cardiometabolic risk factor clustering: prevalence and correlates of 2 phenotypes among US population (NHANES 1999–2004). Archives of Internal Medicine 168, 1617–1624.

Wren, A.M., Seal, L.J., Cohen, M.A., et al., 2001. Ghrelin enhances appetite and increases food intake in humans. Journal of Clinical Endocrinology and Metabolism 86, 5992–5995.

Wyse, C.A., McNie, K.A., Tannahil, V.J., et al., 2008. Prevalence of obesity in riding horses in Scotland. Veterinary Record 162, 590–591.

29

Feeding thin and starved horses

Caroline McGregor Argo

Aetiology

The definition of "acceptable" body condition for horses, ponies and donkeys differs markedly across the globe. In developed countries, where animals are primarily kept by choice, whether directed at breeding, competition or leisure use, expectations for animal welfare are high. Against this background, the presentation of an animal in a poor or emaciated state gives immediate cause for concern while the welfare issues surrounding the all too common and potentially more serious, "over-conditioning" of horses are rarely considered (Fig. 29.1A). Paradoxically, in many developing countries, where the fate of a human family may be inextricably-linked to the working ability of an animal, hardship may impose the acceptance of lower body conditions (Fig. 29.1B).

The presentation of animals in thin or emaciated states is highly emotive (Fig. 29.2). However, extreme loss of body condition (>30% of its "ideal" body weight) may arise as a result of malnutrition, whether through neglect, ignorance or circumstance, focal (e.g., dental disease, dysphagia) or systemic disease (e.g., lymphosarcoma, granulomatous enteritis, parasitism), as a consequence of old age or in feral animals, as a consequence of seasonal changes in the quality and availability of grazing (Dunkel & Wilkins 2004, Ralston 1999, Witham & Stull 1998, Kronfeld 1993). Before treatment options and prognoses can be contemplated, each case must be individually considered. Starvation occurs when animals suffer and become ill from the effects of underfeeding or inappropriate nutrition (Kronfeld 1993). It is an umbrella term, which has been applied equally to animals from which food has been completely and abruptly withdrawn (acute starvation) and to those for which food deprivation has been less severe but prolonged (chronic starvation).

Case evaluation

When starvation is suspected, wherever possible the history of the animal should be explored to gain some understanding of the time course for the loss of body condition. Frequently, changes in body condition are insidious and even large losses in body weight and condition may go undetected until relatively advanced or picked up by a fresh observer (Kronfeld 1993). This is especially true for animals which were overweight or obese prior to feed deprivation (Dugdale et al 2010). Adequacy of nutritional provision or an unwillingness to eat may be suggestive of underlying disease (Kronfeld 1993). High grazing densities, poor growth in young animals and prolonged confinement may be indicators of chronic starvation, where food deprivation may possibly be exacerbated by substantial parasite burdens which further limit the availability of nutrients (Uhlinger 2007). Extra care is warranted when starvation is encountered in heavily pregnant or lactating mares, youngstock, ponies, miniature horses and donkeys. These animals are highly sensitive to starvation and prone to hyperlipidemia which must be clinically addressed before true rehabilitation can begin (Dunkel & Wilkins 2004).

At the outset, clinical priority must focus on arriving at a realistic decision between immediate euthanasia and treatment for the chronically starved animal. An animal in good initial health and body condition may survive a complete withdrawal of food for up to 60 days (Becvarova & Thatcher 2008). However, once the animal has been recumbent for more than 72 h, the prognosis for survival is poor (Becvarova & Thatcher 2008).

Intensive treatment of the recumbent animal may necessitate slinging, intravenous fluid therapy, frequent enteral feeding by nasogastric intubation (Chapter 41) and constant monitoring (Whiting et al 2005). Regrettably therefore, base economics must also play a part in the decision. Not only are these measures expensive but they may further distress an already compromised animal when expectations for success are poor (Whiting et al 2005). Mortality rates of approximately 20% are predicted for severely malnourished animals undergoing rehabilitation, while up to 10 months may be required for surviving animals to regain normal body condition (Whiting et al 2005). An immediate and thorough clinical examination of each animal will help to pinpoint the etiology of weight loss and to identify any concurrent disease or pre-existing conditions. Blood biochemistry screening may aid in the determination of the extent and severity of starvation. Biochemical evaluations should include the evaluation of increased serum concentrations of nonesterified fatty acids, glycerol, total lipids, triglycerides, phospholipids, cholesterol, β-hydroxybutyrate,

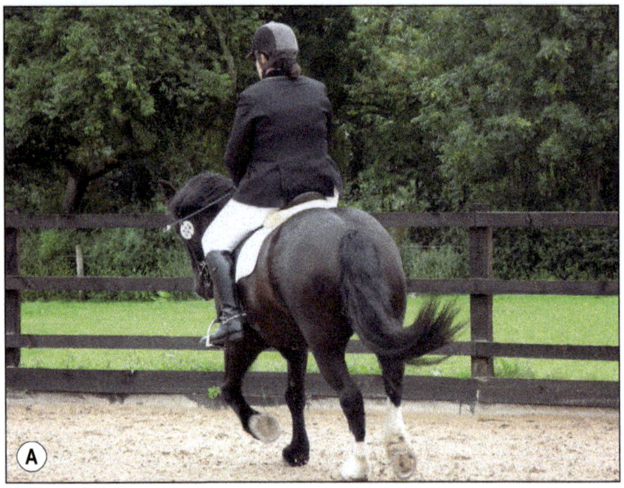

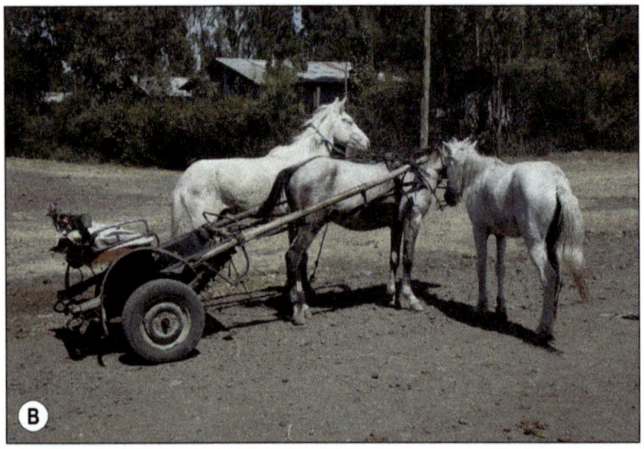

Figure 29.1 The definition of "acceptable" body condition varies widely. A) In "developed" nations, while low body condition is deemed unacceptable the welfare issues associated with obesity are frequently neglected. **B)** Working horses in Ethiopia are in relatively good body condition given the hardships which dominate life in this environment.
Photographs supplied by Prof. D.C. Knottenbelt, University of Liverpool, UK.

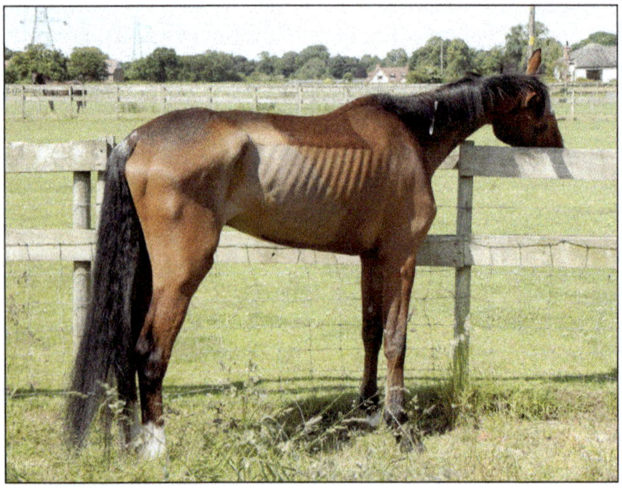

Figure 29.2 The presentation of animals in emaciated states can be highly emotive. Before treatment options and prognoses can be contemplated, each case must be individually considered with respect to its history and the presence of underlying disease.
Photograph supplied by Prof. D.C. Knottenbelt, University of Liverpool, UK.

Box 29.1 Case Evaluation

For emaciated animals, establishing a realistic prognosis for recovery should be the priority.

This should be based on

(a) The duration and rate of body condition loss and / or recumbency.
(b) The extent and treatment prognosis of any underlying disease.
(c) Financial, practical and time constraints

lactate, total and unconjugated bilirubin and cortisol and decreased serum concentrations of magnesium, calcium, potassium and insulin (Durham et al 2004). A clear diagnosis is key to the development of an informed rehabilitation schedule (see Box 29.1).

Pathophysiology of food deprivation

The design of successful rehabilitation protocols demands a clear understanding of the changes which occur during starvation. Food deprivation in previously healthy animals is met by a predictable sequence of metabolic, physiological and behavioral responses designed to conserve body function and ultimately, survival. As a trickle feeder, the free-ranging horse normally spends 50–60% of the day feeding (Ralston 1984) and grazing is interrupted only by regular rest periods with variable indulgence in other activities. Although feed can generally be withheld from otherwise healthy horses for 2–3 days without lasting harm, the physiological responses to food deprivation are initiated within a few hours of the last meal (Dunkel & Wilkins 2004).

Metabolic changes

While the pathophysiology of chronic starvation in the horse is poorly documented, useful inferences can be made from studies in other species. In man, the metabolic responses to starvation are progressive (Emery 2005). Nutrient concentrations in the blood decrease as their consumption by tissues is no longer balanced by absorption from the gastrointestinal tract. Preservation of the central nervous system (CNS), by maintaining the glucose supplies essential for its function, becomes the physiological priority. Within 24 h of the previous meal, as blood glucose concentrations decline further, endocrine mechanisms are activated to conserve blood glucose concentrations (Tresley & Sheean 2008). Plasma concentrations of insulin decrease markedly, while glycogen stored in skeletal muscle and liver is mobilized in response to increased glucagon and catecholamine concentrations (Tresley & Sheean 2008). While catabolized muscle glycogen supports local function, the products of hepatic glycogenolysis are released into the systemic circulation to support function in glucose dependent tissues (erythrocytes, the renal medulla and the CNS; Kraft et al 2005, Ekberg et al 1998). At best however, stored glycogen comprises less than 1% of body mass (Hoffer 2006) (Fig. 29.3).

As the primary defense against starvation, the buffering capacity of glycogen is short-lived and in man, these reserves are depleted within 72 h (Hoffer 2006). As starvation continues, gluconeogenesis is increasingly invoked to maintain

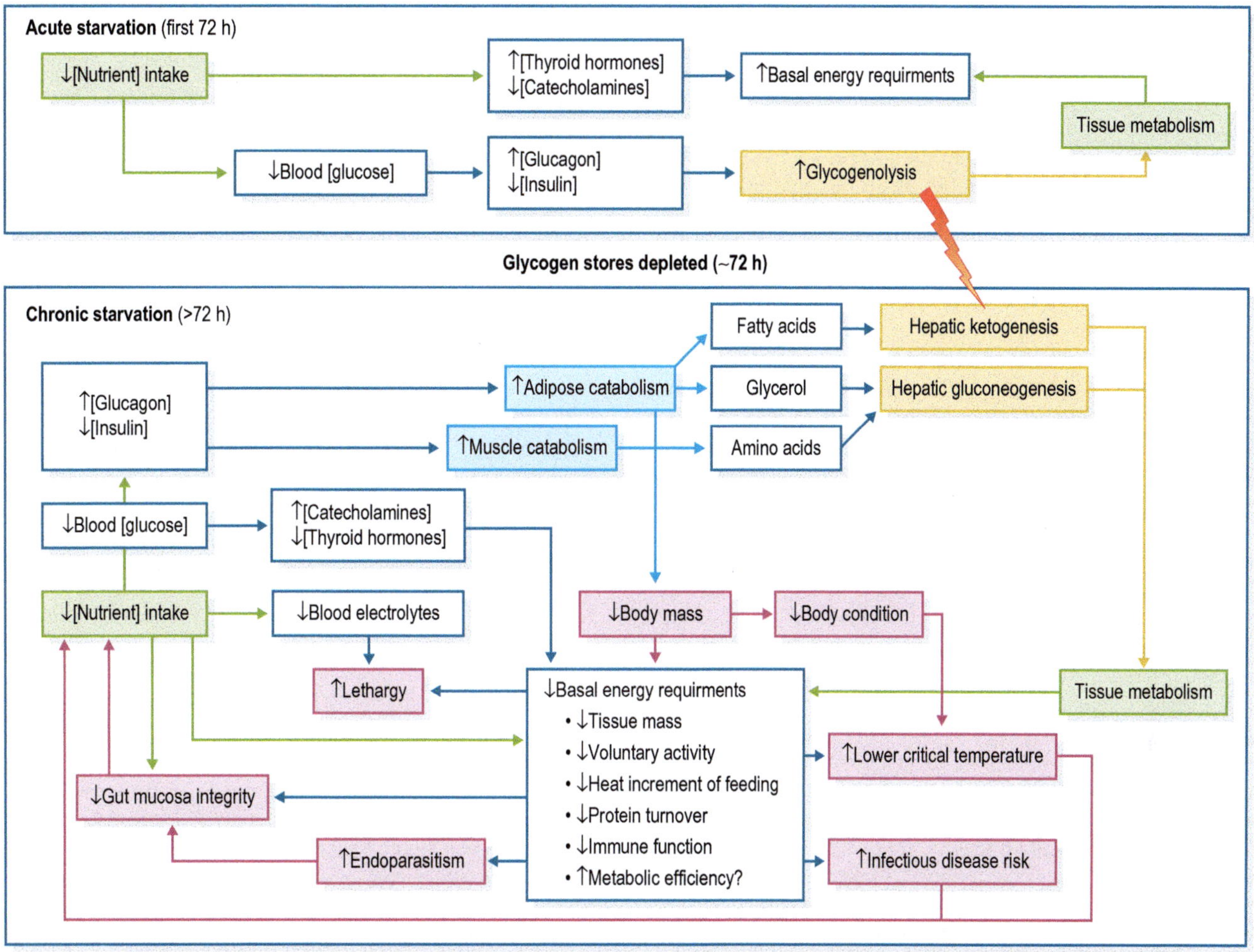

Figure 29.3 Simplified, schematic overview of the major physiological mechanisms invoked in response to short (acute) and prolonged (chronic) starvation. Blue arrows indicate the major pathways through which first, stored body glycogen and later, body tissues are mobilized to support tissue metabolism when nutrient intakes are either markedly reduced or withdrawn (green boxes). Common physical sequelae to chronic starvation in the horse are indicated (pink boxes).

blood glucose concentrations. During early starvation, metabolic energy requirements are increased, both in response to elevated plasma thyroid hormone and catecholamine concentrations and as a direct result of the additional energy requirements for gluconeogenesis (Emery 2005). The transition to gluconeogenesis is fuelled by increased catabolism of stored body fats and proteins from adipose tissue and skeletal muscle. Although amino acids derived from the catabolism of muscle protein and lipolysis-derived glycerol are useful substrates for gluconeogenesis, fatty acids are not (Emery 2005). Hepatic β-oxidation of fatty acids yields ketones, primarily β-OH butyrate, which can also fuel cell metabolism directly through the formation of the Kreb's Cycle precursor, acetyl-coenzyme A (Newsholme & Leech 1983, Hoffer 2006). The potential for gluconeogenic demands to strip body fat and muscle is dramatic – yet as starvation persists further physiological changes serve to protect brain function, while limiting the rate of skeletal muscle loss (Emery 2005). Nonetheless this transition to "emergency" fuels is accompanied by the depletion of serum potassium, phosphorus and magnesium (Tresley & Sheean 2008) (Fig. 29.3).

Over time, neural tissues, which can account for 20% of the glucose oxidized within the body, adapt to decreased glucose availability by progressively using ketones as their primary energy source (Emery 2005). Notably, the horse may be unique in that the rapid development of starvation-induced ketonemia seems absent, especially in the early stages of hypophagia (Naylor 1980). However, in one study, increased ketone concentrations were reported when light-horse mares had been deprived of food for only 48 hours (Sticker et al 1995). Whether this indicates a lack of study or a real, fundamental difference in the ability of the equine CNS to redirect its metabolism to use ketones is unknown. In most species, the ability of the brain to decrease its dependency on glucose is important in limiting the rate of muscle catabolism (Barendregt et al 2008).

Muscle-sparing during chronic food deprivation is further bolstered by a corresponding decrease in whole body metabolism as starvation progresses. This decrease in overall energy requirements is multifactorial. Tissue catabolism directly reduces body mass-related metabolic requirements and structural protein turnover rates may be decreased (Emery 2005). Many of the energy costs of feeding and digestion are eliminated. Chronic starvation or malnutrition is associated with decreased activity levels until only essential movements are performed and these, conducted slowly and with maximum efficiency (Shetty 1999). Further, it is considered that the efficiency of intermediary metabolism may be increased, although the mechanisms which underpin these changes are poorly understood (Shetty 1999) (Fig. 29.3).

Physical changes

As weight loss progresses, sequential changes in the animal's appearance are appreciated. With the goal of achieving weight loss in obese (body condition score; BCS 6.8/9 + 0.5) pony mares, food provision was restricted to 1% of body mass as dry matter of a complete, chaff-based diet for 12 weeks (Dugdale et al 2010). In the first week of dietary restriction, body mass decreased by 4% of outset values before stabilizing at 0.7% of outset body mass in each week thereafter. The dramatic weight loss in the first week was associated with changes in gut fill, readily appreciated as decreased belly girth, and most probably included weight loss resulting from the depletion of glycogen reserves and the attendant water of ligand. Interestingly, weight loss over the 12 weeks was only appreciable as a further decrease in belly or heart girth and was not evident as changes in BCS. The authors conjectured that intra-celomic adipose tissues (omental, mesenteric, and retroperitoneal) may be the most labile and first to be catabolized to meet gluconeogenic demands (Dugdale et al 2010).

The association between body fat content and BCS is nonlinear so, as BCS declines point by point, the quantity of body fat which must be lost to effect each one point change decreases exponentially (Dugdale et al 2010). Continued feed restriction ultimately effects an increasingly rapid decrease in BCS as subcutaneous, inter- and intramuscular adipose reserves are also depleted (Argo et al, in press). Further, as BCS decreases, each unit weight loss may incorporate increasing quantities of lean tissues. A thin animal in BCS2/9 (0 = emaciated to 9 = obese) , already revealing much of its bony architecture to external appraisal, has very little tolerance and only a very small further decrease in body mass may be required to tip the animal towards emaciation. Post-mortem examination of chronically starved and emaciated horses and ponies suggests that following depletion of stored lipid, regional adipose tissues undergo serous atrophy, before these too are lost to visual inspection. Structural adipose bodies, such as those lining the eye socket may be the last to be catabolized (Dugdale et al 2011a, Udo Herzel, personal communication).

Gastrointestinal tract changes

As starvation progresses, evidence in the horse and other species would suggest that food deprivation causes direct effects on the gastrointestinal tract. Protein catabolism may not be restricted to skeletal muscle but may include smooth muscle of the metabolically expensive gut (Emery 2005). Integrity and function of the mucosal surface of the gastrointestinal tract is highly dependent on the uptake of nutrients from digesta (Roberts & Zaloga 2000). In the starved animal, mucosal integrity and function are compromised and villous atrophy in the small intestine may further restrict nutrient absorption during early re-feeding (Emery 2005). Attrition of the digesta–blood barrier may allow systemic invasion of gut bacteria and endotoxins. Decreased gastric volume and delayed gastric emptying are also reported (Magdesian 2003). Gastric ulceration may also arise as a result of continued gastric acid secretion with gastric hypoperfusion and decreased salivary bicarbonate buffering in the absence of feeding (Magdesian 2003) (Fig. 29.3).

Decreased local and systemic immuno-competence may promote endoparasitism, further diverting scarce nutrients from the host and further damaging the integrity of the gut mucosa (Uhlinger 2007). Systemic immunity may be severely compromised within 5 days of the onset of starvation (Naylor & Kenyon 1981) (Fig. 29.3).

Key Points

Chronic starvation and the shift to catabolic metabolism can result in:

- Decreased metabolic rate as a result of decreases in: protein turnover, gut size, gut integrity and digestive function, activity levels and body mass
- Decreased body condition; may only become evident slowly where animals were fat at outset
- Decreased immune status; increased endoparasitism and systemic disease
- Gastric ulceration
- Cold intolerance

Nutritional management of the thin horse

Horses presented in poor or thin body condition, without further indications of underlying disease can simply be offered more food or, where dry matter intake is already maximal, feedstuffs of greater nutritional quality (Whiting et al 2005). In every case, changes to diet quantity and/or quality should be introduced gradually (Stull 2003). These animals are likely to be in a weakened state which may render them less able to defend their social position and access to communal feed supplies and will benefit greatly from separate management, removing competition stress and allowing the level of food intake to be clearly monitored (Kronfeld 1993).

Increasing intakes of good quality hay or haylage is preferred over the rapid introduction of carbohydrate-based cereal concentrates. The insulin response to carbohydrates can be counterproductive, driving essential electrolytes into cells and reducing their availability (Stull 2003). High intakes of concentrate feeds by these compromised animals are likely to overwhelm foregut digestion and impair the recovery of a healthy cecocolonic fermentation (Naylor et al 1984). Where it can be obtained, alfalfa can be provided either as the principal forage (recommended for weanlings) or as a supplement to grass hay intakes as necessary. The increased protein and electrolyte compositions of alfalfa are useful adjuncts to rehabilitation especially for the lactating or growing animal where mineral requirements are increased. For these less-severely malnourished animals, Kronfeld (1993) advised beginning by offering small (~1 kg) hay meals, a few hours apart, over the first 2 days before allowing free access to forages.

In every case, care should be taken to ensure adequate intakes of vitamin and mineral supplements (Lawrence 2008). This is especially important for the correction of vitamin E and vitamin B deficiencies where horses have been kept in stables for very long periods (months to years without access to fresh forage; Lopes & White 2002).

Rehabilitation of the chronically starved horse or pony

Once a decision for rehabilitation has been taken, early care should include removal of the animal to a secure, sheltered and deeply bedded area to promote comfort (Kronfeld 1993). These severely debilitated horses may spend significant proportions of the day recumbent, a mechanism which promotes energy conservation but may exacerbate pressure injuries to skin and muscle. Topical dressings should be used as appropriate. Oral or parenteral antibiosis may jeopardise recovery of the gut microflora and should be avoided unless indicated by over-riding cause. Care should be taken to minimize energy expenditure on thermoregulation. Environmental warming is preferred to heavy rugging, the weight of which can be counterproductive. Modern, lightweight rugs can be useful, both in retaining heat and padding bony protuberances.

A full clinical evaluation should be undertaken to identify any concurrent disease, inform nutritional provision and early treatments and to provide a baseline against which progress can be monitored. Outset BCS should be carefully determined (Henneke et al 1983) and blood samples collected to permit full hematological characterization, characterization of blood electrolyte concentrations, accurate assessment of hydration status, renal and hepatic function, and gut absorptive capacity (Poupard 1993).

Ideally, body mass should be accurately recorded using a weighbridge. Weigh tapes should be used guardedly as these values are readily influenced by changes in gut fill as re-feeding is initiated and parasite burdens are addressed (Kronfeld 1993). A dental examination should be performed and abnormalities corrected; immediately if they are a primary cause of dysphagia or delayed until they can be accomplished with minimal added distress.

Endoparasite burdens may be large and complex. Counterintuitively, the rigorous and early use of broad-spectrum anthelmintics should be avoided. Aggressive treatment may result in colic, extensive mucosal damage and even death (Cheever 2004). Treatment should be used guardedly and only initiated when appetite has been regained and animals begin to show modest weight gain. Fenbendazole has a broader margin of safety and initial treatment with this or another "mild" anthelmintic is recommended for initial use to avoid intestinal obstruction and mucosal trauma arising from a massive die-off. After a further week, a 5-day course of the same drug is recommended. Only when rehabilitation is well-advanced should drugs such as moxidectin and praziquantel to target encysted cyathostomes and tapeworms be applied and even then, initial treatment with a "half-dose" has been advised.

Key Points – Rehabilitation in chronic starvation

- Ensure physical and thermal comfort.
- Rehydrate if necessary.
- Identify and address concurrent disease.
- Delay anthelmintic therapy until appetite is restored
- Beware the refeeding syndrome!

Nutritional management of the chronically starved horse

The journey to emaciation through starvation took time. The path to successful rehabilitation will take even longer. Rushing in with good but ill-considered intentions carries a heavy price. Protocols for re-feeding must account for the fundamental changes that the animal made to its metabolism in order to survive to this point. The dogma which governs re-feeding protocols today, "start low and go slow", was learned at a heavy price in human lives (Keys et al 1950). People and animals in extreme states of emaciation are at high risk of succumbing to the fatal, "refeeding syndrome" (Witham & Stull 1998, Whiting et al 2005, Tresley & Sheean 2008)

The refeeding syndrome

A major factor contributing to the high mortality rates during rehabilitation of severely malnourished animals is the aptly named, refeeding syndrome. This syndrome was first described for the human survivors of prison camps during the Second World War (Keys et al 1950). In chronic starvation, the dependency of the body on glucose metabolism has been minimized. People and animals in this state become exquisitely sensitized to the systemic effects of insulin.

With the abrupt reintroduction of "high glycemic" diets, such as the carbohydrate laden, grain-based feeds for horses, a profound and potentially fatal increase in blood insulin is elicited (Tresley & Sheean 2008). This massive insulin bolus catapults the animals' unprepared cellular machinery from fat and protein catabolic pathways, back to carbohydrate metabolism. This "kick-starting" of cellular glucose uptake inflicts a heavy toll. Intracellular glucose processing obliges cells to take up magnesium, phosphorus, potassium and vitamin B_1 (thiamine), extracellular supplies of which have already been depleted (Tresley & Sheean 2008) (Fig. 29.4).

The dramatic hypophosphatemia, hypokalemia and hypothiaminosis, variously compound to cause respiratory and cardiac depression, cardiac arrhythmia, paralysis, rhabdomyolysis, and confusion (Tresley & Sheean 2008). As the body struggles to regulate the unaccustomed increase in blood glucose, water and sodium are retained. This extracellular volume expansion is the origin of widespread tissue edema, which further exacerbates respiratory and cardiac distress. Death from refeeding syndrome usually occurs within 3–5 days in man (Solomon & Kirby 1990). Two reports of refeeding large groups of starved horses have been published. The earlier study followed 22 horses over 10 days during which 3 horses died, 2 of which had signs consistent with the refeeding syndrome (Witham & Stull 1998). In the second, 9/45 horses died within 19 days of the initiation of refeeding (mean 7.9±6.3 days, range 1–19 days, Whiting et al 2005). Although not significant, this latter study suggested that animals entering rehabilitation programs in BCS <2/9 may have decreased expectations for survival (OR 4.0, 95% CI, 0.82–1.94, Whiting et al 2005) (Fig. 29.4).

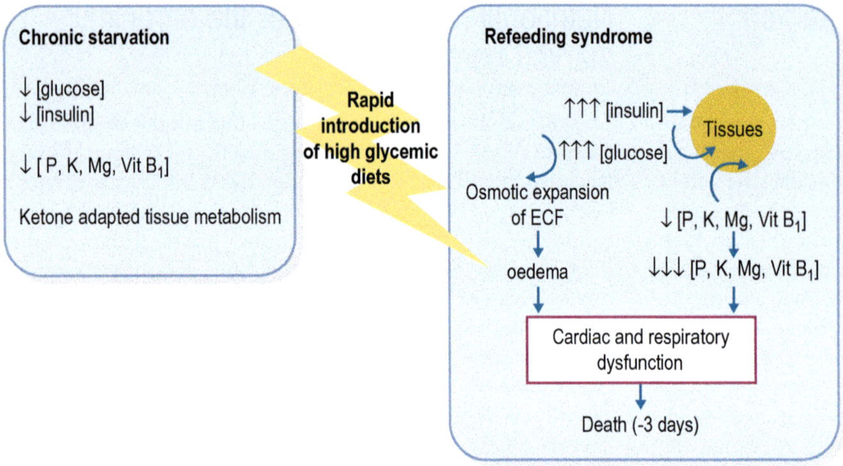

Figure 29.4 Schematic overview of the major mechanisms that contribute to the potentially fatal refeeding syndrome. The dramatic increase in blood glucose results in a massive upsurge in blood insulin concentrations. Obligate cellular uptake of potassium (K), phosphorus (P), magnesium (Mg) and thiamine (vitamin B_1), which accompanies glucose uptake, results in the wholesale depletion of these minerals from the extracellular fluid (ECF) with profound deleterious changes in cardiac and respiratory function. Ketone-adapted tissues in chronically starved animals are not immediately capable of using this "unanticipated" increase in glucose availability. The osmotic consequence of the resultant hyperglycemia is expansion of the ECF compartment. This tissue oedema further compromises cardiorespiratory function and death may occur within 3 days of the initiation of refeeding.

Rehydration protocols

On the first day, priority must be given to restoring hydration status (Kronfeld 1993). Where animals will drink willingly, frequent (every 20–30 minutes), small (2–3 liters) drinks should be offered until the animal no longer drinks greedily, from which point water may be offered ad libitum (Becvarova & Thatcher 2008). For severely malnourished animals, rehydration can be promoted by including salt (0.5–1%) and dextrose (2%) in the initial drinking water (Kronfeld 1993). For animals that will not drink freely, fluids must be administered by nasogastric intubation or intravenously. The route of choice may largely be dictated by circumstance. However, these lethargic and weak individuals are high risk candidates for refeeding syndrome. Establishing intravenous access will more readily allow the monitoring and correction of blood electrolyte imbalances.

Refeeding protocols

Chronically starved, appetent horses

While chronically-starved animals remain standing and are adequately hydrated, they generally remain willing to eat (Becvarova & Thatcher 2008). Enteral feeding is strongly recommended as the optimal route of nutrition to hasten the early resumption of gut integrity, normal nutrient absorption and a functional microflora (Durham et al 2004). Animal rescue organizations have generally adapted feeding-advice from the small number of published studies, which in turn have been developed from human clinical protocols. Commonly, human and equine protocols aim to gradually increase digestible energy (DE) intakes from 0.75 to 1.25 estimated maintenance requirements (based on actual body weight). Low glycemic index foods, such as forages, which do not exceed 20% of the overall dry matter intake as nonstructural carbohydrates are preferred (Becvarova & Thatcher 2008).

Alfalfa hay has been used to good effect as an initial feedstuff (Witham & Stull 1998). Compared to grass hay, alfalfa hays have increased concentrations of DE, protein and minerals which decreases the quantities which must be eaten to achieve target nutrient intakes. Where alfalfa is not available, high quality, leafy grass hays could be used in conjunction with the slow introduction of a low energy, forage-balancer meal to bolster protein, vitamin and mineral intake.

In the earlier study (Witham & Stull 1998), alfalfa was initially offered to meet 75% of predicted maintenance DE requirements (MER) as six small meals, offered every 4 hours over each of the first 3 days. This low level of early intake reflects both the decreased metabolic requirements of the chronically-starved animal and its reduced gastric capacity. Over the following couple of days, as metabolic processes adapted, the size of the 6 daily meals was increased to provide 100% of actual MER requirements. In the second half of this 10 day trial, Alfalfa hay was provided as 3 daily meals and overall provision was increased to 125% of MER.

Other authors have used comparable but less specific regimes. Poupard (1993) advocated the provision of hay and water alone for horses in "very poor" condition, until the horse can support itself, at which time restricted access to "non-lush" grazing was introduced slowly. Horses, stabilized by this early regimen were then fed for weight gain. The feeding of concentrates to supplement ad libitum access to hay and/or non-lush grazing was provided as three daily meals. In the first week, horses were offered 0.5 kg of a molassed, nutrient meal (12% CP) with a cup of bran, and a mineral supplement, mixed and moistened to a liquid form as the first and last meals each day with 0.5 kg of unsupplemented but moistened nutrient meal being given at midday. During the second week, the quantities of concentrate meal were increased to 1.0 kg at each feeding and increased gradually each week thereafter, up to 4 kg of concentrate meal per feeding while the horse remained in "poor condition". After approximately 30 days, if the horse's condition improved to "poor", supplementary feeding was limited to two daily meals.

A strong case can be made that the provision of protein, throughout the entire rehabilitation period, should both be of high biological quality and present in the diet at around 50% in excess of maintenance requirement (Becvarova & Thatcher 2008, NRC 2007). Increased protein quality (optimal amino acid spectrum) and availability recognizes the requirement for lean tissue anabolism and may help to bias the fractionation of surplus dietary energy towards lean tissue regeneration as opposed to storage in adipose deposits. It has been suggested that once horses are consuming consistent intakes of forages and have established good patterns of fecal excretion, forage intakes can be supplemented with linseed meal to provide a further 50% of maintenance requirements. This author recommended that protein provision was continued at this level until rehabilitation was complete (M. Coenen, personal communication). A slightly lower increment in protein provision over maintenance (M + 14%) has previously been recommended (Becvarova & Thatcher 2008). These authors caution that protein provision should only be increased for animals in which normal renal and hepatic function can be demonstrated. It could be conjectured that increased dietary protein could also facilitate muscle anabolism once animals are capable of resuming gentle and increasing levels of daily exercise. However, the anabolic benefits of increased protein feeding can only be evidenced when energy requirements are met from other dietary sources.

The provision of mineral supplements, especially phosphorus, magnesium and potassium, is vital for these animals throughout the early stages of rehabilitation (Becvarova & Thatcher 2008). Deficiencies in the concentrations of these minerals in the peripheral circulation are clearly recognized components of re-feeding syndrome (Witham & Stull 1998). Supplementation of these elements, either as specific feed additives or through the inclusion of phosphorus-rich bran in the re-feeding diet (0.1 to 0.5 kg daily for a 500-kg horse) and/or the relatively mineral-dense alfalfa hays, have variously been recommended.

Box 29.2 Feeding the Chronically Starved Horse

If the gut functions – feed it!

Appetent horses

- Initially (~3 days), alfalfa or good quality grass hay should be offered as small meals, evenly spread throughout the day in quantities not exceeding 75% of estimated daily digestible energy requirements
- Over the following week, forage intake can be gradually increased to 125% of estimated daily DE requirements
- Don't rush rehabilitation. Start low – go slow!

Inappetent horses

- Initially, enteral feeding by nasogastric intubation may be warranted
- Liquidized proprietary horse feeds should be used
- Limit meals to 3–6 liters at intervals of 2–4 hours
- Voluntary feeding should be encouraged throughout and enteral feeding ceased as soon as this becomes established

Chronically starved inappetant horses

For the acutely starved or severely debilitated animal, appetite may be insufficient to enable voluntary feeding and enteral feeding by the nasogastric route becomes essential (Box 29.2). Although total parenteral nutrition (TPN) is available for horses (see Chapter 41), it has been considered both a high risk for re-feeding syndrome and by failing to directly "feed" the gastrointestinal mucosa, may catastrophically delay recovery. Wherever possible, enteral feeding should be prioritized (see Chapter 41).

Although enteral feeding with formulations developed for human subjects has been used with some success, these products are, by design, less suited for the nutritional support of horses, having both low fiber contents and relatively high concentrations of the glycemic compounds which are potential triggers of re-feeding syndrome and laminitis (Lopes & White 2002). More appropriate diets can be formulated from the commercially available, lower-energy pelleted diets marketed as complete feedstuffs for horses (Becvarova & Thatcher 2008). Pellets may require further grinding before soaking to a liquid consistency, compatible with gravitational or pump-assisted flow through the nasogastric tube. Flow through the selected tube should be checked before it is introduced to the animal. As 2–4 hourly feeding intervals of 3–6 liter meals appears to be optimal in the initial days of treatment, it may be preferred that a small diameter nasogastric tube (foal tube; outer diameter, 8 mm) is kept in place to minimize discomfort and veterinary involvement. However, this is not without risk and may inhibit early attempts at voluntary feeding (Hardy et al 1992). Severely starved horses may have decreased stomach capacities and delayed gastric emptying (Naylor et al 1984). Care must be taken to monitor spontaneous reflux before each meal is administered and provision adapted accordingly. Horses, for which required intakes cannot be achieved within 2 days of initiation of enteral feeding, require additional intravenous nutritional support. Vegetable oil (up to 10% of total feed dry matter) has been used to boost the caloric densities of enteral feeds for acutely ill horses and can be useful where gastric capacity is limited. However, dietary oils can further delay gastric emptying and their inclusion must be carefully monitored (Fascetti & Stratton-Phelps 2003). Further details on the parenteral and enteral feeding of compromised horses and ponies can be found in Chapter 41.

Small quantities of hay should always remain within reach and freshly soaked complete feeds should be offered frequently to promote the transition to voluntary self-feeding. Total daily DE and water intakes should be carefully monitored to ensure that in the early stages DE intake approximates 0.75 MER and 60 ml of water/kg BM (Fascetti & Stratton-Phillips 2003). The frequency of nasogastric feeding can be decreased as increasing quantities of foods are voluntarily consumed (Becvarova & Thatcher 2008). Glutamine supplementation of enteral nutrition has been recommended. This amino acid is often considered to be a "non-essential" component of equine nutrition as it is freely synthesized by the normal gastro-intestinal flora. However, glutamine synthesis may be impaired in compromised horses and supplementation may be required to support the direct nutrition of the gastrointestinal mucosa and to re-establish mucosal integrity and function (Lopes & White 2002).

Monitoring rehabilitation

Successful rehabilitation is a long term commitment. Poupard (1993) reported that a period of between 6 and 12 months was required for the chronically starved horse in very poor condition and with no other confounding medical conditions, to reach an acceptable state. When healthy pony mares in thin and moderate condition were allowed ad libitum access to a forage-based diet, weight was gained at approximately 0.35% of outset body mass daily (summer, 0.4% of outset body mass daily; winter, 0.3% daily) (Dugdale et al 2011b). However, under practical conditions, the outset body mass of previously starved animals might be expected to increase by approximately 3–6% over the first few days of rehabilitation as a direct effect of increased gut fill and rehydration of body tissues. Thereafter, once refeeding is established, measurements of body mass might be expected to reflect actual changes in tissue mass. Once maintenance levels of food intake are exceeded (dependent on appetite, ~2 weeks), weight gain will resume. When ad libitum access to forage intake is attained, weight gain should approach 0.3 to 0.4% daily.

For example, an emaciated pony (BCS 1/9), weighing 150 kg at outset, may have an estimated "ideal weight" (based on clinical experience) of 250 kg when in moderate BCS 5/9. The pony enters rehabilitation with an estimated body mass deficit of 100 kg (40%). If the animal regains 5% of its initial body mass as a consequence of refeeding/rehydration, it will still need to gain a further 95 kg. Even if weight is gained at approximately 0.35% of outset body mass daily (0.525 kg) from outset, it might be predicted that a minimum of 6 months (180 days) will be required to reach the desired, moderate BCS. As rehabilitation progresses, the introduction of gentle and increasing exercise to promote the development of muscle mass and limit adipose deposition is warranted when possible. The inclusion of exercise, while potentially slowing overall weight gain, has the potential to contribute greatly to the overall health and longevity of the rehabilitated animal.

In terms of feeding for weight gain, the dogma "start low and go slow" should be remembered throughout. Nonetheless, although slow to instigate in the early stages, once weight gain gathers momentum it can be equally slow to halt. Rigorous, routine monitoring of the animal's body weight and / or body condition, in strict accordance with the scoring system in use (e.g., Henneke et al 1983) and not the "eye" alone, is central to monitoring progress. The current plane of nutrition should be continually reappraised and protocols to promote weight gain must be relaxed as target BCS is approached, if countermeasures against resultant overweight are to be avoided.

References

Argo, C.McG., Curtis, C., Grove-White, D., et al., In press. Weight loss resistance; a further consideration for the nutritional management of obese Equidae. The Veterinary Journal.

Barendregt, K., Soeters, P., Allison, S., et al., 2008. Basics in clinical nutrition: Simple and stress starvation. The European e-Journal of Clinical Nutrition and Metabolism. http://intl.elsevierhealth.com/journals/espen doi:10.1016/j.eclnm.2008.06.006.

Becvarova, I., Thatcher, C.D., 2008. Nutritional management of the starved horse. In: Robinson, N.E., Sprayberry, K.A. (Eds.), Current Therapy in Equine Medicine, sixth ed. Saunders, Philadelphia, pp. 53–58.

Cheever, H., 2004. Equine care in the animal shelter. In: Miller, L., Zawistowski, S. (Eds.), Shelter Medicine for Veterinarians and Staff. Wiley Blackwell, Oxford, pp. 203–208.

Dugdale, A.H.A., Curtis, G.C., Cripps, P., et al., 2010. Effect of dietary restriction on body condition, composition and welfare of overweight and obese pony mares. Equine Veterinary Journal 42 (7), 600–610.

Dugdale, A.H.A., Curtis, G.C., Harris, P.A., et al., 2011a. Assessment of body fat in the pony: I. Relationships between the anatomical distribution of adipose tissue, body composition and body condition. Equine Veterinary Journal 43 (5), 552–561.

Dugdale, A.H.A., Curtis, C., Cripps, P., et al., 2011b. Effect of season and body condition on appetite, body mass and body composition in *ad libitum* fed pony mares. The Veterinary Journal 190, 329–387.

Dunkel, B.M., Wilkins, P.A., 2004. Nutrition and the critically ill horse. The Veterinary Clinics, Equine Practice 20, 107–126.

Durham, A.E., Phillips, T.J., Walmsley, J.P., et al., 2004. Nutritional and clinicopathological effects of post-operative parenteral nutrition following small intestinal resection and anastomosis in the mature horse. Equine Veterinary Journal 36 (5), 390–396.

Ekberg, K., Landau, B.R., Wajngot, A., et al., 1998. Contributions of kidney and liver to glucose production in the postabsorptive state and after 60 h of fasting. Diabetes 48, 292–298.

Emery, P.W., 2005. Metabolic changes in malnutrition. Eye 19, 1029–1034.

Fascetti, A.J., Stratton-Phelps, M., 2003. Clinical assessment of nutritional status and enteral feeding in the acutely ill horse. In: Robinson, N.E. (Ed.), Current Therapy in Equine Medicine, fifth ed. WB Saunders, Philadelphia, pp. 705–710.

Hardy, J., Stewart, R.H., Beard, W.L., et al., 1992. Complications of nasogastric intubation in horses: nine cases (1987–1989). Journal of the American Veterinary Medicine Association 201 (3), 483–486.

Henneke, D.R., Potter, G.D., Krieder, J.L., et al., 1983. Relationship between condition score, physical measurements and body fat percentage in mares. Equine Veterinary Journal 15, 371–372.

Hoffer, L.J., 2006. Metabolic consequences of starvation. In: Shils, M., Olson, J.A., Shike, M., et al. (Eds.), Modern Nutrition in Health and Disease, tenth ed. Lippincott Williams and Wilkins, Baltimore, pp. 741–748.

Keys, A., Brozek, J., Henschel, A., et al., 1950. The Biology of Human Starvation. University of Minnesota Press, Minneapolis.

Kraft, M.D., Btaiche, I.F., Sacks, G.S., 2005. Review of the refeeding syndrome. Nutrition in Clinical Practice 20, 625–633.

Kronfeld, D.S., 1993. Starvation and nutrition of horses: recognition and treatment. Proceedings of the First Conference on Equine Rescue. Santa Barbara, California, USA, 1993. Journal of Equine Veterinary Science 13 (5), 298–303.

Lawrence, L.M., 2008. Updates to the Nutrient Requirements of the Horse: NRC 2007 Guidelines. In: Robinson, N.E., Sprayberry, K.A. (Eds.), Current Therapy in Equine Medicine, sixth ed. Saunders, Philadelphia, pp. 66–72.

Lopes, M.A.F., White II, N.A., 2002. Parenteral nutrition for horses with gastrointestinal disease: a retrospective study of 79 cases. Equine Veterinary Journal 34 (3), 250–257.

Magdesian, G.K., 2003. Nutrition for critical gastrointestinal illness: feeding horses for diarrhoea or colic. The Veterinary Clinics, Equine Practice 19, 617–644.

National Research Council, 2007. Nutrient Requirements of Horses, sixth revised ed. National Academies Press, Washington, DC.

Naylor, M., 1980. Hyperlipemia in horses: Effects of undernutrition and disease. American Journal of Veterinary Research 41 (6), 899–905.

Naylor, J.M., Kenyon, S.J., 1981. Effects of total caloric deprivation on host defence in the horse. Research in Veterinary Science 31, 369–372.

Naylor, J.M., Freeman, D.E., Kronfeld, D., 1984. Alimentation of hypophagic horses. Compendium of Continuing Education 6, 93–99.

Newsholme, E.A., Leech, A.R., 1983. Biochemistry for the Medical Sciences. John Wiley & Sons, Chichester.

Poupard, D.B., 1993. Rehabilitation of horses suffering from malnutrition. Proceedings of the First Conference on Equine Rescue. Santa Barbara, California, USA, 1993. Journal of Equine Veterinary Science. 13 (5), 304–305.

Ralston, S.L., 1984. Controls of feeding in horses. Journal of Animal Science 59, 1354–1361.

Ralston, S.L., 1999. Management of geriatric horses. In: Pagan, J.D., Geor, R.J. (Eds.), Advances in Equine Nutrition, vol. II. Nottingham University Press, Nottingham, UK, pp. 393–396.

Roberts, P.R., Zaloga, G.P., 2000. Enteral nutrition. In: Shoemaker, W.C., Ayres, S.M., Grenvik, A., et al. (Eds.), Textbook of Critical Care, fourth ed. WB Saunders, Philadelphia, pp. 875–898.

Shetty, P.S., 1999. Adaptation to low energy intakes: the responses and limits to low intakes in infants, children and adults. European Journal of Clinical Nutrition 53, S14–S33.

Solomon, S.M., Kirby, D.F., 1990. The refeeding syndrome: A review. Journal of Parenteral and Enteral Nutrition 14, 90–97.

Sticker, L.S., Thompson Jr., D.L., Bunting, L.D., et al., 1995. Feed deprivation of mares: plasma metabolite and hormonal concentrations and responses to exercise. Journal of Animal Science 73, 3696–3704.

Stull, C., 2003. Nutrition for rehabilitating the starved horse. Journal of Equine Veterinary Science 23, 456–459.

Tresley, J., Sheean, P.M., 2008. Refeeding syndrome: recognition is the key to prevention and management. Journal of the American Dietetic Association 108 (12), 2105–2108.

Uhlinger, C.A., 2007. Evidence-based parasitology in horses. Veterinary Clinics, Equine Practice 23, 509–517.

Whiting, T.L., Salmon, R.H., Wruck, G.C., 2005. Chronically starved horses: predicting survival, economic and ethical considerations. Canadian Veterinary Journal 46, 320–324.

Witham, C.L., Stull, C.L., 1998. Metabolic responses of chronically starved horses to refeeding with three, isoenergetic diets. Journal of the American Veterinary Medicine Association 212, 691–696.

30

Hyperlipemia

Andy E. Durham

Hyperlipemia is a life-threatening medical condition seen almost exclusively in pony, donkey and miniature horse breeds. It results from sudden and severe breakdown of body fat stores and nutrition plays a key role in the pathogenesis and treatment of the condition. Intensive therapeutic intervention is an important component in achieving a successful outcome although an overall survival rate of only 56% is reported in six case series published since 1992 (Durham 2006, Hallebeek & Beynen 2001, Mogg & Palmer 1995, Rush-Moore et al 1994, Waitt & Cebra 2009, Watson et al 1992b).

Epidemiology and risk factors

Risk factors for hyperlipemia may be considered in two categories: pre-existing inherent factors that predispose an individual to hyperlipemia; and then precipitating factors that trigger hyperlipemia in predisposed individuals (Table 30-1).

Predisposing factors

Predisposition to hyperlipemia is largely related to insulin resistance (IR) and increased nutritional requirements. Pony, donkey and miniature horse breeds demonstrate a relative insensitivity to insulin that may be further compounded by obesity and a sedentary lifestyle (Jeffcott et al 1986, Reid & Mohammed 1996). IR facilitates mobilization of fat and glycogen stores whenever caloric intake is insufficient (Jeffcott et al 1986, June et al 1992) and thus represents an inherent prolipolytic status that predisposes to hyperlipemia (Breidenbach et al 1999). Mature animals appear predisposed to hyperlipemia (Jeffcott & Field 1985, Reid and Mohammed 1996) perhaps as a result of decreasing insulin sensitivity (Murphy et al 1997) although cases are occasionally encountered in foals and even neonates (Gilbert 1986, Hughes et al 2002, Tan et al 2005). Pregnancy is also associated with IR (Fowden et al 1984) and, moreover, increased nutrient demands that further promote fat mobilization. The latter is also the likely explanation for increased hyperlipemia risk associated with lactation.

Females appear predisposed to hyperlipemia largely due to pregnancy or lactation, although one study found female donkeys to be at twice the risk of males even when not pregnant or lactating (Reid & Mohammed 1996). Examination of data from 135 published cases of hyperlipemia shows 1.5 times as many reproductively inactive females compared with males also supporting that being female is a risk factor independently from pregnancy and lactation (Fig. 30.1). Further unpublished data reveals a significantly higher serum insulin concentration in female than male donkeys supporting IR as a factor in this gender predisposition (N. du Toit, personal communication).

Precipitating factors

Factors known to trigger hyperlipemia in predisposed individuals comprise inadequate feed intake, stress (e.g., feed changes, transportation), pain and disease. The neuroendocrine response to these factors includes increased adrenocorticotrophic hormone, antidiuretic hormone, growth hormone, catecholamines, glucocorticoids and glucagon and suppression of insulin (de Pew et al 1994, Liddell et al 1979, Sticker et al 1995, Stoner 1987). This endocrine milieu favors lipolysis and may trigger hyperlipemia in sick and/or hypophagic subjects.

Primary hyperlipemia occurs in the absence of a precipitating disease process whereas secondary hyperlipemia results from a separate inciting disease, such as enterocolitis, parasitism, colic, and impactions (Mogg & Palmer 1995, Rush-Moore et al 1994, Schotman & Wagenaar 1969, Watson et al 1992b, Waitt & Cebra 2009).

Key Points

- Hyperlipemia is seen mainly in female donkeys, ponies and miniature horses
- Hyperlipemia is closely associated with insulin resistance and factors that result in relative dietary energy deficit

Pathophysiology

Processes controlling fat mobilization

The delivery of fatty acids (FAs) from stored triacylglycerols (TGs) in adipose tissue for oxidation by other cells represents the major energy supply route through the body, especially at times of negative energy balance. This mobilization is achieved by three intercoordinated processes (Fig. 30.2):

1. In adipose tissue: stored TG is hydrolyzed to release free FAs and glycerol into the plasma.

2. In the liver: FAs and glycerol are re-esterified into TGs and exported within very low density lipoprotein particles (VLDLs).
3. In tissues throughout the body (e.g. muscle): TG in VLDLs is hydrolyzed to release FAs which are then absorbed and oxidized as an energy source.

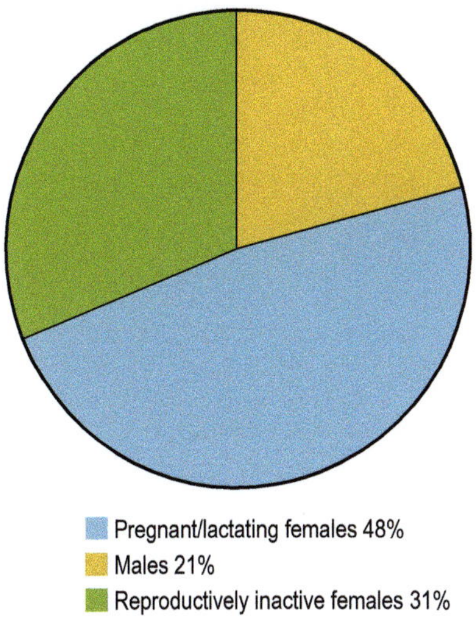

Figure 30.1 Distribution of hyperlipemia cases according to gender and reproductive status. Data derived from 135 published cases (Durham 2006, Gay et al 1978, Jeffcott & Field 1985, Mogg & Palmer 1995, Naylor et al 1980, Oikawa et al 2006, Rush-Moore et al 1994, Waitt et al 2009, Watson et al 1992b).

These three processes are described in further detail below.

Adipose lipolysis

Mechanisms (Fig. 30.2, section 1)

The FAs and glycerol stored in adipose TG are released by the coordinated actions of three enzymes: adipose triglyceride lipase (ATGL), hormone sensitive lipase (HSL), and monoacylglycerol lipase (Vaughan et al 1964, Villena et al 2004, Zechner et al 2009). Following their release, FAs and glycerol may be used for energy by the adipocyte or enter the plasma where they are primarily transported to the liver.

Table 30-1 Factors Associated with Increased Risk of Developing Hyperlipemia

Predisposing factors	Precipitating factors	
	1° hyperlipemia	2° hyperlipemia
Pony/donkey/ miniature horse	Anorexia	Disease
Female	Malnutrition	Pain
Older age	Stressful events	
Pregnancy		
Lactation		
Obesity		
Sedentary lifestyle		

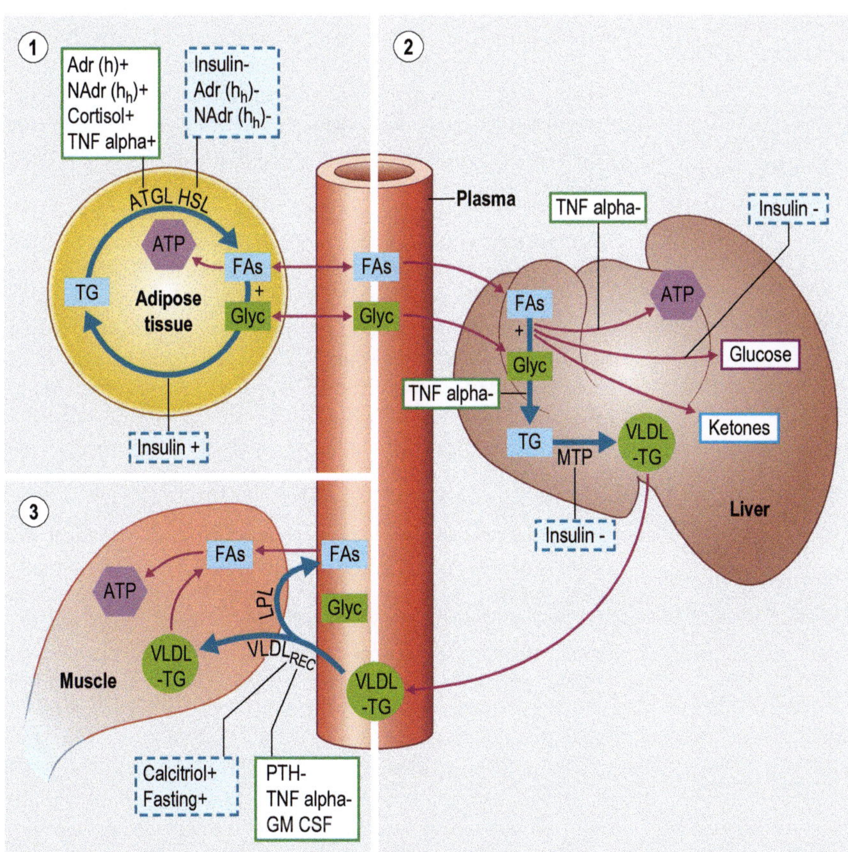

Figure 30.2 Schematic diagram of physiologic and pathophysiologic mechanisms controlling fatty acid and lipid transport. Circled numbers refer to sections in text. ATGL: adipose triglyceride lipase; Glyc = glycerol; HSL = hormone sensitive lipase; LPL = lipoprotein lipase; MTP = microsomal triglyceride transfer protein; $VLDL_{REC}$ = VLDL receptor.

Regulation (Table 30-2a)

ATGL and HSL represent the key, rate-limiting steps in adipose TG hydrolysis and are both closely controlled by the endocrine system. Both ATGL and HSL lipolytic activity is stimulated by catecholamines (beta adrenoreceptors) and inhibited by insulin (Large & Arner 1998). Additional regulatory factors are listed in Table 30-2a (Coppack et al 1994, Large & Arner 1998, Zechner et al 2009). Insulin may further limit FA release from adipose stores by promoting re-esterification of free FAs and glycerol into TG. Regulation of the two enzymes differs slightly in that HSL activity increases during prolonged fasting whereas ATGL is acutely up-regulated following feed withdrawal, probably in response to increased glucocorticoid levels (Villena et al 2004, Zechner et al 2009). Tumor necrosis factor-α (TNF-α) is a potent stimulator of lipolysis during sepsis probably via stimulation of ATGL (Zechner et al 2009).

Hepatic VLDL synthesis and export

Mechanisms (Fig. 30.2, section 2)

Hepatocytes extract most of the circulating FAs and glycerol from the plasma following adipose lipolysis. They may then be oxidized for energy production, used as substrates for gluconeogenesis or ketone synthesis or re-esterified back into TG. Newly synthesized TG is incorporated (along with phospholipids, cholesterol, and apolipoproteins) into VLDL particles enabling transport of hydrophobic lipid in the aqueous plasma medium into which they are secreted.

Regulation (Table 30-2b)

The rate limiting step in hepatic VLDL synthesis is controlled by microsomal triacylglycerol transfer protein (MTP) (Hussain et al 2003). Insulin is a potent inhibitor of MTP and therefore suppresses VLDL synthesis (Kamagate et al 2008). Consistent with this it has been shown that MTP (and therefore hepatic VLDL synthesis) is significantly upregulated during fasting and also in IR states (Bartels et al 2002, Kamagate et al 2008). Increased substrate availability (free FAs and glycerol) following adipose lipolysis induced by fasting is another factor promoting VLDL synthesis (Lewis et al 1995). TNF-α has also been shown to increase hepatic TG synthesis by stimulating FA synthesis by the liver and inhibiting oxidation of FAs thereby increasing substrate for TG synthesis (Chen et al 2009).

Extraction of FAs from plasma VLDL-TG

Mechanisms (Fig. 30.2, section 3)

In peripheral capillary beds (e.g. muscle, fat), VLDL interacts with endothelial lipoprotein lipase (LPL) which releases FAs and glycerol from the TG within. The free FAs enter cells locally to be oxidized as an energy source (or re-esterified in adipose tissue) while most glycerol returns to the liver for further metabolism. An additional mechanism for peripheral VLDL clearance involves the endothelial VLDL receptor which internalizes VLDL particles in their entirety (Takahashi et al 2004).

Regulation (Table 30-2c)

Most LPL exists in adipose tissue and this is stimulated by insulin whereas muscle LPL is upregulated during fasting and exercise (Eckel 1989, Kern 1997, Knapper et al 1995). Heparin and calcitriol both upregulate LPL expression whereas TNF-alpha and parathyroid hormone (PTH) have an inhibitory effect (Chen et al 2009, Querfeld et al 1999, Tornvall et al 1995). It has been suggested in the past that azotemia inhibits LPL in horses although there is no good evidence in support of this (Naylor et al 1980, Vaziri 2009). Regulation of the VLDL receptor appears broadly similar to that of LPL but is also upregulated by thyroid hormones and estradiol and downregulated by granulocyte–macrophage colony-stimulating factor (GM-CSF) (Ishibashi et al 1994, Jokinen et al 1994, Kwok et al 1997, Masuzaki et al 1994).

Key Points

- The flux of FAs and glycerol from adipose stores, via the liver to peripheral tissues, is a key energy supply route and comprises several highly regulated, balanced, interdependent and coordinated enzymatic processes
- FAs and glycerol are released into the plasma from TGs stored in adipose tissue
- Plasma FAs and glycerol are re-esterified back to TG by the liver and secreted into the plasma within VLDL particles
- The TG within plasma VLDL particles is hydrolyzed back to FAs and glycerol in peripheral tissues for use as an energy source

Pathophysiology of hyperlipemia

Hyperlipemia inevitably follows when adipose lipolysis (ATGL- and HSL-dependent) and consequent hepatic VLDL synthesis (MTP- and substrate-dependent) exceeds the rate of clearance of plasma VLDL (LPL- and VLDL receptor-dependent). Risk factors for hyperlipemia (Table 30-1) are likely to be associated with conditions including IR, negative energy balance, increased sympathetic and adrenocortical activity and systemic inflammation. Under such conditions it would be expected that adipose lipolysis and hepatic VLDL synthesis would be increased (Table 30-2a,b, Fig. 30.2). Anorexia increases VLDL clearance by muscle (but not fat), although this process could be antagonized by inflammatory cytokines (Fig. 30.2, Table 30-2c). In a study of hyperlipemic ponies, Watson et al (1992a) found increases in the rates of all three key processes: adipose lipolysis, hepatic VLDL synthesis, *and* VLDL clearance. However, the majority of the cases studied were primary hyperlipemia and it is possible that effects on VLDL clearance could be different in hyperlipemia secondary to inflammatory diseases due to the inhibitory effects of cytokines (TNF-α and GM-CSF) on LPL and the VLDL receptor (Table 30-2c).

In addition to excessive plasma lipid, tissues may also become saturated with fatty infiltration. Amongst these, the liver appears especially prone to lipidosis. As described above, the liver is a key conduit and site for lipid metabolism, extracting and processing adipose tissue-derived free fatty acids and glycerol from the hepatic arterial supply (during fasting) as well as lipid-rich chylomicrons from the hepatic portal venous supply following absorption and synthesis by the intestine (postprandially). The liver's capacity for extraction and synthesis of lipid may outweigh the rate of VLDL secretion leading to hepatic lipidosis and progressive impairment of liver functions.

Table 30-2

(a) Factors Positively and Negatively Influencing Adipose Lipolysis Via Actions on the Lipolytic Enzymes Adipose Triglyceride Lipase (ATGL) and Hormone Sensitive Lipase (HSL)

Stimulate adipose lipolysis (+ATGL,HSL)	Inhibit adipose lipolysis (-ATGL,HSL)
Adrenocorticotropin	Adenosine (A1 receptor)
α-melanocyte stimulating hormone	Catecholamines (alpha$_2$ ARs)
Catecholamines (beta ARs)	Fatty acids
Cholecystokinin	Insulin
Glucagon	Insulin-like growth factor-1
Glucocorticoids	Ketones
Growth hormone	Monoacylglycerols
Parathyroid hormone	Neuropeptide Y (NPY-1 receptor)
Thyrotropin	Nicotinic acid (GPR109A receptor)
Thyroxine	Peptide YY
Tri-iodothyronine	Somatostatin
Tumor necrosis factor-α	

(b) Factors Positively and Negatively Influencing VLDL Synthesis Via Actions on the Hepatic Enzyme Microsomal Triacylglycerol Transfer Protein (MTP)

Stimulate VLDL synthesis (+MTP)	Inhibit VLDL synthesis (-MTP)
Fasting	Insulin
Fatty acids Glycerol	
Insulin resistance	
Tumour necrosis factor-alpha	

(c) Factors Positively and Negatively Influencing VLDL Clearance from the Plasma Via Actions on Endothelial Lipoprotein Lipase (LPL) and VLDL Receptor

Inhibit VLDL clearance (-LPL, VLDL receptor)	Stimulate VLDL clearance (+LPL, VLDL receptor)
Granulocyte–macrophage colony-stimulating factor	Calcitriol
Parathyroid hormone	Exercise (muscle)
Tumor necrosis factor-alpha	Fasting (muscle) Heparin
	Heparin
	Insulin (adipose tissue) Oestradiol
	Estradiol
	Thyroxine
	Tri-iodothryronine

Key Point

- Hyperlipemia results from dysregulation of fatty acid transport mechanisms such that hepatic VLDL synthesis exceeds the capacity for tissue uptake of plasma VLDL

Clinical signs

Many differing clinical signs occur with hyperlipemia (Box 30.1) but inappetance, dullness, depression and weakness are almost invariable. Any clinical signs present might reflect a cause and/or effect of hyperlipemia and this represents a significant diagnostic challenge. When clinical signs result from hyperlipemia per se, they are probably a result of poor peripheral perfusion and fatty infiltration of tissues and organs that may result in multiorgan dysfunction, most frequently affecting the liver and kidneys.

Diagnosis

Blood analysis

Dyslipidemia In hyperlipemia it is expected fundamentally that there will be increased serum concentrations of free FAs, glycerol and VLDL (Fig. 30.2), and therefore increased TGs and cholesterol (contained within VLDLs). Serum or plasma TG concentrations increase many fold higher than the other indicators above and are therefore the analytes of choice in cases of suspected hyperlipemia (Oikawa et al 2006, Naylor et al 1980, Watson et al 1992a). The clinicopathologic definition of hyperlipemia is opaque plasma or serum (Fig. 30.3) with TG concentration >5.6 mmol/l (500 mg/dl). Most clinical cases will have serum or plasma TG concentrations between 6 and 35 mmol/l (530–3100 mg/dl) although values >50 mmol/l (4400 mg/dl) are sometimes seen (Watson et al 1992b). Although two studies of hyperlipemia found an association between TG concentration and failure to survive (Mogg & Palmer 1995, Hallebeek & Beynen 2001), others have not (Durham 2006, Rush-Moore et al 1994, Waitt & Cebra 2009, Watson et al 1992b).

Interestingly sick anorexic horses and healthy donkeys and ponies may sometimes have plasma TG >5.6 mmol/l

Box 30.1 Clinical Signs Seen in Subjects with Hyperlipemia

- Anorexia, adipsia
- Dysphagia
- Colic
- Muscle tremors
- Jaundice
- Pyrexia
- Encephalopathy (depression, circling, head-pressing, nystagmus, convulsions, coma)
- Dull, depressed, weak
- Ataxia
- Reduced fecal output
- Diarrhea
- Ascites
- Abortion
- Rapid weight loss

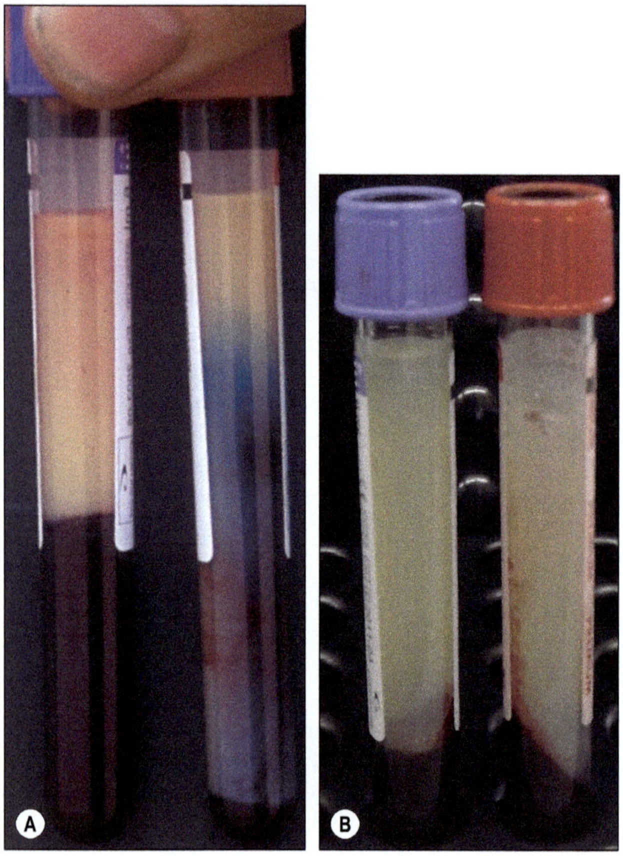

Figure 30.3 Lipemic plasma and serum.

Table 30-3 Common Clinical Problems in Hyperlipemia and Suggested Clinicopathologic Tests

Clinical problem	Clinicopathologic findings
Dehydration	Polycythemia, increased albumin, creatinine, urea, lactate
Anorexia	Increased bilirubin, bile acids, hypokalemia, hypocalcemia
Stress	Neutrophilia, lymphopenia, hypercortisolemia
Insulin resistance	Hyperinsulinemia, hyperglycemia
Hepatic disease/ insufficiency	Increased liver enzymes (e.g., GGT), bile acids, NH_3, hypoglycemia
Renal insufficiency	Azotemia, enzymuria, isosthenuria
Myopathy	Increased CK
Inflammation	Neutrophilia, hyperfibrinogenemia, high SAA

(>500 mg/dl) but maintain translucency of the plasma and without obvious adverse effects of the hypertriglyceridemia (Dunkel & McKenzie 2003, N. du Toit, personal communication).

Further clinical chemistry and hematology A suggested panel of further hematologic and clinical chemistry tests appropriate to common clinical problems associated with hyperlipemia is listed in Table 30-3.

Further diagnostic techniques

Further investigations may be considered in the light of clinical and clinicopathological findings. In cases with increased liver enzymes then ultrasound might indicate hepatomegaly and increased echogenicity associated with hepatic lipidosis although these findings do not rule out a primary hepatopathy. Liver biopsy might be hazardous in an enlarged fatty liver due to the risk of rupture. Further diagnostic considerations based on relative likelihood of identifying primary triggering factors include abdominal ultrasound/radiography and peritoneal fluid and fecal analysis.

Key Points

- Hyperlipemia is defined by opaque serum or plasma with TG concentrations >5.6 mmol/l (>500 mg/dl)
- Most cases of hyperlipemia will have several other abnormal clinicopathologic findings, especially those indicating hepatorenal dysfunction, that might reflect a cause and/or effect of hyperlipemia

Treatment

There are three fundamentally important aspects of therapy in cases of hyperlipemia:

1. Treatment of any identifiable precipitating factors.
2. Treatment of problems resulting from hyperlipemia.
3. Reduction of plasma VLDL.

Treatment of precipitating factors (Table 30-1)

In pregnant mares the induction of parturition might be considered but this may be difficult to achieve safely and could be counterproductive if complications arise. If lactation persists then weaning is wise, although it might become a significant stressor if the mare and foal are physically separated.

The prognosis in cases of secondary hyperlipemia depends heavily on identification and treatment of the primary disease. Investigation and treatment of common predisposing diseases such as dental disease, parasitism, enterocolitis, colon impactions, and bacterial infections is important. Suggested therapeutic products relevant to secondary hyperlipemia are listed in Table 30-4. Use of glucocorticoids might be contemplated for treatment of some conditions (e.g., cyathostominosis, purpura hemorrhagica) although this is controversial. Glucocorticoids promote IR and stimulate lipolysis (Table 30-2, Fig. 30.2) and are therefore generally regarded as contraindicated in hyperlipemia (Watson & Love 1994). However, one study did not find any hypertriglyceridemic effect of glucocorticoids when administered to ponies from which feed was withheld (Freestone et al 1991). Anecdotally, this author's experience of glucocorticoid administration in hyperlipemia cases with primary inflammatory or immune-mediated disease has not given the impression of significant untoward effects although further investigation of their use is required.

Treatment of secondary clinical problems

The main secondary complications of hyperlipemia include hypovolemia, electrolyte imbalances and hepatorenal insufficiency.

Table 30-4 Suggested Empirical Therapeutic Approach to Manage Common Disease Processes Associated with Hyperlipemia

Suspected clinical problems	Suggested product	Suggested dose
Enterocolitis	Di-tri-octahedral smectite	1 g/kg po q 6–12 h
Colon impaction	Mineral oil Nasogastric fluids	0.5–1 l/100 kg by NGT 5 ml/kg/h by indwelling NGT
Parasitism	Moxidectin	0.4 mg/kg PO
Bacterial sepsis	Ceftiofur sodium	2 mg/kg IM q 12 h
Pain	Meloxicam Flunixin	0.6 mg/kg PO/iv q 24 h 1.1 mg/kg PO/IV q 24 h
Gastric ulceration	Omeprazole	2 mg/kg PO q 24 h

Fluid therapy

Intravenous fluid therapy is often indicated to restore fluid, acid–base and electrolyte balance. Intermittent nasogastric intubation or indwelling nasoesophageal tubes[1] may be preferable in gastrointestinal impactions (Lopes 2003) although could be more stressful. It is helpful if efforts are made to warm administered fluids as energy used to warm cold fluids can deplete the recipient of as much as 10% of their caloric requirements. Fluid rates should be calculated to replace pre-existing deficits (most likely 5 to 10% bodyweight) over approximately 6 hours in addition to maintenance requirements (approximately 2 ml/kg/h) plus any ongoing losses if present.

Electrolytes

Sodium and chloride are likely to be plentiful in IV fluids and rarely require further supplementation. Potassium deficits are common in anorexia and can be supplemented in IV fluids by adding 20 mmol/l potassium (= 10 ml/l 15% potassium chloride). Increased amounts can be given where required subject to a maximum infusion rate of 0.5 mmol potassium/kg/hour. Given the lipemic effects of PTH (Table 30-2, Fig. 30.2), restoration of calcium concentrations may be important in hypocalcemic subjects and IV fluids can be supplemented with 10 mmol/l calcium (15 ml/l 40% or 25 ml/l 23% calcium borogluconate). If there are clinical signs of hypocalcemia then increased amounts can be added safely.

Frusemide

Azotemia is common in hyperlipemia, usually a result of hypovolemia although renal failure can be a consequence of dehydration and also lipidosis may compromise renal function further. Azotemia usually improves in response to fluid therapy which should be associated with diuresis. However, if regular urination is not observed then frusemide (1–4 mg/kg IV q 2 hours) should be administered to stimulate diuresis and protect renal function.

Glucose

Markedly depressed subjects with hypoglycemia should be given 10–20 ml IV boluses of 50% glucose to effect, followed by appropriate nutritional support (see below).

Hepatic encephalopathy (HE)

HE should be suspected (along with hypoglycemia) when marked depression and/or neurologic signs are seen and can be treated with orally administered lactulose (0.3 ml/kg q 4–12 hours). Hypertonic 7.2% saline boluses (e.g. 1–2 liters) can be very effective at reducing cerebral edema caused by acute HE but should be used with caution in dehydrated subjects.

Reduction of plasma VLDL

Plasma VLDL is most effectively reduced by restraining further lipolysis and hepatic VLDL synthesis. This can be achieved by providing adequate caloric intake and also possibly by pharmacologic interventions. Stimulating increased VLDL uptake is a further possible benefit of drug therapy.

Nutritional supplementation

Inadequate caloric intake must be addressed in all cases of hyperlipemia. The energy and protein requirements of stabled, sick equids is not known but has been estimated to be approximately 4 kJ/kg/h (1 kcal/kg/h) and 40 mg/kg/h respectively (Durham et al 2004). In this author's experience, good clinical responses can be obtained when nutrition is administered to non-pregnant hyperlipemia cases at rates as low as 2.5 to 3.0 kJ/kg/h (0.6–0.7 kcal/kg/h) (Table 30-5) although some have advocated far higher rates (Golenz et al 1992, Rush-Moore et al 1994). The final trimester of pregnancy may be associated with a 10 to 20% increase in energy requirements (NRC 2007) and this will need to be taken into account in pregnant mares.

Enteral nutrition

Enteral nutrition may be preferred due to low cost and physiologic benefits. Fresh palatable feeds (e.g., grass, carrots, apples, sweet feeds) should always be offered to hyperlipemic subjects. Liquidized gruels of complete pelleted feeds, alfalfa meal or milled oats[2] (Mogg & Palmer 1995, Stratton-Phelps 2004) are theoretically attractive but the practical difficulties of administering adequate quantities to an unwilling recipient limit their usefulness as a sole source of nutritional support. Stabling with an appetent companion might serve as a stimulus to eat (Houpt 1990).

Sugar solutions are easier to administer by mouth or tube although the administration procedure is not without stress. Sugars, such as glucose, galactose and sucrose, typically yield 16 kJ/g (3.8 kcal/g) and therefore 4 to 6 g/kg/day would be required to achieve acceptable energy targets (Table 30-5). This could be administered as 1 g/kg aliquots every 4 to 6 hours but is likely to lead to hyperglycemia. The

[1]Veterinary Enteral Feeding Tube, Mila International Inc., Erlanger Kentucky.

[2]Readibrek, Weetabix Food Company, Kettering, Northamptonshire. Contains 1.5 MJ/kg and 117 g protein/kg.

Table 30-5 Suggested Target Rates for Nutritional Supply of Energy and Protein to Sick, Confined, Nonpregnant, Nonlactating Ponies and Donkeys (Enteral and/or Parenteral)

Bodyweight (kg)	Energy		Protein (g/h)
	kJ/h	kcal/h	
100	250–400	60–100	3–4
150	375–600	90–150	4–6
200	500–800	120–200	6–8
250	625–1,000	150–250	7–10
300	750–1,200	180–300	9–12
350	875–1,400	210–350	10–14
400	1,000–1,600	240–400	12–16

Figures equate to 2.5 to 4.0 kJ/kg/h and 30–40 mg protein/kg/h.

tolerable limit of oral glucose administration is likely to be no more than 3 g/kg/day in most cases of hyperlipemia which is significantly less than estimated requirements.

Liquid diets made for humans could provide higher caloric intakes although high fat content and adverse gastrointestinal effects makes many of them unattractive (Golenz et al 1992, Rush-Moore et al 1994, Stratton-Phelps 2004). Carbohydrate- and protein-rich, low-fat liquid diets are preferable and the use of one such product comprising 12.5% casein and 83% glucose was described by Hallebeek & Beynen (2001) and provided 3.75 kJ/kg/h energy and 33 mg/kg/h protein. This author has used a mixture of 75% glucose and 25% "Casilan 90"[3], administered at 3 to 6 g/kg final mixture per 24 hours in divided doses and the rate adjusted if hyperglycemia progresses. This rate would contribute between 2 and 4 kJ/kg/h energy and 33–55 mg/kg/h protein.

Parenteral nutrition

Administration of lipid-free parenteral nutrition (PN) has proved very effective in promptly normalizing plasma TGs in hyperlipemic subjects (Durham 2006, Rush-Moore et al 1994). The greatest advantage of this technique is that it can be performed with minimal disturbance of the patient. Issues of cost are mitigated by the invariably small size of hyperlipemic subjects and the omission of expensive lipid-emulsion from the PN formula. Parenteral and enteral nutrition are not mutually exclusive alternatives and reasonable efforts should nevertheless be pursued to encourage oral feeding of patients receiving PN.

Some reports describe simple IV dextrose solutions (Mogg & Palmer 1995, Oikawa et al 2006) although glucose and amino-acid mixtures may allow greater caloric supply whilst limiting hyperglycemia (Durham 2006, Rush-Moore et al 1994). This author uses a 50:50 mixture of 50% glucose[4] and 15% amino acid[5]. When administered IV at a typically tolerable rate of 0.5 ml/kg/h, this combined solution provides 2.6 kJ/kg/h energy and 37 mg/kg/h amino acid and invariably leads to a marked decrease in plasma TGs within 6 to 12 hours (Durham 2006). Failure to observe an associated clinical response often indicates that an underlying disease process has not been addressed effectively. Plasma glucose should be measured q 1–4 hours and the rate adjusted (up or down) aiming to maintain plasma glucose between 5–10 mmol/l. Contemporaneous insulin therapy can be used to help limit hyperglycemia and allow greater supply rates of PN (see below).

[3]Casilan 90, Heinz HJ Co Ltd, Hayes, Middlesex. Comprises 88.5% protein, 1% fat and 0.3% carbohydrate and yields 15.5 kJ/g.

[4]Glucose 50%, Fresenius Kabi, Milton Keynes, Northamptonshire. Contains 7.9 kJ/ml.

[5]Aminoven 25, Fresenius Kabi, Milton Keynes, Northamptonshire. Contains 2.5 kJ/ml.

Insulin

Insulin therapy can be used to treat hyperlipemia (Waitt & Cebra 2009) although it is controversial. IR may resist its effects and concerns also exist about inducing hypoglycemia or adverse effects (especially laminitis) with high levels of insulin infusion (0.36 IU/kg/h, Asplin et al 2007). A constant enteral and/or parenteral supply of glucose should always accompany insulin therapy.

Insulin is theoretically helpful for the following reasons:

- Reduction of plasma VLDL (Table 30-2, Fig. 30.2):
  - Suppression of lipolytic hormones (ATGL and HSL)
  - Stimulation of lipogenesis in adipose tissue
  - Suppression of hepatic VLDL synthesis (MTP)
  - Stimulation of VLDL uptake (adipose LPL and VLDL receptors)
- Antihyperglycemic effects enabling higher administration rates of enteral or parenteral nutrition:
  - Stimulation of peripheral glucose disposal
  - Inhibition of hepatic gluconeogenesis.

This author's practice is to commence insulin therapy only when the PN protocol described above leads to plasma glucose concentrations >10 mmol/l. Intravenous infusion of soluble insulin is most effective although requires frequent glucose monitoring. Infusion rates beginning at 0.05 IU/kg/h may be commenced with increases in increments of 0.05 IU/kg/h instituted q 2 hours in cases of persistent hyperglycemia. Alternatively, IM or IV boluses of soluble insulin (e.g., 0.2 IU/kg q 1–6 hours) or longer-acting insulin suspensions (protamine zinc or lente, 0.10 to 0.40 IU/kg q 12–24 hours) can be used.

Heparin

Heparin treatment has been advocated on the basis that it increases LPL activity (Tornvall et al 1995), although experimental evidence suggests that LPL activity may already be maximal in (primary) hyperlipemia (Watson et al 1992a). Theoretically, heparin might be more useful in secondary hyperlipemia cases where there is a greater likelihood of reduced VLDL clearance due to the effects of inflammatory cytokines (Table 30-2c). Doses between 40–250 IU/kg q 6–12 hours have been described.

Further pharmacologic considerations

Dyslipidemia associated with chronic insulin resistance is an important medical problem in humans and is treated with products including statins, fibrates, nicotinic acids, and the insulin sensitizing drugs metformin and thiazolidinediones (Aronoff et al 2000, Backes et al 2005, DeFronzo & Goodman 1995). Many of these products can be associated with adverse effects in people and have not yet been investigated in hyperlipemic horses.

Trilostane, metyrapone and aminoglutethimide inhibit cortisol biosynthesis and have been used for treatment of equine pituitary pars intermedia dysfunction (Durham 2010). They might be indicated if hypercortisolemia is present and serving as a stimulus of lipolysis (Fig. 30.2) although their use in hyperlipemia has not been investigated.

It has been suggested that sedation stimulates food consumption in horses (Houpt 1990). Furthermore, alpha-2 adrenoceptor agonists exert a prompt and potent antilipolytic effect in horses (Fig. 30.2) (Carroll et al 1997, van Dijk et al 2003). Infusion of alpha-2 adrenoceptor agonists merits further study in hyperlipemic subjects although the additional effects of suppression of insulin secretion and stimulating hyperglycemia could be problematic in the management of some cases.

Key Points

- After addressing potential trigger factors and secondary complications, the most important aspect of hyperlipemia management is to increase caloric supply by enteral and/or parenteral routes
- Several drugs including insulin and heparin have potential usefulness to further aid reduction in plasma TGs

Conclusions

Hyperlipemia is a serious metabolic disorder of ponies, donkeys, and miniature horses invariably associated with absolute or relative undersupply of dietary energy. Pregnant and lactating mares are especially predisposed but many underlying disease processes may trigger the condition. Hyperlipemia is acutely life-threatening but can frequently be managed successfully with various nutritional interventions as long as untreatable underlying disease does not exist.

References

Aronoff, S., Rosenblatt, S., Braithwaite, S., et al., 2000. Pioglitazone hydrochloride monotherapy improves glycemic control in the treatment of patients with type 2 diabetes: a 6-month randomized placebo-controlled dose response study. The Pioglitazone 001 Study Group. Diabetes Care 23 (11), 1605–1611.

Asplin, K.E., Sillence, M.N., Pollitt, C.C., et al., 2007. Induction of laminitis by prolonged hyperinsulinaemia in clinically normal ponies. Veterinary Journal 174 (3), 530–535.

Backes, J.M., Gibson, C.A., Howard, P.A., 2005. Optimal lipid modification: the rationale for combination therapy. Vascular Health and Risk Management 1 (4), 317–331.

Bartels, E.D., Lauritsen, M., Nielsen, L.B., 2002. Hepatic expression of microsomal triglyceride transfer protein and in vivo secretion of triglyceride-rich lipoproteins are increased in obese diabetic mice. Diabetes 51 (4), 1233–1239.

Breidenbach, A., Fuhrmann, H., Deegen, E., et al., 1999. Studies on equine lipid metabolism. 2. Lipolytic activities of plasma and tissue lipases in large horses and ponies. Zentralblatt fur Veterinarmedizin A 46 (1), 39–48.

Carroll, G.L., Matthews, N.S., Hartsfield, S.M., et al., 1997. The effect of detomidine and its antagonism with tolazoline on stress-related hormones, metabolites, physiologic responses, and behavior in awake ponies. Veterinary Surgery 26 (1), 69–77.

Chen, X., Xun, K., Chen, L., Wang, Y., 2009. TNF-alpha, a potent lipid metabolism regulator. Cell Biochemistry and Function 27 (7), 407–416.

Coppack, S.W., Jensen, M.D., Miles, J.M., 1994. In vivo regulation of lipolysis in humans. Journal of Lipid Research 35 (2), 177–193.

DeFronzo, R.A., Goodman, A.M., 1995. Efficacy of metformin in patients with noninsulin-dependent diabetes mellitus. The Multicenter Metformin Study Group. New England Journal of Medicine 333 (9), 541–549.

De Pew, C.L., Thompson, D.L. Jr, Fernandez, J.M., et al., 1994. Changes in concentrations of hormones, metabolites, and amino acids in plasma of adult horses relative to overnight feed deprivation followed by a pellet-hay meal fed at noon. Journal of Animal Science 72 (6), 1530–1539.

Dunkel, B., McKenzie, H.C., 2003. Severe hypertriglyceridaemia in clinically ill horses: diagnosis, treatment and outcome. Equine Veterinary Journal 35 (6), 590–595.

Durham, A.E., 2006. Clinical application of parenteral nutrition in the treatment of five ponies and one donkey with hyperlipaemia. Veterinary Record 158 (5), 159–164.

Durham, A.E., 2010. The pharmacological basis for the treatment of endocrinopathic laminitis. Veterinary Clinics of North America Equine Practice 26 (2), 303–314.

Durham, A.E., Phillips, T.J., Walmsley, J.P., et al., 2004. Nutritional and clinicopathological effects of post operative parenteral nutrition following small intestinal resection and anastomosis in the mature horse. Equine Veterinary Journal 36 (5), 390–396.

Eckel, R.H., 1989. Lipoprotein lipase. A multifunctional enzyme relevant to common metabolic diseases. New England Journal of Medicine 320 (16), 1060–1068.

Fowden, A.L., Comline, R.S., Silver, M., 1984. Insulin secretion and carbohydrate metabolism during pregnancy in the mare. Equine Veterinary Journal 16 (4), 239–246.

Freestone, J.F., Wolfsheimer, K.J., Ford, R.B., et al., 1991. Triglyceride, insulin, and cortisol responses of ponies to fasting and dexamethasone administration. Journal of Veterinary Internal Medicine 5 (1), 15–22.

Gay, C.C., Sullivan, N.D., Wilkinson, J.S., et al., 1978. Hyperlipaemia in ponies. Australian Veterinary Journal 54 (10), 459–462.

Gilbert, R.O., 1986. Congenital hyperlipaemia in a Shetland pony foal. Equine Veterinary Journal 18 (6), 498–500.

Golenz, M.R., Knight, D.A., Yvorchuk-St Jean, K.E., 1992. Use of a human enteral feeding preparation for treatment of hyperlipemia and nutritional support during healing of an esophageal laceration in a miniature horse. Journal of the American Veterinary Medical Association 200 (7), 951–953.

Hallebeek, J.M., Beynen, A.C., 2001. A preliminary report on a fat-free diet formula for nasogastric enteral administration as treatment for hyperlipaemia in ponies. Veterinary Quarterly 23 (4), 201–205.

Houpt, K.A., 1990. Ingestive behaviour. Veterinary Clinics of North America Equine Practice 6 (2), 319–337.

Hughes, K.J., Hodgson, D.R., Dart, A.J., 2002. Hyperlipaemia in a 7-week-old miniature pony foal. Australian Veterinary Journal 80 (6), 350–351.

Hussain, M.M., Iqbal, J., Anwar, K., et al., 2003. Microsomal triglyceride transfer protein: a multifunctional protein. Frontiers in Bioscience 8, s500–s506.

Ishibashi, T., Yokoyama, K., Shindo, J., et al., 1994. Potent cholesterol-lowering effect by human granulocyte-macrophage colony-stimulating factor in rabbits. Possible implications of enhancement of macrophage functions and an increase in mRNA for VLDL receptor. Arteriosclerosis, Thrombosis and Vascular Biology 14 (10), 1534–1541.

Jeffcott, L.B., Field, J.R., 1985. Epidemiological aspects of hyperlipaemia in ponies in south eastern Australia. Australian Veterinary Journal 62 (4), 140–141.

Jeffcott, L.B., Field, J.R., McLean, J.G., et al., 1986. Glucose tolerance and insulin sensitivity in ponies and Standardbred horses. Equine Veterinary Journal 18 (2), 97–101.

Jokinen, E.V., Landschulz, K.T., Wyne, K.L., et al., 1994. Regulation of the very low density lipoprotein receptor by thyroid hormone in rat skeletal muscle. Journal of Biological Chemistry 269 (42), 26411–26418.

June, V., Soderholm, V., Hintz, H.F., et al., 1992. Glucose tolerance in the horse, pony and donkey. Journal of Equine Veterinary Science 12 (2), 103–105.

Kamagate, A., Qu, S., Perdomo, G., et al., 2008. FoxO1 mediates insulin-dependent regulation of hepatic VLDL production in mice. Journal of Clinical Investigation 118 (6), 2347–2364.

Kern, P.A., 1997. Potential role of TNFalpha and lipoprotein lipase as candidate genes for obesity. The Journal of Nutrition 127 (9), 1917S–1922S.

Knapper, J.M., Puddicombe, S.M., Morgan, L.M., et al., 1995. Investigations into the actions of glucose-dependent insulinotropic polypeptide and glucagon-like peptide-1(7–36)amide on lipoprotein lipase activity in explants of rat adipose tissue. Journal of Nutrition 125 (2), 183–188.

Kwok, S., Singh-Bist, A., Natu, V., et al., 1997. Dietary regulation of the very low density lipoprotein receptor in mouse heart and fat. Hormone and Metabolic Research 29 (10), 524–529.

Large, V., Arner, P., 1998. Regulation of lipolysis in humans. Pathophysiological modulation in obesity, diabetes, and hyperlipidaemia. Diabetes and Metabolism 24 (5), 409–418.

Lewis, G.F., Uffelman, K.D., Szeto, L.W., et al., 1995. Interaction between free fatty acids and insulin in the acute control of very low density lipoprotein production in humans. Journal of Clinical Investigation 95 (1), 158–166.

Liddell, M.J., Daniel, A.M., MacLean, L.D., et al., 1979. The role of stress hormones in the catabolic metabolism of shock. Surgical Gynecology and Obstetrics 149 (6), 822–830.

Lopes, M.A.F., 2003. Administration of enteral fluid therapy: methods, composition of fluids and complications. Equine Veterinary Education 15 (2), 107–112.

Masuzaki, H., Jingami, H., Yamamoto, T., et al., 1994. Effects of estradiol on very low density lipoprotein receptor mRNA levels in rabbit heart. FEBS Letters 347 (2–3), 211–214.

Mogg, T.D., Palmer, J.E., 1995. Hyperlipidemia, hyperlipemia, and hepatic lipidosis in American miniature horses: 23 cases (1990–1994). Journal of the American Veterinary Medical Association 207 (5), 604–607.

Murphy, D., Reid, S.W.J., Love, S., 1997. The effect of age and diet on the oral glucose tolerance test in ponies. Equine Veterinary Journal 29 (6), 467–470.

National Research Council., 2007. Energy. In: Nutritional requirements of horses, sixth ed. The National Academies Press, Washington DC, pp. 3–33.

Naylor, J.M., Kronfeld, D.S., Acland, H., 1980. Hyperlipemia in horses: effects of undernutrition and disease. American Journal of Veterinary Research 41 (6), 899–905.

Oikawa, S., McGuirk, S., Nishibe, K., et al., 2006. Changes of blood biochemical values in ponies recovering from hyperlipemia in Japan. Journal of Veterinary Medical Science 68 (4), 353–359.

Querfeld, U., Hoffmann, M.M., Klaus, G., et al., 1999. Antagonistic effects of vitamin D and parathyroid hormone on lipoprotein lipase in cultured adipocytes. Journal of the American Society of Nephrology 10 (10), 2158–2164.

Reid, S.W., Mohammed, H.O., 1996. Survival analysis approach to risk factors associated with hyperlipemia in donkeys. Journal of the American Veterinary Medical Association 209 (8), 1449–1452.

Rush-Moore, B., Abood, S.K., Hinchcliff, K.W., 1994. Hyperlipemia in 9 miniature horses and miniature donkeys. Journal of Veterinary Internal Medicine 8 (5), 376–381.

Schotman, A.J., Wagenaar, G., 1969. Hyperlipemia in ponies. Zentralblatt fur Veterinarmedizin A 16 (1), 1–7.

Sticker, L.S., Thompson, D.L., Bunting, L.D., et al., 1995. Feed deprivation of mares: plasma metabolite and hormonal concentrations and responses to exercise. Journal of Animal Science 73 (12), 3696–3704.

Stoner, H.B., 1987. Interpretation of the metabolic effects of trauma and sepsis. Journal of Clinical Patholology 40 (9), 1108–1117.

Stratton-Phelps, M., 2004. Assisted enteral feeding in adult horses. Compendium on Continuing Education for the Practicing Veterinarian 26 (1), 46–49.

Takahashi, S., Sakai, J., Fujino, T., et al., 2004. The very low-density lipoprotein (VLDL) receptor: characterization and functions as a peripheral lipoprotein receptor. Journal of Atherosclerosis and Thrombosis 11 (4), 200–208.

Tan, R.H., Hughes, K.J., Hodgson, D.R., 2005. Hyperlipaemia, neonatal isoerythrolysis and hepatocellular necrosis in a 3-day-old Thoroughbred foal. Australian Veterinary Journal 83 (12), 740–741.

Tornvall, P., Olivecrona, G., Karpe, F., et al., 1995. Lipoprotein lipase mass and activity in plasma and their increase after heparin are separate parameters with different relations to plasma lipoproteins. Arteriosclerosis, Thrombosis and Vascular Biology 15 (8), 1086–1093.

van Dijk, P., Lankveld, D.P., Rijkenhuizen, A.B., et al., 2003. Hormonal, metabolic and physiological effects of laparoscopic surgery using a detomidine-buprenorphine combination in standing horses. Veterinary Anaesthesia and Analgesia 30 (2), 72–80.

Vaughan, M., Berger, J.E., Steinberg, D., 1964. Hormone-sensitive lipase and monoglyceride lipase activities in adipose tissue. Journal of Biological Chemistry 239, 401–409.

Vaziri, N.D., 2009. Causes of dysregulation of lipid metabolism in chronic renal failure. Seminars in Dialysis 22 (6), 644–651.

Villena, J.A., Roy, S., Sarkadi-Nagy, E., et al., 2004. Desnutrin, an adipocyte gene encoding a novel patatin domain-containing protein, is induced by fasting and glucocorticoids: ectopic expression of desnutrin increases triglyceride hydrolysis. Journal of Biological Chemistry 279 (45), 47066–47075.

Waitt, L.H., Cebra, C.K., 2009. Characterization of hypertriglyceridemia and response to treatment with insulin in horses, ponies, and donkeys: 44 cases (1995–2005). Journal of the American Veterinary Medical Association 234 (7), 915–919.

Watson, T.D.G., Love, S., 1994. Equine hyperlipidemia. Compendium on Continuing Education for the Practicing Veterinarian 16 (1), 89–97.

Watson, T.D., Burns, L., Love, S., et al, 1992a. Plasma lipids, lipoproteins and post-heparin lipases in ponies with hyperlipaemia. Equine Veterinary Journal 24 (5), 341–346.

Watson, T.D., Murphy, D., Love, S., 1992b. Equine hyperlipaemia in the United Kingdom: clinical features and blood biochemistry of 18 cases. Veterinary Record 131 (3), 48–51.

Zechner, R., Kienesberger, P.C., Haemmerle, G., et al., 2009. Adipose triglyceride lipase and the lipolytic catabolism of cellular fat stores. Journal of Lipid Research 50 (1), 3–21.

31

Exercise-associated muscle disorders

Patricia A. Harris, José Luis L. Rivero

Muscular disorders unfortunately are not uncommon in the exercising horse, or one that has completed an exercise bout in the last 24 hours or so. These conditions may be associated with a traumatic incidence or the exercise itself. The development of acute muscle pain following exercise, for example, can occur in horses performing strenuous exercise beyond their training adaptation, or as a consequence of repetitive motion injuries (including overtraining/over-use). A training imbalance therefore should be suspected if there is a history of an increase in work intensity without appropriate training, too quick/early return to work following a period of rest, over-training or overload, etc. Such muscular disorders are not commonly associated with a nutritional imbalance and although an appropriate training plus dietary regimen are important in their management they will not be discussed in any further detail in this chapter. Similarly although muscular stiffness and a reluctance to move can be associated with the exhausted horse syndrome this condition will not be discussed in any detail neither will muscle pain or myalgia potentially associated with influenza and other viral diseases. Even though it is not associated with structured exercise, as major outbreaks of atypical myoglobinuria have been reported in Europe and midwestern USA in the recent past a few key points about this condition are given in Box 31.1. This chapter, therefore, concentrates on the equine rhabdomyolysis syndrome (ERS).

Over the years a number of terms have been used to describe horses that develop muscle pain and cramping usually during or after exercise, these include "tying-up, set fast, azoturia, Monday morning disease", etc. It has become clear, however, that these terms really encompass a number of conditions that cause muscular pain rather than signifying one specific disease, hence the term the ERS. In the most common form of ERS some form of exercise is usually the triggering factor for the development of clinical signs. Although exertion *per se* is not always involved, such disorders triggered by exercise are often termed equine exertional rhabdomyolysis (ER), literally the dissolution of striated muscle with exercise.

The ERS affects primarily the muscles of horses of apparently any age, breed or gender and results in the partial or complete inability to move (e.g., signs may range from a show pony that may fail to lengthen when asked, or a racehorse that slows in the closing stages, to an animal that cannot move, or becomes recumbent: Harris 1991). Death can result, although this is rare. The time period between episodes and the severity of the episodes vary between and within individuals (Harris 1991).

Epidemiology and risk factors

ERS according to a number of surveys can affect approximately 5–7% of the thoroughbred racehorse – flat and National Hunt – population, ~8% of polo horses and up to 14% of eventers (MacLeay et al 1999a, McGowan et al 2002a, b, Cole et al 2004, Upjohn et al 2005, Thorpe & Harris 2005). A survey of pleasure horses in Scotland (Mellor et al 2001) suggested a prevalence of 1% and a general survey in Australia concluded that 1.9% of the general equine population over 1 year of age had suffered one or more episodes of ERS during the previous 12 months (Cole et al 2004). In this survey, exercising animals were estimated to be more than 10 times as likely to suffer an episode compared to those not being exercised.

Sufferers have an underlying susceptibility to the condition, which may then be triggered by one or more factors, usually including exercise, resulting in the clinical signs (see Fig. 31.1). The underlying predispositions, as well as the triggering factors, are likely to differ between groups of sufferers – so the measures that may be successful in one individual may not be so successful in another. Sufferers currently may be divided into two groups:

- Those in which the primary underlying susceptibility is intrinsic to the muscle: sometimes referred to as *chronic*.
- Those in which an intrinsic muscle defect does not appear to be present (or to date we have not been able to show that an intrinsic muscle defect is present): sometimes referred to as *sporadic*.

Episodes of ERS may occur intermittently or recurrently in either group but sufferers that fall into the first group tend to first show signs when they are initially asked to work or perform seriously or are being fed increased amounts of feed in anticipation of such a performance. Sufferers in this group therefore tend not to have a history of top class performance before their first episode, although this is not definitive. In addition, as animals between episodes may be "normal", management and performance requirements vary between owners, and horses often have several owners; it may be difficult to determine exactly when the first episode occurred and under what circumstances.

Box 31.1 Atypical Myoglobinuria or Atypical Myopathy

(Whitwell et al 1998, Van der Kolk et al 2010, Van Galen et al 2012 a,b, Votion 2011).

- Typically seen in horses and ponies out at grass, on a low plain of nutrition. Usually not being worked or in light work.
- Sudden onset – often found dead or recumbent – less severe may present with stiffness unrelated to exercise that may rapidly progress to recumbency.
- Metabolic defect may be a multiple acyl-coenzyme A dehydrogenase deficiency, which affects mitochondrial fatty acid energy metabolism. But development is probably multifactorial and may involve mycotoxins/ clostridial toxins in some instances.
- Often preceded by adverse (cold, wet, windy, etc. but no heavy frost) weather conditions. Large outbreaks seem to have occurred following summers, and during autumns, that were significantly warmer than usual.
- One or more animals affected within a group. Others appear to be totally unaffected (but some may be subclinical). Mortality high and can be up to 100% on one pasture. Overall recently estimated at 76%.
- Variable ages – but young (<3 years) and old (>20 years) appear more at risk.
- Usually do not appear to be in distress or pain and will often eat and drink normally (some even appear to be starving) if have access.
- Pulse, temperature, respiration rates can be within acceptable normal limits, even when recumbent, but tachycardia and tachypnea have been reported.
- Can develop respiratory, cardiac, renal and digestive complications.
- CK/AST activities markedly elevated: 10–100 s $\times 10^3$ IU/l.
- Mygolobinuria, ± hypocalcemia (and low ionized calcium especially in terminal stages).
- Inconsistent changes in liver enzymes, Se or glutathione peroxidase (GSHpx) or liver vitamin E levels.
- Biopsy samples taken from postural and/or respiratory muscles and/or myocardium typically show acute segmental necrosis of striated muscle fibers without mineralization.
- No specific treatment currently available (although if associated with *Clostridum* toxin appropriate treatment may be helpful).
- Supportive treatment includes pain management, fluid therapy, administration of calcium, vitamins and antioxidants, plus enhancement of carbohydrate metabolism.
- Recommended to also provide support to apparently unaffected pasture companions (rest, reduce stress, nutritional support, etc.).
- Recent epidemiological work has suggested certain factors within the individual and the environment that seem to increase (e.g., being out at pasture all year, pasture on a steep slope, surrounded by or containing a stream/river or trees especially *Acer pseudoplatanus*, being given hay in fall) or decrease the risk (e.g., being overweight, and regularly vaccinated and given anthelmintic treatment, water provided by a distribution network).
- Certain preventative measures may be helpful especially for pastures with a prior history of deaths (e.g., reduce time out on pasture in spring and autumn, or avoid totally if surrounded by trees especially *Acer pseudoplatanus*, provide water from a distribution network, vaccinate horses regularly, do not allow to get underweight, etc.).

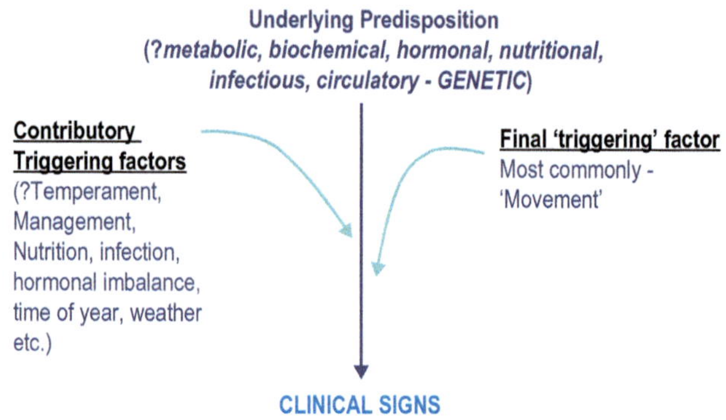

Figure 31.1 Schematic diagram summarizing underlying susceptibility and triggering factors involved in clinical episodes of ERS. Clinical signs occur in horses with either inherited or non-inherited underlying predisposition, being triggered by a combination of factors in which the exercise is usually the most important and definitive factor.

Classification and etiology

An intrinsic muscle defect is not present

Cases of nonintrinsic ERS are usually characterized by a history of adequate performance prior to episodes developing and a successful return to performance following a reasonable period of rest, provision of a balanced, appropriate diet and an appropriate training program. Horses may be of any age, breed or sex and involved in a wide variety of athletic disciplines. Horses can have recurrent episodes of variable severity with inconsistent intervals between them if appropriate changes in the diet and management, etc. are not made (Harris 1991). Episodes of ERS are brought about by external factors which affect muscle function and once corrected complete resolution is possible. In the majority of cases, horses should initially be thought to have nonintrinsic ERS; however, possible intrinsic muscle defects need to be considered if over time multiple episodes of ERS occur despite appropriate management (training and feeding).

This group includes those animals that suffer from this condition mainly due to dietary mismanagement; the most relevant potential conditions are:

- Exercising after a period of over feeding and under exercising.
- Electrolyte imbalances (dietary or individual animal in origin) (see below).
- Provision of too little fiber and too much nonstructural carbohydrate (NSC).
- Inadequate selenium and vitamin E (see below).

In some cases, nutritional supplements have been recommended for ERS not because of a proposed deficiency but because they are postulated, but not proven, to prevent episodes of ERS. These include B vitamins, branched chain amino acids, and chromium.

An initial dietary evaluation determining the approximate daily NSC, oil and forage intake as well as the vitamin, mineral and electrolyte balance may suggest dietary imbalance as a contributing cause. If imbalances appear to exist, a full ration evaluation may be necessary including analysis of hay (or pasture grass) and all complementary and supplementary feeds. Some individuals despite an apparently balanced and adequate intake of electrolytes may have an electrolyte imbalance when assessed by use of fractional urinary electrolyte clearance measurements (Harris & Colles 1988, Harris & Snow 1991, Harris & Gray 1992).

Vitamin E and selenium deficiency

Evidence for a role of vitamin E/Se deficiency in the pathophysiology of ERS has been based on anecdotal reports of supplementation preventing further episodes (Hill 1962, Mansmann et al 1982). These anecdotal findings have not been supported to date by scientific studies. Vitamin E/Se responsive myopathies of sheep and pigs have selective Type I fiber degeneration as compared to the Type II fiber involvement in ERS. However, little is known about the role of free radical induced muscular damage in ERS, delayed onset muscle soreness or even over exertion (Harris & Mayhew 1998).

It is possible that vitamin E/selenium deficiency may be *permissive* to the development of ERS in some circumstances. Measurement of whole blood selenium or glutathione peroxidase activity, as well as serum vitamin E, may be indicated for horses with ERS depending on the diet. It is important to take into account factors such as local geographical areas of selenium deficiency, potentially very low levels of vitamin E in haylages and variable levels in hay. Currently the authors recommend that at least the minimal requirements and preferably an enhanced amount of antioxidants, including vitamin E and Se, are provided to all horses and in particular those with ERS.

The potential for ERS to be associated with a vitamin E/Se deficiency is unlikely when the daily intake of these nutrient is 3–5 IU/kg body weight (BW) for vitamin E depending on exercise load and for Se between 0.003 and 0.006 mg/kg BW.

Electrolyte imbalances

Within this chapter an electrolyte imbalance, as it relates to an individual horse, is taken to represent an inadequate or imbalanced intake or an individual problem with absorption/utilization. It is possible that changes in the intracellular environment within muscle associated with such an electrolyte imbalance may be important. However, there is little published work in this area (Bain & Merritt 1990, Harris & Snow 1991).

Whilst an electrolyte imbalance within the diet may be identified through dietary analysis, an issue within an individual animal may be difficult to determine accurately, One practical way may be to measure urinary fractional excretion (FE) of electrolytes (Harris & Colles 1988, Harris & Gray 1992, McKenzie et al 2002, 2003a), although this at best is only a guide because marked variation can occur due to differences in the core diet, effect of exercise, sampling technique and between individuals as well as within individuals from day to day. Averaging the results of freely voided urine taken on three consecutive days under the same conditions, at the same time of day (pre-exercise and before or >8 h after a concentrate meal, at least 2 weeks after an episode, having been fed a standard ration thought to provide adequate and balanced intake of electrolytes for at least 2 weeks) may increase accuracy. Furthermore, the high calcium crystal concentration of alkaline equine urine requires acidification to accurately assess Ca and Mg content, the high potassium content can interfere with sodium analysis using conventional ion-specific electrodes and results are likely to be unreliable if the urine creatinine concentration is <9000 μmol/l, the pH is 6 or less, blood urea/creatinine are elevated, or there is glucose/hemoglobin present in the urine (Harris & Gray 1992).

Animals without renal disease, that have abnormal FE values while being fed a diet that should provide an adequate and balanced electrolyte content, may have an individual absorption/utilization problem. Such abnormalities (e.g., low or high FE Na values, raised FE PO_4) have been found in some horses and ponies suffering from musculoskeletal problems, in particular the equine rhabdomyolysis syndrome (Harris & Colles 1988, Harris & Snow 1991). Restoration of the FE values to within the expected reference range for the type of diet fed may result in clinical improvement in some but not all animals (see Harris & Snow 1991). It should be noted that no differences in electrolyte status as determined by the FE test was found between thoroughbred horses confirmed to have *the intrinsic muscle defect (RER)* and control horses (McKenzie et al 2002).

Intrinsic muscle defect is present

Some horses develop ERS repeatedly with very little exertion and despite reasonable management practices. Signs are often first apparent at the beginning of training or when horses have developed a reasonable level of fitness or are being fed over a certain level of cereal-based concentrates. Certain breeds of horses appear to have a higher prevalence of ERS and within these breeds specific family lines appear particularly predisposed. This has led to the suggestion that, similar to humans, there are intrinsic inherited defects in muscle function which may predispose horses to such forms of ERS. Documented forms of "intrinsic-defect" ERS include a disorder in muscle contractility or excitation–contraction coupling, which is often referred to as recurrent exertional rhabdomyolysis (RER; Box 31.2) and a defect in carbohydrate storage and/or utilization (polysaccharide storage myopathy [PSSM; Box 31.3]). Other types most probably exist. In both current subgroups a lack of routine daily exercise and a diet high in starch are common predisposing factors for an episode.

Key Points – Exercise-associated myopathies

Intrinsic	Extrinsic (to the muscle)
Underlying muscle defect	Caused by external factors that affect muscle function
Likely to be inheritable	Unlikely to be inherited – unless the external factor is heritable
Examples: PSSM, RER	Examples: electrolyte imbalances, over feeding, under-exercising

Episodes can occur repeatedly, be of variable severity and the time between episodes may not be consistent within or between individuals

Box 31.2 Recurrent Exertional Rhabdomyolysis

(Beech et al 1993, Lopez et al 1995, Lentz et al 1999a,b, 2002, MacLeay et al 1999a, b, c, 2000, Ward et al 2000, Mlekoday et al 2001, Dranchak et al 2005).

- Currently thought to be due to an abnormality in the process of muscle contraction (e.g., the mechanism by which muscle contraction is regulated can be disrupted by excitement and exercise in some susceptible horses). Most likely due to a defect in the regulation of muscle contractility (increased sensitivity of muscle fiber bundles has been shown in vitro to potassium, caffeine and halothane) potentially caused by a defect in skeletal muscle calcium regulation. Recent work, however, suggests that this condition is likely to be caused by a gene/gene alteration that is not yet known to cause similar muscle disease in other species.
- Found mainly in Thoroughbreds, Standardbreds and Arabians.
- RER is reported most frequently in young (two-year-old) fillies in race training. The sex predilection for females does not appear to be as obvious in older horses with RER.
- Commonly suggested triggering factors include:
  - training at a gallop but restraining the horse from reaching top-speed
  - prolonged periods of box rest
  - high grain diets
  - excitement and the presence of a concurrent lameness.
- Incidence of RER may become more frequent as level of fitness increases. Stress is a very common triggering factor. In Standardbreds, ER seems to occur most often after 10–30 min of jogging.
- Horses with RER are typically described as having a nervous temperament and clinical episodes of ER often occur when exercise is accompanied by excitement.
- Most likely to be an inherited condition (possibly autosomal dominant trait with variable expression). It has been suggested that foals of an RER affected stallion or mare would have have at least a 50% chance of inheriting the RER gene. *NB this is modifiable by environmental factors.*

Box 31.3 PSSM

(Valberg et al 1992, 1998, 1999a,b, Valentine et al 1997, 2000, 2001, 2006, Valentine & Cooper 2005, Quiroz-Rothe et al 2002, Annadale et al 2004, 2005, McCue et al. 2006, 2008a,b, 2009a,b, Hunt et al. 2008, Larcher et al. 2008, Barrey et al 2009, Stanley & Piercy 2007, Herszberg et al 2009, Stanley et al 2009).

- The clinical condition is mainly found in Quarter horses and related breeds (e.g., Paints, Appaloosa), Warmbloods and Morgans. Also reported in Anglo-Arabs and Andalusians as well as cob types in the UK. PSSM does not commonly occur in the thoroughbred racehorse if it occurs at all.
- Recent survey suggested that the prevalence of PSSM among overtly healthy Quarter Horses in the US was likely to be between 6 and 12%.
- A prevalence of 33% of all horses outside of draft and Quarter Horse bloodlines and up to 80% of draft horses has been suggested for polysaccharide storage myopathy when amylase-resistant abnormal-polysaccharide is not a required diagnostic criterion.
- Feeding a meal with a high glycemic index produces a lower glucose and insulin response in PSSM Quarter horses compared to normal horses. Thus it appears that such PSSM horses may store a higher proportion of the absorbed glucose after a starch meal in their muscle compared to normal horses. No limitations in the ability of skeletal muscle to metabolize glycogen have been identified in PSSM horses performing anaerobic exercise. However, during submaximal exercise, a defect in substrate flux during metabolism is suggested by stimulation of purine nucleotide metabolism in muscle of PSSM but not healthy horses after 10 min of walk and trot. Muscle cramping with light exercise in PSSM horses may be a result of this defective energy generation in individual muscle fibers.
- In Quarter horses it appears to be associated with abnormal insulin sensitivity but this has not been found in Belgian Warmbloods with PSSM, suggesting that PSSM in these animals may be associated with excessive glycogen synthesis rather than enhanced glucose uptake into muscle cells.
- A missense gain of function mutation (arginine to histidine substitution) in the equine glycogen synthase 1 gene (*GYS1*) has relatively recently been reported in PSSM-affected Quarter Horses, draughts and a variety of other breeds. This mutation causes abnormal increased glycogen synthase activity in skeletal muscle at rest and when activated by glucose-6-phosphate. Hence the increased ratio (of glycogen synthase to branching enzyme activity) in *GYS1*-mutated muscle likely causes abnormal filamentous polysaccharide inclusions to form. This is now referred to as type 1 PSSM to distinguish from those forms of PSSM that are not associated with this genetic mutation (type2 PSSM).
- The precise defect causing the different forms of PSSM is unknown despite numerous biochemical studies. Recent work, at least in the Norman Cob horse breed, concluded that the main disorders seen "could be related to mitochondrial dysfunctions, glycogenesis inhibition and the chronic hypoxia of the PSSM muscles." It has also been suggested that the persistent glycogen synthase activity in type 1 PSSM muscle adversely affects normal muscle energy metabolism during exercise but the actual link between diet, enhanced glycogen synthase activity and muscle cell damage has not been fully elucidated.
- Trigger factors include a change in the exercise routine including unaccustomed stall confinement, being rested for a few days prior to exercise, infection and most importantly the diet. When signs first occur tends to be influenced by the amount of exercise and dietary starch fed.
- Sufferers of this subgroup of ERS tend to have a more calm temperament than the other subgroup and often have persistent elevations of creatine kinase (CK) without these always being associated with clinical signs especially if stable confined. Horses typically are in good (and sometimes overweight) body condition.
- In the Quarter horses and related breeds, and in one warmblood family at least, there appears to be a hereditary basis for PSSM with a dominant mode of inheritance of the *GYS1* mutation although clinical signs of ERS are not always present (depending at least in part on environmental factors).

Clinical signs

Clinical signs usually occur either during or after some form of exercise (as the animal returns home or in the stable/field after exercise). A small number of cases, however, have been reported when the animal is not in work or as it leaves the stable/field at the start of exercise. The main clinical sign is some degree of muscular stiffness, which can be very mild or result in a total inability to move. Recumbency can occur and on rare occasions the condition is fatal. The hind limbs are most commonly affected, usually bilaterally. Firm, swollen muscle groups may be present, especially in the more severely affected animals, but this is not always the case. Palpation of the muscles may or may not be resented. Signs associated with pain and distress may be apparent to a variable extent and attempts have been made to grade the severity of clinical signs (Harris 1991). However, it must be appreciated that temperament can be a very important factor influencing the apparent clinical severity in an individual. Abdominal disturbances can occur at the same time or following an episode of ER. The incidence of myoglobinuria can be difficult to determine, as many owners will not actually see their horse urinate. In the UK, one survey in the early 1990s, suggested that most animals suffered relatively mild episodes in that 38% of cases were stiff, but able to walk, 38% were able to walk with difficulty, 21.5% were unable to walk and 2.5% became recumbent (Harris 1991).

Certain clinical signs are more common with certain subtypes of ERS. In RER, affected animals often experience very frequent episodes with persistent aspartate transaminase (AST) elevations and, as a result, may be retired early from race training. Usually signs are first seen when they become fit. With respect to PSSM sufferers: the clinical signs usually occur 10 to 30 min after the onset of exercise (Firshman et al 2005). Signs are usually first seen at the start of training or after disruption or cessation of their exercise routine. Mild signs include unwillingness to work, reluctance to engage the hindquarters, shifting lameness, stopping and stretching out as if to urinate. Moderately severe signs include a stiff stilted gait, short strides, sweating and firm, painful lumbar and gluteal muscles. More severe cases show excessive sweating, tachypnea, tachycardia, muscle fasciculations, disseminated firm musculature, reluctance or refusal to move and myoglobinuria. Severe cases will show signs within minutes of starting exercise and if they continue to exercise may become unable to stand. Affected animals are often reluctant to exercise. Serum creatine kinase (CK) activity is often persistently elevated despite an extended period of rest. PSSM should be included in the differential diagnosis of "back pain" in competition horses.

Some draft horses and warmbloods appear to suffer from a related condition (sometimes referred to as equine polysaccharide storage myopathy: EPSM) with slightly modified clinical and diagnostic signs (Valentine et al 1997, Valentine 2003, Firshman et al 2005). Reported clinical signs in draft horses include gait abnormalities, progressive muscular weakness, muscle atrophy and recumbency without accompanying elevations in CK activity. In horses which are not exercised few clinical signs, however, may be apparent. Postanesthetic myopathy may be another complication of PSSM in draft breeds. In draft crosses and warmbloods, overt clinical signs of ER may occur less commonly than in Quarter Horses, and in one report the commonest gait abnormalities reported were a reluctance to move forward and engage hindquarters when being ridden and difficulty in picking up the hind feed by hand (Hunt et al 2008). Decreased performance, reluctance to exercise and muscle soreness without evidence of high serum CK are frequent clinical signs in warmbloods.

Key Points – Etiology and risk factors

PPSM	RER
Possibly due to defective energy generation	Due to an abnormality in muscle contraction
More calm	Typically nervous
Often in good condition	May have difficulty maintaining weight
Abnormal insulin sensitivity in Quarter Horses	High incidence in young fillies in training
Associated with feeding grain (sugar/starch rich) diets, commonly seen at the start of training or following a break in training	Risk factors associated with stress e.g., exercising after box rest, excitement, high grain diets, holding back during exercise. Often first seen when fit.
Mainly found in Quarter Horses and related breeds, plus Warmbloods, Morgans, Anglo-Arabs and Andalusians as well as cob types in the UK	Mainly in Thoroughbreds, Standardbreds and Arabians

Diagnosis

Diagnosis of acute ERS is normally based on the clinical history, clinical signs and elevations in serum CK, lactate dehydrogenase (LDH) and AST activity in the absence of underlying liver disease (Harris & Mayhew 1998). The degree of elevation of these enzymes in serum/plasma is dependent mainly upon the severity of muscle damage, the underlying cause (see above), previous history of ERS as well as the length of time that has elapsed between sample collection and the occurrence of muscle damage. Peak values occur in serum approximately 4–6 h, 12 and 24 h for CK, LDH and AST respectively following myonecrosis. Clearance of these enzymes from the bloodstream following rhabdomyolysis occurs rapidly for CK (123±28 min with a plasma clearance of 0.36±0.1 ml/kg/min; Volfinger et al 1994), more slowly for LDH, and is most prolonged for AST (~10 days; Cardinet et al 1967). It has been reported that a three- to fivefold increase in plasma CK activity corresponds to the apparent myolysis of around 20 g of muscle (Volfinger et al 1994).

Confirmation of the *specific* diagnosis of RER involves whole intercostal muscle biopsies and intensive laboratory tests and therefore is rarely undertaken. However, a muscle biopsy is indicated in an animal with several unexplained clinical episodes of ERS. The biopsy site is based on the physiological examination, but epiaxial, gluteal or semimembranosus/semitendinosus muscles are most commonly chosen (Valberg 1999, Quiroz-Rothe et al 2002). Fresh samples can be sent overnight to a suitable laboratory, wrapped in moist but not dripping gauzes (0.9% saline), and chilled (not frozen on icepacks). It is however recommended that specific advice should be obtained, from the receiving diagnostic laboratory, prior to collection and submission. Formalin fixation is less suitable for diagnosis purposes, although it does allow morphological assessment of muscle tissue.

Both electron and optical microscopic lesions found in recurrent cases of ERS are highly variable and depend on severity and the time between the biopsy and the last bout of rhabdomyolysis. The most common consist of polyphasic degenerative and regenerative changes as shown in Fig. 31.2. However, as these changes are nonspecific and reflect the general responses of muscle to injury, many of the recurrent cases of ERS remain in the idiopathic category and a definitive diagnosis of RER due to calcium regulation abnormalities is not possible upon the basis of muscle biopsy and histopathology. Nevertheless, this approach is useful in practice for both confirming myopathy and providing information about severity (Piercy & Weller 2009).

Diagnosis of PSSM is currently definitively confirmed by muscle biopsy, but there is still considerable debate as to the exact criteria for diagnosing an individual as having this disorder. The "gold standard" for diagnosis of PSSM is generally accepted to be the presence of amylase-resistant, periodic acid–Schiff (PAS)-positive, abnormal polysaccharide inclusions in skeletal muscle fibers (Fig. 31.3; Valberg et al 1992, Quiroz-Rothe et al 2002, Ledwith & McGowan 2004, Firshmann et al 2006, Stanley et al 2009). However, others have suggested that excess amylase-sensitive glycogen in the absence of complex polysaccharide may also be used to diagnose PSSM (Valentine et al 1998, 2001, Valentine 2003; see Box 31.4 on PSSM diagnosis). It has been unclear whether horses that have evidence of myopathy with these two histopathologic criteria should be considered with the same disease (Firshmann et al 2006, Stanley & Piercy 2007). In some animals, excessive glycogen may be stored within muscle prior to abnormal PAS-positive, amylase-resistant polysaccharide (De La Corte et al 2002, Valentine et al 2006, Larcher et al 2008). To avoid this confusion, some authors have categorized horses with PSSM into two grades: Grade 1 in which there is histological evidence of myopathy combined with excessive normal (amylase-sensitive) glycogen;

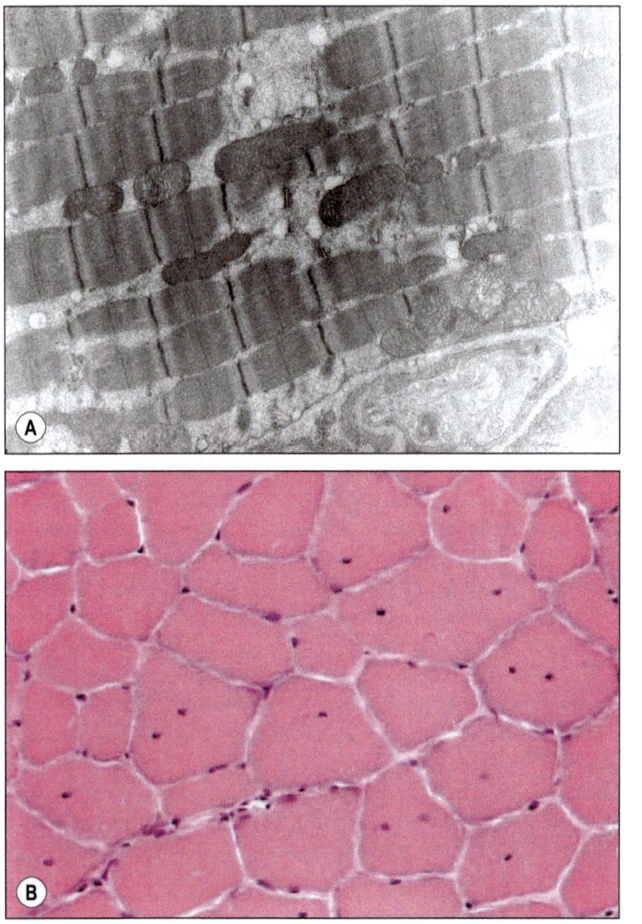

Figure 31.2 Common electron (A, ×16800) and optical (B, H&E, ×200) microscopic lesions found in a gluteal muscle biopsy from a 3-year-old thoroughbred mare with a history of repeated episodes of the equine rhabdomyolysis syndrome. Note the intense myofibrillar degeneration with loss of contractile material in A) and the abundant number of myofibers with internalized nuclei in B).

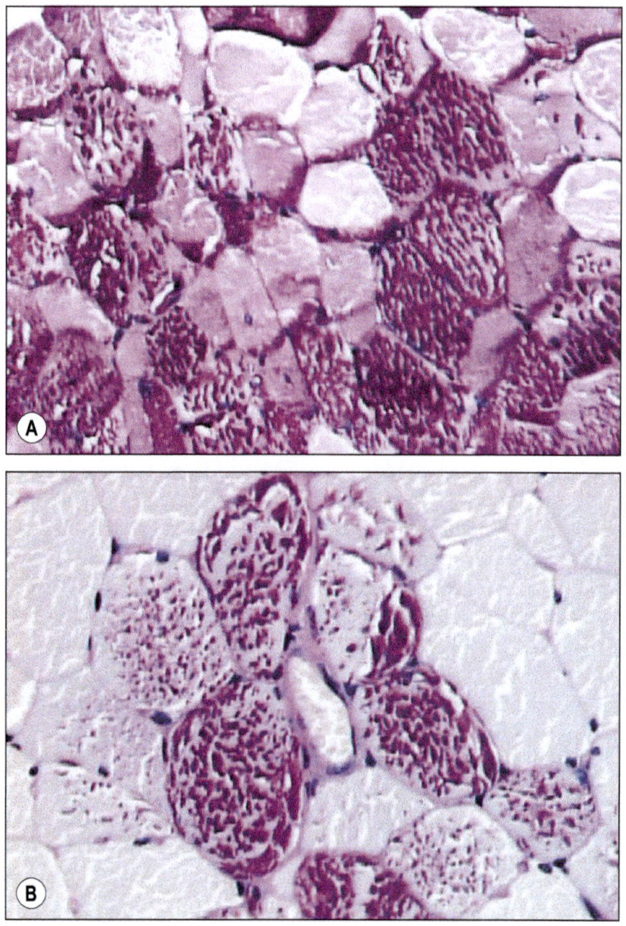

Figure 31.3 Semimembranosus muscle biopsy sample stained with perdiodic acid Schiff (PAS; A), ×200) and PAS following amylase digestion (B), ×400) from a 6-year-old Quarter horse stallion with polysaccharide storage myopathy. Note the abundant pink staining, with granular appearance, inclusions in multiple fibers consistent with abnormal polysaccharide complex.

Box 31.4 PSSM Diagnosis

- The presence of amylase-resistant, abnormal polysaccharide is the most sensitive and specific diagnostic indicator for PSSM in both frozen and formalin fixed sections (this is referred to as Grade 2).
- The levels of glycogen can be up to four times that of normal horses.
- Skeletal muscle fibers from some affected horses shows increased staining for normal amylase-sensitive glycogen, subsarcolemmal vacuoles, necrosis, atrophy and regeneration (this is referred to as Grade 1).
- Important limitations to diagnosing PSSM using amylase resistant polysaccharide include the slow accumulation of amylase-resistant abnormal polysaccharide, which may not be apparent until animals are over 2 yrs of age. Further, the small number of fibers with abnormal polysaccharide in a given biopsy may result in a false negative diagnosis if a sufficiently large muscle sample is not evaluated histologically. Also, evidence suggests that formalin fixation may result in artifactual changes compatible with some described histopathological features of PSSM. See also McCue et al 2009a.
- A diagnosis of Type 1 PSSM can be made by means of a genetic test using hair roots or blood. In horses with ERS or other signs characteristic of PSSM such as weakness, muscle atrophy, pain or stiffness, *GYS1* genotyping should be considered as an option for diagnosis, particularly in horse breeds with an apparent high prevalence of the *GYS1* mutation. In other breeds in which the prevalence is low, or when *GYS1* genotyping is confirmed as normal, muscle biopsy is indicated to further characterize the disorder (see http://www.vdl.umn.edu/ourservices/equineneuromuscular/home.html).
- The form of PSSM caused by a *GYS1* mutation is termed Type1 PSSM to distinguish it from the form of PSSM that is not caused by the *GYS1* mutation, which is called Type 2 PSSM (McCue et al 2009a).

and Grade 2 in which there are histopathologic signs of myopathy together with abnormal (amylase-resistant) polysaccharide (McCue et al 2006, Stanley et al 2009).

Key Points – Diagnostic criteria

	PSSM	RER
Muscle enzyme activities	CK activities may be elevated even when stabled	May have persistent AST elevations due to repeated episodes
Specific diagnosis (confirm with diagnostic laboratory)	Blood test/hair roots (*GYS1* mutation) and/or muscle biopsy Type 1 PSSM is caused by a *GYS1* mutation.	Muscle contracture tests using whole intercostal muscle biopsy – rarely performed
Sub group/ different conditions	Grade 1: histological evidence of myopathy combined with excessive normal (amylase-sensitive) glycogen Grade 2: histopathologic signs of myopathy together with abnormal (amylase-resistant) polysaccharide	

Establishing that ERS is a primary cause of poor performance is challenging when episodes of ER are intermittent and when there is no evident muscle pain or stiffness at the time of presentation. Persistent elevation in AST may indicate previous ER (providing no evidence of liver pathology). However, if serum muscle enzymes are normal, an exercise challenge test may be of value to detect some cases with underlying subclinical ER. At least in the healthy horse, a number of factors influence the extent of any increase in CK and AST activities following exercise and include the intensity and duration of the physical exercise, as well as its nature, plus the fitness, sex, age and possibly diet of the individual animals. The exact nature of the exercise challenge may vary but a sub-maximal exercise test should perhaps be selected for detecting susceptibility to ERS and it should be noted that animals can have an apparently "normal" response to such an exercise test and still suffer an episode of ERS the next time they are ridden or exercised (Harris & Mayhew 1998, Harris 2005).

Key Points

Although the clinical signs of ERS are primarily associated with muscular dysfunction and an unwillingness or inability to move, the primarily underlying susceptibility may or may not be intrinsic to the muscle. The clinical signs, severity and history may be indicative of the underlying etiology but are not necessarily diagnostic. Increasingly sophisticated diagnostic tools are being identified including genetic tests for some subtypes of ERS.

Management and prevention

Treatment depends on the clinical severity but aims to limit further muscle damage, decrease pain and anxiety and most importantly restore and maintain fluid balance plus maximize the chance of an earlier return to work (when appropriate).

There is no single procedure or set of procedures (including diet and management) that can guarantee against further episodes of the ERS. However, appropriate management of susceptible animals, including nutrition, may help to reduce the likelihood or frequency of future episodes. For all sufferers a well-designed exercise program together with a balanced diet, which is suitable for the individual, should be the initial management target. The actual diet which will be the most beneficial to a sufferer will depend on the horse as an individual, and what they are being used for (as influences energy needs), as well as their history with respect to ERS and the likely underlying cause. It is important to note that dietary alterations alone are unlikely to prove successful and must be combined with other changes in management, in particular regular exercise. Minimizing stress and providing regular routines tailored to the individual can also be advantageous. Clinical improvement in signs of ERS can occur within 1 week of the recommended diet change once PSSM or RER horses are on a regular exercise schedule. However, for some individuals the condition may take weeks or months to resolve. In some cases a prolonged period out of work on a low energy ration with permanent (or near permanent) turnout may be required.

Management of those animals *without a known intrinsic muscle problem* will depend on the underlying contributory causes, which are often unique to the individual. An appropriately designed exercise program, plus a nutritionally balanced diet with adequate vitamins and minerals/electrolytes, usually based on forage (with supplemental oil if additional energy is required) and reduced levels of starch and sugar, tends to be the main approach to this group. In individuals the correction of specific electrolyte abnormalities as determined using the fractional electrolyte clearance test might be of value (Harris & Gray 1992).

Horses with mild, repeated nonintrinsic ERS may benefit most from continuing to exercise at a lower intensity for shorter durations while adhering to changes in diet and management. In more severe episodes stall rest and complete confinement are advised for the first 24–72 h until horses are willing to move about without encouragement, signs of muscular pain are not present on palpation and the urine does not contain myoglobin. Continued stall rest, however, is unlikely to be beneficial and may be detrimental. Small paddock turn-out onto pasture that would be suitable for a laminitic-prone animal, in a quiet area, for the majority or at least several hours a day is recommended. Hand walking should be done cautiously, recognizing that the duration of this type of exercise should be short (i.e., initially not for more than 5–10 minutes at a time) and at a very gradual pace. From personal experience it is often beneficial to allow free paddock or arena exercise before hand walking occurs. For horses that continue to suffer episodes during the return to work a more prolonged period of rest with regular and extensive access to a paddock may be required until serum muscle enzyme concentrations are within the normal range or at least the CK is within normal limits and the AST is less than twice normal. Monitoring AST/CK activities during the return to work can be valuable (Harris & Mayhew 1998, Harris 1998, 2005). Continual access to a paddock tends to be beneficial even once back in full training. Training can be resumed very gradually using a regular exercise schedule, which matches the intensity and duration of the exercise to the horses, underlying state of training. Note that for cases of "intrinsic" tying-up this much rest is not recommended (see following sections).

Key Points – General management guidelines

Management (general)

Exercise	• Gradual return to work (amount of rest needed will vary according to individual and underlying cause) • Well-designed exercise program: regular exercise plus paddock turnout
Balanced diet (see examples)	• Balanced diet – with slightly (RER) or markedly reduced starch and sugar intake (PSSM) • Fiber should be the foundation, plus adequate and balanced vitamin/micro- and macronutrient intake • Ensure adequate antioxidant intake
Management	• Regular routines • Reduction of stress – need to tailor to the individual
Paddock turnout	• Regular access to paddock turnout may often be advantageous but avoid paddocks with high NSC pasture plus encourage movement but avoid getting cold or over active

Return to exercise

For pleasure horses, particularly those with PSSM, the return to exercise should be very gradual. If the intensity or duration of exercise is increased too rapidly, horses often develop repeated episodes of ERS. Initial exercise should therefore be limited to a few minutes of uncollected walk. If horses remain calm this may be done in a round pen or on a very long lunge line. Exercise under-saddle may be easier for some owners. However, it should be stressed that even at a walk the duration of exercise initially should be very brief, small circles and steep hills should be avoided. Exercise at an uncollected walk and trot can be increased by a few minutes a day. If the horse seems stiff the exercise session should be terminated. In general, it should usually take 3 weeks to reach 30 minutes of walk and trot. The subsequent length and intensity of exercise can be increased according to the horse's intended athletic pursuit. Quarter Horses with PSSM will often have elevated serum CK activity for 4–6 weeks when they are becoming accustomed to this exercise program. Once horses are fit, it is important to maintain regular daily exercise. Keeping horses with PSSM fit increases oxidative metabolism which enhances the ability to utilize fat for energy metabolism and seems the best prevention against further episodes of ERS. Horses with PSSM are less likely to improve if the only change made is the addition of dietary oil (Hunt et al 2008).

Thoroughbreds with RER horses are often very fit when they develop ERS and require only a few days off before commencing a reduced amount of training. Standardbreds with chronic ERS often benefit from reducing the time spent jogging to less than 20 minutes at a time.

Standardization of regimens

Providing regular routines and management strategies that reduce stress and excitability are particularly important in horses with RER. Strategies include exercising or feeding affected horses first, providing compatible equine company, avoiding negative interactions with horses during riding and training. For some individuals the use of horsewalkers in the return to fitness may not be advisable.

Dietary management

Forage

During the recovery period, decreasing a horse's energy intake is often recommended. Typically as a starting point (depending on body condition score, etc.), aim to feed, 1.5 to 2% BW (on a DM basis) as good quality (with respect to a low mold/spore count, etc.) forage (or an appropriate forage replacer) together with a balanced vitamin/mineral supplement.

As the exercise increases and energy requirements increase the amount of forage being fed can also be increased. The authors currently recommend, from personal experience rather than scientific studies, that for animals prone to ERS wherever possible hay rather than haylage or silage should be fed. This may reflect that weight for weight hay provides more fiber and potassium, more can be fed if energy intake needs to be restricted plus helps support gastric health, and it may help avoid an extra load on the horse's antioxidative capacity. Legume hays may not be an ideal forage. If required alfalfa should be added to the ration gradually as the workload increases but again from personal experience should not be provided at more than 0.4% of BW. For horses with PSSM, forage should have low starch and sugar content - currently would recommend <12% NSC on a dry matter basis - to minimize post-feeding glycemic and insulinemic responses (Borgia et al 2011). Whilst soaking hay will not necessarily result in substantial loss of NSC it may be a helpful supplementary measure (Longland et al 2011).

Which type of complementary feed?

It is very important to note that not giving a "meal" to an ERS horse when all other animals in the yard are being fed can increase stress and should be avoided. Addition of a complementary feed that is high in fiber and has low to moderate starch and high oil content can help to reduce the frequency and severity of episodes of ERS in some cases. Even during the initial recovery phase a small amount can be fed and used as a vehicle for any vitamin and mineral support. If deficiencies in vitamin E, selenium or electrolytes were identified, a gradual introduction of an appropriately balanced diet is best done during the recovery period. The amount of complementary feed and the amount of starch and oil that should/can be supplied will depend on the form of ERS and its severity as well as the horse's energy requirements. Controlled feeding trials have been performed for Quarter Horses with PSSM and Thoroughbreds with RER (MacLeay et al 1999c, McKenzie et al 2003b, Ribeiro et al 2004). Recommendations for other breeds have been extrapolated from these findings or based on clinical experience and extrapolation from owner reports (e.g. Hunt et al 2008).

PSSM

There is evidence that clinical signs of PSSM are more frequent and severe in horses that receive little exercise but are fed moderate to large amounts of NSC from cereal-based feeds (Valberg et al 1997, Valentine et al 2001, Hunt et al 2008). In contrast, feeding a diet with restricted NSC (on a total dietary basis, <10% of digestible energy, DE) with oil providing 6–25% of DE has apparently resulted in either a reduction in muscle glycogen levels and/or clinical improvement of affected horses, with a gradual decrease in the frequency and severity of episodes of muscle pain and underlying damage (Valentine et al 2001b, Firshman et al 2003, McKenzie et al 2003b, Ribeiro et al 2004, Hunt et al 2008). Some oil addition may be advisable for PSSM cases, although the exact amount required has not been confirmed. It has been reported that signs of muscle dysfunction can persist when affected horses are fed an all-forage diet even with a low NSC, whereas diminished clinical signs occur when even a small amount of vegetable oil is added to the diet (McKenzie et al 2003b). In a crossover study, provision of 0.5 kg/day of stabilized rice bran to quarter horses with PSSM resulted in a 20 to 25% decrease in muscle glycogen content compared with the control ration of grass hay (De La Corte et al 1999). There are a number of commercial diets which may be suitable for horses with PSSM. To be effective these diets need to be low in starch as well as high in oil and ideally should have been shown to produce a low insulin (and glycemic) response. To date the potential role that different fatty acid profile may play in the management of these animals has not been evaluated in detail.

RER

A small number of controlled trials have, however, provided evidence that dietary energy source can also be influential with respect to RER in Thoroughbred horses (MacLeay et al 2000, McKenzie et al 2003a). However, the effect of energy source seems to depend on daily DE intake. For RER-affected Thoroughbred horses fed diets that either provided 21.4 MCal/day (~89.5 MJ/day) through a high oil content (2.3 kg/day of stabilized rice bran; 20% DE from fat and 34% DE from NSC) or a high NSC content (2.5 kg/day of sweet feed; 8% DE from fat and 47% DE from NSC), there was no difference in post-exercise serum CK activity. Conversely, when they were fed an energy intake more representative of race horses in training (28.8 MCal ~ 120 MJ/day) through a larger amount of sweet feed (4.5 kg/day; 8% DE from fat and 53% DE from NSC), there was a significant increase in post-exercise serum CK activity (MacLeay et al 2000). A follow up study (McKenzie et al 2003) showed that post-exercise serum CK activity was increased (>3000 U/l) when RER horses were fed a high NSC ration (4.5 kg of sweet feed/day [<5% DE from fat and 45% DE from NSC] but not the lower NSC/high oil ration (4.3 kg fat and fiber concentrate [20% DE from fat, and 9% DE from NSC]).

What about pasture turnout?

For many sufferers of ERS, and in particular PSSM cases, regular pasture turnout (providing regular gentle exercise) can be essential but the pasture itself may be an issue. The author currently recommends that any animal with ERS is treated in a similar way to a laminitic horse: –provided restricted access to grass that could be high in NSC, but is allowed regular access to well managed pasture providing as low an intake of NSC as possible (see Chapters 18 and 27). Although not scientifically evaluated it appears that overall the risk of inactivity with respect to ERS is higher than the risk associated with grass ingestion.

See Boxes 31.5, 31.6 and 31.7 for general and more specific comments on feeding management. Example rations are given in Table 31-1.

Box 31.5 Key Comments on the Management of Any Horse Prone to ERS

- Do not turn the horse out onto lush fast-growing pastures, especially pastures with a high fructan, high starch (e.g., high clover/legume cover) or water-soluble carbohydrate content, but prolonged daily periods out in a sparse paddock is often beneficial.
- Regular daily exercise with some free exercise can be very helpful and even essential in some sufferers – some individuals may be more or less stressed being exercised on their own or in a group – choose the exercise format that causes the least "stress".
- Consider the addition of more digestible fiber sources such as soya hulls and unmolassed sugar beet pulp. These are often most easily provided through an appropriate feed.
- Consider the use of supplementary oil, either through the addition of high oil feedstuffs such as rice bran (but ensure correct overall calcium:phosphorus balance of the diet) or the addition of vegetable oil e.g. corn oil, sunflower or soya oil. Any supplemental oil should be introduced slowly – over several weeks depending on the amount to be added. Recommend feeding not more than 1 ml/kg BW/day without additional advice, although horses may tolerate rations containing up to 20% of oil. There will be individual differences with respect to the type of oil they prefer and the amount they will eat.
- In order to obtain metabolic benefits from the feeding of oil, in addition to those associated with its high energy density and lack of starch content, the oil needs to be fed for several weeks. It is very important to note that oil does not provide any additional protein, vitamins (vitamin E content is variable) and minerals. If the horse is not receiving sufficient, for its workload, from its basal diet, then an appropriate additional balancer may be needed.
- The authors' currently recommend that additional vitamin E should be fed in combination with any supplemental oil. Exact recommendations are not known but an *additional* 1–1.5 IU vitamin E/ml added supplemental oil is the current recommendation (in addition to between 3–5 IU/kg BW depending on exercise load, etc.). Note that 100 ml of oil (~93 g) will provide around 3.5 MJ of energy. Hays and pastures typically contain around 3% or less of oil and commercial feeds should provide the total oil content of their feeds as well as an estimate of the DE.
- It is advisable to try and ensure that the diet provides a sufficient intake of electrolytes in an adequate and balanced manner (appropriate use of the urinary fractional electrolyte excretion test may be valuable in some cases).
- It is advisable to ensure that all horses, but in particular those susceptible to ERS are fed adequate vitamin E (see above) and selenium (between 0.003 and 0.006 mg/kg BW depending on exercise load, etc.).
- Most horses will probably require additional salt especially in hot weather or if working hard.
- Avoid the addition of wheat bran to the horse's diet wherever possible, but certainly avoid large amounts (unbalanced calcium to phosphorus ratio).
- Do not feed in anticipation of an increase in workload – wait until additional energy is needed before increasing intake. On rest days (which should be avoided if possible) any complementary feed intake should be reduced (halved) from the evening before until the evening afterwards. If a more prolonged period of rest is to be given then the type of feed fed should be evaluated and either one of a lower energy density, or forage alone, appropriately supplemented, fed.
- It is important to maintain an adequate vitamin and mineral intake – which may require additional supplementation if on a high forage based diet.
- Reduce workload (and feed intake) but maintain some regular light exercise if a viral infection is thought to be present
- For some horses the use of a horse walker or lunging (may depend on how carried out) may be contraindicated.

Box 31.6 Specific Comments on the Feeding of Horses Prone to RER

- Specific management includes reducing stress and promoting calm behaviour; maintaining exercise and avoiding wherever possible stall rest whilst decreasing the intake of starch/sugar and utilizing dietary oil supplementation when additional energy is required.
- Providing not more than around 2.5 kg of cereal based feed/500-kg horse/day is recommended initially although the exact level of starch/sugar that can be tolerated is individual in nature but tend to recommend less than 20% of the daily DE intake comes from starch and sugar.
- Anecdotal reports suggest that performance may be compromised if feed less than 8–10% starch/sugar as fed in the diet of racehorses but see Chapter 26.
- The beneficial effects of oil supplementation in RER horses may be due to the exclusion of dietary starch rather than specific protective effects of high dietary oil, by making them calmer prior to exercise. For RER horses, the recommendation is to feed at least 15% of the daily DE from oil and ideally around 20% of daily DE if in intensive work.
- For horses undergoing intense exercise, it can be very difficult to achieve this in a palatable form by blending individual components and specialized commercial diets may be required.
- Dantrolene given 1 hour before exercise (and, as recommended by some, to horses that have not been fed their morning feed) may be worth considering (Edwards et al 2003, McKenzie et al 2004) but this is idiopathically hepatotoxic and other factors need to considered before use and with prolonged use.

Box 31.7 Some Specific Comments on the Feeding of Horses Prone to PSSM

- Dietary changes alone may not resolve the condition – successful management often requires dietary change and provision of daily turnout (plus regular exercise).
- Dietary management includes reducing body weight if necessary, and maintaining the starch and sugar intake at a minimum (no cereal grains or added molasses, etc.), use of forage or forage replacers with NSC ≤10–12% and where commercial feeds are provided these should be low in NSC (ideally ≤10%).
- The aim is for the majority of the energy comes from oil and fiber. Aim for at least 15% or less of the total DE to come from starch and sugar and ideally <10% (although this can be difficult to achieve on a DE basis). Additional oil providing >13 and ideally >15% of the total DE intake, should be added as required. There may be some advantage in adding some additional oil in the diet of any PSSM sufferer and for quarter horse PSSM sufferers levels of around 5–10% of the diet as oil, when such levels of energy are required, have been recommended although this needs to be adjusted to the individual (in particular taking into account their weight and BCS).
- A very gradual return to work is needed in these cases once the diet has been adjusted and daily turnout provided. Maintaining a very regular exercise program coupled with maximizing turnout preferably in a field suitable for a laminitis-prone animal is essential in these animals.
- Although 20 or even 25% of DE as oil appears to be recommended especially in the lay-press for horses with PSSM, there are no controlled trials to indicate that this degree of oil supplementation is necessary. In fact, such a diet may result in problems with weight gain, especially in those animals not in hard work with high energy requirements.
- A wide variety of dietary components could be blended to produce a low starch, high oil diet; however, it is extremely important that such diets are balanced to provide adequate protein, vitamin and minerals and palatability. A number of feed companies now manufacture a complete high-fiber, low-starch balanced concentrate. Current recommendations are that it may be advisable to choose one that has been shown at least in some horses to produce a low glucose and insulin response.

Table 31-1 Example Rations for Intrinsic Muscle Defect Sufferers (needs to be adjusted for individual circumstances for guidance only)

	Pleasure horse – occasional exercise	Pleasure horse – occasional exercise	Pleasure horse – occasional exercise
Type of intrinsic muscle defect	RER	PSSM	PSSM
BW	500	500	500
BCS (out of 9)	4–5	5	8
Behavior	Excitable/nervous	OK	Very placid
Estimated DE requirement MJ/day	~ 90 MJ	~90	65 – for maintenance but for weight loss probably only around 50 MJ
Forage (DE)	10 kg (~80 MJ) of a low energy fairly mature hay ~8 MJ/kg as fed	8.75 kg (~70 MJ). NB ideally this should include pasture turnout for as long as possible – but the pasture needs to be low sugar, low yield (as per a laminitic). Appropriate grass management is essential. Management practices such as strip grazing, use of grazing muzzles etc. may be required	~ 7 kg (~56 MJ) of low energy hay. This will need to be provided using double or treble haynets in order to maximize time spent foraging – again ideally time needs to be spent outside moving on appropriate pastures – consider dry lots/turning out into an arena/use of strip grazing/muzzles – ensure water intake/ increasing the exercise load.
Cereals	None	None	None
Cereal based hard feed	None	None	None
Oil – NB oils vary but 100 ml ~93 g	None	300 ml (~11 MJ) vegetable oil in divided doses – gradually added	<100 ml (~3.5 MJ) vegetable oil

Table 31-1 *Continued*

	Pleasure horse – occasional exercise	Pleasure horse – occasional exercise	Pleasure horse – occasional exercise
High-fiber low-starch (starch and sugar content <10%) low energy commercial feed or low mollassed chaff	None	1 kg (~8 MJ) used as a base for the oil – this could be a feed with vitamins and minerals suitable for a laminitic	0.5 kg (~4 MJ) – low mollassed chopped fiber Or to promote weight loss may need to feed a vitamin and mineral providing fiber-based weight loss product with a DE <8 MJ as fed. May need to feed as little as 6 kg per day of this or appropriate low energy hay plus vitamins and minerals. BUT caution re behavioral issues/potential increased risk of gastric ulceration with restricted forage intake.
High-fiber low-starch (starch and sugar – ideally shown to produce a low insulin/glucase response) high oil (10% oil) commercial feed	Nil to 1 kg (~12 MJ) More if weight gain required		
Other	• General vitamin and mineral supplement. • Vitamin E intake at ~1450 IU/day	If the feed does not contain sufficient vitamins and minerals need to supplement with an appropriate level of a general vitamin and mineral supplement. Vitamin E intake at 1900 IU/day	General vitamin and mineral supplement if forage based but not if included in weight loss ration Vitamin E intake at ~1600 IU/day
Comments	NB if other horses are being fed meals providing a small fiber-based meal may help reduce 'stress'	Ideally need to analyze the hay and pasture.	Need to analyze the hay. To promote weight loss no oil should be fed. The ration/management (including exercise protocol) will have to be amended if episodes restart when oil supplementation ceases
% of total DE – using typical actual feeds/forages available.	Oil ~15%; starch and sugar <20%	Oil 20–25%; starch and sugar <15%	Oil >15%; starch and sugar ~15%

Table 31-1 *Continued*

	Pleasure horse – competition exercise PSSM	Pleasure horse – competition exercise RER	Pleasure horse – racelike RER
BW	500	500	500
BCS	6	5	5
Behaviour	Calm	Nervous	Nervous
Estimated DE requirement (MJ/day)	~100	~110	~110
Forage	7 kg	8 kg	8 kg
Cereals	None	None	
Cereal based hard feed	None	None	2.5 kg (with restricted starch and sugar <35%)
Oil (gradually introduce – see text)	500 Mls		540 ml vegetable oil (~0.5 kg)
High fiber low starch (starch and sugar – ideally shown to produce a low insulin/glucose response) high oil (10% oil) commercial feed	3 kg in divided meals mixed with the oil.	5 kg	
Other	Vitamin E intake at 2500 IU/day	Vitamin E intake at 2500 IU/day	Vitamin E intake at 2500 IU/day
Comments	• Would need to reduce oil if weight loss required • Vitamin/mineral/ protein status of the final diet would need to be checked and an appropriate balancer added as required.		• Start at 2.5 kg high cereal based diet if the horse can manage at this level you can increase this gradually until you find the amount that it cannot tolerate – this will be very individual. • Vitamin/mineral/ protein status of the final diet would need to be checked and an appropriate balancer added as required
% of total DE – using typical actual feeds/ forages available	Oil >30%; starch and sugar <15%	Oil ~20–25%; Starch and Sugar ~15%	Oil 25–30%; starch and sugar ~20%

BCS, body condition score; DE, digestible energy.

Key Points – Specific diet requirements

Diet	PSSM	RER
% Total ration DE from starch and sugar	15% or less (ideally <10% but difficult to achieve)	Individually variable: ideally <20%
% Total ration DE from oil	Some oil may be advantageous aim for ideally ≥10% in most cases; potentially >20% may be of value. *NB needs to take into account BCS.* Alternative strategies may be needed if overweight	May not be advantageous until in hard work when used as an alternative energy source to starch. Aim for >15% (and potentially >20% in intensive work)
Additional oil	Fresh, nonrancid, and with professional advice if feeding > 1 ml/kg BW. Add gradually.	
Type of diet	Ideally want evidence that the diet produces a low glucose/insulin response	Some racehorses in typical training may not perform well if feed <10% starch in total diet.
Hay	Hay contains ≤10–12% NSC	Recommend grass hay rather than haylage and possibly avoid high proportion of high starch alfalfa forage.
Pastures	Avoid high sugar, high legume pastures – treat as if a very laminitis-prone animal	
Vitamin E	1–1.5 IU vitamin E/ml added supplemental oil Plus for those animals in no or light work 2–3 IU/kg BW and up to 5 IU/kg BW intake for those animals in intensive work	

Conclusion

Appropriate management procedures and nutrition for horses with ERS can help reduce the likelihood or frequency of episodes of ERS even in those horses with an underlying genetic susceptibility.

References

Annandale, E.J., Valberg, S.J., Mickelson, J.R., et al., 2004. Insulin sensitivity and skeletal muscle glycose transport in horses with equine polysaccharide storage myopathy. Neuromuscl disord 14, 666–674.

Annadale, E.J., Valberg, S.J., Essén-Gustavsson, B., 2005. Effects of submaximal esercise on adenine dinucleotide concentrations in skeletal muscle fibres of horses with polysaccharide storage myopathy. Am J Vet Res 66, 839–845.

Bain, F.R., Merritt, A.M., 1990. Decreased erythrocyte potassium concentration associated with exercise related myopathy in horses. J AM Vet Med Assoc 196, 1259–1261.

Barrey, E., Mucher, E., Jeansoule, N., et al., 2009. Gene expression profiling in equine polysaccharide storage myopathy revealed inflammation, glycogenesis inhibition, hypoxia and mitochondrial dysfunction. BMC Vet Res 5, 29.

Beech, J., Lindborg, S., Fletcher, J.E., et al., 1993. Caffeine contractures, twitch characteristics and the threshold for Ca^{2+}-induced Ca^{2+} release in skeletal muscle from horses with chronic intermittent rhabdomyolysis. Res Vet Sci 54, 110–117.

Borgia, L., Valberg, S., Watts, K., et al., 2011. Glycaemic and insulinaemic responses to feeding hay with different non-structural carbohydrate content in control and polysaccharide storage myopathy- affected horses. J Anim Physiol Anim Nutr 95, 798–807.

Cardinet, G.H., Littrell, J.F., Freedland, R.A., 1967. Comparative investigations of serum creatine phosphokinase and glutamic-oxaloacetic transaminase activities in equine paralytic myoglobinuria. Res Vet Sci 8, 219–226.

Cole, F.L., Mellor, D.J., Hodgson, D.R., et al., 2004. Prevalence and demographic characteristics of exertional rhabdomyolysis in horses in Australia. Vet Rec 155, 625–630.

De la Corte, F.D., Valberg, S.J., Williamson, S., et al., 1999. Enhanced gluscose uptake in horses with polysaccharide storage myopathy (PSSM). Am J Vet Res 60, 458–462.

De la Corte, F.D., Valberg, S.J., Macleay, J.M., et al., 2002. Developmental onset of polysaccharide storage myopathy in Quarter horse foals. J Vet Int Med 16, 581–587.

Dranchak, P.K., Valberg, S.J., Onan, G.W., et al., 2005. Exclusion of linkage of the RYR1, CACNA1S, and ATP2A1 genes to recurrent exertional rhabdomyolysis in Thoroughbreds. Am J Vet Res 67, 1395–1400.

Dranchak, P.K., Valberg, S.J., Onan, G.W., et al., 2005. Inheritance of recurrent exertional rhabdomyolysis in Thoroughbreds. J Am Vet Med Assoc 227, 762–767.

Edwards, J.G.T., Newton, J.R., Ramzan, P.H.L., et al., 2003. The efficacy of dantrolene sodium in controlling exertional rhabdomyolysis in the thoroughbred racehorse. Equine Vet J 35, 707–710.

Firshman, A.M., Valberg, S.J., Bender, J., et al., 2003. Epidemiologic characteristics and management of polysaccharide storage myopathy in Quarter horses. Am J Vet Res 64, 1319–1327.

Firshman, A.M., Baird, J.D., Valberg, S.J., 2005. Prevalence and clinical signs of polysaccharide storage myopathy and shivers in Belgian Draft Horses. J Am Vet Med Assoc 227, 1956–1964.

Firshman, A.M., Valberg, S.J., B Bender, J.B., et al., 2006. Comparison of histopathologic criteria and skeletal muscle fixation techniques for the diagnosis of polysaccharide storage myopathy in horses. Vet Path 43, 257–269.

van Galen, G., Saegerman, C., Marcillaud Pitel, C., 2012a. European outbreaks of atypical myopathy in grazing horses (2006–2009): Determination of indicators for risk and prognostic factors. Equine Veterinary Journal 44, 621–625.

van Galen, G., Marcillaud Pitel, C., Saegerman, C., 2012b. European outbreaks of atypical myopathy in grazing equids (2006–2009): Spatiotemporal distribution, history and clinical features. Equine Veterinary Journal 44, 614–620.

Harris, P.A., 1991. The equine rhabdomyolysis syndrome in the United Kingdom: Epidemiological and clinical descriptive information. Br Vet J 147, 373–376.

Harris, P.A., 1998. Equine rhabdomyolysis syndrome. In: Watson, T. (Ed.), Metabolic and Endocrine Problems of the Horse. W.B. Saunders, London, pp. 75–100.

Harris, P.A., 2005. Feeding and management advice for tying up/azoturia/ Monday Morning disease/equine rhabdomyolysis syndrome. In: Harris, P.A., Mair, T.S., Slater, J.D., et al. (Eds.), Equine Nutrition for All. Proceedings of the1st BEVA & WALTHAM Nutrition Symposium Harrogate, pp. 113–118.

Harris, P.A., Mayhew, I.J., 1998. Musculoskeletal disease. In: Bayly, W., Reed, S. (Eds.), Equine Internal Medicine. WB Saunders, London, pp. 371–427.

Harris, P.A., Colles, C., 1988. The use of creatinine clearance ratios in the prevention of equine rhabdomyolysis. Equine Vet J 20, 459–463.

Harris, P.A., Gray, J., 1992. The use of the urinary fractional electrolyte excretion test to assess electrolyte status in the horse. Equine Vet Educ 4, 162–166.

Harris, P.A., Snow, D.H., 1991. Role of the electrolyte imbalances in the pathophysiology of the equine rhabdomyolysis syndrome. In: Persson, S.G.B., Lindholm, A., Jeffcott, L.B. (Eds.), Equine Exercise Physiology 3. ICEEP Publications, Davis, CA, pp. 435–442.

Herszberg, B., McCue, M.E., Larcher, T., et al., 2009. A GYS1 gene mutation is highly associated with polysaccharide storage myopathy in Cob Normand draught horses. Anim Genet 40, 94–96.

Hill, H.E., 1962. Selenium-vitamin E treatment of tying up in horses. Mod Vet Pract 43, 66.

Hunt, L.M., Valberg, S.J., Steffenhagen, K., et al., 2008. An epidemiological study of myopathies in Warmblood horses. Equine Vet J 40, 171–177.

Larcher, T., Herszberg, B., Molon-Noblot, S., et al., 2008. Polysacharide storage myopathy in Cob Normand draft horses. Vet Pathol 45, 154–158.

Ledwith, A., McGowan, C.M., 2004. Muscle biopsy: a routine diagnostic procedure. Equine Vet Educ 4, 84–89.

Lentz, L.R., Valberg, S.J., Balog, E., et al., 1999a. Abnormal regulation of contraction in equine recurrent exertional rhabdomyolysis. Am J Vet Res 60, 992–999.

Lentz, L.R., Valberg, S.J., Balog, E.M., et al., 1999b. Abnormal regulation of muscle contraction in horses with recurrent exertional rhabdomyolysis. Am J Vet Res 60, 992–999.

Lentz, L.R., Valberg, S.J., Herold, L., et al., 2002. Myoplasmic calcium regulation in myotubes from horses with recurrent exertional rhabdomyolysis. Am J Vet Res 63, 1724–1731.

Longland, A.C., Barfoot, C., Harris, P.A., 2011. Effects of soaking on the water-soluble carbohydrate and crude protein content of hay. Vet Rec 168, 618.

Lopez, J.R., Linares, N., Cordovez, G., et al., 1995. Elevated myoplasmic calcium in exercise-induced equine rhabdomyolysis. Pflugers Arch 430, 293–295.

McCue, M.E., Ribeiro, W.P., Valberg, S.J., 2006. Prevalence of polysaccharide storage myopathy in horses with neuromuscular disorders. Equine Vet J Suppl 36, 340–344.

McCue, M.E., Valberg, S.J., Miller, M.B., et al., 2008a. Glycogen synthase (*GYS1*) mutation causes a novel glycogenosis. Genomics 91, 458–466.

McCue, M.E., Valberg, S.J., Lucio, M., et al., 2008b. Glyocogen synthase 1 (*GYS1*) mutation in diverse breeds with polysaccharide storage myopathy. J Vet Int Med 5, 1228–1233.

McCue, M.E., Armién, A.G., Lucio, M., et al., 2009a. Comparative skeletal muscle histopathologic and ultrastructural features in two forms of polysaccharide storage myopathy in horses. Vet Pathol 46, 1281–1291.

McCue, M.E., Valberg, S.J., Jackson, M., et al., 2009b. Polysaccharide storage myopathy phenotype in quarter horse-related breed is modified by the presence of an RYR1 mutation. Neuromuscul Disord 19, 37–43.

Macleay, J.M., Sorum, S.A., Valberg, S.J., et al., 1999a. Epidemiological factors influencing exertional rhabdomyolysis in thoroughbred racehorses. Am J Vet Res 60, 1562–1566.

Macleay, J.M., Valberg, S.J., Geyer, C.J., et al., 1999b. Heritable basis for recurrent exertional rhabdomyolysis in thoroughbred racehorses. Am J Vet Res 60, 250–256.

MacLeay, J.M., Valberg, S.J., Pagan, J., et al., 1999c. Effect of diet on recurrent exertional rhabdomyolysis in thoroughbred. International Conference on Equine Exercise Physiology 5, Equine Vet J Suppl 30, 458–462.

MacLeay, J.M., Valberg, S.J., Pagan, J.D., et al., 2000. Effect of ration and exercise on plasma creatine kinase activity and lactate concentration in Thoroughbred horses with recurrent exertional rhabdomyolysis. Am J Vet Res 61, 1390–1395.

McGowan, C.M., Fordham, T., Christley, R.M., 2002a. Incidence and risk factors for exertional rhabdomyolysis in thoroughbred racehorses in the UK. Vet Rec 151, 623–626.

McGowan, C.M., Posner, R.E., Christley, R.M., 2002b. Incidence of exertional rhabdomyloysis in polo horses in the USA and the UK in the 1999/2000 season. Vet Rec 150, 535–537.

McKenzie, E.C., Valberg, S.J., Pagan, J.D., et al., 2002. Electrolyte balance in Thoroughbred horses with recurrent exertional rhabdomyolysis consuming diets with varying dietary cation–anion balance. Am J Vet Res 63, 1053–1060.

McKenzie, E.C., Valberg, S.J., Godden, S.M., et al., 2003. Comparison of volumetric urine collection vs single sample urine collection in horses consuming diets varying in cation-anion balance. Am J Vet Res 64, 284–291.

McKenzie, E.C., Valberg, S.J., Godden, S., et al., 2003. Effect of dietary starch, fat and bicarbonate content on exercise responses and serum creatine kinase activity in equine recurrent exertional rhabdomyolysis. J Vet Int Med 17, 693–701.

McKenzie, E.C., Valberg, S.J., Godden, S.M., et al., 2004. The effect of oral dantrolene sodium on post-exercise serum creatine kinase activity in thoroughbred horses with recurrent exertional rhabdomyolysis. Am J Vet Res 65, 74–79.

Mansmann, R.A., Podkonjak, K.R., Jackson, P.D., et al., 1982. Panel report Tying up in horses. Mod Vet Pract 63, 919.

Mellor, D.J., Love, S., Gettinby, G., et al., 2001. Sentinel practice-based survey of the management and health of horses in Northern Britain. Vet Rec 149, 417–423.

Mlekoday, J.A., Mickelson, J.R., Valberg, S.J., et al., 2001. Calcium sensitivity of force production and myofibrillar ATPase activity in muscles from Thoroughbreds with recurrent exertional rhabdomyolysis. Am J Vet Res 62, 1647–1652.

Piercy, R.J., Weller, R., 2009. Muscular disorders of the equine back. In: Henson, F.M.D. (Ed.), Equine back pathology: Diagnosis and treatment. Wiley-Blackwell, Oxford, UK, pp. 168–178.

Quiroz-Rothe, E., Novales, M., Aguilera-Tejero, E., et al., 2002. Polysaccharide storage myopathy in the M Longissimus lumborum of show jumpers and dressage horses with back pain. Equine Vet J 34, 171–176.

Ribeiro, W., Valbery, S.J., Pagan, J.D., et al., 2004. The effect of varying dietary starch and fat content on creatine kinase activity and substrate availability in equine polysaccharide storage myopathy. J Vet Itnern Med 18 (6), 887–894.

Stanley, R.L., Piercy, R.J., 2007. Breed susceptibility in equine polysaccharide storage myopathy. Equine Vet Educ 19, 143–145.

Stanley, R.L., McCue, M.E., Valberg, S.J., et al., 2009. A glycogen synthase 1 mutation associated with equine polysaccharide storage myopathy and exertional rhabdomyolysis occurs in a variety of UK breeds. Equine Vet J 41 (6), 597–601.

Thorpe, P., Harris, P., 2005. Equine rhabdomyolyis syndrome in event horses. In: Proceedings of the 19th Equine Science Society Symposium. Tuscon AZ. Equine Science Society, Champaign IL, pp. 230–231.

Upjohn, M.M., Archer, R.M., Christley, R.M., et al., 2005. Incidence and risk factors associated with exertional rhabdomyolysis syndrome in National Hunt racehorses in Great Britain. Vet Rec 156 (24), 763–766.

Valberg, S.J., Cardinet, III G.H., Carlson, G.P., et al., 1992. Polysaccharide storage myopathy associated with recurrent exertional rhabdomyolyis in horses. Neuromusc Disorders 2, 351–359.

Valberg, S.J., 1999. Spinal muscle pathology. Vet Clin North Am Equine Pract 15, 87–96.

Valberg, S.J., Macleay, J.M., Mickelson, J.R., 1997. Exertional rhabdomyolysis and polysaccharide storage myopathy in horses. Comp Cont Educ. Pract Vet 19, 1077–1086.

Valberg, S.J., Townsend, D., Mickelson, J.R., 1998. Skeletal muscle glycolytic capacity and phosphofructokinase regulation in horses with polysaccharide storage myopathy. Am J Vet Res 59, 782–785.

Valberg, S.J., MacLeay, J.M., Billstrom, J.A., et al., 1999a. Skeletal muscle metabolic response to exercise in horses with "tying-up" due to polysaccharide storage myopathy. Equine Vet J 31, 43–47.

Valberg, S.J., Mickelson, J.R., Gallant, E.M., et al., 1999b. Exertional rhabdomyolysis in Quarter Horses and Thoroughbreds; one syndrome, multiple etiologies. Equine Vet J Suppl. 30, 533–538.

Valentine, B.A., 2003. Equine polysaccharide storage myopathy. Equine VetEduc 15, 254–262.

Valentine, B.A., Cooper, B.J., 2005. Incidence of polysaccharide storage myopathy: necropsy study of 225 cases. Vet Pathol 42, 823–825.

Valentine, B.A., Credille, K.M., Lavoie, J.-P., et al., 1997. Severe polysaccharide storage myopathy in Belgian and Percheron draught horses. Equine Vet J 29, 220–225.

Valentine, B.A., Hintz, H.F., Freels, K.M., et al., 1998. Dietary control of exertional rhabdomyolysis in horses. J Am Vet Med Assoc 212, 1588–1593.

Valentine, B.A., McDonough, S.P., Change, Y.-F., et al., 2000. Polysaccharide storage myopathy in Morgan Arabian and Standardbred related horses and Welsh cross ponies. Vet Pathol 37, 193–196.

Valentine, B.A., Van Saun, R.J., Thompson, K.N., et al., 2001. Role of dietary carbohydrate and fat in horses with equine polysaccharide storage myopathy. J Am Vet Med Assoc 219, 1537–1544.

Valentine, B.A., Flint, T.H., Fisher, K.A., 2006. Ubiquitine expression in muscle from horses with polysaccharide storage myopathy. Vet Pathol 43, 270–275.

Van der Kolk, J.H., Wijnberg, I.D., Westermann, C.M., et al., 2010. Equine acquired multiple acyl-CoA dehydrogenase deficiency (MADD) in 14 horses associated with ingestion of Maple leaves *(Acer pseudoplatanus)* covered with European tar spot (*Rhytisma acerinum*). Mol Genet Metab 101, 289–291.

Volfinger, L., Lassourd, V., Michaux, J.M., et al., 1994. Kinetic evaluation of muscle damage during exercise by calculation of amount of creatine kinase released. Am J Physiol Regul Integr Comp Physiol 266, R434–R441.

Votion, D.-M., 2011. Atypical myopathy. In Proceedings of the European Equine Health and Nutrition Conference. Waregem, Belgium, pp. 115–124.

Ward, T.L., Valberg, S.J., Gallant, E.M., et al., 2000. Calcium regulation by skeletal muscle membranes of horses with recurrent exertional rhabdomyolysis. Am J Vet Res 61, 242–247.

Whitwell, K.E., Harris, P.A., Farrington, P.G., 1988. An outbreak of atypical myoglobinuria. Equine Vet.J 20, 357–363.

32 Developmental orthopedic disease

Ingrid Vervuert, Andrea D. Ellis

Introduction

Developmental orthopedic disease (DOD) is a term used for a cluster of conditions in the growing foal. These conditions are caused by disturbances in the development and maturation of the musculoskeletal system, in particular of the articular and metaphyseal cartilage. DOD is believed to be linked with abnormalities of skeletal growth associated with the conversion of cartilage to bone by the process of endochondral ossification.

In general, DOD incorporates the following spectrum of conditions (adapted from McIlwraith 2001, Jeffcott 2005):

- Physitis
- Osteochondrosis
- Acquired angular limb deformities
- Flexural deformities
- Tarsal bone collapse (synonym: cuboidal bone malformation)
- Cervical vertebral malformation
- Acquired vertebral deformities.

Of these different conditions, osteochondrosis has been the main focus of scientific investigations in horses. The incidence of osteochondrosis in the growing foal can be high, with reported values, depending on the breed and study parameters, of between 10–50% (Stock et al 2005, van Weeren 2006, Wittwer et al 2006). Most breeds of horses are susceptible although ponies and feral horses seem to be much less commonly affected (Jeffcott 2005, Marshall 2007, Lepeule et al 2009). Nonetheless, a recent report documented osteochondrosis of the lateral trochlear ridge in four ponies in which the lesions were similar to those observed at the same site in horses (Voute et al 2011). The heritability of osteochondrosis has been reported to be in the range of (h^2 =) 0.1 to 0.34 for Warmblood horses and between (h^2 =) 0.17 and 0.52 for Standardbred horses (Komm 2010).

All of the conditions included under the DOD umbrella are likely to have a complex multifactorial etiopathogenesis (McIlwraith 2001); however, a number of key factors are commonly thought to be involved, including:

- Rapid growth
- Diet imbalances
- Biomechanical stress or trauma on joint and growth cartilage
- Hormonal factors (e.g. hyperinsulinemia)
- Genetic predisposition.

This multifactorial etiology explains why clear-cut studies showing the induction or prevention of DOD cannot be achieved with small sample populations. Genetic factors seem to be very important in the pathogenesis of osteochondrosis and the identification of so-called quantitative trait loci (QTL) in Hanoverian Warmblood and South German Coldblood horses has emphasized this (Komm 2010).

There are key predilection sites for each of the DOD conditions (Table 32-1). Clinical signs that can be associated with DOD include enlarged growth plates, joint heat, prolonged recumbency, stiffness, lameness, and reduced activity linked to lack of movement/playing (Jeffcott 2005, van Weeren 2006). Clinical signs typically become apparent between birth (although pathological changes may be present prenatally) and 24 months of age (Table 32-1). It is worth noting that whereas the clinical signs associated with angular limb deformities symptoms are external and obvious, for the other manifestations of DOD such as osteochondrosis, no obvious clinical signs may be present.

An overview of the different conditions within the DOD complex is given below, including our current understanding of the involvement of nutrition in their development and prevention.

Etiology and pathology of DOD

A brief summary of the key conditions within the DOD cluster, and their suggested main etiological factors, is given below (for further information see Stashak 2001, Auer and Stick 2006).

Physitis (synonyms: epiphysitis, physiolysis)

Physitis is an abnormality of endochondral ossification in the metaphyseal growth plate (physis), where the structural integrity of the metaphyseal bone is weakened by the disturbance in maturation of the cartilage cells (Jeffcott 2005). Radiographically, physitis may manifest as an irregularity in the growth plate with sclerosis of adjacent bone and an altered metaphyseal contour (Williams et al 1982). Metaphyseal broadening or flaring of the ends of the long bones is a typical feature in the affected growing foal. The enlargement

Table 32-1 Approximate Time of Onset of Key Clinical Signs and the Main Anatomical Sites Involved for Each Condition Within the DOD Complex

Clinical condition	Typical time of onset of signs (months)	Main anatomical sites involved
Physitis	4–12, >24	Distal limbs and stifles joints
Osteochondrosis	3–20	Proximal and distal limbs and cervical spine
Flexural deformities	1–4	Distal forelimbs
Tarsal bone collapse	1–18	Tarsal joints
Cervical vertebral malformation	6–24	Cervical spine
Vertebral abnormalities	6–9	Thoracolumbar spine

Data from Jeffcott 2005.

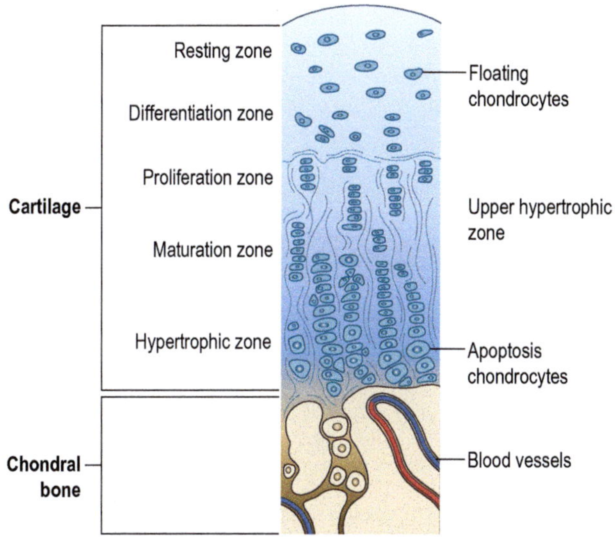

Figure 32.1 Zones of development from articular cartilage to subchondral bone along the growth plates.
Source: A.D. Ellis.

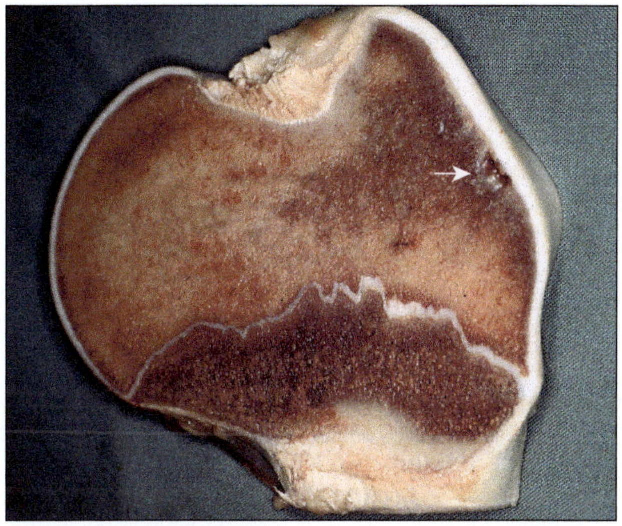

Figure 32.2 OC lesion in the early stage which may "self-repair" or may predispose the horse to further cartilage damage resulting in OCD.
Reproduced with kind permission from van Weeren and Barneveld 1999.

usually presents as a firm swelling and is caused by the formation of new bone. These processes are self-limiting and disappear after closure of the growth plates. Physitis is probably one of the most frequently seen conditions within the DOD complex in Thoroughbred foals (Gee et al 2005). Although the exact etiology of physitis is unknown, high energy intakes which promote rapid growth, traumatic injuries and a genetic predisposition are suggested to be involved (Thompson et al 1988, Gee et al 2005).

Osteochondrosis (OC, synonyms: dyschondroplasia, OCD: osteochondrosis dissecans)

OC is a common disorder of growth cartilage in domestic animals and humans (Komm 2010). In animals, the disorder has been described in pigs, dogs, horses, cattle, cats and rats (Ytrehus et al 2007). It is regarded as the most important cause of leg weakness in swine and it is a frequent cause of lameness in young athletic horses (Ytrehus et al 2007).

OC has been described as a disturbance in the process of endochondral differentiation, proliferation, maturation and eventual ossification in fast-growing animal species and humans (Ytrehus et al 2007). The *first stage of OC development* may be either an impairment of cellular differentiation in the growing cartilage or a failure of maturation and ossification by differentiated chondrocytes low down in the maturation zone (Ytrehus et al 2007, see Fig. 32.1). Either pathway can result in focal lesions that involve areas of cartilage along or just below the otherwise healthy articular cartilage (Fig. 32.2).

The *second stage* includes necrosis of the basal layers of the hypertropic cartilage with subsequent pressure and strain within the joint, giving rise to fissures in the damaged cartilage (Rejnö & Strömberg 1978, Jeffcott & Henson 1998). A *third stage*, which does not always occur, may be the flaking away or fully breaking loose of damaged cartilage fragments - described on X-rays as "joint mice" - and termed osteochondrosis dissecans (OCD - often wrongfully used synonymously with OC).

Osteochondrotic lesions have been reported in many equine joints, but they are most commonly found in the tibiotarsal and femoropatellar joints, and in the dorsal aspect of the distal metacarpus and metatarsus (McIlwraith 2001, van Weeren 2006). In horses, the period during which a lesion develops and possibly regresses is limited to the first months of life. New osteochondrotic lesions rarely develop after the fifth month of life, and lesions that developed in those first five months may be repaired in the following six months (van Weeren & Barneveld 1999, van Weeren 2006).

Several potential etiological factors have been suggested for equine osteochondrosis including rapid growth,

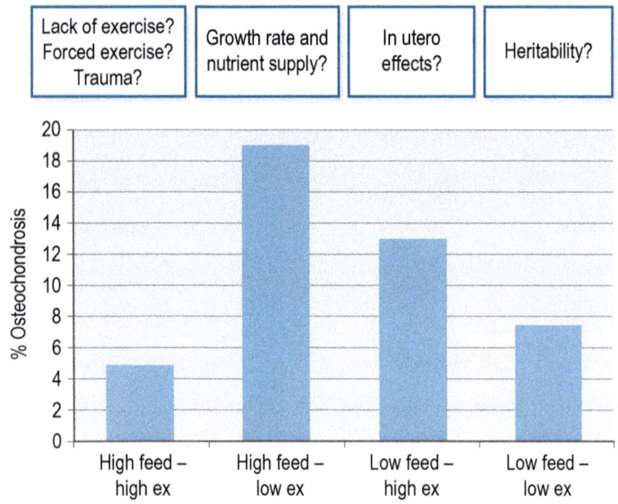

Figure 32.3 Proportion of OC occurrence (radiographic diagnosis) in Dutch Warmblood foals kept according to 4 management systems: high feed, high exercise (ex), low feed and low ex groups (*n*=8 per treatment, adapted from Bruin and Creemers 1994) The gray horizontal overlay highlights factors which may have influenced results due to pre-experimental and experimental influences in such a small sample group.

nutritional imbalances (overfeeding, mineral imbalances and toxicity), endocrine factors, biomechanical stress, trauma or lack of exercise, failure of vascularization and a genetic predisposition (Jeffcott & Henson 1998, Ytrehus et al 2007). One hypothesis for example suggests that cessation of blood supply of the cartilage canal is the primary event in OC (Ytrehus et al 2007). However, recently there has been more focus on the importance of genetic factors (Komm 2010). Candidate genes that may be responsible for osteochondrosis in horses have been identified (e.g., Lampe et al 2009, Wittwer et al 2009).

Results from a study by Bruin and Creemers (1994) are interesting in that they highlight the complex multi-factorial etiology of OC lesions and their possible repair (Fig. 32.3): Dutch Warmblood foals were kept in stables (from 3 months of age) and either exercised on a 20 m diameter horse exerciser (high exercise) or let into a sand paddock (low exercise) for short daily periods. Beside the differences in the level of exercise, foals were also fed one of two feeding levels (high feed vs low feed). In this study the highest incidence of OC was associated with either a high feeding level with a low exercise intensity or a high intensity of exercise in combination with a low feeding level.

There is often a discrepancy between the occurrence of osteochondrotic lesions produced under standardized conditions with a very small number of horses and those osteochondrotic lesions reported under field conditions. For example, osteochondrotic lesions in the growth plates, which were apparently produced through an excessive carbohydrate intake (Glade & Belling 1986), are generally very rare in clinical cases (van Weeren 2006).

Angular limb deformities (synonym: bent legs)

Angular limb deformities represent a deviation of the limb in the sagittal plane. The angulation can arise from any of the physes or the cuboidal bones of the carpus and tarsus. The most common physes involved are those of the distal radius, tibia, metacarpus and metatarsus. The most common deformity is the carpal valgus followed by the fetlock varus, which describes a lateral or medial deviation away from the midline of the carpus or cannon bone respectively. The etiology of angular limb deformities is again complex and thought to be multifactorial. Angular limb deformities are thought to be associated with growth imbalances induced by one of the following defects: joint laxity, irregularities of endochondral ossification of the bones in the carpus or tarsus, excessive exercise, poor confirmation, asynchronous longitudinal growth rate and trauma (Jeffcott 2005). The impact of nutrition has not been investigated.

Flexural deformities (synonyms: contracted tendons, ballerina syndrome)

Flexural deformities are expressed either as a hyperflexion or a hyperextension of a joint region. Flexural deformities are observed in the distal interphalangeal joint, the metacarpophalangeal or metatarsophalangeal joint, the carpal region and rarely the tarsal region (Auer 2006). The forelimbs are more frequently affected. Flexural deformities may be present at birth (congenital deformities) or acquired later in life (acquired deformities). Congenital deformities are thought to be the result of external environmental factors affecting the mare during gestation period (e.g., influenza outbreak, equine goiter, defects in cross-linking of elastin and collagen caused by lathyrism, etc) or other pathological causes such as intrauterine malpositioning (Auer 2006, Charman & Vasey 2008). However, the etiology in many cases remains speculative.

Acquired flexural deformities can be seen in rapidly growing foals, and in association with other painful conditions (Auer 2006). Affected foals are usually on an above-average level of nutrition (Lloyd-Bauer & Fretz 1989). However, the authors did not specify the energy intake. In addition, it has been postulated that an abrupt change from a previously inadequate energy intake to an excessive energy intake may trigger this problem (Auer 2006).

Tarsal bone collapse (synonyms: incomplete ossification of cuboidal bones, cuboidal disease, tarsal bone necrosis)

This condition is associated with collapse of the dorsal aspect of the central and third tarsal bones which causes a flexion deformity of the tarsus (Jeffcott 2005).

Incomplete ossification of the tarsal bones is most frequently associated with a premature birth or as a result of twinning. Foals which are born prematurely would be expected to have a higher propensity for this condition due to the incomplete ossification and reduced cartilage strength. However, the impact of nutrition on tarsal bone collapse has not been investigated.

Cervical vertebral malformation (synonyms: Wobbler disease, equine spinal ataxia)

Cervical vertebral malformation is characterized by malformation or compression of the spinal cord which leads to spasticity, ataxia and incoordination. The two most common syndromes are cervical vertebral instability and cervical static stenosis (Auer & Stick 2006). Cervical vertebral instability is centered in the cranial vertebrae of the neck of young horses. It therefore causes dynamic spinal cord compression and typically affects horses between 4 and 12 months of age (Pool 1993). Cervical static stenosis is located caudally in the neck of horses and is characterized by a closing of the cervical canal causing compression on the spinal cord. Typically, horses start to show the first clinical signs between one and four years of age (Pool 1993). The etiopathogenesis is unknown; however, nutritional imbalances, rapid growth, exercise, gender (males > females), trauma and a genetic predisposition have all been suggested to be factors that could be involved (Auer & Stick 2006). At the present time, none of these possible causes have been confirmed or disproved. It has been demonstrated that dietary restriction and resting young horses with early signs of cervical vertebral malformation may help prevent more severe cervical vertebral abnormalities developing (Mayhew et al 1978, cited by Jeffcott 2005). In addition, proper nutritional balance in the pregnant and lactating mare has been suggested to decrease the occurrence of this disease in foals; and also is a major factor in the treatment of confirmed cases in young, growing horses (Mayhew et al 1978).

Acquired vertebral deformities (synonyms: lordosis, kyphosis)

These conditions describe varying degrees of lordosis and kyphosis, where the vertebral column deviates abnormally in a ventral or dorsal direction respectively. The most common abnormality is kyphosis in the rapidly growing foal which usually occurs post-weaning from 6 to 9 months of age (Jeffcott 2005). Lordosis is usually obvious at birth and the condition can deteriorate as the foal grows. These defects are thought to be the result of fetal malpositioning (Auer & Stick 2006).

Impact of nutrition on DOD

The potential impact of nutrition on DOD, particularly in the area of osteochondrosis research, has attracted much attention and discussion (e.g., Glade & Belling 1986, Ellis 2001, Gee et al 2007). Several epidemiological studies have shown that mares and foals under typical feeding conditions are often fed diets that do not meet the recommended nutritional minimum intake levels (e.g., Winkelsett et al 2005, Lepeule et al 2009).

The two main areas of interest with respect to nutrition and its link with DOD are, first, energy intake, and to a lesser extent protein, and second, minerals (mainly calcium and phosphorus) and trace elements (mainly copper and zinc).

Quantity and quality of energy intake

Rapid growth has been suggested to be a major factor in the development of certain types of DOD (Sandgren et al 1993, Jelan et al 1996, van Weeren & Barnefeld 1999). While final skeletal height is a genetically determined factor, the time period over which an individual achieves its predetermined adult height can be influenced by nutrition. For example, weight and girth gains for ad libitum-fed weanlings and yearlings were higher than those foals fed a restricted diet (Ott & Asquith 1986, Cymbaluk et al 1990). Dietary energy intake and its impact on the incidence of OC have been in the focus of interest for several decades. A high energy intake (150% of NRC level for digestible energy) increased body weight gains and growth rates in weanlings (Thompson et al 1988). It was speculated that skeletal development was impaired by the high growth rate, especially in those cases in which the protein intake was also low (Thompson et al 1988).

Oversupply of energy in the growing foal creates a mismatch between the rates of body weight increase, skeletal growth and micronutrient supply during particular periods of growth as reviewed by Ellis (2001) and Harris et al (2005). However, excess energy and rapid growth should not be considered as being synonymous. Rapid growth may occur due to a genetic predisposition and excess energy intake may not always lead to rapid growth. It is likely that OC develops only when several predisposing factors coexist. This probably accounts for some conflicting reports on the importance of overfeeding and growth (Ellis 2001).

A study by van Tilburg and Ellis (2002) analyzed growth data and radiographic OC scores recorded systematically at a research station between 1994 and 1999. These authors found no correlation between growth rates, withers height and OC scores in 144 Dutch Warmblood foals (30% OC positive) over the period from birth to 12 months. However, OC positive foals showed a higher average daily gain (possible growth spurt?) in the 3 months post weaning (4–6 months of age). Recent large scale epidemiological studies confirm that under typical feeding conditions, body weights and withers heights are not significantly different between OC affected or OC unaffected Warmblood foals (Vervuert et al 2002) or Thoroughbred foals (Jelan et al 1996). The intake of high energy levels (~130% of NRC level vs. 70% of NRC level for digestible energy) was apparently associated with disturbances in growth plate cartilage metabolism (e.g., decreased cartilage hexosamine and hydroxyproline contents) in Thoroughbred weanlings (Glade & Belling 1984, 1986) and widespread lesions, referred to as dyschondroplasia, were reported in growing, exercise restricted, foals (Savage et al 1993a). However, the high energy intake was not associated with an increase in average daily body weight gain (Savage et al 1993a) nor an increase in the daily increase in withers height (Glade & Belling 1986).

Nutritional influence on hormonal regulation of bone growth

Several studies provide evidence that hormonal factors, influenced by the nature of the energy intake (i.e. energy supply and source), may be involved in the etiopathogenesis of DOD (Ralston 1996, Henson et al 1997, Jeffcott & Henson 1998, Treiber et al 2005, Staniar et al 2007). The key hormones involved include insulin, insulin-like growth factors (IGF I and IGF II) and the thyroid hormones (Fig. 32.4).

Insulin, IGF I and IGF II affect endochondral ossification under in vitro conditions in fetal and foal chondrocytes (Henson et al 1997), whereas the in vivo results remain inconclusive (Sloet van Oldruitenborgh-Oosterbaan et al 1999, Verwilghen et al 2009).

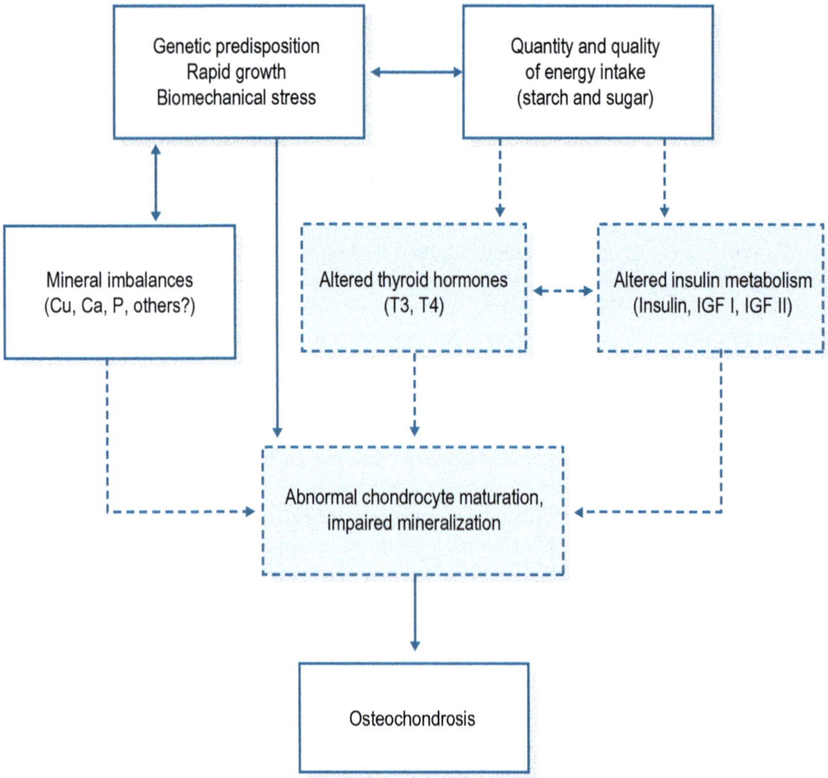

Figure 32.4 Etiological factors involved in equine osteochondrosis.
Adapted from Jeffcott & Henson 1998.

IGF-1 is an important factor for the stimulation of cartilage matrix synthesis by the chondrocytes (Henson et al 1997) and OC lesions in foals have been associated with lower plasma IGF 1 concentrations in comparison with unaffected foals (Sloet van Oldruitenborgh-Oosterbaan et al 1999). In contrast however, Verwilghen et al (2009) found higher plasma IGF 1 concentrations in horses (>15 months) affected with DOD lesions than in healthy horses. They considered this to reflect a repair mechanism within the affected cartilage. In conclusion, more research is needed to elucidate the role of IGF-1, especially the local effects of IGF-1 on bone and cartilage.

Insulin, in vitro, acts as a "survival factor" preventing chondrocyte apoptosis (Henson et al 1997). Diets containing high amounts of easily digestible carbohydrates induced higher postprandial glycemic and insulinemic responses in weanlings affected by OC than in healthy foals (Ralston 1996, Henson et al 1997, Pagan et al 2001, Williams et al 2001, Treiber et al 2005). For example, Treiber et al (2005) found that a group of 9-month-old weanlings that had been provided access from birth to a high sugar and starch feed had a significantly lower insulin sensitivity than the group provided a fat- and fiber-rich complementary feed. Taken together, these findings suggest that chronic elevation of plasma insulin (and/or associated effects) at key stages in the early growth period of horses might trigger imbalances in chondrocyte maturation, thereby delaying the rate of endochondral ossification. However, the Treiber et al (2005) weanling study did not evaluate the effect of diet on the incidence of OC, assessed either by clinical signs of lameness or radiographic evaluation. Data showing an effect on the clinical incidence of OC from feeding fat- and fiber-rich diets instead of traditional starch- and sugar-rich diets are still lacking. Ott et al (2005) did not find that feeding a high starch concentrate intake for 112 days (>30% starch vs. 0% starch) led to a higher incidence of OC in weanlings.

Insulin also shows a strong interaction with the thyroid hormones (T3 and T4). It has been reported, in weanlings, that insulin will stimulate the rapid removal of T4 from the circulation following the ingestion of a high-carbohydrate meal (Glade & Belling 1984, Glade et al 1984). The changes in the hormonal pattern were associated with disturbances in growth plate cartilage metabolism. These results may be of particular interest as thyroid hormones are involved in the final stages of chondrocyte differentiation and the invasion of growth cartilage by blood vessels.

As a result of the studies above and others, feeding diets high in soluble carbohydrates to growing horses have been implicated as a contributing factor to the development of DOD (Ralston 1996, Henson et al 1997, Jeffcott & Henson 1998, Treiber et al 2005, Staniar et al 2007). Therefore the replacement of rapidly digestible carbohydrates with fat and fiber has attracted some attention. The substitution of dietary fat for readily digestible carbohydrates like sugar and starch (SS) decreased postprandial glycemic and insulinemic responses in Thoroughbred weanlings (Staniar et al 2007), but the results on growth factors like IGF-1 are controversial. Staniar et al (2007) found a significant diet-related effect on plasma IGF-1 and average daily gain (both higher in SS foals with seasonal effect), whereas previously Ropp et al (2003) did not find any difference in the circulating serum IGF-1 levels in growing foals with diet. The effect of increasing circulating cholesterol levels, associated with adding 10% oil to the diet, on metabolism also needs further elucidation (Ropp et al 2003). The major limitation of both studies again is the lack of clinical information on osteochondrotic lesions in foals investigated. Much more work is needed to elucidate linkages between diet, insulin/insulin sensitivity and/or other hormones, and bone health.

In the future, metabolic programming of the mare should be an increasing focus of interest as the feeding regimen during gestation might affect fetoplacental development by altering nutrient delivery from maternal to fetal blood. In other species there is some evidence that overnutrition during conception and early embryonic development may contribute to "programming hormone levels" of the fetus (Kwong et al 2000). Fleming (2000) pointed out that growth regulating imprinted genes (IGF-2) may be altered as a consequence of maternal diet. In a study performed by George et al (2009) feeding pregnant mares with a high-starch diet resulted in higher baseline glucose concentrations and a trend for higher baseline plasma insulin levels in their foals when compared to those foals from mares fed a diet containing a low amount of starch. However, insulin sensitivity to an insulin-modified frequently sampled intravenous glucose tolerance test was not different between dietary groups (both fed the low starch diet from ~5 days of age) until day 160. In principle, metabolic programming could be one important factor contributing to the etiopathogenesis of DOD in foals, but research is needed to examine this issue.

Key Points – Energy source and DOD

- Excessive energy intake by growing foals (>130% of digestible energy needs) has been implicated in the pathophysiology of DOD. One hypothesis is that the ingestion of feeds rich in starches and sugars alters endocrine regulation of chondrocyte maturation and apoptosis via effects on insulin, IGF-1 and thyroid hormones.
- The clinical efficacy of replacing dietary starch with alternative energy sources (e.g. oil) on the incidence of osteochondrosis is unknown. Regardless, avoiding large postprandial glycemic and insulinemic responses by reducing the starch intake might be beneficial in helping to mitigate risk of osteochondrosis and other conditions (e.g. gastric ulcers, laminitis).

Protein

Epidemiological studies show that under typical feeding conditions diets are fed that provide excessive, adequate or marginal protein supply to mares and foals (e.g., Winkelsett et al 2005). No significant differences in growth rates, weight gain, height, cannon circumference or in hoof growth and feed utilization were observed in foals which were fed either an adequate or a high protein diet (Savage et al 1993). In accordance with these findings, feeding high protein diets (126% NRC level) to growing foals had no effect on the incidence of dyschondroplasia (Savage et al 1993a). Feeding protein levels well below NRC recommendations (diet: 9% protein vs 14% protein) resulted in markedly depressed growth rates, feed intake and feed utilization by foals (Schryver et al 1987), but osteochondrotic lesions in the foals were not evaluated. In general, a range of 13 to 17% crude protein is recommended as being needed for optimal growth in foals, assuming an adequate energy supply. Such levels of protein have not been associated with an increased risk of OC.

However, whether single amino acids might have a significant impact needs further evaluation in horses. For example, the addition of amino acids (> two- to threefold above recommendation) like methionine, threonine, proline and glycine reduced either the overall OC score or the OC severity score in pigs (Frantz et al 2008). Consistent with these findings, lysine and threonine have been suggested as the two first limiting amino acids for growth in foals (Ott et al 1981, Graham et al 1994, Saastamoinen 1996, Staniar et al 2001). Milk and milk products are rich in lysine and threonine, but amino acids decrease in the mares' milk during lactation, therefore amino acid supply could be marginal during the late suckling period. Supplementation with feed high in protein (e.g., a creep feed with a crude protein content > 16%, soy bean or rape seed meal can provide high amounts of lysine and threonine).

On the other hand, Harris et al (2005) emphasized the possible role of certain amino acids (e.g. leucine, lysine, arginine) in promoting insulin secretion. The ingestion of certain amino acids or proteins may stimulate insulin secretion. For example, studies in humans have demonstrated that the ingestion of soy protein concentrate alone or mixed with glucose increased the insulin response (Moghaddam et al 2006). A significantly higher protein effect was observed in subjects with a large waist circumference.

Up to now, little information is available on the effects of amino acids on insulin secretion in horses. Sticker et al (2001) determined the effects of different amino acid infusions – arginine, aspartic acid, lysine, glutamic acid, and *N*-methyl-D, L-aspartate – in horses. Their main findings were similar to those for humans and showed a significant rise in insulin after the infusion of arginine (0.5 g/kg BW) and lysine. After infusion of arginine, insulin responses were more pronounced in mares than in geldings or stallions. However, currently there is no study directly linking the intake of certain amino acids and the incidence of DOD.

Calcium (Ca), phosphorus (P) and magnesium (Mg)

Ca and P are considered together because they constitute the major part of the mineral content of bone. They are very closely related: a deficiency or an excess of one element will interfere with the proper utilization of the other. The Ca:P ratio in the bone is about 2.0:1. As well as cartilage damage, OC seems to affect bone metabolism for example Firth et al (1999) reported a lower bone mineral density in those foals which developed the most severe OC scores. The involvement of bone metabolism in OC is also reflected by serum osteocalcin, a marker of bone turnover and mineralization. Osteocalcin concentrations have been found to be significantly correlated with the severity of OC in foals during the first months of life (Billinghurst et al 2004, Vervuert et al 2007). The role of Ca in bone metabolism is highlighted in several research papers. For example, Thompson et al (1988) fed weanlings low Ca diets (~35% of Ca requirement for 240 days) which inhibited third metacarpal length and decreased bone mineral content.

Epidemiological studies showed a high incidence of OC in foals and yearlings with low or deficient intakes of Ca and P at this one time point (Knight et al 1985, Winkelsett et al 2005). A deficient level of Ca in the foals' diet is known to inhibit bone growth (Thompson et al 1988); therefore an adequate Ca and P supply to the growing foal is of particular interest (Finkler-Schade et al 1996).

In the past, there has been significant concern about the potential harmful effects of an excessive Ca intake in foals. To date there is no evidence that excessive Ca intake might promote OC lesions (>300% of NRC level, Savage et al 1993), unlike the observations in dogs (Richardson & Zentek 1998). In addition, Thompson et al (1988) found no negative effects on bone density or bone growth in weanlings fed diets for 240 days providing Ca levels that were 2.5-fold higher than the recommended NRC Ca intake as long as adequate P was supplied. Regardless, as with other livestock species, excess Ca in equine diets possibly interferes with the absorption of other essential minerals including phosphorus, magnesium, iron, iodine, zinc and manganese (McDowell 2003). Furthermore, it is important to note that Ca is mainly eliminated by the kidneys and high urinary Ca excretion might predispose for urolithiasis, although there are limited data on this topic.

In contrast to the negligible effects of high Ca intakes (>threefold above requirement) on the incidence of OC, the incidence of dyschondroplasia lesions in foals fed excessive P (388% NRC level for P, 100% NRC level for Ca, Ca:P ratio: 0.3:1) was significantly higher (clinical or radiological findings of dyschondroplasia: 66%, $N = 6$) than in foals fed the adequate control diet (Savage et al 1993). Excessive P in relation to Ca intake interferes with Ca metabolism as Ca absorption or retention is impaired (Schryver et al 1971, Schryver 1975). This in turn may result in the condition of secondary hyperparathyroidism which may lead to increased osteoporosis and subsequent weakening of the subchondral bone. Beside the absolute Ca and P intake, caution is therefore required with respect to the Ca:P ratio of the diet. Ca:P ratios less than 1:1 should be avoided. The authors recommended optimal Ca:P ratio varies in the range of 1.4:1 up to a maximal range of 3:1.

The influence of the dietary anion–cation balance (DCAB) on Ca and P metabolism has received some attention (Baker et al 1993, Wall et al 1993). Rations with a DCAB less than 100 meq/kg dry matter (DM) are acidogenic and result in an enhanced Ca loss via the kidneys. Prolonged consumption of an acidogenic diet (e.g. high amounts of grains DCAB < 100 meq/kg DM) may lead to demineralization of bone; however, precise data on long-term effects are lacking. It is also possible that diets with an excessive P intake may cause an acidogenic situation as P is a strong ion. However, the roughage-to-concentrate ratio appears to contribute to the acidifying effect. Kienzle et al (2006) observed in adult ponies only negligible urinary pH changes with a low DCAB ration, induced by ammonium chloride added to a roughage-based diet. In comparison, there was a significant decrease in urinary pH when the acidogenic diet was added to a more concentrate-based diet (both adjusted to provide an identical DCAB per kg DM).

Milk is a natural source of high-quality Ca and P for foals. Ca and P concentrations in mare milk are relatively constant (Table 32-2). The diet of the mare has not been shown to affect milk Ca and P concentrations. However, according to the recommendations by NRC (2007), mare's milk will not provide sufficient Ca and P for the foal from the beginning of the second/third month of life and therefore Ca and P supplementation by creep feed or a mineral supplement is strongly recommended in the growing foal. For example, mares milk contains around 1.1 g/Ca/l fresh milk (Table 32-2) leading to an average intake of ~19 g/day (at 18 liter intake for a Warmblood foal) and 0.6 g/P/l with an average intake of 11 g/day (equal to a 1.7 ratio). The NRC (2007) recommends a minimum intake for a 4 month old foal (adult weight 600 kg) of 47 g Ca/day and 26 g P/day. Therefore, supplementation is necessary in order to assure correct levels of intake at the current recommended values.

Table 32-2 Mean Mineral Concentrations (mg/kg) in Mare's Milk

Mineral	Colostrum			Milk (>2nd day of lactation)		
	Mean	25	75	Mean	25	75
		Quartile			*Quartile*	
Ca	878	828	910	1035	858	1190
P	676	420	830	602	410	870
Mg	329	140	302	72	54	90
Na	485	340	520	174	130	200
K	1068	928	1162	659	507	877
Cl				278	245	312
S	1025			241	219	267

Data from literature, Coenen et al 2010.

Concentrates and roughages vary widely in their content of Ca and P. In general, Ca concentrations in forages are much greater than those in cereals grains or legume seeds. Cereal grains and legume seeds in contrast are rich in P, and grain by-products, such as rice bran or wheat bran are especially rich in P (Meyer & Coenen 2002). Availability of Ca and P may vary considerably according to their chemical combination or physical association with other compounds in feedstuffs (Meyer & Coenen 2002). Dicalcium phosphate, and monosodium phosphate are highly available to horses (Hintz & Schryver 1972), and alfalfa provides a higher availability of Ca than grass hay (Cuddeford 1994).

Similar to Ca and P, Mg is an integral part in the skeleton, where the Mg is located in the crystal surface (Broadus 1993). To date, there are no data about the impact of Mg on the incidence of DOD. A Mg deficient diet negatively affected Mg content in the bone ash in foals (Harrington 1975), but no osteochondrotic lesions were reported. Although data about the relation between Mg and DOD are lacking, it is important to note that foal requirements are not met by mare's milk. Therefore Mg supplementation by creep feed, legumes like alfalfa or a mineral supplement is recommended in the growing foal >3 months of age.

Key Points – Ca and P nutrition

- Providing an adequate mineral supply is an important consideration in growing foals.
- As mare milk does not provide sufficient Ca and P for the foal from the beginning of the third month of life, and nutrient intake from grass is variable/unknown, additional minerals should be fed to foals.
- Excessive Ca and P intakes should be avoided (>2-fold of requirement). High Ca intakes may adversely affect the availability of other nutrients and the excess Ca must be eliminated via renal excretion.
- A high P intake (>threefold of requirement with an imbalanced Ca:P ratio <1:1) may promote development of osteochondrosis.

Copper (Cu) and zinc (Zn)

The potential role of dietary Cu in the development of cartilage defects in foals has been intensively investigated (e.g., Knight et al 1990, Pearce et al 1998, van Weeren et al 2003, Gee et al 2007). Based on current information, Cu deficiency does appear to be a factor in the pathogenesis of OC in foals. The possible mechanism is thought to be its action via the enzyme lysyl oxidase, a Cu-dependent enzyme that is necessary for collagen synthesis. Cu deficiency results in defective collagen cross-linking in cartilage lesions (Prockop & Tuderman 1982). Davies et al (1996) in addition suggested that Cu inhibits interleukin-1 activity and thereby protects cartilage from synovial-induced damage.

However, Cu supplementation trials have yielded controversial results. Knight et al (1990) looked at post-mortem cartilage changes in foals at 90 and 180 days of age. Mares were fed either 13 or 32 mg/kg DM Cu during the last 3–6 months of gestation and first 3 months of lactation and the foals were given creep feed with either 15 or 55 mg/kg DM from an undisclosed time point but close to the 90-day cut-off. Foals from the low Cu group had more articular and physeal cartilage abnormalities at 180 days than those from the supplemented group. Lesions of OC were only seen in the unsupplemented group. It is important to note that in this study it was not possible to determine the relative influences of the prepartum and postpartum feeding. In addition, a decrease in the prevalence and severity of OC was reported in association with Cu supplementation (25 mg/kg DM vs. 8 mg/kg DM) of weaned foals (Hurtig et al 1993). While all foals in the low Cu group were affected, only five of nine foals developed clinically significant lesions in the high Cu group. In contrast, dietary Cu levels below 10 mg/kg DM (4.4–8.6 mg/kg DM) were not associated with a higher prevalence of OC in Thoroughbred foals raised at pasture (Pearce et al 1998, Gee et al 2007). This confirms that factors other than Cu intake still influence the incidence of OC.

Cu storage in the fetal liver is of great importance for foals' Cu supply during the early month of growth as there is very little Cu in mare's milk (Cu content in mare's milk: 1st day of lactation: 0.76 mg/l, 14th day of lactation: 0.18 mg/l, Grace et al 1999). Cu supplementation of the lactating mare does not increase Cu concentration in the milk (Pearce et al 1998) and foals do not absorb Cu efficiently from their digestive tract in the first months of life (Meyer et al 1982). Hepatic Cu stores provide the foal with its main Cu source during the early postnatal period, especially in those foals which are fed solely milk diets. Fetal liver Cu concentrations of 300 mg/kg DM (Meyer & Tiegs 1995) and 400 mg/kg DM in the liver of newborn foals are suggested to indicate an adequate Cu intake by the pregnant mare (Meyer & Tiegs 1995, Pearce et al 1998).

A decrease in the prevalence and severity of OC has been reported in association with oral Cu supplementation of mares during gestation (Cu sulfate as a thrice weekly dose, equivalent daily dose 0.5 mg Cu/kg BW, ~25–30 mg/kg DM, Pearce et al 1998b). In addition, mare copper supplementation decreased radiographic indices of physitis in the distal third metatarsal bone of the foals at 150 days. Increased Cu intake of the mare during gestation increased Cu storage in the fetal liver, which may be very important for the development of the growing foal (Pearce et al 1998). In addition, a high Cu content in the foals' liver at birth was associated with an improved repair of OC lesions in the foals stifle between the ages from 5 to 11 months (van Weeren et al 2003). It has therefore been suggested that high liver Cu concentrations in foals at birth may promote repair and resolution of some early cartilage lesions (van Weeren et al 2003). Intramuscular Cu supplementation (250 mg calcium Cu edentate) of the mare during late pregnancy, however, had no effect on the liver Cu levels of the foal at birth or 160 days of age and the prevalence of cartilage defects (Gee et al 2007). Thus, parenteral Cu injections cannot be recommended as an alternative to oral Cu supplementation.

Zn may play a secondary role in the pathophysiology of bone disorders by reducing the absorption of Cu, as Zn competes directly for the same transport mechanisms as Cu in the small intestine (McDowell 2003). Furthermore, Zn may impair Cu absorption indirectly by enriching the level of metallothionein, a protein which binds Cu, thereby limiting the transport rate through mucosal cells (McDowell 2003). Although there are very few studies in horses, it seemed that extremely high Zn intakes are necessary to impair Cu absorption e.g. foals fed Zn diets containing either 29 (control) or 250 mg/kg maintained normal serum Cu and Zn concentrations for 14 to 15 weeks, whereas those fed 1000 or 2000 mg Zn/kg became hypocupremic within 5 to 6 weeks and were lame within 6 weeks, owing to cartilaginous disease characteristic of OC (Bridges & Moffitt 1990). Coger et al (1987) found no differences in apparent Cu absorption or tissue concentrations (liver, kidney or spleen) when feeding weanlings either a diet with 38 mg Zn/kg DM (control) or 1170 mg Zn/kg DM for 90 days. In this study, excessive Zn intake resulted in a decrease in apparent Zn absorption from 89% (control diet) to 6% (high Zn diet) which is thought to be the mechanism to avoid Zn toxicosis. Occasionally, Zn poisoning by industrial exposure (e.g. zinc smelter) has been reported to induce generalized osteochondrotic lesions in foals (Gunson et al 1982). Some authors highlight the importance to formulate a correct Zn:Cu ratio in the ration of growing horses (Ellis 2001, Harris et al 2005). However, an optimal ratio, as for Ca and P, has not been validated for the horse. In general, the Zn:Cu ratio should not be wider than 4:1 to 5:1 (Hintz 1996).

Under practical feeding conditions, Cu concentrations in forages vary in the range of 1 to 50 mg/kg depending on soil factors, plant species, stage of maturity, yield, fertilization management, climate and soil pH (Meyer & Coenen 2002). Cereal grains contain Cu in a more narrow range of between 4 and 8 mg/kg, whereas leguminous seeds generally contain Cu in the range between 15 and 30 mg/kg. Zn concentrations in forages are typically less than 60 mg/kg, cereal grains and legumes contain Zn in the range from 15 to 55 mg/kg, with a mean of 30 mg/kg. However, it must be emphasized that biological availability of Zn in grains and legumes is low, apparently related to the high phytate content which is known to bind Zn.

Key Points – Copper nutrition

- Copper status at birth may influence the repair process of existing osteochondrosis lesions in young foals; therefore, oral Cu supplementation of the pregnant mare is recommended to ensure that Cu intake meets current requirements

- Parenteral supplementation of the mare in late pregnancy has no "protective" effect on the development of osteochondrosis in the foal
- The Cu content of mare's milk is low and is not affected by Cu supplementation of the mare
- The negative impact of Zn on Cu availability does not apply under typical feeding conditions

Other trace elements

The impact of other trace elements such as manganese (Mn) or silicon (Si) on the incidence of OC has received little attention in the horse. For example, Mn is involved in proteoglycan metabolism through glycosyl-transferase, which is important in cartilage metabolism. Furthermore, Mn plays a structural role in linking chondroitin sulfate molecules. Mn deficiency has been implicated, but not confirmed, as a cause of skeletal afflictions in newborn foals (Lewis 1996). In pigs, Mn supplementation above recommendation in combination with Cu reduced overall OC scores (Frantz et al 2008).

Si has been speculated to play a role in cartilage and bone metabolism. Feeding pigs a Si containing supplement reduced the overall OC score (Frantz et al 2008). Si supplementation (sodium zeolite A, ~0.1 g Si/kg BW) of lactating mares raised Si concentration in the milk thereby providing Si to the suckling foal (Lang et al 2001). However, bone metabolism as measured by bone markers in blood was not affected in the foals; information on cartilage metabolism was not evaluated in this study. Currently there is no established Si requirement for horses.

Vitamins

Based on work in other animal species including dogs and pigs (Blair et al 1992, Hazewinkel & Tryfonidou 2002), it cannot be excluded that dietary factors such as hyper- or hypovitaminosis A and hyper- or hypovitaminosis D could be of importance in etiopathogenesis of DOD. Vitamin K may be also important in bone growth as Vitamin K is involved in the regulation of bone formation via osteocalcin and its specific interaction with bone hydroxyapatite. However experimental data are lacking in the growing foal.

Vitamin A

Vitamin A has an essential role in the normal metabolism of bone and possibly cartilage. This is indicated by the fact that low and high vitamin A intakes lead to impaired bone mineral density in humans by unknown mechanisms (Combs 2008). Horses with access to pasture consume large amounts of vitamin A through provitamin A carotenoids, mainly beta-carotene. In horses with no access to pasture, the supplementation of retinyl palmitate is strongly recommended (Greiwe-Crandell et al 1997). In pigs, there is evidence that excessive vitamin A levels in the diet significantly reduced the uronic acid concentration in joint cartilage, indicating a reduced concentration of proteoglycans thereby impairing cartilage stability (Blair et al 1992). Feeding pony fillies with excessive levels of vitamin A (12 000 µg retinol/kg BW for 40 weeks) resulted in a retardation of growth and body weight gain (Donoghue et al 1981), but pathological findings related to DOD were not in the scope of this study. Typical feedstuffs for horses like forages or grains do not contain vitamin A, but vitamin A is derived from these feedstuffs by converting provitamin A carotenoids into vitamin A. In roughages like hay, severe losses of carotene can occur due to adverse harvesting conditions and during storage.

The vitamin A content of mare's milk is a function of two factors: the stage of lactation and the vitamin A status of the mare. High amounts of carotenoids and vitamin A can be found in the colostrum, but in the course of lactation vitamin A levels decrease. Levels of beta-carotene in colostrum were 65 times higher compared to milk collected in late lactation while vitamin A was only 8 times higher (Schweigert & Gottwald 1999).

An adequate supply of carotenoids through feeding fresh grass or a visibly green hay of high quality or the addition of carrots is recommended in the broodmare and in the foal after weaning. Excessive vitamin A intake in the growing foal occurs predominantly through excess provision of vitamin A enriched dietary compound feeds/supplements, whereas the risk of toxicity through excess ingestion of carotenoids is thought to be extremely low.

Vitamin D

In humans and many animal species, the action of vitamin D3 (1,25-dihydroxycholecalciferol) on the skeleton can be summarized as stimulating the mineralization of newly formed osteoid and cartilage, associated with positive effects on intestinal Ca absorption and renal Ca reabsorption (Combs 2008). Hazewinkel and Tryfonidou (2002) highlighted the role of low plasma vitamin D3 concentrations in large breed dogs and the impact on disturbances in endochondral ossification during the rapid growth period. These findings have not been confirmed in foals. Plasma vitamin D3 concentrations for example were not different between OC-positive and OC-negative foals (Sloet van Oldruitenborgh-Oosterbaan et al 1999). In general, vitamin D is not required in the diets of mares and foals that are exposed to sunlight, as vitamin D is produced from sterols in the body by the photolytic action of ultraviolet light on the skin (El Shorafa et al 1979a). In ponies deprived of both sunlight and vitamin D, loss of appetite and difficulty in standing were observed (El Shorafa et al 1979a). However, in another study by the same research group, ponies deprived of vitamin D and sunlight for 5 months showed no changes in Ca metabolism when maintained on a ration providing Ca and P intakes according to the then recommended requirements (El Shorafa et al 1979b). More fundamentally, studies in horses suggest that Ca metabolism might be less regulated by the action of vitamin D (physiological ranges) than in other animal species or in humans (Breidenbach et al 1998).

Milk and forages have low vitamin D concentrations, for example, grass hay and alfalfa contain vitamin D only after harvesting and subsequent drying in the sun.

Nutritional recommendations for avoidance of DOD

In general, energy and nutrients should be supplied according to published recommendations. Some key points with regard to the role of nutrition in helping to reduce the risk of osteochondrosis and other aspects of DOD are summarized in Tables 32-3–32-6.

Table 32-3 Feeding the Mare to Help Reduce the Risk of Developmental Orthopedic Disease

Nutrient	Recommendations
Energy and protein status Conception period	Ensure an adequate roughage intake (minimum 1.5 kg DM hay/100 kg BW), limit starch intake <1 g starch/kg BW per meal. Avoid obesity and overfeeding pre- and during conception. Maintenance requirements (unless mare is in work). Ensure minimum nutrient requirements are met.
1–8 months pregnancy	Ensure an adequate roughage intake (minimum 1.5 kg DM hay/100 kg BW), energy supply must be balanced with correct mineral/vitamin levels (see Table 32-4). Stay within maintenance recommendations if mare is not working or is overweight and needs to lose condition. Limit starch intake to <1 g starch/kg BW per meal. Avoid obesity.
9–11 months pregnancy	Ensure an adequate roughage intake (ad libitum feeding recommended); increase levels of nutrients above maintenance (see Table 32-4). Protein intake must meet current recommendations – ensure good quality protein (essential amino acids provided).
Calcium, phosphorus	Primarily ensure minimum intake requirements of Ca and P are met. Stay within recommended ratios of Ca:P at 1.4:1 to 2:1 (maximum 3:1).
Vitamin D	Generally covered by adequate turn-out and sunlight exposure. If exclusively box housing in winter time, vitamin D supplementation is recommended (see Table 32-4).
Copper and Zinc	Meet current recommendations (Cu intake of mare: 0.25–0.40 mg/kg/BW). Owners should assess mare's ration for Zn intake – excess or deficiency should be avoided. In general, the Zn:Cu ratio should not be wider than 4:1 to 5:1. A ratio of 1:1 is acceptable.

Table 32-4 Energy and Nutrient Requirements of the Pregnant or Lactating Mare According to NRC 2007; DE, Protein and Lysine

	Gestation			Lactation		
	1–6 months	7–8 momths	9–11 months	1–3 months	4–5 months	>5 months
MJ/kg BW						
DE	0.142	0.148	0.155	0.264	0.242	0.228
g/kg BW						
Protein	1.26	1.45	1.56	3.06	2.73	2.53
Lysine	0.059	0.062	0.067	0.168	0.147	0.134
Ca	0.040	0.056	0.072	0.120	0.085	0.075
P	0.029	0.041	0.053	0.076	0.051	0.044
Na	0.020	0.020	0.022	0.026	0.024	0.023
K	0.050	0.050	0.052	0.095	0.071	0.067
Mg	0.015	0.0152	0.0154	0.022	0.021	0.017
Cl	0.080	0.080	0.082	0.091	0.091	0.091
mg/kg BW						
Cu	0.20	0.20	0.25	0.22	0.22	0.22
Zn	0.80	0.80	0.80	1.0	1.0	1.0
Mn	0.80	0.80	0.80	1.0	1.0	1.0
Se	0.002	0.002	0.002	0.0025	0.0025	0.0025
IU/kg BW						
Vitamin A	60	60	60	60	60	60
Vitamin D	6.6	6.6	6.6	6.6	6.6	6.6
Vitamin E	1.6	1.6	1.6	2.0	2.0	2.0

DE = digestible energy
Data from Frape 2010. Equine Nutrition and Feeding. Wiley-Blackwell, Oxford, United Kingdom.

Table 32-5 Feeding the Foal to Minimize Risk of Developmental Orthopedic Disease

Nutrient	Recommendations
Energy status Protein	Always provide access to a high quality roughage (e.g., hay, grass) in addition to milk Creep feeding should be strictly balanced with energy requirement – do not allow free access to broodmare mix from dam. Ensure correct lysine levels and minimum protein requirements (see Table 32-6) are always met.
Ca, P	Primarily ensure minimum intake requirements of Ca and P are met. Stay within the recommended range for the ratio of Ca:P, 1.4:1 to 2:1.
Vitamin D	Generally covered by adequate turn-out and sunlight exposure, exclusively box housing in winter time, vitamin D supplementation is recommended (see Table 32-6).
Copper, zinc	Susceptible foals may benefit from an increased Cu intake to around 0.32 mg/kg BW (around 20 mg/kg DM intake) after weaning. Increase zinc with increased Cu intake – keep ratio around 5:1 – as in keeping with ratio of elements in mare's milk.
Vitamin A	Dry silages and old hays may have low content and therefore require supplementation, otherwise little need for additional provision.

Table 32-6 Energy and Nutrient Requirements of the Growing Foal According to NRC 2007; DE, Protein and Lysine (Data from Frape 2010)

Energy and protein	
DE	
Age 4–5 mo	0.192 MJ × BW
Age 6–11 mo	0.172 MJ × BW
Age 12–18 mo	0.163 MJ × BW
Protein	
Age 0–6 mo	(1.44 g × BW) + (512 g × ADG)
Age > 6 mo	(1.44 g × BW) + (844 g × ADG)
Lysine	
Age 0–6 mo	(0.062 g × BW) + (22 g × ADG)
Age > 6 mo	(0.062 g × BW) + (36 g × ADG)
Major elements	
Ca	(0.072 g × BW) + (32 g × ADG)
P	(0.040 g × BW) + (17.8 g × ADG)
Na	0.025 g × BW
K	(0.05 g × BW) + (3.0 g × ADG)
Mg	(0.015 g × BW) + (1.25 g × ADG)
Cl	
Age 0–5 mo	0.033 g × BW
Age 6–11 mo	0.025 g × BW
Age 12–20 mo	0.023 g × BW
Trace elements	
Cu	0.25 mg × BW
Zn	1.0 mg × BW
Mn	1.0 mg × BW
Se	0.0022 mg × BW
Vitamins	
Vitamin A	45 IU × BW
Vitamin D	20 IU × BW
Vitamin E	2 IU × BW

ADG = Average daily weight gain.

References

Auer, J.A., 2006. Diagnosis and treatment of flexural deformities in foals. Clinical Techniques Equine Practice 5, 282–295.

Auer, J.A., Stick, J.A., 2006. Equine Surgery, third ed. WB Saunders Co., Philadelphia.

Baker, L.A., Wall, D.L., Topliff, D.R., et al., 1993. The effect of dietary cation-anion balance on mineral balance in the anaerobically exercised and sedentary horses. Journal Equine Veterinary Science 13 (10), 557–561.

Billinghurst, R.C., Brama, P.A., van Weeren, P.R., et al., 2004. Evaluation of serum concentrations of biomarkers of skeletal metabolism and results of radiography as indicators of severity of osteochondrosis in foals. American Journal Veterinary Research 65 (2), 143–150.

Blair, R., Aherne, F.X., Doige, C.E., 1992. Tolerance of growing pigs for dietary vitamin A, with special reference to bone integrity. International Journal Vitamin Nutrition Research 62 (2), 130–133.

Breidenbach, A., Schlumbohm, C., Harmeyer, J., 1998. Peculiarities of vitamin D and of the calcium and phosphate homeostatic system in horses. Veterinary Research 29 (2), 173–186.

Bridges, C.H., Moffitt, P.G., 1990. Influence of variable content of dietary zinc on copper metabolism of weanling foals. American Journal Veterinary Research 51 (2), 275–280.

Broadus, A.E., 1993. Physiological functions of calcium, magnesium, and phosphorus and mineral ion balance. In: Favus, M.J. (Ed.), Primer on the Metabolic Bone Diseases and Disorders of Mineral Metabolism. Lippincott Raven Publishers, Philadelphia, pp. 41–46.

Bruin, G., Creemers, J., 1994. Het voorkomen van osteochondrose (Dutch); The occurrence of Osteochondrosis, Praktijkonderzoek Veehouderij, Now: Wageningen University Research.

Charman, R.E., Vasey, J.R., 2008. Surgical treatment of carpal flexural deformity in 72 horses. Australian Veterinary Journal 86 (5), 195–199.

Coenen, M., Kirchhoff, S., Kienzle, E., et al., 2010. An update on basic data fort he factorial calculation of energy and nutrient requirements in lactating mares. Übersichten Tierernährung 38, 91–121.

Coger, L.S., Hintz, H.F., Schryver, H.F., et al., 1987. The effect of high zinc intake on copper metabolism and bone development in growing horses. Proceedings 10th Equine Nutrition Physiology Symposium, Fort Collins, CO. Equine Nutrition and Physiology Society, Savoy, IL, pp. 173–178.

Combs, G.F., 2008. The vitamins. Fundamental Aspects in Nutrition and Health, third ed. Elsevier, New York, pp. 95–180.

Cuddeford, D., 1994. Artificially dehydrated lucerne for horses. Veterinary Record 135 (18), 426–429.

Cymbaluk, N.F., Christison, G.I., Leach, D.H., 1990. Longitudinal growth analysis of horses following limited and ad libitum feeding. Equine Veterinary Journal 22 (3), 198–204.

Davies, M.E., Pasqualicchio, M., Henson, F.M.D., et al., 1996. Effects of copper and zinc on chondrocyte behaviour and matrix turnover. Pferdeheilkunde 12, 367–370.

Donoghue, S., Kronfeld, D.S., Berkowitz, S.J., et al., 1981. Vitamin A nutrition of the equine: growth, serum biochemistry and hematology. Journal Nutrition 111 (2), 365–374.

Ellis, A.D., 2001. Osteochondrosis in relation to feeding. Project report VPa-01-11, 1–79.

El Shorafa, W.M., Feaster, J.P., Ott, E.A., et al., 1979a. Effect of vitamin D and sunlight on growth and bone development of young ponies. Journal Animal Science 48 (4), 882–886.

El Shorafa, W.M., Feaster, J.P., Ott, E.A., et al., 1979b. Plasma calcium, phosphorus, magnesium, alkaline phosphatase and 25-OH vitamin D levels in vitamin D-deprived young ponies. Journal Animal Science 49 (Suppl. 1), 239–240.

Finkler-Schade, C., Enbergs, H., Niess, E., et al., 1996. Analyse der Fütterung von Fohlenstuten und Saugfohlen während der Weideperiode in Westfalen. Pferdeheilkunde 12 (3), 251–256.

Firth, E.C., van Weeren, P.R., Pfeiffer, D.U., et al., 1999. Effect of age, exercise and growth rate on bone mineral density (BMD) in third carpal bone and distal radius of Dutch Warmblood foals with osteochondrosis. Equine Veterinary Journal 31 (Suppl.), 74–78.

Fleming, T.P., 2000. Personal communication. Division of Cell Sciences, School of Biological Sciences, University of Southampton, UK.

Frape, D., 2010. Equine Nutrition and Feeding. Wiley-Blackwell, Oxford, United Kingdom.

Frantz, N.Z., Andrews, G.A., Tokach, M.D., et al., 2008. Effect of dietary nutrients on osteochondrosis lesions and cartilage properties in pigs. American Journal Veterinary Research 69 (5), 617–624.

Gee, E., Davies, M., Firth, E., et al., 2007. Osteochondrosis and copper: histology of articular cartilage from foals out of copper supplemented and non-supplemented dams. Veterinary Journal 173 (1), 109–117.

Gee, E.K., Firth, E.C., Morel, P.C., et al., 2005. Articular / epiphyseal osteochondrosis in Thoroughbred foals at 5 months of age: influences of growth of the foal and prenatal copper supplementation of the dam. New Zealand Veterinary Journal 53 (6), 448–456.

George, L.A., Staniar, W.B., Treiber, K.H., et al., 2009. Insulin sensitivity and glucose dynamics during pre-weaning foal development and in response to maternal diet composition. Domestic Animal Endocrinology 37 (1), 23–29.

Glade, M.J., Belling, T.H., 1986. A dietary etiology for osteochondrotic cartilage. Equine Veterinary Science 6, 151–155.

Glade, M.J., Belling, T.H., 1984. Growth plate cartilage metabolism, morphology and biochemical composition in over- and underfed horses. Growth 48, 473–482.

Glade, M.J., Gupta, S., Reimers, T.J., 1984. Hormonal responses to high and low planes of nutrition in weanling thoroughbreds. Journal Animal Science 59 (3), 658–665.

Grace, N.D., Pearce, S.G., Firth, E.C., et al., 1999. Concentrations of macro- and micro-elements in the milk of pasture-fed thoroughbred mares. Australian Veterinary Journal 77 (3), 177–180.

Graham, P.M., Ott, E.A., Brendemuhl, J.H., et al., 1994. The effect of supplemental lysine and threonine on growth and development of yearling horses. Journal of Animal Science 72 (2), 380–386.

Greiwe-Crandell, K.M., Kronfeld, D.S., Gay, L.S., et al., 1997. Vitamin A repletion in thoroughbred mares with retinyl palmitate or beta-carotene. Journal Animal Science 75 (10), 2684–2690.

Gunson, D.E., Kowalczyk, D.F., Shoop, C.R., et al., 1982. Environmental zinc and cadmium pollution associated with generalized osteochondrosis, osteoporosis, and nephrocalcinosis in horses. Journal American Veterinary Medical Association 180 (3), 295–299.

Harrington, D.D., 1975. Influence of magnesium deficiency on horse foal tissue concentraion of Mg, calcium and phosphorus. British Journal of Nutrition 34 (1), 45–57.

Harris, P., Staniar, W., Ellis, A.D., 2005. Effect of exercise and diet on the incidence of DOD. In: Juliand, V., Martin-Rosset, W. (Eds.), The growing horse: nutrition and prevention of growth disorders, EAAP publication No. 114. Wageningen Academic Publishers, Wageningen, pp. 273–290.

Hazewinkel, H.A., Tryfonidou, M.A., 2002. Vitamin D3 metabolism in dogs. Molecular Cell Endocrinology 197 (1–2), 23–33.

Henson, F.M., Davenport, C., Butler, L., et al., 1997. Effects of insulin and insulin-like growth factors I and II on the growth of equine fetal and neonatal chondrocytes. Equine Veterinary Journal 29 (6), 441–447.

Hintz, H.F., 1996. Mineral requirements of growing horses. Pferdeheilkunde 12 (3), 303–306.

Hintz, H.F., Schryver, H.F., 1972. Availability to ponies of calcium and phosphorus from various supplements. Journal Animal Science 34 (6), 979–980.

Hurtig, M.B., Green, S.L., Dobson, H., et al., 1993. Correlative study of defective cartilage and bone growth in foals fed a low-copper diet. Equine Veterinary Journal 16 (Suppl.), 66–73.

Jeffcott, L., 2005. Developemental diseases affecting growing horses. In: Juliand, V., Martin-Rosset, W. (Eds.), The growing horse: nutrition and prevention of growth disorders, EAAP publication No. 114. Wageningen Academic Publishers, Wageningen, pp. 243–255.

Jeffcott, L., Henson, F.M., 1998. Studies on growth cartilage in the horse and their application to aetiopathogenesis of dyschondroplasia (osteochondrosis). Veterinary Journal 156 (3), 177–192.

Jelan, Z.A., Jeffcott, L.B., Lundeheim, N., et al., 1996. Growth rates in Thoroughbred foals. Pferdeheilkunde 3, 291–295.

Kienzle, E., Stürmer, K., Ranz, D., et al., 2006. A high roughage/concentrate ratio decreases the effect of ammonium chloride on acid-base balance in horses. Journal Nutrition 136 (7 Suppl.), 2048S–2049S.

Knight, D.A., Gabel, A.A., Reed, S.M., et al., 1985. Correlations of dietary minerals to incidence and severity of metabolic bone disease in Ohio and Kentucky. Proceedings 31th Annual Convention American Association Equine Practitioners. American Association of Equine Practitioners, Lexington, KY, pp. 445–461.

Knight, D.A., Weisbrode, S.E., Schmall, L.M., et al., 1990. The effects of copper supplementation on the prevalence of cartilage lesions in foals. Equine Veterinary Journal 22 (6), 426–432.

Komm, K., 2010. Fine mapping of quantitative trait loci (QTL) for osteochondrosis in Hanoverian warmblood horses on equine chromosomes (ECA) 2 and 4. Hannover, Tierärztliche Hochschule, Dissertation.

Kwong, W.Y., Wild, A.E., Roberts, P., et al., 2000. Maternal undernutrition during the preimplantation period of rat development causes blastocyst abnormalities and programming of postnatal hypertension. Development 127 (19), 4195–4202.

Lampe, V., Dierks, C., Komm, K., et al., 2009. Identification of a new quantitative trait locus on equine chromosome 18 responsible for osteochondrosis in Hanoverian warmblood horses. Journal Animal Science 87 (11), 3477–3481.

Lang, K.J., Nielsen, B.D., Waite, K.L., et al., 2001. Supplemental silicon increases plasma and milk silicon concentrations in horses. Journal Animal Science 79 (10), 2627–2633.

Lepeule, J., Bareille, N., Robert, C., et al., 2009. Association of growth, feeding practices and exercise conditions with the prevalence of Developmental Orthopaedic Disease in limbs of French foals at weaning. Preventive Veterinary Medicine 89 (3–4), 167–177.

Lewis, L.D., 1996. Feeding and Care of the Horse. Lippincott Williams & Wilkins, Philadelphia.

Lloyd-Bauer, P.M., Fretz, P.B., 1989. Correction of acquired flexural deformity by deep digital flexor tenotomy in a miniature horse. Canadian Veterinary Journal 30 (7), 585–589.

Marshall, M., 2007. Developmental orthopaedic disease in Thoroughbred foals an epidemiological comparison between a stud in Ireland and a stud

in Australia. PhD Thesis, Faculty of Veterinary Science, University of Sydney, Australia.
Mayhew, I.G., Watson, A.C., Heissan, J.A., 1978. Congenital occipitoatlanto-axial malformations in the horse. Equine Veterinary Journal 10, 103–113.
McDowell, L.R., 2003. Minerals in animal and human nutrition, first ed. Elsevier Science BV, Amsterdam Netherlands, pp. 33–100.
McIlwraith, C.W., 2001. Developmental orthopaedic disease (DOD) in horses – A multifactorial process. Proceedings of the 17th Equine Nutrition and Physiology Society, Lexington, Kentucky, May 31–June 2 2001. Equine Nutrition and Physiology Society, Savoy, IL, pp. 2–23.
Meyer, H., Schmidt, M., Lindemann, G., et al., 1982. Prececal and postileal digestibility of elements (Ca, P, Mg) and trace elements (Cu, Zn, Mn) in the horse. Fortschritte in Tierphysiologie Tierernährung 13, 61–69.
Meyer, H., Coenen, M., 2002. Pferdefütterung. Parey Buchverlag, Berlin.
Meyer, H., Tiegs, W., 1995. Cu-Gehalte in der Leber von Foeten und neugeborenen. Fohlen. Pferdeheilkunde 11, 5–11.
Moghaddam, E., Vogt, J.A., Wolever, T.M., 2006. The effects of fat and protein on glycemic responses in nondiabetic humans vary with waist circumference, fasting plasma insulin, and dietary fiber intake. Journal Nutrition 136 (10), 2506–2511.
NRC National Research Council., 2007. Nutrient Requirements of Horses, sixth ed revised. National Academy of Sciences, Washington DC.
Ott, E.A., Asquith, A.L., Feaster, J.P., 1981. Lysine supplementation of diets for yearling horses. Journal of Animal Science 53 (6), 1496–1503.
Ott, E.A., Asquith, R.L., 1986. Influence of level of feeding and nutrient content of the concentrate on growth and development of yearling horses. Journal of Animal Science 62 (2), 290–299.
Ott, E.A., Brown, M.P., Roberts, G.D., et al., 2005. Influence of starch intake on growth and skeletal development of weanling horses. Journal Animal Science 83 (5), 1033–1043.
Pagan, J.D., Geor, R.J., Caddel, S.E., et al., 2001. The relationship between glycaemic response and the incidence of OCD in Thoroughbred weanlings: A field study. American Association Equine Practitioners 47, 322–325.
Pearce, S.G., Firth, E.C., Grace, N.D., et al., 1998a. Effect of copper supplementation on the evidence of developmental orthopaedic disease in pasture-fed New Zealand Thoroughbreds. Equine Veterinary Journal 30 (3), 211–218.
Pearce, S.G., Grace, N.D., Firth, E.C., et al., 1998b. Effect of copper supplementation on the copper status of pasture-fed young Thoroughbreds. Equine Veterinary Journal 30 (3), 204–210.
Pearce, S.G., Firth, E.C., Grace, N.D., et al., 1998c. Effect of copper supplementation on the evidence of developmental orthopaedic disease in pasture-fed New Zealand Thoroughbreds. Equine Veterinary Journal 30 (3), 211–218.
Pool, R.R., 1993. Difficulties in definition of equine osteochondrosis; differentiation of developmental and acquired lesion. Equine Veterinary Journal 16 (Suppl.), 5–12.
Prockop, D.J., Tuderman, L., 1982. Posttranslational enzymes in the biosynthesis of collagen: extracellular enzymes. Methods Enzymology 82 (Pt A), 305–319.
Ralston, S.L., 1996. Hyperglycemia/hyperinsulinemia after feeding a meal of grain to young horses with osteochondrosis dissecans (OCD) lesions. Pferdeheilkunde 3, 320–322.
Rejnö, S., Strömberg, B., 1978. Osteochondrosis in the horse. II. Pathology. Acta Radiologica 358 (Suppl.), 153–178.
Richardson, D.C., Zentek, J., 1998. Nutrition and osteochondrosis. Veterinary Clinics North America Small Animal Practice 28 (1), 115–135.
Ropp, J.K., Raub, R.H., Minton, J.E., 2003. The effect of dietary energy source on serum concentration of insulin-like growth factor-I growth hormone, insulin, glucose, and fat metabolites in weanling horses. Journal Animal Science 81 (6), 1581–1589.
Saastamoinen, M.T., 1996. Protein, amino acid and energy requirements of weanling foals and yearlings. Pferdeheilkunde 3, 297–302.
Sandgren, B., Dalin, G., Carlsten, J., et al., 1993. Development of osteochondrosis in the tarsocrural joint and osteochondral fragments in the fetlock joints of Standardbred trotters. II Body measurements and clinical findings. Equine Veterinary Journal 16 (Suppl.), 48–53.
Stashak, T.S., 2001. Adams Lameness in Horses. Lippincott Williams & Wilkins, Philadelphia.
Savage, C.J., McCarthy, R.N., Jeffcott, L.B., 1993a. Effects of dietary energy and protein on induction of dyschondroplasia in foals. Equine Veterinary Journal 16 (Suppl.), 74–79.
Savage, C.J., McCarthy, R.N., Jeffcott, L.B., 1993b. Effects of dietary phosphorus and calcium on induction of dyschondroplasia in foals. Equine Veterinary Journal 16 (Suppl.), 80–83.
Schweigert, F.J., Gottwald, C., 1999. Effect of parturition on levels of vitamins A and E and of beta-carotene in plasma and milk of mares. Equine Veterinary Journal 31 (4), 319–323.
Schryver, H.F., 1975. Intestinal absorption of calcium and phosphorus by horses. Journal South African Veterinary Association 46 (1), 39–45.
Schryver, H.F., Hintz, H.F., Lowe, J.E., 1971. Calcium and phosphorus inter-relationships in horse nutrition. Equine Veterinary Journal 3 (3), 102–109.
Schryver, H.F., Meakim, D.W., Lowe, J.E., et al., 1987. Growth and calcium metabolism in horses fed varying levels of protein. Equine Veterinary Journal 19 (4), 280–287.
Sloet van Oldruitenborgh-Oosterbaan, M.M., Mol, J.A., Barneveld, A., 1999. Hormones, growth factors and other plama variables in relation to osteochondrosis. Equine Veterinary Journal 31 (Suppl.), 45–54.
Staniar, W.B., Kronfeld, D.S., Wilson, J.A., et al., 2001. Growth of thoroughbreds fed a low-protein supplement fortified with lysine and threonine. Journal Animal Science 79 (8), 2143–2151.
Staniar, W.B., Kronfeld, D.S., Akers, R.M., et al., 2007. Insulin-like growth factor I in growing thoroughbreds. Journal Animal Physiology Animal Nutrition 91 (9–10), 390–399.
Sticker, L.S., Thompson, D.L. Jr, Gentry, L.R., 2001. Pituitary hormone and insulin responses to infusion of amino acids and N-methyl-D,L-aspartate in horses. Journal Animal Science 79 (3), 735–744.
Stock, K.F., Hamann, H., Distl, O., 2005. Prevalence of osseous fragments in distal and proximal interphalangeal, metacarpo- and metatarsophalangeal and tarsocrural joints of Hanoverian Warmblood horses. Journal Veterinary Medicine Series A Physiology Pathology Clincal Medicine 52 (8), 388–394.
Thompson, K.N., Jackson, S.G., Baker, J.P., 1988. The influence of high planes of nutrition on skeletal growth and development of weanling horses. Journal Animal Science 66 (10), 2459–2467.
Treiber, K.H., Boston, R.C., Kronfeld, D.S., et al., 2005. Insulin resistance and compensation in Thoroughbred weanlings adapted to high-glycemic meals. Journal Animal Science 83 (10), 2357–2364.
Van Tilburg, E.M., Ellis, A.D., 2002. Growth rates in Dutch Warmblood horses in relation to osteochondrosis. In: 53rd Proceedings of the European Association of Animal Science, p. 158.
van Weeren, P.R., 2006. Osteochondrosis. In: Auer, J.A., Stick, J.A. (Eds.), Equine Surgery, third ed, Saunders Elsevier, St. Loius, Missouri, pp. 1166–1178.
van Weeren, P.R., Barnefeld, A., 1999. The effect of exercise on the distribution and manifestation of osteochondrotic lesions in the Warmblood foal. Equine Veterinary Journal 31 (Suppl.), 16–25.
van Weeren, P.R., Knaap, J., Firth, E.C., 2003. Influence of liver copper status of mare and newborn foal on the development of osteochondrotic lesions. Equine Veterinary Journal 35 (1), 67–71.
Vervuert, I., Winkelsett, S., Christmann, L., et al., 2007. Evaluation of the influences of exercise, birth date, and osteochondrosis on plasma bone marker concentrations in Hanoverian Warmblood foals. American Journal Veterinary Research 68 (12), 1319–1323.
Vervuert, I., Coenen, M., Borchers, A., et al., 2002. Growth rates and the incidence of osteochondrotic lesions in Hanoverian Warmblood foals. Preliminary data. Proceedings Equine Nutrition Conference Antwerp, Belgium, 21–25 August 2002, p. 39.
Verwilghen, D.R., Vanderheyden, L., Franck, T., et al., 2009. Variations of plasmatic concentrations of Insulin-like Growth Factor-I in post-pubescent horses affected with developmental osteochondral lesions. Veterinary Research Community 33 (7), 701–709.
Voute, L.C., Henson, F.M., Platt, D., et al., 2011. Osteochondrosis lesions of the lateral trochlear ridge of the distal femur in four ponies. Vet Rec 12:168 (10), 265.
Wall, D.L., Topliff, D.R., Freeman, D.W., et al., 1993. The effect of dietary cation-anion balance on mineral balance in the anaerobically exercised horse. Thirteenth Symposium Equine Nutrition Physiology Society, Gainesville, FL. Equine Nutrition and Physiology Society, Savoy, IL, pp. 50–55.
Williams, J.A., Collier, M.A., Ross, M.W., 1982. Physitis in the horse. Modern Veterinary Practice 63, 407–413.
Williams, C.A., Kronfeld, D.S., Staniar, W.B., et al., 2001. Plasma glucose and insulin responses of Thoroughbred mares fed a meal high in starch and sugar or fat and fiber. Journal of Animal Science 79 (8), 2196–2201.
Winkelsett, S., Vervuert, I., Granel, M., et al., 2005. Feeding practice in Warmblood mares and foals and the incidence to osteochondrosis. Pferdeheilkunde 21 (21), 124–127.
Wittwer, C., Hamann, H., Distl, O., 2009. The candidate gene XIRP2 at a quantitative gene locus on equine chromosome 18 associated with osteochondrosis in fetlock and hock joints of South German Coldblood horses. J Heredity 100 (4), 481–486.
Wittwer, C., Hamann, H., Rosenberger, E., et al., 2006. Prevalence of osteochondrosis in the limb joints of South German Coldblood horses. Journal Veterinary Medicine Series A Physiology Pathology Clinical Medicine 53 (10), 531–539.
Ytrehus, B., Carlson, C.S., Ekman, S., 2007. Etiology and pathogenesis of osteochondrosis. Veterinary Pathology 44 (4), 429–448.

33

Oral joint supplements in the management of osteoarthritis

C. Wayne McIlwraith

Introduction

Osteoarthritis (OA) is the single most common cause of lameness in horses (Clegg & Booth 2000) and in one survey, approximately 60% of lameness problems in horses were related to OA (Caron & Genovese 2003). Similarly OA is the most common form of human arthritis, affecting at least 20 million Americans and with its prevalence expected to double over the next two decades (Helmick et al 2008, Lawrence et al 2008). OA involves a complex interaction of biologic and pathologic processes highlighted by eventual degradation of articular cartilage (McIlwraith 1996, 2005). With the US horse population currently estimated to be 7.3 million (AVMA 2007), this means millions of horses currently have this debilitating musculoskeletal condition. Multiple conventional therapies are available for treating OA with the goal of preventing further degradation while restoring function (McIlwraith 2005, Trumble 2005).

Oral joint supplements (OJSs) are a common choice of clients, and have been perceived as a benign treatment for OA in horses (Trumble 2005). The high prevalence of OA in combination with the lack of a definitive cure for OA has probably contributed to the popularity of OJSs among owners, veterinarians, and trainers. These supplements, according to recent market surveys, are the most popular type of nutritional supplements for horses and account for approximately 1/3 (34%) of all equine supplement sales, 1/2 of all pet supplements sold in the US for equine consumption and it is estimated that 49% of all horse owners purchase and administer some form of dietary supplement in their horses (Packaged Facts 2008). In a study of feeding practices in 3-day event horses, the authors found that horses were supplemented with an average of four different oral products daily including electrolytes, plain salt and OJSs (Burk & Williams 2008).

Indications for OJSs

Oral joint supplements are fed to horses for one of two purposes: (1) to treat the lame or make chronically unsound horses sound or (2) to prevent or delay the development of joint problems. The first instance is flawed because often the source of lameness is never diagnosed when the owner or trainer elects to use these oral supplements without consulting a veterinarian. The second premise is hard to disprove but is the basis for high usage of both licensed drugs such as intramuscular Adequan™ and intravenous Legend™, as well as OJSs.

The critical components of articular cartilage are type II collagen fibrils (which provide a structural framework) and extracellular matrix (ECM), which consists of aggrecan molecules and water (Fig. 33.1). The aggrecan molecule consists of aggregations of proteoglycan molecules on a hyaluronan (HA) backbone. The proteoglycan molecule, in turn, consists of a protein backbone with chondroitin sulfate and keratin sulfate side chains. These carry negative charges and due to repulsion as well as some attraction of water provide the compressive resistance to the articular cartilage (McIlwraith 2005). Maintenance of these molecules is critical and some nutraceuticals provide potential building blocks for these molecules. The osteoarthritic process is associated with multiple deleterious mediators from inflamed synovial membrane and trauma as well as being released to initiate a cascade of degradation in the articular cartilage. Interleukin 1 (IL-1) is considered a major cytokine initiating this cascade and this can influence other cells to cause increased release of metalloproteinases, aggrecanase and prostaglandin E_2 (PGE_2). While this negative process can be influenced by certain nutraceuticals in vitro (Fig. 33.2) there is less certainty about their effects in vivo after undergoing digestion.

In 2005 nutraceutical sales reached more than 1 billion for companion animals, and that number was expected to double in the next 3 years. There are more than 100 equine nutraceutical products currently on the market in the US, and such products are used worldwide. This is a disturbing trend for an industry that for the most part, is unregulated by the FDA or other governing bodies, and has weak in vivo scientific basis (Oke & McIlwraith 2008).

Types of OJSs

The majority of joint supplements include glucosamine and/or chondroitin sulfate along with other added ingredients. Historically, the first products available for the horse

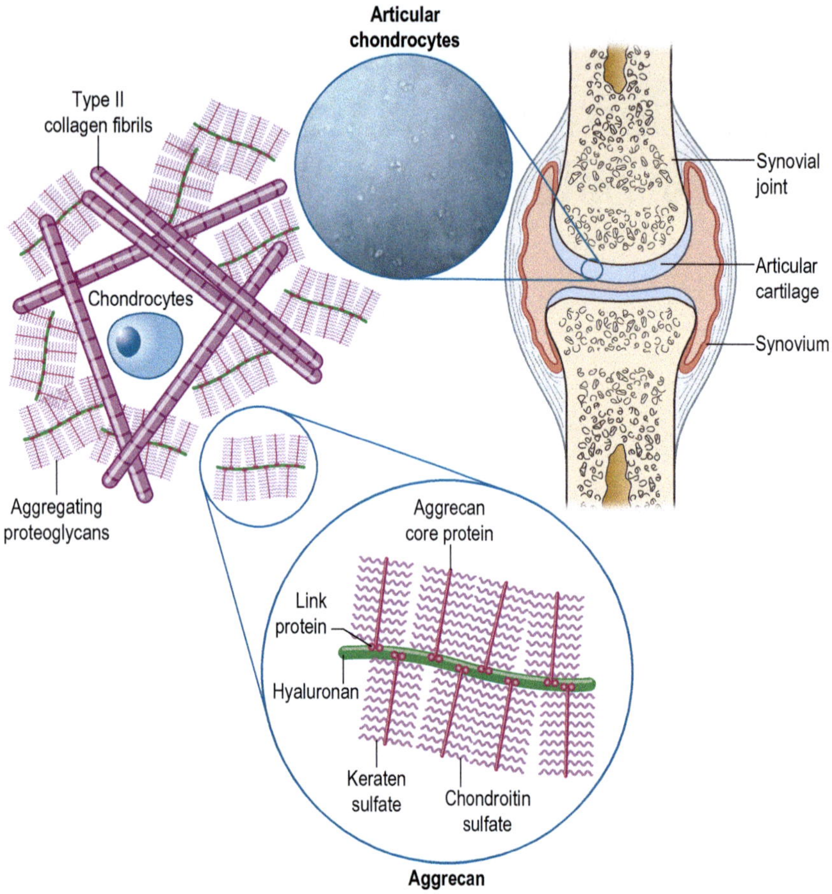

Figure 33.1 A schematic depiction of articular cartilage. The left panel shows the major components including chondrocytes, type II collagen fibrils and aggregating proteoglycans (aggrecans). The aggrecan structure is shown in the bottom panel.

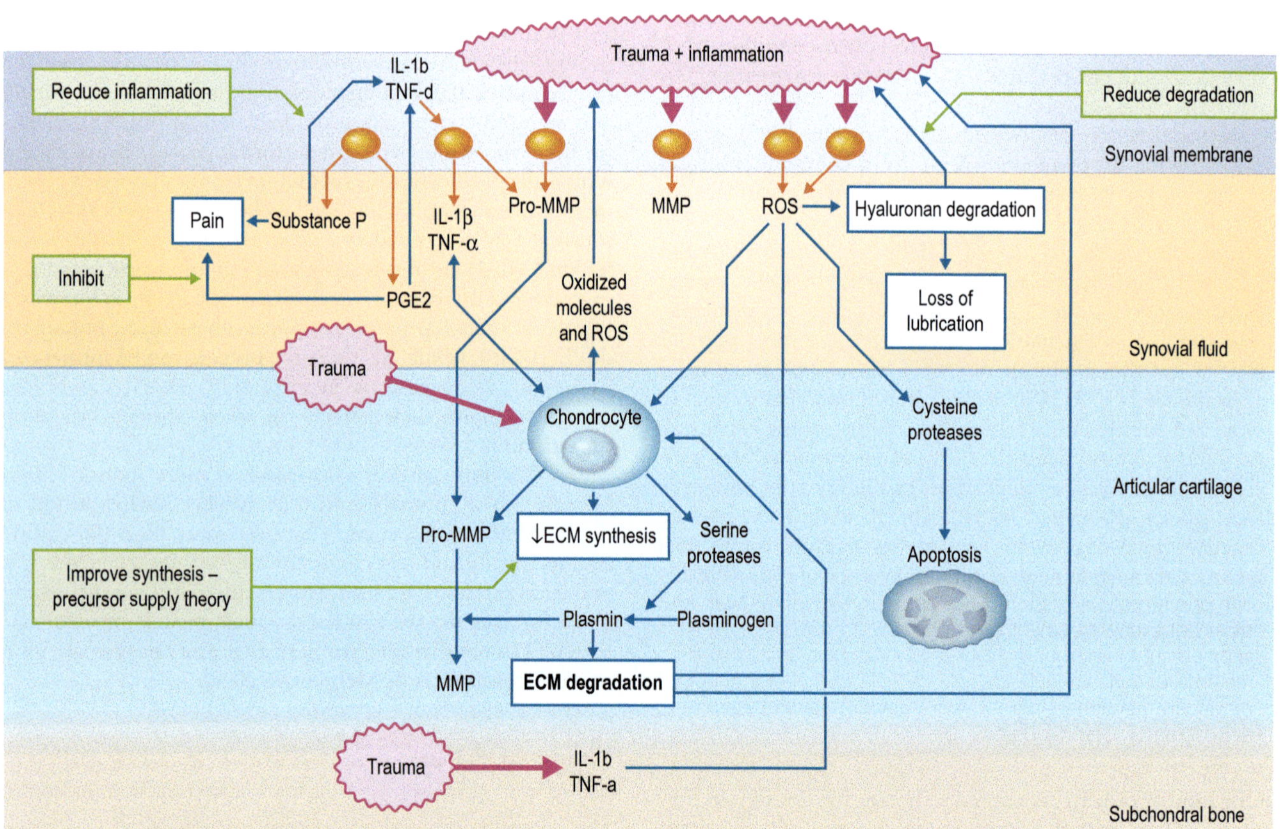

Figure 33.2 A schematic outlining the mechanisms for development of osteoarthritis and the possible mechanisms of action for oral joint supplements in mitigating these processes.

included a chondroitin sulfate product from bovine trachea and a complex of glycosaminoglycans and other nutrients from the sea mussel, *Perna canaliculus*. Glucosamine (GU) is an amino monosaccharide and is the principal component of O-linked and N-linked glycosaminoglycans, and is produced in the body by the addition of amino groups to glucose; this molecule is subsequently acetylated to acetyl glucosamine. Hyaluronan (HA) keratan sulfate and heparan sulfate are composed in part of repeating units of acetyl glucosamine. Chondroitin sulfate (CS) consists of alternating disaccharide units of glucuronic acid and sulfated *N*-acetyl galactosamine molecules and is a principal glycosaminoglycan of aggregating proteoglycan (aggrecan).

Many OJSs have GU and CS as principal components, and may contain additional ingredients including manganese, vitamin C, hyaluronan (hyaluronic acid or HA), polyunsaturated fatty acids (PUFAs), rare earth mineral supplements, unsaponified avocado soy (ASU), cetylmyristoleate, methylsulfonylmethane, and various herbs. With the exception of the latter two (no good equine documentation available), these various products will be discussed below. Box 33.1 discusses the terminology and regulatory issues involved in the use of OSJs.

Glucosamine and/or chondroitin sulfate

Mechanisms of action and in vitro studies

In vitro studies have investigated the effects of glucosamine and CS, individually or in combination, but of course, differ greatly in the source of products, as well as dosages used, in vitro study conditions and responses measured (Dechant & Baxter 2007). Glucosamine and/or CS are thought to counteract cartilage degradation (Sandy et al 1998, Fenton et al 2000, 2002, Grande et al 2000, Lippiello et al 2000, 2002, Nerucci et al 2000, Orth et al 2002, Ilic et al 2003, Mello et al 2004, Dechant et al 2005, Neil et al 2005b) by inhibiting degradative enzymes such as collagenase and aggrecanase (Wright 2001, Lippiello et al 2002, Orth et al 2002, Mello et al 2004, Chan et al 2005), and intermediary mediators, such as nitric oxide, prostaglandin E_2 and nuclear factor kappa B (Bassleer et al 1998a, Fenton et al 2000, 2002, Orth et al 2002, Byron et al 2003, Dodge et al 2005, Largo et al 2003, Mello et al 2004, Nakamura et al 2004, Schlueter et al 2004, Neil et al 2005b). Synthesis of ECM components is thought to be stimulated in the presence of GU and/or CS (Bassleer et al

Box 33.1 Terminology and Regulatory Issues in the Use of Oral Joint Supplements (a US Perspective)

The term nutraceutical was adopted in veterinary medicine from the medical profession and refers to compounds that are neither nutrients nor pharmaceuticals by combining the words "nutrients" (nourishing food or food component) with "pharmaceuticals" (medical drug) (Duren 2005). The nutraceutical category describes a broad list of products sold including nutrients, dietary supplements, functional foods and phytochemicals (including herbs) that are not recognized by the US Food and Drug Administration (FDA) as food or drugs and are intended for the treatment or prevention of disease. The difference between a feed and a nutraceutical is that a nutraceutical is unlikely to have an established nutritive value. Feeds are required to have nutritive value and are accountable, by labeling, for these values. Oral joint supplements fall in between food and drugs and have advantages over either because they are not required to list ingredients or nutrient profiles as required by feeds, and in many cases, intended to treat or prevent disease without first undergoing proper drug approval (Duren 2005).

A supplement was initially defined legally by the Federal Food, Drug and Cosmetic Act (FFDCA), but this was amended in 1994 by the Dietary Supplement Health Education Act (DSHEA). Technically, the DSHEA only covers human products and defines a dietary supplement as a product intended to supplement the diet and contains at least one or more of the following: a vitamin; a mineral; an herb or other botanical; an amino acid; a dietary substance for use to supplement the diet by increasing intakes; or a concentrate, metabolite, constituent, extract or combination of any of the previously mentioned ingredients (McIlwraith 2004). The jurisdiction of veterinary products is primarily the responsibility of the North American Veterinary Nutraceutical Council (NAVNC), which was formed in 1996 to promote and enhance the further quality, safety and long-term effectiveness of nutraceuticals used in veterinary medicine (Trumble 2005). The NAVNC has defined a veterinary nutraceutical as a "non-drug substance that is produced in a purified or extracted form and administered orally to provide agents required for normal bone and body structure and function with the intent of improving the health and well-being of animals" (Booth 2004).

The DSHEA allows manufacturers to make claims with regard to health, structure or function, and nutrient content of a nutraceutical. The Center for Veterinary Medicine allows products to be marketed as nutraceuticals provided they do not claim to treat, cure, or mitigate disease (Trumble 2005); hence, the common practice of advertising of improving joint "health". The FDA perceives veterinary nutraceuticals as unapproved drugs; however, even though they are not labeled or marketed as drugs. The FDA does not regulate these products unless they become unsafe or have labels that claim a drug use and, therefore, there is no requirement to prove safety or efficacy of a nutraceutical. It is the author's opinion that there are two principal issues faced with this regulation: (1) The issue is sufficiently low on the FDA radar screen that there is very little attention paid to it, and (2) There is hardly an incentive for a manufacturer of a nutraceutical to prove efficacy, as such research costs money and a negative result could hurt sales (McIlwraith 2004).

Manufacturers do not have to register themselves or their supplements with the FDA. In general a manufacturer has to comply with the FDA Ingredient Recognition Program, which entails applying for complete ingredient definitions as described by not-for-profit organization of state and federal feed regulators, the Association of American Feed Control Officials (AAFCO) (McIlwraith 2004). There are no requirements of Good Manufacturing Practices (GMPs) for manufactures to guarantee high-quality and batch-to-batch consistency (Oke & McIlwraith 2008) and because there is no post-production monitoring of veterinary nutritional supplements, a myriad of poor quality supplements are available (Oke et al 2006).

1998a,b, Nerucci et al 2000, Noyszewski et al 2001, Lippiello 2003, Dechant et al 2005) by provision of substrate, which may be deficient through dilution or hypermetabolic states (Lippiello 2003); upregulation of gene expression (Grande et al 2000, Dodge & Jimenez 2003); stimulation of cellular receptors and cellular signaling mechanisms, such as CD44 involved in positive feedback (Bassleer et al 1998a, Esford et al 1998, Platt 2001); and inhibition of negative intermediary messengers, such as nuclear factor kappa B, nitric oxide and prostaglandin E_2 (PGE_2) (Bassleer et al 1998a, Fenton et al 2000, 2002, Orth et al 2002, Largo et al 2003, Mello et al 2004, Nakamura et al 2004, Schlueter et al 2004).

The *Precursor Supply Theory* is the most popular explanation regarding the apparent beneficial effects of GU in OA (Oke & Weese 2006). In this theory it is proposed that GU supplies excess basic building blocks for the synthesis of cartilage glycosaminoglycans (GAG) (Fenton et al 2000, Laverty et al 2005, Kelly 1998) and/or bypasses rate-limiting steps in GAG synthesis (Fenton et al 2000, Trumble 2005). In addition, these structure-modifying agents appear to counteract inflammation primarily through their inhibition of intermediate messengers, such as nuclear factor kappa B, nitric oxide and PGE_2 (Bassleer et al 1998a, Fenton et al 2000, 2002, Orth et al 2002, Largo et al 2003, Mello et al 2004, Nakamura et al 2004, Schlueter et al 2004, Neil et al 2005b), that mediate inflammatory responses, in addition to their previously described antianabolic and procatabolic effects. However, these structure-modifying agents have not been found to directly inhibit cyclooxygenase (COX) enzymes, in contrast to many antiarthritic medications (Seaver & Smith 2004). CS has also been shown to affect cell-based inflammatory events by inhibiting chemotaxis, reducing phagocytosis and lysozyme release, and protecting cell membranes from free radical injury (Ronca et al 1998).

It has been pointed out by Dechant and Baxter (2007) that the dosages used to determine the effects of GU and CS on cartilage metabolism in in vitro studies have varied from physiological (μg/ml) to pharmacological (mg/ml) concentrations. Depending on the study, beneficial effects have been reported for dosages as low as 10 μg/ml to as high as 25 mg/ml. Some studies have compared combination treatments to glucosamine or CS alone (Grande et al 2000, Lippiello et al 2000, Orth et al 2002, Dechant et al 2005). Combinations of GU and CS were considered to be the most effective in these studies (Grande et al 2000, Lippiello et al 2000, Orth et al 2002, Dechant et al 2005) and although synergy was suggested by some authors (Lippiello et al 2000), the effect tended to be additive and not synergistic (Dechant & Baxter 2007).

The effects of varying doses of GU and CS alone and in combination on cartilage metabolism in normal and recombinant IL-1α conditioned equine articular cartilage has been evaluated in the author's laboratory using equine cartilage explants (Dechant et al 2005). Articular cartilage explants were allocated randomly to treatment with four doses of GU, CS, or GU + CS in the absence of IL-1 (normal explants) for treatment with four dosages of GU, CS, or GU + CS in the presence of 40 mg/ml recombinant IL-1α (Gibco-Light Technologies, Grand Island, NY, USA) (IL-1 conditioned explants). The patented joint supplements used were SCH-G49GU and TRH122 low molecular weight sodium (Nutramax Laboratories, Edgewood, MD, USA). The treatment groups investigated for both normal and IL-1 conditioned explants were: treatment without GU or CS; four GU concentrations, 12.5, 25, 125 and 250 μg/ml; four CS concentrations, 12.5, 25, 125 and 250 μg/ml; and four GU + CS concentrations 12.5, 25, 125 and 250 μg/ml each of GU and CS (in a 1:1 ratio by concentration). There was no significant negative effect of GU, CS, or GU + CS on normal cartilage explant metabolism. In normal (no IL-1) explants, the most substantial effects observed with the GU, CS and GU + CS treatment were in reducing GAG degradation, without evidence for an advantage of GU + CS compared to GU or CS alone. On the other hand, the highest dosage of GU + CS was more effective than all other treatments in reducing GAG degradation in IL-1 conditioned explants. The ability of GU and CS to protect against cartilage matrix degradation in osteoarthritic and stimulated chondrocytes in cartilage explants have been observed in other in vitro studies (Sandy et al 1998, Fenton et al 2000, 2002, Grande et al 2000, Lippiello 2000, 2002, Nerucci et al 2000, Orth et al 2002, Byron et al 2003). It was also noted that the higher doses of test ingredients (125 and 250 μg/ml) tended to be more effective than the lower dosages (Dechant et al 2005) and these dosage ranges were within the ranges of other in vitro studies. It has been pointed out that high dosages of GU such as 6.5 and 25 mg/ml have been shown to have detrimental effects on cartilage metabolism and chondrocyte viability in studies using bovine articular cartilage explants (De Mattei et al 2002).

Key Points

- Purported mechanisms explaining the role for glucosamine (GU) in osteoarthritis are: (1) provision of substrate for synthesis of cartilage glycosaminoglycans (*precursor supply theory*); and (2) mediation of inflammatory responses
- Chondroitin sulfate (GS) is thought to counteract cartilage inflammatory responses
- There is *in vitro* evidence that GU and CS protect against cartilage matrix degradation

Bioavailability and pharmacokinetics

The obvious flaw with in vitro studies of oral OJSs is that products are tested before undergoing any modification through digestion and absorption. A recent study in which a simulated digestion protocol with ultrafiltration and before testing on cartilage inflammation has been described to test the potential anti-inflammatory and chondroprotective properties of New Zealand green lipped mussel, abalone and shark cartilage (Pearson et al 2007). In this paper the authors showed that shark cartilage in New Zealand green lipped mussels significantly inhibited IL-1-induced PGE_2 synthesis and IL-1-induced GAG release using this useful model for evaluating dietary nutraceuticals in vitro but having the components predigested before testing.

The efficacy of orally administered GU and/or CS depends on the absorption of an oral dose to a sufficient extent to attain therapeutic blood and tissue levels. Studies have also suggested that GU and CS exhibit a high degree of trophism for articular cartilage (Ronca et al 1998, Dodge et al 2005), which means that blood levels may not equate to tissue levels; however, in the absence of good in vivo efficacy studies in the horse, oral bioavailability in the horse provide an important means of extrapolating of results from in vitro studies to the in vivo situation by providing some prediction of fluid and tissue concentrations for GU and CS after oral dosing.

In horses, the oral absorption of 8.0 and 16.9 kDa molecular weight CS was compared because in vitro studies suggested that molecular weight of CS was negatively associated with its permeability across the gastrointestinal tract (Adebowale et al 2000). The oral bioavailability of 8.0 kDa CS was 32% compared to 22% with 16.9 kDa CS (Eddington et al 2001, Du et al 2004). The oral bioavailability of GU hydrochloride in horses was found to be 2.5–5.9% with a large volume of distribution which indicates very poor absorption from the intestinal tract, but extensive tissue uptake (Du et al 2004, Laverty et al 2005). While serum levels of 4.53–6.5 μg/ml for disaccharide fractions of CS (Eddington et al 2001, Du et al 2004) and 10.6 μg/ml for GU (Du et al 2004) were attained, the dose was 5–10 times the typical labeled dose of GU to achieve these levels. Laverty et al (2005) showed that maximum levels of GU serum reached 6 μg/ml (about 1 μg/ml) in the serum and about 0.3–0.71 μM in the synovial fluid after clinically suggested doses of glucosamine hydrochloride were administered orally. It was also found that GU concentrations in the synovial fluid appeared to be relatively stable over time (remaining elevated at 0.1 0.7 μM 12 hours after dosing) in that study (Laverty et al 2005) and Dechant and Baxter suggested that this could indicate minimal utilization of GU by articular tissues. Based on these bioavailability studies it could be concluded that CS has increased potential for efficacy due to greater oral absorption (Eddington et al 2001, Du et al 2004), but it has been pointed out that the CS bioavailability study could be disputed because the assays measured disaccharide fractions of CS, which are not known to be biologically active (Dechant & Baxter 2007).

Claims have been made by suppliers and medical authorities that glucosamine sulfate is superior to glucosamine hydrochloride, but the rationale of this has been questioned (Block et al 2010). In a study of eight female horses, glucosamine sulfate and glucosamine hydrochloride were administered at doses of 20 mg/kg by either intravenous or nasogastric intubation and plasma samples were collected. Glucosamine was assayed by liquid chromatography electrospray tendon mass spectrometry (LCESI/MS/MS). Synovial fluid concentrations of GU were significantly higher at 1 and 6 hours following oral treatment with glucosamine sulfate compared to glucosamine hydrochloride. Twelve hours following oral administration, glucosamine levels in the plasma and the synovial fluid were still significantly higher than baseline glucosamine sulfate preparation but not for the hydrochloride preparation. The conclusion was that higher synovial fluid concentrations of glucosamine were achieved with glucosamine sulfate, but whether this difference translated into a therapeutic effect on the joint tissues remains to be elucidated (Meulyzer et al 2008). In a follow-up paper the same research group demonstrated that joint inflammation (induced with *Escherichia coli* lipopolysaccharide [LPS]) increases GU levels obtained in synovial fluid following oral administration of glucosamine hydrochloride up to fourfold higher than in the clinically normal joints suggested the possibility of an enhanced effect (as synovitis is important in the pathobiology of equine OA) (Meulyzer et al 2009). On the other hand, the maximal GU levels attainable in the synovial fluid in the presence of inflammation based in these studies will likely be in the range of 1–18 μM for both horses and humans and most in vitro studies showing benefits with glucosamine used considerably higher concentrations (Meulyzer et al 2009).

Key Points

- There is some controversy over which substances should be measured in studies on the bioavailability and pharmacokinetics of GU and CS
- In general, the bioavailability of GU and CS appears to be low
- Molecular size of active ingredient, dose and joint inflammatory status may influence delivery to the target site of action

Clinical trials and experimental studies

Horses

Clinical trials and in vivo experimental studies in horses are limited and the results are variable. This was highlighted in a recent review article of 15 in vivo papers published in the equine literature that the authors demonstrated an encouraging trend to manufacturers of these products investing in research, but most not meeting a quality standard that provided sufficient confidence in the results reported (Pearson & Lindinger 2009). Consequently, the overall level of evidence for in vivo demonstration of efficacy is weak. Administration of Cosequin™ (Nutramax Laboratories, Wedgewood, MD) in horses with OA in the distal interphalangeal, metacarpophalangeal, tarsometatarsal, or carpal joints resulted in improvement in lameness grade, flexion test grade and stride length within 2 weeks; however, no further improvement in lameness grade and no significant changes in other variables were seen after 4 weeks (Hanson et al 1997). Twenty-five horses were in the study and there was no placebo group. It has been pointed out by others that although the lack of continued improvement may be attributable to the return of most of the horses in the study to exercise and competition after an initial 2 weeks of treatment, return to previously obtainable performance levels and continuation in a competition career is necessary for a treatment to be considered successful, as well as fulfilling the expectation of the owners of the affected horses (Neil et al 2005a).

Results of other studies using Cosequin have reported no beneficial effects in a chemically induced model of OA (White et al 1994), but it should be recognized that the model is hardly representative of clinical OA. Administration of another product containing GU, glutamic acid, glycine and glucuronic acid (Chondrosulf, IBSA, Lugano, Switzerland) showed results in improvement in vertical ground reaction force and reduction of gait asymmetry in cases of OA of the distal intertarsal or tarsometatarsal joints. In another clinical study, an oral supplement containing 12 000 mg glucosamine sodium sulfate, 12 000 mg glucosamine potassium sulfate, 12 000 mg glucosamine hydrochloride, 300 mg *N*-acetyl-D-glucosamine and 12 000 mg of CS per dose (together with 300 mg of ascorbate and 100 mg of manganese) was given for 2 years to eight horses (Rogers 2006). The author reported that frequency of distal tarsal joint injection decreasing from a mean of 1.7 injections/year prior to supplementation to 0.85 injections/year with supplementation and a notable drop in the injection frequency after 5–8 months of supplementation (Rogers 2006) as an indication of efficacy. However, this study was neither controlled or blinded and relied on the subjective evaluation of lameness (diagnosis of distal tarsal pain/tarsitis by flexion palpation, radiographic and intra-articular anesthesia) by a single veterinarian and trainer.

Humans

Numerous clinical studies have been done with human OA patients. The Glucosamine/chondroitin Arthritis Intervention Trial (GAIT) is the best known and was a multicenter trial assigned 1583 patients to randomly receive 1500 mg of glucosamine; 1200 mg of CS; both GU and CS; 200 mg of celecoxib (Celebrex, Pfizer, New York, NY) or placebo for 24 weeks. Patients randomized to celecoxib had significant improvement in knee pain compared to those randomized to placebo. No statistically significant improvement in knee pain compared to placebo was seen among patients randomized by dietary supplements, although a subset of patients with moderate to severe knee pain at entry who were assigned to the combination of GU and CS seemed to experience some improvement and patients taking CS were found to have statistically significant decrease in knee joint swelling (Clegg et al 2006). A major limitation of the study noted by the authors was the high rate of response to placebo (60%) and the relatively mild degree of OA among the participants. A post-hoc analysis was then undertaken to further assess the observation that patients receiving CS compared to patients who received placebo had improvement in joint swelling (Hochberg & Clegg 2008). The results of this analysis suggested that patients with Kellgren and Lawrence grade II radiographic changes was substantially more responsive to CS than those with Kellgren and Lawrence grade II changes. Also, improvement was more likely to occur in the CS-treated patients with lower WOMAC Function and Stiffness Scores and a numerical trend was seen also in patients with WOMAC Pain Scores.

In another study as part of the GAIT study, progressive loss of joint space (JSW) in patients with knee OA who satisfied radiographic criteria (Kellgren/Lawrence grade II or III and JSW of at least 2 mm at baseline) were studied. The mean JSW loss of 2 years in knees with OA in the placebo group, adjusted for design and clinical factors, was 0.166 mm. No statistically significant difference in mean JSW loss was observed in any treatment group compared with the placebo group. There was a trend towards improvement in the grade II knees. The authors concluded that the power of the study was diminished by the limited sample size, variance of JSW treatment and a smaller than expected loss of JSW (Sawitzke et al 2008).

Wandel and colleagues (Wandel et al 2010) performed a meta-analysis of studies examining the effect of GU, CS or the two in combination on joint pain and on radiological progression of disease in OA of the hip or knee. Ten trials involving a total of 3803 patients were included in the analysis. It was concluded that, compared to placebo, GU, CS, and their combination do not reduce joint pain or have an impact on narrowing of joint space, and the authors recommended that use of GU and CS for treatment of hip or knee OA should be discouraged.

Key Points

- Valid conclusions regarding the efficacy of OJSs in horses are not possible due to a lack of well-designed studies
- Meta-analysis of data from human studies indicates that GU, CS or GU/CS does not reduce joint pain or other clinical signs of OA

Product quality and purity

Due to lack of regulation and oversight, OJS product quality can vary considerably. One study compared labeled claims with laboratory analysis for GU and CS content and found that the measured composition varied significantly (0–115% from labeled claims) (Adebowale et al 2000). Oke et al (2006) analyzed 23 commercially available equine OJSs containing glucosamine, as well as 1 positive (glucosamine hydrochloride) and 3 negative controls. The range of GU free base compared to the amount expected in each product based on the label claim was 0–221.2% with a median of 99.0% and 106% respectively. Of the 23 products included in the study, 9 (39.1%) contained less GU than claimed by the manufacturer and 4 (17.4%) less than 30% of the expected amount of GU (Oke et al 2006). Of the 23 products, only 5 OJSs achieved the recommended dosage (approximately 10 g/GU/day) suggested by the study of Laverty et al (2005). .

Sasha's Blend

Sasha's Blend (New Zealand green lipped mussel, shark cartilage, abalone and *Biota orientalis* lipid extract) is a proprietary mixture of bioactive lipids obtained from New Zealand green lipped mussel (NZGLM) (*Perna canaliculus*), abalone (*Haliotis* sp.), and SKC (*Galorhinus galeus*) and a lipid extract from *Biota orientalis* (Sasha's EQ powder, Interpath Pty Ltd, Australia). Raw ingredients are manufactured in New Zealand with the four constituents being artificially digested in vitro, and an extract of each simulated digest has been evaluated by use of a cartilage explant model of inflammation (Pearson et al 2007). Each constituent has been shown to exert unique effects on the formation of rh-IL-1β-induced PGE_2, GAG and on chondrocyte viability in equine cartilage explants. More recently the product has been tested in 22 healthy horses. Twelve horses were fed 0, 15, 45 or 75 mg of Sasha's Equine Powder (SEQ) (3 horses per treatment) daily for 84 days. Ten other horses received 0 or 15 g of SEQ per day (5 horses per treatment) for 29 days (beginning day −14). One middle carpal joint in each horse was injected twice with IL-1β (10 and 100 ng on day 0 and 1, respectively) and the contralateral joint similarly injected with saline (0.9% NaCl solution). In this study (Pearson et al 2009) administration of the SEQ (up to 75 g/day) to horses for 84 days did not induce any adverse effects. Synovial fluid PGE_2, GAG and protein concentration as well as leukocyte count increased after intraarticular injection of IL-1β (compared to saline injection) in horses that received no SEQ but in horses that were fed SEQ intraarticular IL-1β injections did not induce significant increases in synovial fluid PGE_2 and GAG concentrations. These results suggested that SEQ could be useful in preventing inflammation associated with synovitis and OA in horses.

Hyaluronan (hyaluronic acid)

Intra-articular HA has been used in the horse for many years (Howard & McIlwraith 1996). Oral HA formulated for the horse has been available for 7–8 years and anecdotal reports have suggested that its use has been effective in treating lameness associated with synovial effusion and OA. Hyaluronan has been shown to be absorbed by rats and beagles when administered orally (Schauss et al 2004) but there are no published data from equine studies. Other GAG products such as chondroitin, dermatan and heparan sulfates have also been shown to be absorbed orally in rats and man (Silvestro et al 1994, Dawes et al 1989, 1991, Salartash et al 1999).

A double-blinded, controlled study has been reported in horses where 48 yearlings operated arthroscopically for unilateral or bilateral osteochondritis dissecans (OCD) of the tarsus (yearlings were included only if they had mild or no synovial effusion pre-surgery) (Bergin et al 2006). Twenty-four of the yearlings (27 joints) were treated with 100 mg of HA orally for 30 days postoperatively and 24 (30 joints) with a placebo orally for 30 days. Thirty days post-arthroscopic surgery, a blinded examiner scored the effusion of the dorsomedial tarsocrural joint individually using a scale of 0 to 5 (0 = no effusion, 1 = barely palpable, 2 = palpable effusion (without plantar effusion), 3 = golf ball size effusion with plantar effusion, 4 = tennis ball size effusion with plantar effusion, 5 = greater than tennis ball size effusion with plantar effusion). The mean 30 day effusion score of the HA-treated group (27 joints) was 0.7 while the mean of the 30 day placebo group (30 joints) was 2.05 ($p \leq 0.0001$). Similar results were noted when comparing treated versus placebo for each lesion location, as well as for lesion size. This author feels the results speak for themselves; however, the mechanism of action is certainly less obvious. In a recently conducted survey using the CSU osteochondral fragment model, there was a significant reduction in the PGE_2 levels of the OA joints in horses treated with oral HA compared to both the OA joints of the placebo horses (Frisbie, McIlwraith & Kawcak unpublished data).

Avocado soy unsaponified (ASU)

Avocado/soy bean unsaponifiable (ASU) extracts are produced by extracting the oils from avocados and soy beans, collecting the unsaponifiable fractions (i.e., the oil that remains after hydrolysis and do not form soaps) and combining these in various ratios. This product has been reported to be beneficial in randomized, placebo controlled human trials (Appelboom et al 2001, Maheu et al 1998, Blotman et al 1997). In vitro studies have displayed anabolic, anti-catabolic and anti-inflammatory effects on human chondrocytes. ASU increased the basal synthesis of aggrecan and reversed the IL-1β-induced reduction of aggrecan synthesis by human chondrocytes in alginate beads (Henrotin et al 2003). It also decreased the spontaneous and IL-1 beta-induced production of matrix metalloproteinase (MMP)-3, IL-6 and -8 and PGE_2, while it weakly reversed the IL-1-induced inhibitor of tissue inhibitor of metalloproteinase-1 (TIMP-1) production (Henrotin et al 1998, 2003).

In a blinded and placebo-controlled study using the CSU osteochondral chip fragment model, horses were randomly assigned to two groups with the ASU extract group receiving the supplement mixed with molasses while the placebo group only received molasses from days 0–70. The ASU supplementation did not have a significant effect on pain or lameness, but there was a significant reduction on the degree of macroscopic cartilage erosion and synovial hemorrhage scores in the OA joints compared to placebo controlled joints, as well as s significant decrease in intimal hyperplasia (inflammation) in the synovial membrane. There was also a decrease in the cartilage disease score (Kawcak et al 2007). A significant decrease in cartilage disease indicates that this product could be classified as a disease-modifying osteoarthritic drug (DMOAD). Although the improvements were modest, they were more significant than those seen with other parenteral polysulfated GAG, IV HA and oral HA products tested using the same model of equine OA, at least at the level of articular cartilage change. Unfortunately the ASU extract product used in the CSU equine study cannot be made available in the United States. At present the only ASU product available in North America is sold in combination with GU and CS (Cosequin ASU™, Nutramax Laboratories, Edgewood, MD, USA). Considerable in vitro work has been done with this product, but, as yet, no in vivo efficacy has been reported.

Polyunsaturated fatty acids (PUFAs)

Polyunsaturated fatty acids (PUFAs), at sufficiently high intakes as found in oily fish and fish oils, decrease production of inflammatory cytokines, arachidonic acid-derived eicosanoids (prostaglandins, thromboxanes, leukotrienes, and other oxidized derivatives), other inflammatory agents such as reactive oxygen species and adhesion molecules (Calder 2006). Omega-3 (*n*-3) PUFAs contain α-linolenic acid that is desaturated in the body to produce eicosapentaenoic acid (EPA) and docosahexaenoic acid (DHA) analogs of arachidonic acid (Trumble 2005). In an in vitro bovine cartilage explant model of OA, supplementation with *n*-3 PUFAs showed a decrease in the expression and activity of aggrecanases and MMPs, as well as in the expression of COX-2, IL-1α and tumor necrosis factor-α (Curtis et al 2000). Although there is currently no evidence of efficacy, the potential for usefulness of PUFAs in OA in the horse has led to it being incorporated into some OJSs.

Cetyl myristoleate

Cetyl myristoleate (CM) is another fatty acid that is being used in equine joint supplements. CM is an ester of *cis*-9-tetradecenoic acid (myristoleic acid) and 1-hexadecanol (cetyl alcohol) and is a 14-carbon monounsaturated omega-5 fatty acid (Trumble 2005). CM may act by inhibition of the 5-lipooxygenase pathway, which is responsible for the metabolism of leukotrienes, potent inflammatory mediators, from the arachidonic acid cascade (Bonnet et al 1995). Studies in adjuvant-induced arthritis and collagen-induced arthritis in rats respectively have demonstrated that CM can confer protection and reduce severity of the disease respectively (Diehl & May 1994, Hunter et al 2003). A study in human knee OA has been reported where CM showed improvement in knee flexion and function (Hesslink et al 2002).

A product containing CM, glucosamine hydrochloride, methylsulfonylmethane and hydrolyzed collagen

(Myristol™) was investigated in a blinded-controlled clinical trial with 39 horses. Each horse was scored using AAEP guidelines for lameness, as well as a 0–10 cm Visual Analog Scale (VAS) for lameness at walk, lameness at trot, response to joint flexion, lameness after flexion and quality of life (Keegan et al 2007). Horses were assessed on day 0, 14, 28 and 42 days after treatment. A responder was defined as improving one grade on the AAEP Lameness Scale or 2 cm on the VAS. The Myristol™ treatment group improved significantly more than the placebo group in AAEP Lameness Score, lameness at walk, response to joint flexion, lameness after flexion and quality of life.

Conclusions

Use of OJSs in horses is prevalent worldwide. Although data from in vitro studies indicate that glucosamine and chondroitin sulfate mitigate cartilage degradation, evidence regarding the in vivo efficacy of OJSs is inconclusive, in part due to a lack of well-designed clinical trials.

References

Adebowale, A.O., Cox, D.S., Linang, I., et al., 2000. Analysis of glucosamine and chondroitin sulfate content in marketed products and CACO-2 permeability of chondroitin sulfate raw materials. J Am Nutraceuticals Assoc 3, 37–44.

American Veterinary Medical Association. US Pet Ownership and Demographic Sourcebook (2007 Edition). Center for Info. Management Staff.

Appelboom, T., Schuermans, J., Berbruggen, G., et al., 2001. Symptom modifying effects of avocado/soy bean unsaponifiables (ASU) in knee osteoarthritis. A double-blind, prospective placebo controlled study. Scand J Rheumatol 30, 242–247.

Bassleer, C.T., Combal, J.P., Bougaret, S., et al., 1998a. Effects of chondroitin sulfate and interleukin-1 beta on human articular chondrocytes cultivated in clusters. Osteo Cart 6, 196–204.

Bassleer, C.T., Rovati, L., Franchimont, P., 1998b. Stimulation of proteoglycan production by glucosamine sulfate in chondrocytes isolated from human osteoarthritic articular cartilage in vitro. Osteo Cart 6, 427–434.

Bergin, B.J., Pierce, S.W., Bramlage, L.R., et al., 2006. Oral hyaluronan gel reduces post-operative tarsocrural effusion in the yearling Thoroughbred. Clinical evidence. Equine Vet J 38, 375–378.

Block, J.A., Oegema, T.R., Sande, J.T., et al., 2010. The effects of oral glucosamine on joint health: is a change of research approach needed? Osteo Cart 18, 5–11.

Blotman, F., Maheu, E., Wulwik, A., et al., 1997. Efficacy and safety of avocado/soy bean unsaponifiables in the treatment of osteoarthritis of the knee and hips. A prospective, multi-center, 3-month randomized, double-blind, placebo-controlled trial. Rev Rheum Engl Ed 64, 825–834.

Bonnet, C., Bertin, P., Cook-Moreau, J., et al., 1995. Lipooxygenase products in expression of 5-lipooxygenase and 5-lipooxygenase-activating protein in human cultured synovial cells. Prostaglandins 50, 127–135.

Booth, D.M., 2004. Balancing fact and fiction of novel ingredients: Definitions, regulations and evaluations. Vet Clin North Am Pract 34, 7–38.

Burk, A.O., Williams, C.A., 2008. Feeding management practices and supplement use in top-level event horses. Comp Exercise Physiol 5, 5–93.

Byron, C.R., Orth, M.W., Venta, P.J., et al., 2003. Influence of glucosamine on matrix metalloproteinase expression and activity in lipopolysaccharide-stimulated equine chondrocytes. Am J Vet Res 64, 666–671.

Calder, P.C., 2006. N-3 polyunsaturated fatty acids, inflammation, and inflammatory diseases. Am J Clin Nutrition 83, S1505–S1519.

Caron, J.P., Genovese, R.L., 2003. Principals and practices of joint disease treatment. In: Ross, M.W., Dyson, S. (Eds.), Diagnosis and Management of Lameness in the Horse. Saunders, Philadelphia, 203, pp. 746–764.

Chan, P.-S., Caron, J.P., Orth, M.W., 2005. Effect of glucosamine and chondroitin sulfate on regulation of gene expression of proteolytic enzymes and their inhibitors in interleukin-1-challenged bovine articular cartilage explants. Am J Vet Res 66, 1870–1876.

Clegg, P., Booth, R., 2000. Drugs used to treat osteoarthritis in the horse. In: Practice. 22, 594–603.

Clegg, D.O., Reda, D.J., Harris, C.L., et al., 2006. Glucosamine, chondroitin sulfate, and the two in combination for painful knee arthritis. N Engl J Med 354, 795–808.

Curtis, E.L., Hughes, C.E., Flannery, C.R., et al., 2000. N-3 fatty acids specifically modulate catabolic factors involved in articular cartilage degradation. J Biol Chem 275, 721–724.

Dawes, J., Hodson, B.A., Pepper, D.S., 1989. The absorption, clearance and metabolic fate of dermatan sulfate administered to man – studies using a radio iodinated derivative. Thromb Hemost 62, 945–949.

Dawes, J., McLaren, M., Forbes, C., et al., 1991. The pharmacokinetics of dermatan sulfate MF701 in healthy human volunteers. Br J Coin Pharmacol 32, 361–366.

Dechant, J.E., Baxter, G.M., Frisbie, D.D., et al., 2005. Effects of glucosamine hydrochloride and chondroitin sulfate, alone and in combination, on normal and interleukin-l conditioned equine articular cartilage explant metabolism. Equine Vet J 37, 227–231.

Dechant, J.E., Baxter, G.M., 2007. Glucosamine and chondroitin sulfate as structure modifying agents in horses. Equine Vet Educ 90, 96.

De Mattei, M., Plati, A., Pasello, M., et al., 2002. High doses of glucosamine HCl have detrimental effects on bovine articular cartilage explants cultured in vivo. Osteo Cart 10, 816–825.

Diehl, H.W., May, E.L., 1994. Cetyl myristoleate isolated from Swiss albino mice: an apparent protective agent against adjuvant arthritis in rats. J Pharm Sci 83, 296–299.

Dodge, G.R., Jimenez, S.A., 2003. Glucosamine sulfate modulates the levels of aggrecan and matrix metalloproteinase-3 synthesized by cultured human osteoarthritis articular chondrocytes. Osteoarthritis Cartilage 11 (6), 24–432.

Dodge, G.R., Regatte, R.R., Hall, J.O., 2005. The fate of oral glucosamine traced by BC-labeling in the dog. Osteo Cart 9 (supp B), 541.

Du, J., White, N., Eddington, N.D., 2004. The bioavailability and pharmacokinetics of glucosamine hydrochloride and chondroitin sulfate after oral, intravenous single dose administration in the horse. Bio Pharm Drug Dispos 25, 109–116.

Duren, S., 2005. Oral joint supplements. Panacea or expensive fad? Adv Equine Nutr III, 77–83.

Eddington, N.D., Du, J., White, N., 2001. Evidence of the oral absorption of chondroitin sulfate as determined by total disaccharide content after oral and intravenous administration to horses. Proc Am Ass Equine Pract 47, 326–328.

Esford, L.E., Maiti, A., Bader, S.A., 1998. Analysis of CD44 interactions with hyaluronan in murine L cell fibroblasts deficient in glycosaminoglycan synthesis: a role for chondroitin sulfate. J Cell Sci 111, 1021–1029.

Fenton, J.J., Chlebek-Brown, K.A., Peters, T.L., et al., 2000. Glucosamine HCI reduces equine articular degeneration in explant cultures. Osteo Cart 6, 258–265.

Fenton, J.J., Chlebek-Brown, K.A., Caron, J.P., et al., 2002. Effect of glucosamine on interleukin-1-conditioned articular cartilage. Equine Vet J 34, 219–223.

Grande, D., O'Grady, C., Garone, E., et al., 2000. Chondroprotective and gene expression effects of nutritional supplements on articular cartilage. Osteo Cart 8 (suppl B), 534–535.

Hanson, R., Malley, L.R., Huff, G.K., et al., 1997. Oral treatment with a glucosamine-chondroitin sulfate compound for degenerative joint disease in horses: 25 cases. Equine Pract 19, 16–22.

Helmick, C.G., Felson, D.T., Lawrence, R.C., et al., 2008. For the National Arthritis Data Workgroup. Estimates for the prevalence of arthritis and other rheumatic diseases on the United States. Part I. Arthritis Rheum 58, 15–25.

Henrotin, Y.E., Labasse, A.H., Jaspar, J.M., et al., 1998. Effects of the avocado/soy bean unsaponifiable mixtures on metalloproteinases, cytokines and prostaglandin E_2 production by human articular chondrocytes. Clin Rheumatol 17, 31–39.

Henrotin, Y.E., Sanchez, C., Deberg, M.A., et al., 2003. Avocado/soy bean unsaponifiables increase aggrecan synthesis and reduce catabolic and pro-inflammatory mediator production by human osteoarthritic chondrocytes. J Rheumatol 30, 1825–1834.

Hesslink, Jr., R., Armstrong, D. III, Nagendran, M.V., et al., 2002. Cetylated fatty acids improve knee functions in patients with osteoarthritis. J Rheumatol 29, 1708–1712.

Hochberg, M.C., Clegg, D.O., 2008. Potential effects of chondroitin sulfate on joint swelling: A Gait report. Osteo Cart 16, S22–S24.

Howard, R.D., McIlwraith, C.W., 1996. Hyaluronan and its use in the treatment of equine joint disease. In: McIlwraith, C.W., Trotter, G.W. (Eds.), Joint Disease in the Horse. WB Saunders, Philadelphia, PA, pp. 257–269.

Hunter, Jr., K.W., Galt, R.A., Stehouwer, J.S., et al., 2003. Synthesis of cetyl myristoleate and evaluation of its therapeutic efficacy in a murine model of collagen-induced arthritis. Pharmacol Res 47, 43–47.

Ilic, M.Z., Martinac, B., Handley, C.J., 2003. Effects of long-term exposure to glucosamine and mannosamine on aggrecan degradation in articular cartilage. Osteo Cart 11, 613–622.

Kawcak, C.E., Frisbie, D.D., McIlwraith, C.W., et al., 2007. Evaluation of avocado and soybean unsaponifiable extracts for treatment of horses with experimentally induced osteoarthritis using an equine model. Am J Vet Res 68, 598–604.

Keegan, K.G., Hughes, F., Lane, T., et al., 2007. Effects of an oral nutraceutical on clinical aspects of joint disease in a blinded, controlled clinical trial: 39 horses. Proceedings Am Assoc Equine Pract 53, 252–255.

Kelly, G.S., 1998. The role of glucosamine sulfate and chondroitin sulfates in the treatment of degenerative joint disease. Alt Med Rev 3, 27–39.

Largo, R., Alvarez-Soria, M.A., Diez-Ortego, I., et al., 2003. Glucosamine inhibits IL-1-induced NFkB activation in human osteoarthritic chondrocytes. Osteo Cart 11, 290–298.

Lawrence, R.C., Felson, D.T., Helmick, C.G., et al., 2008. For the National Arthritis Data Workgroup. Estimates for the prevalence of arthritis and other rheumatic diseases on the United States. Part II. Arthritis Rheum 58, 26–35.

Lippiello, L., Woodward, J., Karpman, R., et al., 2000. In vivo chondroprotection and metabolic synergy of glucosamine and chondroitin sulfate. Clin Orthop Rel Res 381, 229–240.

Lippiello, L., Sung Han, M., Henderson, T., 2002. Protective effect of the chondroprotective agent Cosequin DS on bovine articular cartilage exposed in vitro to non-steroidal anti-inflammatory agents. Vet Ther 2, 128–135.

Lippiello, L., 2003. Glucosamine and chondroitin sulfate: biological response modifiers of chondrocytes under simulated conditions of joint stress. Osteo Cart 11, 335–342.

Laverty, S., Sandy, J.D., Celeste, T., et al., 2005. Synovial fluid levels and serum pharmacokinetics in a large animal model following treatment with oral glycosaminoglycan at clinically relevant doses. Arthritis Rheum 52, 181–191.

Maheu, E., Maziers, B., Valat, J.P., et al., 1998. Symptomatic efficacy of avocado/soy bean unsaponifiables in the treatment of osteoarthritis of the knee and hip. A prospective, randomized, double-blind, placebo-controlled, multi-center clinical trial with a 6 month treatment period and a 2 month follow-up to demonstrate a persistent effect. Arthritis Rheum 41, 81–91, 1998.

McIlwraith, C.W., 1996. General pathobiology of the joint in response to injury. In: McIlwraith, C.W., Trotter, G.W. (Eds.), Joint Disease in the Horse. Philadelphia, WB Saunders, pp. 40–70.

McIlwraith, C.W., 2004. Licensed medications, "generic" medications, compounding and nutraceuticals – What is scientifically validated, where do we encounter scientific mistruth, where are we legally? In: Proceedings of the 50th Annual Convention of the American Association of Equine Practitioners, Lexington, KY. American Association of Equine Practitioners, Lexington, KY, pp. 459–475.

McIlwraith, C.W., 2005. From arthroscopy to gene therapy- 30 years of looking in joints. Frank Milne Lecture. Proc Am Assoc Equine Pract 51, 65–113.

Mello, D.M., Nielson, B.D., Peters, T.L., et al., 2004. Comparison of inhibitory effects of glucosamine and mannosamine on bovine articular cartilage degeneration in vitro. Am J Vet Res 65, 1440–1445.

Meulyzer, M., Vachon, P., Beaudry, F., 2008. Comparison of pharmacokinetics of glucosamine in synovial fluid levels following administration of glucosamine sulfate or glucosamine hydrochloride. Osteo Cart 16, 973–979.

Meulyzer, M., Vachon, P., Beaudry, F., et al., 2009. Joint inflammation increases glucosamine levels attained in synovial fluid following oral administration of glucosamine hydrochloride. Osteo Cart 17, 228–234.

Nakamura, H., Shibakawa, A., Tanaka, M., et al., 2004. Effects of glucosamine hydrochloride on the production of prostaglandin E_2, nitric oxide and metalloproteinases by chondrocytes and synoviocytes in osteoarthritis. Clin Exp Rheumatol 22, 293–299.

Neil, K.M., Caron, J.P., Orth, M.W., 2005a. The role of glucosamine and chondroitin sulfate in treatment for and prevention of osteoarthritis in animals. JAVMA 226, 1079–1088.

Neil, K.M., Orth, M.W., Coussens, P.M., et al., 2005b. Effects of glucosamine and chondroitin sulfate on mediators of osteoarthritis in cultured equine chondrocytes stimulated by use of recombinant equine interleukin-l. Am J Vet Res 1861–1869.

Nerucci, E., Fioravanti, A., Cicero, M.R., et al., 2000. Effects of chondroitin sulfate and interleukin-1β, on human chondrocyte cultures exposed to pressurization: a biochemical and morphological study. Osteo Cart 8, 279–287.

Noyszewski, E.A., Wroblewski, K., Dodge, G.R., et al., 2001. Preferential incorporation of glucosamine into the galactosamine moieties of chondroitin sulfates in articular cartilage explants. Arthr Rheum 44, 1089–1095.

Oke, S.L., Aghazadeh-Habashi, A., Weese, J.S., et al., 2006. Evaluation of glucosamine levels in commercial equine oral supplements for joints. Equine Vet J 8, 93–95.

Oke, S.L., Weese, J.S., 2006. Review of glucosamine-containing oral joint supplements: are they effective in the horse? Proc AAEP 2, 574–579.

Oke, S.L., McIlwraith, C.W., 2008. Review of the potential indications and contraindications for equine oral health supplements. Proc AAEP 54, 261–267.

Orth, M.W., Pefers, N., Hawkins, J.L., 2002. Inhibition of articular cartilage degradation by glucosamine-HCl and chondroitin sulfate. Equine Vet J 34, 224–229.

Pearson, W., Lindinger, M., 2009. Low quality of evidence of glucosamine-based nutraceuticals in equine joint disease: Review of *in vivo* studies. Equine Vet J 41, 706–712.

Pearson, W., Orth, M.W., Lindinger, M.I., 2009. Evaluation of inflammatory responses induced via intraarticular injection of interleukin-1 in horses receiving a dietary nutraceutical and assessment of the clinical effects of long-term nutraceutical administration. Am J Vet Res 70, 848–861.

Pearson, W., Orth, M.W., Karrow, N.A., et al., 2007. Anti-inflammatory and chondroprotective effects of nutraceuticals from Sasha's Blend in a cartilage explant model of inflammation. Mol Nutr Food Res 51, 1020–1030.

Platt, D., 2001. The role of disease-modifying agents glucosamine and chondroitin sulfate in the management of equine degenerative joint disease. Equine Vet Educ 13, 206–215.

Packaged Facts, Publishing Division of MarketResearch.com, Inc; 2008 (http://www.packagedfacts.com/pet-supplements-market-c1641).

Rogers, M.R., 2006. The effect of oral glucosamine and chondroitin sulfate supplementation on frequency of intra-articular therapy of the horse tarsus. Intern J Appl Res Vet Med 4, 155–162.

Ronca, E., Palmieri, L., Panicucci, P., et al., 1998. Anti-inflammatory activity of chondroitin sulfate. Osteo Cart 6 (supp A), 14–21.

Salartash, K., Gonze, M.D., Leone-Bay, A., et al., 1999. Oral low-molecular weight heparin and delivery agent prevents jugular venous thrombosis in the rat. J Vasc Surg 30, 526–531.

Sandy, J.D., Garnett, D., Thompson, V., et al., 1998. Chondrocyte-mediated catabolism of aggrecan: aggrecanase dependent cleavage induced by interleukin-l or retinoic acid can be inhibited by glucosamine. Biochem J 335, 59–66.

Sawitzke, E.D., Shi, H., Finco, M.F., et al., 2008. The effect of glucosamine and/or chondroitin sulfate on the progression of knee osteoarthritis. Arthritis Rheum 58, 3183–3193.

Schauss, A.G., Balogh, L., Polyak, A., et al., 2004. Absorption, distribution and excretion of 99 mTechnetium labeled hyaluronan after single oral doses in rats and beagle dogs. FASEB J Abstract 129, 4.

Schlueter, A.E., Orth, M.W., 2004. Further studies on the ability of glucosamine and chondroitin sulfate to regulate catabolic mediators in vitro. Equine Vet J 36, 634–636.

Seaver, B., Smith, J.R., 2004. Inhibition of COX isoforms by nutraceuticals. J Herb Pharmacother 4, 11–18.

Silvestro, L., Lanza, R., Otti, E., et al., 1994. Human pharmacokinetics of glycosaminoglycan using deuterium-labeled and unlabeled substances: evidence for oral absorption. Semin Thromb Hemos 20, 281–292.

Trumble, T.N., 2005. The use of nutraceuticals for osteoarthritis in horses. Vet Clin Equine Prac 21, 575–597.

Wandel, S., Juni, P., Tendal, B., et al., 2010. Effects of glucosamine, chondroitin, or placebo in patients with osteoarthritis of hip or knee: network meta-analysis. British Med J 341, c4675.

White, G.W., Jones, E.W., Hamm, J., 1994. The efficacy of orally administrated sulfated glycosaminoglycan in chemically induced equine synovitis and degenerative joint disease. J Equine Vet Sci 14, 350–353.

Wright, I.M., 2001. Oral supplements in the treatment and prevention of joint diseases: a review of their potential application to the horse. Equine Vet Educ 13, 135–139.

34

Gastric ulceration

Nanna Luthersson, Jenifer A. Nadeau

The horse, as a non-ruminant herbivore, evolved to ingest a high-fiber, low-starch diet through daily (up to 18 h) foraging. Saliva produced in response to chewing helps to buffer gastric acid. Modern management practices including meal feeding, low-fiber/high-concentrate diets, early weaning and intensive training programs with limited opportunity for free movement increases the risk for development of a poorly buffered, acidic gastric environment. These feeding and management practices have been associated with a high prevalence of the equine gastric ulcer syndrome (EGUS) (Vatistas et al 1999a, Lester 2004, Jonsson & Egenvall 2006). EGUS is the term used to describe ulcers in the terminal esophagus, nonglandular stomach, glandular stomach and proximal duodenum (Hammond et al 1986). All ages and breeds of horses are susceptible to EGUS (Luthersson et al 2009a).

Epidemiology of equine gastric ulcers

Prevalence of EGUS varies in adult horses, with Thoroughbreds the predominant breed evaluated. In Thoroughbred racehorses in intensive training, the incidence of gastric ulceration has been reported to be more than 90% in some subpopulations. Severity of ulceration is greatest in animals in training and lesions tend to worsen in severity and number during the training period, particularly at the beginning (Hammond et al 1986, Murray et al 1989, 1996, Vatistas et al 1999a, Jonsson & Egenvall 2006). Prevalence of gastric ulceration in a group of Standardbred racehorses was reported to be 87% (Rabuffo et al 2002). Another study of Standardbred racehorses showed a prevalence of 70% graded as EGUS ≥1 or 42% graded as EGUS ≥2 (Jonsson & Egenvall 2006). Prevalence of gastric lesions in actively competing 3-day event horses was 75% (Michael Murray, unpublished data), 58% in show horses (McClure et al 1999), and 67% in endurance horses after competition (Nieto et al 2004). Although most studies on performance horses report high prevalence of gastric lesions, a prevalence of 40% was found in a group of 156 Western performance horses under heavy use (Bertone 2000). Western performance horses may have fewer lesions due to differences in their management, training and feeding compared to the other groups of horses.

Only a few studies have been carried out on leisure horses and breeding mares. In a post mortem study of retired racehorses, 52% had lesions compared with 37% of pleasure horses (Murray et al 1996). In a study of 80 horses involved in a university riding program, there was a low prevalence of 11% (Chameroy et al 2006). In a study of 201 Danish pleasure/leisure horses 53% (107/201) were graded as having EGUS ≥2 (Luthersson et al 2009a). In a group of pregnant and nonpregnant mares (62) on pasture, an overall prevalence of gastric ulcers was 71% (Le Jeune et al 2009).

Limitations, when comparing studies of EGUS prevalence, include variations in the classification of the ulcers included (in particular the severity level), the number of animals investigated and how the lesions were graded. Slightly different scoring systems have been used in the literature to describe the ulcers. MacAllister et al (1997) reported on both the number of lesions (0–4) and their severity (0–5), whereas Furr and Murray (1989) combined the two to give an overall score value of 0–4. In a study of show horses (McClure et al 1999), the authors used a 0–6 system whereas the EGUS Council Scoring system (Andrews et al 1999) uses a 0–4 system. These differences can significantly affect the prevalence estimates of clinically relevant ulcers, since lower grades of gastric lesions, which reflect minor pathologies such as hyperkeratosis, may or may not be included in the definition of an ulcer. Additionally, some reports include all grades of lesions, while others define clinically significant ulcers and report on their prevalence e.g. ≥ grade 2 according to Luthersson et al in the Danish study (2009a).

Anatomical distribution of gastric ulcers

Ulcers have been identified throughout the stomach. The nonglandular stratified squamous mucosa along the margo plicatus is most commonly affected (Hammond et al 1986, Murray et al 1989, 1996). Prevalence of glandular mucosal lesions is slightly lower than for the squamous lesions, with the pyloric antrum most commonly affected, as illustrated by the Danish study (Luthersson et al 2009a). Ulcerations in the two main regions (squamous or glandular mucosa) might have different etiologies and therefore risk factors. It

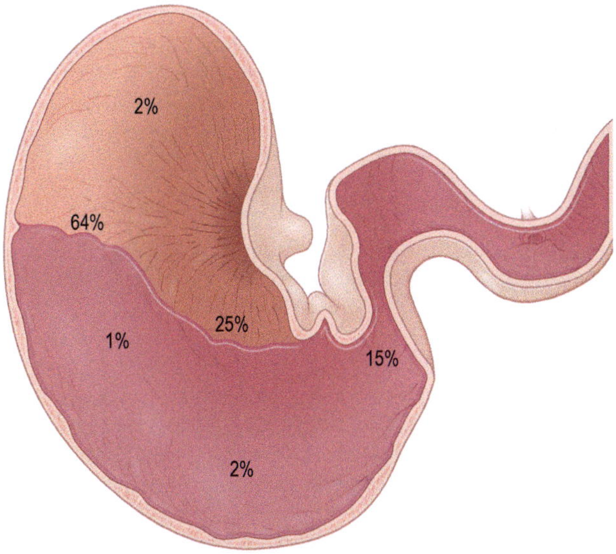

Figure 34.1 A schematic depicting an estimate of the relative distribution of gastric ulcer lesions involving the non-glandular and glandular mucosa.

is the authors' opinion that horses often develop lesions in either the non-glandular or the glandular part of the stomach depending on their "environment". Glandular lesions may be missed by poor endoscopic technique; therefore, the incidence of pathology in this part of the stomach may be greater than previously reported (Andrews et al 2002). Current information on the prevalence of glandular ulcers is limited, but a study of 201 horses showed that 168 horses had visible ulcers (grade 1 and above). Of these, 29 had glandular lesions only, 53 had non-glandular lesions only and 86 had lesions in both regions of the stomach (Luthersson et al 2009a). The most severe lesions in each region were located as shown in Fig. 34.1. Examples of non-glandular and glandular lesions are depicted in Fig. 34.2.

Key Points – Prevalence of EGUS

- In performance horse populations, the reported prevalence of gastric ulceration has ranged from 40% to more than 90%. Few studies have examined EGUS prevalence in leisure and breeding horses
- The nonglandular stratified squamous mucosa along the margo plicatus is the most common site for ulcer lesions
- Severity of lesions is greatest in horses in athletic training; an increase in lesion number and/or severity during training has been reported in Thoroughbred racehorses

Risk factors and pathophysiology

Risk factors for non-glandular and glandular lesions may differ. Lesions in the squamous mucosa mostly reflect peptic injury (HCl and pepsin) to the poorly protected surface of the non-glandular part of the stomach. The primary barriers to HCl in the squamous epithelium are intracellular secretion of bicarbonate ions and the intracellular tight junctions (Orlando 1991, Tobey & Orlando 1991, Orlando et al 1992). These tight junctions are located in the superficial layer of the epithelium, but they only provide a weak barrier as

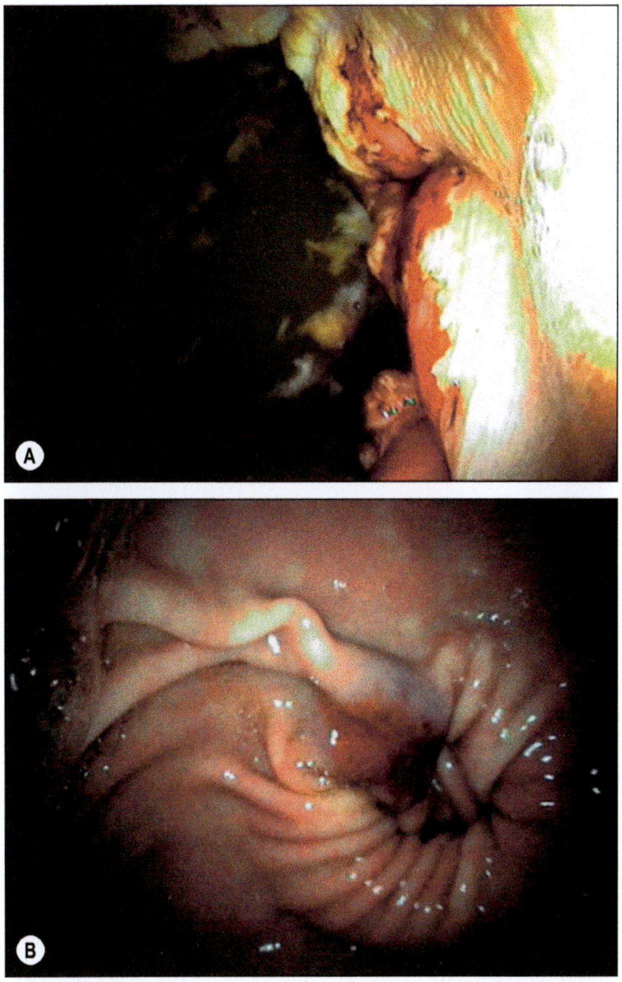

Figure 34.2 Examples of Grade IV non-glandular A) and Grade III glandular B) ulcers. Note the evidence of hemorrhage in both locations.

deeper in the epithelium, the cells transport hydrogen ions intracellularly, resulting in their death when exposed to HCl (Tobey & Orlando 1991). Since there is no surface barrier to HCl and the epithelium has limited ability to prevent peptic injury, there is a limited primary barrier to peptic injury, and prevention effectively relies on limited exposure to acidic gastric secretions (Murray 1999). The glandular mucosa's epithelial cells, through a buffering layer of mucus containing bicarbonate, are protected from direct contact with low pH in the gastric juice. Glandular lesions are thought to result from impaired mucosal defense mechanisms rather than a primary peptic injury. This is supported by the observation that feed deprivation models used to create squamous injury do not produce glandular lesions. Also, when assessing the effect of exercise, only a few glandular lesions were found (Lester et al 2004, Jonsson & Egenvall 2006). Glandular lesions can be successfully induced in horses using excessive administration of non-steroidal anti-inflammatory drugs (NSAIDs) and there is increasing evidence of a bacterial component to glandular ulcer development (Contreras et al 2007, Reed et al 2006). It might therefore be more relevant to divide EGUS into two distinct types: primary squamous ulceration due to increased acid exposure and primary glandular ulceration resulting from failed mucosal defences. Future studies should therefore describe the location of EGUS lesions and analyze non-glandular and glandular EGUS independently to enable the identification of unique risk factors for each anatomical type of lesion.

As discussed above, most investigations in mature horses have been carried out in performance horses, whereas only a few studies have been performed on leisure horses, breeding mares and young horses. Risk factors are therefore focused on typical management practices associated with the management and training of racehorses and competition horses, such as level of training, effect of competition and transportation; meal feeding, fasting, high concentrate diets, low hay diets, and administration of certain drugs. Many of the suggested risk factors are directly associated or can be linked with nutritional practices and it is not always possible to differentiate between these, e.g. transportation often results in a change in feeding and watering regimens.

Age, breed, gender

Age has been identified as a risk factor in some studies. Some studies showed that risk was highest in younger horses, aged 2–6 years (Chameroy et al 2006), while other studies have shown that the risk increases with age (Rabuffo et al 2002). The latter study and its findings relate to racehorses in training and therefore perhaps only reflect a particular age range and use of horses. A study performed on leisure horses showed no association between age and risk of EGUS, nor any effect of breed or gender (Luthersson et al 2009b).

Exercise

Workload has been suggested to be one of the most important risk factors for EGUS. Recent work suggests that horses in light to heavy training for as short as 8 days may be at risk of developing gastric ulcers (White et al 2007). Furthermore, a study in Australia suggested that prevalence in racehorses increased 1.7 times for every week of training (Lester et al 2007). In an earlier study, horses running on a high-speed treadmill showed increased abdominal pressure and decreased stomach volume compared with resting values. It was suggested that contraction of the stomach during exercise allowed acid from the glandular mucosa to reflux up into the nonglandular mucosa resulting in injury to the relatively unprotected nonglandular mucosa – the "acid-splashing" hypothesis (Lorenzo-Figueras & Merrit 2002). Additionally it was found that gastric pH decreased rapidly to < 4 at the beginning of walking, continued to decrease during trotting and galloping, and remained low until the horses returned to a walk. Less marked changes were seen in animals that had been fed prior to being exercised. Horses in intensive training programs are exposed to a longer daily duration of more intense exercise and therefore, potentially an increased duration of acid exposure, possibly contributing significantly to the risk of gastric ulceration. However, all types of work do not necessarily increase the risk of gastric ulcers. A study of pleasure/leisure horses in Denmark showed no apparent effect of workload on the risk of EGUS. None of the animals evaluated were racehorses and even if they were used for equestrian training and competition (dressage or show jumping) exercise workload was less than that of a typical racehorse. This could indicate that only strenuous exercise results in acid injury of the non-glandular mucosa. However, an alternative explanation could relate to the association between starch intake and risk of EGUS (see below). Racehorses typically receive increased amounts of dietary starch in association with increased workload.

Fasting

Horses are continuous but variable gastric acid secreters, and feeding state affects the pH of gastric juice. When feed is withheld from horses before racing or due to the feeding regimen, gastric pH drops rapidly and the nonglandular mucosa is exposed to an acid environment (Vatistas et al 1999b). The pH of gastric juice in horses from which feed was withheld for several hours was 2.0 or less (Murray 1992). In horses fed free-choice timothy hay for 24 hours, mean gastric pH was significantly higher than in fasted horses (3.1 in hay fed vs. 1.5 in fasted) (Murray & Schusser 1989). Intermittent feeding has been shown to both cause and increase the severity of gastric ulcers and has been developed as a reliable model for induction of EGUS (Murray 1994, Murray & Eichorn 1996). Gastric ulceration was induced by alternating 24 hours periods of feed deprivation and ad libitum access to hay, for a total of 96 hours of feed deprivation. The result of this feeding protocol was erosions and ulceration of the nonglandular mucosa of each horse in this study. The non-glandular mucosa, as discussed above, is the most susceptible to this protocol due to its lack of mucosal protective factors.

Pasture turnout

Grazing horses, in general, appear to have a decreased prevalence of EGUS (Murray et al 1989, Hammond et al 1986). Due to a continuous flow of saliva and ingesta, stomach acid is buffered, with pH ≥ 4+ for a large portion of the day (Husted et al 2008). In Thoroughbred racehorses in training, horses with access to some turnout were less likely to have ulceration, and this risk was even lower if they were turned out with other horses (Lester et al 2007). Within seven days, squamous mucosal lesions were induced when horses were taken from pasture to stall confinement with free choice timothy hay and no training (Murray & Eichorn 1996).

Pasture turnout is considered to be advantageous in many reviews but in one study of 62 broodmares (33 pregnant and 29 nonpregnant) kept under similar management on pasture (no details of feeding program given) there was a relatively high ulcer prevalence of ~67% in the pregnant mares and ~76% in the non pregnant mares (Le Jeune et al 2006). This apparently high incidence may reflect dietary management. Additionally there was no effect on intragastric pH of horses housed in a grass paddock, a stall on their own or in a stall with an adjacent companion when fed ad libitum grass hay and grain twice a day (1 kg/100 kg/day), suggesting that housing may not affect gastric pH and that being in a paddock may not provide any benefit (Husted et al 2008). The study of Husted et al (2008) focused only on pH as the primary ulcerogenic factor, whereas other factors might be associated with ulceration. The amount of starch given to each horse per day, for example, was not described. As described below, a high intake of starch may enhance the influence of a low pH by compromising squamous mucosal integrity.

Starch intake

Starch/grain intake has been associated with an increased risk of EGUS in horses. Frank et al (2005) noted a marked increase in ulceration when nonexercising animals were stabled and fed grain at 1% of body weight (BW) (3.7 to 5.1 kg of grain per mare once daily), 1 hour before hay was fed. The remainder of the dietary requirement was met by feeding grass hay. The diet was designed to provide 1.5 times the digestible energy (DE) requirement for maintenance. Exceeding 2 g/kg BW of starch intake per day was associated with an approximately twofold increase in the likelihood of EGUS (severity grade ≥ 2 [out of 5]) and feeding more than 1 g/kg BW of starch per meal was associated with a 2.6 times increase in the likelihood of EGUS ≥ 2 in the non-glandular part of the stomach (Luthersson et al 2009b). In this population, starch intake was independent of workload and as increased level of work was not associated with increased risk the influence of starch on risk of gastric ulcers was significant. The influence of starch on ulcer risk was greatest for nonglandular mucosal lesions.

Vatistas et al (1999b) observed development of ulcers in horses within 14 days of their removal from pasture, stabling (fed 6 kg concentrate feed/day) and entering a simulated training regimen. In another study, dams were supplied with concentrate feed and foals were allowed to eat their dam's food. When more concentrate feed was fed to the mares, lesions in the squamous mucosa were more prevalent and more severe (Taharaguchi et al 2004).

The stomach of the horse has a large, diverse population of microflora when the horse is fed a diet rich in starch or non-structural carbohydrates. The bacteria found in the stomach of the horse include *Streptococcus bovis, Streptococcus equinus, Lactobacillus salivarius, L. mucosae, L. delbrueckii,* and *Mitsuokella jalaludinii* (Al Jassim & Andrews 2009). Volatile fatty acids (VFAs) are produced when carbohydrates are fermented by the microflora within the gastrointestinal tract. VFAs (including acetic, butyric, propionic, and valeric acids), produced by the fermentation of starch/sugar by the gastric microflora, have been shown to reduce mucosal integrity and affect mucosal tissue bioelectric properties (Andrews et al 2006, 2008, Nadeau et al 2003a, b). An in vitro study found that acetic, butyric and propionic acids caused a decrease in barrier function of the squamous mucosa (Nadeau et al 2003a, b). This effect is due to the lipid solubility of these VFAs at pH ≤ 4.0, resulting in VFAs penetrating cells in the non-glandular gastric mucosa, acidifying the cellular contents, inhibiting sodium transport and leading to cellular swelling. Andrews et al (2006) also found that squamous mucosal cells are susceptible to VFA injury in a pH (increased injury with lower pH), dose (higher the dose, greater the damage), and time (longer the tissue is exposed the greater the damage) dependent manner. When the nonglandular gastric mucosa was exposed to lactic acid, tissue permeability was increased but sodium transport was not affected.

High-starch diets are likely to result in higher concentrations of VFA, and, as they are normally associated with lower fiber intakes, more fluid contents within the stomach, and less salivary buffering. Cereals (high starch) tend to be low in calcium and possibly other potential buffering agents, which may also increase risk of ulceration. All of these factors may contribute to the association between starch intake and risk of EGUS.

Forage feeding and type of forage

When fed hay and pasture, horses produced 400–480 g saliva per 100 g dry matter consumed whereas when a concentrate was fed, horses produced approximately half the amount of saliva (206 g saliva per 100 g dry matter consumed; Meyer et al 1985). This would be expected since chewing stimulates saliva production, and horses spend more time chewing forage than they do concentrate feeds. One theory is that saliva produced in sufficient quantities will contribute to the buffering of gastric acid. Without this salivary buffering effect, damage to the gastric mucosa is more likely to occur and lesions (gastric ulcers) may develop.

Free access to fibrous feed (grass or digestible forage) or frequent forage feeding may therefore help reduce the risk of gastric ulceration. Feeding alfalfa hay and grain, however, resulted in higher gastric pH and less peptic injury to the gastric squamous mucosa than feeding bromegrass hay or coastal Bermuda hay with no grain (Nadeau et al 2000, Lybbert et al 2007). This suggests that forage type may also be important. In a recent study (Luthersson et al 2009b), an increased likelihood (4.5 times) of nonglandular gastric ulceration (severity score ≥ 2) was demonstrated when straw was the only forage provided. These horses either had access to straw from their bedding (without any other forage) or were being specifically provided with straw as their forage source with none or very small amounts of hay or haylage (<0.25 kg dry matter (DM)/100 kg BW) in their daily ration. Straw may provide low levels of buffering support due to its low protein and calcium content, plus its physical nature may result in mucosal irritation. In addition, its inclusion at high levels in a ration may affect the nature of the fibrous mat within the stomach, increasing the risk of exposure of the squamous epithelium to acidogenic factors. Additionally, time between forage meals >6 h, compared with more frequent forage feeding with intervals <6 h, increased the likelihood of non-glandular ulcers (Luthersson et al 2009b).

Water intake

It has been shown that horses without access to water in their paddock were more likely to have EGUS ≥ 2 (Luthersson et al 2009b). This association was significant for nonglandular ulcers alone as well as EGUS in all parts of the stomach. Water intake may dilute gastric fluid and therefore increase pH, but other explanations need to be explored.

Electrolyte administration

In a study of endurance horses, paste electrolyte administration by dose syringe resulted in a significant increase in mean ulcer number and severity when compared to placebo administration (Holbrook et al 2005). In the electrolyte treatment group, hyperemia, edema of the oral mucosa, drooping of the lower lip, and ptyalism were noted. Increased risk of ulcers has been shown with electrolyte pastes or hypertonic solutions given orally, but not when electrolytes were mixed in feed or given in lower doses in water (authors' personal observations). More work is needed in this area.

NSAIDs

NSAIDs have long been linked with an increased risk of gastric ulceration in horses (Tomlinson & Blikslager 2003). The NSAIDs phenylbutazone and flunixin meglumine have been shown to induce gastric ulcers in horses, primarily in the glandular mucosa (MacAllister et al 1992). Ulceration may occur as a result of prostaglandin inhibition, which results in reduced mucosal blood flow, decreased mucus production, and increased HCl secretion. Adequate blood flow is necessary to remove hydrogen ions that diffuse through the mucus layer covering the glandular mucosa. Gastric mucosal ischemia may lead to a hypoxia induced cellular acidosis, release of oxygen free radicals, phospholipase and proteases, all of which may damage the cell membrane leading to necrosis.

However, evidence of an association between gastric ulceration and administration of NSAIDs at recommended dosages is lacking (Fennell & Franklin 2009). In a study comparing different NSAIDs alone or in combination (Reed et al 2006), three of the four horses treated with phenylbutazone alone had no nonglandular ulcers while one of the horses had a nonglandular ulcer score of grade 2/4. When treated with phenylbutazone and flunixin meglumine, two horses had a non-glandular ulcer score of grade 2/4, one had a nonglandular ulcer score of grade 3/4 and the horse that had a nonglandular ulcer score of 2 after treatment with phenylbutazone alone had a non-glandular ulcer score of grade 4/4. These results indicate that combination NSAID treatment should be approached with caution. Individual horses will respond differently and there is variability in what may be an acceptable dose and duration of treatment. Horses that are at risk of developing ulcers (e.g., previous history of EGUS) should receive prophylactic administration of anti-ulcer medication and/or be treated with a cyclo-oxygenase-1 sparing NSAID, which are reported to be less toxic to the gastrointestinal tract compared to the more non-selective NSAIDs such as phenylbutazone (Andrews & McConnico 2009).

Key Points – Risk factors for EGUS

- Physical activity/exercise training
- Prolonged feed withholding
- High dietary starch intake (>1 g starch/kg BW per meal or >2 g starch/kg BW per day)
- Inadequate dietary forage (<1.0 kg/100 kg body weight), an interval between forage feedings that exceeds 6 h, or straw as the sole roughage source
- Lack of access to water
- Use of nonsteroidal anti-inflammatory drugs

Potential role of bile acids and bacteria within the stomach

Bile acids

The backflow of duodenal contents is a normal occurrence in horses (Kitchen et al 2000). Some research suggests that refluxed bile salts may contribute to gastric ulceration through an increase in nonglandular mucosal cell permeability to hydrogen ions (Berschneider et al 1999, Vaezi & Richter 1996). Reese & Andrews (2009), however, stated that the effects of bile salts are questionable because the duodenal reflux is less acidic (pH > 4.0) and therefore unlikely to be ulcerogenic (Argenzio 1999).

Bacterial contamination, including *Helicobacter pylori*

Helicobacter pylori is a causative agent of gastric ulcers in humans but there is no conclusive evidence of this in the horse. Squamous and glandular mucosa samples were collected by necropsy from 20 Thoroughbreds and examined for the presence of *Helicobacter* DNA (Contreras et al 2007). Using a Warthin–Starry special stain, spiral-shaped bacteria were found in 2/7 horses with ulcers, 4/5 horses with gastritis and 5/6 horses with both pathologies. *Helicobacter*-like DNA was detected by polymerase chain reaction (PCR) in the squamous and/or glandular mucosa in 2/7 horses with ulcers, 3/5 horses with gastritis, 5/6 horses with both pathologies, and 1/2 horses with normal mucosa. Every sample except one that was positive for the Warthin-Starry stain was PCR positive for the *Helicobacter* assay. The *Helicobacter* genus may colonize the gastric mucosa of horses but its pathogenicity requires further study. In other species, *Helicobacter* species besides *H. pylori* (which is found in the human, macaque, and cat stomach) have been found in the stomach e.g. *H. heilmannii* (in dog, cat, human and monkey; Fox & Lee 1997).

Other bacteria that have been implicated in the inhibition of ulcer healing include *Escherichia coli* and *Lactobacillus* spp. In rats, *E. coli* colonized acetic acid induced gastric ulcers and impaired healing while oral administration of lactulose resulted in an increase in *Lactobacillus* spp. growth and colonization of the ulcer bed (Elliott et al 1998). Secondary bacterial colonization of gastric ulcers in the horse stomach may delay ulcer healing and antibiotic treatment may be indicated.

Clinical signs of EGUS

Potential clinical signs associated with EGUS in adult horses are numerous and often non-specific (Table 34-1). Many signs of gastric ulcers may be attributed to other causes or not recognized as being due to EGUS (e.g. a "picky" appetite). Clinical signs tend to reflect chronic pain and are expressed depending on individual factors such as temperament and workload. Moreover, there does not appear to be a clear relationship between the severity of ulceration and severity of the clinical signs. The authors' opinion is that ulcers in the nonglandular mucosa are better tolerated compared to ulcers in the glandular mucosa. In the nonglandular mucosa, ulcer scores of ≥ 3 are more likely to create obvious clinical signs, whereas in horses with lesions in the glandular mucosa, especially around the pylorus, clinical signs may be seen with lower ulcer scores (≤ 3). A study of 201 Danish pleasure horses showed no relationship between severity of signs and severity of EGUS; additionally, there was no association between body condition score and the incidence of EGUS (Luthersson et al 2009a). On the other hand, a study performed on Thoroughbred racehorses (Lester et al 2007) showed that difficulty in maintaining

Table 34-1 Clinical Signs of Equine Gastric Ulceration Syndrome*

Poor appetite/changed eating behavior	In general feed intake is reduced, but some horses lose appetite for certain components of their diet, such as grain or forage
Weight loss and difficulties in maintaining normal BCS	This weight loss can be a direct consequence of reduced appetite, but it may also represent an increased metabolic rate due to chronic, low-grade pain
Poor hair coat	Horses with EGUS often develop a rough hair coat and look dull, perhaps due to chronic pain and weight loss
Reduced performance	This can be a consequence of negative energy balance and weight loss. In riding horses, such as dressage and show jumping, performance is based on focus and cooperation. In these horses, reduced performance may be a consequence of behavior changes and lack of focus during performance exercise
Behavior changes	Horses with gastric ulceration frequently show signs of changed attitude, either towards other horses or their owners/handlers. They can either develop increased fear and flight responses or become abnormally quiet or dull
Abdominal discomfort	This can be expressed in various ways. Some horses show excessive recumbency and others stretch to urinate frequently. Discomfort on girth tightening is a common sign among riding horses with EGUS
Colic	Acute and severe colic is not associated with gastric ulceration, whereas recurrent colic with mild to moderate pain is more common.
Crib biting	An association has been shown between crib biting and gastric ulceration in horses. Onset of crib biting in foals and younger horses may be a sign of gastric discomfort. In adult horses, crib biting is a stereotypic behavior that is influenced by many factors and cannot be taken as a specific sign of gastric ulceration

BCS, body condition score.
*This is a list of the possible clinical signs in horses with EGUS. These signs are not present in all horses with gastric ulcers. Some horses show several and severe signs, while others show none or very mild signs. Severity of clinical signs and severity of ulcers are not strongly correlated.

body weight was positively associated with squamous mucosal ulceration.

Clinical signs of gastric ulceration in foals tend to be more acute and severe than in adults, but are also commonly non-specific signs of abdominal discomfort (Andrews & Nadeau 1999). The most common clinical signs are colic, poor nursing, diarrhea (usually without fever or other signs of infection), bruxism, ptyalism, dorsal recumbency, and chronic poor condition. Foals with critical illness (e.g., sepsis) are at risk for development of glandular and non-glandular mucosal ulcers. Decreased mucosal blood flow, physiological stress and reduced feed intake may contribute to ulcer development in these circumstances. The etiology and pathophysiology of gastric ulcers in foals may be different compared to adult horses.

Table 34-2 Equine Gastric Ulcer Council Grading System (Andrews et al 1999)

Grade	Appearance of gastric mucosa
0	Intact epithelium
1	Intact mucosa, evidence of hyperkeratosis or hyperemia
2	Small, single or multifocal lesions
3	Large, single or multifocal lesions or extensive superficial lesions
4	Extensive lesions with areas of apparent deep ulceration

Diagnosis of gastric ulceration

The most common, and currently the only reliable method, for diagnosis of gastric ulceration is endoscopy (Andrews et al 1999). In order to reach a mature horse's stomach, an endoscope of at least 200 cm in length is required but a 280–330 cm endoscope is needed to reach the duodenum. The stomach of foals up to 30–40 days in age can be viewed with a 110 cm long endoscope with an outer diameter of 10 mm.

For best results in adult horses, feed should be withheld for at least 12 hours prior to endoscopy to allow sufficient gastric emptying. In foals on a milk diet, a 1–2 h period of fasting is adequate providing the procedure is performed with the foal in lateral recumbency (Jones 2006). By rolling the foal from side to side, the entire mucosa can be examined. In addition, the pylorus and proximal duodenum should be examined. It is important to look at the entire stomach in a systematic way, with accurate documentation of lesion number, severity and location.

As discussed above a number of gastric ulcer scoring systems have been developed. Two of the most popular are included in Tables 34-2 and 34-3 (Andrews et al 1999, MacAllister et al 1997). Most systems score lesions according to number and severity. One study reported that the Equine Gastric Ulcer Council System was quicker and easier to use, more repeatable and greater agreement between examiners when compared to the Number/Severity System (N/S; Bell et al 2007). In the authors' opinion, however, the N/S system is more definitive for grading the number and severity of lesions.

Table 34-3 Number/Severity Scoring System (MacAllister et al 1997)

Grade	Number of lesions	Severity
0	None	Normal
1	1–2 localized lesions	Appears superficial
2	3–5 localized lesions	Deeper structure involved (more than mucosal)
3	6–10 lesions	Multiple lesions and variable severity
4	>10 lesions	Same as Grade 2 but with an active appearance
5	n/a	Same as Grade 4 but with active hemorrhage or adherent blood clot

Nutritional management to reduce risk of gastric ulceration (Box 34.1)

Allowing horses free access to good quality pasture and feeding alfalfa or other high calcium (6–14 mg/g feed on a DM basis) or high protein (17–20% crude protein on a DM basis) forages may help to reduce risk of gastric ulceration. Pasture turnout is preferred to stall confinement as horses on pasture tend to spend more time foraging than horses in a stall, resulting in longer periods of low gastric acidity. Horses fed hay should receive a minimum of 1.0 to 1.5 kg/100 kg BW of long-stem, high quality forage, with hay available throughout the day and night (Videla & Andrews 2009). Additionally, the diet should consist of at least 75% roughage to maintain normal pH balance in the stomach.

Continuous access to pasture forage is preferred for horses at high risk (or with a history) of EGUS but frequent feedings of hay (4–6 meals/day) could be a suitable replacement (Jones 2006). Although one study did show high ulcer prevalence in broodmares kept on pasture (Le Jeune et al 2006), no details of the feeding program were mentioned and the high ulcer incidence may have reflected other aspects of dietary management. Feeding multiple forage types rather than a single forage may help prevent gastric ulceration in some animals by more closely mimicking their varied evolutionary diet and increasing duration and frequency of foraging behavior (Thorne et al 2005).

Overweight horses and ponies at risk of EGUS should receive a minimum amount of high quality forage or a mixture of high quality forage and straw divided into 5–6 portions given at regular intervals (no more than 6 h; Luthersson et al 2009b). Straw should not be the only forage provided as its low protein and calcium contents result in low buffering capacity. Straw may be safely included in the ration at <0.25 kg DM/100 kg BW; in the authors' view this level of straw feeding will not increase risk of impaction colic, cause irritation of the gastric mucosa, or alter the fibrous mat in the stomach.

Grain and grain-based concentrates should be fed sparingly or avoided in horses prone to gastric ulceration (Buchanan & Andrews 2003, Ralston 2007). Volatile fatty acid production in the stomach is greatly augmented when large meals of sweet feed (>2 kg/meal) are ingested. Grains like barley and oats can be substituted to decrease fermentation to VFAs relative to sweet feeds (Buchanan & Andrews 2003). The diet should not exceed 2 g/kg BW of starch intake per day or more than 1 g/kg BW of starch per meal (Frank et al 2005, Luthersson et al 2009b). Also, concentrate meals should not be fed less than 6 h apart (Videla & Andrews 2009). A study of 54 Standardbred racehorses in training found that 75% of horses fed twice daily had gastric ulcers compared to 57.9% of horses fed three times a day (Bezdekova et al 2008). It is therefore recommended that horses be fed at least three times daily to reduce the risk of gastric ulcers.

Vegetable oils such as corn oil may help reduce the risk of gastric ulcers. Ponies fed 45 ml corn oil orally once daily by dose syringe had significantly lower gastric acid output

Box 34.1 General Recommendations to Minimize Risk of EGUS*

- Horses should be fed a forage-based diet. Forage along with a mineral and vitamin supplement is adequate for many horses and ponies.
  - The amount of hay/haylage (as fed) should be a minimum of 1.0 to 1.5 kg/100 kg BW
  - Hay/haylage should be fed frequently or free choice.
- Horses in little or no work as well as "easy keeper" animals may benefit from forages with lower energy content so that the amount fed and the time spent in feeding activity are maximized without promotion of weight gain. Straw should comprise no more than 25% of the forage ration.
- Restrict dietary starch
  - Ideally feed <1 g/kg BW starch/meal and preferably <2 g/kg BW starch per day
  - Examples: 2.5 kg oats (40% starch) for a 500-kg horse = 2 g starch/kg BW; 2.5 kg corn (60% starch) for a 500-kg horse = 3 g starch/kg BW
- Consider adding some chaff, including alfalfa, to grain or sweet feed meals (100–200 g/100 kg BW).
- If additional energy is required, consider the gradual introduction of supplemental vegetable oil (up to 100 ml/100 kg BW) but check the vitamin and mineral balance of the resultant diet.
- Provide pasture turnout whenever possible (although it is important to note that ulcers can occur in pasture managed animals).
- Provide continuous access to water (including horses at pasture).
- Wherever possible and especially in a horse with a known predisposition to EGUS, avoid stressful situations such as travelling long distances, changing environments and long periods of confinement where the horse cannot freely move around. Consider forage provision during transportation and immediately on arrival.
- If horses need to be treated with NSAIDs (such as phenylbutazone or flunixin meglumine), the minimal effective dose should be used. Horses that are predisposed to gastric ulcers should be concurrently treated with antiulcer drugs (omeprazole) at preventive or treatment doses.

*Recommendations are made on an as fed basis.

and increased prostaglandin concentration in their gastric juice when compared to the placebo treatment (Cargile et al 2004). The potential antiulcerogenic properties of three dietary oils were assessed in mares subjected to a feed-fast protocol designed to induce development of ulcers (Frank et al 2005). When compared to placebo (240 ml water/day), corn oil, refined rice bran oil or crude rice bran oil (240 ml of each oil) given daily for 6 weeks did not affect the number and severity of ulcers induced by the 7-day feed-fast protocol that was applied during the last week of each feeding period. Further research is needed to determine the efficacy of dietary oils for management or prevention of EGUS.

Horses should have continuous access to water, including when out in a paddock (Luthersson et al 2009b). With transport to a new location, strategies should be applied to adapt horses to the new water source. Methods to entice water intake include adding apple cider vinegar or another flavour to the new water, adapting the horses to a particular flavor mix before transportation or relocation and then use of this mix in the new water source. Water intake should be monitored. Forage and water should be offered at intervals not to exceed 6 h during transportation. Some authors have also recommended daily administration of omeprazole (4 mg/kg PO) or ranitidine (6.6 mg/kg PO) before, during and after travel to shows or other events (e.g. treatment for 3–4 days before and after transportation; Buchanan & Andrews 2003).

No studies have evaluated the effect of pre-race (or other athletic event) feeding on EGUS. In theory, provision of small amounts of hay within 3–4 h of the event may increase buffering capacity within the stomach and mitigate acid injury of gastric mucosa. In general, grain or grain-based feeds are withdrawn 3–4 h before competition exercise. Water should be made available soon after exercise and hay is usually offered after cool-down.

If horses need to be treated with NSAIDs therapeutically or as a prophylactic and are performing high intensity exercise, travelling, in high-stress environments, or need long term treatment for problems such as arthritis, the minimal dose that effectively controls pain should be used. NSAIDs such as firocoxib and ketoprofen that have minimal effects on the gastrointestinal tract should be considered. Antiulcer medications given at preventative or treatment doses simultaneously with NSAIDS should also be considered (Videla & Andrews 2009).

Medical management

The goal of medical therapy is to relieve pain, eliminate clinical signs and promote ulcer healing. Treatment that increases gastric pH to 4 or more for at least 20 h/day typically quickly decreases clinical signs of pain and facilitates ulcer healing. Many pharmacologic agents are available for treatment of gastric ulcers in humans but few of these drugs have been shown to be effective in the treatment and prevention of EGUS. Antacids, such as aluminum hydroxide and magnesium hydroxide, have a moderate and short-lived effect on gastric pH (Murray & Grodinsky 1992). Histamine type-2 receptor antagonists, such as cimetidine and ranitidine, have poor bioavailability after oral administration, must be given every 6–8 hours, and have poor ability to produce ulcer healing (MacAllister & Sangiah 1993). The most effective drug for treatment of EGUS is the proton pump inhibitor, omeprazole, which binds irreversibly to the parietal cell H^+-K^+ ATPase (proton pump), and thereby blocks secretion of hydrochloric acid. At recommended doses, omeprazole can block acid secretion for 24 h. An equine specific, pH stable form of omeprazole must be used as the human form of omeprazole has poor bioavailability (16%) in horses and duration of acid suppression is insufficient (12 h) (Merrit et al 2002).

Omeprazole has been shown to be an effective treatment for EGUS at a dose of 4 mg/kg orally once daily. Treatment for 28 days in racing animals in full work resulted in 92% improvement and 78% healing of squamous mucosal ulceration (Murray et al 1997) and several other studies have shown high rates of healing at a dose of 4 mg/kg q 24 h. A lower dose of 2 mg/kg q 24 h is effective for the prevention of ulcer recurrence. Glandular ulcer healing rates have not been reported but a longer duration of therapy (28–56 days) may be required.

Coating or binding agents such as sucralfate and bismuth subsalicylate bind to stomach ulcers and promote healing. Used alone, these agents have not been effective in treating EGUS, but may promote healing if used in combination with omeprazole, especially for glandular ulcers (MacAllister 1999). Sucralfate is a hydroxyl aluminum salt of sucrose octasulfate and binds to the negatively charged particles in the ulcer bed, buffering HCl by increasing bicarbonate secretion and stimulating prostaglandin production. The dose of sucralfate when used in combination with other drugs is 20–22 mg/kg PO, q 8–12 h. Bismuth may have a coating effect similar to sucralfate and also reduces or inhibits the activation of pepsin. In humans, bismuth is used as part of the therapy of *Helicobacter pylori* induced gastric ulcers (Brunton 1996). It also may be used in horses with chronic glandular ulceration, at a dose of 2–4 mg/kg PO, q 12 h.

Various feed supplements to treat or prevent gastric ulcers are available, but only a few have been tested in controlled clinical studies. A study of a pectin–lecithin complex (Pronutrin) showed a significant reduction in gastric mucosal lesion scores and the study authors concluded that this product could potentially have a beneficial effect on the healing of gastric ulcers (Venner et al 1999).

Ulcer healing can occur spontaneously if the gastric environment is improved. Amelioration of clinical signs will improve daily feed intake and the increased time spent chewing leads to increased saliva production. A ration of high quality forage hay or haylage (not straw) and limited starch should promote less acidic gastric contents, support healing and reduce the risk of ulcer recurrence.

Many horses in exercise training are maintained on antiulcer medication. In humans there are concerns that long term treatment with antiulcer medications might result in alterations in mineral digestion and increased risk of gastrointestinal infections (Sanduleanu et al 2001). Normal digestive processes in the horse may also be affected by prolonged alterations in gastric pH and in both adult horses and foals the normal barrier function against bacterial colonization in the gastrointestinal mucosa might be reduced (Javsicas & Sanchez 2008).

Different medical management and feeding strategies have been recommended for horses involved in different disciplines (Buchanan & Andrews 2003). A combination of preventative and therapeutic treatments may be needed to prevent or manage gastric ulcers. The general recommendations mentioned earlier should be followed first, since all classes of horses will benefit from them. Even racehorses in hard work can be maintained on a diet significantly lower in starch or even forage-only diets, as shown in a study on Standardbred horses in Sweden (Connysson et al 2006). Reducing the amount of starch in diet and increasing the intake of high quality forage will benefit most horses that cannot be maintained on pasture year round due to climatic conditions, and it can be done without reducing their potential performance.

Conclusions

EGUS has a multifactorial etiology, with a long list of potential risk factors. By following the general recommendations for diet and other aspects of management described in this chapter, it may be possible to prevent or reduce the risk of gastric ulceration despite the influence of individual factors. Although medical treatment of gastric ulcers may be indicated, especially for horses showing severe clinical signs, feeding and management practices should be instituted to help reduce risk of ulcer recurrence.

References

Al Jassim, R.M., Andrews, F.M., 2009. The bacterial community of the horse gastrointestinal tract and its realtion to fermentative acidosis, laminitis, colic, and stomach ulcers. Vet Clinic Equine 25, 199–215.

Andrews, F.M., McConnico, R., 2009. Cause for concern: Evidence that therapeutic dosing of nonselective NSAIDs contributes to gastrointestinal injury. Equine Vet Educ 21, 663–664.

Andrews, F.M., Nadeau, J.A., 1999. Clinical syndromes of gastric ulceration in foals and mature horses. Equine Vet J Suppl. 29, 30–33.

Andrews, F., Bernard, W., Byars, D., et al., 1999. The Equine Gastric Ulcer Council: Recommendations for the diagnosis and treatment of equine gastric ulcer syndrome (EGUS). Equine Vet Educ 11, 262–272.

Andrews, F.M., Reinemeyer, C.R., McCracken, M.D., et al., 2002. Comparison of endoscopic, necropsy and histology scoring of gastric ulcers. Equine Vet J 34, 475–478.

Andrews, F.M., Buchanan, B.R., Smith, S.H., et al., 2006. In vitro effects of hydrochloric acid and various concentrations of acetic, propionic, butyric or valeric acid on bioelectric properties of equine gastric squamous mucosa. Am J Vet Res 67, 1873–1882.

Andrews, F.M., Buchanan, B.R., Elliott, S.B., et al., 2008. In vitro effects of hydrochloric and lactic acids on bioelectric properties of equine gastric squamous mucosa. Equine Vet J 40, 301–305.

Argenzio, R.A., 1999. Comparative pathophysiology of nonglandular ulcer disease: a review of experimental studies. Equine Vet J Suppl 29, 19–23.

Bell R.J.W., Kingston, J.K., Mogg, T.D., 2007. A comparison of two scoring systems for endoscopic grading of gastric ulceration in horses. New Zealand Vet J 55, 19–22.

Berschneider, H.M., Blikslager, A.T., Roberts, M.C., 1999. Role of duodenal reflux in nonglandular gastric ulcer disease of the mature horse. Equine Vet J Suppl 29, 24–29.

Bertone, J.J., 2000. Prevalence of gastric ulcers in elite, heavy use Western performance horses. J Vet Intern Med 14, 366.

Bezdekova, B., Jahn, P., Vyskocil, M., 2008. Gastric ulceration, appetite and feeding practices in Standardbred racehorses in Czech Republic. Acta Vet Brno 77, 603–607.

Brunton, L.L., 1996. Agents for control of gastric acidity and treatment of peptic ulcers. In: Hardmann, J.G., Limbird, L.E., Molinoff, P.B., et al. (Eds.), Goodman and Gilmans's The Pharmacological Basis of Therapeutics, ninth ed. McGraw-Hill, New York, pp. 901–916.

Buchanan, B.R., Andrews, F.M., 2003. Treatment and prevention of equine gastric ulcer syndrome. Vet Clin Equine 19, 575–597.

Cargile, J.L., Burrow, J.A., Kim, I., et al., 2004. Effect of dietary corn oil supplementation on equine gastric fluid acid, sodium, and prostaglandin E_2 content before and during pentagastrin infusion. J Vet Intern Med 18, 545–549.

Chameroy, K.A., Nadeau, J.A., Bushmich, S.L., et al., 2006. Prevalence of nonglandular gastric ulcers in horses involved in a university riding program. J Equine Vet Sci 26, 207 –211.

Connysson, M., Muhonen, S., Lindberg, E.J., et al., 2006. Effects on exercise response, fluid and acid-base balance of protein intake from forage-only diets in Standardbred horses. Equine Vet J Suppl 36, 648–653.

Contreras, M., Morales, A., García-Amado, M.A., et al., 2007. Detection of *Helicobacter*-like DNA in the gastric mucosa of Thoroughbred horses. Lett Appl Microbiol 45, 553–557.

Elliott, S.N., Buret, A., McKnight, W., et al., 1998. Bacteria rapidly colonize and modulate healing of gastric ulcer in rats. Am J Physiol - GI 275, 425–432.

Fennell, L.C., Franklin, R.P., 2009. Do nonsteroidal anti-inflammatory drugs administered at therapeutic dosages induce gastric ulcers in horses? Equine Vet Educ 21, 660–662.

Fox, J.G., Lee, A., 1997. The role of *Helicobacter* species in newly recognized gastrointestinal tract disease of animals. Lab Anim Sci 47, 222–255.

Frank, N., Andrews, F.M. Elliott, S.B., et al., 2005. Effects of dietary oils on the development of gastric ulcers in mares. Am J Vet Res 66, 2006–2011.

Furr, M.O., Murray, M.J., 1989. Treatment of gastric ulcers in horses with histamine type-2 receptor antagonists. Equine Vet. J Suppl. 7, 77–79.

Hammond, C.J., Mason, D.K., Watkins, K.L., 1986. Gastric ulceration in mature Thoroughbred horses. Equine Vet J 18, 284–287.

Holbrook, T.C., Simmons, R.D., Payton, M.E., et al., 2005. Effect of repeated oral administration of hypertonic electrolyte solution on equine gastric mucosa. Equine Vet J 37, 501–504.

Husted, L., Sanchez, L.C., Olsen, S.N., et al., 2008. Effect of paddock vs stall housing on 24 hour gastric pH within the proximal and ventral equine stomach. Equine Vet J 40, 337–341.

Javsicas, L.H., Sanchez, L.C., 2008. The effect of omeprazole paste on intragastric pH in clinically ill neonatal foals. Equine Vet J 40, 41–44.

Jones, S.L., 2006. Gastric ulcer disease. Proceedings of the North American Veterinary Conference, Orlando, Florida, USA, 20, pp. 130–131.

Jonsson, H., Egenvall, A., 2006. Prevalence of gastric ulceration in Swedish Standardbreds in race-training. Equine Vet J 38, 209–213.

Kitchen, D.L., Burrow, J.A., Heartless, C.S., et al., 2000. Effect of pyloric blockade and infusion of histamine or pentagastrin on gastric secretion in horses. Am J Vet Res 61, 1133–1139.

Le Jeune, S.S., Nieto, J.E., Dechant, J.E., et al., 2009. Prevalence of gastric ulcers in Thoroughbred broodmares in pasture: a preliminary study. Vet J 181, 251–255.

Le Jeune, S.S., Nieto, J.E., Dechant, J.E., et al., 2006. Prevalence of gastric ulcers in Thoroughbred broodmares in pasture. Proc AAEP, San Antonio, Texas, USA. American Association of Equine Practitioners, Lexington, KY, 52, p. 264.

Lester, G.D., 2004. Gastrointestinal diseases of performance horses. In: Hinchcliff, K.W., Kaneps, A.J., Geor, R.J. (Eds.), Equine Sports Medicine and Sugery. Saunders, Elsevier Ltd., Philadelphia, 1037–1043.

Lester, G.D., Robertson, I.D., Secomber, C., 2007. Risk factors for gastric ulceration in Thoroughbred racehorses. Proc AAEP, Orlando, Florida, USA. American Association of Equine Practitioners, Lexington, KY, 53, p. 529.

Lorenzo-Figueras, M., Merritt, A.M., 2002. Effects of exercise on gastric volume and pH in the proximal portion of the stomach of horses. Am J Vet Res 63, 1481–1487.

Luthersson, N., Hou Nielsen, K., Harris, P., et al., 2009a. Equine gastric ulceration syndrome (EGUS) in 201 horses in Denmark and the influence of age, sex, temperament, breed and workload. Equine Vet J 41, 619–624.

Luthersson, N., Hou Nielsen, K., Harris, P., et al., 2009b. Risk factors associated with equine gastric ulceration syndrome (EGUS) in 201 horses in Denmark. Equine Vet J 41, 625–630.

Lybbert, T., Gibbs, P., Cohen, N., et al., 2007. Feeding alfalfa hay to exercising horses reduces the severity of gastric squamous mucosal ulceration. In: Proc AAEP, Orlando, Florida, USA. American Association of Equine Practitioners, Lexington, KY, 53, pp. 525–526.

MacAllister, C.G., 1999. A review of medical treatment for peptic ulcer disease. Equine Vet J Suppl. 29, 45–49.

MacAllister, C.G., Sangiah, S., 1993. Effect of ranitidine on healing of experimentally induced gastric ulcers in ponies. Am J Vet Res 54, 1103–1107.

MacAllister, C.G., Sangiah, S., Mauromoustakos, A., 1992. Effect of a histamine H_2 type receptor antagonist (WY 45, 727) on the healing of gastric ulcers in ponies. J Vet Intern Med 6, 271–275.

MacAllister, C.G., Andrews, F.M., Deegan, E., et al., 1997. A scoring system for gastric ulcers in horses. Equine Vet J 29, 430–433.

McClure, S.R., Glickman, L.T., Glickman, N.W., 1999. Prevalence of gastric ulcers in show horses. J Am Vet Med Assoc 215, 256–259.

Merrit, A.M., Sanchez, L.C., Burrow, J.A., et al., 2002. Bioavailability of Gastrogard vs. three generic compounded omeprazole preparations in mature horses. Proc 7th International Colic Research Symposium, Manchester, UK, p. 81.

Meyer, H., Coenen, M., Gurer, C., 1985. Investigations of saliva production and chewing in horses fed various feed. Proc Equine Nutr Physiol Symp Lansing, Michigan, USA. Equine Nutrition and Physiology Society, Savoy, IL, pp. 38–41.

Murray, M.J., 1994. An equine model of inducing alimentary squamous epithelial ulceration. Dig Dis Sci 39, 2530–2535.

Murray, M.J., 1992. Aetiopathogenesis and treatment of peptic ulcer in the horse: a comparative review. Equine Vet J Suppl 7, 68–72.

Murray, M.J., 1999. Pathophysiology of peptic disorders in foals and horses: a review. Equine Vet J Suppl 29, 14–18.
Murray, M.J., Eichorn, E.S., 1996. Effects of intermittent feed deprivation, intermittent feed deprivation with ranitidine administration, and stall confinement with ad libitum access to hay on gastric ulceration in horse. Am J Vet Res 57, 1599–1603.
Murray, M.J., Grodinsky, C., 1992. The effect of famotidine, ranitidine and magnesium hydroxide/aluminium hydroxide on gastric fluid pH in adult horses. Equine Vet J Suppl. 11, 52–55.
Murray, M.J., Schusser, G.F., 1989. Application of gastric pH-metry in horses: measurement of 24 hour gastric pH in horses fed, fasted and treated with ranitidine. J Vet Intern Med 6, 133.
Murray, M.J., Grodinsky, C., Anderson, C.W., et al., 1989. Gastric ulcers in horses: a comparison of endoscopic findings in horses with and without clinical signs. Equine Vet J Suppl 7, 68–72.
Murray, M.J., Schusser, G.F., Pipers, F.S., et al., 1996. Factors associated with gastric lesions in Thoroughbred racehorses. Equine Vet J 28, 368–374.
Murray, M.J., Haven, M.L., Eichorn, E.S., et al., 1997. Effects of omeprazole on healing of naturally-occurring gastric ulcers in Thoroughbred racehorses. Equine Vet J 29, 425–429.
Nadeau, J.A., Andrews, F.M., Mathews, A.M., et al., 2000. Evaluation of diet as a cause of gastric ulcers in horses. Am J Vet Res 61, 784–790.
Nadeau, J.A., Andrews, F.M., Patton, C.S., et al., 2003a. Effects of hydrocholoric, acetic, butyric, and propionic acids on pathogenesis of ulcers in the nonglandular portion of the stomach of horses. Am J Vet Res 64, 404–412.
Nadeau, J.A., Andrews, F.M., Patton, C.S., et al., 2003b. Effects of hydrocholoric, valeric, and other volatile fatty acids on pathogenesis of ulcers in the nonglandular portion of the stomach of horses. Am J Vet Res 64, 413–417.
Nieto, J.E., Snyder, J.R., Beldomenico, P., et al., 2004. Prevalence of gastric ulcers in endurance horses – a preliminary report. Vet J 167, 33–37.
Orlando, R.C., 1991. Esophageal epithelial defense against acid injury. J Clin Gastronenterol Suppl 2 13, S1–S5.
Orlando, R.C., Lacy, E.R., Tobey, N.A., et al., 1992. Barriers to paracellular permeability in rabbit esophageal epithelium. Gastroenterol 102, 910–923.
Rabuffo, T.S., Orsini, J.A., Sullivan, E., et al., 2002. Associations between age, sex and prevalence of gastric ulceration in standardbred racehorses in training. J Am Vet Med Assoc 221, 1156–1159.
Ralston, S.L., 2007. Evidence-based equine nutrition. Vet Clin Equine 23, 365–384.
Reed, S.K., Messer, N.T., Tessman, R.K., et al., 2006. Effects of phenylbutazone alone or in combination with flunixin meglumine on blood protein concentrations in horses. Am J Vet Res 67, 398–402.
Reese, R.E., Andrews, F.M., 2009. Nutrition and dietary management of equine gastric ulcer syndrome. Vet Clin Equine 25, 79–92.
Sanduleanu, S., Jonkers, D., de Bruine, A., et al., 2001. Changes in gastric mucosa and luminal environment during acid-suppressive therapy: a review in depth. Dig Liver Dis. 33 (8), 707–719.
Taharaguchi, S., Okai, K., Orita, Y., et al., 2004. Relation between amounts of concentrated feed given mares and gastric ulcers in foals. J Japan Vet Med Assoc 57, 366–370.
Thorne, J.B., Goodwin, D., Kennedy, M.J., et al., 2005. Foraging enrichment for individually housed horses: practicality and effects on behaviour. Appl Anim Behav Sci 94, 149–164.
Tobey, N.A., Orlando, R.C., 1991. Mechanisms of acid injury to rabbit esophageal epithelium. Gastroenterol 101, 1220–1228.
Tomlinson, J., Blikslager, A., 2003. Role of nonsteroidal anti-inflammatory drugs in gastrointestinal tract injury and repair. J Am Vet Med Assoc 222, 946–951.
Vaezi, M.F., Richter, J.E., 1996. Role of acid and duodenogastroesophageal reflux in gastroesophageal reflux disease. Gastroenterol 111, 1192–1199.
Vatistas, N.J., Sifferman, R.L., Holste, J., et al., 1999b. Induction and maintenance of gastric ulceration in horses in simulated race training. Equine Vet J Suppl 29, 40–44.
Vatistas, N.J., Snyder, J.R., Carlson, G., et al., 1999a. Cross sectional study of gastric ulcers of the squamous mucosa in Thoroughbred racehorses. Equine Vet J Suppl 29, 34–39.
Venner, M., Lauffs, S., Deegen, E., 1999. Treatment of gastric lesions in horses with pectin-lecithin complex. Equine Vet J 31, 91–96.
Videla, R., Andrews, F.M., 2009. New perspectives in equine gastric ulcer syndrome. Vet Clin Nother Am Equine Pract 25, 283–301.
White, G., McClure, S.R., Sifferman, R., et al., 2007. Effects of short-term light to heavy exercise on gastric ulcer development in horses and efficacy of omeprazole paste in preventing gastric ulceration. J Am Vet Med Assoc 230, 1680–1682.

Intestinal disease

Andy E. Durham

Introduction

The National Research Council (NRC) recognizes the importance of both nutritional and behavioral aspects of equine nutrition with their recommendation that carers "efficiently supply dietary ingredients in amounts that will meet the horse's nutrient needs, while still retaining the horse's normal feeding behavior" (NRC 2007c). In the context of performance of many equestrian pursuits, there is, however, an essential incompatibility of these two goals. The requirement for increased energy to fuel performance has generally been met by provision of nutrient-dense diets for which the equine gastrointestinal tract is not well adapted and, furthermore, are associated with restriction of many aspects of normal feeding behavior. In addition to possible adverse consequences on horses' psychological well-being, this imbalance has further negative influences on gastrointestinal health and function.

Diets and feeding behaviors

Dietary causes of intestinal diseases are largely considered to result from intolerance of challenges manifestly distinct from the pressures that shaped evolutionary development of the equine gastrointestinal tract. Although the earliest recognizable equid ancestors browsed on dicotyledonous plants and fruits 55 million years ago, there followed an unimaginably slow evolution into a grazing animal in response to the gradual expansion of grasslands and decline of woodland ecosystems during the Miocene period approximately 18 million years ago (Janis et al 2000). Study of modern feral equids confirms their continuing status as grazers with typically around 90% of dietary intake composed of grasses, sedges and rushes (McInnes & Vavra 1987, Stuska et al 2008). Indeed, grazing is the prime activity of feral horses, ponies and donkeys occupying between 12 and 20 hours per day (Canacoo & Avornyo 1998, Duncan 1980, Kuntz et al 2006, Pratt et al 1986, van Dierendonck et al 1996). Studies of domesticated grazing or hay-fed ponies indicate that voluntary feeding times are no different to values in feral animals and typically around 16 hours per day (Crowell-Davis et al 1985, Sweeting et al 1985), with the majority of forage consumed during the daytime and early evening (Husted et al 2009). Voluntary fasting does not extend longer than 3 to 5 hours in healthy horses (Ralston 1984) and ingestive behavior is significantly increased by social interaction and visibility of other horses (Houpt 1990, Sweeting et al 1985). Ambulatory activity is also an integral part of grazing behavior (Lamoot et al 2005, Ralston 1984). Dietary changes certainly occur in feral horses although most probably in a slow and gradual fashion over several weeks with changes in the seasons and weather influencing quality and quantity of ingested herbage (McInnes & Vavra 1987, Stuska et al 2008).

Along with domestication of the horse came a requirement for improved dietary quality to match the energy expenditure associated with the activities required of them. Although such changes probably began more than 5000 years ago, this is a brief period of time in evolutionary terms. Under modern management systems many horses are fed relatively energy-dense, high-carbohydrate, low-fiber and occasionally high-fat feeds in meals that are often consumed in a relatively short period of time with prolonged periods spent without access to food (Clarke et al 1990, Houpt 1990). When complete pelleted or concentrate diets are offered to horses only around 4 to 10 hours per day is spent feeding (Houpt 1982, Ralston et al 1979) with increased time spent on other behaviors such as wood chewing and coprophagy (Willard et al 1977). Furthermore, many differing choices and sources of preserved forage and concentrate feeds are available to the horse owner creating a greater likelihood of abrupt dietary changes.

Key Points

The equine gastrointestinal tract has gradually evolved in association with:

- A high-fiber, low-starch diet
- A prolonged duration of feeding (>12 hours per day)
- Minimal and gradual changes in dietary composition

Epidemiology and risk factors for intestinal disease

The commonest clinical signs of intestinal disease in horses comprise diarrhea and colic. Colic is generally considered to be the more important of the two presentations in terms

Table 35-1 Estimated Incidence of Intestinal Diseases in USA in 2005 (Data from USDA 2006)

Age group		Colic	Other digestive problems (e.g., diarrhea)
<6 months	% operations affected	2.8	5.7
	% foals affected	4.2	6.3
>6 months	% operations affected	10.4	2.4
	% horses affected	1.9	0.5

Table 35-2 Proportion of All Equine Deaths Related to Colic and Other Digestive Problems in Horses of Different Age Groups in USA in 2005 (Data from USDA 2006)

Age group	Colic	Other digestive problems (e.g. diarrhea)
<30 days	1.5%	6.4%
30 days 6 months	3.4%	8.3%
>6 months	15.2%	3.0%

of prevalence and cause of death in adult horses and the reverse is true in foals (USDA 2006, Tables 35-1 and 35-2). When horses present with diarrhea or colic in equine practice, a precise cause of disease is frequently not identified (Cohen et al 1999, Frederick et al 2009, Kaneene et al 1997, Love et al 1992, Mair et al 1990, Tinker et al 1997). Nevertheless epidemiologic studies have been helpful in highlighting several possible dietary associations with intestinal diseases.

Nutritional risk factors for diarrhea

Although dietary causes of diarrhea are commonly suspected there has been very little investigation of such with far greater research interest in infectious causes (Feary & Hassel 2006). Nutritional factors did not feature in either of two large studies of diarrhoea in adult horses (Love et al 1992, Mair et al 1990) although a specific cause is not identified in many cases in both foals and adults (Frederick et al 2009, Love et al 1992, Mair et al 1990). Nevertheless, several dietary factors are known to be capable of inducing diarrhea such as certain plants (e.g., acorns, blue-green algae, castor beans, heather) and other toxins (e.g., arsenic, selenium, raw linseed oil, propylene glycol) although none are seen commonly or well described (Cohen 2002). Dietary changes such as increased cereal feeding and increased grazing are anecdotally recognized as causes of diarrhea and consistent with this the administration of high doses of grain starch and/or oligofructose consistently induces diarrhea in horses (Rowe et al 1994, van Eps & Pollitt 2006).

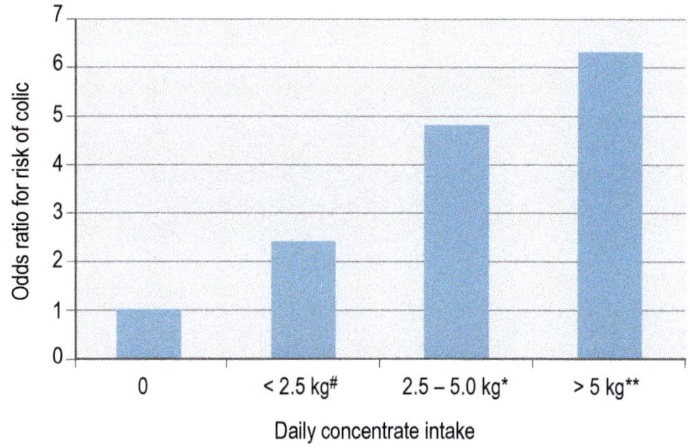

Figure 35.1 **Relationship between concentrate intake and risk of colic in multivariable analysis (# $p = 0.20$; *$p = 0.01$; **$p = 0.004$).**
Data from Tinker et al 1997.

Nutritional risk factors for colic

In contrast to diarrhea, far more epidemiologic investigation of colic has been published, perhaps as a result of its frequently distressing presentation and large economic impact (Traub-Dargatz et al 2001). Aspects of nutrition have featured heavily in such studies (Archer & Proudman 2006). Although epidemiologic studies of specific types of colic have been performed, many have combined all colic cases regardless of diagnosis. The fact that many studies may be unwittingly investigating many different underlying disease processes in various different parts of the gastrointestinal tract, with varying and quite possibly opposite causation, makes it remarkable that significant risk factors can be found. Nevertheless, many nutrition-related risk factors have indeed been identified for equine colic suggesting the existence of common and important pathophysiologic processes culminating in many different painful intestinal diseases. The following describes diet-related risk factors that have been associated with colic in general and also with specific types of colic.

Risk-factors for colic in general

Providing horses with high-starch meals is a common but unnatural feeding practice and several studies have confirmed that the risk of colic significantly increases with higher levels of cereal or concentrate feeding. Such feeding practices are frequently associated with further potential colic risk-factors such as suboptimal forage intake, high levels of exercise, particular breeds of horses and perhaps restricted turnout although multivariate analysis has been applied in several studies to specifically identify causal factors (Fig. 35.1, Table 35-3a) (Hudson et al 2001, Kaya et al 2009, Tinker et al 1997). The consumption of 2.5–5.0 kg of concentrates daily was shown to increase the risk of suffering colic by almost 5 times in one study (Tinker et al 1997), whilst a separate study found a similar quantity of oats to be associated with almost 6 times more colic episodes (Hudson et al 2001). Higher levels of concentrate feeding were even more hazardous with horses fed >5 kg concentrate daily having a greater than 6 times increased risk of colic (Tinker et al 1997). Studies of racing Thoroughbreds

Table 35-3 Nutritional and Diet-Related Factors Found to Increase the Risk of Colic in Multivariate Analyses

(a) Colic in general

Dietary category	Variable	OR	95% CI	*p*	Reference
Concentrates	Fed >5 kg/day concentrate	6.3	1.8–22.0	0.004	Tinker et al 1997
	Fed >2.7 kg/day oats	5.9	1.6–22.0	0.009	Hudson et al 2001
	Fed 2.5–5 kg/day concentrate	4.8	1.4–16.6	0.01	Tinker et al 1997
	No whole grains fed	2.5	1.25–5.0	0.01	Tinker et al 1997
Grazing	No grazing (or recent decrease)	3.0	1.4–6.6	0.007	Hudson et al 2001
Forage	Round bale hay	2.5	1.1–5.6	0.028	Hudson et al 2001
	Coastal grass hay	1.7	1.01–2.70	0.0451	Cohen & Peloso 1996
Dietary changes	Change of hay within previous 2 weeks	9.8	1.2–81.5	0.035	Cohen et al 1999
	Change of hay within previous 2 weeks	4.9	2.1–11.4	<0.001	Hudson et al 2001
	Single change in concentrate in last year	3.6	1.6–5.4	<0.001	Tinker et al 1997
	No grazing (or recent decrease)	3.0	1.4–6.6	0.007	Hudson et al 2001
	Change in concentrate within previous 2 weeks	2.6	0.9–7.2	0.064	Hudson et al 2001
	Multiple changes in concentrate in last year	2.2	1.2–4.1	0.02	Tinker et al 1997
	Multiple changes in hay in last year	2.1	1.2–3.8	0.01	Tinker et al 1997
Other	Diet change within previous 2 weeks	2.2	1.7–2.8	<0.001	Cohen et al 1995

(b) Duodenitis-proximal jejunitis

Dietary category	Variable	OR	95% CI	*p*	Reference
Concentrates	Concentrate fed (per kg)	1.3	1.1–1.6	0.001	Cohen et al 2006
Grazing	Grazing pasture	3.5	1.8–6.8	0.0002	Cohen et al 2006

(c) Enterolithiasis

Dietary category	Variable	OR	95% CI	*P*	Reference
Grazing	No pasture access	6.7	1.4–33.3	<0.05	Hassel et al 2004
	<50% pasture turnout	4.5	1.4–13.9	<0.01	Cohen et al 2000
	No pasture access	2.8	1.1–7.6	0.04	Hassel et al 2008
Forage	Alfalfa >70% of diet	10.8	2.6–44.0	<0.05	Hassel et al 2004
	Oat hay <50% diet	5.0	1.6–14.3	<0.01	Hassel et al 2008
	Alfalfa >50% of diet	4.7	1.4–15.6	0.01	Hassel et al 2008
	Grass hay <50% diet	4.6	1.6–12.5	<0.01	Hassel et al 2008
	Fed any alfalfa hay	4.2	1.3–12.9	0.01	Cohen et al 2000
Other	Carrots fed	2.7	0.98–7.64	0.05	Hassel et al 2008

(d) Colon impaction and displacement

Dietary category	Variable	OR	95% CI	*p*	Reference
Concentrates	Concentrates fed (donkeys)	5.2	1.6–16.4	0.005	Cox et al 2009
Grazing	No pasture access	30.2	25.7–35.5	0.005	Hillyer et al 2002
	No pasture access (donkeys)	3.4	1.3–8.8	0.04	Cox et al 2009

(e) Ileal impaction

Dietary category	Variable	OR	95% CI	*p*	Reference
Forage	Coastal Bermuda grass	4.4	2.1–9.1	<0.05	Little & Blikslager 2002

Table 35-3 *Continued*

(f) Equine grass sickness

Dietary category	Variable	OR	95% CI	*p*	Reference
Grazing	Change of grazing within previous 2 weeks	29.7	6.7–130	<0.001	Wood et al 1998
	No cograzing ruminants*	9.1	4.2–20.0	0.001	Newton et al 2004
	No grass cutting*	8.3	4.5–16.7	<0.001	Newton et al 2004
	Change of grazing within previous 2–3 months	4.1	1.0–16.6	0.048	Wood et al 1998
	Previous cases on premises	2.2	1.4–3.6	0.002	Wood et al 1998

(g) Epiploic foramen entrapment

Dietary category	Variable	OR	95% CI	*p*	Reference
Grazing	Reduction in grazing in previous 28 days	3.7	1.4–9.7	<0.01	Archer et al 2008b
Other	Fed at same time as close companions	4.0	1.3–14.3	0.01	Archer et al 2008b
	No access to mineral/salt lick	2.9	1.1–8.3	0.03	Archer et al 2008b

*Combination of grass cutting and cograzing ruminants may nullify risk reduction.

and Standardbreds reported a mean concentrate intake of 7 to 8 kg/day (up to 13.2 kg/day) (Richards et al 2006, Southwood et al 1993) indicating that an increased incidence of colic is expected as an occupational hazard of competitive racing. It has been suggested that pelleted-, extruded- or sweet-feeds may pose a greater risk than whole grains (Morris et al 1989, Tinker et al 1997) although this is disputed by other studies (Cohen et al 1999, Kaya et al 2009, Little & Blikslager 2002).

Free access to grazing is intuitively beneficial to intestinal health as this both mimics a natural diet and facilitates normal feeding behaviors and associated activities such as gentle exercise and social interaction. Pasture turnout has generally been found to be associated with a reduced risk of colic in comparison to stable confinement. Hudson et al (2001) found that horses that were fully stabled or had a recent reduction in grazing were three times as likely to have colic as those at pasture full time even after controlling for many other associated variables (Table 35-3a), although some studies have found no association between pasture access and colic risk (Cohen et al 1995, Cohen & Peloso 1996, Kaya et al 2009).

When grazing is restricted then preserved forages become the principal supply of fermentable carbohydrate. Some studies have shown no association between the type of hay fed and colic risk (Cohen et al 1995), whereas others have found the choice of hay to have a significant influence on colic (Cohen et al 1999). Feeding coastal grass hay or poor quality hay fed from round bales has been found to increase the risk of colic in general (Table 35-3a) (Cohen & Peloso 1996, Hudson et al 2001). In addition to nutritional quality, the hygienic quality of hay is also a significant consideration. In one study, almost 30% of hays fed to horses that developed colic were of low hygienic quality compared with only 4% of samples fed to control horses (p=0.027, Kaya et al 2009).

Horses appear best adapted to a slow and continual intake of a diet of even quality and dietary changes appear to be poorly tolerated by the equine intestinal tract. Not all studies have confirmed any association between dietary change and colic (Cohen & Peloso 1996, Kaya et al 2009) although this does appear to be among the strongest and most consistently reported risk factors. Events such as changing the batch or type of hay or concentrate, changing stabling conditions, changing the quantity or frequency of feeding and erring from usual feeding times all significantly increase colic risk (Cohen et al 1995, Cohen & Peloso 1996, Tinker et al 1997) and it has generally been found that a recent change in hay or forage is more harmful than a recent change in grain or concentrate (Table 35-3a) (Cohen et al 1999, Hillyer et al 2002, Hudson et al 2001, Little & Blikslager 2002). In a study of horses with chronic intermittent colic, Cohen & Peloso (1996) found diet changes within the 2 week period prior to the colic to be a significant risk factor. After examining many possible aspects and interactions of dietary change, Cohen et al (1999) found that a change of hay in the previous 2 weeks increased the risk of colic by almost 10-fold and was the strongest diet-related risk factor in that study (Table 35-3a). In a separate study, Hudson et al (2001) found a recent dietary change to be associated with a significantly increased risk of colic although a change in hay posed almost double the risk of a concentrate change (Table 35-3a).

Key Points

Episodes of colic have been associated with:

- High levels of cereal feeding (or feeds rich in cereal by-products)
- Limited grazing
- Poor quality forage
- Dietary changes

Risk factors for duodenitis-proximal jejunitis

Although concentrate feeding may increase the risk of colic in general (Tinker et al 1997), the association between concentrate feeding and duodenitis-proximal jejunitis (DPJ) appears to be especially strong (Table 35-3b). In one study, horses with DPJ were receiving a mean concentrate ration of 4.1 kg/day which was significantly greater than the 2.7 kg/day fed to other colic types and lame controls (Cohen et al 2006). In contrast to many other forms of colic, pasture access also represents a strong risk factor for DPJ (Table 35-3b) (Cohen et al 2006). A possible protective effect of feeding Bermuda grass hay against DPJ has been found although this might actually have resulted from other associated variables such as decreased grazing and increased concentrates (Cohen et al 2006, Morris et al 1989). In another study mixed legume-grass hay was more likely to be associated with DPJ cases than other forms of colic (Morris et al 1989).

Risk factors for enterolithiasis

Feeding alfalfa hay represents the strongest risk factor for colon obstruction with enteroliths (Table 35-3c) (Cohen et al 2000, Hassel et al 2004, 2008, Morris et al 1989). In contrast, provision of oat and grass hays has been shown to significantly reduce the risk of enterolith formation even after controlling for reduced alfalfa feeding (Table 35-3c) (Hassel et al 2008). A reduced incidence of enterolithiasis in horses fed Bermuda grass hay has also been suggested (Morris et al 1989). Similarly grazing appears to offer significant protection against enterolithiasis even after controlling for reduced alfalfa consumption (Table 35-3c) (Cohen et al 2000, Hassel et al 2004, 2008). A possible beneficial effect of mineral/vitamin supplementation was also reported for enterolithiasis although this did not reach statistical significance when controlled for other confounding factors (Hassel et al 2008). In contrast, feeding carrots was found to increase the risk of enterolithiasis even in multivariate analysis (Table 35-3c) (Hassel et al 2008).

Risk factors for intestinal impactions

Grazing is a strong protective factor against development of colon impactions and displacements in horses and against colon impactions in donkeys (Table 35-3d, Fig. 35.2) (Cox et al 2009, Dabareiner & White 1995, Hillyer et al 2002). In one large study, horses with colon impactions and displacements were found to be receiving higher concentrate rations than controls although this appeared to be confounded by other factors such as reduced grazing (Hillyer et al 2002). However, in a recent study of colon impactions in donkeys, concentrate feeding remained significantly associated with increased risk of colon impactions even after controlling for other factors such as dental disease, weight loss and reduced grazing (Cox et al 2009).

Feeding coastal Bermuda grass hay compared with timothy, alfalfa, orchard grass or oat hays was the strongest risk factor for ileal impactions in one study (Table 35-3e) (Little & Blikslager 2002) and 11/48 (23%) cases had first received this hay within the previous 3 weeks (Little & Blikslager 2002). Although forage feeding is also very strongly associated with colon impaction and displacements in horses, this may be an indirect effect due to other variables associated with forage such as a reduction in exercise or less grazing time (Hillyer et al 2002). Interestingly, straw feeding in donkeys was not a risk factor for colon impactions and even appeared protective in univariable analysis (Cox et al 2009).

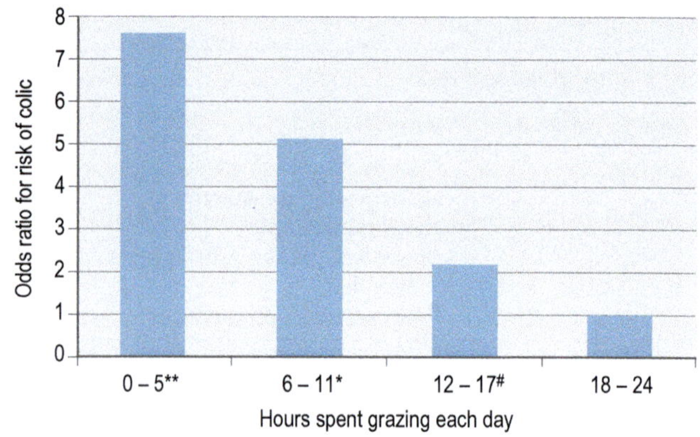

Figure 35.2 Relationship between grazing and risk of colic due to colon impaction or displacement in univariable analysis (significant differences from controls, *$p = 0.004$, **$p < 0.001$, #$p = 0.418$).
Data from Hillyer et al 2002.

Risk factors for equine grass sickness

Aspects of grazing are strongly associated with equine grass sickness (EGS), a condition seen almost invariably in grazing horses (Table 35-3f) (McCarthy et al 2001, Wylie & Proudman 2009). Increased risks of EGS in certain premises and fields have also been demonstrated (Wood et al 1998). A recent change in grazing is recognized as a very strong risk factor for EGS (Doxey et al 1991, Wood et al 1998) and although the risk of EGS is greatest within 2 weeks of a change of grazing, the increased risk of disease is still significant as long as 2–3 months later (Table 35-3f) (Wood et al 1998).

Pasture management practices that significantly reduce the risk of EGS on previously affected premises include pasture cutting, manual feces removal and cograzing with ruminants (Table 35-3f) (Newton et al 2004). However, there appeared to be complex interactions between these practices such that the protective effect of manual feces collection or ruminant cograzing was reduced when combined with pasture cutting (Newton et al 2004). In contrast domestic birds sharing the pasture and use of mechanical paddock sweepers for removal of feces appear to increase the risk of EGS, especially on cut pastures (Newton et al 2004).

Risk factors for epiploic foramen entrapment

Although horses with epiploic foramen entrapment (EFE) spend less time grazing and more time stabled than control horses this may be an indirect relationship related to other factors such as dietary change and increased crib-biting/windsucking behavior in stabled horses (Archer et al 2008a,b). Horses experiencing a reduction in grazing within the previous 28 days were found to have an increased risk of suffering EFE even after controlling for other strong risk factors such as crib biting/windsucking (Table 35-3g) (Archer et al 2008b), although reduced grazing was not identified as a significant risk factor for EFE in a larger international study (Archer et al 2008a). The risk of EFE is reduced by feeding horses at different times from their close associates and also by offering horses mineral or salt licks (Table 35-3g) (Archer et al 2008b).

Risk factors for other types of colic

Along with EGS and DPJ, sand impaction is one of the few types of colic associated with grazing activity although clearly this is unlikely to be related to grass consumption per se (Ragle et al 1989). In addition to its strong association with enterolithiasis, alfalfa hay also represents the strongest risk factor for colic due to blister beetle (cantharidin) toxicity (Helman & Edwards 1997) but appears to decrease the risk of colic due to small intestinal strangulations (Morris et al 1989).

Pathophysiology of nutritional colic and diarrhea

The anatomy and physiology of the equine gastrointestinal tract implies strong adaptation to hindgut fermentation of structural fiber to provide a large supply of energy-rich short chain fatty acids (SCFAs) (Al Jassim & Andrews 2009, NRC 2007a). Starch and sugar intake was likely to be very low in the diet for which horses have evolved, and fructans far more limited than in modern cultivated pasture grasses. Analysis of a typical feral equine diet indeed reveals a very high proportion of cellulose and lignins (e.g., acid detergent fiber [ADF] 50% dry matter [DM]) and relatively low crude protein (e.g. 6% DM) and digestible energy (DE) (e.g. 7 MJ/kg DM) (McInnes & Vavra 1987, Stuska et al 2008). As horses' appetites for forage is limited typically to approximately 2% bodyweight as DM daily, this suggests that their GI tracts are designed for an intake of around 140 kJ DE/kg bodyweight, coinciding with current estimates of equine maintenance energy requirements (127 to 152 kJ DE/kg, NRC 2007b). Consistent with this evolutionary dietary perspective there appears to be a significant disparity between small and large intestinal function in the horse. The equine small intestine is relatively deficient in alpha-amylase (Dyer et al 2002, Richards et al 2004) with a consequent poor capacity for the digestion of starch (Cuddeford 2000, Harris & Arkell 2005, Hintz 2000). In contrast, the fermentative efficiency of the equine large bowel is remarkable and dependent on several fibrolytic bacterial groups including *Clostridium*, *Fibrobacter* and Spirochaetaceae. These bacteria slowly ferment structural carbohydrates to SCFAs, primarily comprising acetate, propionate and butyrate that contribute the major source of energy to forage-fed horses (Al Jassim & Andrews 2009, Daly et al 2001, NRC 2007a). Stability and support of these normal and vital fermentative processes appear key to maintaining intestinal health.

In stark contrast to the high-fiber and limited caloric content of the typical feral diet, the nutritional demands of modern equine activities may require an intake of as much as 290 kJ DE/kg bodyweight (NRC 2007b) which would therefore require a ration energy density of approximately 10 to 15 MJ DE/kg dry matter (DM) even if DM intake increased substantially above 2% bodyweight. The traditional approach to increasing ration energy density has been by increasing provision of sugars and starches although vegetable oils have become more popular in recent years.

Among the most important causal factors to consider in the association between diet and colic or diarrhea is starch arriving in the hindgut after having overwhelmed small intestinal digestion (Fig. 35.3). High-cereal diets are likely to result in significant delivery of starch to the cecum and, additionally, small intestinal transit may be hastened by the more voluminous chyme associated with high starch feeds, further limiting prececal digestibility and increasing hindgut delivery of starch (Clarke et al 1990, Drogoul et al 2001, Metayer et al 2004). In addition to the large population of fibrolytic anaerobes in the hindgut, there is a smaller population of acidophilic, saccharolytic species, including *Bacillus*, *Lactobacillus*, *Streptococcus* and *Mitsuokella* that rapidly hydrolyze starch that has escaped small intestinal digestion, producing lactate and propionate (Al Jassim & Andrews 2009, Hoffman et al 2001, Milinovich et al 2008, Shirazi-Beechey 2008). When horses eat meals rich in starch, the arrival in the hindgut of such a rapidly fermentable carbohydrate initially increases the rate of bacterial multiplication and favors the growth of acidophilic bacteria that generate lactate and result in a fall in pH from the normal 6.7–7.0 to as low as 6.0. This acidification has further effects on bacterial populations including a reduction in fiber-fermenting species, decreased fiber digestibility and decreased SCFA absorption by the colon (Shirazi-Beechey 2008). Consequently further alterations in SCFA profiles occur including reduced acetate, increased proprionate and further increased lactate and decreased pH. The normally highly exclusive intestinal mucosal barrier may be disrupted by low pH leading to systemic absorption of bacterial lipopolysaccharide, exotoxins and vasoactive amines (Bailey et al 2003, Geor & Harris 2007) with subsequent effects on perfusion, pain and intestinal motility. Diarrhea, impaction, inflammation, dysmotility, distension with gas and froth, and subsequent colonic displacement and volvulus are all potential consequences (Clarke et al 1990, de Fombelle et al 2001, Drogoul et al 2001, Hussein et al 2004, Julliand et al 2001, Lopes et al 2004, Potter et al 1992). Fecal pH was less than

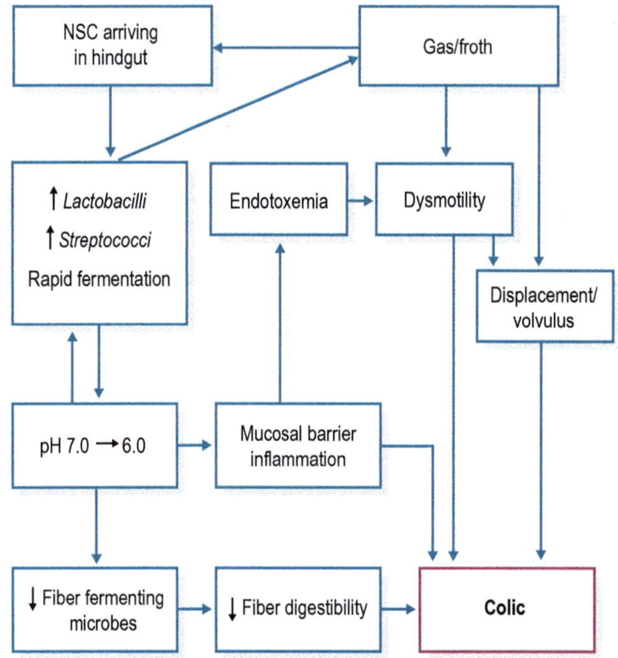

Figure 35.3 Flow diagram depicting the pathophysiologic events triggered by ingestion of excessive non-structural carbohydrate (NSC) including starch and fructan, and culminating with colic.

6.2 in more than a quarter of cereal-fed racehorses in one study (Richards et al 2006) consistent with probable adverse cecocolonic health and function. de Fombelle et al (2001) found that changing the diet from hay only to 70% hay and 30% rolled barley lead to significant alterations in hindgut bacterial flora and VFA concentrations with the potential for provoking colic. These abnormal patterns of increased colonic lactate and decreased fibrolysis have been confirmed within the large intestinal contents of horses with colic (Shirazi-Beechey 2008). Additionally, dietary change is a recognized risk factor for *Salmonella* shedding in hospitalized horses, further implying disturbance of hindgut microflora (Traub-Dargatz et al 1990).

Grass fructans are indigestible oligosaccharides and although there may be some prececal hydrolysis (Longland & Byrd 2006, NRC 2007a) rapid fermentation of any that reaches the hindgut occurs as discussed above for starches. Clearly, grass fructan is a normal nutrient for horses although has the same capacity as starch to induce dysfermentative changes in the cecum and colon. However, there is a marked contrast between the dynamics of gradual ingestion of, say, 1 kg of grass fructan contained in 10 kg DM grass consumed in 16 hours of grazing spread over a day (mean rate of ingestion = 1 g/min) and 1 kg of starch contained in a 3 kg concentrate feed consumed in 10 min (mean rate of ingestion = 100 g/min). Furthermore the former example of an almost continuous slow trickle of fructan ingestion allows for stable adaptation and balancing of the populations of fibrolytic and saccharolytic bacterial species whereas intermittent starch boluses interspersed with forage consumption represent dramatic dietary qualitative changes and may lead to marked and repetitive fluctuations in cecal pH and viability of microbial populations (Harris & Arkell 2005).

However, fructan content of grasses can be markedly variable depending on several factors including grass species, temperature and light exposure creating the potential for large fluctuations in rates of fructan ingestion. For example, fructan content of Meadow Fescue may be undetectable at 11–25°C and as high as 220 g/kg DM grass at 5–10°C (Longland & Cairns 2000). This increases the likelihood of fructan-induced hindgut disturbances when horses are first turned out, moved to a new field or there are changes in the weather (Cohen et al 1999, Huskamp & Kopf 1983, Longland & Byrd 2006, Longland & Cairns 2000). Hoffman et al (2001) showed the largest changes in grass carbohydrate content to occur in the spring and autumn matching seasonal patterns of colic incidence as noted by some studies (Hillyer et al 2001, Traub-Dargatz et al 2001).

Alterations in enteric toxicoinfectious clostridial populations have been etiologically linked with equine grass sickness (Hunter et al 1999) and the increased risk of disease associated with weather patterns, season and recent change of fields is consistent with the potential entero-bacterial destabilizing effect of changes in fructan intake (Hunter et al 1999, McCarthy et al 2001, Wood et al 1998, Wylie & Proudman 2009). Interestingly DPJ is a further intestinal disease that has been associated with increased grazing activity, increased cereal feeding and alterations in intestinal microflora (Cohen et al 2006, Feary & Hassel 2006) and might possibly develop following intestinal microbial disturbance resulting from increased cecal grass fructan delivery as well as cereal starch (Table 35-3b).

Forages especially high in ADF, the most slowly and incompletely fermentable component of structural fiber, increase the risk of colic presumably related to intestinal obstruction with dry fibrous ingesta although this has only been specifically demonstrated for ileal impactions that occur proximal to the sites of fermentative processing (Cohen & Peloso 1996, Hudson et al 2001, Little & Blikslager 2002). Anecdotally however, colon impactions may readily arise in horse breeds fed highly lignified forages such as straw or poor quality hay following employment of this practice as a weight-reduction strategy in obese individuals or in instances of habitual eating of straw bedding in stabled horses. Several studies have indicated breed-associations with digestibility of highly lignified forages. Udén and van Soest (1982) noted considerable variability amongst horses and ponies in cell wall digestibility of timothy grass hay (29.1% cellulose, 8.4% lignin) and found this to be inversely proportional to body size. In a study comparing forages and various breeds, Cuddeford et al (1995) found breed-related effects on ADF digestibility of diets containing oat straw (38.9% ADF) such that donkeys > ponies > Thoroughbreds (Fig. 35.4). Use of straw as a forage source is potentially hazardous, especially in horses, and even the addition of 33% oat straw to an alfalfa diet is associated with a marked decrease in ADF digestibility in horses and ponies (less so in donkeys) (Fig. 35.4).

The risk of colic appears especially high shortly after introducing a new batch of hay in comparison to concentrates (Table 35-3a) (Cohen et al 1999, Hillyer et al 2002, Hudson et al 2001, Little & Blikslager 2002) suggesting that

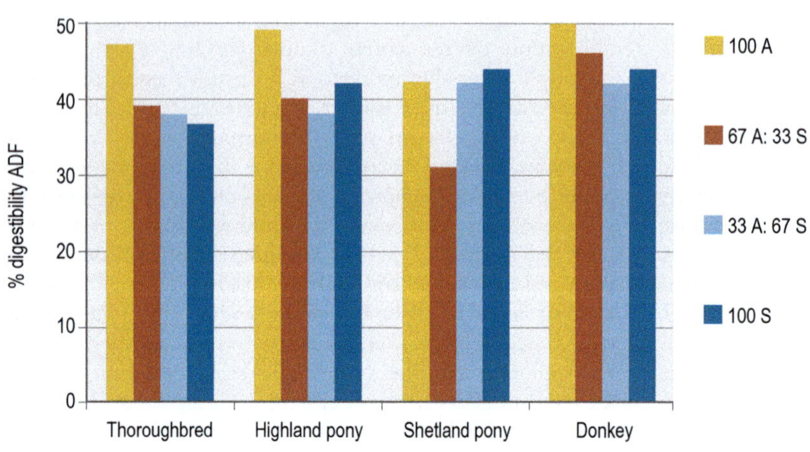

Figure 35.4 Mean apparent digestibility of acid detergent fiber (ADF) in different breeds fed different proportions of alfalfa (A) and oat straw (S) forage.
Data from Cuddeford et al 1995.

maladjustment of fibrolytic bacterial populations to the introduction of new forage sources may be important. The association between changes in forage and colic might also be related to observations that horses only very slowly adapt masticatory efforts when presented with more fibrous forages (Andrea Ellis, personal communication 2011) and that the digestibilities of pure forage sources tend to be higher than when mixed forages are supplied (Cuddeford et al 1995).

The formation of enteroliths is suspected to be favored by an alkaline colonic environment enriched by protein-derived nitrogen and sulfur and also by minerals including calcium, magnesium and phosphorus (Cohen et al 2000, Hassel et al 2004, 2008, 2009). This colonic milieu is strongly favored by feeding alfalfa hay especially when there is no access to grazing or other hay sources (Table 35-3c) (Hassel et al 2004, 2009). It is interesting that unlike many types of colic, increased cereal feeding does not appear to increase the risk of enterolithiasis and increased grass (fructan) intake further reduces the risk of this disease (Hassel et al 2004, 2008). It is possible that modest colonic acidification as a result of cecal delivery of starch and fructan may antagonize the lithogenic processes and one study did find that enterolithiasis cases were fed less cereal than controls although the difference was not significant (Hassel et al 2008). However, feeding vinegar in an attempt to reduce colon pH does not appear to be protective (Hassel et al 2008). Bran feeding might be expected to add further some of the colonic protein and mineral load (especially magnesium and phosphate) but has not been found to affect the risk of enterolithiasis (Hassel et al 2008). The reason why carrots appear to increase the risk of enterolithiasis is thus far unexplained.

Key Points

- Equine digestive anatomy and physiology is consistent with strong adaption to a high fiber, low starch diet and dependence on hindgut fermentation
- Limited pre-cecal digestion of starch is associated with adverse hindgut acidosis at high rates of consumption
- Donkeys and ponies may have greater capacity than horse breeds for fermentation of highly lignified forages

Dietary principles for promoting intestinal health

Intuitively, the health of the equine hindgut should benefit from stability in its fermentative bacterial populations. Disturbance and maladjustment of the hindgut microbes is the probable explanation for the observed causal relationships for several colic risk factors such as high concentrate/cereal feeding, limited grazing time and dietary changes (Table 3-33). Thus a vital principle of equine dietary management is to introduce any changes in a gradual fashion with mixing of the "old" and "new" diet to phase the dietary change over no less than 2 weeks. This can be accomplished with relative ease with concentrate and forage feeding but gradual exposure to grazing is hard to control as intake is unlikely to be linearly related to time at pasture. It was recently indicated that ponies can consume 40% of daily DM intake during 3 hours of pasture access (Ince et al 2005) and that horses can consume up to 1.3% bodyweight as DM in an 8-hour grazing period (Dowler 2009).

Given the limited digestibility of dietary starch it seems intuitively correct to divide concentrate meals into several small feeds. Starch fed to horses in excess of 2 g/kg bodyweight in one meal (e.g., 2 to 3 kg of a cereal-rich concentrate feed for a 500-kg horse) will result in potentially harmful quantities of starch reaching the hindgut especially if inadequately processed barley, maize or wheat products are fed or sudden diet changes occur (Geor & Harris 2007). Consequently it is often suggested that horses should eat no more than 2 g/kg bodyweight of starch per meal (Cuddeford 2000, Hussein et al 2004, Geor 2005, Harris & Arkell 2005). However, even at an intake of 1 g/kg bodyweight per meal there may still be 20% of ingested starch reaching the cecum (Potter et al 1992) suggesting more limited rations are advisable for horses with a history of intestinal disease.

However, despite the logical basis for dividing concentrate meals, there is no clear evidence to support the overall benefits of such a strategy. Although there is evidence of modest nutritional benefit when feeding frequency is increased, the practice may be associated with increased stereotypic behavior in the fed horses and in-contacts (Houpt et al 1988, Clarke et al 1990, Cooper et al 2005, van Weyenberg et al 2007), a strong risk factor for EFE and colon impaction (Archer et al 2008a,b, Hillyer et al 2002). One study that described increased colic risk when feeding high levels of concentrates did not find this risk was controlled when multiple feeds were offered (Tinker et al 1997). Furthermore, it has also been suggested that increased frequency, as well as quantity, of cereal feeding may represent a risk factor for development of gastric squamous mucosal ulceration (Andrews et al 2006). Nevertheless, as a general strategy to improve gastrointestinal health the argument for "little and often" feeding is compelling (Harris 2007). Small and frequent starch boluses are less likely to reach the hindgut than large and infrequent boluses with subsequent benefits to the stability of bacterial populations. The practice of mixing cereal or concentrate feed with forage in large buckets might be an additionally useful strategy to smooth out the peaks and troughs of caecal starch delivery mimicking a natural profile of NSC ingestion in grazing horses.

In comparison with other grains, oats facilitate prececal starch digestion and are the preferred cereal for horses, however cooked processing of barley, maize and wheat significantly improve pre-cecal starch digestibility and make extruded, micronized, steam flaked or popped products more acceptable (Cuddeford 2000). For horses requiring a diet of only moderate energy density, feeds such as sugar beet pulp, soya hulls or almond hulls are attractive as they contain significantly more fiber than cereal-based mixes and may have a digestible energy content approaching that of feeds designed for performance animals (Table 35-4). However, the associated increased water consumption and weight of ingesta associated with high fiber feeds may not suit horses that exercise in short, intense bursts. Relatively high-fat diets have become popular in many equine diets in order to allow energy dense feeds without the undesirable consequences of NSC on the hindgut as described above. Vegetable oils are often fed to horses at rates up to 1 ml/kg bodyweight daily and may typically provide around 34 kJ/ml gross energy. Although this may be inadequate for the

Table 35-4 Comparison of Analysis of 4 Commercially Available Feeds Demonstrating Similarity of Delivery of Fiber-Derived Versus Starch- and Oil-Derived Energy

	Non-molassed sugar beet pulp[a]	Non-molassed sugar beet pulp[b]	High energy cubes[c]	High energy mix[d]
DE MJ/kg	12.4	13.2	12.2	12.8
Protein %	10	10	14	15
Oil %	0.7	0.5	6	6
Fiber %	16	16.5	10	10.5
Starch %	0	1	28	22
Sugar %	5	5	5	4.8

[a]Speedibeet, British Horse Feeds, Ripon, UK; [b]Kwikbeet, Dodson & Horrel, Kettering, UK; [c]Racehorse cubes, Spillers Horse Feeds, Milton Keynes, UK; [d]Power and performance, Allen and Page, Thetford, UK.

supplementation of very hard working horses, it may allow reduction in overall starch content of the ration. For example, the addition of 500 ml vegetable oil to the diet would provide approximately 17 MJ energy and allow removal of around 1.5 kg of typical cereal-rich concentrates. Although one epidemiologic study found no association between oil feeding and colic risk (Cohen et al 1999), vegetable oils have been found to significantly reduce the fibrolytic capacity of the equine hindgut, presumably as a consequence of bactericidal fatty acids produced by fermentation of oil arriving in the hindgut and so higher levels of provision are not advisable (Jansen et al 2002).

Probiotics and prebiotics are popular amongst horse owners, perhaps largely as a result of direct marketing and the assumption that benefits shown in people will also occur in horses. Until recently there had been minimal evidence-based study of probiotics in horses. Appropriate microorganisms should be shown to be able to colonize the equine intestinal tract following oral dosing, not induce any adverse effects and to have a demonstrable benefit on gastrointestinal function under normal and/or disease conditions. Attempts to logically determine potentially beneficial equine-derived bacteria for use in probiotic preparations have proved unsuccessful (Weese et al 2004, Weese & Rousseau 2005) although digestive and health benefits of yeasts of the *Saccharomyces* genus have been shown in both clinical and research scenarios (Desrochers et al 2005, Jouany et al 2008, Medina et al 2002). However, Weese (2002) raised doubts that some probiotic products may not even contain the microbial organisms claimed by the product manufacturer, a concern also described by other authors (Durham 2009). Short chain fructo-oligosaccharides (scFOS) are indigestible oligomers of glucose linked to varying numbers of fructose molecules. Several studies have demonstrated mitigation of adverse effects of carbohydrate overload on the hindgut when horses are pre-fed with small amounts of scFOS (Respondek et al 2008, van Eps & Pollitt 2006).

Given the generally observed reduction in colic risk in association with pasture turnout, this should be encouraged under most circumstances. However, turnout for only a few hours each day may be associated with rapid ingestion of large quantities of grass and a consequent adverse bolus effect of cecal fructan delivery (Ince et al 2005). When followed by a period of stable confinement with hay and concentrate feeds, this may exacerbate the variability and instability of cecocolonic microflora. As a high rate of fructan ingestion is a potential cause of hindgut disturbance in grazing horses, known risk factors for higher fructan levels should be considered as part of horse and pasture management such as grass species (e.g., Timothy lower than Perennial ryegrass), timing of turnout (e.g., lower fructan at night than in the daytime; higher fructan in Spring and Autumn; higher fructan on bright cool days) and pasture treatment (e.g. regular cutting increases fructan content) (Longland & Cairns 2000).

Little information is available on which to base specific recommendations for fiber feeding in horses (Cuddeford 1999). Hintz (2000) suggested that a minimum of 24% neutral detergent fiber (NDF) or 14% ADF might be adequate for gastrointestinal health but a further study suggested that ≥50% NDF may help protect against hindgut disturbance in cereal-fed horses (Drogoul et al 2001). In practice, unknown and variable nutritional quality of forage can confound a logical and informed approach to dietary design although ranges of proprietary haylages often have detailed nutritional declarations. Free access to grass hay or haylage would seem sensible for the promotion of gastrointestinal health and a minimum of 1–1.5% bodyweight of forage (as DM) is usually recommended (Geor & Harris 2007) which is likely to ensure at least 40% NDF and 20% ADF in the overall diet. However, in one study of feeding practices in racehorses it was found that mean roughage provision totalled 3.3±1.4 kg/day for Thoroughbreds and 4.1±1.4 kg/day for Standardbreds, well below this minimum recommended threshold (Southwood et al 1993). Forage should ideally be available at all times with any quantitative restriction being enforced by narrow-weave haynets, double haynets or "haybags". If a change of hay is contemplated as a colic control strategy (e.g. changing from alfalfa to grass hay) then it should be considered that changing the batch of hay is a very strong risk factor for colic (Cohen et al 1999, Hudson et al 2001) and changes should be implemented slowly and gradually.

Diarrhea

There is little specific evidence on which to base feeding advice to minimize diarrhea risk or to manage a horse affected by diarrhea. However, as dietary changes are strongly suspected in the etiology of nutritional diarrhea then the general advice which follows must be considered along with attempts to minimize sudden changes from current dietary quality and quantity.

The possibility of adverse cecal delivery of NSC or oil in feeds may be increased by more rapid intestinal transit times associated with diarrhea and therefore these two dietary components should be firmly restricted in diarrheic horses. Oil should ideally be avoided until diarrhea has resolved and then might be gradually introduced starting at 0.1 ml/kg bodyweight per day and increasing over 2 to 3 weeks to a maximum of 1.0 ml/kg bodyweight per day if weight gain is considered important. As an overall strategy it seems logical to control NSC ingestion to ensure complete small intestinal digestion and absorption. To this end temporary abstinence from grazing (as fructans are indigestible) and limitation of concentrate feeds to no more than 1 g starch per kg bodyweight per meal (e.g., ≤200–300 g concentrate feed per 100 kg bodyweight per meal) is advisable although such feeds could be given every 4 to 6 hours or "trickle-fed" mixed with forage. Additionally a source of easily fermentable fiber such as non-molassed sugar beet pulp, psyllium or soya hulls may be offered along with free access to good quality grass or alfalfa hay. A *Saccharomyces*-containing probiotic product could also be added to the diet.

Abnormal serum concentrations of electrolytes including potassium, sodium, chloride, magnesium and calcium are commonly encountered in cases of diarrhea as a result of decreased absorption, increased losses and perhaps inappetance. Although various formulae exist for specific calculation of deficits and replacement, these do not necessarily translate into straightforward clinical efficacy; and, in this author's experience, responding to identified abnormalities with empirical supplementation in feed or fluid therapy (followed by reassessment of plasma concentrations) is generally equally effective.

Horses are not infrequently encountered that pass normally formed feces along with a separate fecal liquid phase. Although this is rarely associated with health concerns it does cause distress to the horses' carers. In this author's experience many such cases are improved by attention to dentition and improved mastication and the further provision of more highly fermentable fiber such as improving the quality of bulk forage or providing access to non-molassed beet pulp, psyllium or chopped alfalfa products. The association between affected horses and submissive temperament (Zehnder et al 2008) might also support the implementation of individual- rather than group-feeding practices.

Key Points

Dietary strategy suited for most cases of diarrhea includes:

- Avoidance (or limitation) of cereals or cereal-based feeds, pasture grazing, and vegetable oils
- Supply of highly fermentable fiber such as good quality hay, haylage or sugar beet pulp
- Use of *Saccharomyces*-containing probiotics

Colic

Colic encompasses a heterogeneous group of intestinal diseases and it is apparent from inspection of risk factors for various types of colic (Table 35-3) that conflicts may occur whereby implementation of dietary strategies intended to reduce the risk of one type of colic, may increase the risks of another. For example, although increased grazing appears to be protective towards most forms of colic including colon impactions and enterolithiasis (Hassel et al 2008, Hillyer et al 2002, Hudson et al 2001), it increases the likelihood of DPJ (Cohen et al 2006) and grass sickness (Wood et al 1998). Grass cutting has been shown to reduce the risk of equine grass sickness (Newton et al 2004) but is generally associated with increasing grass fructan content (Longland & Cairns 2000) with increased potential for hindgut disturbance. Furthermore, although hays such as alfalfa and Bermuda grass have been associated with increased risk of specific types of colic such as enterolithiasis, DPJ and ileal impaction (Cohen et al 2000, Hassel et al 2008, Little & Blikslager 2002, Morris et al 1989), one study found a significantly lower overall incidence of colic in horses receiving alfalfa, coastal or Bermuda grass hays compared with other types of hay (Cohen et al 1999).

Notwithstanding these potential conflicts, it is usually the case that when horses present with recurrent bouts of colic, the underlying causation is not known and therefore general dietary advice must be offered. Many colic-prone horses may benefit from dietary strategies designed to mimic the diet with which the equid intestinal tract has evolved although the degree to which such diets might be applied will depend heavily on the requirement for continued energy expenditure by working horses or other health concerns such as obesity and laminitis. Grazing is inherently attractive in the colic-prone horse although especially NSC-rich pasture and/or short turnout periods might be counterproductive as boluses of fructan reach the hindgut. Forage should be of good dietary and hygienic quality (e.g., >8 MJ/kg and >8% crude protein), and be freely available in the absence of grass access to sustain a prolonged daily feeding period. Where additional energy is required, then provision of highly fermentable fiber ingredients such as non-molassed sugar beet pulp (e.g. 0.5–4 g dry beet pulp per kg BW daily) or chopped alfalfa (e.g. 2–5 g/kg BW daily) are preferred; and even higher energy density may be achieved if necessary with the addition of judicious amounts of highly digestible starches (e.g., oats, micronized maize) or vegetable oil (<0.5 ml/kg BW daily). It is advisable to divide concentrate meals so that starch is not fed at more than 1 g/kg BW per meal and mixing high-volume fiber concentrates (e.g. beet pulp and alfalfa) with cereal may also promote "trickle feeding". Many high-fiber (>25%), low-starch (<10%) proprietary mixes are also available primarily for non-working and laminitic horses that may also serve as a concentrate supplement for the horse with recurrent colic.

As an example, a 500 kg horse in good to moderate body condition, in light to medium work, with recurrent colic might graze poor to medium quality pasture for at least 12 to 16 hours daily and have free access to good quality hay if stabled. Meals composed of 500 g DM non-molassed sugar beet pulp and 1 kg chopped alfalfa (or mixed chaff) can be offered twice daily supplemented with a small quantity of "ration-balancer" if grazing becomes more limited.

Key Points

In general, a reduction in colic risk might be achieved by:

- Turnout for >12 hours daily
- Free access to good quality forage when pasture grazing is unavailable
- Preferential use of highly fermentable fiber (e.g. sugar beet pulp) and vegetable oils rather than cereals in situations where additional energy is required
- Feeding of *Saccharomyces*-containing probiotics and scFOS prebiotics

The following offers brief evidence-based nutritional advice for the control of certain colic subtypes.

Duodenitis-proximal jejunitis

Dietary factors appear to be important in the cause of DPJ and the risk of disease might be controlled by offering less concentrate feed and also by limiting grazing (Cohen et al 2006). As a general colic-reduction strategy, reduced pasture access is somewhat counterintuitive and further studies of the links between grazing and DPJ might help inform and refine this approach. Increased feeding of hay will necessarily accompany such strategies and Bermuda grass hay has been identified as a possible preference by two studies (Cohen et al 2006, Morris et al 1989). However, it is possible that this strategy could predispose to other types of colic such as impaction.

Enterolithiasis

Alfalfa feeding is consistently the strongest of all recognized risk factors for enterolithiasis and therefore should be avoided or, at least minimized in premises with a history of problems (Cohen et al 2000, Hassel et al 2004, 2008). Replacement with either grazing or non-leguminous hays further reduces the risk (Cohen et al 2000, Hassel et al 2004, 2008). An additional thus far unexplained dietary risk is associated with feeding carrots and therefore these should be avoided pending further study. Vitamin and mineral supplements were associated with half the risk of enterolithiasis in one study although this failed to reach statistical significance (Hassel et al 2008). No effect of wheat or rice bran, vinegar or psyllium feeding has been demonstrated (Hassel et al 2008).

Intestinal impactions and displacements

The greatest risk factors for colon impaction and displacement are non-dietary and include recent transport, crib-biting/windsucking behavior and a recent reduction in exercise (Hillyer et al 2002). Reducing the amount of concentrates fed may help reduce the risks of colon impaction, especially in donkeys (Cox et al 2009, Hillyer et al 2002). Lack of pasture access is a strong risk factor for colon impactions and displacements in horses and so a gradual increase in access to grazing should be encouraged (Hillyer et al 2002).

Although ileal impaction may have important non-dietary risk factors such as tapeworm infestation (Proudman & Holdstock 2000), the feeding of hays especially high in ADF may also predispose to the condition (Little & Blikslager 2002) and therefore grazing and/or good quality grass/alfalfa hays should be fed to susceptible horses.

Horses predisposed to sand colic tend to be grazed on sandy pastures and sand intake may increase when the grazing is sparse or alternatively in wet weather when grass roots may be pulled up and ingested during grazing activity. Additionally, feeding of forage on the ground in sandy pastures or access to sandy ponds and streams might also increase sand consumption. Occasional horses may voluntarily directly ingest large quantities of sand from the ground or from mole hills. Psyllium is often recommended for horses as a preventative strategy for sand colic (Bertone et al 1988, Ragle et al 1989, Ruohoniemi et al 2001) although two separate studies failed to find any beneficial effect of this treatment (Hammock et al 1998, Lieb & Weise 1999). In contrast, two more recent studies supported the use of psyllium and found that fecal sand output was increased in association with administration of 0.5 to 1 g/kg psyllium daily (Hotwagner & Iben 2008, Landes et al 2008). The precise putative mode of action of psyllium is not known although as a feed notable for high levels of readily fermentable fiber it may be that other similar products such as sugar beet pulp might also have a beneficial effect on sand evacuation as well as providing forage so that grazing and sand intake are more restricted.

Equine grass sickness

Evidence-based advice for the reduction of the incidence of this frequently fatal disease has benefited from several epidemiologic studies that have identified prominent diet-related risk factors (Doxey et al 1991, Newton et al 2004, Wood et al 1998). A recent change in fields is the strongest risk factor for this disease (Wood et al 1998) and therefore movements should be strictly avoided in the Spring and early Summer months prior to peak EGS incidence (April to June), especially in otherwise predisposed individuals such as young-adult horses. Avoidance of grazing fields known to have been previously associated with EGS (especially in the previous 2 years) is a helpful albeit frequently impractical step, although might be implemented at least during the high risk season (Wood et al 1998).

Owing to the very strong association between EGS and grazing, various strategies to reduce grass intake are logical. The majority of EGS cases are grazing fulltime and therefore removal from pasture for part of the day is an intuitively reasonable approach. Nevertheless Wood et al (1998) still found that 29% of EGS cases were part-stabled and evidence of the putative benefits of this strategy has not been demonstrated. Supplementary hay feeding is often advised (Gilmour & Jolly 1974, Wylie & Proudman 2009) although also lacks any evidence basis. In fact two large epidemiologic studies found the risk of EGS to be increased by supplementary hay feeding although this may have simply reflected common practices employed on high risk premises (Newton et al 2004, Wood et al 1998). One practice that has been shown to significantly reduce the risk of EGS on previously affected premises is pasture cutting and further possibly beneficial pasture-management strategies include manual feces removal and cograzing with ruminants (Newton et al 2004). However, there appeared to be complex interactions between these practices such that risk of EGS might actually be increased if either manual feces collection or ruminant cograzing were combined with pasture cutting (Newton et al 2004). Avoidance of mechanical paddock sweepers for removal feces and not allowing domestic birds on to pasture is also advisable, especially on cut pastures (Newton et al 2004).

Epiploic foramen entrapment

The greatest risk factors for EFE are crib-biting/windsucking and a previous history of colic (Archer et al 2008a, b). The main dietary risk factor for this disease is a recent decrease in grazing which remains significant even after controlling for possible confounding factors (Archer et al 2008b) and therefore maintenance of unvarying daily time allowed for pasture access may help prevent this disease. The encouragement of grazing and limitation of time spent stabled might indirectly reduce the risk of EFE by decreasing stereotypic behaviors (Hothersall & Nicol 2009). Access to a mineral/salt lick also appears to reduce the risk of EFE and this represents a simple and potentially useful strategy (Archer et al 2008b).

Conclusion

Equine digestive behavior, anatomy and physiology have slowly evolved to accommodate a gradual intake ("trickle feeding") of a high-fiber, low-starch, low-fat diet, composed primarily of grasses, rushes and sedges over a prolonged feeding period with slow and gradual changes in dietary quality. The ideal nutritional strategy for avoidance of intestinal diseases is likely to mimic many aspects of the behavior and dietary supply of the feral animal (Houpt 1990). In practice it will frequently prove difficult (or impossible) to exactly mimic a natural diet and dietary behavior owing to the increased nutritional requirements of working horses and the relatively high nutrient density of available feeds, forages and pasture in comparison to the typical feral diet. Nevertheless, potential dietary risk factors can still be identified and moderated in colic-prone horses as far as is reasonably practical.

References

Al Jassim, R.A., Andrews, F.M., 2009. The bacterial community of the horse gastrointestinal tract and its relation to fermentative acidosis, laminitis, colic, and stomach ulcers. Veterinary Clinics of North America Equine Practice 25 (2), 199–215.

Andrews, F.M., Buchanan, B.R., Smith, S.H., et al., 2006. In vitro effects of hydrochloric acid and various concentrations of acetic, propionic, butyric or valeric acid on bioelectric properties of equine gastric squamous mucosa. American Journal of Veterinary Research 67 (11), 1873–1882.

Archer, D.C., Pinchbeck, G.K., French, N.P., et al, 2008a. Risk factors for epiploic foramen entrapment colic: an international study. Equine Veterinary Journal 40 (3), 224–230.

Archer, D.C., Pinchbeck, G.L., French, N.P., et al., 2008b. Risk factors for epiploic foramen entrapment colic in a UK horse population: a prospective case-control study. Equine Veterinary Journal 40 (4), 405–410.

Archer, D.C., Proudman, C.J., 2006. Epidemiological clues to preventing colic. Veterinary Journal 172 (1), 29–39.

Bailey, S.R., Baillon, M.L., Rycroft, A.N., et al., 2003. Identification of equine cecal bacteria producing amines in an in vitro model of carbohydrate overload. Applied Environment Microbiology 69 (4), 2087–2093.

Bertone, J.J., Traub-Dargatz, J.L., Wrigley, R.W., et al., 1988. Diarrhea associated with sand in the gastrointestinal tract of horses. Journal of the American Veterinary Medical Association 193 (11), 1409–1412.

Canacoo, E.A., Avornyo, F.K., 1998. Daytime activities of donkeys at range in the coastal savanna of Ghana. Applied Animal Behaviour Science 60 (2), 229–234.

Clarke, L.L., Roberts, M.C., Argenzio, R.A., 1990. Feeding and digestive problems in horses. Veterinary Clinics of North America Equine Practice 6 (2), 433–450.

Cohen, N.D., 2002. Toxic colitides. In: Divers, T., Mair, T., Ducharme, N. (Eds.), Manual of Equine Gastroenterology. WB Saunders, London, pp. 417–421.

Cohen, N.D., Gibbs, P.G., Woods, A.M., 1999. Dietary and other management factors associated with colic in horses. Journal of the American Veterinary Medical Association 215 (1), 53–60.

Cohen, N.D., Matejka, P.L., Honnas, C.M., et al., 1995. Case-control study of the association between various management factors and development of colic in horses. Texas Equine Colic Study Group. Journal of the American Veterinary Medical Association 206 (5), 667–673.

Cohen, N.D., Peloso, J.G., 1996. Risk factors for history of previous colic and for chronic, intermittent colic in a population of horses. Journal of the American Veterinary Medical Association 208 (5), 697–703.

Cohen, N.D., Toby, E., Roussel, A.J., et al., 2006. Are feeding practices associated with duodenitis-proximal jejunitis? Equine Veterinary Journal 38 (6), 526–531.

Cohen, N.D., Vontur, C.A., Rakestraw, P.C., 2000. Risk factors for enterolithiasis among horses in Texas. Journal of the American Veterinary Medical Association 216 (11), 1787–1794.

Cooper, J.J., Mcall, N., Johnson, S., et al., 2005. The short-term effects of increasing meal frequency on stereotypic behaviour of stabled horses. Applied Animal Behaviour and Science 90 (3–4), 351–364.

Cox, R., Burden, F., Gosden, L., et al., 2009. Case control study to investigate risk factors for impaction colic in donkeys in the UK. Preventive Veterinary Medicine 92 (3), 179–187.

Crowell-Davis, S.L., Houpt, K.A., Carnevale, J., 1985. Feeding and drinking behavior of mares and foals with free access to pasture and water. Journal of Animal Science 60 (4), 883–889.

Cuddeford, D., 1999. Why feed fibre to the performance horse today? In: Harris, P.A., Gomarshall, G.M., Davidson, H.P.B., et al. (Eds.), Proceedings BEVA Specialist Days on Behaviour and Nutrition. Equine Veterinary Journal Ltd. Harrogate, Yorkshire, UK, pp. 50–54.

Cuddeford, D., 2000. The significance of pH in the hind gut. In: Proceedings of the Third International Conference on Feeding horses, Stoneleigh, Warwickshire, UK, pp. 3–9.

Cuddeford, D., Pearson, R.A., Archibald, R.F., et al., 1995. Digestibility and gastro-intestinal transit time of diets containing different proportions of alfalfa and oat straw given to Thoroughbreds, Shetland ponies, Highland ponies and donkeys. Animal Science 61, 407–417.

Dabareiner, R.M., White, N.A., 1995. Large colon impaction in horses: 147 cases (1985–1991). Journal of the American Veterinary Medical Association 206 (5), 679–685.

Daly, K., Stewart, C., Flint, H., et al., 2001. Bacterial diversity within the equine large intestine as revealed by molecular analysis of cloned 16S rRNA genes. FEMS Microbiology and Ecology 38, 141–151.

de Fombelle, A., Julliand, V., Drogoul, C., et al., 2001. Feeding and microbial disorders in horses: 1-Effects of an abrupt incorporation of two levels of barley in a hay diet on microbial profile and activities. Journal of Equine Veterinary Science 26 (9), 439–445.

Desrochers, A.M., Dolente, B.A., Roy, M.F., et al., 2005. Efficacy of *Saccharomyces boulardii* for treatment of horses with acute enterocolitis. Journal of the American Veterinary Medical Association 227 (6), 954–959.

Doxey, D.L., Gilmour, J.S., Milne, E.M., 1991. A comparative study of normal equine populations and those with grass sickness (dysautonomia) in eastern Scotland. Equine Veterinary Journal 23 (5), 365–369.

Dowler, L.E., 2009. Prediction of hourly pasture dry matter intake in horses. MSc Animal Science Thesis, North Carolina State University, Raleigh, NC, USA.

Drogoul, C., de Fombelle, A., Julliand, V., 2001. Feeding and microbial disorders in horses: 2: Effect of three hay:grain ratios on digesta passage rate and digestibility in ponies. Journal of Equine Veterinary Science 21 (10), 487–491.

Duncan, P., 1980. Time-budgets of Camargue horses. II. Time budgets of adult horses and weaned sub-adults. Behaviour 72 (1–2), 26–49.

Durham, A.E., 2009. The role of nutrition in colic. Veterinary Clinics of North America Equine Practice 25 (1), 67–78.

Dyer, J., Fernandez-Castaño Merediz, E., Salmon, K.S., et al., 2002. Molecular characterisation of carbohydrate digestion and absorption in equine small intestine. Equine Veterinary Journal 34 (4), 349–358.

Feary, D.J., Hassel, D.M., 2006. Enteritis and colitis in horses. Veterinary Clinics of North America Equine Practice 22 (2), 437–479.

Frederick, J., Giguère, S., Sanchez, L.C., 2009. Infectious agents detected in the feces of diarrheic foals: a retrospective study of 233 cases (2003-2008). Journal of Veterinary Internal Medicine 23 (6), 1254–1260.

Geor, R.J., 2005. Diet, feeding and gastrointestinal health in horses. In: Harris, P.A., Mair, T.S., Slater, J.D., et al. (Eds.), Proceedings of the 1st BEVA & Waltham Nutrition Symposia, Harrogate, Yorkshire, UK, pp. 89–94.

Geor, R.J., Harris, P.A., 2007. How to minimize gastrointestinal disease associated with carbohydrate nutrition in horses. In: Proceedings of the American Association of Equine Practitioners Orlando Florida, USA. American Association of Equine Practitioners, Lexington, KY, pp. 178–185.

Gilmour, J.S., Jolly, G.M., 1974. Some aspects of the epidemiology of equine grass sickness. Veterinary Record 95 (4), 77–81.

Hammock, P.D., Freeman, D.E., Baker, G.J., 1998. Failure of psyllium mucilloid to hasten evaluation of sand from the equine large intestine. Veterinary Surgery 27 (6), 547–554.

Harris, P.A. 2007. How should we feed horses - and how many times a day? Veterinary Journal 173 (2), 252–253.

Harris, P.A., Arkell, K., 2005. How understanding the digestive process can help minimize digestive disturbances due to diet and feeding practices. In: Harris, P.A., Mair, T.S., Slater, J.D., et al. (Eds.), Proceedings of the 1st BEVA & Waltham Nutrition Symposia, Harrogate, Yorkshire, UK, pp. 9–14.

Hassel, D.M., Aldridge, B.M., Drake, C.M., et al., 2008. Evaluation of dietary and management risk factors for enterolithiasis among horses in California. Research in Veterinary Science 85 (3), 476–480.

Hassel, D.M., Rakestraw, P.C., Gardner, I.A., et al., 2004. Dietary risk factors and colonic pH and mineral concentrations in horses with enterolithiasis. Journal of Veterinary Internal Medicine 18 (3), 346–349.

Hassel, D.M., Spier, S.J., Aldridge, B.M., et al., 2009. Influence of diet and water supply on mineral content and pH within the large intestine of horses with enterolithiasis. Veterinary Journal 182 (1), 44–49.
Helman, R.G., Edwards, W.C., 1997. Clinical features of blister beetle poisoning in equids: 70 cases (1983–1996). Journal of the American Veterinary Medical Association 211 (8), 1018–1021.
Hillyer, M.H., Taylor, F.G., French, N.P., 2001. A cross-sectional study of colic in horses on thoroughbred training premises in the British Isles in 1997. Equine Veterinary Journal 33 (4), 380–385.
Hillyer, M.H., Taylor, F.G., Proudman, C.J., et al., 2002. Case control study to identify risk factors for simple colonic obstruction and distension colic in horses. Equine Veterinary Journal 34 (5), 455–463.
Hintz, H.F., 2000. Equine nutrition update. In: Proceedings of the American Association of Equine Practitioners San Antonio. American Association of Equine Practitioners, Lexington KY, pp. 62–79.
Hoffman, R.M., Wilson, J.A., Kronfeld, D.S., et al., 2001. Hydrolyzable carbohydrates in pasture, hay, and horse feeds: direct assay and seasonal variation. Journal of Animal Science 79 (2), 500–506.
Hothersall, B., Nicol, C., 2009. Role of diet and feeding in normal and stereotypic behaviors in horses. Veterinary Clinics of North America Equine Practice 25 (1), 167–181.
Hotwagner, K., Iben, C., 2008. Evacuation of sand from the equine intestine with mineral oil, with and without psyllium. Journal of Animal Physiology and Animal Nutrition (Berl) 92 (1), 86–91.
Houpt, K.A., 1982. Gastrointestinal factors in hunger and satiety. Neuroscience and Biobehavioral Reviews 6 (2), 145–164.
Houpt, K.A., 1990. Ingestive behaviour. Veterinary Clinics of North America Equine Practice 6 (2), 319–337.
Houpt, K.A., Perry, P.J., Hintz, H.F., et al., 1988. Effect of meal frequency on fluid balance and behavior of ponies. Physiology and Behavior 42 (5), 401–407.
Hudson, J.M., Cohen, N.D., Gibbs, P.G., et al., 2001. Feeding practices associated with colic in horses. Journal of the American Veterinary Medical Association 219 (10), 1419–1425.
Hunter, L.C., Miller, J.K., Poxton, I.R., 1999. The association of *Clostridium botulinum* type C with equine grass sickness: a toxicoinfection? Equine Veterinary Journal 31 (6), 492–499.
Huskamp, V.B., Kopf, N., 1983. Right dorsal displacement of the large colon in the horse. Equine Practice 5, 20–29.
Hussein, H.S., Vogedes, L.A., Fernandez, G.C., et al., 2004. Effects of cereal grain supplementation on apparent digestibility of nutrients and concentrations of fermentation end-products in the feces and serum of horses consuming alfalfa cubes. Journal of Animal Science 82 (7), 1986–1996.
Husted, L., Sanchez, L.C., Baptiste, K.E., et al., 2009. Effect of a feed/fast protocol on pH in the proximal equine stomach. Equine Veterinary Journal 41 (7), 658–662.
Ince, J., Longland, A., Moore-Colyer, M., et al., 2005. A pilot study to estimate the intake of grass by ponies with restricted access to pasture. British Society of Animal Science Conference. University of York, UK, abstract 109.
Janis, C.M., Damuth, J., Theodor, J.M., 2000. Miocene ungulates and terrestrial primary productivity: where have all the browsers gone? Proceedings of the National Academy of Sciences USA 97 (14), 7899–7904.
Jansen, W.L., Geleen, S.N.J., van der Kuilen, J., et al., 2002. Dietary soyabean oil depresses the apparent digestibility of fiber in trotters when substituted for an iso-energetic amount of corn starch or glucose. Equine Veterinary Journal 34 (3), 302–305.
Jouany, J.P., Gobert, J., Medina, B., et al., 2008. Effect of live yeast culture supplementation on apparent digestibility and rate of passage in horses fed a high-fiber or high-starch diet. Journal of Animal Science 86 (2), 339–347.
Julliand, V., de Fombelle, A., Drogoul, C., et al., 2001. Feeding and microbial disorders in horses: Part 3 – Effects of three hay:grain ratios on microbial profile and activities. Journal of Equine Veterinary Science 21 (11), 543–546.
Kaneene, J.B., Miller, R.A., Ross, W.A., et al., 1997. Risk factors for colic in the Michigan (USA) equine population. Preventive Veterinary Medicine 30 (1), 23–36.
Kaya, G., Sommerfeld-Stur, I., Iben, C., 2009. Risk factors of colic in horses in Austria. Journal of Animal Physiology and Animal Nutrition 93 (3), 339–349.
Kuntz, R., Kubalek, C., Ruf, T., et al., 2006. Seasonal adjustment of energy budget in a large wild mammal, the Przewalski horse (*Equus ferus przewalskii*) I. Energy intake. Journal of Experimental Biology 209 (22), 4557–4565.
Lamoot, I., Callebaut, J., Demeulenaere, E., et al., 2005. Foraging behaviour of donkeys grazing in a coastal dune area in temperate climate conditions. Applied Animal Behaviour Science 92 (1–2), 93–112.
Landes, A.D., Hassel, D.M., Funk, J.D., et al., 2008. Fecal sand clearance is enhanced with a product combining probiotics, prebiotics, and psyllium in clinically normal horses. Journal of Equine Veterinary Science 28 (2), 79–84.
Lieb, S., Weise, J., 1999. A group of experiments on the management of sand intake and removal in the equine. In: Proceedings of the 16th Equine Nutrition and Physiology Symposium, Raleigh, North Carolina. Equine Nutrition and Physiology Society, Savoy, IL, p 257.
Little, D., Blikslager, A.T., 2002. Factors associated with development of ileal impaction in horses with surgical colic: 78 cases (1986–2000). Equine Veterinary Journal 34 (5), 464–468.
Longland, A.C., Byrd, B.M., 2006. Pasture nonstructural carbohydrates and equine laminitis. Journal of Nutrition 136 (suppl. 7), 2099S–2102S.
Longland, A.C., Cairns, A.J., 2000. Fructans and their implications in the aetiology of laminitis. In: Proceedings of the Third International Conference on Feeding horses, Stoneleigh, Warwickshire, UK, pp. 52–55.
Lopes, M.A., White, N.A., Crisman, M.V., et al., 2004. Effects of feeding large amounts of grain on colonic contents and feces in horses. American Journal of Veterinary Research 65 (5), 687–694.
Love, S., Mair, T.S., Hillyer, M.H., 1992. Chronic diarrhea in adult horses: a review of 51 referred cases. Veterinary Record 130 (11), 217–219.
Mair, T.S., de Westerlaken, L.V., Cripps, P.J., et al., 1990. Diarrhoea in adult horses: a survey of clinical cases and an assessment of some prognostic indices. Veterinary Record 126 (19), 479–481.
McCarthy, H.E., Proudman, C.J., French, N.P., 2001. Epidemiology of equine grass sickness: a literature review (1909–1999). Veterinary Record 149 (10), 293–300.
McInnes, M.L., Vavra, M., 1987. Dietary relationships among feral horses, cattle, and Pronghorn in southeastern Oregon. Journal of Range Management 40 (1), 60–66.
Medina, B., Girard, I.D., Jacotot, E., et al., 2002. Effect of a preparation of *Saccharomyces cerevisiae* on microbial profiles and fermentation patterns in the large intestine of horses fed a high fiber or a high starch diet. Journal of Animal Science 80 (10), 2600–2609.
Metayer, N., Lhote, M., Bahr, A., et al., 2004. Meal size and starch content affect gastric emptying in horses. Equine Veterinary Journal 36 (5), 436–440.
Milinovich, G.J., Burrell, P.C., Pollitt, C.C., et al., 2008. Microbial ecology of the equine hindgut during oligofructose-induced laminitis. The ISME Journal 2 (11), 1089–1100.
Morris, D.D., Moore, J.N., Ward, S., 1989. Comparison of age, sex, breed, history and management in 229 horses with colic. Equine Veterinary Journal (suppl.) 7, 129–132.
National Research Council., 2007a. Carbohydrates. In: Nutrient Requirements of Horses, sixth ed. National Academies Press, Washington, pp. 34–43.
National Research Council., 2007b. Energy. In: Nutrient Requirements of Horses, sixth ed. National Academies Press, Washington, pp. 3–33.
National Research Council., 2007c. Feeding behavior and general considerations for feeding management. In: Nutrient Requirements of Horses, sixth ed. National Academies Press, Washington, pp. 211–234.
Newton, J.R., Hedderson, E.J., Adams, V.J., et al., 2004. An epidemiological study of risk factors associated with the recurrence of equine grass sickness (dysautonomia) on previously affected premises. Equine Veterinary Journal 36 (2), 105–112.
Potter, G.D., Arnold, F.F., Householder, D.D., et al., 1992. Digestion of starch in the small or large intestine of the equine. Europische Konferenz uber die Ernahrung des Pferdes. PferdeHeilkunde Sonderheft 1, 107–111.
Pratt, R.M., Putman, R.J., Ekins, J.R., et al., 1986. Use of habitat by free-ranging cattle and ponies in the New Forest, Southern England. Journal of Applied Ecology 23 (1), 539–557.
Proudman, C.J., Holdstock, N.B., 2000. Investigation of an outbreak of tapeworm-associated colic in a training yard. Equine Veterinary Journal (suppl.) 32, 37–41.
Ragle, C.A., Meagher, D.M., Lacroix, C.A., et al., 1989. Surgical treatment of sand colic. Results in 40 horses. Veterinary Surgery 18 (1), 48–51.
Ralston, S.L., 1984. Controls of feeding in horses. Journal of Animal Science 59 (5), 1354–1361.
Ralston, S.L., Van den Broek, G., Baile, C.A., 1979. Feed intake patterns and associated blood glucose, free fatty acid and insulin changes in ponies. Journal of Animal Science 49 (3), 838–845.
Respondek, F., Goachet, A.G., Julliand, V., 2008. Effects of dietary short-chain fructooligosaccharides on the intestinal microflora of horses subjected to a sudden change in diet. Journal of Animal Science 86 (2), 316–323.
Richards, N., Choct, M., Hinch, G.N., et al., 2004. Examination of the use of exogenous alpha amylase and amyloglucoside to enhance starch digestion in the small intestine of the horse. Animal Feed Science and Technology 114 (1–4), 295–305.
Richards, N., Hinch, G., Rowe, J., 2006. The effect of current grain feeding practices on hindgut starch fermentation and acidosis in the Australian racing Thoroughbred. Australian Veterinary Journal 84 (11), 402–407.
Rowe, J.B., Lees, M.J., Pethick, D.W., 1994. Prevention of acidosis and laminitis associated with grain feeding in horses. Journal of Nutrition 124 (12 Suppl), 2742S–2744S.
Ruohoniemi, M., Kaikkonen, R., Raekallio, M., et al., 2001. Abdominal radiography in monitoring the resolution of sand accumulations from the large colon of horses treated medically. Equine Veterinary Journal 33 (1), 59–64.
Shirazi-Beechey, S.P., 2008. Molecular insights into dietary induced colic. Equine Veterinary Journal 40 (4), 414–421.
Southwood, L.L., Evans, D.L., Bryden, W.L., et al., 1993. Nutrient intake of horses in thoroughbred and standardbred stables. Australian Veterinary Journal 70 (5), 164–168.
Stuska, S., Pratt, S.E., Beveridge, H.L., et al., 2008. Nutrient composition and selection preferences of forages by feral horses: the horses of Shackleford

Banks, North Carolina. http://www.nps.gov/calo/parkmgmt/upload/Nutrient%20Composition%20and%20Selection%20Preferences.pdf.

Sweeting, M.P., Houpt, C.E., Houpt, K.A., 1985. Social facilitation of feeding and time budgets in stabled ponies. Journal of Animal Science 60 (2), 369–374.

Tinker, M.K., White, N.A., Lessard, P., et al., 1997. A prospective study of equine colic risk factors. Equine Veterinary Journal 29 (6), 454–458.

Traub-Dargatz, J.L., Kopral, C.A., Seitzinger, A.H., et al., 2001. Estimate of the national incidence of and operation-level risk factors for colic among horses in the United State, spring. 1998. to spring 1999. Journal of American Veterinary Medical Association 219 (1), 67–71.

Traub-Dargatz, J.L., Salman, M.D., Jones, R.L., 1990. Epidemiologic study of salmonellae shedding in the feces of horses and potential risk factors for development of the infection in hospitalized horses. Journal of American Veterinary Medical Association 196 (10), 1617–1622.

Udén, P., van Soest, P.J., 1982. Comparative digestion of timothy (*Phleurn pratense*) fibre by ruminants, equines and rabbits. British Journal of Nutrition 41, 267–272.

United States Department of Agriculture, 2006. Part I: Baseline reference of equine health and management, 2005. http://www.aphis.usda.gov/vs/ceah/ncahs/nahms/equine/equine05/equine05_part1.pdf.

van Dierendonck, M.C., Bandi, N., Batdorj, D., et al., 1996. Behavioural observations of reintroduced Takhi or Przewalski horses (*Equus ferus Przewalskii*) in Mongolia. Applied Animal Behaviour Science 50 (2), 95–114.

van Eps, A.W., Pollitt, C.C., 2006. Equine laminitis induced with oligofructose. Equine Veterinary Journal 38 (3), 203–208.

van Weyenberg, S., Buyse, J., Janssens, G.P., 2007. Digestibility of a complete ration in horses fed once or three times a day and correlation with key blood parameters. Veterinary Journal 173 (2), 311–316.

Weese, J.S., 2002. Microbiologic evaluation of commercial probiotics. Journal of American Veterinary Medical Association 220 (6), 794–797.

Weese, J.S., Anderson, M.E., Lowe, A., et al., 2004. Screening of the equine intestinal microflora for potential probiotic organisms. Equine Veterinary Journal 36 (4), 351–355.

Weese, J.S., Rousseau, J., 2005. Evaluation of *Lactobacillus pentosus* WE7 for prevention of diarrhea in neonatal foals. Journal of American Veterinary Medical Association 226 (12), 2031–2034.

Willard, J.G., Willard, J.C., Wolfram, S.A., et al., 1977. Effect of diet on cecal pH and feeding behavior of horses. Journal of Animal Science 45 (1), 87–93.

Wood, J.L.N., Milne, E.M., Doxey, D.L., 1998. A case-control study of grass sickness (equine dysautonomia) in the United Kingdom. Veterinary Journal 156 (1), 7–14.

Wylie, C.E., Proudman, C.J., 2009. Equine grass sickness: epidemiology, diagnosis, and global distribution. Veterinary Clinics of North America Equine Practice 25 (2), 381–399.

Zehnder, C., Pfister, K., Gerhards, H., et al., 2008. Field study on risk factors for free faecal water in pleasure horses. In: Proceedings of 12th Congress of the European Society of Veterinary and Comparative Nutrition, Vienna, Austria, p. 130.

36

SECTION E Clinical Nutrition

Urinary tract disease

Harold C. Schott II

Dietary management of equine patients with urinary tract disorders can improve quality of life and, for some conditions (e.g., urolithiasis), may limit recurrence of disease. Patients with acute kidney injury (AKI) and acute renal failure (ARF) often have a decreased appetite during the onset of these problems and nutritional support may include enteral and parenteral nutrition in an attempt to attenuate negative energy and protein balances that could prolong disease course and complicate recovery. Equids with chronic kidney disease (CKD) often have weight loss or a decrease in body condition as one of their main clinical problems. Improvement of body condition by ensuring adequate energy and protein intake is therefore essential for long-term management of CKD. Finally, lower urinary tract disease syndromes, including urolithiasis and bladder paralysis accompanied by accumulation of sabulous urine sediment, are challenging conditions to manage because equids normally excrete large amounts of calcium crystals in urine. Although dietary dissolution of cystoliths is rarely possible, dietary changes to attenuate crystalluria may limit stone recurrence and accumulation of urine sediment in equids with bladder paralysis.

Acute kidney injury and acute renal failure

Fortunately, ARF remains an uncommon problem in horses. Nevertheless, it is a serious disorder that if not properly recognized and managed often has a poor outcome. Reversible AKI usually develops as a complication of another disease process that causes hypovolemia and decreased renal perfusion (colic, colitis, hemorrhage, or exhaustive exercise). This may progress to ARF if renal hypoperfusion is not recognized and treated appropriately (Geor 2007). Treatment with nephrotoxic medications including aminoglycoside antibiotics, oxytetracycline (especially when administered at high dosages for correction of flexural deformities in neonatal foals), and nonsteroidal anti-inflammatory drugs (NSAIDs) as well as exposure to endogenous pigments (myoglobin or hemoglobin) or heavy metals (mercury, cadmium, zinc, arsenic, and lead) or excessive administration of vitamin D or vitamin K_3 can also cause AKI and ARF (Schmitz 2007). Hemodynamically-induced AKI is often associated with oliguria (urine output <0.5 ml/kg for >6 hours) whereas urine production with nephrotoxin-associated AKI often remains normal (non-oliguric AKI).

Clinical signs in horses with AKI and ARF most commonly reflect the primary disease process: for example, colic, diarrhea, or restricted gait and pigmenturia due to rhabdomyolysis (Geor 2007). Oliguria or anuria followed by development of edema in the face of appropriate fluid therapy are alarm signs for ARF. More subtle clinical signs that should prompt investigation of AKI in non-oliguric patients include more severe lethargy and inappetance than would typically be expected with the primary disease.

When these clinical signs are observed, serum biochemical analysis is indicated to assess for azotemia as well as alterations in serum electrolyte concentrations and acid-base balance. Azotemia is the term used to describe increases in blood urea nitrogen (BUN) and creatinine (Cr) concentrations detected on a serum chemistry profile; thus, azotemia is a laboratory diagnosis. Azotemia can be prerenal in origin, consequent to decreases in renal blood flow (RBF) and glomerular filtration rate (GFR) or can be due to primary (intrinsic) ARF or disruption of the urinary tract (post-renal failure) (Bayly 1991). The term "prerenal failure" has been used to describe reversible increases in BUN and Cr associated with renal hypoperfusion. Serum electrolyte concentrations are generally within reference ranges and urine specific gravity is increased (>1.025 but often approaching 1.045–1.050) with prerenal failure, due to maintenance of concentrating ability (Brobst et al 1977, Grossman et al 1982). Although use of this term is firmly entrenched in both the human and veterinary medical literature, it likely contributes to a lack of recognition of subclinical renal damage that accompanies a number of medical and surgical conditions. This can be attributed to a large renal functional reserve capacity. In many patients with reversible azotemia, changes in glomerular and tubular function and integrity can be demonstrated by proteinuria and cast formation, impaired concentrating ability (urine specific gravity of 1.015–1.025 in a markedly dehydrated patient), and increases in urine sodium concentration (>20 mmol/l) and excretion (Seanor et al 1984).

To increase awareness of subclinical renal damage in patients with decreased RBF and GFR, the term acute kidney injury has been introduced in human and, subsequently, small animal medicine. AKI has been defined as an increase in Cr of as little as 0.3 mg/dl (≈25 μmol/l) within 24–48 hours of onset of disease or hospital admission, even when the upper limit of the reference range may not be exceeded (Mehta et al 2007, Lattanzio & Kopyt 2009). Further evidence to support subclinical renal damage with AKI includes the abnormal urinalysis findings mentioned above as well as biochemical analysis of urine to detect increased enzyme activity (e.g., urine gamma glutamyl transferase activity to urine Cr ratio [IU/g × 0.01] exceeding 25, indicative of sloughing of proximal tubule epithelial cells into the tubule lumen) (Adams et al 1986) and, in other species, detection of novel urine biomarkers such as kidney injury molecule-1 (Han et al 2008).

Metabolic changes accompanying AKI and ARF

Before nutritional management is discussed, it is useful to review the metabolic changes that accompany ARF. However, because there is little published information on this subject in horses, extrapolation from other species is necessary.

Oxygen consumption, a measure of energy expenditure, in patients with uncomplicated ARF is similar to that of healthy individuals. In contrast, oxygen consumption may increase by 20–30% in patients with sepsis or multiple organ dysfunction syndrome (MODS) complicated by ARF (Schneeweiss et al 1990). Thus, energy requirements are determined more by the primary disease process than ARF.

Most patients with ARF have a poor appetite, leading to a negative energy balance. A decreased carbohydrate intake and depletion of hepatic glycogen stores in ARF leads to increased oxidation of fatty acids to meet energy demands. Increased mobilization of triglycerides to support this process is accompanied by development of hyperlipidemia with increased triglyceride content of plasma lipoproteins, especially very low density lipoproteins (VLDLs) and low density lipoproteins (LDLs) (Druml et al 1985). These lipid abnormalities in ARF are a consequence of impaired lipolysis by both hepatic triglyceride lipase and peripheral lipoprotein lipase, with metabolic acidosis further inhibiting the latter (Druml et al 1985). Despite prolonged insulin action due to decreased renal clearance, as well as decreased hepatic insulin degradation, maximal insulin-stimulated glucose uptake by muscle is decreased and muscle glycogen synthesis is impaired, supporting tissue resistance to insulin (May et al 1985). Consequently, both hypertriglyceridemia and hyperglycemia are common findings in patients with ARF.

Next, protein catabolism leading to a sustained negative nitrogen balance is a hallmark of ARF. In addition to inadequate intake, metabolic effects of uremic toxins along with metabolic acidosis cause accelerated protein degradation and impaired amino acid uptake by muscle cells. Release of cytokines and proteases during a systemic inflammatory response, coupled with increased secretion of catecholamines and glucocorticoids, also contribute to protein catabolism. Further, insulin-stimulated muscle protein synthesis is suppressed with ARF, again due to accelerated protein catabolism and insulin resistance. Another important mechanism of protein breakdown with ARF is stimulation of hepatic gluconeogenesis from amino acids (Druml 1998). Glucose administration to healthy subjects completely suppresses hepatic gluconeogenesis from amino acids; however, in patients with ARF hepatic gluconeogenesis can only be partly suppressed by glucose infusion, an effect mediated by a glucocorticoid dependent pathway (Cianciaruso et al 1991). Thus, no matter what nutritional support is provided to patients with ARF, it is impossible to fully counteract a negative nitrogen balance during the acute stage of ARF.

Nutritional management of AKI and ARF

Nutritional support for human patients with AKI and ARF is focused on limiting protein and energy wasting that commonly accompanies renal failure (Druml 2005, Fiaccadori et al 2008, Fiaccadori & Cremaschi 2009). Benefits of nutritional support include promoting tissue repair and supporting immune function, with the ultimate goal of reducing mortality. The enteral route is preferred; however, concurrent partial or total parenteral nutrition (TPN) is often required to meet nutritional needs, especially in patients in which the primary disease precludes enteral feeding. As described above, human patients with AKI or ARF are prone to developing hyperglycemia and hypertriglyceridemia as well as electrolyte and acid-base derangements. Judicious administration of intravenous (IV) fluids is the mainstay therapy to maintain hydration and normalize serum electrolyte concentrations and acid-base balance. A detailed discussion of fluid therapy is beyond the scope of this chapter and interested readers are referred to recent reviews (Langston 2008, Prowle et al 2010, Schrier 2010). Human, as well as companion animal, patients in which renal replacement therapy is pursued, by either intermittent peritoneal dialysis or hemodialysis, may derive benefits from greater control of uremia; however, fluid exchange procedures may further challenge macronutrient and micronutrient losses (Fiaccadori & Cremaschi 2009, Bloom & Labato 2011). Similar principles should also apply to nutritional support of horses with AKI and ARF.

In equids with AKI or ARF, the initial approach to nutritional support consists of offering a variety of highly palatable feeds to encourage voluntary intake, with fresh grass (that may need to be cut and brought to the patient) often the most readily accepted feedstuff. When patients remain completely anorectic for 48 hours or more, forced enteral feedings are recommended to provide energy and protein (Carr & Holcombe 2009). Enteral feedings can be made by pulverizing and moistening commercially available pelleted feeds (complete "senior" feeds are preferred due to their typically higher fiber content). Administration of 1 kg of feed in 6–8 liters of water via a nasogastric tube six to eight times a day can provide 15 to 18 Mcal (30–36 kcal/kg/day), essentially meeting maintenance energy requirements for a 500 kg horse (Carr & Holcombe 2009; see Chapter 41). Alternatively, low residue diets designed for humans (Vital HN™, Osmolite™) or horses (Critical Care Meals™, Platinum Enteral Immunonutrition Formula™, WellSolve Well-Gel™) can also be provided as liquid formulations through smaller diameter indwelling nasogastric tubes (Sweeney & Hansen 1990, Buechner-Maxwell et al 2003). Unfortunately, these commercial "liquid diets" are considerably more expensive and have not been documented to be of greater benefit than complete pelleted feeds, providing feeding of the latter is tolerated.

In human patients with AKI, nutritional support has targets of at least 1.5 g/kg protein and 30 kcal/kg non-nitrogen calories with lipids providing 30–35% of total calories per day (Fiaccadori et al 2008). Although no data exist for equids with AKI or ARF, these goals would seem reasonable targets as well, perhaps with a lower percentage of calories derived from fat because most equids would likely be less adapted to fat in their diets. Fat limitation may be even more important to consider in patients that are predisposed to hyperlipidemia (e.g., ponies, Miniature horses, donkeys, and burros) or that have grossly lipemic plasma prior to nutritional supplementation. Generally, enteral feeding with pelleted feeds or commercial low residue diets should also provide an adequate amount of protein; however, protein catabolism will not be completely attenuated in patients with ARF for the reasons described above. A further benefit of providing enteral nutrition is local nutrient delivery to enterocytes, thereby helping to maintain their function as well as integrity of the intestinal mucosal barrier (Carr & Holcombe 2009).

In addition to being cautious about the amount of fat added to the diet, the type of fat supplemented may also have an impact on severity of renal damage. Specifically, although study findings are somewhat conflicting, supplements rich in omega-3 polyunsaturated fatty acids (PUFA), as compared to fat supplements that are largely omega-6 PUFA, have been documented to slow progression of CKD in human and small animal patients (Fassett et al 2010, Roudebush et al 2010). However, recent data suggest that short-term feeding of omega-3 PUFA may also be "renoprotective" during AKI. For example, mice that were fed an omega-3 PUFA-enhanced diet (fish [menhaden] oil with 28% omega-3 PUFA, providing 5% of total calories) as compared to mice that had been fed a diet with corn oil (2% omega-3 PUFA, providing 5% of total calories) for 4 weeks had dramatically improved survival following experimental renal ischemia (Hassan & Gronert 2009). Novel omega-3 PUFA-derived autacoids, in particular protectin D1, appear to exert potent anti-inflammatory effects and limit neutrophil influx during the acute inflammatory response (Hassan & Gronert 2009). Despite the fact that acute dietary supplementation with omega-3 PUFA to equids at the onset of AKI and ARF may have little or no immediate renoprotective effect, their use in nutritional support may still be preferred over supplementation with vegetable oils that contain minimal omega-3 PUFA.

When enteral feeding is either not possible (e.g., with nasogastric reflux due to ileus) or not well tolerated (e.g., produces colic signs), TPN will need to be pursued. There have been no investigations of altering common TPN formulations of dextrose, amino acids, and lipid emulsions for supportive care of horses with ARF; thus, a recommended approach would be to initiate TPN with routine formulations (Carr & Holcombe 2009) with close monitoring of serum glucose and triglyceride concentrations. In patients with significant hyperglycemia (>200 mg/dl ≈10 mmol/l) or hyperlipidemia (triglycerides >500 mg/dl ≈6 mmol/l), it would seem prudent to initiate TPN using formulations with reduced amounts of dextrose and lipid and to monitor changes in these values over the initial few hours of administration. To facilitate use of TPN in patients with ARF, it may be useful to initially prepare TPN in smaller volumes (e.g., 1–2 liters) until a formulation that is reasonably well tolerated is found. Finally, because uremia can increase the risk of gastrointestinal ulceration, equids with ARF should receive concurrent anti-ulcer drugs, preferably a proton pump inhibitor, in an attempt to limit development of gastric ulcers.

As equine patients are recovering from AKI and ARF and appetite is returning, it is important to once again offer a variety of palatable feedstuffs to encourage voluntary intake. Further, if turn out to a small grass paddock is available, it should be used for several hours each day. Horses recovering from ARF do not necessarily need to have IV fluid therapy maintained until azotemia has fully resolved, especially if they are willing to voluntarily drink adequate (50 ml/kg/day) or even increased amounts of water. Further, maintenance IV fluids can be administered during the part of the day that patients are stalled. Some equids recovering from AKI and ARF may continue to waste sodium and chloride in their urine for several weeks until tubular function fully recovers. Offering salt water (0.45% NaCl solution) as well as plain water may be an effective management tool to replace ongoing electrolyte losses in urine. Fractional electrolyte clearance (excretion) values can be calculated after measuring electrolyte and creatinine concentrations in urine and serum samples collected within a few hours of each other to determine whether patients continue to waste sodium and chloride. In this author's opinion, clearance values greater than 1.5% for sodium and 2% for chloride would be considered increased in the recovery period (in the absence of electrolyte supplementation) and would prompt offering a hypotonic saline solution to drink (always with plain water also available) or addition of loose salt to a concentrate feed meal (5 g of NaCl per 100 kg body weight twice a day). It should also be mentioned that interpreting fractional clearance values in these patients can be difficult because they may remain increased for 48–72 hours after discontinuing IV fluid therapy or when supplemental NaCl is provided in water or feed.

Key Points

- Energy and protein malnutrition along with hyperglycemia and hyperlipidemia are common problems with acute renal failure
- Because acute kidney injury and acute renal failure are typically consequences of other primary diseases, nutritional support for recovery from the renal insult must also address nutritional requirements for the primary disease
- The initial approach to nutritional support includes offering a variety of feedstuffs, especially fresh grass, to encourage voluntary feed intake
- In anorectic horses, enteral and parenteral nutrition are often required to attenuate energy and protein malnutrition

Chronic kidney disease

Although chronic renal failure (CRF) is also fairly uncommon in equids (Schott et al 1997), the primary management challenge is maintenance of body condition of affected horses. Thus, nutritional support is a key aspect of long-term care.

A change in terminology has also recently been adopted in human and small animal medicine for patients with chronic renal disease. Rather than describing patients as having CRF (typically an end stage problem), the term chronic kidney disease has been introduced to shift attention to detection of earlier stages of chronic renal disease (Winearls & Glassock 2009; http://www.iris-kidney.com/guidelines/en/staging_ckd.shtml). Although CKD by nature is a progressive disorder, earlier recognition and intervention may slow rate of progression and thereby prolong life and, for people and small animals, delay the need for renal replacement therapy (Finco et al 1999, Ruggenenti et al 2001).

In contrast to human and small animal patients in which glomerular disease, accompanied by proteinuria, is a common cause of CKD, most horses with CKD have tubulointersitial disease, termed chronic interstitial nephritis (CIN). In some instances, a history of neonatal disease, a serious medical or surgical problem, or treatment with nephrotoxic medications may be associated with subsequent onset of CIN but often a precipitating cause or event is not recognized. Less commonly, anomalies of development (renal agenesis or hypoplasia, renal dysplasia, or polycystic kidney disease) may be the cause of CKD in equids (Schott 2007). Horses with CKD are often presented for evaluation of weight loss; however, for horses in competition, loss of condition, decreased performance, and a dull hair coat may be earlier complaints before weight loss becomes evident. Additional findings may include mild ventral edema, polyuria and polydipsia (PU/PD), excessive dental tartar and halitosis (associated with gingivitis attributed to urease producing bacteria that result in excess ammonia production), and a uremic or "fishy" odor to the hair coat (as urea can also be eliminated through sweat glands) (Schott et al 1997). Regardless of the presenting complaint, a diagnosis of CKD is generally made by detection of azotemia and isosthenuria (urine with a tonicity similar to plasma and a specific gravity ranging from 1.008–1.014), typically in a euhydrated patient. Depending on the diet being consumed, hypercalcemia is also sometimes found in equids with CKD (Leroy et al 2011) and the combination of azotemia, hypercalcemia, and isosthenuria is essentially pathognomonic for CKD in equids. Further clinical evaluation often includes transabdominal ultrasonographic imaging that may reveal increased echogenicity of the renal parenchyma, consistent with interstitial fibrosis, and nephrolithiasis providing further support that the disease is chronic in nature (Schott 2007).

Chronic kidney disease, in humans and potentially horses, is accompanied by retention of nearly 100 solutes normally excreted in urine and their toxic effects exerted over time comprise the uremic syndrome (Vanholder & Glorieux 2003, Almeras & Argilés 2009). These solutes are largely derived from protein catabolism and can be divided into three categories: (1) small water-soluble compounds (<500 Da); (2) protein-bound solutes (also mostly <500 Da); and (3) "middle molecules" (>500 Da). Effects of these compounds vary in both concentration and tissue-dependent characteristics and knowledge about toxic effects of many of these compounds remains limited. When individual solutes are experimentally administered to healthy subjects, adverse clinical signs are rarely observed. However, when a number of these uremic toxins accumulate in human patients with CKD, their combined effects produce lethargy, altered mentation, decreased appetite, and a number of other adverse effects on many body systems (Vanholder & Glorieux 2003, Almeras & Argilés 2009). Both urea and creatinine are included in the first group of small molecules, however, urea is generally considered the more toxic of the two compounds. An early multicenter, prospective study (The National Cooperative Dialysis Study, initiated in the United States in 1976; Sargent & Gotch 1975) that applied pharmacokinetic principles to determine timed average urea concentrations (TAC_{urea}) in humans receiving hemodialysis for CKD found that patients receiving more intensive dialysis, producing a TAC_{urea} value of 50 mg/dl (≈18 mmol/l), had lower morbidity and fewer hospitalizations for complications of CKD than patients receiving less intensive dialysis, producing a TAC_{urea} value of 90 mg/dl (≈32 mmol/l) (Sargent & Gotch 1975). Similarly, it has been the author's experience that equids with mild CKD and BUN concentrations <55–60 mg/dl (≈20 mmol/l) show minimal signs of the uremic syndrome. However, once BUN exceeds 75–100 mg/dl (≈27–35 mmol/l), equids generally show more clinical signs of uremia. Thus, an important goal of nutritional support in CKD is to minimize excess protein intake that could result in higher BUN concentrations.

The progressive loss of nephron function that is characteristic of CKD precludes complete remission of disease. However, many horses with early CKD may be able to continue in performance or live as pets for months to years with appropriate management. Fluid therapy is sometimes initiated in equids when CKD is first recognized in an attempt to lower the magnitude of azotemia. Short-term (2–3 days) fluid support is most rewarding in patients with an acute exacerbation of CKD and should be pursued in patients that have recently had a decrease in appetite or other clinical problems that may have caused dehydration. Patients that respond with an increase in urine output and a decrease in the magnitude of azotemia have a more favorable prognosis than patients in which weight gain, development of edema, and minimal change in BUN and Cr are observed. Equids that respond favorably to fluid therapy may also need this treatment repeated whenever another problem results in dehydration or at times when more severe lethargy or decreases in appetite are observed.

Nutritional management of CKD

Therapeutic diets for small animal veterinary patients with CKD have been in use for over 60 years. These so-called "renal diets" have less protein, phosphorus, and sodium contents in comparison to typical maintenance diets and may also have increased buffering capacity, soluble fiber, vitamins, antioxidants, and omega-3 PUFA (Roudebush et al 2010). In a prospective study of dogs with CKD, feeding a renal diet markedly decreased signs of uremia. Furthermore, dogs fed the renal diet had a median survival time that was three times longer than that for dogs fed a commercial maintenance diet (Jacob et al 2002). Clearly, nutritional management is an important tool for prolonging survival of patients with CKD.

Nutritional management of equids with CKD has the primary goal of improving and maintaining body condition for as long as possible. As with ARF, this involves offering multiple feedstuffs and frequent meals to encourage adequate energy intake, with a target of 30 kcal/kg/day. Appetite and feed selected by affected equids can vary from day to day with good quality grass pasture remaining the most preferred feed. Thus, ideal management for horses with CKD involves providing pasture access for as much of the year as possible. When dry forage must be fed, grass hays are preferred over legumes due to the lower protein and calcium contents of the former. However, if appetite for grass hay is poor and the patient is willing to eat alfalfa or another legume, the latter forages should be offered to provide energy intake. Further, horses that are offered an initial flake of a legume hay will sometimes continue eating grass forage after the legume has been finished. To ensure adequate energy intake, feeding concentrate feeds is often required in addition to free choice forage intake. Oats have long been recommended for horses with CKD due to their palatability, energy content, and high digestibility. Other concentrate feeds that would be appropriate to help meet energy requirements would include pelleted senior feeds that are higher in fiber content as well as pelleted feeds high in fat. Again, concentrate feedstuffs may need to be varied from day to day to encourage intake. As with AKI and ARF, gastrointestinal ulceration can be a component of the uremic syndrome with CKD necessitating treatment with anti-ulcer medications in horses with a decreased appetite (horses with a good appetite are less likely to need antiulcer medications).

Over the past several decades restricting dietary protein intake by human and veterinary patients with CKD was thought to have beneficial effects; however, the current recommendation is to provide an adequate, but not excessive, amount of dietary protein to meet requirements while maintaining a neutral nitrogen balance. In horses with CKD, a dietary protein intake of 1.0–1.5 g/kg/day would be a reasonable goal. Adequacy of dietary protein intake can be indirectly assessed by monitoring the BUN to Cr ratio: values greater than 15 (mg/dl) or 0.075 (μmol/l:mmol/l) suggest excessive protein intake while values less than 10 (mg/dl) or 0.05 (μmol/l:mmol/l) may indicate inadequate protein intake. Because glomerular disease accompanied by proteinuria is uncommon in horses, additional protein intake to replace urinary protein losses is rarely required in horses. However, if total serum protein and albumin concentrations are decreased, equids with CKD should be assessed for proteinuria, preferably by measuring urine protein to urine Cr ratio (normal value <1 with units of mg/dl for each measurement). An elevated urine protein to urine Cr ratio (>2) would support glomerulonephritis and additional dietary protein, as well as anti-inflammatory medications to limit proteinuria, may be necessary.

Proatherogenic dyslipidemias, characterized by high triglycerides and low high density lipoproteins, are a significant problem in people with CKD and require treatment with statins and other medications (Harper & Jacobson 2008). Fortunately, cardiovascular diseases that affect human patients are rare in horses and, therefore, medical management of hyperlipidemia in equids with CKD is rarely necessary, although patients with advanced CKD may develop grossly lipemic plasma (Naylor et al 1980). Furthermore, for equids in the earlier stages of CKD, fat supplementation can be useful to increase caloric intake and maintain body condition. As discussed with ARF, supplementation with products rich in omega-3 PUFA can slow progression of spontaneously occurring CKD in humans and small animal patients (Fassett et al 2010, Roudebush et al 2010). Despite the fact that similar data is lacking in equids with CKD, a comparative approach makes it logical to recommend supplementation with fat products that are also high in omega-3 PUFA (alpha-linolenic-acid) in this species. Crushed or soaked flaxseed yielding flaxseed oil (also known as linseed oil), flaxseed meal products, as well as other commercial supplements rich in omega-3 PUFA are options for horses with CKD. Although an optimal "dose" has not been established, 225–335 g (8–12 ounces, providing 2–3 Mcal) is the typical amount of flaxseed meal fed daily and other commercial supplements should be fed according to label directions. Finally, it warrants mention that pasture grass is also rich in omega-3 PUFA such that there may be less benefit of fat supplementation on a diet that is largely based on pasture, other than provision of additional calories. In this situation, the type of fat used likely has less of an impact on progression of CKD and palatability may be the most important determinant of what product is used.

In addition to lower protein content, renal diets for small animal patients with CKD are also lower in phosphorus content because renal phosphate excretion is reduced with CKD. Furthermore, intestinal phosphate binders are often administered to patients with CKD to limit hyperphosphatemia and renal secondary hyperparathyroidism, metabolic disturbances that further contribute to progression of CKD (Finco et al 1999, Roudebush et al 2010). Although hyperphosphatemia may accompany ARF in equids, horses with CKD more commonly have serum phosphorus concentrations near or below the lower limit of the reference range (Schott et al 1997). Thus, nutritional management to limit intake of phosphorus does not seem to be of as much concern in equids. Unlike humans and small animals, equids with CKD may have markedly increased serum calcium concentrations, both total and ionized (Schott et al 1997, Leroy et al 2011). Further, the magnitude of hypercalcemia appears to be directly related to dietary calcium intake. This unusual and nearly pathognomonic clinicopathologic abnormality for CKD in equids appears to be a consequence of species differences in calcium homeostasis. Specifically, hormonal control of intestinal calcium absorption appears to be poor in equids (Breidenbach et al 1998) and increasing dietary calcium intake leads to proportional increases in both calcium absorption and elimination in urine (Schryver et al 1970). Thus, a decrease in urinary calcium excretion with CKD, in the face of continued intestinal absorption, leads to higher serum calcium concentrations. Clinically, decreased calcium excretion can be appreciated by reduced amounts of crystals in urine of horses with CKD. Of interest, the author has never observed adverse effects (e.g., tissue mineralization, altered neuromuscular function) of hypercalcemia in equids with CKD.

Sodium restriction is another feature of human and small animal diets for patients with CKD (Roudebush 2010, Wright & Cavanaugh 2010). Increased sodium (salt) intake may exacerbate hypertension, proteinuria, and edema in patients with CKD as well as increase production of oxygen radicals that may directly damage renal vasculature and tubules and contribute to progression of CKD. In the author's experience, equids with stable CKD do not have increased urinary sodium concentrations (>50 mmol/l) and fractional sodium clearance values are typically normal (<1%). Thus, adding salt to the diet of equids with CKD (although advocated by this author in the past to increase voluntary water intake) could possibly do more harm than good and is no longer recommended. Because ongoing membrane damage by oxygen radicals appears to be another mechanism contributing to progression of CKD, supplementation with antioxidants (vitamin C, vitamin E, carotenoids, and others) has also been pursued (Brown 2008). In a small study, feeding a renal diet with additional antioxidants to dogs with spontaneous CKD resulted in decreases in oxidative stress and serum Cr concentration (Brown 2008). Whether antioxidant supplementation to equids with CKD would be beneficial remains unknown, especially for animals with access to fresh grass that already contains abundant antioxidants.

In the later stages of CKD, progressive uremia suppresses appetite. Thus, "appetite-stimulating" medications, usually anabolic steroids, are sometimes administered to horses with CKD. The author has had little success using anabolic steroids for appetite stimulation. However, in humans with CKD undergoing dialysis, administration of growth hormone and androgens has improved visceral protein stores, muscle mass, and strength, especially when combined with resistance exercises (Dong & Ikizler 2009). Thus, it may be worthwhile to add a small amount of forced exercise (hand-walking several times a week) to the management regimen of equids with CKD because exercise could have the dual benefits of appetite stimulation and preservation of muscle mass. In small animal patients with CKD, dedicated owners may elect to have percutaneous feeding tubes placed for supplemental enteral nutrition in the later stages of CKD. Although it would not be strongly recommended, use of a small diameter indwelling nasogastric tube and supplemental enteral nutrition with liquid diets could also be pursued in select cases of advanced CKD in horses. Another intervention that has decreased morbidity and improved quality of life in humans with CKD is administration of synthetic erythropoietin to limit anemia (Covic et al 2008). Unfortunately, an equine analog of erythropoietin is not currently available and use of either the human or canine products is not recommended in equids.

Finally, it should not be surprising that the prognosis for long-term survival with CKD is related to the magnitude of the decrease in GFR, which is best reflected by Cr. In the author's experience, most equids with a Cr <3 mg/dl (≈260 μmol/l) maintain a reasonably good attitude, appetite, as well as body condition and simply require additional water intake, although access to pasture is strongly recommended for these patients. Once Cr exceeds 5 mg/dl (≈440 μmol/l); however, progression of CKD accelerates and signs of uremia (lethargy and weight loss) tend to worsen over a period of months. Another negative prognostic indicator appears to be heavy proteinuria (urine protein to urine Cr ratios >3) as CKD in horses with glomerulonephritis tends to deteriorate more rapidly than patients with CIN. Thus, nutritional management may have its greatest life-prolonging effect in equids with Cr values from 2–5 mg/dl (180–440 μmol/l), although the recommendations provided should be pursued for all horses with CKD. Finally, due to the variable nature of progression, each case should be handled on an individual basis with the emphasis on maintenance of body condition until humane euthanasia becomes necessary.

Key Points

- Maintenance of body condition is the primary nutritional goal for equids with CKD and can likely prolong survival for months to years
- The approach to nutritional support of equids with CKD includes offering a variety of feedstuffs, especially fresh grass, to encourage voluntary feed intake
- Adequacy of dietary protein intake can be monitored by the BUN to Cr ratio
- Fat supplements rich in omega-3 PUFA are recommended for equids with CKD and can be fed to provide up to 20% of daily calories as long as hyperlipidemia is not present
- Due to species variations in calcium homeostasis, hypercalcemia is a nearly pathognomion finding in horses with CKD yet adverse clinical effects of hypercalcemia have not been described
- Restriction of phosphorus intake does not seem to be as critical in horses with CKD as in human or small animal patients with CKD
- Supplemental sodium (salt) feeding to horses with CKD is not recommended

Urolithiasis

Despite the fact that horses excrete much greater amounts of calcium crystals in urine than dogs and cats, the prevalence of urolithiasis is surprisingly less common in equids (DeBowes 1988, Laverty et al 1992, Dusterdieck-Zellmer 2007). Male horses, especially geldings, are predisposed to urolithiasis (75% of all cases), but a breed predisposition has not been described. This sex predilection has been attributed to the shorter, distensible urethra of the mare, which likely permits voiding of small calculi (DeBowes 1988, Dusterdieck-Zellmer 2007). Uroliths are most common in the urinary bladder (60%), although they may also develop in the kidneys (12%), ureters (4%), and urethra (24%) (Laverty et al 1992).

Two steps are required for urolith formation: precipitation of urinary crystals (nucleation) and crystal growth. Factors that contribute to nucleation include supersaturation of urine, genetics associated with excretion of larger amounts of calcium (hypercalciuria) or oxalates (hyperoxaluria); and urine stasis (Evan 2010). Crystal growth is subsequently enhanced or limited by presence of various amounts of promoters and inhibitors, respectively, in urine. Because calcium carbonate and calcium oxalate crystals are normally present in equine urine, inhibition of crystal growth is the more important factor in limiting development of uroliths in equids. The most important inhibitor of crystal growth in equids is likely the large amount of mucus that is normally secreted into the renal pelvis and proximal ureter. This helps to maintain the crystals in suspension and limits aggregation.

Since normal urine of most species is typically supersaturated, spontaneous nucleation rarely leads to urolith formation. Rather, stasis of urine flow, as intermittently occurs in the renal pelvis and bladder, increases the chance of contact between crystalloid material and uroepithelium and subsequent aggregation and crystal growth (Evan 2010). More importantly, damage to uroepithelial surfaces results in local activation of inflammatory and clotting pathways, producing a nidus for crystal adherence (See & Williams 1992). Desquamated epithelial cells, leukocytes, or necrotic debris may also provide a nidus for crystal growth at more distal sites in the urinary tract. Uroepithelial damage from a variety of causes is likely an important factor for development of uroliths in horses. For example, after urinary tract

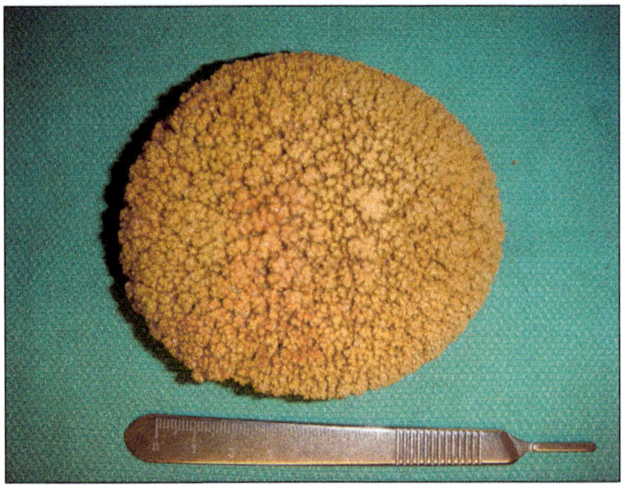

Figure 36.1 Typical appearance of a urolith removed from the bladder of a horse.

instrumentation (e.g., catheterization, endoscopy), areas of traumatized uroepithelium are rapidly covered with a fine layer of crystalline material. Fortunately, this material usually dissolves spontaneously unless complicated by urinary tract infection. Similarly, papillary necrosis with NSAID toxicity appears to be a risk factor for development of nephrolithiasis in equids (Ehnen et al 1990). Once crystal growth has been initiated around a nidus, equine urine has the further disadvantage of being alkaline, favoring crystallization of most urolith components, especially calcium carbonate (Dusterdieck-Zellmer 2007).

In equids there are two basic forms of uroliths and both are composed primarily of calcium carbonate crystals with lesser amount of magnesium, ammonium, and phosphate (DeBowes 1988). Most are yellow-green, spiculated stones that can easily be fragmented (Fig. 36.1). Less commonly, uroliths are gray-white, smooth stones that are more resistant to fragmentation. The latter stones often contain increased amounts of phosphate. Examination of the cut surface of equine uroliths by scanning electron microscopy reveals a pattern of irregular, concentric bands around a core suggesting that calculus growth occurs by accretion of pre-existing crystals rather than by de novo crystal formation at the urolith's surface (Neumann et al 1994). Gaps between adjacent crystals result in porosity to the urolith. Porosity can also make uroliths fragile, providing a therapeutic advantage in that many stones can be crushed or fragmented before surgical or manual removal (DeBowes 1988, Dusterdieck-Zellmer 2007). Although not yet documented, it is likely that there are genetic risk factors for urolithiasis in equids as a recurrence rate of 45% was reported in one large retrospective report (Laverty et al 1992). Thus, nutritional management of horses with urolithiasis is primarily instituted to limit the chance of recurrence once the initial diagnosis has been made and the urolith(s) removed by various manual or surgical procedures.

Neurological diseases resulting in bladder paralysis, that frequently manifest as overflow incontinence, can be complicated by accumulation of a large mass of urine sediment in the ventral aspect of the bladder. This condition, termed sabulous urolithiasis, can be confused with cystolithiasis (Holt & Mair 1990, Schott 2006). Important differences detected during rectal palpation include a large bladder with bladder paralysis, while most cases of cystolithiasis have a small bladder due to dysuria and more frequent urination. Further, in equids with sabulous urolithiasis, the accumulated urine sediment can usually be indented with firm digital pressure and urine can easily be expressed when pressure is placed on the bladder during palpation. In contrast, true cystoliths are firm and nonindentable. Although differentiation between a cystolith and sabulous urolithiasis is often straightforward in horses with neurological disease, bladder paralysis may be idiopathic (without other neurological deficits) in nearly a third of male equids in which the problem is detected (Schott 2006). In these animals, it is important to differentiate between the two disorders because surgical treatment of sabulous urolithiasis is not indicated. Rather, when sabulous urolithiasis is detected in horses with or without neurological disease, the preferred treatment is bladder lavage, rather than a cystotomy, to remove the excessive urine sediment. In addition, antimicrobial treatment for ascending urinary tract infection is often necessary along with dietary management to limit production and accumulation of urine sediment.

Nutritional management of urolithiasis

Dietary dissolution of struvite (ammonium magnesium phosphate) cystoliths and urethral plugs has been a mainstay therapy in dogs and cats for several decades and commercial diets have been developed for this specific purpose (Osborne et al 1999). These diets are canned food products (allowing for increased moisture intake) with lower contents of protein, magnesium, and phosphorus. Lower protein intake decreases urinary urea excretion, thereby decreasing substrate availability for urease producing bacteria to form ammonia. The diets are also higher in salt content to promote increased water intake and urine output (to lower urine specific gravity and decrease urine supersaturation) and are formulated to produce acidic urine (to decrease struvite crystal precipitation and growth) (Osborne et al 2008b). Feeding these diets to affected small animals often results in stone dissolution and relief of clinical signs with in weeks to a few months. However, only about half of the bladder stones in these species are primary struvite uroliths. Other types of uroliths include calcium oxalate stones (most common) with urate and cystine uroliths being minor contributors (Osborne et al 2008b). Unfortunately, calcium oxalate stones are not as amenable to dietary dissolution, although commercial diets lower in protein and calcium content are available to decrease the risk of recurrence after stone removal. Furthermore, urinary acidification actually increases urinary calcium excretion in small animals and is counterproductive for treatment of calcium oxalate urolithiasis. Thus, these latter diets are not designed to acidify urine. Clearly, optimal dietary modification for management of urolithiasis varies with the type of urolith.

Fortunately, nutritional management of urolithiasis in equids is more straightforward because nearly all stones are calcium carbonate uroliths (Mair & Osborne 1986, Osborne et al 2008a). The principles of nutritional management of urolithiasis in equids are similar to those in other species and include: (1) decreasing the intake of minerals comprising uroliths (primarily calcium); (2) decreasing urine supersaturation; and (3) acidifying the urine to decrease crystal formation, depending on crystal type. In addition, appropriate antimicrobial therapy for urinary tract infection, when present, should be pursued (Remillard et al 1992). Unfortunately, dietary dissolution of equine cystoliths by following these principles is rarely successful, likely due to the size of the stones when the diagnosis is initially made. As previously mentioned, these nutritional recommendations are most useful following initial diagnosis and removal of uroliths with a goal of decreasing the risk of recurrent stone formation.

To the author's knowledge, there is only one report detailing long-term dietary management of recurrent cystolithiasis in a gelding, after repeated surgical treatment (Remillard et al 1992). In this report, the initial approach after the second surgical intervention was to limit calcium intake by feeding a grass hay diet (calcium 0.4% of dry matter [DM] intake). Within 3 months several small cystoliths had again developed prompting a third surgical intervention. The diet was modified to an oat hay diet (calcium 0.2% of DM intake) that produced an elevated serum parathyroid concentration, consistent with a diet that would be considered calcium deficient. Nevertheless, another cystic calculus developed within 6 months, prompting a fourth surgical procedure. Subsequently, urinary acidification was added to the oat hay diet by administration of ammonium chloride (100 mg/kg, PO, q 12 h) but this treatment only reduced urine pH to 6.5. The urinary acidifying agent was changed to ammonium sulfate at a higher dose (175 mg/kg, PO, q 12 h) and a urine pH of near 5.0 was maintained for a 7-month treatment period. The gelding was reported to remain free of further cystolithiasis during the period of urinary acidification and for at least another year on the oat hay diet alone. Although the gelding had free access to a trace mineral salt block throughout the treatment course, additional loose salt was never supplemented in this case due to concerns that it could increase urinary calcium excretion. This case report clearly demonstrates the challenges of recurrent cystolithiasis in horses and again raises the question of whether or not this gelding had increased susceptibility due to a higher rate of urinary calcium excretion or lack of urinary inhibitors of crystal aggregation. Further, despite feeding a diet that ultimately produced a neutral to slightly negative calcium balance, urine osmolality remained high (1350 mOsm/kg) and urinary acidification had to be instituted to decrease urine pH to limit crystal formation. It warrants mention that the horse had to be dosed orally twice a day due to low palatability of ammonium sulfate. In addition, long-term feeding of a marginal calcium balance diet may not be desirable.

In an attempt to make long-term dietary management of recurrent cystolithiasis or sabulous urolithiasis more practical, another approach has been to add pelleted anionic salt supplements to the diet to acidify the urine. Anionic supplements (e.g., SoyChlor® and BioChlor®) were originally developed to limit development of milk fever and other periparturient metabolic disorders in dairy cattle by producing a mild acidifying effect in both blood and urine (Goff 2008). Most diets fed to livestock have a positive dietary cation–anion balance (DCAB) that tends to produce a mild metabolic alkalosis. Metabolic alkalosis predisposes cows to milk fever by altering the conformation of the parathormone receptor, making it less responsive to the increases in parathormone that accompany hypocalcemia (Goff 2008). Thus, the goal of supplementation with anionic salts is to produce a mild metabolic acidosis that is accompanied by a corresponding decrease in urine pH. Because addition of anions as either ammonium chloride or ammonium sulfate tends to decrease palatability by increasing ammonia, careful mixing of hydrochloric acid into protein pellets has become the standard approach for decreasing DCAB for dairy rations. Nevertheless, these anionic supplements must be introduced slowly over a few days to minimize any decrease in feed intake and they are typically only fed for 3–4 weeks prior to parturition to decrease the risk of periparturient metabolic disorders. Further, the acidifying effects of these supplements tend to be somewhat short-lived as metabolic adaptations over several weeks lessen the acidifying effect of these supplements (Goff 2008).

In horses, incorporation of an organic soy product rich in chloride and sulfate ions into a pelleted feed to produce a DCAB of 85 mEq/kg of DM has been successfully used to subtly decrease blood pH and induce aciduria (urine pH of 5.0–5.5), as compared to a control diet with a DCAB of 190 mEq/kg of DM that resulted in a urine pH of 8.0 (McKenzie et al 2002). More importantly, the authors reported a substantial reduction in the amount of urine sediment (crystals) in horses with low urine pH when fed the low DCAB diet. Although this study was not designed to evaluate the effects of aciduria on urolithiasis, it demonstrated that decreasing DCAB can be an effective means to acidify equine urine and limit crystalluria. In the author's experience with a limited number of cases, feeding horses (~500 kg) 0.5 kg of a commercial anionic pellet designed for dairy cattle twice daily has effectively decreased urine pH to values less than 6.0. Although no adverse effects were observed with supplementation over several months, only about half of the horses willingly consumed the supplement. Further, in two horses in which the supplement was used in an attempt to dissolve a bladder stone, no change in cystolith size was apparent after 3 months of supplementation. This experience, although limited, emphasizes that urinary acidification is most likely to be of greatest benefit to decrease the risk of recurrence of urolithiasis or accumulation of sabulous deposits in horses with bladder paralysis.

In summary, dietary recommendations to decrease the risk of recurrence of urolithiasis or accumulation of sabulous sediment in horses with bladder paralysis include limiting calcium intake, making management changes to increase water intake (to limit urine supersaturation), and feeding anionic supplements to acidify urine. Limiting calcium intake is best accomplished by feeding forages that are lower in calcium; specifically, by feeding grass and oat hays as compared to legume hays or using pasture grass as the primary forage source. Although horse owners may raise concerns about the "hardness" or calcium content of water sources offered to affected horses, it is important to recognize that the amount of calcium ingested in water is negligible in comparison to that ingested in forage. Next, grazing pasture may also be the best way to increase dietary water content and limit urine supersaturation. Alternately, salt supplementation may also increase voluntary water intake by some, but not all equids. Finally, urinary acidification (with a target urine pH of 5.5 or lower) by feeding anionic supplements may also be of benefit to limit urine crystal formation.

Key Points

- Uroliths in horses are primarily composed of aggregates of calcium carbonate crystals and most commonly develop in the bladder of male horses
- Accumulation of excessive urine sediment, termed sabulous urolithiasis, may occur in horses with bladder paralysis and can mimic cystolithiasis
- Dietary dissolution of equine uroliths or sabulous debris is rarely successful
- The recurrence rate for urolithiasis may exceed 40%
- Dietary recommendations to limit the risk of recurrence of urolithiasis include feeding a lower calcium diet combined with pasture turn out or salt supplementation to limit urine supersaturation
- Feeding a supplement with a low cation-anion balance (anionic supplement) may decrease urine pH and limit formation of urine crystals, and thereby limit the risk of stone recurrence or accumulation of sabulous urine sediment

References

Adams, R., McClure, J.J., Gossett, K.A., et al., 1986. Evaluation of a technique for measurement of γ-glutamyltransferase in equine urine. Am J Vet Res 46, 147–150.

Almeras, C., Argilés, À., 2009. The general picture of uremia. Semin Dial 22, 329–333.

Bayly, W.M., 1991. A practitioner's approach to the diagnosis and treatment of renal failure in horses. Vet Med 86, 632–639.

Bloom, C.A., Labato, M.A., 2011. Intermittent hemodialysis for small animals. Vet Clin North Am: Small Anim Pract 41, 115–133.

Breidenbach, A., Schlumbohm, C., Harmeyer, J., 1998. Peculiarities of vitamin D and of the calcium and phosphate homeostatic system in horses. Vet Res 29, 173–186.

Brobst, D.F., Grant, B.D., Hilbert, B.J., et al., 1977. Blood biochemical changes in horses with prerenal and renal disease. J Equine Med Surg 1, 171–177.

Brown, S.A., 2008. Oxidative stress and chronic kidney disease. Vet Clin North Am: Small Anim Pract 38, 157–166.

Buechner-Maxwell, V.A., Elvinger, F., Thatcher, C.D., et al., 2003. Physiological responses of normal adult horses to a low-residue diet. J Equine Vet Sci 23, 310–317.

Carr, E.A., Holcombe, S.J., 2009. Nutrition of critically ill horses. Vet Clin North Am: Equine Pract 25, 93–108.

Cianciaruso, B., Bellizzi, V., Napoli, R., et al., 1991. Hepatic uptake and release of glucose, lactate, and amino acids in acutely uremic dogs. Metabolism 40, 261–290.

Covic, A., Seica, A., Gusbeth-Tatomir, P., et al., 2008. Hemoglobin normalization trials in chronic kidney disease: what should we learn about quality of life as an end point? J Nephrol 21, 478–484.

DeBowes, R.M., 1988. Surgical management of urolithiasis. Vet Clin North Am: Equine Pract 4, 461–471.

Dong, J., Ikizler, T.A., 2009. New insights into the role of anabolic interventions in dialysis patients with protein energy wasting. Curr Opin Nephrol Hypertens. 8, 469–475.

Druml, W., 1998. Protein metabolism in acute renal failure. Miner Electrolyte Metab 24, 47–54.

Druml, W., 2005. Nutritional management of acute renal failure. J Ren Nutr 15, 63–70.

Druml, W., Zechner, R., Magometschnigg, D., et al, 1985. Post-heparin lipolytic activity in acute renal failure. Clin Nephrol 23, 289–293.

Duesterdieck-Zellmer, K.F., 2007. Equine urolithiasis. Vet Clin North Am: Equine Pract 23, 613–629.

Ehnen, S.J., Divers, T.J., Gillette, D., et al., 1990. Obstructive nephrolithiasis and ureterolithiasis associated with chronic renal failure in horses: Eight cases (1981–1987). J Am Vet Med Assoc 197, 249–253.

Evan, A.P., 2010. Physiopathology and etiology of stone formation in the kidney and the urinary tract. Pediatr Nephrol 25, 831–841.

Fassett, R.G., Gobe, G.C., Peake, J.M., et al., 2010. Omega-3 polyunsaturated fatty acids in the treatment of kidney disease. Am J Kidney Dis 56, 728–742.

Fiaccadori, E., Cremaschi, E., 2009. Nutritional assessment and support in acute kidney injury. Curr Opin Crit Care 15, 474–480.

Fiaccadori, E., Parenti, E., Maggiore, U., 2008. Nutritional support in acute kidney injury. J Nephrol 21, 645–656.

Finco, D.R., Brown, S.A., Brown, C.A., et al., 1999. Progression of chronic renal disease in the dog. J Vet Intern Med 13, 516–528.

Geor, R.J., 2007. Acute renal failure in horses. Vet Clin North Am: Equine Pract 23, 571–591.

Goff, J.P., 2008. The monitoring, prevention, and treatment of milk fever and subclinical hypocalcemia in dairy cows. Vet J 176, 50–57.

Grossman, B.S., Brobst, D.F., Kramer, J.W., et al., 1982. Urinary indices for differentiation of prerenal azotemia and renal azotemia in horses. J Am Vet Med Assoc 180, 284–288.

Han, W.K., Walker, S.S., Johnson, A., et al, 2008. Urinary biomarkers in the early diagnosis of acute kidney injury. Kidney Int 73, 863–869.

Harper, C.R., Jacobson, T.A., 2008. Managing dyslipidemia in chronic kidney disease. J Am Coll Cardiol 51, 2375–2384.

Hassan, I.R., Gronert, K., 2009. Acute changes in dietary Ω-3 and Ω-6 polyunsaturated fatty acids have a pronounced impact on survival following ischemic renal injury and formation of renoprotective docosahexaenoic acid-derived protectin D11. J Immunol 182, 3223–3232.

Holt, P.E., Mair, T.S., 1990. Ten cases of bladder paralysis associated with sabulous urolithiasis in horses. Vet Rec 127, 108–110.

Jacob, F., Polzin, D.J., Osborne, C.A., et al, 2002. Clinical evaluation of dietary modification for treatment of spontaneous chronic renal failure in dogs. J Am Vet Med Assoc 220, 1163–1170.

Langston, C., 2008. Managing fluid and electrolyte disorders in renal disease. Vet Clin North Am: Small Anim Pract 38, 677–697.

Lattanzio, M.R., Kopyt, N.P., 2009. Acute kidney injury: new concepts in definition, diagnosis, pathophysiology, and treatment. J Am Osteopath Assoc 109, 13–19.

Laverty, S., Pascoe, J.R., Ling, G.V., et al., 1992. Urolithiasis in 68 horses. Vet Surg 21, 56–62.

Leroy, B., Woolums, A., Wass, J., et al, 2011. The relationship between serum calcium concentration and outcome in horses with renal failure presented to referral hospitals. J Vet Intern Med 25, 1426–1430.

Mair, T.S., Osborne, R.S., 1986. Crystalline composition of equine urinary calculi. Res Vet Sci 40, 288–291.

May, R.C., Clark, A.S., Goheer, M.A., et al., 1985. Specific defects in insulin-mediated muscle metabolism in acute uremia. Kidney Int 28, 490–497.

McKenzie, E.C., Valberg, S.J., Godden, S.M., et al, 2002. Plasma and urine electrolyte and mineral concentrations in Thoroughbred horses with recurrent exertional rhabdomyolysis after consumption of diets varying in cation-anion balance. Am J Vet Res 63, 1053–1060.

Mehta, R.L., Kellum, J.A., Shah, S.V., et al, 2007. Acute Kidney Injury Network: report of an initiative to improve outcomes in acute kidney injury. Crit Care 11, R31–R38.

Naylor, J.M., Kronfeld, D.S., Acland, H., 1980. Hyperlipemia in horses: effects of undernutrition and disease. Am J Vet Res 41, 899–905.

Neumann, R.D., Ruby, A.L., Ling, G.V., et al., 1994. Ultrastructure and mineral composition of urinary calculi from horses. Am J Vet Res 55, 1357–1367.

Osborne, C.A., Lulich, J.P., Polzin, D.J., et al, 1999. Medical dissolution and prevention of canine struvite urolithiasis. Twenty years of experience. Vet Clin North Am: Small Anim Pract 29, 73–111.

Osborne, C.A., Albasan, H., Lulich, J.P., et al., 2008a. Quantitative analysis of 4468 uroliths retrieved from farm animals, exotic species, and wildlife submitted to the Minnesota Urolith Center: 1981–2007. Vet Clin North Am: Small Anim Pract 39, 65–78.

Osborne, C.A., Lulich, J.P., Forrester, D., et al., 2008b. Paradigm changes in the role of nutrition for the management of canine and feline urolithiasis. Vet Clin North Am: Small Anim Pract 39, 127–141.

Prowle, J.R., Echeverri, J.E., Ligabo, E.V., et al., 2010. Fluid balance and acute kidney injury. Nat Rev Nephrol 6, 107–115.

Remillard, R.L., Modransky, P.D., Welker, F.H., et al., 1992. Dietary management of cystic calculi in a horse. J Eq Vet Sci 12, 359–363.

Roudebush, P., Polzin, D.J., Adams, L.G., et al., 2010. An evidence-based review of therapies for canine chronic kidney disease. J Small Anim Pract 51, 244–252.

Ruggenenti, P., Schieppati, A., Remuzzi, G., 2001. Progression, remission, and regression of chronic renal diseases. Lancet 19 (357), 1601–1608.

Sargent, J.A., Gotch, F.A., 1975. The analysis of concentration dependence of uremic lesions in clinical studies. Kidney Int Suppl (2), 35–44.

Schmitz, D.G., 2007. Toxins affecting the urinary system. Vet Clin North Am: Equine Pract 23, 677–690.

Schott, H.C., 2006. Urinary incontinence and sabulous urolithiasis: chicken or egg? Equine Vet Educ 8, 17–19.

Schott, H.C., 2007. Chronic renal failure in horses. Vet Clin North Am: Equine Pract 23, 593–612.

Schott, H.C., Patterson, K.S., Fitzerald, S.D., et al., 1997. Chronic renal failure in 99 horses. Proc Annu Conv Am Assoc Equine Pract 43, 345–346.
Schneeweiss, B., Graninger, W., Stockenhuber, F., et al, 1990. Energy metabolism in acute and chronic renal failure. Am J Clin Nutr 52, 596–601.
Schrier, R.W., 2010. Fluid administration in critically ill patients with acute kidney injury. Clin J Am Soc Nephrol 5, 733–739.
Schryver, H.F., Craig, P.H., Hintz, H.F., 1970. Calcium metabolism in ponies fed varying levels of calcium. J Nutr 100, 955–964.
Seanor, J.W., Byars, T.D., Boutcher, J.K., 1984. Renal disease associated with colic in horses. Mod Vet Pract 65, A26–A29.
See, W.A., Williams, R.D., 1992. Urothelial injury and clotting cascade activation: Common denominators in particulate adherence to urothelial surfaces. J Urol 147, 541–548.
Sweeney, R.W., Hansen, T.O., 1990. Use of a liquid diet as the sole source of nutrition in six dysphagic horses and as a dietary supplement in seven hypophagic horses. J Am Vet Med Assoc 197, 1030–1032.
Vanholder, R.C., Glorieux, G.L., 2003. An overview of uremic toxicity. Hemodial Int 7, 156–161.
Winearls, C.G., Glassock, R.J., 2009. Dissecting and refining the staging of chronic kidney disease. Kid Int 75, 1009–1014.
Wright, J.A., Cavanaugh, K.L., 2010. Dietary sodium in chronic kidney disease: a comprehensive approach. Semin Dial 23, 415–421.

37

SECTION E Clinical Nutrition

Hepatic insufficiency

Andy E. Durham

The equine liver constitutes approximately 1% of bodyweight in the horse (Sisson 1975) and plays a key role in many aspects of equine nutrition including synthetic, storage, processing and digestive functions pertaining to all major and many minor nutrients. Failure of the liver to accomplish its many roles may lead to disturbance of nutrient availability and homeostasis potentially leading to several clinical nutritional problems including those listed in Table 37-1.

There is no reason to suspect that the dietary requirements of horses suffering from compensated liver disease differ from normal horses and specific dietary change is unnecessary in such cases other than perhaps screening for potential dietary hepatotoxins. However if compromise of normal hepatic functions is suspected on the basis of clinical (e.g. weight loss, photodermatitis) or clinicopathological (e.g., increased serum bile acid concentration, hypoalbuminemia) evidence then dietary manipulations should be considered. Dietary management has been shown to significantly improve morbidity and mortality in human patients with liver failure (Alberino et al 2001, Manguso et al 2005) and might be expected to be equally important in equine cases. Unfortunately there is a scarcity of good quality data to help provide evidence-based nutritional guidelines for hepatic insufficiency in horses. Extrapolation of information derived from other species is a poor substitute for specific equine evidence but might be considered and applied cautiously in the absence of the latter.

Metabolic consequences of hepatic insufficiency

The prime fundamental metabolic considerations important for dietary formulation in hepatic insufficiency cases comprise protein-energy malnutrition and the putative interactions between diet and hepatic encephalopathy (HE).

Protein-energy malnutrition

Relative deficiency in both dietary protein and energy (protein-energy malnutrition) is commonly recognized in human patients with hepatic insufficiency (Caregaro et al 1996) and weight loss is also one of the most frequently observed signs in horses with hepatic failure (McGorum et al 1999, Durham et al 2003a). Several factors may lead to protein-energy malnutrition including inappetance, mild fat malabsorption and insulin resistance. Insulin resistance is a common feature of hepatic failure in humans (Arakawa et al 2004) and horses (A.E. Durham unpublished data) and reduces tissue glucose uptake and glycogen synthesis (Blei et al 1982, Petrides et al 1994). Consequent depletion of normal glycogen reserves creates a greater reliance on gluconeogenesis in the absence of constant dietary intake and this is also facilitated by an insulin resistant status (Owen et al 1983). Gluconeogenesis relies upon substrates including amino acids from protein degradation and glycerol from lipolysis leading to a general catabolic status and an abnormal reliance on body protein for energy (Swart et al 1988). It has been shown that an overnight fast in a cirrhotic patient is metabolically similar to 2 or 3 days of total starvation in normal subjects (Owen et al 1983). Ultimately functional impairment of hepatic gluconeogenesis in an end-stage failing liver may have dire consequences on plasma and tissue glucose homeostasis with hypoglycemia a probable result (West 1996).

Hepatic encephalopathy

Dietary protein has long been implicated in the pathophysiology of HE as a potential source of neurotoxic ammonia, mercaptans, oxyphenol and aromatic amino-acids (AAAs) that might generate "false neurotransmitters" (Balo & Korpassy 1932, Philips et al 1952, Schwartz et al 1954, Fischer et al 1976, Marchesini et al 1990, Holecek 2010). Recent evidence especially implicates degradation of dietary glutamine by intestinal glutaminase in the generation of systemic hyperammonemia (Romero-Gómez et al 2009). In the past the apparent association between proteins, amino acids and HE has been used to advocate the use of low-protein diets in subjects with hepatic insufficiency with or without HE (Schwartz et al 1954, Sherlock et al 1956). Intuitively however, protein-restricted diets can only reduce protein-derived neurotoxins if they provide enough energy and protein to prevent endogenous proteolysis. Furthermore, more recent human studies have indicated that normal to high protein diets are generally well tolerated (especially with concurrent lactulose therapy) and that protein restriction simply promotes catabolism of endogenous protein and might actually facilitate HE (Kearns et al 1992, Morgan et al 1995). In 1997 an evidence-based consensus guideline from the European Society of Enteral and

Table 37-1 Nutritional/Metabolic Problems Associated with Hepatic Insufficiency

Carbohydrate	Protein	Fat	Other
Insulin resistance Decreased glycogen storage Increased gluconeogenesis (early-catabolic) Decreased gluconeogenesis (end-stage-hypoglycemia)	Insulin resistance Catabolism of body protein Hypoalbuminemia (mild) Decreased clotting factors Decreased AAA metabolism Hepatic encephalopathy	Insulin resistance Catabolism of adipose stores Malabsorption of fat (mild)	Decreased vitamins A, D, E, K Decreased Zn, Ca, Mg, P Increased Fe, Cu, Mn

AAA = aromatic amino acids.

Parenteral Nutrition (Plauth et al 1997) advocated the abandonment of protein restricted diets for humans with hepatic insufficiency with or without HE. More recently a randomized trial further demonstrated that even transient protein restriction does not benefit patients during an episode of HE (Córdoba et al 2004).

Several studies in humans have shown that patients with HE are improved when animal protein is replaced by vegetable protein in the diet (Amodio et al 2001) and it might be supposed therefore that the debated encephalopathic risks associated with dietary protein in other species may not be as significant in herbivores such as the horse. Possible reasons why vegetable protein might be less likely to provoke HE include: higher arginine content (important for conversion of ammonia to urea); lower methionine content (source of mercaptans); lower tryptophan content (source of oxyphenol and tryptamine); lower tyrosine and phenylalanine content (sources of several false neurotransmitters); and lower nitrogen assimilation due to retention by colonic flora and associated higher dietary fiber promoting higher fecal bulk and nitrogen losses (Weber et al 1985, Bianchi et al 1993, Amodio et al 2001). Interestingly the ratio of branched chain amino acids (BCAAs) to AAAs tends to be lower (i.e., theoretically less favorable) in cereals and pulses (3.28 and 2.89) compared with meat and fish (3.49 and 3.18) casting doubt on the importance of this analyte (Amodio et al 2001). However, not all studies have found vegetable protein to be significantly beneficial, although the use of vegetable protein is generally favored by dieticians in people with HE on the balance of available evidence (Blendis 1989, Amodio et al 2001). Therapeutic use of BCAA supplementation has been investigated in several human studies but the overall specific benefit remains equivocal (Als-Nielsen et al 2003, Marchesini et al 1990). Glutamine supplementation would appear inadvisable in the face of hepatic failure given its association with hyperammonemia (Romero-Gómez et al 2009).

Oral administration of lactulose, a nonabsorbable disaccharide, results in mild hindgut acidosis decreasing microbial generation of ammonia and increasing ionization to ammonium thus reducing absorption (Kircheis & Häussinger 2002). In this author's experience oral lactulose administration at 0.3 ml/kg q 6–24 h is effective in the treatment and prophylaxis of acute and chronic HE in horses and also remains popular in human cases despite absence of a strong evidence-basis (Als-Nielsen et al 2004). The product is suitable for long-term administration (months to years) and is rarely associated with adverse effects such as soft feces.

Key Points

- Metabolic changes occurring in hepatic failure promote a catabolic status
- There is little if any logical basis to restrict dietary protein in cases of hepatic insufficiency

Dietary principles in hepatic insufficiency

Basic features of the ration

Adequate digestible energy and protein consumption is very important in order to help preserve body proteins and fat stores. In human cirrhosis cases the recommended daily energy and protein intakes are respectively 147–168 kJ/kg bodyweight (BW) and 1.2 to 1.5 g/kg BW daily (Plauth et al 2006). These correspond to a small increase above field maintenance requirements for healthy horses (National Research Council [NRC] 2007a,c) and appear to be reasonable targets for horses with hepatic insufficiency subject to body condition. In human cirrhotic patients, frequent meals are recommended in order to avoid the prompt catabolic effects of fasting in the presence of probable insulin resistance and depleted glycogen reserves. Although more slow and gradual nutrient assimilation is likely to be associated with the equine fermentative alimentary tract in comparison to humans, free access to grass and/or forage interspersed with frequent small concentrate meals seem logical in order to limit catabolism and gluconeogenesis.

Grazing and forage

Grazing should be encouraged for several hours (e.g., 10–14 hours) each day although monitoring of intake and clinical signs becomes more difficult with 24-hour turnout. Short periods of turnout may also be undesirable however as sudden gorging on grass may be disruptive to the stability of hindgut flora and promote ammoniagenesis. Night-time turnout might be considered in subjects with photodermatitis. Where grass is limited or unavailable then grass hay or haylage should be available at all times. Leguminous hays generally provide greater dietary energy and protein and might be useful in cases with significant weight loss although the putative encephalopathic risks of their higher protein content makes them generally inadvisable as the main source of dietary forage if signs of HE have been observed.

Concentrate feeding

Supplementary concentrate feeds may be used to enhance and balance a forage-based diet as well as providing a means for administration of therapeutic agents if required. Provision of a glucose source such as cereal-starch is intuitively helpful to restrain gluconeogenesis although highly glycemic meals may be undesirable in the face of probable insulin resistance. Standard proprietary low-to-medium energy and protein mixes or cubes (e.g., 8–10 MJ/kg digestible energy and 8–10% crude protein) might be used, or a ration formulated from highly fermentable fiber such as sugar beet pulp or chopped alfalfa and inclusion of some starch-rich ingredients (e.g., micronized maize) or molasses to provide glucose and reduce gluconeogenesis as well as improving palatability of the ration. Wheat bran might also be considered if appetite is poor. Any cereal-based feeds should be divided into at least four to six daily meals or perhaps mixed with forage in large buckets (especially during the night) to promote "trickle feeding" and stability in colon fermentation and to reduce possible surges in insulin and ammoniagenesis. In order to promote stability of hindgut flora, starch should not be fed at greater than 1 g/kg BW per meal which is equivalent to feeding a 500-kg horse <3.3 kg of a 15% starch mix/cube or <0.75 kg of micronized maize (assuming 67% starch).

Addition of vegetable oil to the diet is a useful means of providing both dietary energy (typically 34 kJ/ml) and essential fatty acids and supplementation is logical in equine hepatic insufficiency to compensate for possible fat malabsorption. Although biliary secretions play an important role in fat digestion, malabsorption of high levels of dietary fat does not appear to be a large concern in most cases of hepatic insufficiency in dogs and humans (Jenkins et al 1976, Okita 2004). In human cirrhotic patients, dietary fat content comprising between 20–28% of total dietary energy is recommended (Okita 2004) which would equate to a very high-fat diet in horses. Routine inclusion of 0.1 ml/kg BW vegetable oil might be appropriate for most cases of hepatic insufficiency in horses and levels as high as 0.75 to 1.0 ml/kg BW could be a useful means of increasing dietary energy as long as palatability is not unduly decreased and evidence of fat malabsorption (diarrhea or steatorrhea) is not seen.

Assuming a dietary intake of 2% BW daily as dry matter, the target dietary protein range of 1.2 to 1.5 g/kg is quite low in the context of generally available equine feeds equating to a protein content in the overall ration of just 6.0 to 7.5%. This is less than the crude protein (CP) content of most horse-feeds creating a likelihood of mild to moderate protein excess. This is a potential concern in horses showing signs of HE but is of no real consequence in horses showing other signs of hepatic insufficiency. Despite reassuring findings in the context of dietary protein intake and HE in humans outlined previously, avoidance of large quantities of dietary ingredients known to be particularly protein-rich (e.g., alfalfa, brewers grains, cottonseed, soya, linseed) is still generally advisable in horses with HE. However, in terms of limiting endogenous protein catabolism, the quality as well as quantity of dietary protein is clearly important and therefore use of judicious amounts of the above high-protein feeds or perhaps a proprietary "feed balancer" might be useful in circumstances where forage quality is particularly poor. The pathogenetic relevance of dietary BCAA:AAA ratio is unclear, and, given the widely accepted benefits of vegetable protein in human patients, may not be a great concern in equine diets. Nevertheless, it might be of interest to consider that the protein in oats, wheat, soya and beet pulp are relatively rich in AAAs (albeit lower than meat-protein [Amodio et al 2001]), whereas grass and legume hays, wheat bran, maize and milo (sorghum) have a relatively high BCAA content (Divers et al 1988, Ralston 1988).

Vitamin and mineral supplementation

Where the diet is primarily forage-based, supplementation with vitamins and minerals may be advisable. Reduced absorption and storage of fat-soluble vitamins (A, D, E, and K) are a concern in hepatic insufficiency (Jenkins et al 1976, Plauth et al 1997) although water-soluble vitamins (e.g., vitamins B and C) are unlikely to become deficient in horses consuming appropriate rations. Recommended daily maintenance intakes of vitamins A, D and E in healthy horses are 30 IU/kg BW, 6.6 IU/kg BW and 1.0 IU/kg BW respectively (NRC 2007d) and provision of double these maintenance requirements appears reasonable in hepatic insufficiency and is well below known toxic levels in horses and people (Geubel et al 1991, NRC 2007d). Where dietary oil supplementation is practiced then further vitamin E provision may be wise (e.g., 1–2 IU/ml oil). Vitamin K requirements are not known in horses although normal equine diets may typically provide between 0.05–0.4 mg/kg BW daily (NRC 2007d) and therefore ensuring intake toward the upper end of this range appears sensible.

Hepatic insufficiency in people is frequently associated with reduced serum concentrations of calcium, magnesium, phosphorus and zinc; and increased concentrations of iron, copper and manganese (Arakawa et al 2004). The frequent inclusion of iron in proprietary equine micronutrient supplements is of special concern owing to its known capacity for hepatotoxicity in horses (Mullaney & Brown 1988, Edens et al 1993) and the frequent finding of excessive iron in equine liver biopsies (Durham et al 2003b). Selection of iron-free and copper-free products is recommended. Low plasma zinc concentrations (especially in relation to increased copper) are common and regarded as pathophysiologically important in fibroplasia and ammonia detoxification in human hepatic insufficiency and cirrhosis (Arakawa et al 2004). Recommended daily zinc intake in normal horses is 0.8 mg/kg BWT (NRC 2007b) and supplementation is a consideration if plasma zinc concentration is low (<10 micromole/L) and/or plasma copper concentration is high (>20 μmol/l) (Wichert et al 2002).

Specific ration examples for horses with hepatic insufficiency include 12 hours per day grazing (subject to problems with photosensitization) with ad libitum good quality grass hay or haylage when off pasture; supplemented with 0.5 to 1 kg/100 kg BW low to medium energy proprietary mixes or cubes divided into no less than four meals per day. If weight loss is apparent then additional energy might be supplied by gradually (over 2 weeks) replacing the mix or cubes with equal weights of soaked sugar beet pulp and micronized maize. Addition of vegetable oil at 0.1 to 0.5 ml/kg BW may also be used to supply greater dietary energy. Vitamin supplementation with A, D and E should be added to ensure at least NRC recommendations described above. If or when the horse is deemed to have regained adequate hepatic function (based on clinical and clinicopathological indices) then a gradual return to a normal diet is recommended.

Key Points

Grazing and good quality grass hays should be made available continuously although high levels of leguminous forages might be inadvisable

- Small and frequent concentrate meals are helpful to provide a constant glucose supply to deter catabolism and gluconeogenesis

Adequate supply of fat soluble vitamins (A,D,E,K) and zinc warrants particular attention in cases of hepatic insufficiency

Parenteral nutrition

Given the metabolic intolerance of fasting which typifies hepatic failure, parenteral nutrition may sometimes be required as a temporary measure in inappetant or hypophagic acute or chronic hepatic insufficiency cases. Advised protocols are beyond the scope of this publication and the interested reader is referred to Chapter 41 in this book and other recent reviews (Plauth & Schuetz 2009, Plauth et al 2009, Magdesian 2010).

Conclusions

Dietary changes are not required for horses with compensated liver disease but should be applied in horses where there is suspicion of compromise of hepatic functions. Key elements of feeding the horse with hepatic insufficiency comprise avoidance of fasting and provision of a well balanced diet with adequate digestible energy and protein to prevent catabolism of body tissues. Although once widely advocated, dietary protein restriction is inappropriate and should be avoided although particularly high-protein diets may be unwise in horses showing signs of HE. Supplementation of certain micronutrients such as fat-soluble vitamins and zinc are probably beneficial whilst avoiding additional provision of potential hepatotoxins such as iron and copper.

References

Alberino, F., Gatta, A., Amodio, P., et al., 2001. Nutrition and survival in patients with liver cirrhosis. Nutrition 17 (6), 445–450.

Als-Nielsen, B., Gluud, L.L., Gluud, C., 2004. Non-absorbable disaccharides for hepatic encephalopathy: systematic review of randomized trials. British Medical Journal 328 (7447), 1046–1050.

Als-Nielsen, B., Koretz, R.L., Kjaergard, L.L., et al., 2003. Branched-chain amino acids for hepatic encephalopathy. Cochrane Database of Systematic Reviews 1, CD001939.

Amodio, P., Caregaro, L., Pattenò, E., et al., 2001. Vegetarian diets in hepatic encephalopathy: facts or fantasies? Digestive and Liver Disease 33 (6), 492–500.

Arakawa, Y., Moriyama, M., Arakawa, Y., 2004. Liver cirrhosis and metabolism (sugar, protein, fat and trace elements). Hepatology Research 30S, 46–58.

Balo, J., Korpassy, B., 1932. The encephalitis of the dog with Eck fistula fed on meat. Archives of Pathology 13, 80–87.

Bianchi, G.P., Marchesini, G., Fabbri, A., et al., 1993. Vegetable versus animal protein diet in cirrhotic patients with chronic encephalopathy. A randomized cross-over comparison. Journal of Internal Medicine 233 (5), 385–392.

Blei, A.T., Robbins, D.C., Drobny, E., et al., 1982. Insulin resistance and insulin receptors in hepatic cirrhosis. Gastroenterology 83 (6), 1191–1199.

Blendis, L.M., 1989. Nutritional management of patients with chronic liver disease. Baillières Clinical Gastroenterology 3 (1), 91–108.

Caregaro, L., Alberino, F., Amodio, P., et al., 1996. Malnutrition in alcoholic and virus-related cirrhosis. American Journal of Clinical Nutrition 63 (4), 602–609.

Córdoba, J., López-Hellín, J., Planas, M., et al., 2004. Normal protein diet for episodic hepatic encephalopathy: results of a randomized study. Journal of Hepatology 41 (1), 38–43.

Divers, T.J., Bernard, W.V., Reef, V.B., 1988. Equine liver disease and liver failure - causes, diagnosis and treatment. In: Proceedings of the 10th Bain-Fallon Memorial Lectures. Adelaide, Australia, 23–27 May, 1988. Artarmon, NSW, Australia, pp. 35–46.

Durham, A.E., Newton, J.R., Smith, K.C., et al., 2003a. Retrospective analysis of historical, clinical, ultrasonographic, serum biochemical and haematological data in prognostic evaluation of equine liver disease. Equine Veterinary Journal 35 (6), 542–547.

Durham, A.E., Smith, K.C., Newton, J.R., et al., 2003b. Development and application of a scoring system for prognostic evaluation of equine liver biopsies. Equine Veterinary Journal 35 (6), 534–540.

Edens, L.M., Robertson, J.L., Feldman, B.F., 1993. Cholestatic hepatopathy, thrombocytopenia and lymphopenia associated with iron toxicity in a thoroughbred gelding. Equine Veterinary Journal 25 (1), 81–84.

Holecek, M., 2010. Three targets of branched-chain amino acid supplementation in the treatment of liver disease. Nutrition 26 (5), 482–490.

Fischer, J.E., Rosen, H.M., Ebeid, A.M., et al., 1976. The effect of normalization of plasma amino acids on hepatic encephalopathy in man. Surgery 80 (1), 77–91.

Geubel, A.P., DeGalocsy, C., Alves, N., et al., 1991. Liver damage caused by therapeutic vitamin A administration: estimate of dose related toxicity in 41 cases. Gastroenterology 100 (6), 1701–1709.

Jenkins, D.J., Gassull, M.A., Leeds, A.R., et al., 1976. The relation of impaired vitamin A and E tolerance to fat absorption in biliary diversion. International Journal for Vitamin and Nutrition Research 46 (2), 226–230.

Kearns, P.J., Young, H., Garcia, G., et al., 1992. Accelerated improvement of alcoholic liver disease with enteral nutrition. Gastroenterology 102 (1), 200–205.

Kircheis, G., Häussinger, D., 2002. Management of hepatic encephalopathy. Journal of Gastroenterology and Hepatology 17 (suppl.3), S260–S267.

Magdesian, K.G., 2010. Parenteral nutrition in the mature horse. Equine Veterinary Education 22 (7), 364–371.

Manguso, F., D'Ambra, G., Menchise, A., et al., 2005. Effects of an appropriate oral diet on the nutritional status of patients with HCV-related liver cirrhosis: A prospective study. Clinical Nutrition 24 (5), 751–759.

Marchesini, G., Dioguardi, F.S., Bianchi, G.P., et al., 1990. Long-term oral branched-chain amino acid treatment in chronic hepatic encephalopathy. Journal of Hepatology 11 (1), 92–101.

McGorum, B.C., Murphy, D., Love, S., et al., 1999. Clinicopathological features of equine primary hepatic disease: a review of 50 cases. The Veterinary Record 145 (5), 134–139.

Morgan, T.R., Moritz, T.E., Mendenhall, C.L., et al., 1995. Protein consumption and hepatic encephalopathy in alcoholic hepatitis. Journal of the American College of Nutrition 14 (2), 152–158.

Mullaney, T.P., Brown, C.M., 1988. Iron toxicity in neonatal foals. Equine Veterinary Journal 20 (2), 119–124.

National Research Council., 2007a. Energy. In: Nutrient Requirements of Horses, sixth ed. National Academies Press, Washington, pp. 3–33.

National Research Council., 2007b. Minerals. In: Nutrient Requirements of Horses, sixth ed. National Academies Press, Washington, pp. 69–108.

National Research Council., 2007c. Protein and amino acids. In: Nutrient Requirements of Horses, sixth ed. National Academies Press, Washington, pp. 54–68.

National Research Council., 2007d. Vitamins. In: Nutrient Requirements of Horses, sixth ed. National Academies Press, Washington, pp. 109–127.

Okita, M., 2004. Chronic hepatic disease and dietary instruction. Hepatology Research 30S, 92–95.

Owen, O.E., Trapp, V.E., Reichard, G.A., et al., 1983. Nature and quantity of fuels consumed in patients with alcoholic cirrhosis. Journal of Clinical Investigation 72 (5), 1821–1832.

Petrides, A.S., Vogt, C., Schulze-Berge, D., et al., 1994. Pathogenesis of glucose intolerance and diabetes mellitus in cirrhosis. Hepatology 19 (3), 616–627.

Phillips, G.B., Schwartz, R., Gabuzda, G.J., et al., 1952. The syndrome of impending hepatic coma in patients with cirrhosis of the liver given certain nitrogenous substances. New England Journal of Medicine 247 (7), 239–246.

Plauth, M., Schuetz, T., 2009. Hepatology - Guidelines on Parenteral Nutrition, Chapter 16. German Medical Science 7, 1–12.

Plauth, M., Merli, M., Kondrup, J., et al., 1997. ESPEN guidelines for nutrition in liver disease and transplantation. Clinical Nutrition 16 (2), 43–55.

Plauth, M., Cabré, E., Riggio, O., et al., 2006. ESPEN Guidelines on Enteral Nutrition: Liver disease. Clinical Nutrition 25 (2), 285–294.

Plauth, M., Cabré, E., Campillo, B., et al., 2009. ESPEN Guidelines on Parenteral Nutrition: hepatology. Clinical Nutrition 28 (4), 436–444.

Ralston, S.L., 1988. Equine clinical nutrition: specific problems and solutions. Compendium of Continuing Education for the Practicing Veterinarian 10, 356–363.

Romero-Gómez, M., Jover, M., Galán, J.J., et al., 2009. Gut ammonia production and its modulation. Metabolic Brain Disease 24 (1), 147–157.

Schwartz, R., Phillips, G.B., Seegmiller, J.E., et al., 1954. Dietary protein in the genesis of hepatic coma. New England Journal of Medicine 251 (17), 685–689.

Sherlock, S., Summerskill, W.H.J., Dawson, A.M., 1956. Treatment and prognosis of hepatic coma. Lancet 2, 689–694.

Sisson, S., 1975. Equine digestive system. In: Getty, R., (Ed.), Sisson and Grossman's The Anatomy of the Domestic Animals, fifth ed, vol 1. WB Saunders Company, London, pp. 454–497.

Swart, G.R., van den Berg, J.W., Wattimena, J.L., et al., 1988. Elevated protein requirements in cirrhosis of the liver investigated by whole body protein turnover studies. Clinical Science (London) 75 (1), 101–107.

Weber, F.L., Minco, D., Fresard, K.M., et al., 1985. Effects of vegetable diets on nitrogen metabolism in cirrhotic subjects. Gastroenterology 89 (3), 538–544.

West, H.J., 1996. Clinical and pathological studies in horses with hepatic disease. Equine Veterinary Journal 28 (2), 146–156.

Wichert, B., Frank, T., Kienzle, E., 2002. Zinc, copper and selenium intake and status of horses in Bavaria. Journal of Nutrition 132 (6 Suppl 2), 1776S–1777S.

38

Nutritional considerations in grass sickness, botulism, equine motor neuron disease and equine degenerative myeloencephalopathy

Bruce McGorum, Robert S. Pirie, John A. Keen

Grass sickness

Grass sickness (GS, equine dysautonomia) is a multisystem neuropathy characterized by damage to autonomic, enteric and somatic neurons. GS has a high mortality rate (>95%) and significant welfare and financial consequences. An identical disorder occurs in dogs, cats, hares, rabbits, llamas (Symonds et al 1995, Whitwell 1997, Lewis et al 2009) and possibly in sheep (Pruden et al 2004).

Epidemiology and risk factors

GS occurs throughout most Northern European countries, with the highest incidence, estimated at 1–2% of horses per annum, being in Northeast Scotland. GS also occurs in Chile, Argentina, Falkland Islands (termed *mal seco*) and Colombia (termed *tambora*). Interestingly, despite significant movement of horses between United Kingdom, Ireland, and North America, only one case of GS is reported from North America (Wright et al 2010), and the authors are aware of only a few unpublished cases having occurred in Ireland. This suggests that the occurrence of GS is more dependent on the presence or absence of an environmental factor than on direct transmission of a contagious agent between horses. The temporospatial clustering of GS cases is consistent with involvement of contagious or other spatially and temporally localized processes such as local climate and/or pasture management practices (French et al 2005). Most risk factors for GS (Table 38-1) are consistent with it being a toxico-infection with a resilient soil borne organism, such as *Clostridium botulinum*, to which horses may develop immunity.

As the name suggests, GS almost exclusively affects horses that eat fresh herbage, either because they are grazing or because they receive freshly cut herbage when stabled. The risk of GS is greater when horses are grazing full-time than part-time (Gilmour & Jolly 1974), however, even short duration grazing, such as grazing verges while ploughing or while walking in hand, is considered sufficient to induce GS (Begg 1936). All but 2 of 183 GS cases reported by Wood et al (1998) were grazing for at least part of the day, and one of these nongrazing GS cases had been at pasture 1 week previously, while the other case was not confirmed by histological examination of autonomic neurons. There are, however, previous references to GS affecting stabled horses that had no apparent access to fresh herbage (Nairn 1922, Pool 1928, Guthrie 1940), including a group of pit ponies that ate only cereal, bran, and hay (Forsyth 1941). Guthrie (1940) suggested that such cases could result from ingestion of the putative causal toxin in hay or in soil which was adherent to the turnips which were fed to some stabled horses. The latter is consistent with recent proposals that soil, rather than grass, may be the source of the causal agent (Wood et al 1999, Bohnel et al 2003). Unfortunately, these early reports of GS in housed horses are largely anecdotal reports that were not confirmed by histological examination of autonomic neurons. More convincingly, Lannek et al (1961) reported GS in 7 of 36 stabled horses in Sweden which had no access to fresh herbage, with GS being confirmed by histological examination of autonomic ganglia in 1 case. A possible link with ingestion of linseed (*Linum usitatissimum*) was investigated, but not proven. The occurrence of dysautonomia in housed cats (Symonds et al 1995) and caged rabbits (Whitwell 1997), which likely results from the same neuronal insult as GS (Whitwell 1997), indicate that these diseases can occur in the absence of access to soil, pasture or fresh herbage.

Etiology

While there is increasing evidence that GS is a toxicoinfection with *C. botulinum* types C or D (see McGorum & Pirie 2009 for review of evidence), definitive proof is currently lacking. Alternative hypotheses include *Clostridium perfringens* enterotoxicity (Ochoa & Velandia 1978, Gilmour et al 1981) and mycotoxicosis (Robb et al 1997). Cyanide toxicity, resulting from ingestion of cyanogenic glycosides in white clover (*Trifolium repens*) (Gordon 1934, Greig 1942, Lannek et al 1961, McGorum & Anderson 2002), can be discounted as a cause of GS because the authors have observed GS in horses grazing pastures which have no cyanogenic plants. Toxicity from ingestion of alsike clover (*Trifolium hybridum*) (Tocher et al 1923) or tormentil (*Potentilla tormentilla*) (Nairn 1922) has also been discounted as a cause of GS.

C. botulinum serotypes A, B, C, D and E and their neurotoxins have been identified in soil and herbage from GS-affected premises (Bohnel et al 2003). While the presence of botulinum neurotoxins (BoNT) on freshly cut grass appears to contradict the strict anaerobic nature of *C. botulinum*, it is hypothesized that the bacterium may survive and produce toxins within the protective biofilm coating the leaf surface. The diversity of serotypes identified in the soil was

Table 38-1 Factors that Increase the Risk of GS

Horse factors	Young age (peak incidence in 2–7-year-olds), although GS is rare in foals <6 months old Good to fat body condition Low serum concentrations of IgG to surface antigens of *C. botulinum* type C and *C. novyi* type A, and to *C. botulinum* type C neurotoxin complex toxoid Lack of recent history of cograzing with a GS-affected horse
Premise factors	Geographical location GS occurs more commonly on sand or loam soils than on chalk soils High soil nitrogen content Large number of horses on premise Stud farms and livery/riding establishments Recent occurrence of GS on premise Rearing of domesticated birds on premise
Management factors	Grazing or feeding freshly cut grass Recent stressful procedures, dietary change and/or movement of pasture Use of ivermectin as ultimate and penultimate anthelmintics Mechanical removal of feces from pastures increases the risk of GS while manual removal of feces reduces the risk Frequent chain harrowing Lack of grass cutting Soil disturbance such as digging drainage channels Lack of supplementary feeding with hay or haylage Lack of cograzing with ruminants
Other factors	Season, with peaks in spring and autumn Cool (7–11°C), dry weather in preceding 10–14 days

Data from Gilmour & Jolly 1974, Doxey et al 1991a,b, Wood et al 1998, Hunter & Poxton 2001, McCarthy et al 2004, Newton et al 2004.

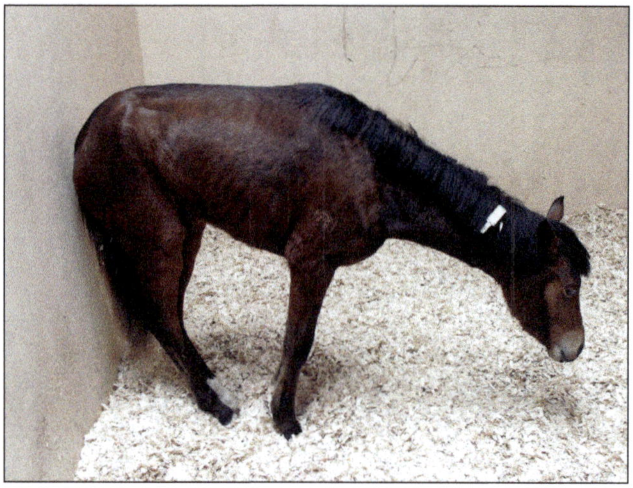

Figure 38.1 Chronic GS case with marked weight loss and a "tucked up" abdomen. The base narrow stance, low head carriage and leaning against the stable wall are suggestive of generalized myasthenia.

considered as evidence that they were introduced from external sources, such as animal or bird feces or organic fertilizers, rather than representing the geo-specific types of *C. botulinum* which are normally found in different types of soil (Smith & Sugiyama 1988). If GS is indeed a toxicoinfectious form of botulism, the longevity of botulinum spores in soil (Mitscherlich & Marth 1984) may explain the frequent recurrence of GS on some premises.

Plants collected from fields immediately after an outbreak of GS had reduced antioxidant and weak pro-oxidant activities, increased concentrations of fructose and low-molecular-weight phenolic compounds, significantly more of one amino acid zone (probably valine), significantly less tartaric acid, and a non-significant decrease in ascorbic acid content, when compared with control plants (McGorum et al 2000). This suggests that plants from GS premises may be under oxidative stress, possibly due to chilling, drought or fungal colonization. It is theoretically possible that the altered biochemical content of ingested plants may contribute, directly or indirectly, to the development of GS. Horses with acute GS have alterations in blood/plasma concentrations of several antioxidants, consistent with oxidative stress, the acute phase response and/or the secondary metabolic complications of GS (McGorum et al 2003). While this study found no evidence of systemic macromolecular oxidative damage, macromolecular oxidative damage occurring at the neuronal level could theoretically contribute to GS. Horses with acute GS also have hyperglycemia (Stewart et al 1940) and hyperlipidemia (Milne et al 1990), presumably reflecting negative energy balance. They also have perturbations in plasma amino acid profile resembling those of severe protein malnutrition (McGorum & Kirk 2001). In addition, horses with GS and cograzing healthy horses had depletion of the plasma sulfur amino acids cyst(e)ine and methionine which may indicate xenobiotic exposure.

Clinical signs and diagnosis

Clinically, GS occurs in acute, sub-acute and chronic forms, reflecting the severity and duration of clinical signs, most of which are attributable to autonomic dysfunction. These include dysphagia, generalized ileus, patchy sweating, salivation, ptosis, rhinitis sicca and tachycardia. The clinical signs and diagnosis of GS are described in detail elsewhere (Pirie 2006, McGorum & Pirie 2009) and are illustrated in Figs 38.1–38.3).

Prevention of GS

Until the cause of GS is known, it is difficult to give sound advice regarding disease prevention. While attempts to eliminate the risk factors listed in Table 38-1 should theoretically reduce the statistical probability of a horse developing GS, prevention of GS on high risk premises is probably achieved only by permanently stabling horses and feeding a diet free from freshly cut herbage. This control measure, however, is rarely used because of practical, economic and welfare considerations. Furthermore, occasional cases have

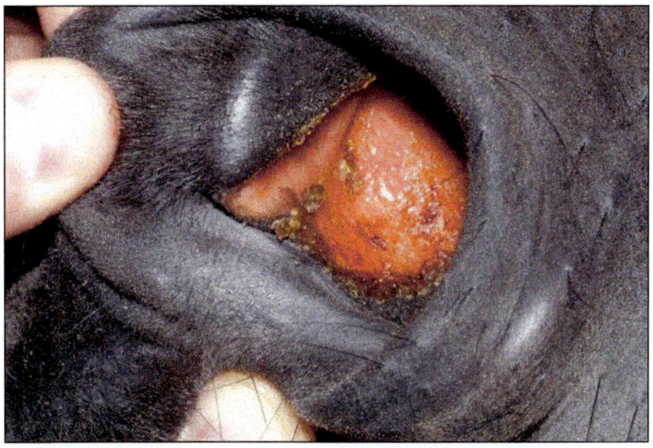

Figure 38.2 Rhinitis sicca, which is considered pathognomonic for GS.

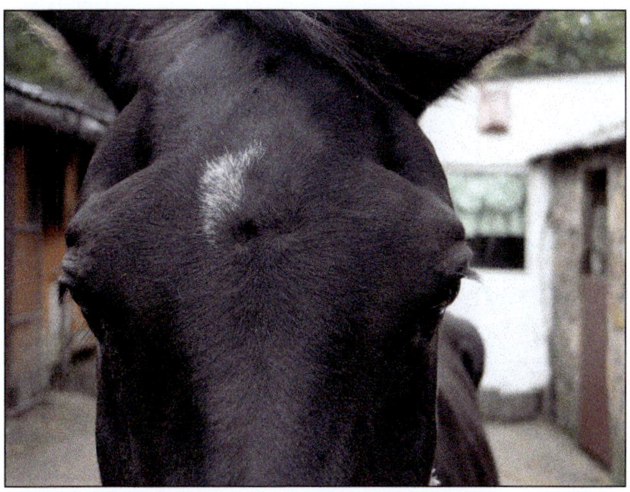

Figure 38.3 Bilateral ptosis is a common feature of GS. This is most easily identified by observing the downward direction of the upper eyelashes in this horse's right eye. Application of topical phenylephrine to this horse's left eye has restored normal eyelash direction, thereby aiding recognition of ptosis.

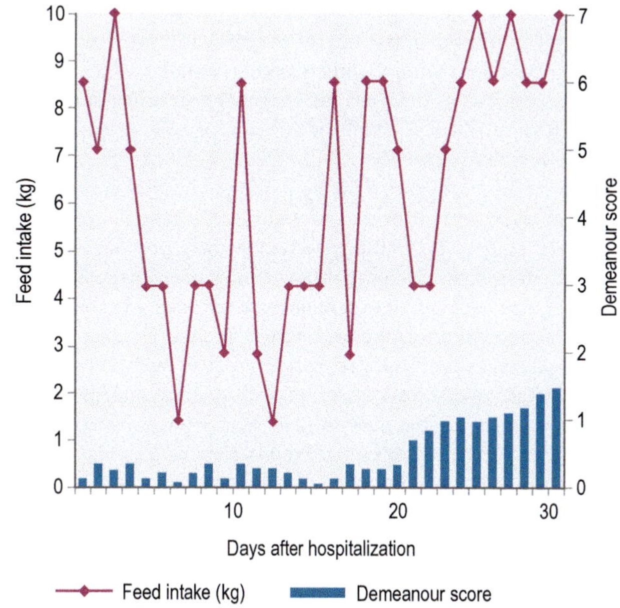

Figure 38.4 Graph illustrating the marked temporal variation in feed intake (kg) and demeanour score in a horse with chronic GS. Both variables improve towards the end of the hospitalization period.

been reported in stabled horses (vide supra). Following the discovery of an association with weather (Doxey et al 1991a), some owners of high-risk premises stable their horses when dry weather with a temperature of 7–11°C has persisted for 10 consecutive days. Stabling is particularly recommended for new horses that are moved onto high-risk premises. If certain fields are considered high-risk for GS, they can be grazed by sheep or cattle, especially in spring. If GS occurs in a group of horses, it is generally recommended that the co-grazing horses are stabled for 2–4 weeks, or moved to another field, because they are otherwise at increased risk of developing GS.

Management of GS

Horses with acute or subacute GS should be euthanized on humane grounds once a confident diagnosis is made, because these forms are invariably fatal. Some horses with chronic GS survive with intensive nursing care (Doxey et al 1995a). Owners should be aware, however, that the survival is largely determined by the severity of nerve damage and the associated complications, rather than the quality of the veterinary and nursing care. Consequently, even with the best care, an affected horse may not survive. As there is no specific antidote or drug treatment to reverse nerve damage, nursing care can only address the common complications of gastrointestinal dysfunction, anorexia, weight loss, dysphagia, dehydration and rhinitis sicca. Analgesics, omeprazole, intestinal prokinetics, fluids, electrolytes and probiotics are commonly administered, but their efficacy is unknown. The reader is directed to other texts for detailed information on management of chronic GS (Milne 1996, McGorum et al 2009). Cisapride, an intestinal prokinetic drug which reduces gastrointestinal transit time in chronic GS (Milne et al 1996), is currently rarely used because of its limited availability, safety concerns and high cost and because its effect on survival rate is unknown. Unfortunately, administration of the antioxidant acetylcysteine, the appetite stimulant brotizolam or a laxative/antioxidant extract from *Aloe vera*, did not give a measurable increase in case survival (Fintl & McGorum 2002).

Nutritional support is essential to counteract the marked cachexia which characterizes GS. Unfortunately depression, poor appetite, dysphagia, colic and pain associated with esophageal and gastric ulceration limit the quantity and nature of food that is ingested. Indeed, few horses eat well for more than four days consecutively (Doxey et al 1995b; Fig. 38.4). Ideally, a high-energy, high-protein diet, which is palatable and readily swallowed, should be fed in small amounts frequently throughout the day (4–5 feeds per day). In practice, however, the selection of food offered is usually dictated by the individual horse's preferences, which unfortunately change regularly, rather than being based on nutritional requirements. Feeds are often offered warm or tepid in the early stages to improve palatability. It is worth offering feeds of different consistency to determine which is preferred, although most horses prefer a mix of soup consistency made by thoroughly soaking pellets in water or dilute molasses. As affected horses rarely eat sufficient conserved forage, particularly if they are dysphagic, they should be allowed frequent short duration access to grazing or offered freshly cut grass. Hay or haylage should be avoided if the horse has a tendency to develop esophageal choke. In the early stages, particularly when horses are depressed, hand feeding from a raised bucket may encourage eating. Hooking the feed bucket on a stable door may also encourage horses to eat and take an interest in their environment.

Most horses that have a realistic chance of survival do not require prolonged administration of fluids and/or feeds via intravenous or nasogastric routes. Short-term nasogastric feeding of pellet slurries has proved beneficial in some cases, but this procedure is poorly tolerated by some horses with severe rhinitis sicca. Extreme care should be taken when administering food by stomach tube to horses with GS because administration of large quantities of high energy, high protein food can induce frequently fatal intestinal bacterial overgrowth, diarrhea and toxemia. Consistent with this observation, small intestinal bacterial overgrowth, commonly with *C. perfringens,* is one of the major gastrointestinal manifestations of human dysautonomia (Chelimsky & Chelimsky 2003). This is a consequence of gastrointestinal dysmotility and loss of peristalsis which is an important defense against small intestine bacterial colonization (Husebye 2005, Connor & di Lorenzo 2006). The authors have used continuous enteral feeding with Fresubin HP Energy liquid tube feed in four horses with chronic GS. This liquid feed, formulated for treatment of catabolic human patients, was administered via an indwelling narrow bore nasogastric tube (Mila 18 FG), using an Applix Smart pump (Fig. 38.5). As the tube was inserted via a stab incision through the skin overlying the nostril, the horse was able to graze and eat with the feeding system *in situ.* All three horses had improved demeanour, voluntary food intake and fecal output, without evidence of clinically significant small intestinal bacterial overgrowth or metabolic and electrolyte disturbances resulting from the re-feeding syndrome. Further evaluation in additional cases is required to determine whether this treatment affects case outcome. Inability to maintain the nasogastric tube in situ in some horses appears to be the main limitation of this technique. Close monitoring was required to prevent the tube blocking and the pump dislodging. Parenteral nutrition (see Chapter 41), sometimes in combination with insulin administration, has been used successfully to manage horses with chronic GS for between a few days and several weeks (Andrew Durham, personal communication 2010).

Key Points – Grass Sickness (GS)

- GS is a multisystem neuropathy, presenting predominantly as gastrointestinal and autonomic dysfunction
- While the etiology is unproven, increasing evidence suggests it may be a toxic-infectious form of botulism type C or D
- Acute and subacute GS is invariably fatal, while horses with chronic GS may recover with intensive nursing care and nutritional support

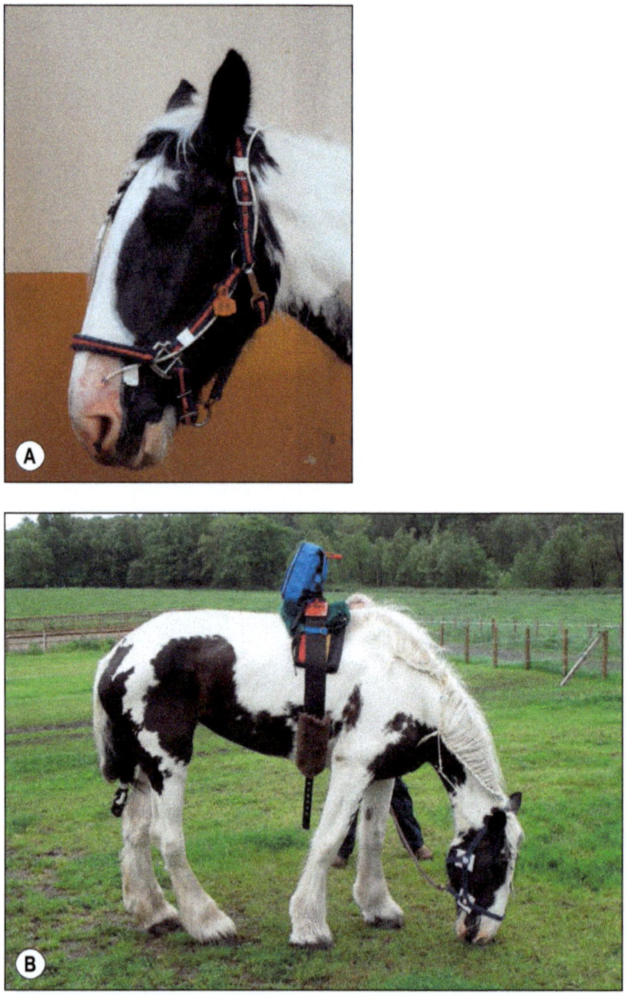

Figure 38.5 (A and B) Chronic GS case with continuous enteral liquid feeding system in situ.

Botulism

Botulism is a neuromuscular disorder causing generalized flaccid paralysis. It is caused by botulinum neurotoxins (BoNTs) from *C. botulinum*, a Gram-positive, strictly anaerobic, spore forming bacterium found ubiquitously in soil and occasionally in the intestinal tract of birds and animals.

Epidemiology and risk factors

Equine botulism has been associated with four (A, B, C and D) of the seven (A–G) serotypes of *C. botulinum*, all of which cause an identical clinical disease. Although botulism occurs worldwide, there are geographical differences in the prevalence of equine botulism and in the serotypes which cause disease in horses. In North America, equine botulism is most commonly attributed to serotype B, and less commonly to types A and C (Kinde et al 1991, Wichtel & Whitlock 1991, Whitlock & Buckley 1997, Schoenbaum et al 2000, Weese 2009). *C. botulinum* grows optimally in anaerobic environments with neutral or alkaline pH, and is inhibited at pH <4.5. BoNT is produced during stationary and growth phases and during bacterial lysis, and optimally at pH 5.7

to 6.2 and when protein concentration is high (Stringer et al 1999). BoNT is inactive until cleaved by bacterial or host proteases.

The three modes of intoxication are ingestion of preformed toxin in contaminated food (forage poisoning), production of toxin within the gastrointestinal tract following ingestion of bacteria or spores (toxicoinfectious botulism or shaker foal syndrome) and production of BoNT from bacteria contaminating wounds (wound botulism). Catastrophic and costly outbreaks of botulism can occur following ingestion of contaminated feeds (Kinde et al 1991). Botulism in adult horses is most commonly due to ingestion of preformed BoNT/B in poorly conserved silage, haylage, hay and straw (Mitchell et al 1939, Ricketts et al 1984, Divers et al 1986, Haagsma et al 1990, Kinde et al 1991). Forage is often contaminated with soil containing *C. botulinum* spores during harvesting, but clostridia germinate and grow only if the pH is suitable and there is high water content. In good quality silage, microbial fermentation of water soluble carbohydrates produces organic acids, mainly lactic, which lowers the pH to a level which inhibits growth of clostridia. The pH does not drop sufficiently if the forage has low soluble carbohydrate content. While pH ≤4.5 usually inhibits clostridial growth, inhibition may not occur at this pH if the forage has excessively high water content. For this reason, and because clostridia grow in very wet conditions, wet preserved forages pose a risk for botulism. Wet forage should be prewilted under good weather conditions to ensure sufficient acid production to inhibit *C. botulinum*. It is generally recommended that bagged forage is consumed within 3–7 days of opening the bag because, once the bag is opened, aerobic microbial putrefaction degrades organic acids, increasing the pH and permitting growth of *C. botulinum*. Large bags may pose increased risk of botulism, because they will be consumed more slowly after opening, especially if they are used to feed a single horse. Forage ensiled in plastic bags should be discarded if the bag is punctured, unless it can be consumed within 3–7 days of the puncture. Since some feeds which have been linked with outbreaks of equine botulism have an abnormal odor or appearance consistent with putrefaction (Ricketts et al 1984, Hunter et al 2002), such feeds should not be offered to horses. Unfortunately as this is not a consistent finding, normal smell and appearance do not guarantee that a feed is safe for horses.

Type C botulism is typically associated with contamination of feeds with decaying animal or bird carcasses. Unfortunately, ingestion of as little as 50–100 g of hay contaminated by a decaying carcass may be lethal for a horse (Muller 1963). Type C botulism is also associated with ingestion of bird feces, soil or dirt, and ingestion of bacteria that were transmitted to feed troughs by birds that had scavenged animal carcases (Heath et al 1990, Whitlock et al 1997, Schoenbaum et al 2000). Since poultry manure often contains *C. botulinum* types C and D, it should not be applied to fields that are grazed by horses or to fields which are used for production of hay or haylage.

Shaker foal syndrome is a toxico-infectious form of botulism which most commonly affects rapidly growing 1–2 month old foals, and occasionally adult horses, in certain geographical areas (Swerczek 1980a,b). Experimental oral challenges with botulinum spores indicate that necrotic gastrointestinal lesions and stress are prerequisites for development of this disease. An additional risk factor for this disease is ingestion of large volumes of fat and protein rich milk from mares which are fed fat and protein rich diets. Toxico-infectious botulism is also one of the proposed causes of grass sickness (vide supra).

Etiology and pathophysiology

BoNTs cause generalized neuromuscular dysfunction by blocking acetylcholine release through the cleavage of SNARE proteins which are involved in synaptic vesicle exocytosis at neuromuscular junctions, peripheral cholinergic nerve terminals in autonomic ganglia and postganglionic parasympathetic nerve terminals. BoNTs do not inhibit function of peripheral sensory nerves and central neurons. Horses appear to be particularly sensitive to BoNTs (Swerczek 1980a), which are amongst the most potent identified biological protein toxins.

Clinical signs

Clinical signs of botulism reflect generalized myasthenia and autonomic dysfunction (described in detail in McGorum 2003, Whitlock 2009). Generalized flaccid paralysis causes exertional muscle tremors and abnormalities in posture and gait, progressing to tetraparesis and ultimately tetraparalysis with death due to paralysis of respiratory muscles. Bulbar dysfunction, often an early feature of botulism, causes ptosis, pupillary dilatation, weakness of the tongue, cheeks, masticatory muscles, pharynx and larynx. This may cause dysphagia, quidding, drooling of saliva, nasal regurgitation of food and water, soft palate displacement, dysphonia and aspiration pneumonia. Tongue weakness is readily evident as a reduction in the normally strong retraction that follows gentle withdrawal of the tongue. Offering the horse food and water can aid detection of weakness of the muscles of prehension, mastication and deglutition. Inability to swallow food typically occurs prior to inability to swallow water. Flaccidity of the tail and anus are common. Ileus, constipation, urine retention and colic may occur. Clinical signs commence several hours to several days after toxin ingestion, and may progress slowly or very rapidly. Sudden, unexplained death may herald the onset of an outbreak.

Diagnosis

A presumptive diagnosis of botulism is commonly made based on historic and clinical data, and by elimination of other diagnoses (described in detail in McGorum 2003, Whitlock 2009). A definitive diagnosis of botulism is rarely achieved. The diagnosis is supported by culture of *C. botulinum* from feed, gastrointestinal contents or tissues, or by detection of BoNT in feed, serum, plasma or gastrointestinal contents. However, such analyses must be interpreted with caution, since BoNT is rarely detected in serum or plasma because horses are particularly susceptible to extremely low quantities of this exquisitely potent toxin (Swerczek 1980a). Furthermore, bacteria and BoNT are occasionally detectable in intestinal contents and feces from healthy horses. A diagnosis of botulism is supported by demonstration of brief, small amplitude, overly abundant motor unit action potentials on needle electromyography of appropriate muscles.

There are no pathognomonic gross or histological post mortem features for botulism.

Management

Potential sources of BoNT, such as silage, should be removed. Early administration of specific antitoxin, available only in some countries, can markedly increase survival rates (described in detail by Whitlock 2009). Fenicia et al (2002) recommended that metronidazole and penicillin are not administered to cases of toxicoinfectious or wound botulism, because lysis of intraluminal clostridia may release BoNT. Furthermore, metronidazole pretreatment predisposed mice to develop clinical botulism following oral challenge with botulinum spores, presumably because it favored intestinal colonization by *C. botulinum* (Wang & Sugiyama 1984). Broad-spectrum antimicrobials are commonly administered to counteract secondary infections resulting from aspiratioh or from decubital ulcers. Foals with respiratory failure may be managed by mechanical ventilation and oxygen supplementation. Good nursing care is essential to success, to prevent decubital and corneal ulcers, to maintain nutrition and fluid and electrolyte balance and to minimize aspiration pneumonia. While horses with mild dysphagia may manage to eat soaked pellet diets, especially if they are offered at a height to facilitate swallowing, additional nutritional support is commonly required. Milk replacement may be administered to affected foals via indwelling nasogastric tubes. Adults may be fed liquid diets via indwelling nasogastric tubes or pellet slurries via nasogastric intubation (see Chapter 41). Administration of fluid via a nasogastric tube often overcomes the requirement for intravenous fluid administration. Short-term parenteral nutrition may be beneficial, but is costly and rarely required. Constipation may be managed by administering liquid paraffin, fluids and electrolytes. Ocular lubricants should be used to prevent corneal ulceration. Drugs that potentiate neuromuscular blockade including aminoglycosides, procaine, tetracyclines, and magnesium based laxatives should be avoided. Horses that survive botulism have a complete, but often protracted, recovery.

Prevention

Husbandry practices which can reduce the risk of botulism are outlined in Box 38.1. Effective botulinum vaccines are available in many countries, but provide only strain specific immunity (see Whitlock 2009 for detailed information).

Key Points – Botulism

- Botulinum neurotoxins cause generalized neuromuscular and autonomic dysfunction
- Botulism results from ingestion of preformed toxin in contaminated food (forage poisoning), production of toxin within the gastrointestinal tract following ingestion of bacteria or spores (toxicoinfectious botulism or shaker foal syndrome) or production of toxin from bacteria contaminating wounds (wound botulism)
- A diagnosis of botulism is commonly made based on historic and clinical data, because laboratory confirmation of the disease can prove problematic
- Disease control involves optimizing management practices (avoidance of sources of toxin, especially by optimal preparation, storage and feeding of forages) and vaccination

Box 38.1 Measures to Control Botulism

- Avoid feeding decaying forage and feeds
- Avoid inclusion of soil when cutting grass for hay, haylage or silage production, by cutting grass at >7 cm height. A crude ash content > 10% DM likely indicates soil contamination.
- Discard bagged forage if the bag is punctured, unless the forage can be consumed within 3–7 days of the puncture
- Ensure that all bagged forage is consumed within 3–7 days of opening the bag
- Avoid contamination of feeds with animal and bird carcases and feces
- Dispose of animal carcases appropriately
- Good vermin control
- Do not apply poultry manure to fields which are grazed by horses or which are used for hay, haylage or silage production
- Horses in endemic areas should be vaccinated if vaccines are available

Equine motor neuron disease (EMND)

EMND, first described in 1990, is associated with low vitamin E status, and is characterized by oxidative damage to somatic lower motor neurons, especially those supplying highly oxidative type I muscle fibers (Cummings et al 1990, 1993). EMND is rare in horses less than 2 years old.

Epidemiology, risk factors and etiopathogenesis

While the etiopathogenesis of EMND remains incompletely understood, its association with low vitamin E status is evidenced by all affected horses having plasma/serum vitamin E levels consistent with deficiency, and by experimental induction of EMND by prolonged feeding of a vitamin E-deficient diet (Divers et al 1994, Mohammed et al 1994, DeLaRuaDomenech et al 1995a,b, 1997a,b, McGorum et al 2006). Lipopigment accumulation in retinal pigment epithelium and spinal cord capillary endothelium is also consistent with oxidative damage associated with deficiency of vitamin E which protects against lipid peroxidation (Cummings et al 1995, Riis et al 1999). In North American cases, and most European cases, low vitamin E status likely reflects prolonged inadequate intake of fresh green herbage, which is a rich source of dietary antioxidants including vitamin E. However 40% of EMND horses in a European study (McGorum et al 2006) had part- or full-time access to grass-based pasture at the onset of EMND, suggesting that, in these cases, the low vitamin E status and EMND were attributable to factors other than lack of green herbage. Unfortunately, no intrinsic, managemental or environmental risk factors were identified for EMND in these grazing horses. It is likely that many, if not all, of the grazing horses that developed EMND had a dietary intake of vitamin E that was adequate to meet normal equine requirements, since most pasture grasses supply more than the minimum National Research Council daily estimate of the vitamin E requirement for adult horses (Hintz 1992, 1994, DeLaRua-Domenech et al 1997b). Furthermore, it is stated that vitamin

E supplementation is not required for horses that are consuming fresh herbage or are grazing pasture (Blakley & Bell 1994). One explanation for the low vitamin E status of grazing EMND horses is ingestion of forage with low vitamin E content, however this is unlikely because the herbage was typical of pastures used to graze horses and in some instances the pasture was described as lush. While it is stated that horses with access to green forage for less than 3 months per year may have low vitamin E concentrations (Divers et al 2001), the precise daily duration of access to pasture that is required to ensure adequate dietary intake of vitamin E is unknown and likely to be highly variable, since it will be dependent on numerous horse (age, breed, exercise level, unidentified heritable factors) and pasture (herbage type and quantity, season, growth conditions) factors (Blythe et al 1991a, Blakley & Bell 1994, DeLaRua-Domenech et al 1997a). The low vitamin E status of grazing EMND horses may reflect failure of absorption or retention of dietary vitamin E. In this respect, studies on equine degenerative myeloencephalopathy suggest there may be a familial predisposition towards low bioavailability of vitamin E (Mayhew et al 1987). Failure to absorb vitamin E may be due to intestinal epithelial absorptive dysfunction, a lack of bile, pancreatic enzymes and dietary fats, or to the presence of competing factors within the intestine, such as high levels of dietary polyunsaturated fats (Machlin 1984). Consistent with this possibility, oral vitamin E supplementation of EMND horses produced inconsistent increases in plasma vitamin E (Divers et al 2001) compared with normal horses (Blakley & Bell 1994). Furthermore, human vitamin E deficiency disorders which lead to neurodegeneration affect primarily patients with significant gastrointestinal or metabolic disorders that reduce vitamin E bioavailability (Satya-Murti et al 1986). Further investigation of grazing EMND horses using an oral vitamin E absorption test is warranted. Alternatively, the reduced vitamin E concentrations in grazing EMND cases may reflect excessive utilization of vitamin E due to exposure to environmental oxidants such as iron, cadmium and lead (Dabbagh et al 1994, DeLaRuaDomenech et al 1997a, Hijova et al 2004, Saly et al 2004). Importantly, it is unlikely that the grazing horses developed EMND as a sole consequence of inadequate dietary vitamin E intake, since horses develop EMND only after prolonged (at least 14 months) feeding of a severely vitamin E deficient diet (Divers et al 2002). A causal role for mechanisms which are not directly linked to low vitamin E status in North American EMND cases was supported by the observation that, after adjusting for the effects of plasma vitamin E levels, factors including age, turnout type and size, predominant type of concentrate fed and rabies vaccination status contributed significantly to the overall likelihood of EMND (DeLaRuaDomenech et al 1997a,b). These findings suggest that EMND is a multifactorial disorder. Causal factors proposed for the related disorder human amyotrophic lateral sclerosis include excess iron and copper, and occupational exposure to lead, solvents and chemicals (Chancellor et al 1993), but this association remains unproven and other studies failed to show this association (Bergomi et al 2002). Evidence supporting involvement of trace element toxicosis in EMND includes similarities in the clinicopathological features of EMND and lead toxicosis (Sojka et al 1996), and the presence of elevated levels of copper in spinal cords from EMND cases (Polack et al 2000).

Horses with EMND have lower serum glucose concentrations than controls following oral and intravenous glucose administration, possibly because of enhanced glucose utilization by muscle (Benders et al 2005).

Clinical signs

Clinical signs are largely attributable to myasthenia of postural muscles which contain a high component of Type I myofibers. Consequently, horses with EMND are unable to lock their passive stay apparatus, and appear weaker when standing than when moving. They may have an elevated tailhead due to neurogenic atrophy and subsequent contracture of the sacrocaudalis dorsalis medialis muscles. EMND results in muscle tremors, muscle atrophy particularly affecting the neck, back and pelvic limbs, increased time spent in recumbency, shortened stride length and shifting body position when standing. Horses with EMND often show progressive weight loss for 1 month prior to the onset of muscular weakness, despite having a normal to increased appetite. They may have coprophagy and hyperhidrosis. Fundic examination may reveal a mosaic pattern of dark yellow to dark brown lipofuschin deposits in the tapetum and at the tapetal–nontapetal junction (Riis et al 1999).

Diagnosis

A diagnosis of EMND should not be discounted on the basis of a horse having access to lush pasture. The diagnosis is supported by a low serum alpha-tocopherol concentration (<1.5 mg/l), although low levels may also occur in apparently healthy horses and in horses with nutritional myodenegeration. EMND is confirmed premortem by histological examination of biopsies of the sacrocaudalis dorsalis medialis muscle and spinal accessory nerve (Jackson et al 1996, Valentine et al 1998). Both techniques have a sensitivity and specificity approximating 90% when assessed by a suitably experienced pathologist.

Management and prevention

Horses with EMND should receive a readily available form of vitamin E (DL-alpha-tocopherol, 5000–10 000 IU per day PO) and access to fresh green forage. There is a theoretical but unproven risk for high-doses of vitamin E to adversely vitamin A, D, and/or K status. It is prudent to supplement all horses on the management system, since it is likely that other horses have subclinical disease. Dimethylsulfoxide, vitamin C and corticosteroids may be administered in the acute phase, but their efficacy is unknown. Exercise should be avoided until horses recover. Approximately 40% of EMND horses improve within 6 weeks of treatment, 40% stabilize but remain disfigured, while 20% are euthanized due to further deterioration (Divers & Mohammed 2009). Athletic function rarely recovers.

Key Points – Equine Motor Neuron Disease (EMND)

- EMND is associated with low vitamin E status, and is characterized by oxidative damage to somatic lower motor neurons, especially those supplying highly oxidative type I muscle fibers

- Most cases are attributable to inadequate intake of fresh green forage, but some horses at pasture develop the disease
- Vitamin E supplementation and provision of fresh green forage may be beneficial in some cases

Equine degenerative myeloencephalopathy (EDM)

EDM is a diffuse, progressive degenerative disease of select areas of the spinal cord and brainstem. Like EMND, it is associated with a deficiency of vitamin E and possibly other dietary antioxidants (Mayhew et al 1987, Blythe et al 1991a,b, Blythe & Craig 1992a,b, Cummings et al 1995). The horse's age at the time of the neurological insult appears to determine whether vitamin E deficiency leads to EMND or EDM. EDM appears to reflect an insult to the developing nervous system, since it most commonly affects horses less than 2 years old, while EMND affects older horses. It would be reasonable to assume that horses slightly older than 2 years old may develop both EDM and EMND, but interestingly only very few cases with clinical signs and lesions of both diseases have been observed (Caroline Hahn, personal communication 2010). Neurodegenerative lesions resembling EDM were induced experimentally in two foals which were subjected to vitamin E deprivation from the last trimester of gestation to 6 months of age (Mayhew 2008).

Epidemiology, risk factors and etiology

EDM typically affects young growing horses that are reared in dirt lots and fed diets lacking in vitamin E, such as heat-treated pellets and sun-dried forage. However, as with EMND, EDM may affect horses that are continuously on pasture (Blythe et al 1991b). EDM may affect many animals in a management group. A familial and likely hereditary basis, possibly associated with low bioavailability of vitamin E, is reported in several breeds (Mayhew et al 1987, Blythe et al 1991a,b, Mayhew 2008). Additional risk factors include exposure to wood preservatives, particularly creosote, and insecticides (Dill et al 1989a,b, 1990), indicating that environmental oxidants may also be involved in some cases.

Clinical signs

EDM results in symmetrical weakness, ataxia and hypometria of pelvic limbs or all four limbs (Blythe & Craig 1992b, Mayhew 2008). Clinical signs typically have an insidious onset and are progressive, but acute onset may occur.

Diagnosis

Diagnosis is based on clinical signs, signalment, historic information and elimination of other diagnoses (reviewed by Blythe & Craig 1992b). Serum concentrations of vitamin E are low in EDM cases and other horses in the same management system, unless they have been recently fed diets containing vitamin E or have received vitamin E supplementation.

Management and prevention

Vitamin E supplementation (described earlier for EMND) may stabilize clinical signs, but is usually not curative (Mayhew 2008). Provision of fresh green forage and administration of vitamin E (DL-alpha-tocopherol, 5–10 000 IU per day PO) to in-contact horses and pregnant and nursing mares may prevent development of further clinical cases.

Key Points – Equine Degenerative Myeloencephalopathy (EDM)

- EDM is a diffuse, progressive degenerative disease of select areas of the spinal cord and brainstem
- EDM, like EMND, is associated with a deficiency of vitamin E, and possibly other antioxidants
- Vitamin E supplementation and provision of fresh green forage may be beneficial in some cases

References

Begg, G.W., 1936. Grass disease in horses. Vet Rec 48, 655–662.

Benders, N.A., Dyer, J., Wijnberg, I.D., et al., 2005. Evaluation of glucose tolerance and intestinal luminal membrane glucose transporter function in horses with equine motor neuron disease. Am J Vet Res 66, 93–99.

Bergomi, M., Vinceti, M., Nacci, G., et al., 2002. Environmental exposure to trace elements and risk of amyotrophic lateral sclerosis: A population-based case-control study. Environ Res 89, 116–123.

Blakley, B.R., Bell, R.J., 1994. The vitamin A and E status of horses raised in Alberta and Saskatchewan. Can Vet J 35, 297–300.

Blythe, L.L., Craig, A.M., 1992a. Equine degenerative myeloencephalopathy. Part I: clinical signs and pathogenesis. Comp Cont Educ Pract Vet 14, 1215–1221.

Blythe, L.L., Craig, A.M., 1992b. Equine degenerative myeloencephalopathy. Part II: diagnosis and treatment. Comp Cont Educ Pract Vet 14, 1633–1636.

Blythe, L.L., Craig, A.M., Lassen, E.D., et al., 1991a. Serially determined plasma alpha-tocopherol concentrations and results of the oral vitamin E absorption tests in clinically normal horses and in horses with degenerative myeloencephalopathy. Am J Vet Res 52, 908–911.

Blythe, L.L., Hultgren, B.D., Craig, A.M., et al., 1991b. Clinical, viral, and genetic evaluation of equine degenerative myeloencephalopathy in a family of Appaloosas. JAVMA 198, 1005–1013.

Bohnel, H., Wernery, U., Gessler, F., 2003. Two cases of equine grass sickness with evidence for soil-borne origin involving botulinum neurotoxin. J Vet Med B 50, 178–182.

Chancellor, A.M., Slattery, J.M., Fraser, H., et al., 1993. Risk factors for motor neuron disease – a case control study based on patients from the Scottish motor neuron disease register. J Neurol Neurosurg Psych 56, 1200–1206.

Chelimsky, G., Chelimsky, T.C., 2003. Evaluation and treatment of autonomic disorders of the gastrointestinal tract. Semin Neurol 23, 453–458.

Connor, F.L., Di Lorenzo, C., 2006. Chronic intestinal pseudo-obstruction: assessment and management. Gastroenterol 130, S29–S36.

Cummings, J.F., de Lahunta, A., George, C., et al., 1990. Equine motor neuron disease – A preliminary report. Cornell Vet 80, 357–379.

Cummings, J.F., de Lahunta, A., Summers, B.A., et al., 1993. Pathological findings in equine motor neuron disease. J Neuropath Exp. Neurol 52, 278.

Cummings, J.F., de Lahunta, A., Mohammed, H.O., 1995. Endothelial lipopigment as an indicator of α-tocopheral deficiency in two equine neurodegenerative disorders. Acta Neuropathol 90, 266–272.

Dabbagh, A.J., Mannion, T., Lynch, S.M., et al., 1994. The effect of iron overload on rat plasma and liver oxidant status *in vivo*. Biochem J 300, 799–803.

DeLaRuaDomenech, R., Mohammed, H.O., Atwill, E.R., et al., 1995a. Epidemiologic evidence for clustering of equine motor neuron disease in the United States. Am J Vet Res 56, 1433–1439.

DeLaRuaDomenech, R., Mohammed, H.O., Cummings, J.F., et al., 1995b. Incidence and risk factors of equine motor-neuron disease – an ambidirectional study. Neuroepidemiol 14, 54–64.

DeLaRuaDomenech, R., Mohammed, H.O., Cummings, J.F., et al., 1997a. Association between plasma vitamin E concentration and the risk of equine motor neuron disease. Vet J 154, 203–213.

DeLaRuaDomenech, R., Mohammed, H.O., Cummings, J.F., et al., 1997b. Intrinsic, management, and nutritional factors associated with equine motor neuron disease. J Am Vet Med Assoc 211, 1261–1267.

Dill, S.G., Hintz, H.F., deLahunta, A., et al., 1989a. Plasma and liver copper values in horses with equine degenerative encephalomyelopathy. Can J Vet Res 53, 29–32.

Dill, S.G., Kallfelz, F.A., deLahunta, A., et al., 1989b. Serum vitamin E and blood glutathione peroxidase values in horses with degenerative encephalomyelopathy. Am J Vet Res 50, 166–168.

Dill, S.G., Correa, M.T., Erb, H.N., et al., 1990. Factors associated with the development of equine degenerative encephalomyelopathy. Am J Vet Res 51, 1300–1305.

Divers, T.J., Bartholemew, R.C., Messick, J.B., et al., 1986. *Clostridium botulinum* type B toxicosis in a herd of cattle and a group of mules. JAVMA 188, 382–386.

Divers, T.J., Mohammed, H.O., Cummings, J.F., et al., 1994. Equine motor neuron disease – findings in 28 horses and proposal of a pathophysiological mechanism for the disease. Equine Vet J 26, 409–415.

Divers, T.J., de Lahunta, A., Hintz, H.F., et al., 2001. Equine motor neuron disease. Equine Vet Educ 13, 63–67.

Divers, T.J., de Lahunta, A., Hintz, H.F., et al., 2002. Equine motor neuron disease – update. Proceedings of the 20th Amer Coll Vet Internal Med, pp. 202–203.

Divers, T.J., Mohammed, H.O., 2009. Equine motor neuron disease. In: Robinson, N.E., Sprayberry, K.A. (Eds.), Current Therapy in Equine Medicine 6. Ch 133. Elsevier, St. Louis, pp. 615–617.

Doxey, D.L., Gilmour, J.S., Milne, E.M., 1991a. The relationship between meteorological features and equine grass sickness (dysautonomia). Equine Vet J 23, 370–373.

Doxey, D.L., Gilmour, J.S., Milne, E.M., 1991b. A comparative study of normal equine populations and those with grass sickness (dysautonomia) in eastern Scotland. Equine Vet J 23, 365–369.

Doxey, D.L., Milne, E.M., Harter, A., 1995a. A recovery of horses from dysautonomia (grass sickness). Vet Rec 137, 585–588.

Doxey, D.L., Tothill, S., Milne, E.M., et al., 1995b. Patterns of feeding and behaviour in horses recovering from dysautonomia (Grass sickness). Vet Rec 137, 181–183.

Fenicia, L., Da Dalt, L., Anniballi, F., 2002. A case of infant botulism due to neurotoxigenic *Clostridium butyricum* type E associated with *Clostridium difficile* colitis. Eur J Clin Microbiol 21, 736–738.

Fintl, C., McGorum, B.C., 2002. Evaluation of three ancillary treatments in the management of equine grass sickness. Vet Rec 151, 381–383.

Forsyth, A.A., 1941. Grass disease in a coalmine. Vet J 97, 26–28.

French, N.P., McCarthy, H.E., Diggle, P.J., et al., 2005. Clustering of equine grass sickness cases in the United Kingdom: a study considering the effect of position-dependent reporting on the space-time K-function. Epidemiol Infect 133, 343–348.

Gilmour, J.S., Brown, R., Johnson, P., 1981. A negative serological relationship between cases of grass sickness in Scotland and *Clostridium perfringens* type A enterotoxin. Equine Vet J 13, 56–58.

Gilmour, J.S., Jolly, G.M., 1974. Some aspects of the epidemiology of equine grass sickness. Vet Rec 95, 77–81.

Gordon, A., 1934. Enterotoxaemia in herbivorous animals – its possible bearing on grass sickness in horses. The Veterinary Record 14, 1016–1036.

Greig, J.R., 1942. Grass sickness in horses, a review of the present knowledge of the disease with particular reference to the nature of the causal agent. Trans Highland Agric Soc Scot 54, 1–27.

Guthrie, W.J., 1940. Grass sickness in horses. J Royal Agric Soc 100, 50–59.

Haagsma, J., Haesebrouck, F., Devriese, L., et al., 1990. An outbreak of botulism type B in horses. Vet Rec 127, 206.

Heath, S.E., Bell, R.J., Chrino-Trejo, M., 1990. Feed-trough dirt as a source of *C. botulinum* type C intoxication in a group of farm horses. Can Vet J 31, 13–19.

Hijova, E., Nistiar, F., Kuchta, M., 2004. Influence of acute cadmium exposure on plasma antioxidant parameters in rats. Bul Vet Inst Pulawy 48, 155–157.

Hintz, H.F., 1992. Nutritional requirements. In: Robinson, N.E. (Ed.), Current Therapy in Equine Medicine. WB Saunders Co, Philadelphia, pp. 715–716.

Hintz, H.F., 1994. Nutrition and equine performance. J Nutr 124, 2723S–2729S.

Hunter, J.M., Rohrbach, B.W., Andrews, F.M., et al., 2002. Round bale grass hay: a risk factor for botulism in horses. Compend Cont Educ (Pract Vet) 24, 166–169.

Hunter, L.C., Poxton, I.R., 2001. Systemic antibodies to *Clostridium botulinum* type C: do they protect horses from grass sickness (dysautonomia)? Equine Vet J 33, 547–553.

Husebye, E., 2005. The pathogenesis of gastrointestinal bacterial overgrowth. Chemotherapy 51, 1–22.

Jackson, C.A., de Lahunta, A., Cummings, J.F., et al., 1996. Spinal accessory nerve biopsy as an ante mortem diagnostic test for equine motor neuron disease. Equine Vet J 28, 215–219.

Kinde, H., Bettey, R.L., Ardans, A., et al., 1991. *Clostridium botulinum* type-C intoxication associated with consumption of processed alfalfa hay cubes in horses. JAVMA 199, 742–746.

Lannek, N., Lindberg, P., Persson, F., et al., 1961. A grass disease enzootic in stable-fed horses with an investigation of the aetiological role of the food. Vet Rec 73, 601–603.

Lewis, C.A., Bozynski, C.C., Johnson, G.C., et al., 2009. Colonic impaction due to dysautonomia in an alpaca. J Vet Int Med 23, 1117–1122.

Machlin, L.J., 1984. Handbook of Vitamins: Nutritional, biochemical and clinical aspects. Marcel Dekker, New York. pp. 129

Mayhew, I.G., Stowe, H.D., Derksen, F.J., et al., 1987. Equine degenerative myeloencephalopathy – a vitamin E deficiency that may be familial. J Vet Internal Med 1, 45–50.

Mayhew, I.G., 2008. Nutritional diseases. In: Mayhew, I.G. (Ed.), Large Animal Neurology, second ed. John Wiley & Sons, Chichester, pp. 360–373.

McCarthy, H.E., French, N.P., Edwards, G.B., et al., 2004. Why are certain premises at increased risk of equine grass sickness? A matched case-control study. Equine Vet J 36, 130–134.

McGorum, B.C., 2003. Diffuse skeletal muscle weakness. In: Robinson, N.E. (Ed.), Current Therapy in Equine Medicine 5. WB Saunders, London, Chapter 14.2, pp. 740–745.

McGorum, B.C., Anderson, R.A., 2002. Bio-markers of cyanide exposure in horses with grass sickness. Vet Rec 151, 442–445.

McGorum, B.C., Kirk, J., 2001. Equine dysautonomia (grass sickness) is associated with alterations in plasma amino acid concentrations, and depletion in plasma sulphur amino acids. Equine Vet J 33, 473–477.

McGorum, B.C., Pirie, R.S., 2009. Equine grass sickness. In: Robinson, N.E. (Ed.), Current Therapy in Equine Medicine 6. Saunders Elsevier, St Louis, Chapter 81, pp. 361–365.

McGorum, B.C., Fry, S.C., Wallace, G.W., et al., 2000. Properties of herbage in relation to equine dysautonomia: biochemical composition, antioxidant and prooxidant actions. J Agric Food Chem 48, 2346–2352.

McGorum, B.C., Wilson, R., Pirie, R.S., et al., 2003. Systemic concentrations of antioxidants and biomarkers of macromolecular oxidative damage in horses with grass sickness. Equine Vet J 35, 121–126.

McGorum, B.C., Mayhew, I.G., Amory, H., et al., 2006. Horses on pasture may be affected by equine motor neuron disease. Equine Vet J 38, 47–51.

McGorum, B.C., Milne, E.M., Pirie, R.S., et al., 2009. Management of chronic grass sickness horses. E-booklet (http://www.worldhorsewelfare.org/information/press-releases)

Milne, E.M., 1996. Clinical diagnosis and management of acute and sub-acute grass sickness. Equine Vet Educ 8, 71–73.

Milne, E.M., Doxey, D.L., Gilmour, J.S., 1990. Serum-lipids and lipoproteins in equine colic and grass sickness. Res Vet Sci 48, 170–174.

Milne, E.M., Doxey, D.L., Woodman, M.P., et al., 1996. An evaluation of the use of cisapride in horses with chronic grass sickness (equine dysautonomia). Br Vet J 152, 537–549.

Mitchell, C.A., Walker, R.V.L., McKercher, D.G., 1939. Isolation of *Cl. botulinum* from oat grain. Can J Comp Med 3, 245–247.

Mitscherlich, E., Marth, E.H., 1984. Microbial survival in the environment. Springer, Berlin, pp. 91–113.

Mohammed, H.O., Cummings, J.F., Divers, T.J., et al., 1994. Epidemiology of equine motor-neuron disease. Vet Res 25, 275–278.

Muller, J., 1963. Equine and bovine botulism in Denmark. Bull Off Int Epizoot 59, 1374.

Nairn, W., 1922. Grass disease in the horse. Vet Rec 450–456.

Newton, J.R., Hedderson, E., Adams, V.J., et al., 2004. An epidemiological study of risk factors associated with the recurrence of equine grass sickness (dysautonomia) on previously affected premises. Equine Vet J 36, 105–112.

Ochoa, R., Velandia, S.D., 1978. Equine grass sickness, serological evidence of association with *Clostridium perfringens* type A enterotoxin. Am J Vet Res 39, 1049–1051.

Pirie, R.S., 2006. Grass sickness. Clin Tech Eq Prac 5, 30–36.

Polack, E.W., King, J.M., Cummings, J.F., et al., 2000. Concentrations of trace minerals in the spinal cord of horses with equine motor neuron disease. Am J Vet Res 61, 609–611.

Pool, W.A., 1928. Grass disease in horses. Vet Rec 8, 23–34.

Pruden, S.J., McAllister, M.M., Schultheiss, P.C., et al., 2004. Abomasal emptying defect of sheep may be an acquired form of dysautonomia. Vet Pathol 41, 164–169.

Ricketts, S.W., Greet, T.R., Glyn, P.J., et al., 1984. Thirteen cases of botulism in horses fed big bale silage. Equine Vet J 16, 515–518.

Riis, R.C., Jackson, C., Rebhun, W., et al., 1999. Ocular manifestations of equine motor neuron disease. Equine Vet J 31, 90–91.

Robb, J., Doxey, D., Milne, E.M., et al., 1997. The isolation of potentially toxigenic fungi from the environment of horses with grass sickness and mal seco. In: Hahn, C., Gerber, V., Herholz C., et al. (Eds.), Proceedings of 1st International Workshop on grass sickness, EMND and related disorders. Bern, Switzerland 26–27 October 1995, pp. 52–54

Saly, J., Baranova, D., Pesek, L., et al., 2004. Effect of lead on health and productivity of layers. Bull Vet Inst Pullawy 48, 75–80.

Satya-Murti, S., Howard, L., Krohel, G., et al., 1986. The spectrum of neurologic disorder from vitamin E deficiency. Neurology 36, 917–921.

Schoenbaum, M.A., Hall, S.M., Glock, R.D., et al., 2000. An outbreak of type C botulism in 12 horses and a mule. J Am Vet Med Assoc 217, 365–368.

Smith, L.D.S., Sugiyama, H., 1988. Botulism: The organism, its toxins, the disease, second ed. Thomas Books, Springfield, IL,

Sojka, J.E., Hope, W., Pearson, D., 1996. Lead toxicosis in 2 horses: Similarity to equine degenerative lower motor neuron disease. J Vet Int Med 10, 420–423.

Stewart, J., Gordon, W.S., McCallum, J.W., 1940. Grass sickness in horses – biochemical investigation. Vet Rec 52, 237–243.

Stringer, S.C., Haque, N., Peck, M.W., 1999. Growth from spores of nonproteolytic *Clostridium botulinum* in heat-treated vegetable juice. Appl Environ Microb 65, 2136–2142.

Swerczek, T.W., 1980a. Experimentally induced toxico-infectious botulism in horses and foals. Am J Vet Res 41, 348–350.

Swerczek, T.W., 1980b. Toxico-infectious botulism in foals and adult horses. JAVMA 176, 217–220.

Symonds, H.W., Thompson, H., Nash, A., et al., 1995. A cluster of cases of feline dysautonomia (Key-Gaskell syndrome) in a closed colony of cats. Vet Rec 136, 353–355.

Tocher, J.F., Tocher, J.W., Brown, W., et al., 1923. Grass sickness investigation report. Vet Rec 3, 37–45, 75–89.

Valentine, B.A., Divers, T.J., Murphy, D.J., et al., 1998. Muscle biopsy diagnosis of equine motor neuron disease and equine polysaccharide storage myopathy. Equine Vet Educ 10, 42–50.

Wang, Y., Sugiyama, H., 1984. Botulism in metronidazole-treated conventional adult mice challenged orogastrically with spores of *Clostridium botulinum* type A or B. Infect Immun 46, 715–719.

Weese, J.S., 2009. Clostridial diseases. In: Robinson, N.E. (Ed.), Current Therapy in Equine Medicine 6. Saunders Elsevier, St Louis, pp. 158–166

Whitlock, R.H., 2009. Botulism (shaker foal; forage poisoning). In: Smith, B.P. (Ed.), Large Animal Internal Medicine, fourth ed. Mosby, St Louis, pp. 1096–1101.

Whitlock, R.H., Buckley, C.A., 1997. Botulism. Vet Clin North Am 13, 107.

Whitlock, R.H., Sandigo, E.J., 1997. Type C botulism in New Mexico horses: an outbreak. In: Trock, S.C., et al. (Eds.), Proceedings 40th Annu Meet Am Assoc Vet Lab Diagn, pp. 61.

Whitwell, K., 1997. Histopathology of grass sickness – comparative aspects of dysautonomia in various species (equine, feline, canine, leporids). In: Hahn, C., Gerber, V., Herholtz, C., et al. (Eds.), Grass Sickness, Equine Motor Neurone Disease and Related Disorders. Equine Veterinary Journal Limited, Newmarket, UK, pp. 52–54.

Wichtel, J.J., Whitlock, R.H., 1991. Botulism associated with feeding alfalfa hay to horses. J Am Vet Med Assoc 199, 471–472.

Wood, J.L.N., Milne, E.M., Doxey, D.L., 1998. A case control study of grass sickness (equine dysautonomia) in the United Kingdom. Vet J 156, 7–14.

Wood, J.L.N., McGorum, B.C., Mayhew, I.G., 1999. Equine dysautonomia: has grass been blamed unfairly all this time? Equine Vet J 31, 451–452.

Wright, A., Beard, L., Bawa, B., et al., 2010. Dysautonomia in a six-year old mule in the United States. Equine Vet J 42, 170–173.

39

Feeding management pre- and post-surgery

Tim Mair

Introduction

General anesthesia in the horse has a much higher mortality and morbidity than most other species. The confidential enquiry into perioperative equine fatalities (CEPEF) (Johnston et al 1998, 2002) recorded a mortality rate of 1.6%, which decreased to 0.9% when anesthesia for colic surgery and obstetrical procedures was excluded. Another study of mortality during elective procedures from a single center recorded a death rate of 0.063% (Mee et al 1998), and a more recent study from one large veterinary hospital in Kentucky recorded a rate of fatalities directly related to anesthesia of 0.12%, rising to 0.24% with the inclusion of horses killed or dying within 7 days post general anesthesia (Bidwell et al 2007). Sick and shocked horses that require emergency surgery (primarily horses affected by colic) carry a higher mortality rate (1.9%) (Johnston et al 2002). Mee et al (1998) found that mortality associated with general anesthesia was 4.25 times more likely for emergency procedures not associated with colic than for similar procedures carried out electively; emergency general anesthesia for colic carried an increased risk of mortality of 9.86 times that of elective cases. In another study, pre-operative and anesthesia-related variables associated with intra- and postoperative mortality were assessed in 774 surgical colic cases; cardiovascular compromise, level of pain, age, and breed were all shown to be associated with the risk of mortality (Proudman et al 2006). Various metabolic and endocrine changes occur during anesthesia and surgery in horses, and these may have profound, albeit temporary, effects on the nutritional status of the horse. Feeding practices around the time of surgery, and the underlying disease status of the horse, will also have important implications to the metabolic condition.

Hormonal and metabolic changes associated with general anesthesia and surgery

Horses develop a stress response to anesthesia and surgery, which results in numerous endocrine, humoral and metabolic changes designed to restore or maintain homeostasis (Wagner 2009). Among other effects, the stress response results in the activation of the adrenocortical system, redistribution of blood flow, mobilization of substrates such as glucose and free fatty acids, and activation of the immune system (Muir 1990). The interaction between nutritional status and feeding practices with the stress response in horses undergoing surgery and anesthesia has received little attention, but is likely to be significant.

The degree of stress imposed by anesthesia and surgery is difficult to quantify. Traditional approaches include measuring physiological parameters such as heart rate and plasma cortisol concentrations. In humans, anesthesia without surgery does not produce a stress response, but surgery does, and the magnitude of the cortisol response varies with the severity of the surgical procedure (Traynor & Hall 1981). In contrast, inhalation anesthesia alone in normal horses is associated with a marked increase in plasma cortisol (Taylor 1985, 1998, Luna & Taylor 1995, 2001, Robertson et al 1996, Luna et al 1997, 1999). Relatively benign surgical procedures in horses, such as arthroscopic surgery, produce only minor and short-lived further increases in cortisol (Robertson et al 1990). Horses affected by serious intestinal diseases causing colic have pre-existing hypercortisolemia (Hoffsis & Murdick 1970, Hodson et al 1986, Santschi et al 1991, Hinchcliff et al 2005, Edner et al 2007, Sherlock & Mair 2008). Although abdominal surgery is also known to cause increases in serum cortisol levels (Taylor 1985, Stegmann & Jones 1998), the surgery itself causes only slight increases in the stress response above that already induced by the disease and anesthesia.

The cortisol reaction contributes to a variety of protective responses (Zaloga & Marik 2001, Wagner 2009) including: (i) maintenance of blood pressure by increasing the synthesis of catecholamines, sensitizing smooth muscle cells to the effects of catecholamines, and by inhibiting vasodilation by decreasing nitric oxide synthesis; (ii) increasing the provision of nutrients through stimulating hepatic gluconeogenesis and decreasing peripheral utilization of glucose (which result in hyperglycemia), increasing protein catabolism and decreasing protein synthesis, and promoting lipolysis; and (iii) prevention of an excessive inflammatory reaction in response to injury by stabilizing lysosomal membranes, decreasing capillary permeability and by altering the expression of pro- and anti-inflammatory cytokines. Glucocorticoids also stimulate tissue cells to produce lipocortins (peptide hormones that interact with the immune system to decrease production of prostaglandins, thromboxanes and leukotrienes) and decrease the migration of inflammatory cells into tissues (Muir 1990). The long-term effects of increased circulating cortisol levels for prolonged periods of time can include delayed wound healing, muscle wasting, immune deficiencies, and increased susceptibility to infection. Lipocortin also inhibits prostaglandin production in the gastrointestinal tract, which might promote gastrointestinal ulceration (Breazile 1987).

In addition to a cortisol response, anesthesia and surgery result in other endocrine and metabolic responses, including increases in circulating catecholamines (Robertson 1987, Wagner et al 1990) and changes in insulin and glucose levels. The pre-anesthetic and anesthetic induction drugs can also affect insulin responses and glucose metabolism (Robertson 1987). Alpha-2-adrenergic agents (such as xylazine) can inhibit insulin release by stimulating alpha-2-adrenoceptors in pancreatic beta cells, thereby resulting in hyperglycemia (Thurmon et al 1982). Feed intake pre- and post-surgery will also affect the insulin response, with fasting resulting in a suppression of the insulin response, and refeeding enhancing insulin release (Robertson 1987, Taylor 1989, Robertson et al 1990). Surgery in humans generally causes hyperglycemia (Clarke 1973), but in horses this response appears to be more variable, and some anesthetic drugs may actually result in hypoglycemia (Robertson 1987, Taylor 1989, Robertson et al 1990).

Plasma concentrations of non-esterified fatty acids are also affected by stress and surgery. Increased sympathetic activity associated with pain or fear will cause lipolysis and an increase in non-esterified fatty acid concentration (Snow 1979), but decreased sympathetic activity associated with sedation and anesthesia may have the opposite effect. The insulin response will also affect nonesterified fatty acid concentration because insulin is antilipolytic; suppression of insulin therefore tends to cause an increase in nonesterified fatty acid concentration. Preoperative fasting is also likely to increase nonesterified fatty acid concentration, but this may fall once the horse is sedated, and in the immediate postoperative period the concentration may be normal or low (Robertson 1987, Robertson et al 1990).

As in humans, the stress response in horses to anesthesia and surgery is temporary and is unlikely to be clinically relevant in healthy individuals undergoing surgical treatment. However, severely malnourished humans suffer more serious complications following abdominal and thoracic surgery, and preoperative total parenteral nutrition may be beneficial in these patients (Veterans Affairs Total Parenteral Nutrition Cooperative Study Group 1991). The significance of the stress response to anesthesia and surgery in malnourished horses has received little attention.

Perioperative glucose regulation and control

Development of hyperglycemia in humans after major surgery is common and is modulated by many factors. These include perioperative metabolic state, intraoperative management of the patient, and neuroendocrine stress response to surgery. Acute insulin resistance also develops

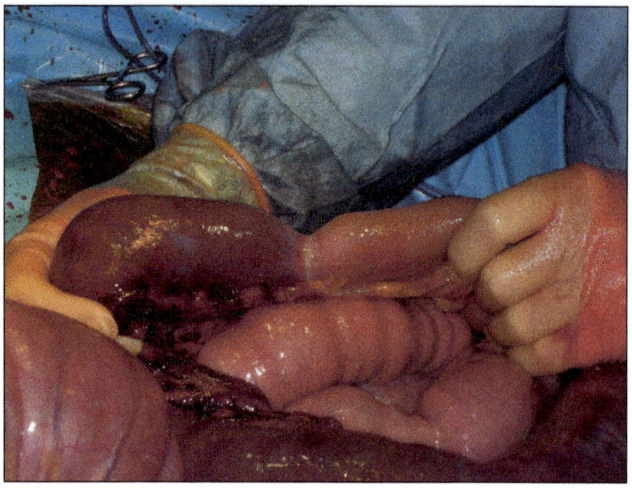

Figure 39.1 Intraoperative view of small intestinal strangulation (the intestine to the left is strangulated).

perioperatively and contributes significantly to hyperglycemia, which is associated with poor outcomes in critically ill post-surgical patients (Bochicchio et al 2005a, b). Many studies have shown that intensive insulin therapy can combat insulin resistance, decrease blood glucose levels, and induce anabolic processes, thus, decreasing morbidity and mortality. Initial studies in humans demonstrated improved outcomes in critically ill, postsurgical patients who received intensive glycemic control (IGC) including insulin therapy. These results were quickly extrapolated to other clinical areas, and IGC was enthusiastically recommended in the perioperative period. However, recent prospective trials have not been able to show the benefit of IGC (Finfer et al 2009); neither an appropriate therapeutic glycemic target nor the true efficacy of perioperative glycemic control has been fully determined. IGC also increases the risk of hypoglycemia significantly, which is not inconsequential in critically ill patients (Akhtar et al 2010).

The use of insulin therapy in critically ill horses and horses after surgery has received relatively little attention. Endotoxemia and the systemic inflammatory response syndrome are frequent consequences of many gastrointestinal diseases (including strangulating obstructions and colitis) (Fig. 39.1) in horses (Bryant & Moore 2008). Endotoxin has been shown to decrease insulin sensitivity in horses (Toth et al 2008). The pathophysiology and systemic manifestations of endotoxemia in horses and sepsis in humans are very similar and the maintenance of normoglycemia with the use of insulin in endotoxemic horses may contribute to a significant reduction in morbidity and mortality. With the use of controlled delivery pumps and regular blood glucose monitoring, maintenance of normoglycemia with a constant rate infusion of insulin is an achievable goal in equine critical care, especially in neonates (Sykes & Furr 2005). In adult horses with acute colic, hyperglycemia has been found to be common, and severe hyperglycemia has been shown to be associated with a worse prognosis for survival (Hollis et al 2007, Hassel et al 2009); these observations suggest that glycemic control in adult horses during and after colic surgery may also warrant investigation.

Key Points

- Anesthesia and surgery can induce several metabolic and endocrine alterations, including increases in circulating cortisol and catecholamines, hyperglycemia and insulin resistance
- This stress response is temporary and unlikely to be clinically relevant in healthy animals undergoing surgical treatment but may exacerbate disturbances in horses with critical illness such as surgical colic. Additionally, poor nutritional status at the time of surgery may impact the extent of endocrine and metabolic derangements due to surgery and anesthesia.

Feeding management pre-surgery

Most authors recommend withholding food but not water for 6 to 12 hours prior to inducing general anesthesia (Taylor & Clarke 2007, Robertson & Scicluna 2009). The justification for preoperative starvation is that it reduces gut content and increases the functional residual capacity of the lung. This may help oxygenation, but the beneficial effect is probably very limited, as it is impossible to empty the gastrointestinal tract completely. Starvation beyond 12 to 18 hours is likely to induce significant stress and metabolic derangements.

Relatively short periods of perioperative fasting can have significant effects on the metabolic status of systemically healthy horses. However, the effects on physiological functions are minor. Reinprecht et al (2007) studied the metabolic and clinical effects of feed deprivation in 20 horses subjected to orthopedic surgery. The patients were fasted from 12 hours before until 4 hours after surgery. Plasma glucose and free fatty acids increased after surgery and returned to pre-operative levels 72 hours after surgery. A significant rise in segmented granulocytes occurred 24 hours after surgery. Serum aspartate amino transferase (AST) reached its highest activity 24 hours after surgery, whereas creatine kinase (CK) activities were highest at 2 hours after surgery. Abdominal sounds were significantly reduced until 24 hours after surgery, although appetite was not depressed.

Although the metabolic and clinical effects of preoperative starvation in systemically healthy horses are short-lived and unlikely to be clinically significant, horses affected by acute abdominal disease requiring surgery (i.e., surgical colic) are compromised due to the disease, often starved for long periods of time and sometimes exposed to the stress of long trailer rides. Edner et al (2007) studied some metabolic parameters in 20 healthy horses given anesthesia alone and 20 horses undergoing abdominal surgery for colic, and found that the post-anesthetic period was associated with increased lipolysis and weight loss in the horses with colic. Plasma cortisol, free fatty acids, glycerol, glucose, lactate and creatine kinase (CK) were elevated and serum phosphate and potassium were lower in colic horses before anesthesia. Anesthesia and surgery resulted in a decrease in plasma free fatty acids and glycerol in colic horses whereas levels increased in healthy horses. During anesthesia plasma lactate and phosphate both increased in both groups. In the colic horses, plasma lactate continued to rise after surgery. Plasma free fatty acids and glycerol increased for 8 hours after standing in the colic horses. In both groups serum CK increased and phosphate decreased after anesthesia. By day 7 after anesthesia most parameters were similar in both groups. However, colic horse lost on average 8% of their initial body weight. These results suggest that the colic horses were in a negative energy balance for the first week after surgery.

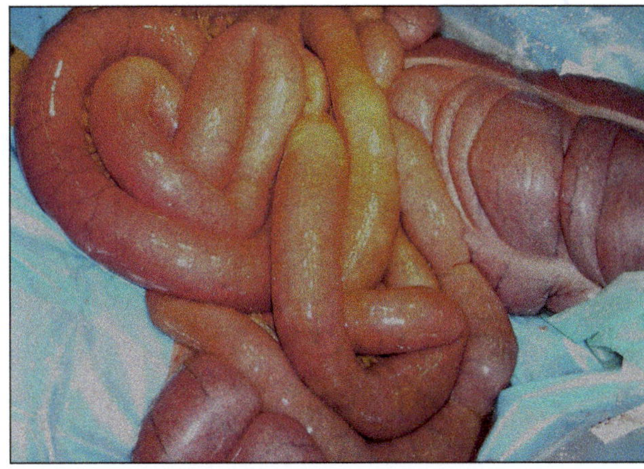

Figure 39.2 **Intraoperative view showing diffusely distended small intestine due to postoperative ileus.**

Postoperative colic and ileus

Postoperative ileus (the failure of effective aboral propulsion of gastrointestinal tract contents) (Fig. 39.2) is a well-recognized clinical entity in horses (Becht & Richardson 1981, Adams 1988, Little et al 2001, Senior et al 2004). Postoperative ileus affecting the stomach and small intestine is manifested as pain, toxemia and gastric reflux, and is a major postoperative complication following colic surgery, especially surgery involving ischemic damage to the small intestine (Edwards & Hunt 1985, Hunt et al 1986, MacDonald et al 1989, Van der Velden & Klein 1993, Proudman et al 2002, Blikslager et al 1994, Freeman et al 2000, Cohen et al 2004, Mair & Smith 2005, Garcia-Seco et al 2005). Mortality rates between 13 and 86% have been reported for this condition (Hunt et al 1986, Blikslager et al 1994), and the condition is also associated with increased duration of hospital stay and increased costs to owners (French et al 2002). The etiology and pathogenesis of postoperative ileus following intestinal surgery are unclear, although current theories suggest that intestinal inflammation associated with the primary disease, intestinal distension and surgical trauma to the small intestine is likely an important factor (Koenig & Cote 2005, Doherty 2009).

Postoperative colic unassociated with colic surgery or other types of abdominal surgery is recognized as a clinical problem in horses. For example, Mircica et al (2003) reported that five of 84 horses showed signs of "gastrointestinal discomfort" following nonabdominal surgery, an incidence of nearly 6%. The majority of postanesthetic colic cases occur within 72 hours of anesthesia (Senior et al 2004). There are several possible causes; recent changes in management (including recent transport, changes to exercise routine and dietary changes) are recognized as important risk factors for many types of naturally-occurring colic (Tinkler et al 1997, Cohen et al 1999, Hillyer et al 2002), and similar factors are probably associated with post-operative colic. Sympathetic nervous activity involving the release of endogenous catecholamines increases as part of the perioperative nocifensive and stress responses to surgery (Weismann 1990). These and exogenous catecholamines decrease gut motility in man (Steinbrook 1998). One study demonstrated an increased prevalence of postanesthetic colic in horses undergoing surgery compared to those anesthetized for noninvasive procedures (i.e., magnetic resonance imaging) (Andersen et al 2006).

In humans, postoperative ileus is known to affect all parts of the gastrointestinal tract after surgery, but different segments are not equally susceptible (Woods et al 1978, Livingston & Passaro 1990). Motility of the large intestine of horses may also be adversely affected by general anesthesia (Gerring 1992). General anesthesia depresses gut motility and the development of post-operative colic is not considered unusual (Taylor & Clarke 2007). This may vary from transient mild discomfort to more severe colic and impaction of segments of the large intestine. Development of impaction of the large colon has been associated with several factors, including stall confinement after musculoskeletal injury and hospitalization for reasons other than gastrointestinal tract disease. In one study, 19 of 147 horses with impaction of the large colon had undergone general anesthesia and arthroscopy prior to developing impaction (Dabareiner & White 1995). Cecal impaction has also been associated with hospitalization, surgery and the administration of anesthetic agents (Ross et al 1985, Collatos & Ronano 1992). Anesthetic and analgesic drugs may have marked depressant effects on gut motility, and may be important factors in the development of these conditions. Starvation depresses gut motility and may also predispose to impaction and other forms of colic. For example, starvation for 18 hours and the use of a muzzle preoperatively was blamed as the likely cause of colic in six horses after non-abdominal surgery (Jones et al 1991).

There appear to be very few published studies that have evaluated factors affecting postoperative fecal production in horses, and the effects of pre- and postoperative feeding practices on return of bowel function after anesthesia remain largely unknown. Little et al (2001) found that reduced fecal output following surgery unrelated to the gastrointestinal tract (defined as ≤ 3 defecations per 24-hour period after surgery) was associated with age ≥5 years old, orthopedic procedures of >60 minutes' duration and no phenylbutazone therapy after surgery. 12% of the total number of horses in the study developed postoperative colic, all of which demonstrated reduced fecal output. These results support the view that colic can occur as a complication of surgery for problems that do not involve the gastrointestinal tract and suggest that there is an intermediate clinical phase manifested as reduced fecal output before overt signs of colic are seen.

An increased risk of post-operative colic may also occur with the use of opioids in the anesthetic protocol, although the results of several retrospective studies have conflicted: Mircica et al (2003) did not find an association whereas Senior et al (2004) did show that morphine was a risk factor for postanesthetic colic. Senior et al (2004) reviewed the records of 496 orthopedic operations on 428 horses to estimate the prevalence of, and identify the risk factors for, the development of colic in horses after surgery. Fourteen of the horses developed colic; eight of them were undiagnosed, three were classified as impactions, one as tympanic colic of the colon, one as incarceration of the small intestine in the epiploic foramen, and one as left dorsal displacement of the colon in the nephrosplenic space. Morphine was associated with a fourfold increased risk of colic compared with the use of no opioid or butorphanol, and out-of-hours surgery was also associated with an increased risk. This association between the use of morphine and postoperative colic probably results from opioid-suppression of normal gut motility. Morphine is mainly a μ-agonist (Branson & Gross 2001), and it has been shown that μ-receptor agonists can decrease the propulsive motility and cause sphincter closure in the gastrointestinal tract (Sojka et al 1988, Roger et al 1994). Postoperative colic is most likely to occur with higher doses, and probably prolonged systemic administration.

In addition to anesthetic and analgesic drugs, other factors such as preoperative starvation and the administration of other drugs around the time of surgery are likely to be important in the etiopathogenesis of postoperative colic (Taylor & Clarke 2007). A multicenter prospective case-control study of post anesthetic colic was reported by Senior et al (2006). The estimated mean prevalence of colic in the study population was 5.2%; however the prevalence varied between each of the four participating centers. The most commonly diagnosed cause of colic was large intestinal impaction. Multivariable analyses showed that the center involved and the type of surgery performed were associated with an increased risk of postanesthetic colic. Preoperative food deprivation and the use of opioid drugs were confounding factors.

Key Points

- Postoperative ileus is a major complication following colic surgery, especially when there has been ischemic damage to the small intestine
- Postoperative colic not associated with colic surgery or other types of abdominal surgery also occurs in horses. The severity of colic may vary from transient mild discomfort to impaction of segments of the large intestine
- Anaesthetic and analgesic drugs depress gut motility, and may be important factors in the development of these postoperative complications
- There is very little information on the impact of feeding practices pre- and/or post-surgery on risk for development of postoperative complications

Postoperative feeding management

There appears to be a wide variation in opinion between different surgeons and hospitals with respect to the timing of reintroduction of feed postoperatively. Most horses undergoing nonabdominal surgery or simple intestinal surgery (such as management of intestinal displacements without enterotomy) will recommence partial enteral feeding within 6 to 12 hours of recovery from anesthesia (Spier & Meagher 1989, Durham 2005, White 2009). However, following small intestinal resection and anastomosis (Fig. 39.3), horses are frequently starved for longer lengths of time. In one study of surgical colic cases, postoperative feed withdrawal for more that 10 days was reported in some cases (Cohen et al 2004) and in another study of 30 horses subjected to small intestinal resection and anastomosis, feed

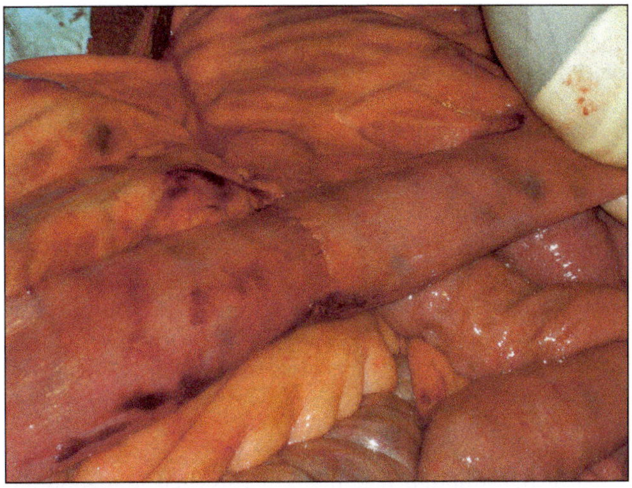

Figure 39.3 End-to-end small intestinal anastomosis (intraoperative view).

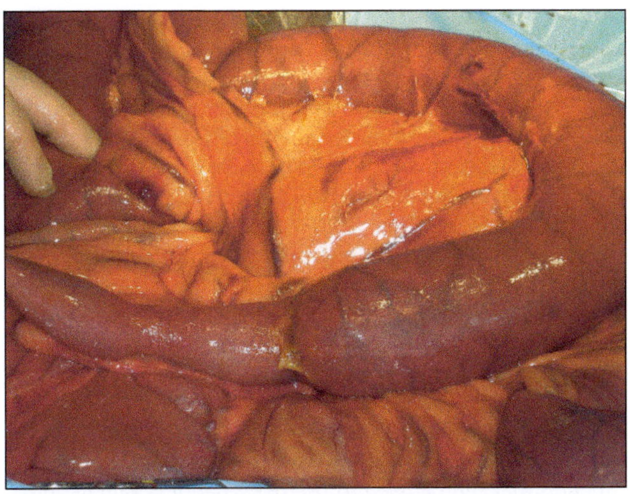

Figure 39.4 Impaction of food at an end-to-end small intestinal anastomosis (intraoperative view).

was withheld for a mean duration of 76 hours (range 48 to 91 hours) (Durham et al 2003). The rationale for starving horses after small intestinal surgery is to protect the anastomosis, allowing it time to heal before being stressed by food, and to prevent intestinal impaction (Fig. 39.4) and ileus. However enteral feeding is crucial to the maintenance of the gastro-intestinal mucosa (Ralston 2002), and in human research there is no evidence that bowel rest and a period of starvation are beneficial for healing of wounds and anastomotic integrity (Silk & Menzies Gow 2001). Indeed, it has been shown that early feeding has beneficial effects with regard to enterocyte function, wound healing, anastomotic strength and gastro-intestinal motility (Haydock & Hill 1986, Schroeder et al 1991).

Several studies have demonstrated biochemical evidence of negative energy balance (including increased serum triglyceride concentrations) in horses following routine starvation after colic surgery (Milne et al 1990, Protopapas 2000, Edner et al 2007). Nutritional deprivation has been shown to cause deleterious effects on gastrointestinal permeability, morphology and function in numerous species (Hughes & Dowling 1980, van der Hulst et al 1998, MacFie 2000). Starvation causes a reduced metabolic rate via a number of mechanisms, including a reduction in circulating insulin which in turn reduces the conversion of thyroxine (T_4) to triiodothyronine (T_3). This is a protective process as reducing the metabolic rate conserves energy, thereby prolonging life. However, other effects of starvation are more detrimental; they include depression of the immune system, decreased synthesis of proteins such as albumin, atrophy of intestinal villi and reduction of digestive enzyme activity. In addition, muscle atrophy and weakness occur due to the breakdown of protein as an energy source. Starvation as a consequence of illness will therefore delay healing, increase the risk of infection, reduce the effectiveness of antibiotic therapies and cause weakness and lethargy. Following colic surgery this could lead to an increased risk of adhesions and wound complications, an increase in the length of hospitalization and reduced postoperative survival (Ralston 2002).

At present the nutritional requirements of horses following colic surgery are largely unknown. During the immediate postoperative period, a 15–20% reduction in energy demand for digestion is likely (Geor 2007). The basal energy requirement for stall-confined horses is estimated to be approximately 100 kJ/kg/day, which represents approximately 70% of the maintenance requirement at pasture (Pagan & Hintz 1986, White 2009), but this will be balanced by increased energy demands caused by stress of the disease and surgery (Durham et al 2004). An estimated energy requirement during the initial post-operative period of approximately 100 kJ/kg/day digestible energy (DE) has been suggested (Durham 2005). As feeding and exercise are increased in the later postoperative period, so the energy demands will increase, but these will be mitigated by the reducing metabolic consequences of the surgery and the primary disease. When the horse is allowed access to pasture (usually at around 8 weeks after surgery), the daily energy requirements are likely to be similar to the estimated field maintenance requirement of normal horses (approximately 140–150 kJ/kg/day) (Durham 2005). A protein requirement of 1 g crude protein per 100–200 kJ DE has been suggested for normal adult horses at rest (Hansen et al 1988, Divers 1991, Rooney 1998), and this amount has been suggested as a reasonable estimate of protein requirement in horses in the immediate post-operative period (Durham 2005). Adequate energy from carbohydrates or fat is needed to prevent utilization of protein for energy during the postoperative period. It has been suggested that horses that are not ingesting 50% of their maintenance requirement for 48–72 hours should have nutritional support (Dunkel & McKenzie 2003, Magdesian 2003); however, the long-term detrimental effects for a relatively short period of negative energy balance after colic surgery have not been evaluated.

Parenteral nutrition has been used to treat the negative energy balance following gastro-intestinal surgery in horses (Lopes & White 2002, Durham et al 2004). However Durham et al (2004) showed that parenteral nutrition does not have a strong beneficial influence on short or long-term survival. These findings along with the high cost and associated risks, such as thrombosis, increased insulin resistance, hyperglycemia, sepsis, etc. of parenteral nutrition mean other methods are needed to reduce the length of time these surgical patients spend in negative energy balance; early enteral feeding is one such method. The primary energy source utilized by enterocytes is glutamine obtained from the lumen, not from the plasma, and this is one reason why enteral feeding may be more beneficial than parenteral nutrition. However, in horses that develop postoperative ileus or in other cases where enteral feeding is not possible, parenteral nutrition may be required.

Generally the basis of feeding practice in postoperative laparotomy patients is derived from a subjective assessment of clinical experience rather than scientific information (Spier & Meagher 1989). Studies in human patients have shown that many of the concerns regarding early feeding are unfounded. Early enteral feeding (within 24 hours of surgery) in humans following intestinal resection and anastomosis has been demonstrated in numerous studies to be safe and associated with a shorter period of ileus (Zhou et al 2006, Feo et al 2004, Lewis et al 2001, Stewart et al 1998, Reissman et al 1995, Seenu & Goel 1995, de Aquilar-Nascimento & Goelzer 2002). Surgical injury itself increases resting energy expenditure and protein loss, and intake of energy and protein after gastrointestinal surgery fall often below what is required in the post-operative recovery period (Keele et al 1997). The benefits of early postoperative feeding are not confined to malnourished patients, and in human studies reduced nutritional intake has been shown to predispose patients to complications (Keele et al 1997). Studies in rats showed an increase in collagen synthesis at the anastomosis and laparotomy sites in the animals that were not starved after small intestinal resection, thereby actually leading to faster healing and reduced dehiscence rates (Kiyami et al 1999). The reduction in ileus is thought to be caused by the gastro-colic reflex, distension of the intestine and a direct improvement in enterocyte function due to nutrient supply (Ross et al 1990, Naylor et al 2006). Numerous studies have shown that feeding stimulates increased intestinal sounds in horses (Ehrhardt and Lowe 1987, Naylor et al 2006) as well as increasing the frequency, intensity and duration of intestinal myoelectrical complexes (Clarke et al 1990, Ross et al 1990, Merritt et al 1995).

Most hay or grass is not evaluated for nutrient content, so the daily energy and protein intake frequently is not known for horses being fed hay/grass in the postoperative period. The use of pellet feeds that contain sources of fiber (e.g., "senior feed" products) allows more accurate calculation of energy and protein intake (White 2009). Other "complete horse feed" pellets often contain grains, thereby increasing soluble carbohydrate concentrations, which in some cases may be advantageous but this must be balanced against the risk of excessive gas production and altering the flora in the cecum and colon (and an increased risk of laminitis). Oral liquid diets made for humans have been used in horses but these contain no fiber, and their use increases the risk of colitis and laminitis (Buechner-Maxwell et al 2003). Other liquid diets made for horses (consisting of alfalfa pellets, dextrose, vegetable oils and amino acids) have been shown to be capable of maintaining body condition in horses but also increase the risk of laminitis and diarrhea (Naylor et al 1984).

The optimum feeding regime for horses following colic surgery has not been determined, and this will vary depending on the primary disease process, type of surgery, presence or absence of post-operative complications (including postoperative ileus), etc. In most cases a forage-based diet of hay or fresh grass is chosen and fed as soon as medical judgment suggests ingested food can be tolerated (White 2009). Alternatives include pellet-type feeds consisting of alfalfa or total diet feeds. After surgery for simple large colon obstructions, water is generally offered immediately, and grass hay, alfalfa hay or fresh grass is routinely fed from 6 to 12 hours after surgery (White 2009). Approximately 0.5 kg of hay can be fed every 3 hours, which allows monitoring of the horse and intestinal motility. Ad libitum feeding can usually be started 24 hours after the start of feeding. Following surgery for small intestinal diseases, water or food is generally not offered until gastric reflux has ceased and there is evidence of progressive gastrointestinal motility; however, post-operative ileus may not become apparent until 12–36 hours after surgery, and waiting this long until allowing consumption of water or food may have detrimental effects.

Early (by 6 hours) post-operative feeding following all forms of colic surgery, including small intestinal resection and anastomosis, has been recommended by several surgeons (Snyder & van Hoogmoed 2000, Freeman et al 2000). However, there is little published information about the effects of early enteral nutrition following small intestinal surgery, and the optimum type of feed, quantity and precise timing of feeding are largely unknown. Although feeding can be a stimulus for intestinal motility, early feeding can also result in pain and accumulation of fluid and ingesta in the stomach and small intestine in some cases (White 2009). Prior to offering food, many surgeons recommend offering small amounts of water (e.g., 1 liter) every hour until the horse is no longer thirsty, then offering hay or a pellet feed (up to 0.5 kg) every 3 hours, increasing over 24 to 48 hours until ad libitum hay or a full ration of pellets (based on the basal energy requirements of the horse) can be fed (White 2009). If early feeding is introduced following small intestinal surgery, the cessation of oral intake may be required if the horse subsequently shows signs of pain or ileus. At this time, there appear to be no objective measures of bowel function that can be used to predict when it is safe to allow enteral feeding after small intestinal surgery, and the decision of when, how much and how often to feed an individual horse following surgery needs to be made on a case by case basis.

Key Points

- Although opinion varies on the timing of reintroduction of enteral feeding after surgery, most horses undergoing non-abdominal surgery or simple intestinal surgery can begin to ingest feed within 6 to 12 hours of recovery
- Some clinicians also recommend an early (within 6–8 hours) reintroduction to feeding in horses that have undergone small intestinal resection and anastomosis, unless there are clear contraindications such as postoperative ileus
- A forage-based diet (e.g., high-quality hay or soaked hay cubes or pellets) is recommended for the first 5–7 days post-surgery followed by a gradual return to normal diet. Cereal grains and grain-based feeds should be avoided until 10–14 days after intestinal surgery

Practical approach to feeding pre- and post-surgery

The following guidelines are based on the author's own recommendations for feeding horses before and after surgery. These recommendations are based on experience rather than good scientific evidence, and are used as guidelines only; every case should be considered on its own merits.

Pre-surgical starvation

For routine elective surgical procedures, starvation for 6 to 12 hours is undertaken. The horse is allowed free access to water. Non-edible bedding should be used (or a muzzle fitted) to stop the horse from ingesting bedding material. In most cases of emergency surgery, preoperative starvation is not an issue since the horse's condition necessitates surgery regardless of the nutritional status. In animals where gastric distension may be present (primarily horses affected by pyloric or small intestinal obstruction), decompression by passage of a nasogastric tube should be undertaken immediately prior to induction of general anesthesia.

Post-surgical feeding

Nongastrointestinal surgery

For non-gastrointestinal surgery, feeding is resumed as soon as the horse has made a full recovery from the anesthesia and clinical assessment indicates normal alimentary tract function (within 4 to 6 hours of cessation of anesthesia in most horses).

Dental surgery

In most cases no specific dietary modifications are required following dental procedures such as tooth extractions. However, in horses where there is significant periodontal disease, feeding roughage with short fiber length such as chaffed hay or straw is recommended in order to reduce the risk of food impactions within periodontal pockets. Depending on the extent and nature of the disease, such dietary modification may be necessary long-term. For geriatric horses with severe dental abnormalities and/or numerous missing teeth, feeding of slurry made from pelleted "complete feeds" with a high fiber content may be necessary as an alternative to feeding hay.

Esophageal surgery

For surgical procedures involving full thickness wounds of the esophageal wall (esophagotomy, esophageal resection and anastomosis, etc.), food and water are withheld for 48 hours after surgery, and maintenance intravenous fluid therapy instituted. After this time, depending on the health of the esophageal wound, slurries of soaked high-fiber pellets or "complete feed" pellets can be fed orally. Hay or other roughage should not be fed until such time as the esophageal wound has healed (as assessed by esophagoscopy and/or radiography). For cases where there is devitalized esophageal wall or an open esophageal perforation (that is being left to heal by secondary intention), the horse should be fed by an indwelling feeding tube (assisted enteral feeding - see Chapter 41) that can be placed via the nose, via the esophageal wound or via an esophagostomy (Fig. 39.5). Indwelling or repeated nasogastric intubation can cause iatrogenic damage to the nasal cavity, pharynx and esophagus, and horses being fed in this way should be closely monitored for these complications as well as having their general hydration status monitored (i.e., monitoring packed cell volume, total serum protein concentration, electrolytes, urination, etc.). Purpose-made enteral feeding tubes are better than standard nasogastric tubes, but a tube with a 12 mm internal diameter is needed for most enteral diets containing fiber (fiber-free enteral diets [such as human formulations] can be administered through a smaller tube but these have been associated with diarrhea and laminitis and use of these formulations is not recommended for more than a few days). Indwelling tubes can usually be left in place safely for 7–8 days. The end of the tube should be placed in the stomach rather than the distal esophagus, and the end should be open-ended rather than fenestrated (to prevent it from becoming clogged with food). Several formulations of enteral diets have been published (Naylor et al 1984, Fascetti & Stratton-Phelps 2003) (see Chapter 41). The rate of administration of these diets should be gradually increased over a 3–5 day period. In most cases, approximately one quarter of the final volume of feed is administered for one to two days, then one half for the next one to two days, then three quarters for one to two days followed by the total volume (Geor 2008). The daily volume of food should ideally be administered in four to six batches with a maximum volume of 6–8 liters per feed (including approximately one liter of water to flush the tube after administering the feed). Pelleted feeds should be soaked in warm water to soften them before mixing in a blender (each batch of feed should be prepared freshly). Prior to administering each batch of feed, assessment to detect gastric reflux should be made - the presence of more than 1 liter of gastric reflux is an indication to withhold enteral feeding until the reflux has subsided.

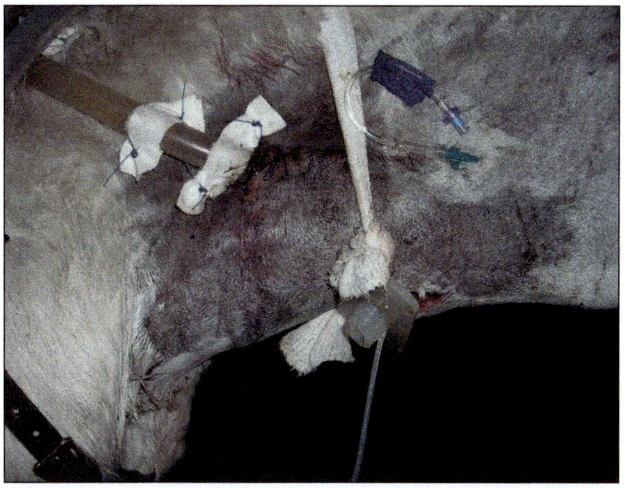

Figure 39.5 Indwelling esophagostomy tube (this horse also has a tracheostomy tube).

Gastric and small intestinal surgery

Gastric surgery is rarely undertaken in adult horses other than rare cases of primary gastric impaction treated by gastrotomy (Owen et al 1987, Kellam et al 2000). However, firm, dehydrated gastric impactions can occur secondarily to small intestinal obstructions. Although these impactions usually resolve spontaneously after surgical resolution of the primary disease and when the horse has been adequately rehydrated, some surgeons recommend routine postoperative gastroscopy following surgery for small intestinal obstructions, and advocate repeated fluid and mineral oil administration (via nasogastric tube) until the impaction has passed before allowing access to solid food.

As described above, the author prefers to feed horses early after colic surgery, provided that adequate bowel function is present. Assessment of bowel function is not easy, but careful monitoring of the heart rate, intestinal sounds and ultrasonographic evidence of small intestinal motility should all be undertaken routinely. Feeding is not undertaken or is stopped if there is evidence of ileus. This author does not perform routine nasogastric intubation after small intestinal surgery unless there is suspicion of ileus (as shown by increasing heart rate, abdominal pain or immotile distended small intestine observed by ultrasonography). Early feeding is believed to stimulate bowel function as well as maintaining the health of the intestinal tract. For small intestinal obstructions, whether these are simple obstructions (such as ileal impaction or proximal enteritis) (Fig. 39.6) or strangulating obstructions necessitating resection and anastomosis, water (1 to 2 liters) is usually offered within 4–6 hours of surgery or within 4–6 hours of cessation of gastric reflux in horses that have been affected by postoperative ileus. Water is offered every hour initially to test gastrointestinal function. In uncomplicated cases, food is offered as soon as 6–12 hours after surgery. In most cases, a handful of grass or hay is offered approximately every hour. If there are no signs of complications, a small feed is usually offered at 12–18 hours. This will usually consist of a small amount (up to approximately 0.5 kg) of grass hay or alfalfa or a complete pelleted feed with or without a small quantity of wheat bran (or a combination of these feeds). Such feeds are offered every 2–3 hours. After the next 24 hours, the volume of each feed is steadily increased and the frequency decreased over 3 to 5 days. Grazing for short periods (5–10 minutes two to three times a day) can also be introduced after 3–4 days. Grain-concentrate feeds are avoided for the first 10–14 days after surgery, but thereafter the horse should be able to resume a normal feeding regimen.

In horses where there is particular concern about the functionality of an anastomosis, a soft, low-bulk ration (e.g., fresh grass, or mashes/slurries of grass nuts/alfalfa pellets/complete diet pellets) should be fed for the 3 to 4 days prior to introducing hay. Molasses may be added to the diet to increase palatability. A similar diet can be fed in horses that demonstrate colic after food is re-introduced after small intestinal surgery (that might indicate impaction or "sludging" of food at the anastomosis).

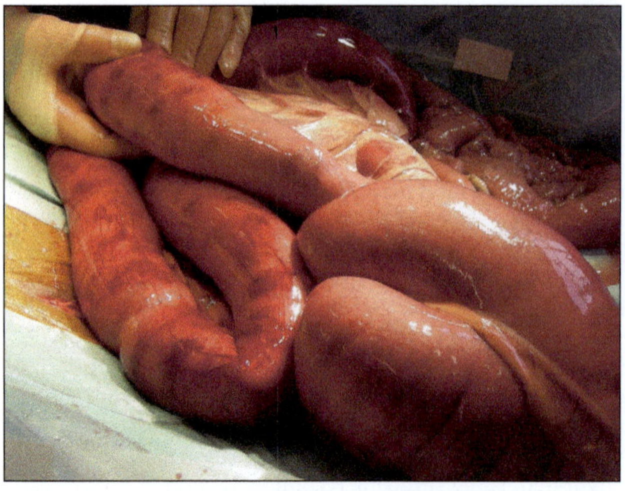

Figure 39.6 Intraoperative view of anterior enteritis.

Horses that develop postoperative ileus or with anterior enteritis cannot tolerate enteral feeding until such time as bowel function returns. Intensive fluid therapy is required to maintain fluid and electrolyte balance, and regular nasogastric intubation (every 3 hours) is needed to decompress the stomach. Whilst horses can tolerate starvation for several days under these circumstances, parenteral nutrition should be considered if the ileus persists more than 2 to 3 days.

Large intestinal surgery

The feeding regime for horses following large intestinal surgery is similar to that following small intestinal surgery, except feeding is carried out sooner, and good quality forage (grass hay or alfalfa) is considered important. Horses undergoing large intestinal surgery are at a particular risk of developing diarrhea, but this risk is decreased by feeding grass hay. Most horses are offered water at about 4–6 hours after surgery. Small handfuls of hay or grass are offered from about 6–8 hours after surgery, and fed every hour thereafter. Grazing in hand for 5 to 10 minutes three times a day is allowed from 12 to 24 hours after surgery.

Small colon surgery

Surgery of the small colon is perceived as having a higher complication rate than surgery of other regions of the intestinal tract. Reasons include restricted surgical access, the high bacterial content of the distal intestine, the relatively dehydrated and coarse nature of the fecal balls, and the relatively high activity of collagen-degrading enzymes. For these reasons, attempts should be made to limit stresses placed on colotomies or anastomoses of the small colon for the first few days after surgery. These include emptying the large colon at the time of surgery and feeding a soft, low-bulk ration (e.g., fresh grass, or mashes/slurries of grass nuts/alfalfa pellets/complete diet pellets) initially. In some cases mineral oil is also administered by nasogastric tube for the first 2 days after surgery.

Intestinal surgery in foals

Enteral feeding of foals with colic or abdominal distension is contraindicated and intravenous fluid and dextrose therapy is required to prevent fluid and electrolyte imbalances, and hypoglycemia. Nursing from the mare can be prevented by separating the mare and foal by a partition or by the use of a muzzle. Following intestinal surgery, similar considerations to the adult are needed to determine the optimum time to reintroduce oral feeding, but in most cases with intestinal distension, enteritis or intestinal resection, enteral rest for at least 48 hours is recommended; earlier return to oral feeding may induce ileus. Parenteral nutritional support is required if enteral rest for longer than 48 hours is necessary. When feeding is reintroduced, approximately 100 ml of water or dextrose solution is administered every 2 hours. The volume offered is slowly increased until a volume of 350–400 ml is administered. Once this volume is achieved and assuming that the foal tolerates this volume, a 50:50 mixture of water and milk/milk replacer is given.

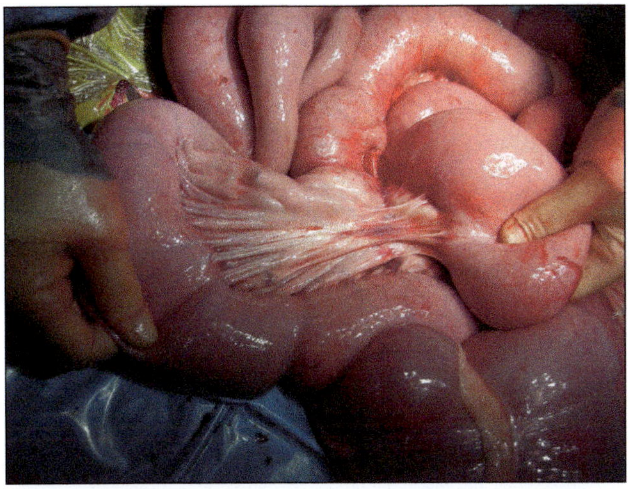

Figure 39.7 Intraoperative view of intestinal and mesenteric adhesion following previous intestinal surgery.

The strength of the milk solution is slowly increased over several feeds until full strength milk/milk replacer is used.

Feeding horses with adhesions or food intolerance after colic surgery

Intra-abdominal adhesions (Fig. 39.7) are common complications following intestinal surgery, especially small intestinal surgery. These can predispose affected horses to recurrent episodes of abdominal pain. Some horses also seem to develop food intolerance associated with motility disorders, possibly relating to damage to the smooth muscle of the bowel or the neurological control of bowel function. These horses may benefit from a low residue diet fed in several feeds per day. The following recipe is used by the author (derived from recommendations from the University of Liverpool - Dr Debbie Archer, personal communication): For a 500 kg horse - "pasture mix" (flaked cereals) (up to 4 kg/day), unmolassed sugar beet (500 g/day), chopped alfalfa grass hay (1 kg/day), wheat bran (500 g), and as much grass as possible if the horse can be turned out.

Summary

General anesthesia in the horse has a much higher mortality and morbidity than most other species. Sick and shocked horses that require emergency surgery (primarily horses affected by colic) carry the highest mortality rate (1.9%). Various metabolic and endocrine changes occur during anesthesia and surgery in horses (including a cortisol response, an increase in circulating catecholamines, and changes in insulin levels), and these may have profound, albeit temporary, effects on the nutritional status of the horse. Feeding practices around the time of surgery, and the underlying disease status of the horse, have important implications to the metabolic condition. Most authors recommend withholding food but not water for 6 to 12 hours prior to inducing general anesthesia in order to reduce gut content and increase the functional residual capacity of the lung. Starvation beyond 12 to 18 hours is likely to induce significant stress and metabolic derangements. Horses affected by acute abdominal disease requiring surgery (i.e., surgical colic) are compromised due to the disease, often starved for long periods of time and sometimes exposed to the stress of long trailer rides. Horses undergoing abdominal surgery for colic undergo increased lipolysis and weight loss compared with healthy horses. Colic horses are usually in a negative energy balance for the first week after surgery. There appears to be a wide variation in opinion between different surgeons and hospitals with respect to the timing of reintroduction of feed postoperatively. Most horses undergoing nonabdominal surgery or simple intestinal surgery will recommence partial enteral feeding within 6 to 12 hours of recovery from anesthesia. However, following small intestinal resection and anastomosis, horses are frequently starved for longer lengths of time, because of concern that feeding will place the anastomosis under increased stress and risk of failure. However, there is little evidence to support this contention, and in other species it has been shown that early feeding has beneficial effects with regard to enterocyte function, wound healing, anastomotic strength and gastrointestinal motility. For these reasons, some surgeons favor early feeding (within 6–8 hours) of horses after all forms of colic surgery (unless there are reasons not to do so such as postoperative ileus). In most cases a forage-based diet of hay or fresh grass is chosen and fed as soon as medical judgment suggests ingested food can be tolerated. Alternatives include pellet-type feeds consisting of alfalfa or total diet feeds. Postoperative ileus is a major postoperative complication following colic surgery, especially surgery involving ischemic damage to the small intestine. Postoperative ileus precludes enteral feeding, and horses affected by this disorder require intensive intravenous fluid therapy and repeated nasogastric intubation; parenteral nutrition may be required if the ileus persists longer that 2–3 days.

References

Adams, S.B., 1988. Recognition and management of ileus. Vet Clinics N Am: Equine Pract 4, 91–104.

Akhtar, S., Barash, P.G., Inzucchi, S.E., 2010. Scientific principles and clinical implications of perioperative glucose regulation and control. Anesth Analg 110, 478–497.

Andersen, M.S., Clark, L., Dyson, S.J., Newton, J.R., 2006. Effects of perianaesthetic morphine on the prevalence of colic in horses after general anaesthesia for MRI or nonabdominal surgery. Equine Vet J 38, 368–374.

Becht, J.L., Richardson, D.W., 1981. Ileus in the horse: clinical significance and management. Proc. Am. Ass Equine Pract 27, 291–297.

Bidwell, L.A., Bramlage, L.R., Rood, W.A., 2007. Equine perioperative fatalities associated with general anesthesia at a private practice - a retrospective case series. Vet Anaesth Analg 34, 23–30.

Blikslager, A.T., Bowman, K.F., Levine, J.F., et al., 1994. Evaluation of factors associated with postoperative ileus in horses: 31 cases (1990–1992). J Am Vet Med Assoc 205, 1748–1752.

Bochicchio, G.V., Sung, J., Joshi, M., et al., 2005a. Persistent hyperglycemia is predictive of outcome in critically ill trauma patients. J Trauma 58, 921–924.

Bochicchio, G.V., Salzano, L., Joshi, M., et al., 2005b. Admission preoperative glucose is predictive of morbidity and mortality in trauma patients who require immediate operative intervention. Am Surg 71, 171–174.

Branson, K.R., Gross, M.E., 2001. Opioid agonists and antagonists. In: Adams, H.R. (Eds.), Veterinary Pharmacology and Therapeutics, eighth ed. Iowa State University Press, Ames, USA. pp. 268–298.

Brezile, J.E., 1987. Physiologic basis and consequences of distress in animals. J Am Vet Med Ass 191, 1212–1215.

Bryant, C.E., Moore, J.N., 2008. Systemic inflammatory response syndrome: endotoxaemia reconsidered. In: White, N.A., Moore, J.N., Mair, T.S. (Eds.), The Equine Acute Abdomen. Teton New Media, Jackson, WY, USA, pp. 192–200.

Buechner-Maxwell, V.A., Elvinger, C.D., Murray, M.J., et al., 2003. Physiologic response of normal adult horses to a low-residue liquid diet. J Equine Vet Sci 23, 310–317.

Clarke, R.S.J., 1973. Anaesthesia and carbohydrate metabolism. Br J Anaesth 45, 237–241.

Clarke, L.L., Roberts, M.C., Argenzio, R.A., 1990. Feeding and digestive problems in horses. Physiologic responses to a concentrated meal. Vet Clin North Am: Equine Pract 6, 433–450.

Cohen, N.D., Gibbs, P.G., Woods, A.M., 1999. Dietary and other management factors associated with colic in horses. J Am Vet Med Ass 215, 53–60.

Cohen, N.D., Lester, G.D., Sanchez, L.C., et al., 2004. Evaluation of risk factors associated with development of postoperative ileus in horses. J Am Vet Med Ass 225, 1070–1078.

Collatos, C., Ronano, S., 1992. Cecal impaction in horses: causes, diagnosis and medical treatment. Compend Contin Educ Pract Vet 15, 976–981.

Dabareiner, R.M., White, N.A., 1995. Large colon impaction in horses: 147 cases (1985–1991). J Am Vet Med Assoc 206, 679–685.

De Aquilar-Nascimento and Goelzer, 2002. Early feeding after intestinal anastomosis: risks or benefits? Rev Assoc Med Bras 48, 348–352.

Divers, T.J., 1991. Perioperative partial/total parenteral nutrition. Proc Am Coll Vet Surg 1, 306–308.

Doherty, T.J., 2009. Postoperative ileus: pathogenesis and treatment. Vet Clinics N Am: Equine Pract 25, 351–362.

Dunkel, B., McKenzie, H.C., 2003. Severe hypertriglyceridaemia in clinically ill horses: diagnosis, treatment and outcome. Equine Vet J 35, 590–595.

Durham, A.E., 2005. How to feed the convalescent horse following intestinal surgery. In: Proceedings of The 1st BEVA & Waltham Nutrition Symposia. pp. 79–87.

Durham, A.E., Phillips, T.J., Walmsley, J.P., et al., 2003. Study of the clinical effects of postoperative parenteral nutrition in 15 horses. Vet Rec 153, 493–498.

Durham, A.E., Phillips, T.J., Walmsley, J.P., et al., 2004. Nutritional and clinicopathalogical effects of post-operative parenteral nutrition following small intestinal resection and anastomosis in the mature horse. Equine Vet J 36, 390–396.

Edner, A., Nyman, G., Essen-Gustavsson, B., 2007. Metabolism before, during and after anaesthesia in colic and healthy horses. Acta Vet Scand 49, 34.

Edwards, G.B., Hunt, J.M., 1985. An analysis of the incidence of postoperative ileus (POI) and an assessment of the predisposing factors. Proc Equine Colic Res Symp 2, 307–312.

Ehrhardt, E.E., Lowe, J.E., 1987. Lengthy electronic auscultation of the equine abdomen to monitor the effects of analgesics, sedatives and other drugs. Proc Am Ass Equine Pract 33, 525–538.

Fascetti, A.J., Stratton-Phelps, M., 2003. Clinical assessment of nutritional staus and enteral feeding in the acutely ill horse. In: Current Therapy in Equine Medicine, fifth ed. Elsevier, Philadelphia, pp. 705–710.

Feo, C.V., Romanini, B., Sortini, D., et al., 2004. Early oral feeding after colorectal resection: a randomised controlled study. ANZ J Surg 74, 298–301.

Finfer, S., Chittock, D.R., Su, S.Y., et al, 2009. Intensive versus conventional glucose control in critically ill patients. N Engl J Med 360, 1283–1297.

Freeman, D.E., Hammock, P., Baker, G.J., et al, 2000. Short- and long-term survival and prevalence of post-operative ileus after small intestinal surgery in the horse. Equine Vet J Suppl 32, 42–51.

French, N.P., Smith, J., Edwards, G.B., et al., 2002. Equine surgical colic: risk factors for postoperative complications. Equine Vet J 34, 444–449.

Garcia-Seco, E., Wilson, D.A., Kramer, J., et al, 2005. Prevalence and risk factors associated with outcome of surgical removal of pedunculated lipomas in horses: 102 cases (1987–2002). J Am Vet Med Ass 226, 1529–1537.

Geor, R.J., 2007. How to feed horses recovering from colic. Proc Am Ass Equine Pract 52, 196–201.

Geor. R.J., 2008. Nutritional management of the colic patient. In: White, N.A., Moore, J.N., Mair, T.S. (Eds.), The Equine Acute Abdomen. Teton New Media, Jackson, WY, pp. 403–415.

Gerring, E.L., 1992. Management of intestinal ileus in horses. Compend Contin Educ Pract Vet 15, 1102–1103.

Hansen, T.O., White, N.A., Kemp, D.T., 1988. Total parenteral nutrition in four healthy adult horses. Am J Vet Res 49, 122–124.

Hassel, D.M., Hill, A.E., Rorabeck, R.A., 2009. Association between hyperglycemia and survival in 228 horses with acute gastrointestinal disease. J Vet Intern Med 23, 1261–1265.

Haydock, D.A., Hill, G.L., 1986. Impaired wound healing in surgical patients with varying degrees of malnutrition. J Parenter Enteral Nutr 10, 550–554.

Hillyer, M.H., Taylor, F.G.R., Proudman, C.J., et al., 2002. A case control study of simple colonic obstruction and distension colic in the horse. Equine Vet J 34, 455–463.

Hinchcliff, K., Rush, B., Farris, J., 2005. Evaluation of plasma catecholamine and serum cortisol concentrations in horses with colic. J Am Vet Med Assoc 227, 276–280.

Hodson, N., Wright, J., Hunt, J., 1986. The sympatho-adrenal system and plasma levels of adrenocorticotropic hormone, cortisol and catecholamines in equine grass sickness. Vet Rec 118, 148–150.

Hoffsis, G., Murdick, P., 1970. The plasma concentration of corticosteroids in normal and diseased horses. J Am Vet Med Assoc 157, 1590–1594.

Hollis, A.R., Boston, R.C., Corley, K.T.T., 2007. Blood glucose in horses with acute abdominal disease. J Vet Intern Med 21, 1099–1103.

Hughes, C.A., Dowling, R.H., 1980. Speed of onset of adaptive mucosal hypoplasia and hypofunction in the intestine of parenterally fed rats. Clin Sci 59, 317–327.

Hunt, J.M., Edwards, G.B., Clarke, K.W., 1986. Incidence, diagnosis and treatment of postoperative complications in colic cases. Equine Vet J 18, 264–270.

Johnston, G.M., Taylor, P.M., Holmes, M.A., et al., 1998. Confidential enquiry of perioperative equine fatalities (CEPEF -1): Preliminary results. Equine Vet J 27, 193–200.

Johnston, G.M., Eastment, J.K., Wood, J.L.N., et al., 2002. The confidential enquiry into perioperative equine fatalities (CEPEF): mortality results of phases 1 and 2. Vet Anaesth Analg 29, 159–170.

Jones, R.S., Edwards, G.B., Brearley, J.C., 1991. Commentary on prolonged starvation as a factor associated with post operative colic. Equine Vet Educ 3, 16–18.

Keele, A.M., Bray, M.J., Emery, P.W., et al., 1997. Two phase randomised controlled clinical trial of postoperative oral dietary supplements in surgical patients. Gut 40, 393–399.

Kellam, L.L., Johnson, P.J., Kramer, J., et al., 2000. Gastric impaction and obstruction of the small intestine associated with persimmon phytobezoar in a horse. J AmVet Med Ass 216, 1279–1281.

Kiyami, T., Efron, D.T., Tantry, U., et al., 1999. Effect of nutritional route on anastomatic healing in the rat. J Gastrointest Surg 3, 441–446.

Koenig, J., Cote, N., 2005. The effect of inflammation of the equine jejunum on motilin receptors and binding of erythromycin lactobionate. In: Proc. 8th Int.Equine Colic Res.Symp., Quebec City, Canada, pp. 80–81.

Lewis, S.J., Egger, M., Sylvester, P.A., et al., 2001. Early enteral feeding versus 'nil by mouth' after gastrointestinal surgery: systematic review and meta-analysis of controlled trials. Br Med J 323, 773–776.

Little, D., Redding, W.R., Blikslager, A.T., 2001. Risk factors for reduced post-operative fecal output in horses: 37 cases (1997–1998). J Am Vet Med Ass 218, 414–420.

Livingston, E.H., Passaro, E.P. Jr., 1990. Postoperative ileus. Dig Dis Sci 35, 121–132.

Lopes, M.A., White, N.A., 2002. Parenteral nutrition for horses with gastro-intestinal disease: a retrospective study of 79 cases. Equine Vet J 34, 250–257.

Luna, S.P.L., Taylor, P.M., 1995. Pituitary-adrenal activity and opioid release in ponies during thiopentone/halothane anaesthesia. Res Vet Sci 58, 35–41.

Luna, S.P.L., Taylor, P.M., 2001. Cardiorespiratory and endocrine effects of endogenous opioid antagonism by naloxone in ponies anaesthetized with halothane. Res Vet Sci 70, 95–100.

Luna, S.P.L.,Taylor, P.M., Massone, F., 1997. Midazolam and ketamine induction before halothane anaesthesia in ponies: cardiorespiratory, endocrine, and metabolic changes. J Vet Pharmacol Ther 20, 153–159.

Luna, S.P.L., Taylor, P.M., Brearley, J.C., 1999. Effects of glucose infusion on the endocrine, metabolic, and cardiorespiratory responses to halothane anaesthesia of ponies. Vet Rec 145, 100–103.

MacDonald, M.H., Pascoe, J.R., Stover, S.M., et al., 1989. Survival after small intestinal resection and anastomosis in horses. Vet Surg 18, 415–423.

MacFie, J., 2000. Enteral versus parenteral nutrition: the significance of bacterial translocation and gut barrier function. Nutrition 16, 606–611.

Magdesian, K.G., 2003. Nutrition for clinical gastrointestinal illness: feeding horses with diarrhea or colic. Vet Clin N Am: Equine Pract 19, 617–644.

Mair, T.S., Smith, L.J., 2005. Survival and complication rates of 300 horses undergoing surgical treatment of colic. Part 2. Short-term complications. Equine Vet J 37, 303–309.

Mee, A.M., Cripps, P.J., Jones, R.S., 1998. A retrospective study of mortality associated with general anaesthesia in horses: emergency procedures. Vet Rec 142, 307–309.

Merritt, A.M., Panzer, R.B., Lester, G.D., et al., 1995. Equine pelvic flexure myoelectric activity during fed and fasted states. Am J Physiol 269, G262–G268.

Milne, E.M., Doxey, D.L., Gilmour, J.S., 1990. Serum lipids and lipoproteins in equine colic and grass sickness. Res Vet Sci 48, 170–174.

Mircica, E., Clutton, R.E., Kyles, K.W., et al., 2003. Problems associated with perioperative morphine in horses: a retrospective case analysis. Vet Anaesth Analg 30, 147–155.

Muir, W.W., 1990. The equine stress response to anaesthesia. Equine Vet J 22, 302–303.

Naylor, J.M., Freeman, D.E., Kronfeld, D.S., 1984. Alimentation of hypophagic horses. Comp Contin Educ Pract Vet S93–S99.

Naylor, J.M., Poirier, K.L., Hamilton, D.L., et al., 2006. The effects of feeding and fasting on gastrointestinal sounds in adult horses. J Vet Intern Med 20, 1408–1413.

Owen, R.A., Jagger, D.W., Jagger, F., 1987. Two cases of equine primary gastric impaction. Vet Rec 121, 102–106.

Pagan, J.D., Hintz, H.F., 1986. Equine energetics. I. Relationship between body weight and energy requirements in horses. J Anim Sci 63, 815–821.

Protopapas, K., 2000. Studies on the role of nutrition and metabolic disturbances following equine colic surgery. DVetMed Thesis, University of London.

Proudman, C.J., Smith, J.E., Edwards, G.B., et al., 2002. Long-term survival of equine surgical colic cases. Part 1: patterns of mortality and morbidity. Equine Vet J 34, 432–437.

Proudman, C.J., Dugdale, A.H., Senior, A.M., et al, 2006. Pre-operative and anaesthesia-related risk factors for mortality in equine colic cases. Vet J 171, 89–97.
Ralston, S.L., 2002. Nutritional support after alimentary tract surgery. In: Mair, T., Divers, T., Ducharme, N. (Eds.), Manual of Equine Gastroenterology. W.B Saunders, Edinburgh, pp. 196–198.
Reinprecht, B., Hackl, S., Reisinger, R., et al, 2007. Metabolic and clinical traits in horses undergoing feed deprivation for elective orthopaedic surgery. Berl MunchTierazl Wochenschr 120, 134–140.
Reissman, P., Teoh, T.A., Cohen, S.M., et al., 1995. Is early oral feeding safe after elective colorectal surgery? A prospective randomized trial. Ann Surg 222, 73–77.
Robertson, J.T., Scicluna, C., 2009. Preoperative evaluations: general considerations. In: Muir, W.W., Hubbell, J.E. (Eds.), Equine Anesthesia. Monitoring and Emergency Therapy, second ed. Elsevier, St Louis, Missouri, pp. 121–130.
Robertson, S.A., 1987. Some metabolic and hormonal changes associated with general anaesthesia and surgery in the horse. Equine Vet J 19, 288–294.
Robertson, S.A., Steele, C.J., Chen, C., 1990. Metabolic and hormonal changes associated with arthroscopic surgery in the horse. Equine Vet J 22, 313–316.
Robertson, S.A., Malark, J.A., Steele, C.J., 1996. Metabolic, hormonal and hemodynamic changes during dopamine infusions in halothane anesthetized horses. Vet Anesth 25, 88–97.
Roger, T., Bardon, T., Ruckesbusch, Y., 1994. Comparative effects of mu and kappa opiate agonists on the cecocolic motility in the pony. Can J Vet Res 58, 163–166.
Rooney, D.K., 1998. Clinical nutrition. In: Reed, S.M., Bayly, W.M. (Eds.), Equine Internal Medicine. W.B. Saunders Co., Philadelphia, pp. 216–250.
Ross, M.W., Martin, B.B., Donawick, W.J., 1985. Cecal perforation in the horse. J Am Vet Med Assoc 187, 249–253.
Ross, M.W., Cullen, K.K., Rutkowski, J.A., 1990. Myoelectric activity of the ileum, cecum, and right ventral colon in ponies during interdigestive, nonfeeding, and digestive periods. Am J Vet Res 51, 561–566.
Santschi, E., LeBlanc, M., Weston, P., 1991. Progestagen, oestrone sulphate and cortisol concentrations in pregnant mares during medical and surgical disease. J Reprod Fertil Suppl 44, 627–634.
Senior, J.M., Pinchbeck, G.L., Dugdale, A.H.A., et al., 2004. Retrospective study of the risk factors and prevalence of colic in horses after orthopaedic surgery. Vet Rec 155, 321–325.
Senior, J.M., Pinchbeck, G.L., Allister, R., et al, 2006. Post anaesthetic colic in horses: a preventable complication? Equine Vet J 38, 479–484.
Seenu, V., Goel, A.K., 1995. Early oral feeding after elective colorectal surgery: is it safe? Trop Gastroenterol 16, 72–73.
Sherlock, C., Mair, T., 2008. Serum cortisol concentrations in horses with colic. In: Proceedings of the 9th International Equine Research Colic Symposium. Liverpool, UK, pp. 96–97.
Schroeder, D., Gillanders, L., Mahr, K., et al., 1991. Effects of immediate postoperative enteral nutrition on body composition, muscle function, and wound healing. J Parenter Enteral Nutr 15, 376–383.
Silk, D.B.A., Menzies Gow, N., 2001. Post operative starvation after gastrointestinal surgery. Early feeding is beneficial. Br Med J 323, 761–762.
Snow, D.H., 1979. Metabolic and physiological effects of adrenoceptor agonists in the horse. Res Vet Sci 27, 372–378.
Snyder, J.R., van Hoogmoed, L., 2000. Postoperative care, prevention and treatment of ileus. Proc Eur Coll Vet Surg 9, 157–160.
Sojka, J.E., Adams, S.B., Lamar, C.M., et al., 1988. Effect of butorphanol, pentazocine, meperidine, or metoclopramide on intestinal motility in female ponies. Am J Vet Res 49, 527–529.
Spier, S.J., Meagher, D.M., 1989. Perioperative medical care for equine abdominal surgery. Vet Clin N Am: Equine Pract 5, 429–443.
Steinbrook, R.A., 1998. Epidural anesthesia and gastrointestinal motility. Vet Anesth Analg 86, 837–844.
Stegmann, G.F., Jones, R.S., 1998. Perioperative plasma cortisol concentrations in the horse. J S Afr Vet Ass 69, 137–142.
Stewart, B.T., Woods, R.J., Collopy, B.T., et al., 1998. Early feeding after elective open colorectal resections: a prospective randomized trial. Aust N Z J Surg 68, 125–128.
Sykes, B.W., Furr, M.O., 2005. Equine endotoxaemia – a state-of-the-art review of therapy. Aust Vet J 83, 45–50.
Taylor, P.M., 1985. Changes in plasma cortisol concentrations in response to anaesthesia in the horse. In: Proceedings of the 2nd International Congress of Veterinary Anesthesiologists, Sacramento. pp. 165–166.
Taylor, P.M., 1989. Equine stress response to anaesthesia. Br J Anaesth 63, 702–709.
Taylor, P.M., 1998. Adrenocortical and metabolic responses to dobutamine infusion during halothane anaesthesia in ponies. J Vet Pharmacol Ther 21, 282–287.
Taylor, P.M., Clarke, K.W., 2007. Handbook of Equine Anaesthesia. Saunders, Elsevier, Edinburgh, pp. 134.
Thurmon, J.C., Neff-Davis, C., Davis, L.E., et al., 1982. Xylazine hydrochloride-induced hyperglycemia and hypoinsulinemia in thoroughbred horses. J Vet Pharmacol Ther 5, 241–245.
Tinkler, M.K., White, N.A., Lessard, P., et al, 1997. Prospective study of equine colic risk factors. Equine Vet J 29, 454–458.
Toth, F., Frank, N., Elliott, S.B., et al., 2008. Effects of intravenous endotoxin challenge on glucose and insulin dynamics in horses. Am J Vet Res 69, 82–88.
Traynor, C., Hall, G.M., 1981. Endocrine and metabolic changes during surgery: anaesthetic implications. Br J Anaesth 53, 153–160.
Van den Velden, M.A., Klein, W.R., 1993. The effects of cisapride on the restoration of gut motility after surgery of the small intestine in horses: a clinical trial. Vet Quarterly 15, 175–179.
Van der Hulst, R.R., von Meyenfeldt, M.F., van Kreel, B.K., et al, 1998. Gut permeability, intestinal morphology, and nutritional depletion. Nutrition 14, 1–6.
Veterans Affairs Total Parenteral Nutrition Cooperative Study Group, 1991. Perioperative total parenteral nutrition in surgical patients. N Engl J Med 325, 525–532.
Wagner, A.E., 2009. Stress associated with anesthesia and surgery. In: Muir, W.W., Hubbell, J.A.E. (Eds.), Equine Anesthesia. Monitoring and Emergency Therapy. second ed. Saunders, Elsevier, St.Louis, pp. 101–108.
Wagner, A.E., Bednarski, R.M., Muir, W.W., 1990. Hemodynamic effects of carbon dioxide during intermittent positive-pressure ventilation in horses. Am J Vet Res 51, 1922–1929.
Weismann, C., 1990. The metabolic response to stress: an overview and update. Anesthesiology 73, 308–327.
Woods, J.H., Erikson, L.W., Condon, R.E., et al., 1978. Postoperative ileus: a colonic problem? Surgery 84, 527–533.
White, N.A., 2009. Colic treatment and post-colic nutrition. In: Pagan, J.D. (Eds.), Advances in Equine Nutrition IV. Nottingham University Press, Nottingham, pp. 327–345.
Zaloga, G., Marik, P., 2001. Hypothalamic-pituitary-adrenal insufficiency. Crit Care Clin 17, 25–41.
Zhou, T., Wu, X.T., Zhou, Y.J., et al., 2006. Early removing gastrointestinal decompression and early oral feeding improve patient's rehabilitation after colorectostomy. World J Gastroenterol 12, 2459–2463.

40

Feeding orphan and sick foals

Sarah J. Stoneham

Introduction

It is essential to understand the nutrition of the healthy neonatal foal in order to manage the nutrition of a neonate compromised either by disease or loss of the dam. For the purposes of this chapter the foal under a month of age will be discussed.

The neonatal foal has a high metabolic rate and low hepatic glycogen reserves that only last a few hours (Ousey 2003). Newborn foals are dependent on frequent ingestion of good quality colostrum and then milk. Foals that fail to nurse even for a few hours will rapidly become hypoglycemic, hypovolemic, hypothermic and start to break down body tissue to meet their metabolic needs. During the first week of life, healthy foals suckle five to seven times per hour with each bout lasting just under 2 minutes (Carson & Wood Gush 1983). Over the first month of life, the frequency and duration of the suckling bouts decreases as the foals suckle more efficiently.

Ingestion of adequate quantities of good quality colostrum within the first few hours of life is essential for transfer of maternally derived immunoglobulins (*transfer of passive immunity*). Thoroughbred mares produce an average of 1–2 liters of colostrum. For maximum efficiency of this specialized but short-lived process for transfer of colostral antibodies, foals should ingest colostrum within 4 hours of birth. Colostrum provides immunoglobulins, complement, lysozyme and lactoferrin and large numbers of B-lymphocytes that are essential for the development of the foal's immune system. It also contains growth factors and hormones important for development and maturation of the gastrointestinal tract. Ingestion of the non-nutrient factors in colostrum plays a vital role in the preparation of the gut of the newborn foal for digestion of enteral feed (Ousey 2006).

During the first 24 hours post partum foals consume about 15% of their bodyweight as milk (8 liters for a 50-kg foal); this increases to 12–15 liters by the end of the first week of life (Ousey et al 1996). The first month of life is a period of very rapid growth. Thoroughbred foals gain 1.5–2 kg/day (Jelan et al 1996, Martin Rosset & Young 2007), and most Thoroughbred foals will have doubled their birthweight by a month of age. Growth rate in healthy foals is breed, age and month of birth dependent (Chapter 12 provides data on normal growth rates of foals).

From about 2 days of age foals begin nibbling feed, grass and hay copying the feeding behavior of the dam. They start being able to digest solid feed from about 3 weeks of age. Levels of lactase and cellobiase increase in the fetus until birth (Roberts 1975) and then steadily decline from 4 months of age reflecting the change in the foal's nutrient sources. Hind gut fermentation is not fully established until foals are 3–4 months of age.

It is well established that in order to produce a sound, healthy athlete a smooth growth curve should be maintained rather than periods of restriction and compensatory growth. Although moderate restriction in growth can be compensated for to some extent, capacity for compensation decreases with age. In general, differences in growth rates have little influence on mature size after the rapid neonatal growth phase is completed (Martin Rosset 2005). The reader is referred elsewhere in this book for a more complete discussion on foal growth and development (Chapter 12).

The orphan foal

The management of an orphan foal will depend on the age at which the foal loses its dam. In the author's experience foals <2 months of age require a milk -based diet in order to maintain a satisfactory growth curve. The older the foal, the smaller the proportion of milk required in the diet.

The author considers fostering to a nurse mare to be the best option for foals less than 6–8 weeks of age. Although this option may be considered labour intensive and expensive initially, it is likely to provide the most satisfactory outcome for the foal in the long term.

Short-term options

The most common causes of orphan foals are death of the mare, rejection by the mare or persistent agalactica. The situation is often sudden and, for non-professionals, unexpected so they are frequently unprepared. Good short-term management of the nutritional needs of the foal will allow time for the best long term option to be put in place.

What to feed

First, in newborn foals it is important to ensure ingestion of adequate quantities of good quality colostrum. In foals >18 hours of age, blood samples should be taken to determine immunoglobulin G concentrations. Mare milk replacers are available worldwide and are preferred when mare's milk is

Table 40-1 Comparison of the Energy (Digestible Energy [DE]) and Nutrient Composition of Mare's Milk First Month of Lactation with Alternatives on As Fed Basis (Lucas 1991; Jennifer Ousey, Personal Communication)

	Protein g/100 ml	Fat g/100 ml	Ca:P	Lactose g/100 ml	Gross DE MJ/l
Mares' milk (early lactation)	3.3	2.9	1.7:1	6.9	2.4
Goats' milk	3.8	4.4	1.2:1	4.9	2.5
Cows' milk	3.3	3.7	1.28:1	4.8	2.5
Mare milk replacer (average)	3.1	1.7		7.1	3.07–3.84

not available. If mare milk replacers are not immediately available, either unmodified goat milk or semi skimmed (2% fat) cow milk with 20 g/l of dextrose added can be used. Sugar (sucrose) should not be used as young foals lack the enzymes to digest sucrose (Table 40-1).

How to feed

Ousey (1999, 2003) recommends that foals under 2 days of age are fed hourly, then every 2 hours for a further 12 days, after which there should be a gradual decrease in the frequency and increase in the volume fed such that by 8 weeks of age the foal is receiving four feeds daily.

Once healthy foals have got used to milk replacer appetite tends to be greater than requirements and foals fed ad libitum tend to have excessive daily weight gain.

In the authors' experience, an average daily gain (ADG) >2 kg/day is excessive for a Thoroughbred foal up to 30 days of age (see Chapter 12). For other breeds, data on ADG should be consulted. Farm-specific data on foal growth rates provides the best guide. Alternatively, many international feed companies are able to provide optimum growth curves for various breeds. To avoid excessive or erratic growth rate, the foal should be weighed at least weekly, with feeding rates adjusted as needed.

Mare milk replacer prepared per manufacturer's instructions tends to have a higher energy density than mare's milk, so smaller volumes are required than would be the case for a foal suckling from its dam. Feeding a more dilute milk replacer solution at higher volume than recommended during the initial few days will help the orphan foal adapt to milk replacer. The author usually reduces the quantity of milk powder added to each liter of water by about 25% and increases the volume fed each day by the same percentage. Over the course of several days these dilutions and volumes can be changed in line with manufacturer's recommendations. Alternatively it can be made up to provide an energy density similar to that of mare's milk (2.13 MJ/l).

Foals digest mare's milk very efficiently (e.g. gross energy [GE] digestibility of 97–99%). However, GE digestibility is lower (approximately 90%) for the first few days of feeding when foals are provided mare milk replacer (Ousey 2006).

Fostering

Foster mares provide the ideal solution for an orphan foal. However, there are several things to consider in selecting a potential foster mare:

- Temperament – it is important that there is no risk of injury to the foal or personnel;
- Disease risk – the mare should be screened for risk of EHV 1, strangles and other infectious disease; and
- Stage of lactation – if there is a significant disparity between the stage of lactation and foal age it may be necessary to consider mineral supplementation as milk mineral levels change throughout lactation.

Fostering is a labour intensive process that may take several days. It is most likely to succeed with experienced, patient and confident personnel. Successful fostering usually requires someone to be with or close to the mare and foal at all times during the first 1–2 days. The use of a fostering crate or gate will allow the foal to be left unattended with the mare. However, the foal should remain under observation with someone available to quickly intervene if necessary.

There are several techniques for fostering foals that depend on personal experience. Some tips that the author has found useful include:

1. Withhold milk from the foal for 1–2 hours prior to introduction to the foster mare.
2. Use sedation for the mare.
3. Ensure the mare has easy access to a plentiful supply of hay/feed and water.
4. Have plenty of assistance available when the foal is first introduced to the mare.
5. In some cases carefully fitted hobbles may be helpful.
6. Strip the mare's udder and cover the foal with her milk.
7. Don't allow the mare to sniff the foal until a bond is established.
8. Take the mare outside to hand graze her with the foal close by.

Kelly (1999) provides further details of fostering techniques.

Hand rearing

If a suitable foster mare is not available, foals can be successfully hand reared. Although foals reared on milk replacer or goat's milk grow and develop satisfactorily, long-term behavioural problems can develop unless they are carefully managed.

Manufacturers of mare milk replacer provide guidelines on quantities of milk to be fed. With newborn foals it is sensible to gradually increase the quantities fed over the first few days and follow directions regarding the concentration of replacer used. Naylor and Bell (1985) suggest that milk replacer should be fed at 10–15% dilution which is greater than recommended by some manufacturers, although over the last few years, manufacturer's recommendations have changed to be more in line with this recommendation.

It is important to maintain high standards of hygiene with the preparation of the milk, and utensils used for preparation and feeding. Any unused prepared milk should be stored in a refrigerator until the next feed.

It is preferable to teach the foal to drink from a bucket so that the milk can be put in the stable and the foal left to feed. This minimizes the association between feeding and the handlers. It is preferable for the foal to drink smaller quantities at frequent intervals rather than fewer large feeds, which are more likely to overwhelm the digestive system. Episodes of feeding-associated diarrhea are common as the foal's digestive system adapts to mare milk replacer. The use of probiotics can be helpful.

Little evidence on the efficacy of probiotics for treatment or prevention of on infectious diarrhea is available. The author prefers preparations made specifically for horses but does not recommend probiotics for use in foals under 24 hours of age or in foals with compromise to the integrity of the mucosal barrier of the gastrointestinal tract. If an episode of diarrhea persists, reducing the concentration of milk replacer may help in some instances. However it is important not to overlook other possible causes of diarrhea.

Foal creep rations designed for use in foals under 3 months of age are available. These feeds are designed to be readily digested by young foals with immature hindgut fermentative capacity and usually contain a significant proportion of milk pellets. These can be introduced from a few days of age. Manufacturers' recommendations should be followed; however a rule of thumb for feeding concentrates to foals is 450 g per day per month of age up to a maximum of 3 kg per day. It is recommended to consult with an equine nutritionist when these feeds are used to ensure appropriate nutrition.

Fresh, clean water should always be available together with grass and/or good quality hay. In the author's experience, haylage feeding can induce diarrhea in younger foals.

Exercise is extremely important in the development of a sound healthy individual and therefore it is important to ensure that orphan foals receive adequate exercise. Some owners prefer to manage these foals in a stable with no turnout, a practice that should be discouraged. If a paddock is unavailable a large barn may be suitable providing there is a suitable footing and dust levels are not excessive.

Orphan foals often become excessively "humanized"; this usually results in serious behavioral problems as the foal matures. Orphan foals should be treated in the same way as foals with their dams, and the company of humans must not replace that of horses.

The author considers it essential that orphan's foals be provided an equine companion without delay. An old, quiet pony mare or gelding is a suitable companion. The foal and companion can be turned out together once acquainted and, when housed (e.g., in a stall), a partition can allow them to be fed separately yet maintain social contact. With an older foal it may be possible to keep them with the group of mares and foals they had previously been with if weaning from the paddock has started. However the safety of this will depend on the temperament of the orphan and others in the group.

Gastric ulcer syndrome

Although the use of prophylactic antiulcer medication in sick neonatal foals remains controversial the author routinely uses prophylactic antiulcer medication in orphan foals. Whether the foal is fostered or hand reared, the loss of the mother and changes in management for the young foal are undoubtedly stressful. The choice of drug will depend on age of foal, assessment of risk and licensed products available to the clinician. The most commonly used drugs are omeprazole, ranitidine and sucralfate.

Monitoring growth and development

It is important to monitor weight and height regularly and compare to standard growth curves for breed and sex. The use of condition scoring is also a useful technique. Similar growth curves can be expected for hand-reared foals to those reared on mares (Cymbaluk et al 1993). However in the author's experience it is a common complication for inexperienced personnel to feed hand-reared foals to appetite, which tends to produce excessive growth rates and associated problems (e.g., physitis). As mentioned, it is important to adjust feeding in accordance with growth rate.

One study found that fostered Thoroughbred foals grew more rapidly than those reared on their dams by 0.0366 kg/day. The authors suggested that the nurse mares (e.g., part and pure bred Tennessee Walkers) are selected for their mothering and milk producing ability, whereas Thoroughbred dams are selected on race performance (Willard et al 2005). In the UK, cobs or larger ponies are most commonly used as foster mares, selected principally for placid temperament and mothering ability.

Key Points – Feeding orphan foals

- Plan short-term feeding for the orphan foal, considering:
  - Colostrum for foals under 18 hours of age
  - Mare milk replacer or goats milk
  - Frequency and quantity of feeding are age dependent
- Fostering vs. hand rearing
  - Fostering is preferable and the most cost-effective
- Hand rearing
  - Avoid humanization
  - Calculate nutritional/feed requirements
- Monitor growth and development

Sick neonatal foals

Requirements of the sick neonatal foal

Healthy foals aged 1–4 days spend approximately 12 hours standing and active, increasing to nearly 14 hours per day by day 7, whereas sick foals are often recumbent for much of the time. This behavioral difference reduces energy expenditure by approximately two thirds. On the other hand, environmental temperatures below the lower critical temperature (24°C in sick foals) will increase metabolic rate and so can increase energy requirements for maintenance (Ousey 1997, Ousey et al 1997).

Although studies on the requirements of sick foals are sparse, research suggests that the energy requirements of sick neonatal foals are considerably less than their healthy counterparts. Studies of immature foals and foals with perinatal asphyxia syndrome showed they have a lower metabolic rate, requiring only 260–290 kJ/kg/day (13–14.5 MJ/day for a 50 kg foal) compared to 540–600 kJ/kg/day for healthy foals (Ousey et al 1996, Ousey 2003).

A recent study using indirect calorimetry in sick foals reported energy requirements of approximately 188 kJ/kg/day (Paradis 2001). Historically, it was thought that conditions such as sepsis and systemic inflammatory response syndrome (SIRS) in young as well as mature patients produced a hypermetabolic state and therefore increased energy requirements. However, recent studies (Taylor et al 2003, Turi et al 2001) in children have refuted this theory, finding that children do not become hypermetabolic during critical illness. Turi et al (2001) speculated that this is due to diversion of energy for growth into the recovery process.

Recent studies in humans having found that the overfeeding of critically ill patients has an adverse affect on outcome (Dandona et al 2005). Similarly, McKenzie & Geor (2009) have suggested a conservative approach to calorie provision for sick neonatal foals. Providing excess carbohydrate can result in hyperglycemia, which may increase production of proinflammatory cytokines and increase production of CO_2, which can worsen hypercapnia in foals with respiratory compromise. Excessive dietary protein increases protein catabolism which can produce azotemia, while excessive feeding of lipids results in hypertriglyceridemia. One study reported that triglyceride concentrations >200 mg/l (>2.25 mmol/l) were associated with non-survival in neonatal foals receiving parenteral nutrition (Myers et al 2009).

Mare's milk has high carbohydrate (lactose) content. Insulin secreted by the beta cells in the pancreas is essential for regulation and homeostasis of blood glucose in the face of high carbohydrate intake. Maturation of beta cells in the pancreas occurs very late in gestation and is dependent on the prepartum cortisol surge which prepares the fetus for birth in the few days before parturition (Holdstock et al 2004, Fowden et al 2005).

Foals that have not been subjected to this cortisol surge often exhibit insulin resistance and have poor regulation of blood glucose concentrations (e.g., premature/dysmature foals, foals delivered by early caesarean section). Various disease processes such as sepsis can also result in a degree of insulin resistance or low levels of insulin secretion.

Buechner-Maxwell and Thatcher (2004) have suggested that crude protein requirements for neonates are 4–6 g protein/100 non-protein calories. However, other authors have recommended a lower protein requirement (2–5 g/kg/day) for foals with normal plasma protein concentrations, and a higher rate of provision (6.5 g/kg/day) for sick neonates that are hypoproteinemic (Stratton-Phelps 2008). The criteria for diagnosis of hypoproteinemia will depend on factors such as foal age, disease process, and laboratory reference ranges.

It is important not to overlook the intake of colostrum by newborn foals. In foals <18–24 hours old, the mechanism for transfer of immunoglobulins across the small intestine may still be operational. Each case must be evaluated as to whether enteral supplementation with high quality colostrum may be appropriate. After 24 hours of age supplementation via the enteral route is no longer indicated.

Neonatal diseases that affect gastrointestinal function

Immaturity

Development of the gastrointestinal tract may be affected by prematurity or intrauterine growth retardation (IUGR). Wang et al. (2005) have shown that IUGR significantly alters intestinal growth and morphology, and endocrine homeostasis in piglets; this in turn contributes to lower growth rates. The lack of maturity of the beta cells in the pancreas often results in insulin resistance and hyperglycemia.

Many immature foals are unable to digest milk and, if fed enterally, will develop ileus, gastric distension and colic. Gastric distension will increase pressure on the diaphragm and compromise respiratory function.

It is advisable to avoid enteral nutrition until normal progressive gut sounds are audible and meconium is being passed; there should be no evidence of abdominal distension or gastric reflux. Even if enteral feeding is considered inappropriate, small volumes of colostrum 5–10 ml/h (or mare's milk if no colostrum is available) are important in furthering gastrointestinal growth and maturation.

Perinatal asphyxia syndrome (PAS)

Perinatal hypoxia tends to affect the organs of high blood flow (i.e. central nervous system, kidney, and gut). So, as with immature foals, the enteral route should only be used once normal gut function has been confirmed. One should be cautious about allowing these foals to suck a bottle or the mare as the suck reflex is frequently affected. Therefore, although they may be keen to nurse, if the suckle reflex is poorly coordinated there is increased risk for development of aspiration pneumonia. In these cases, if enteral feeding is appropriate, a bowl, bucket or indwelling feeding tube should be used.

Sepsis/septic shock

Neonatal foals in septic shock are usually not nursing and rapidly become recumbent. These foals often have unstable blood pressure and blood glucose concentrations. In the author's experience, caution with enteral feeding is advisable until the foal has been stabilized and started to recover. These foals may develop stress induced hyperglycemia. Acute illness can result in insulin resistance, hyperglycemia and glucose intolerance. The mechanism of this insulin resistance has not been elucidated but the counter regulatory hormones (e.g., catecholamines, cortisol, glucagons, and growth hormone) are likely involved. Proinflammatory cytokines stimulate release of these counter regulatory hormones. Insulin receptor signaling is also affected in sepsis (Van den Berghe 2004). Hyperglycemia may further increase production of proinflammatory cytokines.

Colic/enterocolitis/ileus

Colic in the neonatal foal can be either medical or surgical. It is important to determine the likely cause prior to deciding the most appropriate route of feeding. In most cases the foal will be either partially or completely "off suck". Enteral feeding is usually contraindicated when there is an obstruction of the gut. The exception to this is meconium retention; the author has found that provided there is not marked abdominal distension or ileus, suckling from the mare is not contraindicated. However if the foal is "off suck" enteral feeding should be withheld. Enteral feeding also is contraindicated when ileus is detected, as it is likely to worsen the condition.

In young foals with severe enterocolitis a period of enteral rest is often required and parenteral nutrition should be instituted early in the course of the condition. The disease process often produces a marked hypoproteinemia in these foals.

However the benefits of milk, which provides some protection against infection by enhancing mucosal immunity and some protection against gastric ulceration, should not be overlooked. Therefore, consideration should be given to small-volume milk feedings, with close monitoring of gastrointestinal indicators of intolerance.

Lactose intolerance

Lactose intolerance is a recognized cause of diarrhea in the foal. It is most commonly seen as a secondary intolerance associated with Rotavirus infection. Foals can develop secondary intolerance following any disease affecting the small intestine and it has been recognized as a cause of persistent diarrhea following infection with *Clostridium difficile*.

Secondary intolerance is usually temporary and resolves once the small intestinal mucosa specifically the lactase producing cells have repaired. It can be treated by the provision of lactase orally (the author uses one or two 125 mg lactase tablets, six to eight times daily, for a 50–70 kg foal).

Key Points – Feeding sick neonatal foals

- Avoid over-feeding. Sick, minimally active foals have lower energy requirements than healthy, active foals
- Consider how the disease process affects gastrointestinal function

Enteral feeding

Enteral feeding is considered preferable to parenteral feeding as it encourages preservation of the gastrointestinal mucosa, encourages development of the gastrointestinal tract and reduces the risk of sepsis related to bacterial translocation (Chandra 1999). However, as discussed above, there are certain conditions when enteral feeding is counterproductive or it is not possible to meet the foal's nutritional requirements via the enteral route.

Assessment of gastrointestinal function

To determine whether enteral feeding is appropriate (Box 40.1) for a particular foal a careful assessment of the gastrointestinal tract should be made.

Box 40.1 When to Avoid Enteral Feeding

1. Gastric reflux
2. Absence or decreasing progressive gut sounds
3. Increasing abdominal distension
4. Evidence on ultrasound of gastric distension or ileus
5. Suspicion of sepsis, septic shock, prematurity or perinatal asphyxia syndrome
6. Colic associated with ileus

Assessment of gastrointestinal function should include:

1. Evaluation of abdominal distension. Serial measurements of abdominal circumference at a specific point can help to make this a more objective assessment.
2. Abdominal auscultation, systematic auscultation of gut sounds.
3. Check for gastric reflux.
4. Check for the passage of meconium/milk feces as appropriate.
5. Ultrasound evaluation of the abdomen may be helpful in assessing gastric emptying and development of ileus.

These factors combined with the stability of the foal's clinical condition will help determine whether the foal is likely to tolerate enteral feeding. When selecting the most appropriate feeding regimen for a foal it is important to consider the effect various disease processes may have on gastrointestinal function as inappropriate feeding can prolong recovery or produce further problems such as ileus, colic, unstable blood glucose concentrations, all of which may worsen the prognosis for the foal.

What to feed

Mare's milk provides trophic substances for normal growth and development of the gastrointestinal tract, the physiological stimulus for metabolic regulation, and helps to maintain mucosal integrity (Ousey 1999). It is also efficiently digested. This makes it the best source of nutrition for enteral feeding. It is usually possible to obtain milk from the dam if she is available. Alternatively, previously frozen donor mare's milk can be used. It is important to pay attention to hygiene when collecting and storing mare's milk for feeding sick foals as they are highly susceptible to infection.

If no mare's milk is available, either goat's milk, mare milk replacer or 2% cow milk (with 20 g/l dextrose added) can be used, as previously discussed. If mare's milk replacer is to be used the author has found it preferable to feed it at a reduced concentration and gradually increase the strength over several days.

Enteral feeding of sick foals

It is important to carefully assess the strength and coordination of the suckle reflex, and only if these are normal should a sick foal be allowed to nurse (from a mare or nipple bottle). The author prefers that inexperienced carers feed the foal via a bowl rather than a nipple bottle. It takes only a little patience and encouragement for most foals to feed from a bowl and subsequently a bucket.

If the suck reflex is weak or poorly coordinated the use of an indwelling feeding tube (14 French 130 cm, Mila International) is preferred. The use of an indwelling tube allows the foal to be fed smaller volumes more frequently, rather than overwhelming the digestive system with large bolus feeds necessitated by repeated passage of a larger bore nasogastric tube.

When placing a feeding tube, it is important to be well prepared with all the necessary equipment on-hand. The foal should be adequately restrained, either standing or in sternal recumbency. Due to the narrow gauge of the tube there is no cough reflex if the tube is placed in the trachea. In many foals the tube can be palpated in the esophagus

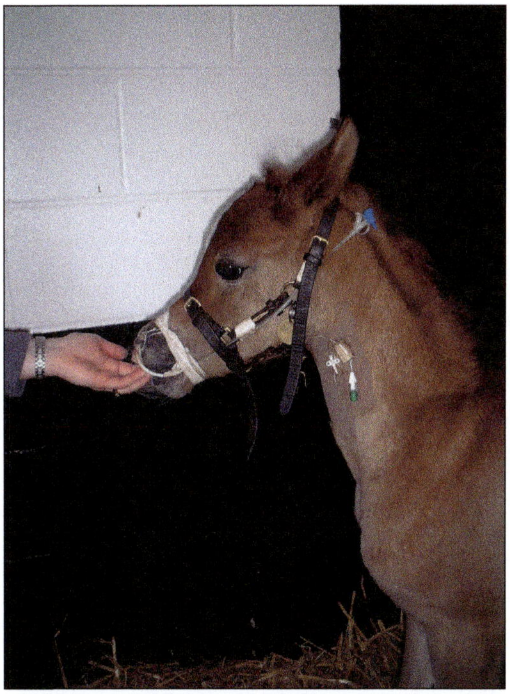

Figure 40.1 **A neonatal foal with a small bore, indwelling feeding tube (14 French 130 cm, Mila International,) placed via the left nostril. The tube is sutured to the nostril and then taped to the halter/head collar.**

(which is often mobile in the young foal). However, if in doubt, radiography or endoscopy can confirm correct placement of the tube in the esophagus. The author favours placement to the distal esophagus rather than into the stomach. Once in place the tube may be sutured to the nostril and then taped on to the head or head collar (see Fig. 40.1).

The feeding tube should be replaced daily and high standards of hygiene maintained during feeding. This is particularly important as these foals are often receiving medication for prevention of gastric ulceration, which will increase gastric pH (low gastric pH is one of the important defence mechanisms against infection of the gastrointestinal tract). The feeding tube should be plugged to avoid aspiration of air into the stomach.

It is important to explain the feeding protocol to carers. Before feeding it is critical to check that the tube is still in place and there is no reflux. Milk should be delivered by gravity flow and a small amount of water should be administered at the end of feeding to clear the tube. It is essential that the foal is in sternal recumbency or standing during the administration of milk. The author prefers the foal to be standing for feeding as soon as it is possible.

How much to feed

When starting to feed a sick newborn foal with milk, a rate of 2 ml/kg/h is a reasonable starting point; if this amount is well tolerated the feeding rate can be slowly increased to 4 ml/kg/h over the first day. Over the next 5 or so days, the feeding rate can be increased gradually to normal intake of approximately 23% body weight. The rate of increase should be based on clinical assessment of each individual case. It is important to continually monitor gastrointestinal function by assessment of abdominal distension, passage of feces, gastric reflux and abdominal auscultation.

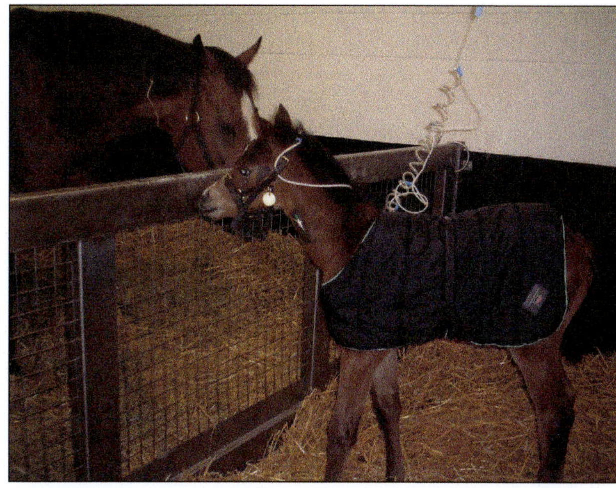

Figure 40.2 **Use of a partition within a box stall allows maintenance of the mare–foal bond even in situations where the sick foal is not feeding from the mare.**

The indwelling feeding tube does not interfere with development of the suckle reflex and can be left in place until the foal is sucking normally from the mare.

Mare management

If the foal is not nursing from the mare (or nursing activity is decreased), it is important to take care of the mare's udder. If left, mares may stop lactating or develop mastitis rapidly. The mare should be milked every 2–3 hours; if the milk is to be stored the udder should be clean, and a clean container used for the collection of milk. It is also important that the person milking the mare washes their hands prior to milking. The milk should then be frozen or stored in a fridge immediately. Some mares may require small doses of oxytocin to encourage milk let down (0.5 IU of oxytocin given IV or IM is usually sufficient). Nutrition of the mare should be appropriate to the stage of lactation to encourage milk production such that the nutritional demands of the foal can be met as it recovers. It is also important whenever possible to maintain the mare-foal bond even in situations where the sick foal is not feeding from the mare (see Fig. 40.2).

Key Points – Enteral feeding

- Confirm that gastrointestinal function is not compromised
- Reassess gastrointestinal function regularly
- Mare's milk is the most appropriate feed
- Feed by bowl or indwelling tube
- Start at a rate of 2 ml/kg/hr and gradually increase
- Take care of the mare's udder

Parenteral nutrition

There have been considerable advances in the use of parenteral nutrition in sick neonatal foals and it has increasingly become accepted as an integral part of treatment in foals where the nutritional needs of the foal cannot be met via the enteral route. It is generally accepted that neonatal foals can be maintained on dextrose solutions for 12–24 hours but foals requiring parenteral nutrition for 24 hours or more require amino acids, dextrose, and in most cases, lipids. The use of lipid containing solutions increases the cost of therapy but allows calorie density of the solutions to be increased and it is easier to maintain blood glucose concentrations within the normal range (4–9 mmol/l).

The advent of simple formulations (Hansen 1990, McKenzie & Geor 2009) has made the use of parenteral nutrition more feasible in clinical practice. In both human and equine neonatal medicine the importance of minimal enteral feeding of newborn patients receiving parenteral nutrition is well recognized. The importance of hormones, growth factors and other substance found in milk in the normal development of the gastrointestinal tract of the newborn has already been discussed. In practical terms this means providing 5–10 ml/foal/h of fresh mare's milk via an enteral feeding tube.

Formulation

There are four possible approaches to formulation of parenteral nutrition solutions:

1. The relatively simple formulation based on recommendations by Hansen (1990) which has been used in Newmarket. Although Hansen (1990) describes three levels of formulation the author has found the starting level (see Example 1) to be practical in the short and medium term. It aims to provide glucose at a rate similar to that provided to the fetus in late gestation by placental blood flow. This formula is suitable for most cases, although individuals with severe hypoproteinemia may benefit from an increase in amino acid provision to 3–4 g/kg/day.

Example 1: Parenteral nutrition regimen for 50-kg foal using day 1 formula (Hansen 1990, Ousey 2003)

Glucose 10 g/kg/day = 500 g = 1000 ml 50% glucose (provides 7 mg/kg/min)

Amino acids 2 g/kg/day = 100 g = 1176 ml of 8.5% amino acid solution

Lipds 1 g/kg/day = 50 g = 500 ml 10% lipids

Total volume = 2676 ml

Total 2675 ml/24 h = 111 ml /h

Provides 54 kcal/kg/day

Provided there are no additional losses neonatal foals have a fluid requirement of 4–5 ml/kg/h so a 50-kg foal requires a total of 4.8–6 liters of fluid in 24 hours. Therefore, additional isotonic fluid will be required. Plasma, and fluids used in drug administration should be included in calculation of total fluids administered each day. The addition of isotonic fluids will reduce the hypertonicity of the parenteral nutrition mix, thereby reducing the risks of endothelial damage.

Start the infusion at a rate of 37 ml/h, If blood glucose remain stable and within the normal range for 4 hours the rate of infusion can be increased to 74 ml/h, and if blood glucose level remains within normal limits for a further 4 hours the rate can be increased to 111 ml/h.

2. Alternatively the more precise requirements of the foal can be calculated. This method has recently been well described (Buechner-Maxwell & Thatcher 2006).

Example 2: Formulation for a 50-kg foal with severe hypoproteinemia (Buechner-Maxwell & Thatcher 2006)

Specific requirements for normoglycemic and hypoproteinemic foals

Step 1: Calculate non-protein energy requirements

30 kcal/kg/day

So 50×30 = 1500 kcal/day

Step 2: Calculate protein requirement and energy generated from protein

This foal is hypoproteinemic so will be given protein at high end of the recommended range

4–6 g/100 non-protein calories

1500 kcal/day × 6 g protein/100 kcal non-protein calories = 90 g protein

Each gram of protein provides 4 kcal DE

So 90×4 = 360 kcal

So total calories 1500+360=1860 kcal

This provides 37.2 kcal/kg/day

Step 3: This foal is normoglycemic so parenteral nutrition can be formulated using 60% glucose and 40% lipids to provide non-protein calories. If the foal was hyperglycemic prior to starting parenteral nutrition, non-protein calories could be provided by 40% glucose and 60% lipids.

So 60% non-protein calories to be provided by glucose

1500 kcal×60%=900 kcal

1 ml of 50% glucose provides 1.7 kcal

900/1.7=530 ml 50% glucose

40% non-protein calories to be provided by lipid

1500 kcal×40%=600 kcal

1 ml 20% lipid provides 2 kcal

600 kcal/2=300 ml 20% lipid

Step 4: Calculate volume of amino acids

90 g protein required

1 ml of 8.5% amino acid solution contains 0.085 g protein

90 g/0.085=1058.8 ml 8.5% amino acid solution

Step 5: So, the parenteral nutrition solution for a 24-hour period comprises:

530 ml 50% glucose

300 ml 20% lipid emulsion

1059 ml 8.5% amino acid solution

Total volume=1889 ml

Step 6: Calculate the glucose concentration 265/1889=14%

265 g glucose in a volume of 1889 ml=14% glucose in TPN solution

Sick foals may be at risk from vascular injury with solutions >10% glucose so the parenteral nutrition solution could be diluted further with isotonic crystalloids to produce a 10% glucose solution

To give a 10% solution total volume would be 2650 ml

So 2650 ml−1889 ml=761 ml isotonic crystalloids required to produce a 10% glucose solution

Step 7: Final infusion rate 2650 ml/24 h=110 ml/h

Step 8: Calculate additional fluids required to meet total daily fluid requirement of foal.

4–5 ml/kg/h =4.8–6 liters

3. McKenzie & Geor (2009) suggest a simplified approach using one of two standard solutions and calculating infusion rate based on meeting caloric requirements of the foal. Formula 1 is most suitable for short-term use and Formula 2, which contains lipids, is more suitable for long-term use.

Example 3a:

Parenteral nutrition for a 50-kg foal with using Formula 1 (no lipids)

Formula 1 (McKenzie & Geor 2009)

1500 ml 50% dextrose

1500 ml 8.5% amino acids

This provides 1.02 kcal/ml

So the caloric requirement for 50-kg foal (40–60 kcal/kg/day) =

50 kg×50 kcal =2500 kcal

24 hour requirement of Formula 1: 2500 kcal/1.02 kcal/ml=2451 ml

So infusion rate 2451 ml/24 h=102 ml/h

Example 3b:

Parenteral nutrition for 50-kg foal using Formula 2

Formula 2 (McKenzie & Geor 2009)

1500 ml 50% dextrose

500 ml 20% lipids

2000 ml 8.5% amino acids

This provides 1.08 kcal/ml

So the caloric requirement of a 50-kg foal (40–60 kcal/kg/day) =

50 kg×50 kcal =2000 kcal/day

24-h requirement of Formula 2: 2500 kcal/1.08 kcal/ml=2315 ml

So the infusion rate = 2315 ml/24 h = 96 ml/h

4. Outside the hospital setting the use of glucose, amino acid and lipid solutions available as a premix (see Tables 40-2 and 40-3) may be useful for providing short-term partial parenteral nutrition. This does not require stocks of all three solutions and appropriate mixing equipment. This approach is practical for foals that are relatively metabolically stable (e.g., those that have had gastrointestinal surgery or those foals that it is not possible to meet their requirements via the enteral routine and require parenteral support to remain in a positive energy balance). The requirements can be calculated using methods in the above examples.

Practical considerations

It is recommended that parenteral nutrition solutions be administered through a dedicated central catheter. Delivery can be via a single or dual lumen catheter. In practical terms, jugular catheters are preferable for the administration of parenteral nutrition solutions in neonatal foals.

Polyurethane catheters should be a minimum of 13–20 cm in length (see Table 40-4). Following aseptic catheter placement, an extension set should be connected to the catheter and the area carefully padded and bandaged. High standards of hygiene are essential when dealing with the catheter and parenteral nutrition solutions as they provide an ideal environment for bacterial contamination. With careful management long term catheters can be left in place for 7–10 days; however infusion sets should be changed every 24 hours.

Solutions should be prepared under aseptic conditions, preferably in a laminar flow hood. The bags containing the solutions should be protected from light as amino acid solutions can be degraded by exposure to light. Parenteral nutrition should be administered via an electric infusion pump and it is essential to deal with any interruptions in flow of the solution as a matter of urgency as the foal will become dependent on a continuous flow of nutrients.

Administration rate

The total amount of parenteral nutrition solution to be administered in 24 hours is calculated and an hourly rate calculated. When starting to administer parenteral nutrition, the author starts at a rate one-third of the final rate and then monitors blood glucose hourly for 3–4 h. If glucose concentration remains within normal limits (4.0–9.0 mmol/l), the rate is increased to two-thirds of final rate and again blood glucose is monitored hourly and if it remains within normal limits the rate is increased again after a further 3–4 h.

Table 40-2 Components for Parenteral Nutrition Solutions Used in Europe

Glucose 50%	Baxter Healthcare, Thetford, UK
Amino acids 15%	Intrafusin22, Fresenius-Kabi AG, Bad Homburg, Germany
Lipids 20% &10%	Intralipid 20% and 10% Fresnius-Kabi AG, Bad Homburg Germany
Mixing bag	Freka-Mix Fresenius Kobi AG, Bad Homburg, Germany

Table 40-3 Constituents of Multi Chamber Parenteral Premix Solutions Available in Europe

	Amino acids	Glucose	Non protein calories	Protein calories	Lipid
Clinimix N920E (Baxter Healthcare)	28 g/l	100 g/l	400 kcal/l	110 kcal/l	0
Kabiven Central (Fresnius-Kabi)	34 g/1026 ml	100 g/1026 ml	800 kcal/1026 ml	100 kcal/1026 ml	40 g/1026 ml

Table 40-4 Catheters Suitable for Long-Term Use in Neonatal Foals

Catheter type	Manufacturer
16 g 13 cm single lumen over needle polyurethane	Mila International, Florence, KY, USA
16 g 20 cm single lumen over the wire polyurethane	Mila International, Florence, KY, USA, Arrow International Inc., Reading PA USA
7fr (14 g/18 g) double lumen over the wire polyurethane	Arrow International Inc., Reading PA, USA

If the foal becomes hyperglycemic the rate of infusion should be reduced and blood glucose monitored. If blood glucose concentrations return to the reference range after 2–3 hours, this infusion rate is continued and increased more slowly. However, if the hyperglycemia persists insulin infusion may be indicated (see section on insulin therapy). Once blood glucose concentrations are stable monitoring interval can be increased to 4–6 hourly.

As the foal recovers there should be a gradual switch from parenteral to enteral nutrition. As enteral feeding is gradually increased, lipids are removed from the parenteral nutrition mix for 12–24 hours after which the infusion rate of the glucose/amino acid mix is halved for a further 12–24 hours. Blood glucose concentrations should be monitored during this weaning period, as there is a risk of hypoglycemia.

Insulin therapy

Hyperglycemia is a relatively common complication of parenteral nutrition often as a result of some degree of insulin resistance, low insulin secretion or stress-induced hyperglycemia. As a result it can be difficult to maintain blood glucose concentrations within an acceptable range (4–9 mmol/l).

If reducing the parenteral nutrition infusion rate by up to 50% fails to reduce blood glucose levels after 2–3 hours the use of continuous-rate insulin infusion should be considered. Once insulin infusion has been started interruption in flow of parenteral nutrition infusion should be considered an emergency as it can result in severe hypoglycemia. There is an approximately 90 minute lag in the response to insulin infusion due to the gradual saturation of cellular insulin receptors (McKenzie & Geor 2009). This must be considered when assessing response to any changes in infusion rate of either insulin or parenteral nutrition solutions.

The literature reports a wide range of starting infusion rates, Stratton-Phelps (2008) recommends starting at 0.01 IU normal human insulin/kg/h, i.e., 5 IU/50 kg/foal/h, whereas McKenzie & Geor (2009) recommend 0.07 IU/kg/h, i.e., 35 IU for a 50 kg foal/h. The author favors starting at the lower rate, unless the hyperglycemia is severe and nonresponsive to reduction in the rate of parenteral nutrition administration, in which case a rate of 0.02 IU/kg/h is used initially.

Blood glucose should be monitored every hour once insulin infusion has started until a steady state has been achieved. If the foal becomes hypoglycemic 0.25–0.5 g/kg of 50% glucose can be administered slowly over about 5 minutes and insulin infusion rate dropped or stopped. Blood glucose should be checked every 30–60 minutes.

Monitoring

Regular close monitoring of the foal is essential to reduce the risk of complications and allow early intervention should any problem occur. The frequency of monitoring can be reduced as the foal becomes stable and is maintained on an unchanged feeding regimen (Box 40.6).

Key Points – Parenteral feeding

- Young foals unable to tolerate enteral feeding for >24 hours should be fed by the parenteral route
- Calculate requirements, formulate parenteral nutrition solution and the rate of administration appropriate to the condition of the foal and the clinical setting
- Use a dedicated catheter, prepare solutions aseptically and use electric infusion pump.
- Monitor foal frequently to avoid common complications

Box 40.6 Clinical Monitoring of Foals Receiving Parenteral Nutrition

1. Blood glucose
   2–6 hourly
2. Urine glucose
   2–6 hourly
3. Serum creatinine
   24–48 hourly
4. Serum proteins
   12–48 hourly
5. Serum electrolytes
   12–24 hourly
6. Serum triglycerides
   24 hourly
7. Lipemia
   24 hourly
8. Bodyweight
   Daily
9. Catheter site
   12 hourly

Complications

Most foals that require parenteral nutrition have multiple problems; many are at "high risk" of developing infection and are metabolically compromised. In a recent review of 45 cases of sick foals under 14 days of age receiving parenteral nutrition. Krause & McKenzie (2007) reported that disease severity was positively associated with complications associated with the administration of parenteral nutrition and their occurrence was also associated with an increased risk of non-survival.

Some of the more commonly seen complications associated with parenteral nutrition include:

1. *Catheter site infection/thrombophlebitis*: Aseptic catheter placement, the use of an extension set, use of a dedicated line either using a dual lumen catheter or a separate catheter help to reduce the risk of infection. The catheter should be checked twice daily. The catheter site should be examined for signs of inflammation, swelling or exudation. Ultrasonography can also be used if a problem is suspected.

2. *Persistent hyperglycemia*: Some degree of insulin resistance is not uncommon in premature and septic foals, perhaps due to immature pancreatic beta cells or stress induced hyperglycemia. A recent study of critically ill neonatal foals reported blood glucose levels >10 mmol/l were associated with non survival to hospital discharge (Hollis et al 2008). Reducing the infusion rate and then increasing it more slowly may overcome the problem, however if hyperglycemia persists the use of insulin infusion should be considered.

    When trying to stabilize blood glucose in these foals it is important to change one element at a time and allow enough time for the change to be effective. A period of 2–3 hours should be allowed for equilibration. So if reducing the infusion rate has failed to reduce blood glucose levels after 2 hours then insulin infusion should be started at 0.01 IU/kg/h and blood glucose monitored for 2–3 hours before any further changes are made. If hyperglycemia persists, either the infusion rate of parenteral nutrition can be further reduced or insulin infusion rate increased. Re-formulation of the nutrition solution using a ratio of 60% lipids to 40% dextrose is another approach to the management of persistent hyperglycemia (see example 2 for calculations).
3. *Hypertriglyceridemia/hyperlipemia*: This is a relatively common complication particularly when high percentages of lipids are included in the mix. If triglyceride levels remain >0.6 mmol/l the amount of lipid in the mix should be reduced, blood glucose should be monitored closely as reducing or removing lipid from the mix can result in less stable blood glucose levels. If triglyceride concentrations are above 5 mmol/l, lipid should be removed from the mix.

References

Buechner-Maxwell, V., Thatcher, C.D., 2004. Parenteral nutrition and the equine patient: Case Presentation. Proc. 22nd ACVIM.

Buechner-Maxwell, V., Thatcher, C.D., 2006. Neonatal Nutrition in Equine Neonatal Medicine A case based Approach, Paradis MR (Ed.). Saunders Elsevier, Philadelphia.

Carson, K., Wood-Gush, D.G.M., 1983. Behaviour of Thoroughbred foals during nursing. Equine Vet J 15, 257–262.

Chandra, R.K., 1999. Nutrition and immunology: from clinic to cellular biology and back again. Proc Nutr Soc 58 (3), 681–683.

Cymbaluk, N.F., Smart, M.E., Bristol, F.M., et al., 1993. Importance of milk replacer intake and composition in rearing orphan foals. Can. Vet J 34, 479–486.

Dandona, P., Mohanty, P., Chaudhuri, A., et al., 2005. Insulin infusion in acute illness. J Clin Invest 115, 2069–2072.

Fowden, A.L., Gardner, D.S., Ousey, J.C., et al., 2005. Maturation of pancreatic beta-cell function in the fetal horse during late gestation. J Endocrinol 186, 467–473.

Hansen, T.O., 1990. Nutritional support: parenteral feeding. In: Koterba, A.M., Drummond, W.H., Kosch, P.C. (Eds.), Equine Clinical Neonatology. Lea & Febiger, Philadelphia.

Holdstock, N.B., Allen, V.L., Bloomfield, M.R., et al., 2004. Development of insulin and proinsulin secretion in newborn pony foals. J Endocrinol 181, 469–476.

Hollis, A.R., Furr, M.O., Magdesian, K.G., et al., 2008. Blood glucose concentrations in critically ill neonatal foals. J Vet Intern Med 22 (5), 1223–1227.

Jelan, Z.A., Jeffcott, L.B., Lundeheim, N., et al., 1996. Growth rates in Thoroughbred foals. Pferdeheilkunde 12 (3), 291–295.

Lucas, D.M., 1991. A role for practical nutrition in the management of developmental orthopaedic disease. Equine Vet Educ 3, 76–79.

Kelly, A.J., 1999. Practical tips on fostering. Proc. BEVA specialist days on behaviour and nutrition.

Krause, J.B., McKenzie, H.C., 2007. Parenteral nutrition in foals: a retrospective study of 45 cases (2000–2004). Equine Vet J 39 (1), 74–78.

Martin-Rosset, W., 2005. Growth and development in the equine EAAP no. 114 p5–21. Wageningen Academic Pub.

Martin-Rosset, W., Young, B., 2007. Energy and protein requirements and feeding of the suckling foal, EAAP no 120. Wageningen Academic Publishers, Wageningen, pp. 221–243.

McKenzie, H.C., Geor, R.J., 2009. Feeding management of sick neonatal foals. Vet Clinics N Am. Equine 25, 93–108.

Myers, C.J., Magdesian, K.G., Kass, P.H., et al., 2009. Parenteral nutrition in neonatal foals: clinical description, complications and outcomes in 53 foals (1995–2005). Vet J 181 (2), 137–144.

Naylor, J.M., Bell, R., 1985. Raising the orphan foal. Vet Clin N Am: Equine Pract 1, 169–178.

Ousey, J.C., 1997. Thermoregulation and the energy requirement of the newborn foal, with reference to prematurity. Equine Vet J Suppl 24, 104–108.

Ousey, J.C., 1999. How to feed the sick foal. Proc. BEVA specialist days on behaviour and nutrition.

Ousey, J.C., 2003. Feeding the newborn foal in health and disease. Equine Vet Educ Manual 6, 50–54.

Ousey, J.C., 2006. Physiology and metabolism in the newborn foal with reference to orphaned and sick foals, EAAP no 120. Wageningen Academic Publishers, Wageningen, pp. 187–201.

Ousey, J.C., Holdstock, N., Rossdale, P.D., et al., 1996. How much energy do sick neonatal foals require compared with healthy foals? Pferdeheilkunde 12 (3), 231–237.

Ousey, J.C., Prandi, S., Zimmer, J., et al., 1997. Effects of various feeding regimens on the energy balance of equine neonates. Am J Vet Res 58 (11), 1243–1251.

Paradis, M.R., 2001. Nutrition and indirect calorimetry in neonatal foals. Proc 19th ACVIM Denver, CO, 19, 245.

Roberts, M.C., 1975. The development and distribution of mucosal enzymes in the small intestine of the fetus and young foal. J Reprod Fert Suppl 23, 717–723.

Stratton-Phelps, M., 2008. Nutritional management of the hospitalised horse. The Equine Hospital Manual. Blackwell Publishing, pp. 261–311.

Taylor, R.M., Cheeseman, P., Preedy, V., et al., 2003. Can energy expenditure be predicted in critically ill children? Pediatr Crit Care Med 4, 176–180.

Turi, R.A., Petros, A.J., Eaton, S., et al., 2001. Energy metabolism of infants and children with systemic inflammatory response syndrome and sepsis. Ann Surg 233 (4), 581–587.

Van den Berghe, G., 2004. How does blood glucose control with insulin save lives in intensive care? J Clin Invest 144 (9), 1187–1195.

Wang, T., Huo, Y.J., Shi, F., et al., 2005. Effects of intrauterine growth retardation on development of the gastrointestinal tract in neonatal pigs. Biol Neonate 88, 66–72.

Willard, J.G., Williams, J.L., Willard, J.C., et al., 2005. The effect of age of dam on birth weight and growth of Thoroughbred foals. The growing horse: nutrition and prevention of growth disorders, EAAP No 14. Wageningen Academic Publishers, Wageningen, pp. 65–66.

41

SECTION E Clinical Nutrition

Assisted enteral and parenteral feeding

Elizabeth A. Carr

Introduction

The field of equine critical care has made many advances in the last few decades. Equine intensive care facilities are common in most referral hospitals and early recognition of disease coupled with more proactive and intensive therapy has resulted in increased success rates in the treatment of many surgical and medical diseases. Despite the significant changes in the way we approach the treatment of critical illness it is still relatively uncommon that we consider the nutritional status of the patient in our initial therapeutic plan. The nutritional status of a human prior to hospitalization, as well as early nutritional intervention during hospitalization, has clearly been linked to morbidity and mortality (Robert & Zaloga 2000, Ward 2003). Malnutrition has been shown to negatively impact survival, immune function, wound healing, and gastrointestinal function in humans as well as in animal models and most likely negatively affects numerous other processes (Keusch 2003, Robert & Zaloga 2000, Schroeder et al 1991, Studley 1936, Windsor & Hill 1988). Early nutritional intervention, whether by enteral or parenteral feeding, has been shown to improve measured outcomes in multiple human and animal studies. Unfortunately, it can be difficult to assess nutritional status of a horse prior to admission as information regarding intake and previous body condition may be lacking. However, a poor body condition or a history of recent weight loss can be indicators of inadequate nutritional intake. Despite the lack of data in the equine field, extrapolation from human medicine would strongly suggest that early nutritional support would likely decrease morbidity and mortality and improve long term recovery in the equine patient as well. This chapter discusses the metabolic consequences of food deprivation, the pathologic metabolic responses seen with illness, and the indications for, as well as the types of nutritional supplementation. Nutritional requirements will be mentioned when different from those of normal horses. Otherwise the reader is directed to other chapters in this book for more specific information on the core nutritional needs in the horse.

Effects of feed deprivation

Protein/calorie malnutrition

The average, healthy adult horse can apparently tolerate food deprivation (protein/calorie malnutrition (PCM) or simple starvation) for 24 to 72 hours with few systemic effects. The following description of metabolic alterations during starvation is derived from research in humans or other species unless otherwise stated. A decline in blood glucose concentration can occur with feed deprivation. Insulin concentrations decrease and energy demands are initially met via glycogenolysis resulting in an increase in the breakdown of liver glycogen stores. During the first hours to days of starvation glycogen stores are mobilized from various tissues (liver, kidney, muscle) for glucose production. Lipid mobilization is triggered by alterations in insulin/glucagon levels and the activity of hormone sensitive lipase. As glucose becomes limiting many body tissues begin to rely on fatty acid oxidation and the production of ketone bodies as energy sources. Glycerol produced from lipid degradation, lactate from the Krebs cycle and amino acids provided from muscle tissue breakdown continue to be utilized for gluconeogenesis to provide energy to glucose dependent tissues (central nervous system and red blood cells). This response to starvation correlates with an increase in circulating levels of growth hormone, glucagon, epinephrine, leptin and cortisol and a decrease in insulin and thyroid hormones. These hormone fluxes are an afferent stimulus for the hypothalamic response to starvation resulting in an increased drive to eat and a decrease in energy expenditure. Metabolism slows in an effort to conserve body fuels and the body survives primarily on fat stores, sparing lean tissue until such a time as re-feeding occurs (Hill 1992).

While no single definition of PCM, cachexia or malnutrition exists, a history of loss of 10–20% body mass is used by some authors to define cachexia (Corish & Kennedy 2000). Individuals with pre-existing PCM are at a disadvantage when intake is restricted due to surgery or illness. In both humans and laboratory animals nutritional supplementation has been shown to positively influence both survival and morbidity during critical illness (Stapleton et al 2007). Early nutritional supplementation should strongly be considered in horses presenting with preexisting PCM.

Catabolic response to injury and inflammation

In contrast to PCM, in humans and laboratory animals, the metabolic response to injury (critical illness, sepsis, trauma, surgical manipulation, etc. is characterized by an increased metabolism and the onset of a catabolic process leading to excessive breakdown of tissue proteins. This metabolic state is the result of a complex interaction of inflammatory cytokines (interleukin (IL)-1, IL-2, IL-6, tumor necrosis factor

(TNF)-α and γ-interferon) released at the site of injury or inflammation, circulating hormones released in response to stress and injury (hypothalamic-pituitary-adrenal axis), and neurotransmitters (sympathoadrenal axis) (Romijn 2000). Infusion of cytokines, including IL-6 and TNF-α, results in release of corticotrophin, cortisol, epinephrine and glucagon resulting in an increase in the resting metabolic rate and lipolysis (Stouthard et al 1995, Van der Poll et al 1991). TNF-α activation of NFκB results in stimulation of proteolytic pathways (Langhans 2002). In response to injury there is increased metabolic activity of the brain. Afferent nerve activity and brain stimulation can result in autonomic nerve stimulation with direct effects on hormone secretion, for example, splanchnic nerve stimulation as a result of injury results in increased glucagon secretion and hyperglycemia (Bloom & Edwards 1975). Afferent nerve activity from the injured site also results in hypothalamic-pituitary activation increasing activity of cortisol, catecholamines, growth hormone, aldosterone and ADH (Romijn 2000). In humans, prolonged infusions of glucagon, cortisol and epinephrine resulted in increased protein breakdown and elevated resting metabolic rate (Bessey et al 1984). Prolonged elevation in cortisol is associated with onset of insulin resistance. In addition, peripheral nerve endings have been shown to exist on adipocytes; stimulation of which results in increased lipolysis. These responses are designed to provide endogenous substrates for gluconeogenesis, wound healing, immune cell replication and synthesis of acute phase. While this response is beneficial, long-term muscle breakdown results in loss of muscle strength and function and compromise to the patient's overall health.

During illness or after trauma, food intake frequently falls. However, despite this decline in intake the adaptive responses to starvation do not occur. Hepatic gluconeogenesis continues and rapid protein catabolism occurs. There is an increased mobilization of stored fuels and metabolic cycling resulting in heat production and energy depletion. Insulin resistance develops and hyperglycemia may occur despite the absence of food intake. In severe metabolic stress the body appears to preferentially utilize amino acids from the breakdown of skeletal muscle proteins as a metabolic fuel, in contrast to PCM where fat is the principal source of energy. The adaptive switch to fat utilization is limited due, in part, to increased concentrations of circulating insulin. The result is an increase in lean tissue breakdown, visceral organ dysfunction secondary to loss of structural and enzymatic proteins, impaired wound healing (due to loss of precursors for wound healing) and immunosuppression (Romijn 2000, Sternberg et al 2000). Nitrogen losses during this catabolic response can be as high as 20–30 g/day versus 4–5 g/day in the same human experiencing PCM (Rafael & Mora 1999). Muscle weakness and increased morbidity result from excess protein breakdown as well as muscle disuse due to inactivity. As sodium and water retention are a component of this response (thought to be the result of a fall in the activity of the sodium/potassium pump (Na/K-ATPase) and cortisol induced fluid retention, weight loss and muscle wasting frequently goes unnoticed (Vanhorebeek & Van den Berghe 2004). Cytokine production results in behavioral changes including anorexia and decreased activity. Food deprivation during this hypermetabolic/catabolic state results in a much greater loss of lean muscle mass and visceral protein than would be expected during simple starvation. The metabolic adaptations to starvation in a healthy human can result in a 75% decrease in protein loss whereas the metabolic responses to critical illness result in an increase in energy and protein metabolism.

Nutritional supplementation will reverse the catabolic processes occurring during simple starvation but will not completely reverse those occurring during metabolic stress because as long as tissue injury persists catabolic processes are maintained. In the critically ill patient protein catabolism continues despite protein supplementation in the diet. The goals of nutritional support in critical illness should be to save life, preserve and improve cellular function and speed recovery (Powell-Tuck 2007). More recently, research in nutritional therapy has been focused on attenuating the metabolic response to stress, preventing oxidative cellular injury and favorably modulating the immune response with the ultimate goal being to reduce disease severity, complications and length of stay and improve outcome.

Key Points

- The metabolic response to prolonged protein/calorie malnutrition (starvation) in healthy individuals includes a fall in metabolic rate with sparing of body proteins and a switch by many tissues to the utilization of fat for energy
- The catabolic response to injury or inflammation may include an increased metabolic rate, continued utilization of protein and glucose as fuels despite a fall in nutritional intake
- Nutritional supplementation will not completely reverse the increased catabolism seen with injury and inflammation

Nutritional support

The need for nutritional support in the horse will depend on a number of factors. The healthy adult horse with a body condition score of 4 to 6/9 (Henneke system) with a minor injury or undergoing an elective surgery rarely requires nutritional supplementation even if the patient is unable or unwilling to eat for a few days. However, regardless of the type and complexity of the illness or injury, early nutritional support should be strongly considered in patients with increased metabolic demands, such as young growing animals, individuals presenting with a prior history of malnutrition or hypophagia, patients with underlying metabolic abnormalities that could worsen with feed deprivation and individuals with an illness such as severe trauma, sepsis or strangulating bowel obstructions that results in excess losses (ex-albumin loss through a compromised gastrointestinal tract) and an increased metabolic rate. Underweight horses (BCS of 3.5 out of 9 or less though this depends on the breed and individual characteristics) should ideally receive nutritional support early in the disease process rather than waiting to see if the individual will begin to eat on his/her own volition. Obese or over conditioned individuals particularly pony breeds, miniature horses and donkeys as well as lactating mares are at risk for developing hyperlipemia and should receive nutritional support if their serum triglycerides are above normal reference values (see Chapter 30). Older horses, or individuals diagnosed with equine Cushing's syndrome or equine metabolic syndrome are insulin resistant and may be at greater risk for developing hyperlipemia, and fatty infiltration of their liver. Depending on the severity and type of underlying disease process and individual characteristics (breed, body condition) these individuals may develop severe hyperlipemia (triglycerides >500 mg/dl or >5.6 mmol/l) within days of onset. The combination of illness and metabolic effects of hyperlipemia can worsen the individual's inappetance creating a vicious cycle. Consequently, if feed deprivation is prolonged (in some cases as little as 1–2 days of anorexia can result in moderate to severe hyperlipemia) or there is a concern regarding the individual's desire or ability to eat, early intervention is indicated to prevent more severe malnutrition.

Nutritional needs of the sick or injured horse

While the energy requirements of horses of various ages, stages of growth and activity levels have been determined and equations are available to calculate these needs, the energy and protein requirements for the hospitalized, sick equine patient are not known and likely vary depending on disease state, environment and level of fitness of the individual. Historically, multipliers have been used to estimate the energy requirements in certain conditions including severe sepsis, trauma or burn injuries. However, the increased metabolic demand of illness or surgical trauma and recovery is likely to be balanced by the inactivity and decreased metabolic demands of digestion of the patient during hospitalization. Consequently, these multipliers likely overestimate the caloric requirement of certain illnesses. Studies in the human ICU and in sick neonatal foals suggest that the metabolic energy needs may fall more closely within the range of the resting to maintenance energy requirements of normal, healthy individuals (Cerra et al 1997, Paradis 2001, Stapleton et al 2007). The exceptions to this are individuals with extreme trauma, burns or severe sepsis, surgical conditions that require intestinal resection and patients with large areas of devitalized tissue (e.g., clostridial myositis patients that undergo multiple fasciotomy procedures). When estimating the energy requirements of the majority of other equine patients resting energy requirements are an acceptable target. Resting energy requirements (RER) are defined as the amount of energy needed to maintain an individual (no weight gain or loss) in a thermoneutral environment without the metabolic demands of digestion. Maintenance energy requirements include the demands of digestion in this equation and are ~30% higher than resting energy requirements. Resting energy requirements will vary slightly depending on the size of the horse but can be estimated using ~22–23 kcal/kg/day (92–96 kJ/kg/day) for the average full size horse. Maintenance energy requirements (as digestible energy) can be estimated using 30–35 kcal/kg/day. If a patient tolerates nutritional supplementation at resting energy requirements the feeding rate (i.e., calories/kg/day) can be gradually increased if needed.

Protein requirement

The maintenance protein requirement of the healthy adult horse is estimated at approximately 0.5–1.5 g/kg/day (see Chapter 6). The needs of a growing foal are higher and may approach 7 g/kg/day during maximum growth periods (Oftedal et al 1983); additionally the lysine requirements of growing horses are higher than for mature horses. During critical illness or severe injury protein catabolism and utilization of amino acids as a source of fuel continue despite the presence of other energy stores. Consequently, when calculating protein requirements in human patients it is recommended to provide the higher end of the estimated need (Cerra et al 1997, Powell-Tuck 2007). Another consideration is supplementation of nonessential amino acids that may improve outcome in illness. In humans, glutamine is considered a conditionally essential amino acid and is used as a fuel for enterocytes and other rapidly dividing cells (Lacey & Wilmore 1990). In periods of inappetance the majority of glutamine is produced by mobilization of muscle stores (Gamrin et al 1996). Glutamine release during critical illness may act as a cell signaling molecule regulating the inflammatory and immune response, however, in periods of illness when glutamine requirements may actually increase endogenous sources may be inadequate resulting in relative glutamine deficiency (Wischmeyer 2007). In laboratory animals, glutamine has been shown to be critical in maintaining gut wall integrity, immune function and antioxidant supplies (Wischmeyer 2007). Glutamine supplementation has been shown to improve clinical outcome in both laboratory and human studies (Novak et al 2002). In humans, glutamine supplementation at 0.2 g/kg/day is recommended when using the parenteral route. The amount and ideal route of glutamine supplementation has not been determined in the horse. In one study glutamine improved mucosal restitution in an oxidant injured equine colon model (Rotting et al 2004). Other recommendations for amino acid supplementation include branched chain amino acids and arginine supplementation. Arginine is a precursor to nitric oxide an important vasodilating agent, upregulates immune function, secretion of several hormones and may reduce ischemia-reperfusion injury (Potenza et al 2001, Ruth 1998). Studies looking at specific amino acid supplementation in critically ill or injured horses are currently lacking. Parenteral amino acid solutions that contain nonessential amino acids are available. When feeding by the enteral route, protein needs can be met by feeding a complete feed (which generally contain nonessential or conditionally essential amino acids) or by addition of specific amino acids to a component diet. For example, Critical Care Meals for horses (MD's Choice, Louisville, TN) provides a separate component that contains glutamine, arginine and other non-essential amino acids. Alternatively, glutamine can be purchased separately and added to a diet though recommendations for amounts are currently not available. Caution may be required in horses with liver failure as some studies in humans have demonstrated that deamination of glutamine is a major contributor to hyperammonemia (Romero-Gomez et al. 2009).

Routes of nutritional support

The choice whether to use the enteral or parenteral route of feeding can be summarized by the simple statement "if the gut works use it." While there is conflicting data regarding the pros and cons of parenteral feeding verses enteral feeding, it is clear that enteral feeding has some distinct benefits. Enteral nutrients provide the majority of nutrition to the gut which is responsible for 15–35% of the total body oxygen consumption and protein turnover (Stoll et al 1998). Enteral feeding offers the advantage of maintaining the gastrointestinal tract, and is generally less expensive. Enteral feeding has been shown to improve gut barrier integrity, gut mass, protein content, motility, and function in piglets (Burrin et al 2000). The complete absence of enteral nutrition results in mucosal atrophy, increased gut permeability and enzymatic dysfunction in critically ill human patients (Hernandez et al 1999). Even small amounts of enteral feeding may provide benefits. In a neonatal piglet model, provision of 5–10% of nutritional needs by enteral feeding resulted in improved intestinal motility and lactose digestion and decreased mucosal permeability. Enteral provision of 20% of energy and nutrient needs for normal growth prevented loss of gut protein mass whereas 40–60% of nutritional needs were needed to maintain normal gastrointestinal growth (Burrin et al 2000).

The enteral route of nutritional support is simpler as there is less concern of fluid and electrolyte overload and this route allows fiber feeding, which cannot be achieved parenterally. That said, clinicians are often hesitant to use the enteral route in horses with gastrointestinal disorders. In the critically ill patient with poor perfusion and decreased oxygen delivery to the tissues the gastrointestinal tract is one of the most vulnerable organs to ischemia. Decreased oxygen delivery has been shown to increase mucosal permeability resulting in increased translocation of bacteria and absorption of bacterial toxins (Luyer et al 2004, Saito et al 1987). Inflammatory mediators, produced in the gut as a result of ischemia, are absorbed across the damaged mucosa and enter the portal and systemic circulations; this absorption has been implicated in the onset of septic shock or multi-organ failure (Rokyta et al 2003). Inflammation and enterocyte injury can result in decreased motility and nutrient absorption. In this situation institution of forced enteral feeding may result in colic, bacterial overgrowth, diarrhea and other complications. Because digestion increases the metabolic activity of the enterocytes enteral feeding during states of poor oxygen delivery may actually worsen the oxygen debt and ischemic injury. In contrast, enteral nutrition has been shown to increase total hepatosplanchnic blood flow in healthy patients resulting in greater oxygen delivery to the mucosa suggesting that enteral feeding may be beneficial in the poorly perfused gut (Rokyta et al 2003). In a rat *Escherichia coli* sepsis model, enteral feeding of glucose resulted in improved intestinal perfusion rates (Gosche et al 1990). Given this conflicting information, the decision on the route of administration of supplemental nutrition must be determined on a case-by-case basis, with consideration of the primary disease condition, the status of the gastrointestinal tract, and individual clinician preference. The enteral route is always preferred when the gastrointestinal tract is functional. However, patients with overwhelming bowel ischemia, inflammation, high risk of ileus or intestinal resection may not always be the best candidates for enteral nutrition and may be better off started on parenteral nutrition while they are gradually reintroduced to enteral nutrition.

Enteral nutrition

Types of enteral nutrition can vary from normal feedstuffs (i.e., grains, hay and complete pelleted diets), slurry diets composed primarily from normal feedstuffs, and liquid component diets that allow the clinician to tailor the feeding regimen by adding fiber, vitamins and minerals and conditionally essential amino acids separately (Tables 41-1–41-3). In horses with decreased appetite or complete anorexia the choices are limited to those diets that can be administered through a nasogastric tube. Complete pelleted feeds offer several advantages – they are relatively inexpensive, meet the maintenance nutrient requirements of the adult horse, and contain sources of fiber. Fiber is beneficial in increasing colonic blood flow, enzymatic activity and colonic mucosal cell growth and absorption (Scheppach 1994). Disadvantages of pelleted diets lie principally in the difficulty involved in giving them via nasogastric intubation. Both human and equine liquid formulations are available and have been used as enteral nutrition support in horses (Golenz et al 1992, Hallebeek & Beynen 2001, Hardy 2003, Sweeney & Hansen 1990). Alternatively, diets prepared using specific components have been described (Naylor et al 1984). Corn oil (or other non-rancid, palatable vegetable oil) may be added to the diet to increase the caloric content but should be added gradually (increasing the intake by ¼–½ cup or 60–120 ml daily not to exceed 2 cups or 500–600 ml total daily intake for a 500-kg horse) to prevent feed refusal and/or diarrhea. Oil should not be added to the ration of hyperlipemic patients. The use of human products (Osmolite and Vital HN) in the mature horse can be very expensive and has been associated with diarrhea and laminitis (though cause and effect are not clear). Consequently, they are rarely used and generally not recommended. Liquid diets can be given by continuous flow

Table 41-1 Nutritional Content of Selected Commercial Liquid Diets

	Vital HN*	Osmolite*	Critical care meals/ packet
Cal/l	1000	1008	1066
Protein	41.7 g/dl	40 g/dl	12%
Fat	10.8 g/dl	34 g/dl	1%
Carbohydrate	185 g/l	135.6 g/l	73%

*Product formulated for human use

Table 41-2 Composition of an Enteral Diet Used for Long-Term Tube Feeding of Healthy Horses (Coenen 1986).

	%		DM g/kg
Alfalfa meal	32.8	ash	84
Corn starch, processed	26.8	protein	85
Sugar	22.0	fat	38
Skim milk powder	9.6	fiber	106
Oil (corn or soy)	3.9	Ca	13.2
Vitamin supplement	1.23	P	9.3
Ca-phosphate	0.95	Na	9.1
Na-phosphate	1.92	K	9.5
MgO	0.29		
NaCl	0.5		

Table 41-3 Composition of and Feeding Schedule for the "Naylor Diet"

Constituents	Day 1	Day 2	Day 3	Day 4	Day 5	Day 6	Day 7
Electrolyte mixture	230	230	230	230	230	230	230
Water (liters)	21	21	21	21	21	21	21
Dextrose (grams)	300	400	500	600	800	800	900
Dehydrated cottage cheese (grams)	300	450	600	750	900	900	900
Dehydrated alfalfa meal (g)	2000	2000	2000	2000	2000	2000	2000
Energy (non protein calories), kcal	7400	8400	9400	10400	11800	11800	12200

From Naylor, J.M., Freeman, D.E., Kronfield, D.S.,1984. Alimentation of hypophagic horses. Comp Cont Educ Pract Vet 6:S93–S99.

through an indwelling small-bore (18F) nasogastric feeding tube (Mila International, Erlanger, KY), or via periodic passage of a nasogastric tube and administration of larger meals. When using pelleted diets, the author recommends that 1 kg of a pelleted complete feed be soaked in approximately 4 liters of water. Once this water has been absorbed, an additional 2 liters of water are added to form a slurry that can be administered via a large bore (external diameter 305 cm) nasogastric tube. Slurry diets made from complete pelleted feeds will not pass through a nasogastric tube using gravity alone. Instead, the slurry should be administered by use of a marine supply bilge pump. If a bilge pump is not available or a large bore tube cannot be passed, pulverizing the pellets prior to adding water may improve gravity flow. The horse should be checked for the presence of gastric reflux prior to administration and the slurry should be pumped slowly with attention paid to the horse's attitude and reaction. As the stomach volume of a mature, 450-kg horse is approximately 9 to 11 liters, the volume of each feeding should not to exceed 6–8 liters per feeding for 450–500-kg horses. The volume fed should be adjusted for smaller horses. Studies in healthy horses have shown that the feeding of liquid diets is associated with increased intestinal transit time and decreased pre-cecal starch and fat digestion (Coenen 1986). Therefore, avoidance of high starch (>25% DM) and high fat (>6% DM) diets is recommended, with the use of highly digestible carbohydrate sources (e.g. processed corn starch).

Long-term placement of nasogastric tubes is not without the risk of complications (Naylor et al 1984). Small bore, 18F, softer (polyurethane) tubes are recommended if intubation is prolonged as they are better tolerated by the patient but generally preclude the use of slurry diets (Mila International, Erlanger, KY). Alternatively, intermittent placement of a nasogastric tube is effective in decreasing complications but can be difficult, and at times traumatic to the patient. When instituting enteral feeding, particularly in a horse with prolonged anorexia, it is best to start gradually increasing the amount fed over several days (Table 41-4). A maximum of 50% of calculated requirements should be fed in the first 24 hours; if the horse tolerates this level of supplementation the amount can be increased over the next few days until the target feeding rate is achieved. Rapid changes in feed amount such as feeding 100% of required intake the first day in an animal that has not eaten for 3–5 days can be associated with colic or diarrhea, particularly with liquid diets made for humans or high fat diets. In addition, the use of liquid diets formulated for humans has been associated with laminitis though cause and effect was not clear (Lopes & White 2002, Naylor et al 1984).

Table 41-4 A Suggested Assisted Enteral Feeding Schedule for a 450-kg Horse

Day 1	Day 1	Day 2	Day 3	Maintenance (1–1.5% BW)
Number of meals	2–3	3–4	4–6	4–6
Complete feed (kg)/meal	0.5 kg	0.75	0.75–1.0	1.0–1.25
Water (l)/meal	4–6	4–6	6–8	6–8

Creation of an esophagotomy should be considered when prolonged nutritional support is likely to be required or when medical or surgical conditions prevent passage of a nasogastric tube. Esophagotomy can be performed in a standing, sedated animal and once in place allows frequent intubation and feeding while avoiding the trauma and discomfort associated with repetitive nasogastric intubation. Once the animal has recovered and its appetite has returned, tube feeding can be discontinued to allow the esophagotomy incision to heal by second intention.

Esophagotomy (rewritten with permission from John Stick [Stick 2011])

The skin over the left jugular furrow is prepared for surgery in the desired area. The esophagus is occasionally located on the right side of the trachea and should be approached over the right jugular furrow in those horses. Passage of a nasogastric tube facilitates identification of the esophagus at surgery. A 5-cm skin incision is made ventral to the vein. The esophagus is sharply incised longitudinally for 3 cm down to the indwelling nasogastric tube. The nasogastric tube is removed and a polyethylene nasogastric tube (with an outer diameter of 14 to 24 mm) is placed into the stomach through the esophagostomy. Failure to place the tube into the stomach allows easy dislodgement. Care should be taken to ensure that the end of the tube is placed into both the elastic inner layer and the inelastic outer muscle layer of the esophagus. Difficulty in tube placement is usually an indication that the incision in the muscle layer is inadequate to accommodate the diameter of the tube. Sutures can be placed in the mucosa to form a seal around the tube but probably are unnecessary because they do not prevent leakage of saliva. The tube should be secured firmly, first with butterfly tape bandages sutured to the skin and then with elastic tape bandages. Tubes of large diameter are preferred; they should be capped between feedings and flushed with water after each meal to maintain patency.

An esophagotomy tube should remain in place for a minimum of 7 to 10 days to permit granulation tissue to form a true stoma. A longer period is necessary if the tube is placed in an area of rupture. When the tube is removed and normal feeding resumed it is recommended to place feed at the level of the withers to decrease the amount of swallowed feed lost through the stoma. The stoma will heal spontaneously after tube removal and fistula formation is rare.

Key Points

- Enteral nutrition provides intraluminal nutrition to the gastrointestinal tract and has been shown in other species to improve gut barrier integrity, gut mass, protein content, motility and function
- Enteral feeding should be increased gradually with careful assessment of gastric residuals prior to bolus feeding
- Enteral nutrition can be tailored using complete feeds or specific components diets
- An esophagotomy should be considered whenever long-term force feeding is needed as it can decrease the risk of complications associated with nasogastric intubation

Parenteral nutrition

The major advantage of parenteral nutrition (PN) is its ability to supply nutrition when the enteral route is unavailable and to be able to tailor the types of nutrition provided for each individual animal. Parenteral nutrition has been shown to decrease weight loss particularly lean body mass, improve wound healing, immune function and outcome in human and animal studies when the enteral route cannot be utilized (Peter et al 2005). Parenteral nutrition can be used to provide partial nutritional support (PPN) or total nutritional support (TPN). In the adult horse it is most commonly used to supply partial nutrition when oral intake is insufficient or the oral route cannot be used. Horses with proximal enteritis, colitis, postoperative ileus, esophageal lacerations or obstructions can receive nutritional support until resolution of the underlying problem allows re-institution of adequate enteral feeding (1.5% body weight or ~23 kcal/kg day [96 kJ/kg/day]). Recumbent or dysphagic animals at risk for aspiration pneumonia, individuals with pre-existing protein/calorie malnutrition, increased energy demands (late gestation, early lactation and young, growing animals), metabolic derangements resulting in hyperlipemia, and completely anorexic animals or those with prolonged decreased feed consumption (less than 25% maintenance for several days) should also be considered as candidates for partial or total parenteral nutrition.

There has been a significant amount of information published in recent years evaluating the pros and cons of PN. Much of the impetus has come from the desire to determine if there is a negative effect of relying on PN as the sole nutritional source. While the results of studies vary it appears that the major disadvantage lies in the loss of the beneficial effect of enteral nutrition on maintaining gut function and mass. Parenteral nutrition is more expensive than enteral feeding both in terms of supplies and time. In humans, the parenteral route may also be associated with an increased risk of infection, although results are contradictory (Peter et al 2005, Gramlich et al 2004). Published reports of PN use in horses primarily consist of case reports with little information evaluating the benefits and risks of parenteral nutrition (Durham 2003, Durham 2006, Greatorex 1975, Hansen et al 1988, Hoffer et al 1977).

In a retrospective study examining 79 equine cases of gastrointestinal disease treated with parenteral nutrition the most common complication of PN was hyperglycemia (Lopes & White 2002). Four horses developed thrombophlebitis. Because no comparison was made between PN-treated individuals and controls the authors were unable to determine if PN affected outcome.

Formulating parenteral nutrition

Depending on the desired goals and duration of supplementation solutions containing various amounts of carbohydrate, amino acids, lipids, vitamins, electrolytes and minerals can be formulated. Carbohydrates and lipids are used to meet the horse's energy needs, preventing breakdown of endogenous protein for energy, and allowing the administered amino acids to be used for wound healing and immune functions. Carbohydrate is commonly provided using 50% dextrose solutions. These solutions are hyperosmolar (2525 mOsm/l) and should be infused through a central line or large peripheral vein (jugular vein) to reduce the risk of thrombophlebitis. Dextrose provides 3.4 kcal/g or 170 kcal/100 ml (50 g) of 50% dextrose.

Lipids are recommended to provide the remainder of non-protein calories. Lipids are isotonic and can be infused separately in a peripheral vein or combined with other components. Lipids come in 10 and 20% emulsion and are composed principally of safflower and soybean oil, egg yolk phospholipids and glycerin. Lipids should be added to the solution last to avoid destabilization of the emulsion due to an acidic environment. Some clinicians mix PN solutions in isotonic crystalloids to provide fluid support as well as nutritional support. When doing so it is best to separate the lipid component as the presence of divalent cations can result in destabilization of the emulsion. Many clinicians are reluctant to use lipids in PN solutions due to the costs and risks associated with destabilization as well as metabolic consequences that may develop (hyperlipemia, fatty liver, lipid thromboembolism). It can be difficult to provide total energy requirements without lipids especially in insulin resistant patients or patients with systemic inflammation as these individuals appear to have a harder time regulating blood glucose. Lipids are very calorie dense containing 9 kcal/g. While recommendations vary, lipids can be added to provide 30–60% of the non-protein calories in a PN solution. The addition of lipids to PN is beneficial in patients with persistent hyperglycemia or hypercapnia reducing the dependency on glucose as the principal energy source. Lipids should be avoided in horses with known hyperlipemia or in horses suspected of being lipid intolerant. Lipid intolerance can be seen in patients with systemic inflammation, sepsis or underlying metabolic derangements and triglyceride levels should be monitored regularly.

Amino acid preparations are available in several concentrations; 8.5% and 10% solutions are most commonly used in veterinary medicine. They are approximately twice the osmolarity of plasma and are acidic and should be mixed with dextrose prior to adding the lipid component to prevent destabilization of the lipid emulsion. Solutions containing both essential and conditionally essential amino acids, including glutamic acid would seem to be preferable though no data on the benefits of conditionally essential amino acids in horses is available. As already discussed, while resting energy requirements should be used when calculating caloric needs for adult animals, protein requirements should be determined using maintenance requirements of approximately 0.7 g/kg/day or higher. While there is no clear data on the benefits of a higher protein supplementation, current recommendations in humans are to provide protein in excess of the normal daily requirement because of the higher protein catabolism seen with injury or inflammation. The ratio of non-protein calories to nitrogen should be at least 100:1 in the final solution to limit the use of protein as an energy source. This can be calculated using the conversion of 1 g of nitrogen to 6.2 g of protein. Protein provides ~4 kcal of energy per gram of protein and 100 ml (10 g) of 10% amino acid solution contains 40 kcal.

Additional components may be added to parenteral nutrition or given separately including electrolyte solutions, vitamin and mineral supplements. The vitamin and mineral requirements of the critically ill horse are unknown but published recommendations for healthy horses (NRC 2007) can be used when determining feeding rates. Multivitamin supplements for humans are available and can be added directly to PN solutions. If possible, however, it is best to limit the amount of additives to PN solutions to avoid contamination or lipid destabilization. Based on information in humans it is strongly recommended to supplement water-soluble B vitamins daily as deficiencies can exacerbate problems associated with refeeding (Marinella 2005). Though horses synthesize some of the B vitamins in their gastrointestinal tract chronic inappetance or long-term use of antimicrobials may affect synthesis. Parenteral B vitamins are light sensitive; when added to crystalloids the fluids need to be protected from sunlight. Some vitamins are best given orally (vitamins C and E) or added to separate crystalloid solutions (B vitamins). Vitamin C is also produced by the horse and a need for supplementation has not been documented. However, some authors recommend oral supplementation in sick horses with recommendations of 10–20 g per horse per day (Ralston 1990). Fat-soluble vitamins such as vitamins E, D, and A, are stored in body tissue and generally do not need daily supplementation. However, the antioxidant benefits of vitamin E may make it worth providing oral supplementation early in illness. Recommended doses of oral vitamin E vary significantly from 40 IU/horse/day to 500 IU/kg/day. Minerals, if required, are best supplemented in separate crystalloid solutions since divalent cations may destabilize lipid emulsions. While trace mineral requirements for sick animals are not known trace mineral supplementation is rarely performed except in patients receiving parenteral nutrition as their sole nutritional source for prolonged periods (>7 days).

Preparation of parenteral nutrition should be performed under a laminar flow hood (or a clean surface away from drafts or excessive dust) using aseptic techniques. Lipids should be added last to prevent destabilization of the emulsion in acidic solutions. Parenteral solutions are an excellent media for growth of bacteria and ideally should be used within 24 hours of preparation. Prior to use they should be kept in a dark, cool area away from direct sunlight to minimize degradation and loss of vitamins (when these have been added to the solution). Over time lipid emulsions will destabilize and oxidize therefore they should not be stored for prolonged periods. The shelf life of a lipid solution will vary depending on the type of lipids and the size of the emulsion so manufacturer's recommendations should be used when determining shelf life. Because PN solutions are hyperosmolar delivery through a central venous or jugular catheter is recommended. Because of the increased risk of sepsis associated with parenteral feeding, a separate catheter or portal should be designated for parenteral nutrition only. In the authors' clinic, a 14-gauge double-lumen catheter (Arrow catheter, Reading, PA) is used with one port designated for administration of parenteral nutrition. Catheter placement and line maintenance should be performed using strict aseptic technique and it is currently recommended that all lines be changed daily and that connections should not be broken after changes. The administration of PN solutions should not be stopped suddenly; if the animal needs to be moved it is best to continue administration during the transfer. Gradual introduction of parenteral nutrition is recommended to decrease risk of complications. It is recommended to use an intravenous infusion pump to ensure that the rate of infusion is consistent. We generally start with an infusion rate targeting ~25% of the daily requirement. The most common complication associated with PN is hyperglycemia and blood glucose concentrations should be determined before increasing the rate of infusion. If blood glucose concentrations are within reference ranges then the rate can be increased by an additional 25% every 4–8 hours. In the author's experience most horses will develop mild hyperglycemia that corrects without treatment. Horses with persistent hyperglycemia may require insulin infusions to control the hyperglycemia and allow continued infusion of the nutrient solution.

Complications associated with parenteral nutrition

Hyperglycemia both at admission and during hospitalization has been associated with an increased risk of complications including infections and renal failure, longer hospital stays, and reduced survival in humans and horses with critical illness or injury (Capes et al 2000, Johnston et al 2007). In a landmark prospective, randomized, controlled clinical trial of humans admitted to the ICU tight glycemic control using intensive insulin therapy during hospitalization was associated with a significant improvement in morbidity and mortality compared to the more traditional, less stringent glycemic control (Van den Berge et al 2001). Tight glycemic control (maintained between 80–110 mg/dl compared to 180–200 mg/dl) decreased the incidence of infections, acute renal failure, days of mechanical ventilation, and improved neurologic outcome in brain injury patients (Langouche & Van den Berge 2006). Additional studies some using less stringent glucose control have found similar results (Krinsley 2004, Van den Berge et al 2006). As previously mentioned, hepatic gluconeogenesis is upregulated during the acute phase of critical illness. Insulin resistance and loss of exercise associated uptake of glucose as well as the increased production of glucose are thought to result in hyperglycemia. Normal cells down regulate glucose transporters during periods of hyperglycemia to protect against glucose toxicity (Klip et al 1994). During inflammation this protective response is lost, allowing glucose to enter the cell along a steep concentration gradient (Pekala et al 1990, Shikman et al 2001). Elevated intracellular glucose concentrations have been associated with increased oxidative stress, mitochondrial dysfunction and altered energy metabolism (Van den Berghe 2004). The use of insulin therapy to maintain blood glucose levels within the normal range has been shown to have the added benefit of correcting dyslipidemias (Mesotten et al 2004). Additional reported beneficial effects of maintaining euglycemia include improved immune function due to improved phagocytosis (Rassias et al 1999), decreased glycosylated non-functional immunoglobin (Black et al 1990), and blunting of the catabolic process (Derde et al 2010, Weekers et al 2003).

While extrapolation to a different species with different underlying diseases should always be performed cautiously it would seem prudent to try to maintain blood glucose concentrations within or close to normal range. It is unclear at this time if strict glycemic control is better than a less-stringent control. In cases where hyperglycemia persists the use of intensive insulin infusions is recommended to attempt to normalize the blood glucose concentration.

Lipid infusions have been associated with allergic reactions, hyperlipemia, alterations in liver function and fat embolism. The risk of fat embolization is higher in larger droplet emulsions or in emulsions that have been stored too long and have begun to destabilize. While solutions containing lipids are very useful in providing additional calories their use needs to be determined on a case-by-case basis. Lipids should be avoided in patients with a predisposition to or pre-existing hyperlipemia or underlying liver dysfunction. Thrombocytopenia, coagulopathy, fat embolization, thrombocytopenia, coagulopathies and alterations in cellular immunity are reported with lipid infusions. Triglyceride levels and platelet counts should be monitored regularly when lipids are added to PN solutions.

Additional complications reported with PN include hyperammonemia and elevations in serum urea nitrogen due to excess protein catabolism, hypercapnia due to excess carbohydrate metabolism, thrombophlebitis due to hypertonicity and pulmonary embolism (thought due to destabilized lipid emulsions) and sepsis (Durham et al 2003, 2004, Jeejeebhoy 2001, Lopes & White 2002, Sternberg et al 2000).

Monitoring

It is recommended to monitor blood glucose at least every 4 to 6 hours when starting parenteral nutrition and to adjust the rate to try to maintain blood glucose within or close to the established normal ranges. If significant hyperglycemia (>180 mg/dl) develops and persists for more than 2–4 hours the infusion should be slowed or insulin infusion begun. If costs are a concern blood values may be monitored less frequently once steady state has been achieved. In addition daily assessment should include serum electrolytes, $PvCO_2$, blood urea nitrogen, triglycerides and ammonia and liver function during the acclimation period. If possible the horse should be weighed daily. Once a steady state has been reached the frequency of blood monitoring can be decreased however, the same approach should be used when discontinuing parenteral nutrition.

The most common reason for instituting PN is the unwillingness or inability of a patient to ingest feed. If the latter, palatable feeds should be offered even during PN therapy to try to stimulate appetite. Once a patient has begun to readily ingest and tolerate a reasonable amount of food (25% normal intake or more) and has a steady appetite, parenteral nutrition can be gradually discontinued. Decreasing the supplement by 25% every 4–8 hours is generally well tolerated. Frequent monitoring of blood glucose during withdrawal (every 4 hours) is warranted, particularly in foals due to the risk of transient hypoglycemia. An example of how to calculate parenteral nutrition requirements is found in Box 41.1.

Box 41.1 Adult Horse Parenteral Nutrition

PN formulation:

1000 ml 50% dextrose*	(500 g dextrose)=	1700 kcal
1000 ml 10% amino acids (AA)	(100 g AA) =	400 kcal
500 ml 20% lipids	(100 g lipids)=	1000 kcal
2.5 liters in one bag	3100 kcal/bag	

One bag = 1240 kcal/l or 1.24 kcal/ml

Maintenance energy requirements:

For horses less than 600 kg = 34 kcal/kg/day

For horses greater than 600 kg = 31 kcal/kg/day

Protein requirements 0.5 to 1.5 g/kg day:

Goal of 1 g/kg/day

Example 1: 500-kg horse needs 17 000 kcal/day and 500 g protein

17000/3100 = 5.5 bags per day or 12.5 liters/day= ~500 ml/h

5.5 bags = 550 g protein

Example 2: 600-kg horse needs 18 600 kcal/day and 600 g protein

18600/3100 = 6 bags/day or 15 liters/day= 625 ml/h

6 bags = 600 g protein.

1 g nitrogen = 6.2 g protein

100 g protein/ bag = 16.1 g nitrogen

2700 kcal non-protein calories/bag

2700/16.1 = 167 non-protein kcal/g protein (within 100–200 kcal/g desired)

*1 liter of 50% dextrose can be purchased in a 2 liter bag to allow addition of other components.

**Should have 100–200 g of non-protein kcalories per gram nitrogen.

Key Points

- Parenteral nutrition allows provision of nutritional support when the enteral route is unavailable
- Parenteral nutrition allows supplementation to be tailored to the individual animal's needs
- Parenteral nutrition must be handled with strict aseptic technique and should be gradually introduced and discontinued to prevent metabolic consequences

Conclusion

It is clear that nutritional support is an important adjunct to medical therapy in the sick, injured or debilitated equine patient. What is not clear is the optimal route, composition, or amounts of support. The enteral route should be chosen whenever possible to maximize the benefits to the gastrointestinal tract as well as the patient as a whole. Complete or partial parenteral nutrition is most useful as a bridge during recovery and transition to enteral feeding in the horse. While the exact caloric requirement for sick, debilitated horses is unknown estimates are available to use as a target for nutritional supplementation. Research in humans and laboratory animals suggests that even a little nutritional support is beneficial and the reader is encouraged to consider nutritional support whether enteral or parenteral in any anorexic, chronically debilitated or sick equine patient.

References

Bessey, P.Q., Watters, J.M., Aoki, T.T., et al., 1984. Combined hormonal infusion simulates the metabolic response to injury. Annals of Surg 200, 264–281.

Black, C.T., Hennessey, P.J., Andrassy, R.J., 1990. Short-term hyperglycemia depresses immunity through nonenzymatic glycosylation of circular immunoglobulin. J Trauma 30, 832–833.

Bloom, S.R., Edwards, A.V., 1975. The release of pancreatic glucagons and inhibition of insulin in response to stimulation of sympathetic innervation. J Physiol 253, 157–173.

Burrin, D.G., Stoll, B., Jiang, R., et al., 2000. Minimal enteral nutrient requirements for intestinal growth in neonatal piglets: how much is enough? Am J Clin Nutr 71, 1603–1610.

Capes, S.E., Hunt, D., Malmberg, K., et al., 2000. Stress hyperglycaemia and increased risk of death after myocardial infarction in patients with and without diabetes: a systematic overview. Lancet 2000 355, 773–778.

Cerra, F.B., Rios Benitez, M., Blackburn, G.L., et al., 1997. Applied Nutrition in ICU Patients: A Consensus Statement of the American College of Chest Physicians. Chest 111, 769–778.

Coenen, M., 1986. Verdaulichkeit und praecaaecale Passage einer suspendierfähigen Diät in Abhängigkeit von der Applikationsform, (spontane Futteraufnahme bzw. flüssig per Sonde) [Digestibility and precaecal passage of a special diet in dependence on the route of application (spontaneous oral feed intake vs. tube feeding as liquid diet suspended in water)] J. Anim. Physiol. a. Anim. Nutr. 56, 104–107.

Corish, C.A., Kennedy, N.P., 2000. Protein-energy undernutrition in hospital in-patients. Brit J Nutr 83, 575–591.

Derde, S., Vanhorebeek, I., Ververs, E., et al., 2010. Increasing intravenous glucose load in the presence of normoglycemia: effect on outcome and metabolism in critically ill rabbits. Crit Care Med 38, 602–611.

Durham, A.E., 2006. Clinical application of PN in 5 ponies and 1 donkey in the treatment of hyperlipaemia. Vet Rec 158, 159–164.

Durham, A.E., Phillips, T.J., Walmsley, J.P., et al., 2004. Nutritional and clinicopathological effects of post operative parenteral nutrition following small intestinal resection and anastomosis in the mature horse. Eq Vet J 36, 390–396.

Durham, A.E., Phillips, T.J., Walmsley, J.P., et al., 2003. Study of the clinical effects of postoperative parenteral nutrition in 15 horses. Vet Rec 153, 493–498.

Gamrin, L., Essen, P., Forsberg, A.M., et al., 1996. A descriptive study of skeletal muscle metabolism in critically ill patients: Free amino acids, energy-rich phosphates, protein, nucleic acids, fat, water and electrolytes. Crit Care Med 24, 575–583.

Golenz, M.R., Knight, D.A., Yvorchuk-St Jean, K.E., 1992. Use of a human enteral feeding preparation for treatment of hyperlipemia and nutritional support during healing of an esophageal laceration in a miniature horse. J Am Vet Med Assoc 200, 951–953.

Gosche, J.R., Garrison, R.N., Harris, P.D., et al., 1990. Absorptive hyperaemia restores intestinal blood flow during *Escherichia coli* sepsis in the rat. Arch of Surg 125, 1573–1576.

Gramlich, L., Kichian, K., Pinilla, J., et al., 2004. Does enteral nutrition compared to parenteral nutrition result in better outcomes in critically ill adult patients? A systematic review of the literature. Nutr 20, 843–848.

Greatorex, J.C., 1975. Intravenous nutrition in the treatment of tetanus in horses. Vet Rec 97, 21.

Hallebeek, J.M., Beynen, A.C., 2001. A preliminary report on a fat-free diet formula for nasogastric enteral administration as treatment for hyperlipaemia in ponies. Vet Quart 23, 201–205.

Hansen, T.O., White, N.A., Kemp, D.T., 1988. Total parenteral nutrition in four healthy adult horses. Am J Vet Res 49, 122–124.

Hardy, J., 2003. Nutritional Support and Nursing Care of the Adult Horse in Intensive Care. Clin Tech Eq Prac 2, 193–198.

Hernandez, G., Velasco, N., Wainstein, C., et al., 1999. Gut mucosal atrophy after a short enteral fasting period in critically ill patients. Jof Crit Care 14, 73–77.

Hill, G.L., 1992. Understanding protein energy malnutrition. In: Hill, G.L. (Ed.), Disorders of Nutrition and Metabolism in Clinical Surgery. Understanding and Management. Churchill Livingstone, London, pp. 71–83.

Hoffer, R.E., Barber, S.M., Kallfelz, F.A., et al., 1977. Esophageal patch grafting as a treatment for esophageal stricture in a horse. J Am Vet Med Assoc 171, 350–354.

Jeejeebhoy, K.N., 2001. Total parenteral nutrition: Potion or poison? Am J Clin Nutr 74, 160–163.

Johnston, K., Holcombe, S.J., Hauptman, J.G., 2007. Plasma lactate as a predictor of colonic viability and survival after 360 degrees volvulus of the ascending colon in horses. Vet Surg 36, 563–567.

Keusch, G.T., 2003. The history of nutrition: Malnutrition, infection and immunity. J Nutr 133, 336S–340S.

Klip, A., Tsakiridis, T., Marette, A., et al., 1994. Regulation of expression of glucose transporters by glucose; a review of studies in vivo and in cell culture. FASEB J 8, 43–53.

Krinsley, J.S., 2004. Effect of an intensive glucose management protocol on the mortality of critically ill adult patients. Mayo Clin Proc 79, 992–1000.

Lacey, J.M., Wilmore, D.W., 1990. Is glutamine a conditionally essential amino acid? Nutr Rev 48, 297–309.

Langhans, W., 2002. Peripheral mechanisms involved with catabolism. Curr Opin Clin Nutr Metab Care 5, 419–426.

Langouche, L., Van den Berghe, G., 2006. Glucose metabolism and insulin therapy. Crit Care Clin 22, 119–129.

Lopes, M.A.F., White, N.A., 2002. Parenteral nutrition for horses with gastrointestinal disease: a retrospective study of 79 cases. Eq Vet J 34, 250–257.

Luyer, M.D., Jacobs, J.A., Vreugdenhil, A.C., et al., 2004. Enteral administration of high fat nutrition before and directly after hemorrhagic shock reduces endotoxemia and bacterial translocation. Ann of Surg 239, 257–264.

Marinella, M.A., 2005. Refeeding syndrome and hypophosphatemia. J Intensive Care Med 20, 155–159.

Mesotten, D., Swinnen, J., Vanderhyodonc, F., et al., 2004. Contribution of circulating lipids to the improved outcome of critical illness by glycemic control with intensive insulin therapy. J Clin Endocrinol Metab 89, 219–226.

Naylor, J.M., Freeman, D.E., Kronfeld, D.S., 1984. Alimentation of hypophagic horses. Comp Contin Educ of the Pract Vet 6, S93–S99.

Novak, F., Heyland, D.K., Avenell, A., et al., 2002. Glutamine supplementation in serious illness: a systematic review of the evidence. Crit Care Med 30, 2022–2029.

NRC, 2007. Nutrient Requirements of Horses, sixth ed. The National Academies Press, Washington DC.

Oftedal, O.T., Hintz, H.F., Schryver, H.F., 1983. Lactation in the Horse: Milk Composition and Intake by Foals. J Nutr 113, 2196–2206.

Paradis, M.R., 2001. Nutrition and indirect calorimetry in neonatal foals, In Proceedings of 19th Annual Veterinary Medical Forum of the American College of Veterinary Internal Medicine, Denver, CO May.

Pekala, P., Marlow, M., Heuvelman, D., et al., 1990. Regulation of hexose transport in aortic endothelial cells by vascular permeability factor and tumor necrosis factor-alpha but not by insulin. J Biol Chem 265, 18051–18054 2001 p 245–7.

Peter, J.V., Moran, J.L., Phillips-Hughes, J., 2005. A meta analysis of treatment outcomes of early enteral versus early parenteral nutrition in hospitalized patients. Crit Care Med 33, 260–261.

Potenza, M.A., Nacci, C., Mitolo-Chieppa, et al., 2001. Immunoregulatory effects of L-arginine and therapeutical implications. Curr Drug Targets Immune Endocr Metabol Disord 1, 67–77.

Powell-Tuck, 2007. Nutritional interventions in critical illness. Proc Nutr Soc 66, 16–24.

Rafael, J.F., Mora, M.D., 1999. Malnutrition: Organic and Functional Consequences. World J Surg 23, 530–535.

Ralston, S.L., 1990. clinical nutrition of adult horses. In: Turner AS (Ed.). Clinical Nutrition Veterinary Clinics of North America Equine Practice 6, 339–354.

Rassias, A.J., Marrin, C.A., Arruda, J., et al., 1999. Insulin infusion improves neutrophil function in diabetic cardiac surgery patients. Anesth Analg 88, 1011–1016.

Roberts, P.R., Zaloga, G.P., 2000. Enteral nutrition. In: Shoemaker, W.C., Ayres, S.M., Grenvick, A., et al. (Eds.), Textbook of Critical Care, fourth ed, WB Saunders, Philadelphia, pp. 875–898.

Rokyta, R., Matejovic, M., Krouzecky, A., et al., 2003. Enteral nutrition and hepatosplanchnic region in critically ill patients: Friends or foes? Physiol Res 52, 31–37.

Romero-Gomez, M., Jover, M., Galan, J.J., et al., 2009. Gut ammonia production and its modulation. Metab Brain Dis 24, 147–157.

Romijn, J.A., 2000. Substrate metabolism in the metabolic response to injury. Proc Nutr Soc 59, 447–449.

Rotting, A.K., Freeman, D.E., Constable, P.D., et al., 2004. Effects of phenylbutazone, indomethacine, prostaglandin E2, butyrate, and glutamine on restitution of oxidant-injured right dorsal colon of horses in vitro. Am J Vet Res 65, 1589–1595.

Ruth, E., 1998. The impact of L-arginine-nitric oxide metabolism on ischemia/reperfusion injury. Curr Opin Clin Nutr Metab Care 1, 97–99.

Saito, H., Trocki, O., Alexander, J.W., et al., 1987. The effect of route of nutrient administration on the nutritional state, catabolic hormone secretion, and gut mucosal integrity after burn injury. J Parent and Ent Nutr 11, 1–7.

Scheppach, W., 1994. Effects of short chain fatty acids on gut morphology and function. Gut 35 (supplement), S35–S38.

Schroeder, D., Gillanders, L., Mahr, K., et al., 1991. Effects of immediate postoperative enteral nutrition on body composition, muscle function and wound healing. J of Parent Enteral Nutr 15, 376–383.

Shikhman, A.R., Brinson, D.C., Valbracht, J., et al., 2001. Cytokine regulation of facilitated glucose transport in human articular hondrocytes. J Immunol 167, 7001–7008.

Stapleton, R.D., Jones, N., Heyland, D.K., 2007. Feeding critically ill patients: What is the optimal amount of energy? Crit Care Med 35 (supplement), 535–540.

Sternberg, J.A., Rohovsky, S.A., Blackburn, G.L., et al., 2000. Total parenteral nutrition for the critically ill patient. In: Shoemaker, W.C., Ayres, S.M., Grenvick, A., et al. (Eds.), Textbook of Critical Care, fourth ed. WB Saunders, Philadelphia, pp. 898–908.

Stick, J.A., 2011. Esophagus. In: Auer, J.A., Stick, J.A., (Eds.), Equine Surgery, fourth edition. Saunders Elsevier, St Louis, MO, pp. 367–388.

Stoll, B., Henry, J., Reeds, P.J., et al., 1998. Catabolism dominates the first-pass intestinal metabolism of dietary essential amino acids in milk protein-fed piglets. J Nutr 128, 606–614.

Stouthard, J.M.L., Romijn, J.A., Van der Poll, T., et al., 1995. Endocrine and metabolic effects of interleukin-6 in humans. Am Jof Physiol 268, E813–819.

Studley, H.O., 1936. Percentage weight loss: A basic indicator of surgical risk in patients with chronic peptic ulcer. J Am Med Assoc 106, 458–460.

Sweeney, R.W., Hansen, T.O., 1990. Use of a liquid diet as the sole source of nutrition in six dysphagic horses and as a dietary supplement in seven hypophagic horses. J Am Vet Med Assoc 197, 1030–1032.

Van den Berghe, G., Wilmer, A., Hermans, G., et al., 2006. Intensive insulin therapy in medical intensive care patients. N Engl J Med 354, 449–461.

Van den Berghe, G., 2004. How does blood glucose control with insulin save lives in intensive care? J Clin Invest 114, 1187–1195.

Van den Berghe, G., Wouters, P., Weekers, F., et al., 2001. Intensive insulin therapy in critically ill patients. N Engl J Med 345, 1359–1367.

Van der Poll, T., Romijn, J.A., Endert, E., et al., 1991. Tumor necrosis factor mimics the metabolic response to acute infection in healthy humans. Am J Physiol 261, E457–465.

Vanhorebeek, I., Van den Berghe, G., 2004. Hormonal and metabolic strategies to attenuate catabolism in critically ill patients. Curr Opin in Pharm 4, 621–628.

Ward, N., 2003. Nutrition support to patients undergoing gastrointestinal surgery. Nutr J 2, 1–5.

Weekers, F., Giulietti, A.P., Michalaki, M., et al., 2003. Metabolic, endocrine, and immune effects of stress hyperglycemia in a rabbit model of prolonged critical illness. Endocrinology 144, 5329–5338.

Windsor, J.A., Hill, G.L., 1988. Risk factors for post operative pneumonia: The importance of protein depletion. Annals Surg 208, 209–214.

Wischmeyer, P.E., 2007. Glutamine: Mode of action in critical illness. Crit Care Med 35 (supplement), 541–544.

Appendix: Nutritional requirements, recommendations and example diets

Examples of typical rations and how the nutrients they provide match with the requirement data given in Tables A1–A5 (based on NRC 2007) are shown in Figs A1–A5. In each case the average composition of typical feedstuffs and typical German commerical supplements and feeds have been used. Brief comments are then given with regard to these example diets (note that these are *real-world* examples of rations that are commonly fed to horses).

As a guide to the figures, a value of 1 means that the nutrients provided by that diet would meet the NRC requirements. A value of 2 indicates that the diet is providing twice the requirement level and a value of 0.5 means that only 50% of the requirement is met. In each case, the amount of the daily intake of each nutrient from different ration components is represented by different colours of the column bars. The nutrient composition of the compound/complementary feeds and mineral supplements used in these examples are presented in Table A6.

Maintenance

Basing the ration for a 500 kg horse at maintenance on grass hay, salt and a forage balancer (vitamin–mineral) supplement gives the nutrient profile depicted in Fig. A1A. Note the following:

- It should be clear that a healthy horse cannot lose bodyweight (BW) on such a diet unless hay quantity is restricted or of very poor (straw-like) quality.
- An average hay-based diet with 8% crude protein (CP) can provide sufficient protein for horses at maintenance. For some animals – especially those recovering from illness or being fed very mature hays or during seasons when hays are known to have much lower protein content – additional protein with an improved amino acid profile may be required. Some forage balancers do provide additional protein with a good amino acid profile.
- Even though the hay chosen has a low Ca content (3 g/kg) it would provide sufficient Ca to meet NRC requirements. However, the amount of Ca provided only just reaches the lower end of PH's more optimal recommendations given in Table A1. For horses that have been previously been in exercise work and now undergoing stall/box rest, PH recommends additional Ca.
- The intake of sodium and several trace elements will be below the recommended requirements unless a forage balancer is provided.
- In this example, salt is provided through supplementation but for many horses the provision of a salt block may be sufficient.
- Potassium in forage is commonly >20 g/kg dry matter (DM); this results in a daily over-consumption of potassium, which does not appear to cause health problems.
- Good hay (green color, harvested without rain and no heating (>~40°C) during post harvest fermentation) contains plenty of β-carotene; 15 mg is used here as an average value. Assuming that 1 mg carotene is converted to 400 IU vitamin A, there is an apparent very high intake of vitamin A. However: (1) the level in hay may be reduced due to oxidation of the carotene (inferior harvesting condition, post mature hay, or long storage [>1 year]); and (2) horses appear able to decrease the rate of conversion to vitamin A when excess carotene is consummed.

In Fig. A1A the grass hay is replaced by a legume hay (mature) but the vitamin-mineral supplement is the same as in Fig. A1A. It should be noted that this commercially available supplement is lower than most in its calcium content (10%) but not as low as one would ideally recommend for a legume hay-based ration.

- Adding a general mineral supplement supplies trace elements not otherwise provided but, especially if not specifically designed for alfalfa forage, there is a risk that such supplements will increase the macro element intake to levels far in excess of requirements (although intake may not reach overt toxic levels, especially in the case of P, the excess intake will substantially increase the environmental load).
- Many mineral supplements contain >10% Ca, which is certainly not required for an alfalfa hay-based ration. Ideally the forage balancer should be designed at least to support either a grass hay or a legume hay based ration.
- Unfortunately, many vitamin–mineral supplements contain inadequate levels of some trace elements and, in particular, Vitamin E. In this example, providing 100 g/day of the commercial supplement (which is more than the manufacturer's recommended intake levels) only just met Zn and Cu requirements providing the hay had average levels of these nutrients. The relatively low proportion of the daily intake provided by the forage (green component of the column) shows the importance of the forage balancer (blue component).

  It is important to note that if all the β-carotene in the hay was destroyed by oxidation, the supplemental vitamin A provided by the vitamin and mineral supplement would be sufficient to cover requirements. The apparent oversupply is not an issue as relatively little is ingested as preformed vitamin A.

Conclusion

Most hays will be suitable as a maintentance diet but will require trace element supplementation in most cases to

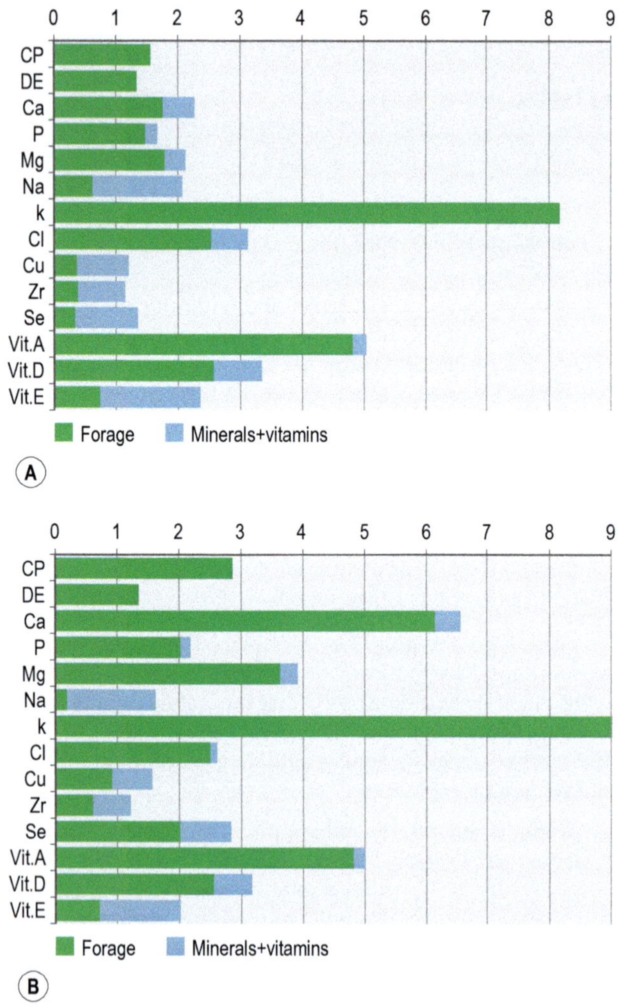

Fig. A1 **Energy and nutrient provision by a ration designed for a 500-kg horse at maintenance.**

(A) Based on average grass hay:
- 12 kg hay, average meadow hay, 8% CP as fed
- 30 g NaCl
- 100 g forage balancer – trace element/vitamin supplement (Cu 800, Zn 3000, Se 10 mg/kg; vitamin.A 35 000 IU/kg, vitamin E 8000 mg/kg)
- No concentrates (energy providing feeds).

(B) Legume hay based:
- 12 kg legume forage hay, mature
- 30 g NaCl
- 80 g mineral supplement

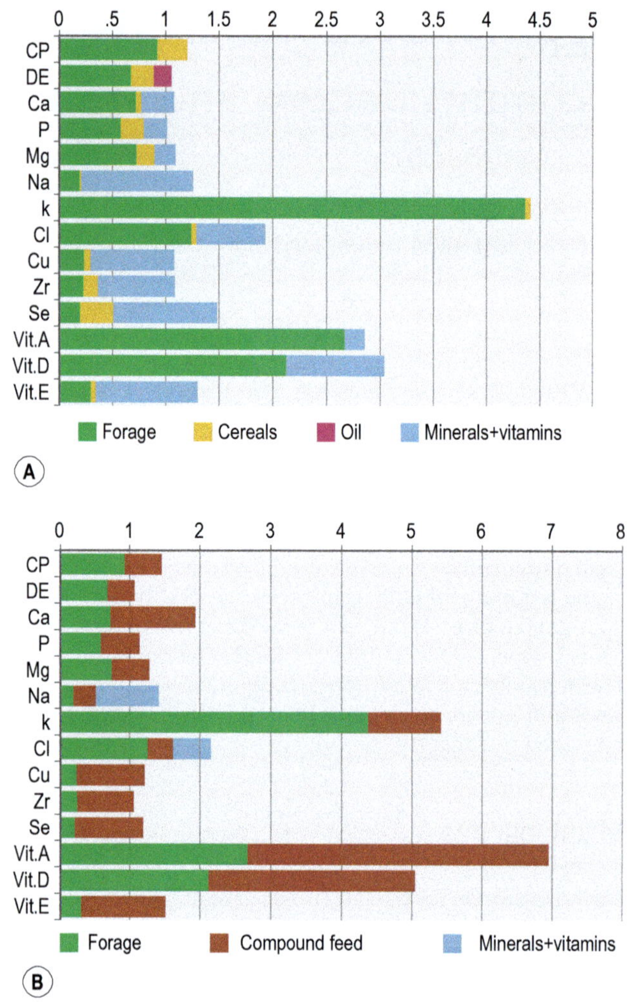

Fig. A2 **Energy and nutrients provision by a ration designed for a 500-kg horse in hard work.**

(A) Home mix of grass hay, cereal grain, oil, a balancer supplement, and salt:
- 10 kg hay (average meadow hay)
- 2 kg oats
- 0.5 kg oil
- 120 g vitamin-mineral forage balancer
- 60 g NaCl

(B) Hay plus compound feed for exercise:
- 10 kg meadow hay
- 4 kg compound feed
- 60 g NaCl (represented by the gray part of Na and Cl column)

provide the required intake of all nutrients. Depending on the protein quality, amino acid supplementation may or may not be required. Under certain circumstances vitamin supplementation may be required (e.g., preserved forage that has been stored for a prolonged period of time will have low vitamin A and/or vitamin E [especially haylage/silage]). Additional macro elements (apart from sodium) are not normally required, although some nutritionists (PH) would recommend increased Ca intakes for stall/box rested animals.

Exercise

Figure A2 illustrates a typical hay + grain + oil + vitamin/mineral supplement combination as the basic model for feeding an intensively exercising horse.

The example in Fig. A2A includes 0.5 kg soy bean oil, which helps to limit starch intake.

- The green part of the energy column indicates the relative proportion of energy that the hay provides – it will depend on the hay being fed and in practice the actual value is often greater than the theoretical table value.
- As CP provision is >1 it can be assumed that there is a surplus in essential amino acids; this may not always be the case especially if poor quality hay or unusual protein sources are fed.
- As with the maintenance example, mineral supplementation (especially the trace elements) is required to meet requirements.
- Without additional NaCl the sweat related requirements in Na and Cl cannot be met. However, the

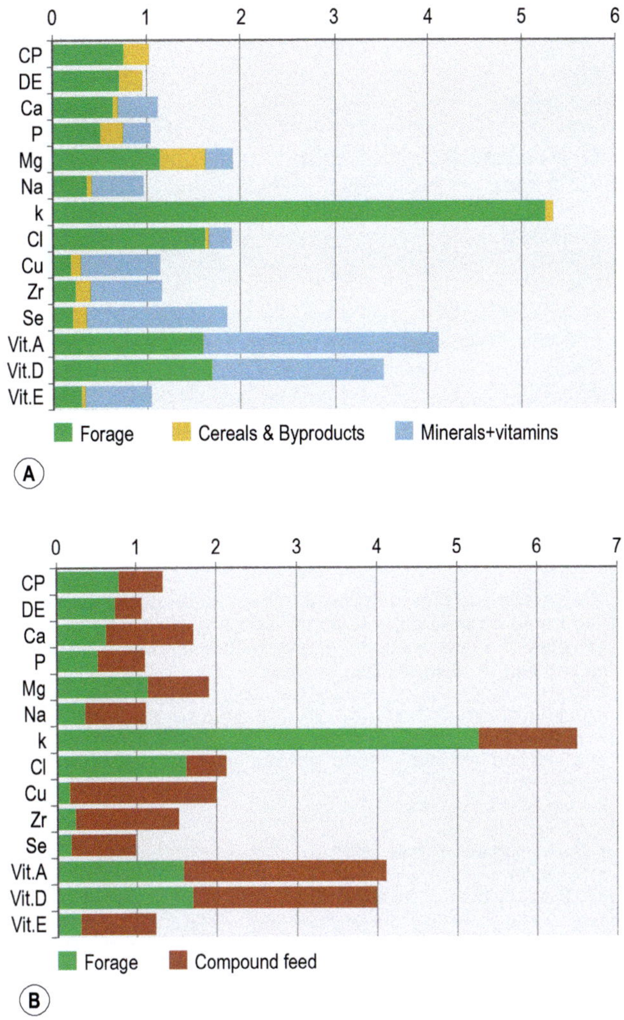

Fig. A3 Energy and nutrients provision by a ration designed for a 500-kg mare in the last month of pregnancy.

(A) Hay + grain + supplements:
- 8 kg hay
- 1 kg barley
- 0.5 kg linseed meal (solvent extracted)
- 150 g vitamin–mineral supplement

(B) Hay + compound feed.
- 8 kg meadow hay + 2.5 kg compound feed (18% CP)

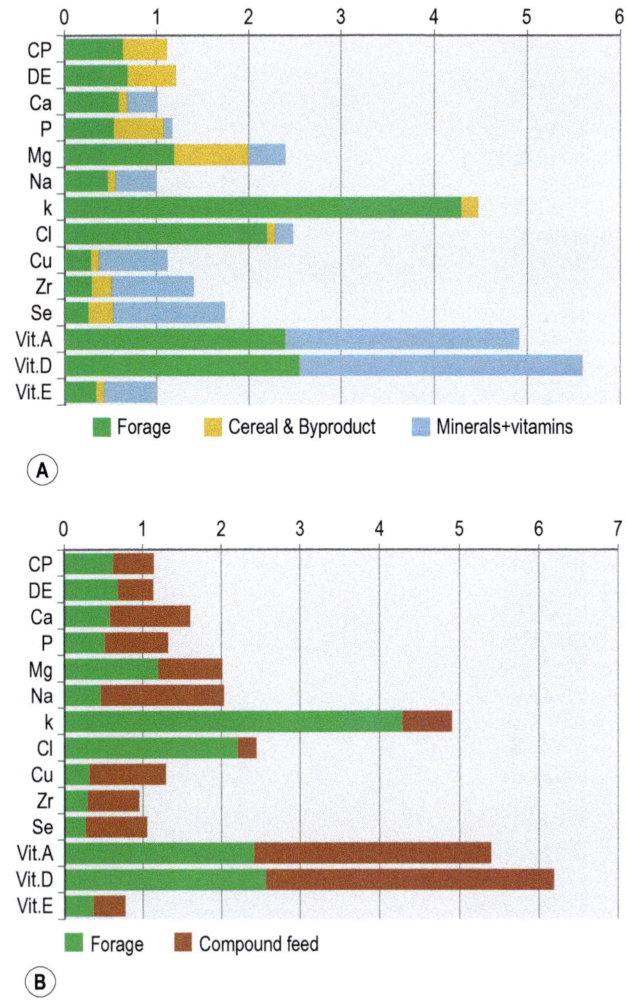

Fig. A4 Energy and nutrients provision by a ration designed for a 500-kg horse in the 2nd month of lactation.

(A) Hay + grain + protein feed + supplements:
- 12 kg meadow hay
- 4 kg corn, flaked
- 1 kg linseed (solvent extracted)
- 150 g vitamin–mineral supplement

(B) Hay + compound feed:
- 12 kg meadow hay
- 5 kg compound feed, 16% CP

mineral supplement should not be selected on the basis of NaCl provision; Na and Cl supplementation should be addressed through the addition of salt with reference to sweat production (see also Chapter 14).

Figure A2B represents the alternative to a home mixed ration – a hay plus commercial compound feed ration.

- The compound feed should replace the grain and the mineral supplement; but NaCl should be provided separately.
- The quality of the overal ration again will depend on the feeding value of hay in a similar way to Fig. A2A except that the amino acid profile of the overall diet will typically be superior when compared to the grain-based ration.
- This German compound feed, in common with many commercial feeds, provides an oversupply of vitamin A even if all the β-carotene in the hay has been lost.
- The ration also oversupplies vitamin D (even for the more optimal recommendations by PH for stabled horses).
- However, the vitamin E intake is marginal (on a NRC basis and low with respect to PH's more optimal recommendations).

Pregnant mare

Figure A3 illustrates example rations for a pregnant mare.

- An important consideration is the contribution of the chosen forage to total protein intake. Data on the protein content of the forage is therefore critical. The addition of a protein-rich source (in this case linseed) helps to ensure that protein quality is in an appropriate range. However, many grass forages or meadow hays are below the CP content of the hay used in this

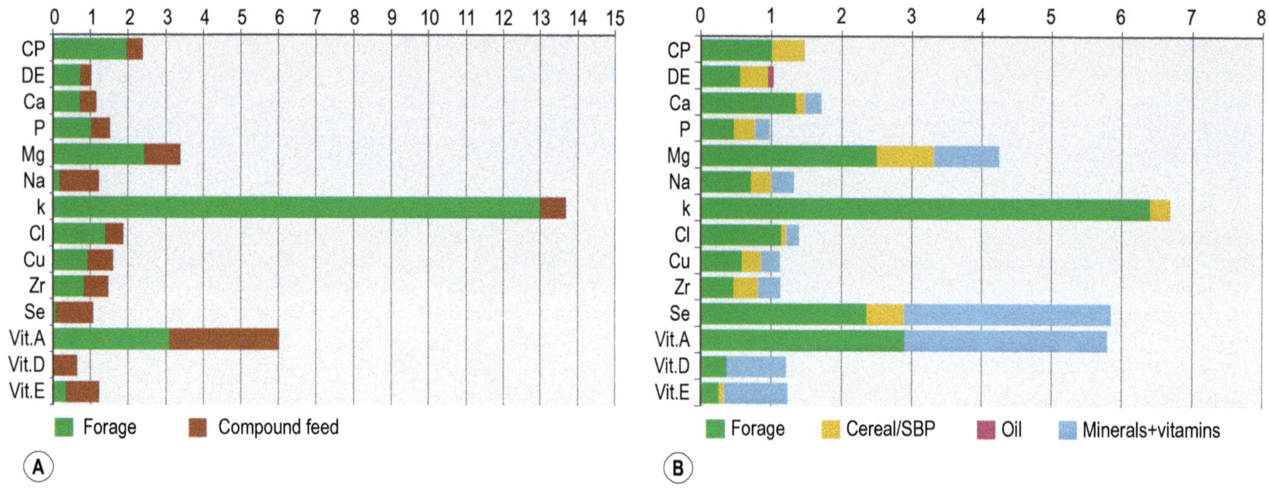

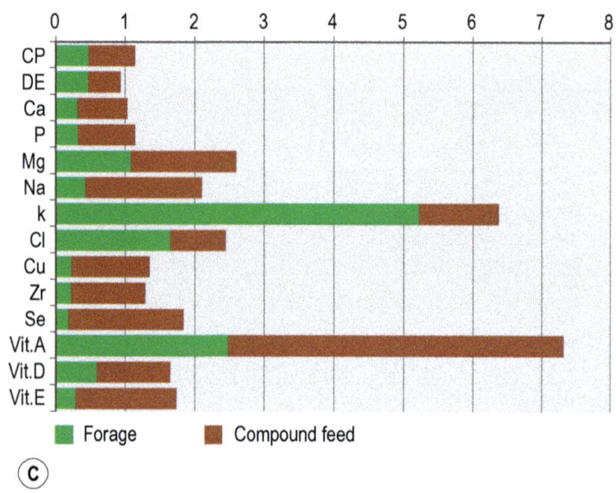

Fig. A5 Energy and nutrient provision by a ration designed for (500-kg horse when adult) a 6 month weanling at about 225 kg BW (a value of 1 means supply equals recommendation, a value > 1 means supply exceeds requirements).

(A) Pasture + compound feed – expected DM intake from pasture about 2% of BW:
- 25 kg grass
- 1.5 kg compound feed (for a growing foal)

(B) Home mix:
- 4 kg alfalfa hay (early cut)
- 1.5 kg oats
- 0.5 kg sugar beet pulp (SBP)
- 0.1 kg oil
- 0.2 kg soy bean solvent extract
- 80 g vitamin–mineral supplement

(C) Hay + compound feed:
- 4 kg meadow hay
- 2.5 kg compound feed

example (frequently <10% CP as fed) and therefore protein (and amino acid intake) can become marginal or deficient unless adequate amounts of a protein providing supplement of a suitable quality are provided.

- Another key area of concern for the pregnant animal is copper – the Cu content of hays vary considerably and many can be significantly lower than used in these examples and may result in deficient intake, especially if PH's more optimal Cu intake is the target.
- An appropriate vitamin–mineral supplement is essential for adequate trace element supply if a fortified compound feed is not fed.
- Again the quantity of vitamins that need to be supplied by the vitamin-mineral supplement will vary to some extent according to the vitamin content of the forage, time of year and access to pasture etc. Old stored hay, for example, can be very low in vitamins A and E.

Lactating mare

Figures A4A and A4B reflect the requirements for lactating mares.

- Lactating mares have a high dry matter intake (DMI). Hay can easily be provided at >10 kg/day for a 500-kg lactating mare and intakes of around 15 kg are common (Fig. A4A).
- The milk yield requires extra protein and typically around 50% of protein and energy will come from grain-based and protein-rich feeds. The actual quantities of these feeds will depend on the feeding value of the forage.
- It is not possible to ensure an adequate mineral and trace element intake without a supplement.
- It is important to know the Ca content of the forage in order to select a supplement with the required Ca concentration (levels in commercial products typically vary from <10 up to 25%).
- Again the quantity of vitamins that need to be supplied by any vitamin-mineral supplement will vary to some extent according to the vitamin content of the forage, time of year and access to pasture etc. Old stored hay for example can be very low in vitamins A and E.
- A compound feed can substitute the grain + protein feed + vitamin-mineral supplement combination, and often results in a more convenient ration. Such feeds typically include soy bean, linseed products, or comparable byproducts from peanut, cottonseed or other seeds, all of which are high in protein and starch.

The CP of the compound feed should be about 16% (Fig. A4B).

Weanling

Figure A5 depicts typical rations for a weanling at 6 months of age.

- Many foals are out at pasture around weaning time (Fig. A5A).
- If feeding preserved forages, highly fermentable fiber should be a major characteristic of rations for foals close to weaning. Early cut meadow hay or alfalfa are preferred sources, combined with feeds rich in pectins like sugar beet pulp (Fig. A5B).
- Oil provides non starch energy and also helps to maintain palatability and reduces dust – helping to minimize wastage and loss of mineral compounds.
- The protein requirements for growth will not be covered by forage of average quality. As mentioned before, the feeding value of hay dictates the need for grain and protein supplements (when linked with the type and breed of animal, desired rate of growth, etc.).
- Amino acid intake of the diet is key. *Note:* Information on protein quality of the forage is needed for accurate dosing of supplementary protein feeds. Late cut hay may be low in protein but, more importantly, low in protein quality.
- The selection of mineral supplements or compound feeds should avoid vitamin excess.
- Again, most forage will induce a high K intake (many fold higher than the requirement). Foals, like adult horses, that are kept outside are unlikely to need high vitamin D supplements. Common supplements also result in unnecessarily high vitaimin A provision. Average pasture ensures sufficient carotene supply (see the example for vitamin A intake when 1 mg carotene within grass is converted to 400 IU vit. A in Fig. A5A – which clearly shows that the grass alone would supply sufficient vitamin A).
- Vitamin–mineral supplementation via a specific product or through a commercial compound feed will be required.
- For selecting a mineral supplement for a certain type of forage it is helpful to know the calcium, copper and zinc content. Many products are high in calcium and therefore not well balanced for legume based forage ration (e.g., alfalfa hay).
- The diet in Fig. A5B is based on the typical feed materials that are available on a predominantly cattle production focussed farm. The mineral supplement used here is low in Ca as some restriction of additional Ca provision is indicated for diets including alfalfa (or other legume forage).
- The diet for a weanling can be simplified by use of a compound feed in addition to pasture or hay (Fig. A5C).

Table A1 Daily Maintenance Nutrient Requirements (RQ)s and Recommendations (RC) for a 500-kg Horse According to North American (NRC 2007) and German (GEH 2013) Authorities, as Well as More Optimal Recommendations (OR) of One of the Editors (PH)

	NRC (RQ)	GEH (RC)	This book (RQ/RC)	PH (OR)	Editor's comments
Energy (MJ) NB: DE or ME	DE: 64–76 MJ Depending on basal activity level, cum temperament. NB NRC in Mcal. 1 Mcal = 4.184 MJ	ME: 55 MJ NB: GEH use MJ ME per kg metabolic BW differentiated for type of animal (MJ/kg $BW^{0.75}$); pony (0.4), Warmblood (0.52), Thoroughbred (0.64)	Depends on system used	Base on NRC but adapt to individual	The best judge of absolute energy requirement is the horse – feed to the individual e.g. • if it is too fat then it is receiving too much energy! • if it is too excitable then need to evaluate energy sources and training/management practices, etc. Requirements/need for complementary feed may change with time according to environmental conditions, availability of grass during any turnout, nature of the forage, time spent at maintenance, exercise level prior to any box rest, whether ill, etc. The lower end of these ranges can be hard to achieve practically especially when providing grass turnout. Need to adjust forage energy level to try to maximize time spent foraging – very mature forages/highly silicated forages especially if provided solus may increase the risk of impaction colic in some individuals. Think of ways to environmentally enrich any stable especially during prolonged box rest – e.g., use of mirrors.
CP (g)	540–720	(317 g of prececally digestible protein = protein soluble in neutral detergent; assuming an average prececal digestibility of 0.7 results in an estimate of) ~ 453 g CP	540–720	550–750	Protein quality, i.e., amino acid profile is as, if not more, important than total intake. Can exceed upper recommended levels if providing high intakes of legume hays, e.g., alfalfa see Chapter 6. If stabled for long periods good stable management is required especially if excess protein given. In silages (and to a lesser extent in haylages) part of CP undergoes proteolysis, up to 60% of nitrogen can be present as non-protein-nitrogen without any sign of spoilage. Results in actual protein value being far less to the horse.
Lysine (g)	23.2–31	(27 g of prececally digestible lysine assuming 0.7 for digestibility as for CP gives) 39 g for gross lysine	23.2–31	30	In weight loss scenarios our current advice is to ensure adequate protein esp key amino acids to try and minimize skeletal muscle loss (plus increase exercise if possible). Balancing/maximizing forage intake using mature forages increases the risk of an inadequate intake of lysine.
Ca (g)	20	17	17	37.5–50	Stabled horses at rest may lose bone mineral content and therefore may require proportionally more Ca, although any additional calcium may not automatically reverse the effects of de-conditioning. An excessive calcium intake (i.e. 4-5-fold × requirements) has no advantages and may be undesirable.

Table A1 *Continued*

	NRC (RQ)	GEH (RC)	This book (RQ/RC)	PH (OR)	Editor's comments
P (g)	14	12	12	22.5–30	Ratio of Ca:P may be as important as total amount – aim between 1.5–2:1. Effects of phytase on P-availability practically appears to be negligible.
Mg (g)	7.5	5.5	5.5	10–15	No scientific evidence that higher magnesium intakes either reduce the risk of laminitis or promote calm behavior.
K (g)	25	15	25	25+	On forage based maintenance diets should be impossible not to provide sufficient K. No evidence higher intakes (as provided by forage-based rations) has any negative effects under normal circumstances.
Na (g)	10	2.8	2.8	10 (–15)	Providing free salt or a salt block in an easily accessible place may be sufficient. Monitor use. Do not use mineral blocks formulated for other species. NB up to 15 g for those losing 3 liters of sweat/day through any activity/environmental conditions, etc.
Cl (g)	40	40 (1.6 accordingly the strict factorial approach)	40	40	Cl provision of 80 mg/kg BW/day will support Cl homeostasis and not promote the development of metabolic alkalosis. Intake levels based purely on factorial methods will be too low.
Cu (mg)	100	106	106	100–150	Recommend that not >30% of the total dietary intake of trace elements comes from chelated mineral sources.
I (mg)	3.5	2.1	1.1	2	Iodine levels from NRC appear too high. Very difficult to assess iodine intakes from organic materials. Seaweeds contain very variable and sometimes very high levels of I.
Fe (mg)	400	420	420	400–450	Some mineral sources contain high levels of iron contamination. Rare to have an inadequate intake of iron.
Mn (mg)	400	420	420	400–450	Unlikely to have an inadequate intake of Mn under practical circumstances.
Se (mg)	1	1.1	1.1	1.5–2	Especially if on box rest due to illness etc. may be helpful to maintain above minimum levels of antioxidants. >1 mg/100 kg BW may increase the risk of hoof quality issues.
Zn (mg)	400	420	420	400–450	Cu:Zn ratio in the diet may be important – current advice is to try and maintain around 3.5–4.5:1.

Table A1 *Continued*

	NRC (RQ)	GEH (RC)	This book (RQ/RC)	PH (OR)	Editor's comments
Vitamin A (IU)	15K	16K	16K	40K (vitamins A/β-carotene)	Of the 40K ~ half i.e., 20K to come from preformed vitamin A ideally, especially if being fed preserved forages. Risks are with over provision of vitamin A rather than excessive ingestion of the precursor β-carotene. More mature forages may have lower β-carotene levels. Stored forages may have lower β-carotene levels.
Vitamin D (IU)	3.3K	3.2K	3.2K	5K	May not be important to add if out at grass in sunshine but likely to be required if stabled. Recent work in other species suggest vitamin D to have a wider influence than previously thought.
Vitamin E (IU)	500	530	530 (increase under certain circumstances see Vitamin Chapter)	1000–1500	No known risks of the higher intakes and may help provide additional support especially to the convalescent/stressed animal. Silage, haylage and hay levels of vitamin E can be very low. Diets with additional oil supplementation plus those that include haylages/silages require additional vitamin E support (at least 1 IU/ml of supplemental oil).
Thiamin (mg)	30	32	32	32	Although theoretically the horse should obtain sufficient B vitamins from the diet and microbial production, under certain conditions this may not be adequate (e.g., stressed animals, those on a low forage diet or any with a disturbed gastrointestinal tract microbiota).
Riboflavin (mg)	20	21	21	NRC	
Others					Especially if box rested for long periods need to promote good hoof quality – through hygiene, etc. Some animals with poor hooves may benefit from biotin at 3–5 mg/100 kg BW for many months. Additional vitamin C may be of value if lung health is compromised. Additional folic acid may be advantageous in animals without access to fresh forage – folate supplementation should be carried out with caution in horses treated with dihydrofolate reductase inhibitors (for EPM).

BW, body weight; CP, crude protein; DE, digestible energy; EPM, equine protozoal myeloencephalitis; ME, metabolizable energy.
K = ×1000.

Table A2 Nutrient Requirements (RQ)s and Recommendations (RC) for a 500-kg Horse in Exercise Training, according to North American (NRC 2007) and German (GEH 2013) Authorities, as Well as More Optimal Recommendations (OR) of One of the Editors (PH)

	NRC (RQ)	GEH (RC)	This book (RC)	PH (OR)	Editor's comments
Energy (MJ) NB: DE or ME	DE: 84–144 MJ MJ Based on one of 4 levels of exercise. NB: NRC in Mcal. 1 Mcal ~ 4.184 MJ	ME: 60–140 MJ NB: GEH use MJ ME per kg metabolic BW Calculation based on heart rate (HR), 60 min: walk, HR 90 >13.5 MJ trot, HR 130 >28.2 MJ canter, HR 170 >49.8 MJ or for 4 min at HRmax >26.7 MJ	Depends on system used	Based on NRC but adapt to individual	The best judge of absolute energy requirement is the horse – feed to the individual • if it is too fat then it is receiving too much energy! • if it is too excitable then need to evaluate energy sources and training/management practices, etc. Very difficult to determine individual animal exercise level – owner perceptions vary considerably, individual metabolism plays a role, as does temperament during and after exercise. Requirements/need for complementary feed may change with environmental conditions, availability of grass during any turnout, nature of the forage, body condition, rider fitness, etc. Forage should remain the foundation of any diet even in the very intensively exercising animals – consider less mature forages, more highly digestible fiber sources (e.g., soya hulls, sugar beet) see Chapter 17. Difficult to keep starch intakes <1 g/kg BW/meal if use cereals fed solus – consider >2 meals/day, mixed feeds, use of oil addition etc.
CP (g)	699–1004	Maintenance + 20% 380 g precaecally digestible CP corresponding to 545 g CP	699–1004	750–1500	Protein quality, i.e., amino acid profile is as, if not more, important than total intake. Ensure adequate water intake and stable hygiene. Exact extra needs are unknown, elevated feed intake will often cover those extras. Horses with inferior training response and loss in BW may profit from additional quality CP from appropriately processed linseed or soy bean meal.
Lysine (g)	30–43	46 g Maintenance + 20% See CP	30–43	30–50	Allow up to 0.1 g/kg BW in hard/intensive exercise and training so as not to limit muscle development and repair plus to try and ensure adequate general amino acid composition to the diet.
Ca (g)	30–40	20.4 (Maintenance + 20%; a surplus ensures the coverage of increased bone metabolism)	21	45 g + 0.2 g/l sweat loss	May need to provide higher amounts when first go into training (up to 60 + g) in particular when being concurrently stabled following free paddock exercise.

Table A2 *Continued*

	NRC (RQ)	GEH (RC)	This book (RC)	PH (OR)	Editor's comments
P (g)	18–29	14.4 (maintenance + 20%, see above)	15	25–30 + (hard work) needs to be in proportion with Ca	Ratio of Ca: P may be as important as total amount – aim between 1.5 – 2:1. May be an advantage to increase when first go into training (~35 +g) Sweat loss negligible.
Mg (g)	9.5–15	6.6 (maintenance + 20%)	6.5	15 + 0.125 g/l sweat loss	May help when first go into training (~20 g).
K (g)	28.5–53	Maintenance + 1.65 g/kg sweat = 31.5 g for 1–2 h exercise with 10 liters sweat	24 (10 l sweat)	Minimum of 35+ at least 0.5 g/l sweat loss	Potential not to provide sufficient K if on low forage intakes especially if exchange grass hay weight for weight with haylage. Need to replenish potassium lost in sweat especially post exercise (through forage based intake plus potassium containing supplements). A good balanced diet with adequate electrolyte content needs to be fed post exercise.
Na (g)	14–41	Maintenance + 3.9/kg sweat; amount r; corresponding to 41.7 g for 1–2 h exercise with 10 liters of sweat; amounts related to 10 liters sweat equals 100 g NaCl and needs to be distributed over 2–3 days	43 (10 l sweat)	15 + 1.2 g (endurance type work) or + 2 g (occasional hard work)/l sweat loss	Providing free salt or a salt block in an easily accessible place may be sufficient unless in hard work or with high sweat losses. Do not use mineral blocks formulated for other species. Monitor use. Sodium intake based on pure replacement factorial method overestimates sodium intake especially if one tries to replace all that is lost around the time of loss rather than over the 2–3 days as recommended by GEH. A good balanced diet with adequate electrolyte content needs to be fed for several days post exercise.
Cl (g)	47–93	Maintenance + 5.35 g/kg sweat; corresponding to 93.5 g for 1–2 h exercise with 10 liters of sweat; amounts related to >10 liters sweat need to be distributed over 2–3 days. See Na.	56 (10 l sweat)	40 +~3 g/l sweat	Replacement should be covered if adequate Na and K provided by NaCl and KCl.
Cu (mg)	100–125	106	106	125–175	
I (mg)	3.5–4.4	2.1	2.1	2–3	Iodine levels from NRC appear too high and are largely based on one short-term stepwise study that may not be applicable to the field situation. From personal experiences levels of 0.4 µg/BW should be adequate. Very difficult to assess iodine intakes from organic materials. Seaweeds contain very variable and sometimes very high levels of I.

Table A2 *Continued*

	NRC (RQ)	GEH (RC)	This book (RC)	PH (OR)	Editor's comments
Fe (mg)	400–500	420	420	500–625	Some mineral sources contain high levels of iron contamination. Rare to have an inadequate intake of iron. Anemia in exercising animals is rarely if ever due to iron deficiency.
Mn (mg)	400–500	480	420	500–700	
Se (mg)	1–1.25	1.1	1.5	2–3	Especially if on box rest due to illness, etc. may be helpful to maintain above minimum levels of antioxidants. Rec not > 0.01 mg/kg BW.
Zn (mg)	400–500	530	420	500–700	Cu:Zn ratio in the diet may be important – current advice is to try and maintain around 3.5–4.5:1.
Vitamin A (IU)	22.5K	24K	24K	50K (mix vitamin A and β-carotene)	Around 30K to come as preformed vitamin A. Risks are with over provision of vitamin A rather than excessive ingestion of the precursor β-carotene. More mature forages may have lower β-carotene levels. Stored forages may have lower β-carotene levels.
Vitamin D (IU)	3.3K	3.2K	3.2	5K	May not be important to add if out at grass in sunshine but likely to be required if stabled.
Vitamin E (IU)	800–1000	1100	530–1060	1500–2500	Haylage and hay levels of vitamin E can be very low. Higher intakes may be advantageous re oxidative stress of exercise/ immune support. Recommend not >10 IU/kg BW unless specific clinical reason.
Thiamin (mg)	30–62.5	63	32–64	65	
Riboflavin (mg)	20–25	21	21	25	
Others					Additional vitamin C may be of value if respiratory compromised (e.g., when stabled/lung inflammation/ RAO).

BW, body weight; CP, crude protein; DE, digestible energy; ME, metabolizable energy; RAO, recurrent airway obstruction.
K = ×1000.

Table A3 Daily Nutrient Requirements (RQ)s and Recommendations for a 550-kg Mare at 10 Months of Pregnancy, (RC) according to North American (NRC 2007) and German (GEH 2013) Authorities, as Well as More Optimal Recommendations (OR) of One of the Editors (PH)

	NRC (RQ)	GEH (RC)	This book (RQ/RC)	PH (OR)	Editor's comments
Energy (MJ) NB: DE or ME	DE: 84.5 MJ Allowing for 0.52 kg/ day ADG. NB: NRC in Mcal 1 Mcal ~ 4.184 MJ	ME: 71.7 MJ for day 305 of gestation; energy and nutrient requirements follow an exponential growth curve of the fetus with day of gestation as determining variable; energy of fetus is derived by fetal heart rate NB: GEH use MJ ME per kg metabolic BW	Depends on system used	Base on NRC but adapt to individual	The best judge of absolute energy requirement is the horse – feed to the individual. Early obesity in young mares may lead to placental restriction and lowered birth weights – but not proven. Mares that are too fat at parturition may provide less milk than anticipated to the foal – possible compensatory growth post weaning in her offspring. Mares that are too thin at parturition may build up own reserves during early lactation – again possible compensatory growth post weaning in her foal. Foals of mares fed reduced energy or protein levels during pregnancy and then adequate amounts during lactation – may not necessarily be smaller at birth but tend to grow more slowly during the 1st month but by 6 months of age can have the same overall weight gain as foals from mares that had not been restricted during late pregnancy – suggesting potentially too rapid growth in this period. Need to feed the mare during pregnancy for her own requirements as well as the fetus – e.g., young mares may still be growing themselves – thin mares may need to put on weight. If the mare gains less than 10% during pregnancy it is likely that she will utilize some of her own body stores to meet demands, which may not be an issue if she was in an adequate to good body condition beforehand but can be if this was not the situation. Many mares put on weight in mid gestation and do not need further weight gain during the latter part of gestation – unless as discussed above need to put on condition themselves. Need to try and ensure start to introduce the feed that will be provided during lactation before parturition. Poor quality forage is very unlikely to provide sufficient energy (and other key nutrients) for the pregnant mare especially from mid and during late gestation. Beware of starving an obese mare due to the potential risk of hyperlipemia and beware of overfeeding a thin mare especially with high starch diets (increased risk of laminitis, etc.). It is important to consider the nature of the forage being provided as well as its nutritional content, e.g., beware in certain countries fescue with endophyte fungus – (remove from areas at least 90days prior to foaling); hybrid sorghum/Sudan grasses can increase the risk of cystitis syndrome/ prussic acid poisoning etc.

Table A3 *Continued*

	NRC (RQ)	GEH (RC)	This book (RQ/RC)	PH (OR)	Editor's comments
CP (g)	841	500 prececal digestible protein corresponds to 715 g CP	841	~1000	Protein quality, i.e., amino acid profile is as if not more important than total intake.
Lysine (g)	36	30	36	40	
Ca (g)	36	41	41	~50 +	Ratios of protein and calcium requirements to energy intake are not identical in pregnancy to those at maintenance – so one cannot just increase the amount of the basal diet to match energy needs. Over 80% of the magnesium and 90% of the calcium and phosphorus content are deposited in the 8th–11th months. For most mares a compound, manufactured, appropriately fortified feed, specifically designed for the purpose can be advantageous especially in mid/the last third of pregnancy.
P (g)	26	29	28	32	Ratio of Ca:P may be as important as total amount – aim between 1.5–2:1.
Mg (g)	8	6.0	5.8	12.5–15	
K (g)	26	15.7	25	25+	On forage based maintenance diets should be impossible not to provide sufficient K.
Na (g)	11	4.0	4.0	15	Providing free salt or a salt block in an easily accessible place may be sufficient. Monitor use. Do not use mineral blocks formulated for other species.
Cl (g)	41	41 (2 g accordingly strict factorial approach)	41	40+	
Cu (mg)	125	106	110	150–200	Nearly half the copper, zinc and manganese accumulation in the newborn foal occurs, in the 10th month of gestation. Cu supplementation during pregnancy may be important re helping to reduce risk of nutritional associated DOD. Pasture and forage vary considerably in their nutritional content and yet in most pregnant mares these provide the bulk of the diet. Ideally monitor so that the diet can be appropriately fortified for the individual circumstances. Even if additional energy and protein not needed a vitamin–mineral supplement (+ lysine) likely to be required. Advise a maximum of 30% of any trace element intake should come from chelated sources.

Table A3 *Continued*

	NRC (RQ)	GEH (RC)	This book (RQ/RC)	PH (OR)	Editor's comments
I (mg)	4	2.1	2.1	2–3	Iodine levels from NRC appear too high. Seaweeds contain very variable and sometimes very high levels of I. Too much or too little iodine can lead to goiter. Rec lower upper limit than NRC for the pregnant mare at 3 mg/100 kg BW.
Fe (mg)	500	530	530	NRC	Some mineral sources contain high levels of iron contamination. Rare to have an inadequate intake of iron.
Mn (mg)	400	420	420	600–750	
Se (mg)	1	1.6	1.55	2–3	Higher intakes of vitamin E and selenium to the mare during the periparturient period may beneficially influence colostrum concentrations of immunoglobulins.
Zn (mg)	400	530	530	600–750	Cu : Zn ratio in the diet may be important – our current advice is to try and maintain around 3.5–4.5 : 1.
Vitamin A (IU)	30K	32K	32K	60K	Some suggest β-carotene source may influence conception rates but controversial.
Vitamin D (IU)	3.3K	5.3K	3.2–5.3K	~7K (NRC 1989 ~2.5% DM intake)	Especially if inside during the winter.
Vitamin E (IU)	800	1100	1000	1600–2500	Higher intakes of vitamin E and selenium to the mare during the periparturient period may beneficially influence colostrum concentrations of immunoglobulins.
Thiamin (mg)	30	32	30	30	
Riboflavin (mg)	20	21	20	20	
Others					Further recommendations from the literature include. Folic acid ~ 1.1–1.3 mg/kg DM in pregnant mares.

BW, body weight; CP, crude protein; DE, digestible energy; DOD, developmental orthopedic disease; ME, metabolizable energy.
K = ×1000.

Table A4 Nutrient Requirements (RQ)s and Recommendations (RC) for a 500-kg Mare in the 2nd Month of Lactation, according to North American (NRC 2007) and German (GEH 2013) Authorities, as Well as More Optimal Recommendations (OR) of one of the Editors (PH)

	NRC (RQ)	GEH (RC)	This book (RQ/RC)	PH (OR)	Editor's comments
Energy (MJ) NB: DE or ME	DE: 133 Allows for 16.2 kg milk/day. NB: NRC in Mcal. 1 Mcal ~ 4.184 MJ	ME: 109–105 MJ for day 28 – day 60 of lactation; peak of lactation at about day 30 NB: GEH use MJ ME per kg metabolic BW	Depends on system used	Base on NRC and adapt to individual	The best judge of absolute energy requirement is the horse – feed to the individual. Milk yield (~2–4% BW) is influenced by: • Mare's innate ability • Feed consumption in late gestation • Water availability • Intake of energy and nutrients during lactation • Quality of forage • Stage of lactation. All nutrient and energy requirements depend on the actual amount of milk produced and the amount deposited within the milk. The concentrate proportion of the feed required will vary according to the individual and the quality of the feed being provided. A very heavy milker may need 1.75% BW as concentrates (non-forage portion) although more typical may be 0.75–1.25% especially if on good pasture. Increasing the starch providing concentrate proportion of the diet will increase the milk yield, but decrease the fat and protein content of the milk. Ratios of protein and calcium requirements to energy intake are not identical in lactation to those at maintenance – so one cannot just increase the amount of the basal diet to match energy needs. For most mares a compound, manufactured, appropriately fortified feed, specifically designed for the purpose can be advantageous during lactation.
CP (g)	1530	870–780 g prececal digestible CP corresponds to 1243–1115 g CP	1530	1600–1800	Protein quality i.e., amino acid profile is as if not more important than total intake. Really depends on milk yield, etc.
Lysine (g)	84.4	61–54	84.4	50–60	NRC 2007 Lysine recommendations are much higher than NRC 1989 (then 50 g) – mares were fed such levels without any apparent issues. Can be difficult to provide such high levels of lysine in typical diets and rare to do so.
Ca (g)	58.9	52–45	53	70–82.5	The amount of calcium deposited in early lactation is around 1.2 g/kg milk and around 0.8 g/kg milk in late lactation. Pasture and forage vary considerably in their nutritional content and yet in most horses these provide the bulk of the diet. Ideally regularly monitor these so that the diet can be appropriately fortified for the individual circumstances.
P (g)_	38	37–31	30	45–55	Ratio of Ca : P may be as important as total amount – aim between 1.5–2 : 1.

Table A4 *Continued*

	NRC (RQ)	GEH (RC)	This book (RQ/RC)	PH (OR)	Editor's comments
Mg (g)	11	8–7.5	8.4	15	
K (g)	48	27–26	20.4	50+	
Na (g)	13	7–6.4	7	~20	Providing free salt or a salt block in an easily accessible place may be sufficient. Monitor use. Do not use mineral blocks formulated for other species.
Cl (g)	45.5	45–44 (6 g accordingly strict factorial approach)	45 (NB factorial much lower)	45	Early lactation: 89–93 mg/kg BW/day.
Cu (mg)	125	106	106	125–150	Milk contains relatively low levels of copper & zinc and there is little effect of Cu supplementation on milk content.
I (mg)	4.4	2.1	2.2	2–3	Iodine levels from NRC appear too high. Iodine is concentrated across the placenta and in the milk: the most vulnerable are foals from highly supplemented mares. Rec lower upper limit than NRC for the pregnant mare at 3 mg/100 kg BW. Seaweeds contain very variable and sometimes very high levels of I.
Fe (mg)	625	530	530	NRC	Some mineral sources contain high levels of iron contamination. Rare to have an inadequate intake of iron.
Mn (mg)	500	420	420	600–750	
Se (mg)	1.25	1.6	1.6	2–3	
Zn (mg)	500	530	530	600–750	Cu:Zn ratio in the diet may be important – our current advice is to try and maintain around 3.5–4.5:1.
Vitamin A (IU)	30K	32K	32K	60–90K NB ~ 30K from vitamin A – rest from β-carotene sources	There is minimal transference across the placenta of vitamin A and therefore foals are born with a relative vitamin A deficiency. This may lead to problems especially if mares are fed a vitamin A-deficient diet, the colostrum levels are low or if the foals fail to suckle adequately.
Vitamin D (IU)	3.3K	5.3K	5.3K	5–9K based NRC 1989 allowing 3% DM intake	Likely to be outside but supplementation required if not. Toxicity is possible so beware of over supplementing.
E (IU)	1000	1100	1100	1600–2500	
Thiamin (mg)	37.5	32	32	40	
Riboflavin (mg)	25	21	21	25	
Others					Further recommendation. Folic acid ~1.1 mg/kg DM in lactating mares.

BW, body weight; CP, crude protein; DE, digestible energy; ME, metabolizable energy.
K = ×1000.

Table A5 Daily Nutrient Requirements (RQ)s and Recommendations (RC) for a 215-kg Weanling (6 Months of Age) Growing at 0.72 kg/day, According to North American (NRC 2007) and German (GEH 2013) Authorities, as Well as More Optimal Recommendations (OR) of One of the Editors (PH)

	NRC (RQ)	GEH (RC)	This book (RQ/RC)	PH (OR)	Editor's comments
Energy (MJ) NB: DE or ME	DE: 49 Growing at 0.72 kg/day NB: NRC in Mcal 1 Mcal ~ 4.184 MJ	ME: 42 MJ NB: GEH use MJ ME per kg metabolic BW	Depends on system used	Base on NRC but consider individual circumstances	The best judge of absolute energy requirement is the horse – feed to the individual. NB: BW equations for adults are not appropriate for foals. A validated BCS system is not available for foals. Growth rate of the weanling will be affected by • its genetic potential in particular, • its growth rate while suckling, • level of weaning stress and • nutrient intake (protein and energy). Requirements for supplemental feed will change with environmental conditions, availability of grass during any turnout, activity levels in field (e.g., colts tend > fillies; groups tend > individuals). In the first year post weaning, non-forage/concentrate or supplemental feed intake should not exceed 70% of total daily intake. For many horses and ponies, far lower concentrate intakes may be preferable, and more commonly found. From around 2–3 months of age often need to increase the level of supplementary feed (fed in addition to forage) as the quality and quantity of the mare's milk decreases (as a guide between 0.2–0.45 kg of supplementary feed/month of age until weaning depending on the breed, individual, rate of growth and type of feed). The foal at weaning must be able and accustomed to eating solid supplementary feed. Consider gradual weaning processes (as less stressful).

Table A5 *Continued*

	NRC (RQ)	GEH (RC)	This book (RQ/RC)	PH (OR)	Editor's comments
CP (g)	676	400 g prececal digestible CP corresponding to 570 g CP	676	700–800 depending on growth rate and quality of protein	Protein quality i.e. amino acid profile is as if not more important than total intake. The foal will require proportionally less protein and amino acids but more energy as it grows (as an increasing proportion of the daily gain is fat and less is muscle).
Lysine (g)	29	25–28	29	35–40	Protein quality is important (intake of key amino acids such as lysine and threonine) e.g., ~170 mg lysine/kg BW/day for weanlings. Threonine at least 80% of the lysine.
Ca (g)	39	35 for 700 g daily gain with 16.8 g Ca/kg	26	42	The minimum requirement = requirement for maintenance + requirement for growth. Foals growing at a rapid rate deposit greater quantities of bone, muscle and fat than their slower growing counterparts – so need more minerals and amino acids to support this growth.
P (g)	21.5	23 for 700 g daily gain with 8.3 g P/kg	22	23	Ratio of Ca: P may be as important as total amount – aim for 1.5–2:1.
Mg (g)	4.1	4 for 700 g daily gain with 0.4 g Mg/kg	5	7	
K (g)	13	9.4 for 700 g daily gain and 2 g K/kg	10	15+	On forage based maintenance diets should be impossible not to provide sufficient K.
Na (g)	5	3 for 700 g daily gain with 2.7 g Na/kg	5	5–10	Do not use mineral blocks formulated for other species.
Cl (g)	20.1	18 for 700 g gaily gain with 1.2 g Cl/kg (2 g accordingly strict factorial approach)	20	20	
Cu (mg)	54	62	60	100–125	Copper supplementation may not be the "magic bullet" suggested by some in the past as far as DOD is concerned *but*. Rec to maintain a good copper and zinc intake and balance throughout gestation and growth. Rec not more than 30% of total intake of any trace elements is provided in an organic form.

Table A5 *Continued*

	NRC (RQ)	GEH (RC)	This book (RQ/RC)	PH (OR)	Editor's comments
I (mg)	1.9	1	1.0	1	Iodine levels from NRC appear too high. Very difficult to assess iodine intakes from organic materials. Seaweeds contain very variable and sometimes very high levels of I.
Fe (mg)	270	450	300	270	Some mineral sources contain high levels of iron contamination. Rare to have an inadequate intake of iron.
Mn (mg)	216	225	220	325	
Se (mg)	0.54	0.8	0.8	1	Caution re IM injections of Se. Provide adequate vitamin E/Se to avoid selenium-associated muscular issues.
Zn (mg)	216	225	220	300–400	Cu : Zn ratio in the diet may be important – current advice is to try and maintain around 3.5–4.5 : 1.
Vitamin A (IU)	10K	17K	17K	21K	Risks are with over provision of vitamin A rather than excessive ingestion of the precursor β-carotene. More mature forages may have lower β-carotene levels. Stored forages may have lower β-carotene levels.
Vitamin D (IU)	5K	3.9K	3.9– 6.2K	5K	Although may not be as essential for Ca metabolism as other species may be very important for other reasons to ensure vitamin D intake is adequate especially if foals stabled.
Vitamin E (IU)	434	560	560	750–1000	Important to provide adequate vitamin E to reduce the risk of vitamin E/Se responsive myopathy.
Thiamin (mg)	16.2	17	17	17	Some suggest up to 25.
Riboflavin (mg)	11	11	11	11	Some suggest up to twice this.
Others					Vitamin K may be important for bone health and may not be as bioavailable as previously thought.

BW, body weight; CP, crude protein; DE, digestible energy; DOD, developmental orthopedic disease; ME, metabolizable energy.
K = ×1000.

Table A6 Nutrients in Forages and the Commercial Products Used for the Calculations in the Example Diets (as Fed)

	CP	CF	Dig. CP	DE	Ca	P	Mg	Na	K	Cl	Cu	Zn	Se	Vitamin A	Vitamin D	Vitamin E
	g	g	g	MJ	g	g	g	g	g	g	mg	mg	mg	IU	IU	mg
Pasture, temperate grass, cool season	53	5	40	1.9	1.1	0.9	0.4	0.04	7.0	1.0	2	7	0.01	1200	0	6
Hay, meadow	80	17	46	7.6	2.9	1.7	1.1	0.5	17.0	8.3	3	12	0.03	6000	700	30
Hay, alfalfa, early cut (NDF 42% DM)	170	22	118	9.0	13.0	2.0	3.0	1.0	21.0	6.0	8	25	0.02	7040	440	26
Hay, legume, mature (NDF 51% DM)	149	13	104	7.8	10.2	2.3	2.3	0.2	20.0	8.0	8	20	0.16	6000	700	30
Compound feed for exercise	110	30	77	10.4	12.0	4.0	2.0	2.0	10.0	6.0	30	100	0.3	24000	2400	300
Compound feed for pregnancy	180	40	140	11.2	15.0	6.0	2.3	3.3	12.7	8.0	90	200	0.3	30 000	3000	300
Compound feed for lactation	160	62	123	11.8	12.0	6.0	1.8	4.0	6.0	2.4	25	66	0.2	18 000	2400	200
Compound feed for growth	180	40	141	11.7	11.0	7.0	2.5	3.4	6.0	6.2	24	90	0.35	18 750	2000	250
Forage balancer (Figs A1A and A2A)					100.0	25.0	25.0	30.0		60.0	800	3000	10.00	350 000	25000	8000
Vitamin–mineral supplement for pregnant mares (Fig. A3)					100.0	50.0	15.0	40.0		65.0	700	2000	10.0	500 000	40000	3700
Vitamin–mineral supplement for lactation (Fig. A4)					125.0	27.0	30.0	36.0		64.0	600	3000	10.0	500 000	67000	3500
Vitamin–mineral supplement for growth (Fig. A5)					100.0	50.0	48.0	20.0		40.0	175	850	20.0	350 000	50000	5000

BW, body weight; CF, crude fiber; Dig. CP, crude protein; DE, digestible energy; ME, metabolizable energy; NDF, neutral detergent fiber.
Note that pasture is assumed to be in the vegetative state with 200 g DM/kg.

Glossary

Coarse mix. A common form of bagged feed for horses comprising a mixture of flaked, rolled or cracked cereals together with pellets and other ingredients.

Complementary feedingstuff. An EU definition describing a compound feed which has a high content of certain substances but which, by reason of its composition, is sufficient for a daily ration only if used in combination with other feed or forage.

Complete feed. Compound feed which, by reason of its composition, is sufficient for a daily ration.

Compound feed. Mixture of at least two feed materials, whether or not containing feed additives, for oral animal feeding in the form of complete or complementary feed.

Concentrate. Term commonly used to describe the non-forage component(s) of an equine diet.

Control measure. Any action and activity that can be used to prevent or eliminate a food safety hazard.

Critical Control Point (CCP). A step at which control can be applied and is essential to prevent or eliminate a food safety hazard or rescue it to an acceptable level.

Critical limit. A criterion that separates acceptability from unacceptability.

Good Manufacturing Practice. Describes basic sanitary conditions and practices in a manufacturing site; includes: plant facilities, maintenance, cleaning and housekeeping, pest control, material handling and training.

Hazard Analysis Critical Control Point (HACCP). A system that identifies, evaluates and controls hazards which are significant for food safety.

Hazard. A biological, chemical or physical agent in, or condition of, food with the potential to cause an adverse health effect.

Hazard Analysis (in HACCP). The process of collecting and evaluating information on hazards and conditions leading to their presence to decide which are significant for food safety and therefore should be addressed in the HACCP plan.

Safe Food. Food that does not cause harm to the consumer when it is prepared and/or eaten according to its intended use.

Straights. Single ingredients in processed or unprocessed forms (e.g. rolled oats, sugar beet pulp).

Supplements. Commonly used colloquial term describing mixtures of additives for oral feeding to horses, typically administered in small doses and offered in feed or separately, and intended for a specific benefit beyond normal nutritional needs (but not including legally defined drugs.)

Sweet feed. Similar to coarse mix (see above), term commonly used in the US.

Index

Page numbers followed by "f" indicate figures, "t" indicate tables, and "b" indicate boxes.

H